D1583106

Paediatric and Adolescent Gynaecology

A Multidisciplinary Approach

This book provides a multidisciplinary overview of developmental anomalies, disorders and intersex conditions. These are complex conditions that demand high standards of care and treatment by all healthcare professionals involved with the management of these psychological, medical and surgical problems. This textbook, which involves leading international experts from a wide range of disciplines, aims to distil their wealth of expertise and to provide the best possible advice and recommendations concerning medical intervention. Another important theme is the psychological well-being of the patient, the need for informed consent and the right to know one's diagnosis. Patients and their families expect high standards of care, communication and consultation, and this book will help doctors to achieve this.

In addition to covering the management of disorders of development, comprehensive sections discuss menstrual cycle abnormalities, polycystic ovary syndrome, gynaecological cancer the late effects of childhood cancer and fertility preservation, dermatological conditions and infections.

Emphasizing as it does the multidisciplinary approach to healthcare, the book will be essential reading for specialists in paediatric and adolescent gynaecology, reproductive endocrinologists, paediatric and plastic surgeons, and clinical geneticists.

Paediatric and Adolescent Gynaecology

A Multidisciplinary Approach

Editor-in-chief

Adam H. Balen

Department of Reproductive Medicine,
Leeds General Infirmary, Leeds

Co-editors

Sarah M. Creighton

The Elizabeth Garrett Anderson and
Obstetric Hospital, University
College London Hospitals, London

Melanie C. Davies

Reproductive Medicine Unit,
University College London Hospitals, London

Jane MacDougall

Department of Obstetrics and Gynaecology,
Addenbrooke's Hospital, Cambridge

Richard Stanhope

Institute of Child Health, London

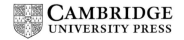

CAMBRIDGE
UNIVERSITY PRESS

PUBLISHED BY THE PRESS SYNDICATE OF THE UNIVERSITY OF CAMBRIDGE
The Pitt Building, Trumpington Street, Cambridge, United Kingdom

CAMBRIDGE UNIVERSITY PRESS
The Edinburgh Building, Cambridge CB2 2RU, UK
40 West 20th Street, New York, NY 10011–4211, USA
477 Williamstown Road, Port Melbourne, VIC 3207, Australia
Ruiz de Alarcón 13, 28014 Madrid, Spain
Dock House, The Waterfront, Cape Town 8001, South Africa

http://www.cambridge.org

© Cambridge University Press 2004

This book is in copyright. Subject to statutory exception
and to the provisions of relevant collective licensing agreements,
no reproduction of any part may take place without
the written permission of Cambridge University Press.

First published 2004

Printed in the United Kingdom at the University Press, Cambridge

Typefaces Utopia 8.5/12 pt. and Dax   *System* LaTeX 2_ε [TB]

A catalogue record for this book is available from the British Library

ISBN 0 521 80961 4 hardback

Every effort has been made in preparing this book to provide accurate and up-to-date information which is in accord with accepted standards and practice at the time of publication. Nevertheless, the authors, editors and publisher can make no warranties that the information contained herein is totally free from error, not least because clinical standards are constantly changing through research and regulation. The authors, editors and publisher therefore disclaim all liability for direct or consequential damages resulting from the use of material contained in this book. Readers are strongly advised to pay careful attention to information provided by the manufacturer of any drugs or equipment that they plan to use.

Although case histories are drawn from actual cases, every effort has been made to disguise the identities of the individuals involved.

Every effort has been made to reach copyright holders; the publishers would like to hear from anyone whose rights they have unknowingly infringed.

The publisher has used its best endeavors to ensure that the URLs for external websites referred to in this book are correct and active at the time of going to press. However, the publisher has no responsibility for the websites and can make no guarantee that a site will remain live or that the content is or will remain appropriate.

Contents

Contributors

Kerstin Albertsson-Wikland
Endocrine Division
Sahlgrenska University Hospital
Göteborg
Sweden

Julie Alderson
Department of Adolescent Psychology
Ashley Wing
St James' Hospital
Leeds LS9 7TF
UK

Adam H. Balen
Department of Reproductive Medicine
Leeds General Infirmary
Leeds LS2 9NS
UK

Leith A. Banney
Department of Dermatology
Addenbrooke's Hospital
Cambridge CB2 2SW
UK

Marie-Louise Barrenäs
Department of Paediatrics
University of Göteborg
East Hospital
416 85 Göteborg
Sweden

Peter R. Brinsden
Bourn Hall Clinic
Bourn
Cambs CB3 7TR
UK

Fergus Cameron
Department of Endocrinology and Diabetes
   and Centre for Hormone Research
Murdoch Children's Research Institute
Royal Children's Hospital
Flemington Rd
Parkville
Melbourne
Victoria 3052
Australia

Polly Carmichael
Department of Psychological Medicine
Great Ormond Street Hospital
Great Ormond St
London WC1N 3JH
UK

Alan Cooklin
Department of Child and
   Adolescent Psychiatric Services
North House
The Middlesex Hospital
Cleveland St
London W1T 3AA
UK

Gerard S. Conway
University College Hospital London
Huntley St
London WC1E 6AU
UK

Sophie Christin-Maitre
Hospital Saint-Antione
184 rue du Faubourg Saint-Antoine
75012 Paris
France

Rosamund Cox
Kettering General Hospital
Rothwell Rd
Kettering
Northants NN16 8UZ
UK

Sarah Creighton
The Elizabeth Garrett Anderson
   and Obstetric Hospital
University College London Hospitals
London WC1E 6AU
UK

Hilary O. D. Critchley
Section of Obstetrics and Gynaecology
Department of Developmental
   and Reproductive Sciences
University of Edinburgh
37 Chalmer's St
Edinburgh EH3 9ET
UK

Peter Cuckow
Great Ormond Street Hospital for Children
   and The Institute of Urology
The Middlesex Hospital
London W1N 8AA
UK

Alfred Cutner
Elizabeth Garrett Anderson Hospital
Huntley St
London WC1E 6AU
UK

Melanie C. Davies
Reproductive Medicine Unit
University College London Hospitals
London WC1E 6DH
UK

Colin Davis
Department of Gynaecology
St Bartholomew's and the Royal London Hospitals
London E1 1BB
UK

Rose de Brun
Department of Radiology
Great Ormond Street Hospital for Children
London WC1N 3JH
UK

David Dunger
Department of Paediatrics
Addenbrooke's Hospital
Cambridge CB2 2SW
UK

D. Keith Edmonds
Department of Gynaecology
Institute of Obstetrics and Gynaecology
Hammersmith Hospital
London W12 0NN
UK

Joanna L. Fried
Columbia Presbyterian Medical Center
622 West 168th St
New York
NY 10032
USA

Julie Glanville
Department of Reproductive Medicine
Clarendon Wing
Leeds General Infirmary
Leeds LS2 9NS
UK

Margaret Hall-Craggs
Department of Radiology
UCH Hospitals Trust
Mortimer St
London W1N 8AA
UK

Charles Hanson
Department of Obstetrics and Gynaecology and
    Institute of the Health of the Woman and Child
University of Göteborg
East Hospital
416 85 Göteborg
Sweden

Melissa Hines
Department of Psychology
City University
Northampton Square
London EC1V 0HB
UK

Ieuan A. Hughes
Department of Paediatrics
Addenbrooke's Hospital
Cambridge CB2 2SW
UK

Ilpo Huhtaniemi
Department of Physiology
University of Turku
Kiinamyllynkatu 10
20520 Turku
Finland

Jarmo Jääskeläinen
Department of Paediatrics
Addenbrooke's Hospital
Cambridge CB2 2SW
UK

Howard S. Jacobs
Emeritus Professor of Reproductive Endocrinology
Middlesex Hospital
London W1N 8AA
UK

Per-Olaf Janson
Department of Obstetrics and Gynaecology and
    Institute of the Health of the Woman and Child
University of Göteborg
East Hospital
416 85 Göteborg
Sweden

Christopher J. H. Kelnar
Section of Child Life and Health
Department of Developmental
    and Reproductive Sciences
University of Edinburgh
20 Sylvan Place
Edinburgh EH9 1UW
UK

Berit Kristöm
Göteborg Paediatric Growth Research Centre
Institute of the Health of the Woman and Child
University of Göteborg
East Hospital
416 85 Göteborg
Sweden

Clementina La Rosa
Department of Paediatric Endocrinology
Great Ormond Street Hospital for
    Children and The Middlesex Hospital
London W1N 8AA
UK

Jerome Levallet
Department of Biochemistry
University of Caen
14032 Caen
Spain

Lih Mei Liao
Department of Psychology
University College Hospital
London WC1E 6AU
UK

Gillian Lockwood
Midland Fertility Service
Aldridge
UK

Tito Lopes
Queen Elizabeth Hospital
Sheriff Hill
Gateshead
Tyne-and-Wear
UK

Jane MacDougall
Department of Obstetrics and Gynaecology
Addenbrooke's Hospital
Cambridge CB2 2SW
UK

Nadia Micali
Eating Disorders Unit
Maudsley Hospital
Denmark Hill
London SE5 8AZ
UK

Catherine L. Minto
Academic Department of Obstetrics
   and Gynaecology
UCH 86-96
Chenies Mews
London WC1E 6AU
UK

Anders Möller
Department of Psychology
University of Göteborg
Göteborg
Sweden

Pierre Mouriquand
Department d'Urologie Pediatrique
29 Rue Soeur Bouvier
69322 Lyon
Cedex 05
France

Azad Najmaldin
Department of Paediatric Surgery
St James University Hospital
Leeds LS2 9NS
UK

Helen M. Picton
Department of Obstetrics and Gynaecology
University of Leeds
UK

Eleonora Porcu
Reproductive Medicine Unit
Institute of Obstetrics and Gynaecology
University of Bologna
Via Masserenti
Bologna 13-40138
Italy

Russalind Ramos
Columbia Presbyterian Medical Center
622 West 168th St
New York
NY 10032
USA

Sarah Ramsden
Department of Child and Adolescent
   Psychiatric Services
North House
The Middlesex Hospital
Cleveland St
London W1T 3AA
UK

Anthony J. Rutherford
Department of Obstetrics and Gynaecology
Leeds General Infirmary
Leeds LS2 9NS
UK

Christopher Schelvan
Department of Radiology
UCH Hospitals Trust
Mortimer St
London W1N 8AA
UK

Margaret Simmonds
Androgen Insensitivity Syndrome
   Support Group (AISSG)
www.medhelp.org/www/ais

Andrew Sinclair
Murdoch Children's Research Institute
Royal Children's Hospital
Flemington Rd
Parkville
Melbourne
Victoria 3052
Australia

Craig Smith
Department of Endocrinology
   and Diabetes and Centre for Hormone
   Research
Murdoch Children's Research Institute
Royal Children's Hospital
Flemington Rd
Parkville
Melbourne
Victoria 3052
Australia

Richard Stanhope
Department of Paediatric Endocrinology
Great Ormond Street Hospital
   for Children, The Middlesex Hospital
   and the Institute of Child Health
30 Guilford St
London WC1N 1EH
UK

Jane C. Sterling
Department of Dermatology
Addenbrooke's Hospital
Cambridge CB2 2SW
UK

Manuel Tena-Sempere
Department of Physiology
University of Córdoba
14004 Córdoba
Spain

Nikesh Thiruchelvam
The Institute of Child Health
30 Guilford St
London WC1N 1EH
UK

Angela B. Thompson
Department of Haematology
Royal Hospital for Sick Children
17 Millerfield Place
Edinburgh EH9 1LF
UK

Cristina Traggiai
Department of Paediatric Endocrinology
Great Ormond Street Hospital for Children
   and The Middlesex Hospital
London W1N 8AA
UK

Janet Treasure
Department of Psychiatry
Thomas Guy House
Guys Campus
London SR1 9RT
UK

Hamish B. Wallace
Department of Haematology
Royal Hospital for Sick Children
17 Millerfield Place
Edinburgh EH9 1LF
UK

Gary L. Warne
Department of Endocrinology
   and Diabetes
Royal Children's Hospital
Parkville
Melbourne
Victoria 3052
Australia

Michelle P. Warren
Columbia Presbyterian
  Medical Center
622 West 168th St
New York
NY 10032
USA

Peter Webster
Eating Disorders Unit
Maudsley Hospital
Denmark Hill
London SE5 8AZ
UK

Kerstin Wilhelmsen-Landin
Endocrine Division
Sahlgrenska University Hospital
Göteborg
Sweden

Paul Wood
Kettering General Hospital
Rothwell Rd
Kettering
Northants NN16 8UZ
UK

Christopher R. J. Woodhouse
The Institute of Urology
The Middlesex Hospital
London WC1N 3JH
UK

Stefano Venturoli
Reproductive Medicine Unit
Institute of Obstetrics and Gynaecology
University of Bologna
Via Masserenti
Bologna 13-40138
Italy

Preface

The management of intersex conditions and anomalies of the development of the female genitalia can only be properly achieved with appropriate input from a number of health professionals. Furthermore, the needs of the individual may change over time and so both the patient and her family must be provided with a seamless transition between the various stages of care – from the diagnosis, which may be in early infancy or in the teenage years, through childhood, adolescence and then to adulthood. Therefore, although intersex conditions are rare, it is imperative that they are managed in centres by a multidisciplinary team that includes paediatric surgeons, urologists (often paediatric and adult), plastic surgeons, endocrinologists, specialist nurses, psychologists and also the gynaecologist. The role of the gynaecologist is to help to coordinate the transition from childhood through adolescence and then womanhood and to help with issues relating to sexual function and sexual identity, endocrinology and fertility. It is during the difficult time of adolescence that the patient usually first realises that there are serious problems and it is often the specialist gynaecologist who helps her to understand the diagnosis and requirements for management. The support of a skilled nurse and clinical psychologist is invaluable at this time.

The Department of Health in the UK is currently reviewing the national provision of services for the management of intersex. Parathentically, those units that have the skills to manage intersex conditions also have the appropriate facilities to treat complex developmental anomalies of the Müllerian tract (for example cervical and vaginal agenesis). Disorders of sexual development may result in ambiguous genitalia or anomalies of the internal genital tract; they can be caused by genetic defects, abnormalities of steroidogenesis, and dysynchrony during organogenesis. Age of presentation will depend upon the degree of dysfunction caused.

In addition to an understanding of normal and abnormal development, it is essential that the health professional has knowledge of all aspects of adolescent gynaecological health, including the causes of menstrual cycle disturbances and pelvic pain, polycystic ovary syndrome, premature ovarian failure, gynaecological cancers and the reproductive sequelae of childhood cancer. An awareness of the range of dermatological conditions and infections is also required.

In this book we have synthesized the experience of a multinational and multidisciplinary collection of authors who have gained considerable experience in the diagnosis and management of developmental disorders of sexual differentiation. We provide the reader with an overview of normal development and function and then provide both general guidance on the multiple facets of management together with detailed descriptions of specific conditions. We have highlighted areas of uncertainty and controversy. There is still much work to be done in unravelling the pathogenesis and genetics of many conditions, their prevalence and epidemiology, and also when and how best to treat. The book is a contemporary overview and is aimed at all healthcare professionals who may have to participate in the care of patients with anomalous sexual development and all aspects of gynaecological, reproductive and sexual health.

Adam H. Balen

Part I

Normal development

Embryology of the female genital tract

Fergus Cameron and Craig Smith

Murdoch Children's Research Institute, Royal Children's Hospital, Melbourne, Australia

Introduction

Regardless of their sex, all human embryos initially develop a common set of genital structures. A pair of primordial gonads, the genital ridges, appear in both males and females during the sixth week of embryonic life. Two associated ducts develop, the Müllerian and Wolffian ducts, while presumptive external genitalia appear as folds of cloacal tissue. The fate of these undifferentiated internal and external structures depends upon the genetic sex of the embryo. In individuals with an XY sex chromosome constitution, the genital ridges become testes. Hormones released from the developing testes masculinize the internal ducts and external genitalia. Sertoli cells of the fetal testes synthesize anti-Müllerian Hormone (AMH; also known as Müllerian inhibitory substance), which induces Müllerian duct regression. Meanwhile, testosterone secretion from Leydig cells induces Wolffian duct differentiation into vas deferens, and virilization of the external genitalia into penis and scrotum. Testis differentiation is initiated by the *SRY* gene (sex-determining region of the Y chromosome). In individuals with an XX sex chromosome constitution, *SRY* is absent and the genital ridges differentiate as ovaries rather than testes. Furthermore, in the absence of AMH and testosterone, the ducts follow alternative developmental paths. In the absence of AMH, the Müllerian ducts are free to differentiate into the Fallopian tubes, uterus and upper portion of the vagina. In the absence of testosterone, the Wolffian ducts regress. The external genitalia of female embryos differentiate into clitoris and labia.

Since gonadal and genital tract development occur in the absence of *SRY* and male hormones in XX embryos, female has traditionally been considered the "default" pathway of sexual differentiation. This chapter will focus on differentiation of the female internal ducts (genital tract) during embryogenesis, with some consideration of gonadal and external genital formation.

Development of the genital and urinary systems

The genital system develops in close association with the urinary system. The entire urogenital system is derived from intermediate mesoderm early in embryogenesis. Formation of the urinary system depends upon the coordinated differentiation of ductal epithelium and nephrogenic mesenchyme. From the first of these are derived the genital tracts, ureters and renal collecting ducts, and from the latter the nephrons in both the mesonephric (embryonic) and metanephric (definitive) kidneys. Several transcription factors and growth factors are implicated in the control of kidney development. Mouse knockout studies have identified one important gene, *Pax-2*, which is required for the differentiation of the intermediate mesoderm into nephric structures (Torres et al., 1995). Mice homozygous for *Pax-2* were found to lack kidneys, ureters and both male and female internal genital tracts (Torres et al., 1995). The *PAX* genes (in humans; *Pax* in mice) specify transcription factor proteins that turn on other genes, playing a part in specification of cell fate during embryogenesis. Another gene, *WT1*, is expressed in the mesenchyme and required for its differentiation into the primitive kidney (Kreidberg et al., 1993). *WT1* encodes a zinc finger transcription factor and is responsible for inhibiting cell proliferation. *WT1*, therefore, operates as a tumour suppressor, and mutations in this gene cause paediatric renal tumours (Wilms' tumours). The tyrosine kinase receptor gene c-*ret* is necessary for ureter

Paediatric and Adolescent Gynaecology, ed. Adam Balen et al. Published by Cambridge University Press.
© Cambridge University Press 2004.

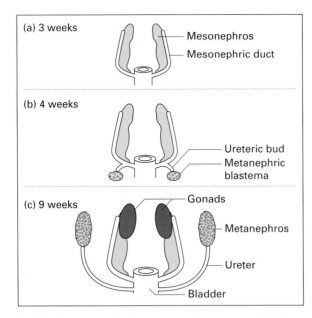

Fig. 1.1. Development of the urinary system in human embryos.

growth (Schuchardt et al., 1994) and *Wnt-4* is essential for metanephric tubule formation (Stark et al., 1994).

Under normal circumstances, the embryonic nephrons, mesonephri, appear after four weeks of gestation and are drained by a pair of mesonephric ducts. These grow caudally into the posterior wall of the urogenital sinus. The ureteric buds arise from the distal mesonephric ducts at five weeks of gestation and their presence stimulates the adjacent intermediate mesoderm to differentiate into the definitive (metanephric) kidneys (Grobstein, 1955) (Fig. 1.1). At between eight and twelve weeks of gestation, the secretion of testosterone by testicular Leydig cells stimulates the mesonephric (Wolffian) ducts to transform into the vasa deferentia (Moore, 1988). In the absence of testosterone, the mesonephric ducts will regress. The region of the vas deferens proximal to the testis differentiates into the epididymis and at around approximately 12 weeks of gestation unites with the rete testis. Seminal vesicles sprout from the distal mesonephric duct at 10 weeks of gestation, and from these, under the influence of dihydrotestosterone, the prostate and bulbourethral glands develop (Larsen, 1993).

AMH is the first molecule to be synthesized and secreted by Sertoli cells (Tran et al., 1977). It is first seen at the time of seminiferous tubule organization and persists until the commencement of puberty (Josso et al., 1990; Tran et al., 1977, 1981). The role of AMH is unclear after sexual dimorphism has been achieved, which in humans is at 6–8 weeks of gestation (Josso et al., 1977), with the Müllerian ducts having undergone complete regression by

10 weeks of gestation (Jirasek, 1971; Josso et al., 1977). Despite cloning of a putative AMH type II receptor (belonging to the serine/threonine kinase receptor superfamily; Grootegoed et al., 1994), the basis for this progressive regression is unknown (Hunter, 1995). Studies of freemartinism indicate that AMH (derived from a twin male calf) is responsible for bovine sex reversal in female calves (Vigier et al., 1987). This would seem to imply that AMH receptors exist in the developing gonad regardless of karyotype.

External genitalia

Between the fifth and seventh weeks of embryonic life, the cloacal folds, a pair of swellings adjacent to the cloacal membrane, fuse anteriorly to form the genital tubercle. The perineum develops and divides the cloacal membrane into the anterior urogenital membrane and the posterior anal membrane. The cloacal folds anteriorly form the urethral folds. Another pair of swellings, this time within the cloacal membrane, form the labioscrotal folds (Larsen, 1993). At this stage, no sexual dimorphism of the external genitalia has occurred and the structures are all bipotential.

In males, the endoderm-lined urogenital sinus develops into the genital tubercle and forms the urethral groove. This will eventually become the penile urethra. The urogenital membrane ruptures in the seventh week, exposing the urogenital sinus to liquor, and the genital tubercle begins to form the phallus. Whereas testosterone is required for the differentiation of the mesonephric ducts, its metabolite, dihydrotestosterone, is necessary for male differentiation of the urogenital sinus and external genitalia (Fisher, 1992). The labioscrotal folds fuse in the midline, commencing posteriorly, to form the scrotum, and the penile urethra becomes enclosed within the shaft of the penis. The inguinal canal develops by the third month and testicular descent occurs through this to the scrotum between seven and nine months of gestation (Larsen, 1993). Formation of the male external genital duct structures is dependent on placental chorionic gonadotrophin (hCG), which stimulates Leydig cells to secrete testosterone and its metabolites. Enlargement of the formed genitals in the second and third trimesters is dependent upon gonadotrophin-stimulated testosterone release (Grumbach and Conte, 1992). These gonadotrophins are follicle-stimulating hormone (FSH) and luteinizing hormone (LH).

Female internal genital duct structures

The female reproductive tract differentiates from a pair of embryonic ducts, the Müllerian ducts (Fig. 1.2). Since

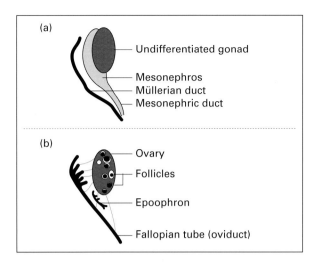

Fig. 1.2. Development of the female reproductive tract. In females, the Müllerian ducts give rise to the Fallopian tubes (oviduct), while the mesonephric ducts regress, leaving vestiges called the epoophron. Only one side of the reproductive tract is shown.

they develop adjacent to the mesonephric ducts, they are sometimes also called the paramesonephric ducts. The Müllerian ducts appear in both sexes during the sixth week of embryogenesis, arising by invagination of a cord of coelomic epithelium extending from the urogenital sinus to the third thoracic segment (Byskow and Hoyer, 1988). In the absence of AMH, the distal tips fuse prior to contact with the pelvic urethra. This becomes the uterovaginal canal, the unfused segments becoming the Fallopian tubes (Moore, 1988). The inferior fifth of the vagina arises from a pair of urethral swellings (sinuvaginal bulbs).

In the female, as in the male, the external genital derivatives consist of the genital tubercle, the urogenital sinus, the urethral folds and the labioscrotal folds. In the absence of testosterone, there is no fusion of the labioscrotal folds and no elongation of the genital tubercle (Larsen, 1993). The genital tubercle bends inferiorly and becomes the clitoris. The urethral folds develop as the labia minora and the labioscrotal folds as the labia majora. The urogenital sinus becomes the vestibule of the vagina. The external genitalia are recognizably female at the end of 12 weeks of gestation (Moore, 1988).

Abnormalities of genital tract differentiation

In humans and other mammals, sexual differentiation is essentially determined by the presence or absence of male sex hormones. Consequently, disorders of sex differentiation can be divided into 46,XY individuals, with a deficiency or resistance to male sex hormones, or 46,XX individuals, with an excess of male sex hormones. These can be further subdivided into biosynthetic defects of male sex hormone synthesis/metabolism and sex hormone receptor defects. The term "pseudohermaphroditism" is used to describe those whose external genitalia are at odds with their karyotype, gonadal morphology and internal genitalia. Abnormalities in male sexual differentiation (male pseudohermaphroditism) are caused by deficient testosterone production or a resistance to its actions (Bale et al., 1992; Federman and Donahoe, 1995). With regard to testosterone synthesis, some of the biosynthetic defects affect both glucocorticoids and androgens. These include cholesterol side-chain cleavage deficiency, 17α-hydroxylase/17,20-lyase deficiency and 3β-hydroxysteroid dehydrogenase deficiency (Grumbach and Conte, 1992). All of these conditions are autosomal recessive. In a 46,XY individual, they present with female or ambiguous genitalia. The gonads have a normal testicular morphology and Müllerian duct structures are absent. Wolffian duct structures are absent or hypoplastic in the first two and normal in the last (Grumbach and Conte, 1992).

Defects in the gene for the LH receptor (Kremer et al., 1995; Latronico et al., 1996), resulting in Leydig cell hypoplasia and male pseudohermaphroditism, have also been described. Affected individuals have been found to be homozygous for mutations in the gene for the LH receptor that give rise to normal binding of the ligand but an absence of any increased production of cAMP (Kremer et al., 1995). A deficiency in 17β-hydroxysteroid dehydrogenase results in a 46,XY individual with female or ambiguous external genitalia, normal testes, absent Müllerian duct structures and hypoplastic Wolffian duct structures (Grumbach and Conte, 1992). Deficiency of 5α-reductase, another autosomal recessive condition, results in a deficiency of dihydrotestosterone, with normal internal virilization and inadequate external virilization. Individuals with 46,XY have ambiguous external genitalia, normal Wolffian duct structures and lack Müllerian duct structures, although the testes are morphologically normal.

Absent or malfunctioning androgen receptors (complete or partial androgen insensitivity syndrome, respectively) result in an unambiguous external female phenotype in the former and an ambiguous phenotype in the latter. Wolffian duct structures are absent or hypoplastic and Müllerian duct structures are absent (Migeon et al., 1981). Testes are characterized by the presence of hyperplastic Leydig cells, which are organised into adenomatous clumps. Affected individuals usually suffer from oligospermia or azoospermia (Ferenczy and Richart, 1972; O'Leary, 1965).

Persistent Müllerian duct syndrome

Deficiencies in AMH production or a resistance to its action will result in 46,XY individuals with internal and external male genital duct structures with the retention of Müllerian duct structures (persistent Müllerian duct syndrome) (Josso et al., 1991). The diagnosis is often made only once the Müllerian duct structures are discovered at the time of inguinal hernia repair, abdominal surgery or orchidopexy. There is an association with undescended testes and this is consistent with the putative role of AMH in testicular descent (Hutson et al., 1990). (However, AMH null mutant mice have normal, descended testes (Behringer 1995)). The allele for AMH is located on the short arm of chromosome 19 and some cases have been shown to have been associated with homozygous mutations of this gene (Knebelmann et al., 1991). Other patients have been found to have normal amounts of bioactive AMH, implying an AMH receptor defect (Knebelmann et al., 1991).

Anomalies of female genital development

Developing 46,XX embryos may be exposed to androgens from several sources. These include exogenous androgens either ingested (progestogens, testosterone) or produced by the mother (ovarian and adrenal tumours, maternal congenital adrenal hyperplasia (CAH), virilizing luteoma of pregnancy), which cross the placental circulation (Jones, 1981; Kirk et al., 1990; New, 1992). Female pseudohermaphroditism has also been described with placental aromatase deficiency (Shozu et al., 1991). Exposure prior to 12 weeks of gestation will result in labial fusion, whereas later exposure will result only in clitoromegaly (Grumbach and Conte, 1992).

Approximately half of the 46,XX individuals with disordered sexual differentiation are due to virilizing neonatal CAH (New et al., 1989). Biosynthetic defects in cortisol production result in excessive adrenal stimulation by adrenocorticotrophic hormone. This, in turn, causes an excessive production of C19 androgens from precursors that would have otherwise have been destined for cortisol synthesis. There are three autosomal recessive conditions that result in such an outcome in 46,XX embryos.

The commonest form of CAH results from 21α-hydroxylase deficiency. Defects in adrenal 21α-hydroxylation

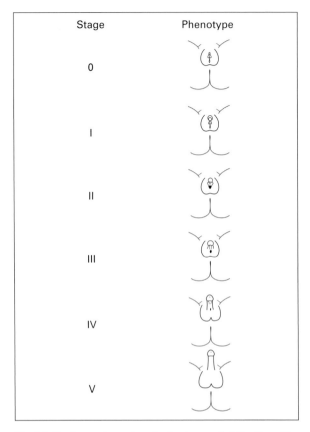

Fig. 1.3. Prader staging system for the degree of virilization of the external genitalia. 0, normal female external genitalia; I, female external genitalia with clitoromegaly; II, clitoromegaly with partial labial fusion forming a funnel-shaped urogenital sinus; III, increased phallic enlargement and complete labioscrotal fusion forming a urogenital sinus with a single opening; IV, complete scrotal fusion with urogenital opening at the base or on the shaft of the phallus; V, normal male external genitalia.

result in deficient aldosterone and cortisol production and excessive production of 17-hydroxyprogesterone, androstenedione and testosterone. This is the commonest form of CAH, with an approximate incidence of 1 in 10–15 000 (New et al., 1989). In embryonic 46,XY patients, the excess testosterone production in itself is of no consequence. Patients with a 46,XX karyotype can be born with all degrees of virilization of the external genitalia, ranging from isolated clitoromegaly to full fusion of the labioscrotal folds associated with a urethra terminating on the tip of the phallus. Prader developed a scoring system by which this degree of virilization could be quantified (von Prader, 1954; Fig. 1.3). Homozygous male and female patients with 21α-hydroxylase deficiency will commonly have varying degrees of salt loss and predisposition to life-threatening addisonian crises.

Embryonic 46,XX virilization associated with hypertension occurs in 11β-hydroxylase deficiency. This is 20 times less common than 21α-hydroxylase deficiency (Rosler et al., 1982). In this condition, homozygotes for the mutant allele have an endocrine profile similar to that seen in 21α-hydroxylase deficiency: decreased aldosterone and cortisol production with an increase in C19 androgens. The main difference is that the enzymatic block occurs further along the synthetic cascade and that one of the immediate precursors (deoxycorticosterone) has its own inherent mineralocorticoid activity. Deoxycorticosterone is produced in excess and a hypertensive state results. These patients do not usually experience hypotensive, hypoglycaemic crises (Grumbach and Conte, 1992).

Whilst 3β-hydroxysteroid dehydrogenase deficiency usually results in 46,XY pseudohermaphroditism, it can also cause clitoromegaly in the 46,XX fetus. This is thought to be the result of peripheral conversion of C19 steroids to testosterone by hepatic 3β-hydroxysteroid dehydrogenase, which has a distinct genetic control from the adrenal and testicular enzyme (Grumbach and Conte, 1992). Heterogeneity is evident in the phenotype of this disease, as it is in the other forms of CAH, with both salt-losing and non-salt-losing forms described (Bongiovanni, 1962; Pang et al., 1983).

Defects in 46,XX sex differentiation not associated with androgen defects occasionally occur in association with malformations of the intestine and urinary tract. These can involve persistence of a primitive cloaca, may be accompanied by renal failure and are often incompatible with life (Carpentier and Potter, 1959; Gearhart and Rock, 1989). Unlike other forms of 46,XX virilization, the internal genital ducts are often affected, suggesting an early defect in mesenchymal differentiation. The description of one such patient with a chromosomal breakpoint in the region of *PAX-2* has provided further evidence of this (Seaver et al., 1994).

Summary

Female genital tract ontogeny occurs as a consequence of gonadal determination and subsequent sexual differentiation. Internal genital duct development is intimately associated with the development of the urinary system, both anatomically and genetically. Disorders of female genital tract differentiation can be associated with gonadal dysgenesis, disorders of gonadal/adrenal hormone production, renal malformation and cloacal anomalies.

REFERENCES

Bale P M, Howard N J, Wright J E (1992). Male pseudohermaphroditism in XY children with female phenotype. *Pediatr Pathol* 12, 29–49.

Behringer R R (1995). The mullerian inhibitor and mammalian sexual development. *Philos Trans R Soc Lond B Biol Sci* 350, 285–288.

Bongiovanni A M (1962). The adrenogenital syndrome with deficiency of 3β-hydroxysteroid dehydrogenase. *J Clin Invest* 41, 2086–2092.

Byskow A G and Hoyer P E (1988). Embryology of mammalian gonads and ducts. *The Physiology of Reproduction*, pp. 265–302. Raven Press, New York.

Carpentier P J and Potter E L (1959). Nuclear sex, genital malformation in 48 cases of renal agenesis with special reference to nonspecific female pseudohermaphroditism. *Am J Obstet Gynecol* 78, 235–258.

Federman D D, Donahoe P K (1995). Ambiguous genitalia: etiology diagnosis and therapy. *Adv Endocrinol Metab* 6, 91–116.

Ferenczy A, Richart R M (1972). The fine structures of the gonads in the complete form of testicular feminization syndrome. *Am J Obstet Gynecol* 113, 399–409.

Fisher D A (1992). Endocrinology of fetal development. *Williams' Textbook of Endocrinology*, 8th edn, pp. 1049–1077. Saunders, Philadelphia, PA.

Gearhart J P, Rock J D (1989). Female pseudohermaphroditism; unusual variants and their management. *Adolesc Pediatr Gynecol* 2, 3–9.

Grobstein C (1955). Tissue interactions in the morphogenesis of the mouse metanephros. *J Exp Zool* 130, 319–340.

Grootegoed J A, Baarends W M, Themmen A P (1994). Welcome to the family: the anti-mullerian receptor. *Mol Cell Endocrinol* 100, 29–34.

Grumbach M M, Conte F A (1992). Disorders of sex differentiation. *Williams' Textbook of Endocrinology*, 8th edn pp. 853–951. Saunders, Philadelphia, PA.

Hunter R H F (1995). *Sex Determination, Differentiation and Intersexuality in Placental Mammals*. Cambridge University Press, Cambridge.

Hutson J M, Williams M P L, Fallat, M E, Attah A (1990). Testicular descent: new insights into its hormonal control. *Oxford Rev Reprod Biol* 12, 1–56.

Jirasek J E (1971). *Development of the Genital System and Male Pseudohermaphroditism*. Johns Hopkins Press, Baltimore, MD.

Jones H W J (1981). Nonadrenal female pseudohermaphroditism. *The Intersex Child: Pediatric and Adolescent Endocrinology*, pp. 65–79. Karger, Basel.

Josso N, Picard J-Y, Tran D (1977). The antimullerian hormone. *Rec Prog Horm Res* 33, 117–167.

Josso N, Legeai L, Forest M G, Chaussain J L, Brauner R (1990). An enzyme-linked immunoassay for anti-Mullerian hormone: a new tool for the evaluation of testicular function in infants and children. *J Clin Endocrinol Metab* 70, 23–27.

Josso N, Boussin L, Knebelmann B, Fekete C N, Picard J Y (1991). Anti-mullerian hormone and intersex states. *Trends Endocrinol Metab* 2, 227–233.

Kirk J M, Perry L A, Shard W S (1990). Female pseudohermaphroditism due to a maternal adrenocortical tumour. *J Clin Endocrinol Metab* 70, 1280–1284.

Knebelmann B, Boussin L, Guerrier D et al. (1991). Anti-Mullerian hormone Bruxelles: a nonsense mutation associated with the persistent Mullerian duct syndrome. *Proc Natl Acad Sci USA* 88, 3767–71.

Kreidberg J A, Sariola H, Loring J M et al. (1993). *WT-1* is required for early kidney development. *Cell* 74, 679–691.

Kremer H, Kraaij R, Toledo S P A et al. (1995). Male pseudohermaphroditism due to a homozygous missense mutation of the luteinizing hormone receptor gene. *Nat Genet* 9, 160–164.

Larsen W J (1993). *Human Embryology*. Churchill Livingstone, New York.

Latronico A C, Anasti J, Arnhold I J et al. (1996). Brief report: testicular and ovarian resistance to luteinizing hormone caused by inactivating mutations of the luteinizing hormone-receptor gene. *N Engl J Med* 334, 507–512.

Migeon C J, Brown T R, Fichman K R (1981). Androgen insensitivity syndrome. *The Intersex child: Pediatric and Adolescent Endocrinology*, pp. 171–202. Karger, Basel.

Moore K L (1988). *The Developing Human: Clinically Orientated Embryology*. Saunders, Philadelphia, PA.

New M I, White P C, Pang S, Dupont B, Speiser P (1989). The adrenal hyperplasias. In Schriver, C R, Beaudet A, Sly W, Valle D eds., *The Inherited Basis of Molecular Disease*, 6th edn, pp. 1881–1917. McGraw-Hill, New York.

New M I (1992). Female pseudohermaphroditism. *Sem Perinatol* 16, 299–318.

O'Leary J A (1965). Comparative studies of the gonad in testicular feminization and cryptorchidism. *Fertil Steril* 16, 813–819.

Pang S, Levine L S, Stoner E et al. (1983). Nonsalt-losing congenital adrenal hyperplasia due to 3β-hydroxysteroid dehydrogenase deficiency with normal glomerulosa function. *J Clin Endocrinol Metab* 56, 808–818.

Rosler A, Liberman E, Sack et al. (1982). Clinical variability of congenital adrenal hyperplasia due to 11β-hydroxylase deficiency. *Horm Res* 16, 133–141.

Schuchardt A, D'Agati V, Larsson-Blomberg L, Constantini F, Pachnis V (1994). Defects in the kidney and enteric nervous system of mice lacking the tyrosine kinase receptor. *Nature* 367, 380–383.

Seaver L H, Grimes J, Erickson R P (1994). Female pseudohermaphroditism with multiple caudal anomalies: absence of Y-specific DNA sequences as pathogenetic factors. *Am J Med Genet* 51, 16–21.

Shozu M, Akasofu K, Takenori T, Kubota Y (1991). A new cause of female pseudohermaphroditism: placental aromatase deficiency. *J Clin Endocrinol Metab* 72, 560–566.

Stark K, Vainio S, Vassileva G, McMahon A P (1994). Epithelial transformation of metanephric mesenchyme in the developing kidney regulated by *Wnt-4. Nature* 372, 679–683.

Torres M, Gomez-Pardo E, Dressler G R, Gruss P (1995). *Pax-2* controls multiple steps of urogenital development. *Development* 121, 4057–4065.

Tran D, Meusy-Desolle N, Josso N (1977). Anti-Mullerian hormone as a functional marker of foetal Sertoli cells. *Nature* 269, 411–412.

(1981). Waning of anti-Mullerian activity: an early sign of Sertoli cell maturation in the developing pig. *Biol Reprod* 24, 923–931.

Vigier B, Watrin F, Magre S, Tran D, Josso N (1987). Purified bovine AMH induces a characteristic freemartin effect in fetal rat prospective ovaries exposed to it in vitro. *Development* 100, 43–55.

von Prader A (1954). Der genitalbefund beim Pseudohermaproditismus femininus des kongenitalen adrenogenitalen Syndroms Morphologie Hausfigkeit Entwicklung und Vererbung der verschiedenen Genitalformen. *Helv Pediatr Acta* 9, 231–248.

2

Molecular genetics of gonad development

Andrew Sinclair and Fergus Cameron

Murdoch Children's Research Institute, Royal Children's Hospital, Melbourne, Australia

Introduction

Sex determination involves the commitment of the embryo to follow either a male or female developmental pathway. The key step in this process is the development of the undifferentiated embryonic gonads into either testes or ovaries. In humans, sex is determined at the moment of fertilization by the constitution of the sex chromosomes. Two X chromosomes result in ovaries and a female phenotype while an X and Y constitution produces testes and male development.

It has been known for some time that the Y chromosome carries a dominant testis-determining gene, which causes the undifferentiated embryonic gonad to develop as a testis. The masculinizing effect of the testis results from the secretion of the hormones testosterone and anti-Müllerian hormone (AMH; also known as Müllerian inhibitory substance, MIS). AMH causes regression of the embryonic female Müllerian ducts. In the absence of the Y chromosome (and absence of the testis-determining gene), ovaries will develop. Interestingly, female development will still occur in the absence of ovaries or their hormonal products. Consequently, the decisive event in sex determination is whether or not a testis develops. In humans and other mammals, sex determination can be equated with testis determination.

This chapter describes what we know of the genes that control human gonad development and how alterations in these genes can cause sex-reversed phenotypes. The Y-linked testis-determining gene *SRY* and others in this complex developmental network, such as *SOX9, WT1, SF1, DAX1* and *DMRT1*, are discussed. (The nomenclature used for these genes depends on the species, for example *SRY* in humans and *Sry* in mice; the protein products are designated SRY and Sry, respectively.) Mutations, translocations and deletions of these genes are described and related to a range of gonadal and sex-reversed phenotypes. Finally, a developmental gene network describing the control of testis determination is presented.

SRY: the testis-determining gene

The Y-linked *SRY* (sex-determining region, Y) gene initiates the developmental process leading to testis determination. *SRY* was isolated by analysis of Y chromosome fragments translocated to the X chromosome in XX sex-reversed male patients with testicular tissue (Sinclair et al., 1990). *SRY* maps to the short arm of the human Y chromosome, near the pseudoautosomal region. Mutations were detected in the *SRY* gene of XY females (for a more detailed clinical description of these patients see Table 2.1) indicating that *SRY* is required for normal testis development (Berta et al., 1990; Jäger et al., 1990). Finally it was demonstrated that mice transgenic for *Sry* developed into sex-reversed males, despite an XX karyotype (Koopman et al., 1991). Consequently, among Y-derived sequences, *SRY* is both required and sufficient for male sex determination.

It was hoped the isolation of *SRY* would lead to an unravelling of the molecular genetic pathway leading to testis development. However, it is now 12 years since the discovery of SRY and still we know relatively little about how this gene is regulated and how it activates a complex developmental network. The properties of the *SRY* gene have made such analysis difficult. The binding site recognized by the SRY protein is also shared by many other proteins (Harley

Paediatric and Adolescent Gynaecology, ed. Adam Balen et al. Published by Cambridge University Press.
© Cambridge University Press 2004.

Table 2.1. Genes associated with abnormal testicular development in humans

Gene	Human chromosome	Clinical phenotype	Aetiology
SRY	Yp11.1	XX male	90% caused by X/Y translocation
		XY female	15% SRY mutation
		True hermaphrodite	SRY mutation
SOX9	17q24	XY female, campomelic dysplasia	Mutation of SOX9 (haploinsufficiency)
		XX male	Duplication of SOX9 (overexpression)
DAX1	Xp21.3	Adrenal hypoplasia hypogonadotrophic hypogonadism	Mutation of DAX1
		XY female	Duplication of DAX1 (overexpression)
SF1	9q34	XY female, adrenal failure	Mutation of SF1 (haploinsufficiency)
WT-1	11p13	XY female with either Denys–Drash or Frasier syndrome	Deletion or mutation of WT1 (haploinsufficiency)
DMRT1	9p24.3-pter	XY female	Deletion of region including DMRT1 (haploinsufficiency?)
XH2	Xq13	XY female	Mutation of XH2
WNT-4	1p35	XY female	Duplication of WNT-4 (overexpression)

Note: Adapted from Veita et al., 2001.

et al., 1994) and is present in the regulatory regions of many genes, most of which do not have roles in sex determination. As yet we still do not know the in vivo target of SRY.

SRY structure

The human *SRY* gene contains a single exon encoding a protein of 204 amino acid residues, including a central 79 residue motif, the HMG box (**h**igh **m**obility **g**roup) (Clépet et al., 1993). The HMG motif is capable of sequence-specific DNA binding and bending, both of which are critical for SRY function (Giese et al., 1992). These properties suggest that SRY may function as an "architectural" transcription factor; these factors are thought to act by changing the chromatin structure in the regulatory regions of target genes, allowing the assembly of regulatory complexes (Koopman, 2001). The HMG domain also contains signal motifs required for transporting the SRY protein into the nucleus, where it can regulate transcription (Poulat et al., 1995; Südbeck and Scherer, 1997). The nonHMG box regions of SRY are not well conserved between different mammalian species. Striking differences between mouse and human SRY protein exist, particularly at the C-terminal. In the mouse, the C-terminal of Sry is 252 amino acid residues long (human is only 69 residues) and contains a glutamine/histidine-rich domain that mediates *trans*-activation in vitro. No such region has been identified in human SRY protein, suggesting that it

may act as a repressor rather than an activator of transcription (Ramkissoon and Goodfellow, 1996). This has led to the conclusion that the HMG box is the only part required for SRY function. However, it has recently been demonstrated in mouse that nonHMG box regions are required for Sry function. Curiously, these nonHMG box regions of mouse Sry are not shared with other mammals. This suggests that mouse and human SRY proteins may interact with different cofactors (Koopman, 2001).

SRY expression

In male mouse embryos, *Sry* is expressed only in the genital ridge in a narrow developmental window. *Sry* is briefly expressed within the pre-Sertoli cells of male mouse gonads at the onset of testis differentiation (between 10.5 and 12.5 days postconception (dpc)) (Koopman et al., 1990; Lovell-Badge, 1992). It appears that the role of *SRY* is to act as a molecular switch, stimulating Sertoli cell formation and consequent testis determination. By contrast, in humans, SRY shows more widespread expression. In humans, SRY is expressed at 41 days postovulation (dpo), peaks at 44 dpo and persists at low levels throughout the embryonic period and beyond (Hanley et al., 2000). Human *SRY* is expressed in a variety of nongonadal embryonic and adult tissues (Clépet et al., 1993). Its function in these tissues is unclear, and the transcript may be inactivated in nongonadal sites.

However, XY females with mutations in *SRY* do not display any other phenotypes, suggesting *SRY* action is restricted to the testis.

SRY regulation and function

The factors regulating *SRY* expression during testis differentiation are unknown. Evidence suggests that genes involved in early gonad development, such as the Wilms' tumour gene (*WT1*), may activate *SRY*. Recently, it was shown that specific isoforms of *WT1* can activate *Sry* in mice, both in vitro and in vivo (Hammes et al., 2001; Hossain and Saunders, 2001). The SRY promoter region lacks an obvious TATA box, but is GC rich and contains putative regulatory response elements upstream of the transcription initiation site. The sequence motif recognized by the SRY protein, AACAAAG, is also present in the region of the transcription start site of the *SRY* gene itself, implying possible autoregulation (Vilain et al., 1992). Cell migration experiments with normal and *Sry*-transgenic gonads suggest multiple roles for *Sry*. These include induction of mesonephric cell migration into the ridges to surround resident germ and Sertoli cells within the developing cords (Capel et al., 1999; Martineau et al., 1997), proliferation of cells within the ridges (Schmahl et al., 2000), and the induction of Sertoli cell differentiation (Tilmann and Capel, 1999).

SRY mutations: XY females

Mutations in *SRY* have been found in 10–15% of XY females with complete gonadal dysgenesis. All but two reported cases of 46,XY females with complete gonadal dysgenesis have mutations in the HMG box, highlighting its crucial functional role (Cameron and Sinclair, 1997). The two exceptions are a deletion 5′ to the HMG box (McElreavey et al., 1992) and a point mutation 3′ to the HMG box, which results in a truncated protein (Tajima et al., 1994). Y chromosome deletions and translocations have also been reported but these are rarer (Schafer, 1995). The gonads in these patients appear as ovaries with the same gonadal phenotype as in patients with 45,X Turner's syndrome (Schafer, 1995). Only gonadal tissues appear to be affected, even though (mutant) *SRY* is expressed in other somatic tissues of the body. There are several cases of familial mutations of *SRY* associated with 46,XY complete gonadal dysgenesis (e.g. Berta et al., 1990; Jäger et al., 1990). Mutant SRY protein from these familial cases shows a range of effects from normal to substantially reduced binding. By contrast, all de novo SRY mutants showed abolition of sequence-specific DNA binding (Harley et al., 1992). This loss of binding in the familial cases suggests that these mutations are conditionally sex reversing. Although the mechanism is unknown, it is likely that SRY is required at a threshold level in order to be functional. Any sequence changes that reduce SRY expression or activity may alter its ultimate functional impact. As only 15% of XY females with complete gonadal dysgenesis have a mutation in *SRY*, it implies that 85% carry a mutation in some other gene involved with the testis pathway.

SRY translocation: XX males

By contrast, 80% of XX males can be accounted for by the translocation of Y-derived sequences to the X chromosome (Ferguson-Smith, 1966). Almost all these patients test positive for the presence of SRY. The amount of Y sequence DNA present varies from as little as 35 kb (Sinclair et al., 1990) to over 75% of the Y chromosome short arm. The degree of masculinization shows a correlation with the amount of Y sequence present (Ferguson-Smith et al., 1990) and most have no disability other than infertility. Approximately 20% of XX males lack any detectable Y sequence including the region for *SRY* (Palmer et al., 1989). The majority of these patients have ambiguous genitalia but have an otherwise male phenotype (Ferguson-Smith et al., 1990). Sex reversal in this instance could be explained by a gene downstream from *SRY* undergoing a mutation that results in its constitutive expression, although this would be a rare event. Alternatively, SRY may act by repressing an inhibitor of male development. In this scenario, XX males (lacking *SRY*) may have a recessive (loss of function) mutation in this inhibitory gene so that it can no longer switch off downstream male-determining genes (McElreavey et al., 1993).

SRY mutations: XX true hermaphrodites

True hermaphrodites contain both ovarian and testicular gonadal tissue. The majority do not have any Y chromosomal material. Some XX true hermaphrodites have been shown to carry translocated Y sequences, including *SRY* on one X chromosome. Random X chromosome inactivation will result in different cells being either testis determining (through *SRY*) or ovarian determinating (because of absence of *SRY*). The most common cause of true hermaphroditism is 46,XX/46,XY mosaicism (Schafer, 1995).

SOX9, a key sex-determining gene

The isolation of *SRY* revealed a related gene family, the *SOX* (*SRY*-related HMG box) genes (Gubbay et al., 1990;

Sinclair et al., 1990). There are more than 20 of these genes, which seem to play a role in a variety of developmental processes.

Campomelic dysplasia, sex reversal and *SOX9*

The role of *SOX9* in testis determination was discovered as a result of its association with the bone dysmorphic syndrome *campomelic dysplasia* (CD). Patients with this syndrome have a number of skeletal and extraskeletal abnormalities, such as bowing of the long bones, brachydactyly and micrognathia. While 46,XX individuals with CD have normal ovaries, 75% of 46,XY patients with CD are sex-reversed females with either partial or complete gonadal dysgenesis (Cooke et al., 1985). External genitalia range from completely female without ambiguity to a male phenotype with minor ambiguities (Houston et al., 1983). Tommerup and colleagues (1993) analysed patients with CD with translocations of chromosome 17 and were able to map the locus causing both CD and sex reversal to 17q24.3–25.1. *SOX9* was subsequently identified within this critical region (Foster et al., 1994; Wagner et al., 1994).

SOX9 mutations

Sex-reversed patients with CD have mutations in *SOX9*, implying a role in both skeletal and testis development. In most cases, only one allele is mutated, suggesting that haploinsufficiency of *SOX9* is responsible (Cameron and Sinclair, 1997). As appears to be the case with *SRY*, gene dosage may be critical for normal *SOX9* function. Mutations in the *SOX9* HMG box result in impaired DNA-binding ability of the SOX9 protein (Meyer et al., 1997). In contrast to *SRY* mutations, loss-of-function mutations in *SOX9* have been identified throughout the open reading frame of the gene. Most of these mutations result in a protein with a truncated C-terminus, implying that this region is critical for SOX9 function. Indeed, a conserved *trans*-activation domain has been identified within amino acid residues 402 to 509 of the human SOX9 protein (Südbeck et al., 1996). This suggests that *SOX9* specifies a classic transcription factor with both a DNA binding and *trans*-activation domain capable of upregulating other genes. There are three classes of *SOX9* mutation: those that affect the *SOX9* HMG box and impair DNA binding (Foster et al., 1994; Wagner et al., 1994); those that affect transcriptional *trans*-activation (Südbeck et al., 1996); and translocation breakpoints in regulatory regions upstream of *SOX9* that reduce or abolish transcription (Wirth et al., 1996).

The HMG box of *SOX9* contains two independent nuclear localization signals (Südbeck and Scherer, 1997). In mice, Sox9 protein is initially cytoplasmic in the genital ridges of both sexes prior to 11.5 dpc but moves to the nucleus at later stages of testes development (Morais da Silva et al., 1996). It has been suggested that some factor(s) interact with the nuclear localization signal to mediate this change in subcellular Sox9 localization (Koopman, 2001). No mutations in the nuclear localization signals have been reported in patients with CD.

Three lines of evidence suggest that gain-of-function mutations involving *SOX9* can induce a male phenotype in XX humans and mice. First, a 46,XX sex-reversed male patient has been described with a duplication of the chromosomal region carrying *SOX9*. Presumably, duplication and the associated overexpression of *SOX9* account for this sex reversal (Huang et al., 1999). Such submicroscopic duplications of *SOX9* may explain some of the *SRY*-negative 46,XX males. Second, Bishop and colleagues (2000) have reported a mouse insertional mutant (Odsex) that appears to disrupt the regulatory region of *Sox9* and derepresses its expression. Consequently, *Sox9* fails to be downregulated in XX genital ridges, resulting in male development. Third, Vidal et al. (2001) have reported XX sex reversal in transgenic mice overexpressing *Sox9* in the genital ridges. These three observations suggest that *SOX9* induces Sertoli cell differentiation, resulting in testis formation and subsequent male development.

Embryonic expression of *Sox9*

Only male-to-female sex reversal has been observed in patients with CD. This implies that mutations in *SOX9* prevent testicular but not ovarian development, and that *SOX9* lies within the testis-determining pathway. In mouse embryos, *Sox9* is expressed in mesenchymal precursors during chondrogenesis, consistent with its proposed role in skeletal development, and in the indifferent gonads of both sexes (10.5 dpc). Expression is subsequently upregulated during testis differentiation and extinguished during ovary differentiation (Morais da Silva et al., 1996). This sexually dimorphic expression profile is also seen in embryonic chicken gonads (Kent et al., 1996), implying an important conserved role for *Sox9* in vertebrate testis determination. In humans, the expression profile of *SOX9* follows a similar pattern to *SRY* (Hanley et al., 2000). Immunohistochemical staining has shown that the Sox9 protein is localized in the nuclei of developing Sertoli cells in the male gonad (Morais da Silva et al., 1996). This suggests that Sox9 acts as a regulator of Sertoli cell differentiation. Given the importance of Sertoli cells for testis formation,

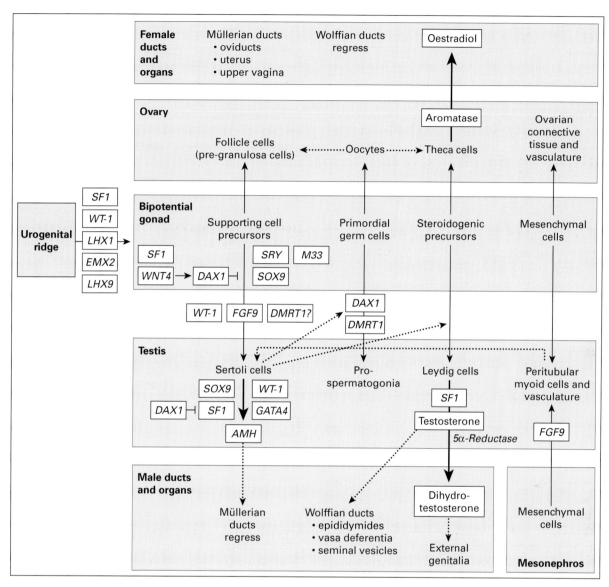

Fig. 2.1. The developmental network controlling gonad formation. Gene and cellular interactions during gonadal development. Pathways of cellular differentiation and/or migration are indicated by thin white arrows, biosynthetic pathways by thick white arrows, and hormonal or unknown signalling pathways by dashed arrows. Genes or gene products are shown in boxes. The nomenclature used is that for humans. DMRT1? is shown in a dashed box indicating its position in this pathway is not known. (Modified from Koopman, 2001.)

it is understandable that mutations in *SOX9* cause sex reversal.

SOX9 regulation and targets

SRY and SOX9 are both HMG box-containing proteins and recognize the same binding motif in vitro. Like SRY, SOX9 is thought to act as a transcription factor, but unlike SRY, SOX9 has a putative *trans*-activation domain at its C-terminus (Südbeck et al., 1996; reviewed in Schafer and Goodfellow,

1996). Although definitive data are lacking, it is possible that SRY could directly regulate *SOX9* expression in the Sertoli cell lineage. If so, *SOX9* could provide the missing link between *SRY* and *AMH* (see section on AMH regulation). It is known that SOX9 causes upregulation of *AMH* (Fig. 2.1 and below). However, AMH is produced by the Sertoli cells and all the evidence indicates that SOX9 has some role in Sertoli cell differentiation. Given that *SOX9* is expressed much earlier in development, it presumably regulates some as yet unknown factor in testis determination. One target gene for mouse Sox9 in the developing skeletal system has already been identified. Several lines of in vivo and in vitro evidence indicate that the Sox9 protein directly regulates expression of the gene for collagen type IIa in mouse chondrocytes (Bell et al., 1997; Ng et al., 1997). While type II collagen is not expressed in embryonic gonads, Sox9 might regulate the expression of similar extracellular matrix proteins during testis formation (collagen type V, laminin, etc.). Some *SOX9* mutations result in CD with sex reversal (75% of XY infants with CD) and others result in bone dysplasia (CD) alone without XY sex reversal. One explanation for the lower frequency of sex reversal is that the majority of fetuses with CD develop ovotestes, which resolve to either testes or ovaries after birth. No cases of *SOX9* mutations resulting in sex reversal without CD have been reported (Koopman, 2001; Meyer et al., 1997) and the distribution of sex-reversing mutations in human *SOX9* does not indicate any part of the protein has a specific role in sex determination (Cameron and Sinclair, 1997).

DMRT1: duplications of 9p and 46,XY gonadal dysgenesis

Deletions of the tip of human chromosome 9p have been shown to be associated with sex reversal and XY gonadal dysgenesis. Many of the patients with 9p deletions also have associated complex phenotypic features including external genital and craniofacial abnormalities resulting from monosomy or an unbalanced translocation (Veitia et al., 2001). Recently, a gene was discovered that maps to 9p and is a candidate autosomal testis-determining gene.

Sex-determining mechanisms appear to be very different in vertebrates and invertebrates. So it was surprising to find a family of genes related by a DMdomain (DNA-binding motif) that plays a sex specific role across the different phyla. The *Drosophila dsx* (doublesex) gene and the *Caenorhabditis elegans mab-3* gene share the DM domain and both genes are involved with the differentiation of sex specific structures such as the peripheral nervous system and yolk protein development. A search for DM-related genes in humans revealed the *DMRT1* (**DM**-**r**elated **t**ranscription factor **1**) gene. *DMRT1* maps to the distal short arm of human chromosome 9 (Raymond et al., 1998). *DMRT1* is upregulated specifically in the male genital ridge in humans (Moniot et al., 2000), mice and chickens (Raymond et al., 1999a; Smith et al., 1999). *DMRT1* expression occurred in the Sertoli cell lineage in addition to in the germ cells of the developing testes. In the chicken, *DMRT1* mapped to the Z chromosome, raising the possibility of a

dosage-related male sex-determining mechanism in that species (Nanda et al., 1999). *DMRT1* is expressed at very high levels specifically in the chicken male gonad, more than could be explained by the twofold difference in gene dosage between males (ZZ) and females (ZW). These observations are consistent with an important role for *DMRT1* in vertebrate sex determination. Despite these data, intensive searches have failed to reveal any mutations in *DMRT1* in patients with XY gonadal dysgenesis. Furthermore, *DMRT1* maps just outside a 500 kb region that has been identified as the smallest region involved with XY female gonadal dysgenesis (Calvari et al., 2000). It is possible that *DMRT1* has distal regulatory regions that overlap this minimal region.

In humans, a related gene, *DMRT2*, as well as several other unrelated genes, map to the human 9p interval associated with XY sex reversal (Raymond et al., 1999b). The large deletions of chromosome 9 seen in sex-reversed XY female patients would presumably remove a number of genes from this region, so it is not possible to assess the specific role of *DMRT* using such patients. However, *Dmrt2* in mice is expressed during somite development and not in developing genital ridges, suggesting that a role in sex determination is unlikely. The function of *Dmrt1* in mice was explored using a gene-specific deletion. *Dmrt1* knockout mice do not show a sex-reversed phenotype (Raymond et al., 2000), suggesting either that *Dmrt1* is not a male sex-determining gene or that other related genes can compensate the male sex-determining function of *Dmrt1* in mice. It is not yet known how many members are in the *DMRT* gene family, nor whether any of these are expressed during gonadal development.

DAX1: dosage-sensitive sex reversal

Duplications of the short arm of the X chromosome (Xp21.3) can cause XY female sex reversal. This led to the suggestion that a **d**osage-**s**ensitive **s**ex-reversing (*DSS*) gene must reside on the X chromosome. It was postulated that two active copies of this gene in an XY individual might override normal testis development, resulting in XY female sex reversal. Analysis of Xp21 microduplications in several patients defined a critical 160 kb *DSS* region (Bardoni et al., 1994). Deletions of this region do not affect testis development but result in *adrenal hypoplasia congenita* (AHC) and hypogonadotrophic hypogonadism (HH) (Muscatelli et al., 1994). Within the DSS region a novel candidate gene was identified: *DAX1* (**D**SS-**A**HC-critical region of the **X** chromosome, gene **1**), encoding an orphan nuclear receptor (Zanaria et al., 1994). The protein is unusual in that it contains a putative ligand-binding domain but lacks the zinc finger DNA-binding motif typical of other nuclear receptors. Instead, it has an N-terminal domain comprising three and one half repeats of a 65 amino acid residue motif domain rich in alanine and glycine (Zanaria et al., 1994). The Dax1 protein localizes to the nucleus in mice and, like other nuclear receptors, is expected to regulate the expression of specific target genes. Zanaria et al. (1994) found that DAX1 bound to retinoic acid response elements (RERs) in vitro, mediating retinoic acid *trans*-activation. *DAX1* is normally likely to be subject to X chromosome inactivation, as individuals with Klinefelter's syndrome (XXY) are male, not sex-reversed females.

Loss-of-function mutations in *DAX1* cause AHC and HH (Muscatelli et al., 1994) but it was not clear if *DAX1* was also responsible for dosage-sensitive sex reversal. In an effort to create a mouse model for DSS, Swain et al. (1998) produced transgenic mice with multiple copies of *Dax1*. However, sex reversal was only seen when *Dax1* was overexpressed on a mouse background (*Mus poschiavinus*) with a weak *Sry* allele. This suggests that *Dax1* acts antagonistically to *Sry* to prevent testis development (Swain et al., 1998). It also indicates that the mouse is less sensitive to gene dosage than humans. *Dax1* expression in mice is downregulated with testis differentiation but persists in the developing ovary (Swain et al., 1998). These observations suggest a role for *Dax1* either in promoting ovarian development or in suppressing testis development when duplicated or overexpressed. The recent production of mice with mutated *Dax1* allows us to distinguish between these possibilities. Surprisingly, XX mice lacking *Dax1* developed ovaries and were fertile (Yu et al., 1998). This indicates that *Dax1* acts as an antitestis gene rather than having a role as an ovarian determining gene (Fig. 2.1). These knockout mice further revealed roles for *Dax1* in spermatogenesis, with lack of *Dax1* in males causing degeneration of the testicular germinal epithelium and sterility (Yu et al., 1998). In both sexes, mice lacking *Dax1* had compromised endocrine cell development. In normal circumstances, *DAX1* appears to play a key role in gametogenesis and endocrine development rather than sex determination.

FGF9: mesenchymal proliferation, mesonephric migration and Sertoli cell differentiation

The family of fibroblast growth factors (FGFs) regulates a range of developmental processes. One of them, FGF9, has been implicated in gonadal development. Mice lacking the gene *Fgf9* have a range of phenotypes from testicular hypoplasia to complete male-to-female sex reversal (Colvin et al., 2001). It is possible that, in humans, mutations altering *FGF9* signalling may account for some cases of XY sex

reversal. In mouse embryonic gonads, *Fgf9* is expressed just after the onset of *Sry* at 10.5 dpc. This is consistent with Fgf9 acting downstream from Sry. Mice null for *Fgf9* showed impaired Sertoli cell development. This suggests that Fgf9 could directly induce three specific functions of Sertoli cells: specification, proliferation and differentiation (Colvin et al., 2001). Sertoli cells appear to facilitate testis determination by allowing germ cells to enter mitotic arrest (Burgoyne et al., 1988a,b). Lack of peritubular myoid cells or mesenchyme could also cause sex reversal because these cells stimulate Sertoli cell differentiation (Colvin et al., 2001). Mice lacking Fgf9 also showed a reduction in cells proliferating in the coelomic epithelium. Normally there is a burst of proliferation in the coelomic epithelium from 11.3 to 11.5 dpc (Schmahl et al., 2000). This suggests that Fgf9 may control this cell proliferative phase. Finally, exogenous Fgf9 given to Fgf9-deficient mice induced mesonephric migration into the testes. This suggests that Fgf9 acts as a chemotactic factor for migrating mesonephric cells (Colvin et al., 2001). Induction of mesonephric migration resulted in cord formation and *Sox9* expression while blocking migration inhibited the formation of testicular cords (Tilmann and Capel, 1999). In many respects, Fgf9 can mediate multiple Sry-dependent processes. Fgf9 appears to affect early steps in testis development, including Sertoli cell development, gonadal cell proliferation and mesonephric cell migration (Fig. 2.1).

Steroidogenic factor 1: regulator of steroidogenesis and gonad differentiation

Steroidogenic factor 1 (SF1; also known as Ad4BP) is an orphan nuclear receptor and a key regulator of steroidogenic enzymes. As such SF1 plays a crucial role in both gonadal and adrenal development (Ingraham et al., 1994). *SF1* is expressed in all primary steroidogenic tissues, including the adrenal cortex, Leydig cells of the testis and ovarian follicles (Parker and Schimmer, 1997). In the mouse embryo, *Sf1* is expressed in the gonads of both sexes between 9 and 12 dpc. *Sf1* then shows continued expression throughout testis development but is downregulated during ovarian development. In mouse testis, *Sf1* expression becomes localized in both Sertoli and Leydig cells (Ikeda et al., 1994). Like other nuclear receptors, *SF1* encodes a conserved zinc finger DNA-binding domain and a ligand-binding domain (Wong et al., 1996). A highly conserved putative *trans*-activation domain called AF2 is present at the C-terminus. These data indicate that SF1 has a role in both the formation of the gonadal primordium and in subsequent sexual differentiation (Fig. 2.1). SF1 is also expressed at other sites in the developing embryo, including the hypothalamus and in pituitary gonadotrophs, indicating that it functions at several levels of the reproductive axis (Ingraham et al., 1994; Parker and Schimmer, 1997).

In addition to its function in mature gonads, SFI plays a role in gonadal differentiation during embryogenesis. Null mutant $Sf1$ knockout mice (XX and XY) lack both adrenal glands and gonads. These mice develop as phenotypic females but die after birth from adrenal failure. Detailed analysis of these mice showed that in the absence of $Sf1$ the genital ridge displayed arrested development and then atrophied (Luo et al., 1994). A mutation in human $SF1$ is associated with XY sex reversal and adrenal failure (Achermann et al., 1999). A target for SF1 appears to be AMH, which contains an SF1-binding site in its promoter. SF1 and AMH proteins are coexpressed in Sertoli cells during testis formation and it has been shown both in vitro and in vivo that SF1 is required to upregulate AMH (Giuili et al., 1997; Shen et al., 1994). Mutation of the SF1-binding site in the AMH promoter in vivo resulted in decreased levels of AMH expression (Arrango et al., 1999). DAX1 also inhibited transcriptional inactivation of SF1 and in so doing compromised steroidogenesis (Ito et al., 1997; Zazopoulos et al., 1997). SF1 can induce $DAX1$ expression by interaction with $DAX1$ upstream promoter elements (Burris et al., 1995). This completes an interactive circle of $SF1$ and $DAX1$ expression and repression. SF1 appears to act at three important steps in the sex-determining cascade. The first is in the early establishment of the bipotential gonad, prior to SRY expression; the second is in the upregulation of AMH during testis differentiation, and the third is in regulating steroid synthesis in Leydig and theca cells (Koopman, 2001).

Wilms' tumour 1: multiple roles in sex determination

$WT1$ is an oncogene associated with a paediatric kidney cancer (Wilms' tumour). $WT1$ encodes a zinc finger protein that is thought to act as a transcription factor (Call et al., 1990). Heterozygous mutations affecting the zinc finger domain of WT1 result in patients with Denys–Drash syndrome, characterized by renal failure and genital abnormalities, including XY female sex reversal (Pelletier et al., 1991a). Frasier syndrome, also associated with XY female sex reversal, has been shown to result from a mutation in a splice donor site in $WT1$, causing loss of a specific isoform of WT1 (Barbaux et al., 1997). Patients with Frasier syndrome are characterized by late-onset but progressive

glomerulopathy and 46,XY gonadal dysgenesis, with streak gonads but normal female external genitalia (Veitia et al., 2001).

In mouse, $Wt-1$ is expressed from 9 dpc in the undifferentiated gonads and mesonephros (developing kidney) of both males and females. In the developing mouse embryo, $Wt1$ is expressed at the same time as $Sf1$ (Pelletier et al., 1991b). Targeted disruption of $Wt1$ in mice resulted in failure of kidney, ovary and testis development. This suggests that $Wt1$ acts early in urogenital development (possibly in conjunction with $Sf1$) to ensure proper formation of the indifferent embryonic gonad (Fig. 2.1). $Wt1$ does not appear to be required for $Sf1$ expression as $Sf1$ is still expressed in $Wt1$ knockout mice. However, $Wt1$ may contribute to $Sf1$ upregulation (Parker et al., 1999). Another study suggests that the WT1 protein can regulate $DAX1$ expression by binding to a GC-rich sequence in the promoter (Kim et al., 1999).

The mutations in $WT1$ that result in XY females in both Denys–Drash and Frasier syndrome indicate that $WT1$ plays an additional role in testis development. Human $WT1$ comprises 10 exons and produces a range of different transcripts using alternative splice sites and translation start sites. It is thought that the different isoforms of WT1 play a variety of different functions. A specific isoform of WT1 (the same isoform abolished by the $WT1$ mutations in Frasier syndrome) appears to interact with SF1 to upregulate AMH expression in the testis (Arrango et al., 1999). Recently, Hossain and Saunders (2001) have shown that $Wt1$ can regulate the expression of Sry in vitro. $In\ vivo$ experiments by Hammes et al. (2001) demonstrated that Sry levels fall in the absence of specific isoforms of Wt1 (WT1+KTS), causing abolition of $Sox9$ and Amh expression and XY sex reversal. It appears that the WT1+KTS isoform is essential for high levels of Sry expression in the male embryonic gonad (Hammes et al., 2001).

$LIM1$ ($LHX1$), $LHX9$ and $EMX2$: formation of the genital ridge?

The mouse homeo-paired box gene $Lim1$ (also known as $Lhx1$) appears to play a role in kidney and gonad development. Targeted disruption of $Lim1$ results in mice completely lacking head structures and in early death. Surviving fetuses also lack kidneys and gonads. $Lim1$ is expressed in early urogenital ridge development in both the mesonephros and metanephros (Shawlot and Behringer, 1995). It is assumed that in humans LIM1 acts at the same level as SF1 and WT1 in the formation and maturation of the genital ridges but its role in gonad development is not clear as the lethality of knockout $Lim1$ embryos makes such analysis difficult (Koopman, 2001) (Fig. 2.1).

Lhx9 is another member of the Lim homeobox domain family of transcription factors with a potential role in gonad development. $Lhx9$ is expressed in the epithelial and mesenchymal cells of the urogenital ridges of embryonic mice at 9.5 dpc, later localizing to the interstitial regions as differentiation occurs. In mutant mice lacking Lhx9, germ cells seem to migrate normally, but somatic cells of the genital ridge fail to proliferate normally and a discrete gonad fails to form (Birk et al., 2000). In the absence of testosterone and AMH, these mice develop as phenotypic females. In addition, the levels of Sf1 are considerably reduced in mice lacking $Lhx9$, implying that $Lhx9$ lies upstream of $Sf1$ (Fig. 2.1). This suggests that $Lhx9$ permits cell proliferation, $Sf1$ expression and is essential for the formation of the indifferent gonad (Birk et al., 2000). Mutations in many other genes involved with early gonadal development ($Sf1$, $Wt1$ and $Lim1$) are associated with major defects in other organs. However, in mice carrying an $Lhx9$ null mutation, only gonadal development is affected. It is possible that mutations in $LHX9$ might be responsible for some forms of gonadal agenesis (early regression of gonads of both sexes) in humans (Birk et al., 2000).

Another homeobox-containing transcription factor, $Emx2$, is expressed in mesonephric tubules, coelomic epithelia, Wolffian ducts and the genital ridges. Targeted removal of $Emx2$ resulted in mice with poorly developed gonads and their mesonephric tubules and Wolffian ducts degenerated (Miyamoto et al., 1997). Every indication is that Emx2 acts early in urogenital ridge maturation but is likely to act downstream of Wt1 as Wt1 is unaffected in mice with mutant Emx2 (Koopman, 2001).

M33: an intermediate between SRY and SOX9?

The mouse gene $M33$ has also been implicated in gonadal development. $M33$ shows similarity to the $Drosophila$ polycomb group of genes (PcG). Mice with targeted disruption of $M33$ showed retarded gonad development associated with varying degrees of XY sex reversal (Katoh-Fukui et al., 1998). Sry was expressed normally in these $M33$ mutant mice but $Sox9$ expression was reduced. This suggests that M33 may act as an intermediate between Sry and Sox9 or acts cooperatively with Sry to activate or repress downstream genes directly (Fig. 2.1) (Koopman, 2001). In $Drosophila$, PcG proteins regulate the coordinate expression of homeotic genes. So another potential role for M33 may be to regulate Hox gene expression in the mammalian urogenital ridge.

X-linked mental retardation with α-thalassaemia and XY sex reversal

X-linked mental retardation with α-thalassaemia (ATR-X syndrome) is an X-linked disorder with severe mental retardation, characteristic facial features, α-thalassaemia, genital abnormalities and several other congenital anomalies. Mutations in $XH2$, encoding a putative DNA helicase, are responsible for the ATR-X syndrome (Gibbons et al., 1995). $XH2$ maps to Xq13.3 and potentially acts by disrupting chromatin structure, allowing access for DNA regulatory molecules. The level of gonadal dysgenesis in affected individuals is variable, in some instances leading to complete male-to-female sex reversal and female gender assignment, suggesting a role for $XH2$ in testis development (Ion et al., 1996). The absence of Müllerian ducts in ATR-X patients suggests that AMH has been expressed from the Sertoli cells in the testis. Mutations in $XH2$, therefore, appear to disrupt testis development after the action of SRY and the differentiation of Sertoli and Leydig cells but prior to testis organization. XH2 must function downstream from SRY and AMH in the testis-determining pathway (Pask and Graves, 2001).

GATA4

GATA4 is a transcription factor with a role in gonadal development and differentiation. In mouse embryos, $Gata4$ is expressed at 11.5 dpc in somatic but not the germ cell lineage of the developing gonads of both sexes. Later in development (13.5 dpc) $Gata4$ is downregulated in the ovary but continues to be expressed in the nuclei of newly differentiated Sertoli cells (Koopman, 2001; Viger et al., 1998). GATA4 also appears to act in synergy with SF1 in the regulation of AMH (Tremblay and Viger, 1999; Viger et al., 1998).

Regulation of anti-Müllerian hormone

AMH is synthesized in the Sertoli cells; it is one of the first proteins produced by the developing testis. AMH causes regression of the Müllerian ducts within the male embryo, which would otherwise develop as oviducts, uterus and upper vagina. Within the small regulatory region of the AMH gene, binding sites have been identified for SOX9 and SF1 (de Santa Barbara et al., 1998; Giuili et al., 1997; Shen et al., 1994). SOX9 and SF1 bind to adjacent sites in the regulatory region of AMH and cause significant upregulation of AMH expression. In mice, mutation of the Sox9- or Sf1-binding sites in the Amh regulatory region causes abolition or diminution, respectively, of *Amh* expression (Arrango et al., 1999). SOX9 appears to be essential for initiating *AMH* expression. SF1 physically interacts with the adjacent SOX9 protein to cause significant upregulation of AMH transcript levels. A specific isoform of WT1 also appears to physically interact with SF1 to upregulate AMH expression synergistically (Arrango et al., 1999). As a counter to this, DAX1 has been shown in vitro to repress the synergistic action of SF1 and WT1 on the *AMH* promoter (Nachtigal et al., 1998). This suggests that the normal upregulation of AMH expression would be blocked when there is an abnormal double dose of the gene *DAX1* and its product is present in high levels in the testis, resulting in XY sex reversal. The normal role of DAX1 in the ovary may be to prevent the expression of *AMH*. One member of the GATA family of transcription factors, GATA4, is found in the developing gonads. A GATA4-binding site is also present in the *AMH* regulatory region. It is thought the GATA4 protein may bind this site and interact with SOX9 to regulate *AMH* expression (Tremblay and Viger, 1999; Viger et al., 1998). The role of WT1 and GATA4 on *AMH* regulation has not been confirmed in vivo. However, it is clear that SOX9 and SF1 are required to upregulate *AMH* expression (Fig. 2.1). While AMH is required for sex-specific differentiation of the reproductive tract, the absence of AMH does not affect testis development.

WNT-4: ovarian development and testis suppression

Wnt-4, a member of the *Wnt* gene family encoding signalling molecules, appears to be required for ovarian development and acts to suppress testis formation. *Wnt-4* is initially expressed in the genital ridge and mesonephros of both sexes but as sex-specific gonadal differentiation proceeds it is downregulated in the testis but maintained in the ovary (Vainio et al., 1999). Male (XY) mice lacking *Wnt-4* develop normal testes and Wolffian duct derivatives. By contrast, females (XX) lacking *Wnt-4* are masculinized as the Müllerian duct is absent and the Wolffian duct is similar to that of a male. Furthermore, the ovaries of female mice with mutated *Wnt-4* express genes coding for enzymes normally associated with testosterone production. Finally, the ovaries of these mice display a marked decrease in oocyte development (Vainio et al., 1999). The *Wnt-4* mutant mice imply that steroid cell precursors of Leydig and theca cells must be present in the indifferent gonad of both males and females. As the testis develops more rapidly than the ovary, the Leydig cells can begin producing testosterone as soon as testis cords form in the embryo. By contrast,

the theca cells in the ovary are not steroidogenically active until birth (Vainio et al., 1999). These data suggest that in normal XX females high levels of *Wnt-4* expression act in the indifferent genital ridge to repress testosterone production in the precursors of Leydig cells, allowing theca cells to develop eventually. Presumably, the downregulation of *Wnt-4* expression allows testosterone biosynthesis from Leydig cells to proceed in normal (XY) males (Vainio et al., 1999). Consequently, *Wnt-4* appears to have three distinct functions in the female pathway: formation of the Müllerian duct, suppression of Leydig cell development in the indifferent genital ridge, and postmeiotic maintenance of oocytes in the ovary (Fig. 2.1).

The human orthologue *WNT-4* has been isolated and maps to human chromosome 1p35, a region that is analogous to mouse chromosome 4q (Jordan et al., 2001). In mice, distal chromosome 4q is known to be implicated in XY sex reversal. A sex-reversed XY female patient has been described with a duplication of *WNT-4* and overexpression of the gene (Jordan et al., 2001). In mice, both *Wnt-4* and *Dax1* are downregulated in the developing testis (at 11.5 and 12.5 dpc, respectively) but both genes continue to be expressed in the ovary. Jordan and colleagues used *Sf1* and *Wnt-4* to transfect mouse Leydig and Sertoli cell lines and demonstrated that Wnt-4 upregulates *Dax1* expression. They speculate that Dax1 then exerts an antagonistic effect on *Sry*, preventing testis development and causing sex reversal. In humans, *WNT-4* and *DAX1* may act in concert to prevent testis formation and promote female development (Jordan et al., 2001).

Summary

The molecular genetics of gonad development must involve an ordered cascade of events. Since the isolation of *SRY* in 1990, several other genes have been identified that are critical for normal gonad development. These genes and their known and potential interactions point to a complex developmental network with multiple positive and negative regulatory elements (Fig. 2.1). The formation of gonads involves a range of different cell types, which need to be coordinated by a series of signalling molecules, receptors, signal transduction systems and transcription factors (Koopman, 2001). We know that some individual genes act at multiple points in gonad development, playing several different regulatory roles. At this stage, our understanding of the exact relationships between key regulatory genes such as *SRY* and *SOX9* is unknown, let alone all their downstream targets. At present, only a small proportion of sex-reversed patients can be explained by defects in the known testis genes. Clearly, more genes involved with gonad development wait to be discovered. The challenge for the future is both to identify new genes and to piece together their interactions in order to gain a more complete insight into the molecular genetics of gonad development.

REFERENCES

Achermann J C, Ito M, Hindmarsh P C, Jameson J L (1999). A mutation in the gene encoding steroidogenic factor-1 causes XY sex reversal and adrenal failure in humans. *Nat Genet* 22, 125–126.

Arrango N A, Lovell-Badge R, Behringer R R (1999). Targeted mutagenesis of the endogenous mouse *Mis* gene promoter: *in vivo* definition of genetic pathways of vertebrate sexual development. Cell 99, 409–419.

Barbaux S, Niaudet P, Gubler M-C et al. (1997). Donor splice-site mutations in WT1 are responsible for Frasier syndrome. *Nat Genet* 17, 467–469.

Bardoni B, Zanarai E, Guioli S et al. (1994). A dosage sensitive locus at chromosome Xp21 is involved in male to female sex reversal. *Nat Genet* 7, 497–501.

Bell D, Leung K H, Wheatley S C et al. (1997). SOX9 directly regulates the type-II collagen gene. *Nat Genet*, 16, 174–178.

Berta P, Hawkins J R, Sinclair A H et al. (1990). Genetic evidence equating SRY, the testis determining factor. *Nature* 348, 448–450.

Birk O S, Casiano D E, Wassif CA et al. (2000). The LIM homeobox gene *Lhx9* is essential for mouse gonad formation. *Nature* 403, 909–912.

Bishop C E, Whitwhort DJ, Qin Y et al. (2000). A transgenic insertion upstream of *Sox9* is associated with dominant XX sex reversal in the mouse. *Nat Genet* 26, 490–494.

Burgoyne P S, Buehr M, Koopman P, Rossant J, McLaren A (1988a). Cell-autonomous action of the testis-determining gene: Sertoli cells are exclusively XY in XX ↔ XY chimaeric mouse testes. *Development* 102, 443–450.

Burgoyne P S, Buehr M, McLaren A (1988b). XY follicle cells in ovaries of XX ↔ XY female mouse chimaeras. *Development* 104, 683–688.

Burris T P, Guo W, Le T, McCade E R B (1995). Identification of a putative steroidogenic factor-1 response element in the DAX-1 promoter. *Biochem Biophys Res Commun* 214, 576–581.

Call K M, Glaser T, Ito C Y et al. (1990). Isolation and characterisation of a zinc finger polypeptide gene at the human chromosome 11 Wilms' tumor locus. *Cell* 60, 509–520.

Calvari V, Bertini V, de Grandi A et al. (2000). A new submicroscopic deletion that refines the 9p region for sex reversal. *Genomics* 65, 203–212.

Cameron F, Sinclair A H (1997). Mutations in *SRY, SOX9* and testis-determining genes. *Hum Mutat* 9, 388–395.

Capel B, Albrecht K H, Washburn L L, Eicher E M (1999). Migration of mesonephros cells into the mammalian gonad depends on Sry. *Mech Dev* 84, 127–131.

Clépet C, Schafer A J, Sinclair A H, Palmer M S, Lovell-Badge R, Goodfellow P N (1993). The human SRY transcript. *Hum Mol Genet* 2, 2007–2012.

Colvin J S, Green R P, Schmahl J, Capel B, Ornitz D M (2001). Male to female sex reversal in mice lacking fibroblast growth factor 9. *Cell* 104, 875–889.

Cooke C T, Mulcahy M T, Cullity G J, Watson M, Sprague P (1985). Campomelic dysplasia with sex reversal: morphological, cytogenetic studies of a case. *Pathology* 17, 526–529.

de Santa Barbara P, Bonneaud N, Boizet B et al. (1998). Direct interaction of SRY-related protein SOX9 and steroidogenic factor 1 regulates transcription of the human anti-Müllarian hormone gene. *Mol Cell Biol* 18, 6653–6665.

Ferguson-Smith M A (1966). X-Y chromosomal interchange in the aetiology of true hermaphrodites and XX Klinefelter's syndrome. *Lancet* ii, 475–476.

Ferguson-Smith M A, Cooke A, Affara N A, Boyd E, Tolmie J L (1990). Genotype–phenotype correlations in XX males and their bearing on current theories of sex determination. *Hum Genet* 84, 198–202.

Foster J W, Dominguez-Steglich M A, Guioli S et al. (1994). Campomelic dysplasia and autosomal sex reversal caused by mutations in an SRY-related gene. *Nature* 372, 525–530.

Gibbons R, Picketts D J, Villard L, Higgs D R (1995). Mutations in a putative global transcriptional regulator cause X-linked mental retardation with α-thalassemia (ATR-X syndrome). *Cell* 80, 837–845.

Giese K, Cox J, Grosschedl R (1992). The HMG domain of lymphoid enhancer factor 1 bends DNA and facilitates assembly of functional nucleoprotein structures. *Cell* 69, 185–195.

Giuili G, Shen W-H, Ingraham H A (1997). The nuclear receptor SF-1 mediates dimorphic expression of Müllerian inhibiting substance *in vivo. Development* 124, 1799–1807.

Gubbay J, Collignon J, Koopman P et al. (1990). A gene mapping to the sex determining region of the mouse Y chromosome is a member of a novel family of embryonically expressed genes. *Nature* 346, 245–250.

Hammes A, Guo J-K, Lutsch G et al. (2001). Two splice variants of the Wilms' tumour 1 gene have distinct functions during sex determination and nephron formation. *Cell* 106, 319–329.

Hanley N A, Hagan D M, Clement-Jones M et al. (2000). *SRY, SOX9* and *DAX1* expression patterns during human sex determination and gonadal development. *Mech Dev* 91, 403–407.

Harley V R, Jackson D I, Hextall P J et al. (1992). DNA binding activity of recombinant SRY from normal males and XY females. *Science* 255, 453–456.

Harley V R, Lovell-Badge R, Goodfellow P N (1994). Definition of a consensus DNA binding site for SRY. *Nucl Acid Res* 22, 1500–1501.

Hossain A, Saunders G F (2001). The human sex-determining gene *Sry* is a direct target of Wt1. *J Biol Chem* 276, 16817–16823.

Houston C S, Optiz J M, Spranger J W et al. (1993). The campomelic syndrome: review. *Am J Med Genet* 15, 3–28.

Huang B, Wang S, Ning Y, Lamb A N, Bartley J (1999). Autosomal XX sex reversal caused by duplication of *SOX9*. *Am J Med Genet* 87, 349–353.

Ikeda Y, Shen W-H, Ingraham H A, Parker K L (1994). Developmental expression of mouse steroidogenic factor 1 an essential regulator of steroid hydroxylases. *Mol Endocrinol* 8, 654–662.

Ingraham H, Lala D S, Ikeda Y et al. (1994). The nuclear receptor steroidogenic factor 1 acts at multiple levels of the reproductive axis. *Genes Dev* 8, 2302–2312.

Ion A, Telvi L, Chaussain J L et al. (1996). A novel mutation in the putative DNA helicase XH2 is responsible for male-to-female sex reversal associated with an atypical form of the ATR-X syndrome. *Am J Hum Genet* 58, 1185–1191.

Ito M, Yu R, Jameson J L (1997). DAX-1 inhibits SF-1-mediated transactivation via carboxy-terminal domain that is deleted in adrenal hypoplasia congenita. *Mol Cell Biol* 17, 1476–1483.

Jäger R J, Anvret M, Hall K, Scherer G (1990). A human XY female with a frameshift mutation in the candidate testis determining gene SRY. *Nature* 210, 352–354.

Jordan B K, Mansoor M, Ching S T et al. (2001). Up-regulation of WNT-4 signalling and dosage sensitive sex reversal in humans. *Am J Hum Genet* 68, 1102–1109.

Katoh-Fukui Y, Tsuchiya R, Shiroishi T et al. (1998). Male-to female sex reversal in M33 mutant mice. *Nature* 393, 688–692.

Kent J, Wheatley S C, Rews J E, Sinclair A H, Koopman P (1996). A male-specific role for *SOX9* in vertebrate sex determination. *Development* 122, 2813–2822.

Kim J, Prawitt D, Bardeesy N et al. (1999). The Wilms' tumor suppressor gene (WT1) product regulates *Dax-1* gene expression during gonadal differentiation. *Mol Cell Biol* 19, 2280–2299.

Koopman P (2001). *sry, sox9* and mammalian sex determination. In *Genes, Mechanisms in Vertebrate Sex Determination*, Scherer G, Schmid M, eds., pp. 25–56. Birkhauser, Basel Switzerland.

Koopman P, Münsterberg A, Capel B, Vivian N, Lovell-Badge R (1990). Expression of a candidate sex-determining gene during mouse testis determination. *Nature* 348, 450–452.

Koopman P, Gubbay J, Vivian N, Goodfellow P N, Lovell-Badge R (1991). Male development of chromosomally female mice transgenic for *Sry*. *Nature* 351, 117–121.

Lovell-Badge R (1992b). The role of *SRY* in mammalian sex determination. In *Post-Implantation Development in the Mouse*, Chadwick D J, Marsh J, eds., pp. 162–182. John Wiley, New York.

Luo X, Ikeda Y, Parker K L (1994). A cell-specific nuclear receptor is essential for adrenal, gonadal development and sexual differentiation. *Cell* 77, 481–490.

McElreavey K, Vilain E, Abbas N, Herskowitz I, Fellous M (1992). XY sex reversal associated with a deletion 5′ to the SRY HMG box in the testis-determining region. *Proc Natl Acad Sci USA* 89, 11016–11020.

McElreavey K, Vilain E, Abbas N, Herskowitz I, Fellous M (1993). A regulatory cascade hypothesis for mammalian sex determination: SRY represses a negative regulator of male development. *Proc Natl Acad Sci USA* 90, 3368–3372.

Martineau J, Nordqvist K, Tilman C, Lovell-Badge R, Capel B (1997). Male-specific cell migration into the developing gonad. *Curr Biol* 7, 958–968.

Meyer J, Sudbeck P, Held M et al. (1997). Mutational analysis of the *SOX9* gene in campomelic dysplasia and autosomal sex reversal: lack of genotype/phenotype correlations. *Hum Mol Genet* 6, 91–98.

Miyamoto N, Yoshida M, Kuratani S, Matsuo I, Aizawa S (1997). Defects of urogenital ridge development in mice lacking *Emx2*. *Development* 124, 1653–1664.

Moniot B, Berta P, Scherer G, Sudbeck P, Poulat F (2000). Male specific expression suggests a role of DMRT1 in human sex determination. *Mech Dev* 91, 323–325.

Morais da Silva S, Hacker A, Harley V, Goodfellow P, Swain A, Lovell-Badge R (1996). *Sox9* expression during gonadal development implies a conserved role for the gene in testis differentiation in mammals and birds. *Nat Genet* 14, 62–68.

Muscatelli F, Strom T M, Walker A P et al. (1994). Mutations in the *DAX-1* gene give rise to both X-linked adrenal hypoplasia congenita and hypogonadotrophic hypogonadism. *Nature* 372, 672–676.

Nachtigal M W, Hirokwaw Y, Enjeart-VanHouten D L, Flanagan J N, Hammer G D, Ingraham H A (1998). Wilms' tumor 1 and Dax1 modulate the orphan nuclear receptor SF-1 in a sex specific gene expression. *Cell* 93, 445–454.

Nanda I, Shan Z, Schartl M et al. (1999). 300 million years of conserved synteny between chicken Z and human chromosome 9. *Nat Genet* 21, 258–259.

Ng L-J, Wheatley S, Muscat G E O et al. (1997). SOX9 binds DNA, activates transcription, coexpresses with type II collagen during chondrogenesis in the mouse. *Devel Biol* 183, 108–121.

Palmer M S, Sinclair A H, Berta P et al. (1989). Genetic evidence that *ZFY* is not the testis-determining factor. *Nature* 342, 937–939.

Parker K L, Schimmer B P (1997). Steroidogenic factor 1: a key determinant of endocrine development and function. *Endocr Rev* 18, 361–377.

Parker K L, Schedl A, Schimmer B P (1999). Gene interactions in gonadal development. *Annu Rev Physiol* 61, 417–433.

Pask A, Graves J A M (2001). Sex chromosomes, sex determining genes. In *Genes, Mechanisms in Vertebrate Sex Determination*, Scherer G, Schmid M, eds., pp. 71–95. Birkhauser, Basel Switzerland.

Pelletier J, Bruening W, Kashtan C E et al. (1991a). Germline mutations in the Wilms' tumor suppressor gene are associated with abnormal urogenital development in Denys–Drash syndrome. *Cell* 67, 437–447.

Pelletier J, Schalling M, Buckler A, Rogers A, Haber D A, Housman D (1991b). Expression of the Wilms' tumor gene *wt-1* in the murine urogenital system. *Gene Dev* 5, 1345–1356.

Poulat F, Girad F, Chevron M-P et al. (1995). Nuclear localisation of the testis determining gene product SRY. *J Cell Biol* 128, 737–748.

Ramkisoon Y, Goodfellow P N (1996). Early steps in mammalian sex determination. *Curr Biol* 6, 316–321.

Raymond C S, Shamu C E, Shen M M et al. (1998). Evidence for evolutionary conservation of sex-determining genes. *Nature* 391, 691–695.

Raymond C S, Kettlewell J R, Hirsch B, Bardwell V J, Zakower D (1999a). Expression of *Dmrt1* in the genital ridge of mouse and chicken embryos suggests a role in vertebrate sexual development. *Dev Biol* 215, 208–220.

Raymond C S, Parker E D, Kettlewell J R et al. (1999b). A region of human chromosome 9p required for testis development contains two genes related to known sexual regulators. *Hum Mol Genet* 8, 989–996.

Raymond C S, Murphy M W, O'Sullivan M G, Bardwell V J, Zakower D (2000). *Dmrt1*, a gene related to worm and fly sexual regulators, is required for mammalian testis differentiation. *Genes Dev* 14, 2587–2595.

Schafer A J (1995). Sex determination, its pathology in man. In *Advances in Genetics*, Vol. 33, Hall J C, Dunlap J C, eds., pp. 275–329. Academic Press, San Diego, CA.

Schafer A, Goodfellow P N (1996). Sex determination in humans. *BioEssays* 18, 955–963.

Schmahl J, Eicher E M, Washburn L L, Capel B (2000). *Sry* induces cell proliferation in the mouse gonad. *Development* 127, 65–73.

Shawlot W, Behringer R (1995). Requirement for Lim1 in head organiser function. *Nature* 374, 425–430.

Shen W-H, Moore C C D, Ikeda Y, Parker K L, Ingraham H A (1994). Nuclear receptor steroidogenic factor 1 regulates the Müllerian inhibiting substance gene: a link to the sex determination cascade. *Cell* 77, 651–661.

Sinclair A H, Berta P, Palmer M S et al. (1990). A gene from the human sex-determining region encodes a protein with homology to a conserved DNA-binding motif. *Nature* 346, 240–244.

Smith C A, McClive P J, Western P S, Reed K J, Sinclair A H (1999). Conservation of a sex determining gene. *Nature* 402, 601–602.

Südbeck P, Scherer G (1997). Two independent nuclear localisation signals are present in the DNA-binding high mobility group domains of SRY and SOX9. *J Biol Chem* 272, 27848–27852.

Südbeck P, Leinhard Schmitz M, Baeuerle P A, Scherer G (1996). Sex reversal by loss of the C-terminal transactivation domain of human *SOX9*. *Nat Genet* 13, 230–232.

Swain A, Narvaez V, Burgoyne P, Camerino G, Lovell-Badge R (1998). *Dax1* antagonizes Sry action in mammalian sex determination. *Nature* 391, 761–767.

Tajima T, Nakae J, Shinohara N, Fujieda K (1994). A novel mutation localised in the 3′ non-HMG box region of the SRY gene in 46XY gonadal dysgenesis. *Hum Mol Genet* 3, 1187–1189.

Tilmann C, Capel B (1999). Mesonephric cell migration induces testis cord formation and Sertoli cell differentiation in the mammalian gonad. *Development* 126, 2883–2890.

Tommerup N, Schempp W, Meinecke P et al. (1993). Assignment of an autosomal sex reversal locus (*SRA1*), campomelic dysplasia (CMPD1) to 17q24.3-q25.1. *Nat Genet* 4, 170–173.

Tremblay J J, Viger R S (1999). Transcription factor GATA-4 enhances Müllerian inhibiting substance gene transcription through a direct interaction with nuclear receptor SF-1. *Mol Endocrinol* 13, 1388–1401.

Vainio S, Heikkila M, Kispert A, Chin N, McMahon A P (1999). Female development in mammals is regulated by Wnt-4 signalling. *Nature* 397, 405–409.

Veitia R A, Salas-Cortes L, Ottolenghi C, Pailhoux E, Cotinot C, Fellous M (2001). Testis determination in mammals: more questions than answers. *Mol Cell Endocrinol* 179, 3–16.

Vidal V I, Chaboissier M-C, de Rooij D G, Schedl A (2001). Sox9 induces testis development in XX transgenic mice. *Nat Genet* 28, 216–217.

Viger R S, Mertineit C, Trasler J M, Nemer M (1998). Transcription factor GATA-4 is expressed in a sexually dimorphic pattern during mouse gonadal development and is a potent activator of the Müllerian inhibiting substance promoter. *Development* 125, 2665–2675.

Vilain E, Fellous M, McElreavey K (1992). Characterisation and sequence of the 5′ flanking region of the human testis-determining factor *SRY*. *Meth Mol Cell Biol* 3, 128–134.

Wagner T, Wirth J, Meyer J et al. (1994). Autosomal sex reversal and campomelic dysplasia are caused by mutations in and around the *SRY*-related gene *SOX9*. *Cell* 79, 1111–1120.

Wirth J, Wagner T, Meyer J et al. (1996). Translocation breakpoints in three patients with campomelic dysplasia and autosomal sex reversal map more than 130 kb from *SOX9*. *Hum Genet* 97, 186–193.

Wong M, Ramayya M S, Chrousos G P, Driggers P H, Parker K L (1996). Cloning and sequence analysis of the human gene encoding steroidogenic factor 1. *J Mol Endocrinol* 17, 139–147.

Yu R N, Ito M, Saunders T L, Camper S A, Jameson J L (1998). Role of Ahch in gonadal development and gametogenesis. *Nat Genet* 20, 353–357.

Zanaria E, Muscatelli F, Bardoni B et al. (1994). An unusual member of the nuclear hormone receptor superfamily responsible for X-linked adrenal hypoplasia congenita. *Nature* 372, 635–641.

Zazopoulos E, Lalli E, Stocco D M, Sassone-Corsi P (1997). DNA binding and transcriptional repression by DAX1 blocks steroidogenesis. *Nature* 390, 311–315.

3

Gonadotrophin receptors

Manuel Tena-Sempere[1], Jerome Levallet[2] and Ilpo Huhtaniemi[3]

[1] Department of Physiology, University of Córdoba, Spain
[2] Department of Biochemistry, University of Caen, France
[3] Department of Physiology, University of Turku, Finland

Introduction

Physiological and biochemical studies have established the role of gonadotrophins and their receptors in great detail in the regulation of reproductive functions. However, structural studies of genes for the gonadotrophin subunits and gonadotrophin receptors have provided reproductive endocrinologists with improved tools to study normal and pathological functions of the hypothalamic–pituitary–gonadal (HPG) axis. In this chapter, we review the current concepts of normal and pathological functions of the gonadotrophin receptors for luteinizing hormone (LH) and follicle-stimulating hormone (FSH). Amongst the most intriguing novel findings in this field are the recently discovered activating and inactivating mutations in gonadotrophin receptor genes. They corroborate and extend our knowledge of clinical consequences of gonadotrophin resistance and inappropriate gonadotrophin action. The information obtained from human mutations has been complemented by animal models with disrupted or inappropriately activated gonadotrophin ligand or receptor genes (transgenic and knockout mice). These clinical and experimental genetic disease models form a powerful tool for exploring the physiology and pathophysiology of gonadotrophin function and provide good examples of the use of molecular biological approaches to explore the pathogenesis of diseases.

LH and FSH play a crucial role in reproductive functions. Their effects on specific gonadal target cells are mediated by their cognate receptors, the LH receptor (R) and FSHR. This chapter reviews key information about structure, function and physiological and pathophysiological correlates of the gonadotrophin receptors. Although the main emphasis is on receptor function in women, animal data and findings in males are presented when they are relevant for understanding the general principles of gonadotrophin receptor function.

Physiology of gonadotrophin receptor function

LH and FSH are essential regulatory signals in the control of gonadal function and their cognate receptors are key elements in the regulatory network that controls development and function of the reproductive axis. Therefore, several factors have to be considered when assessing the normal and pathological function of gonadotrophins. In addition to the secretion of gonadotrophins, the expression of their receptors is of crucial importance.

Biological actions of gonadotrophins in the female ,

Gonadotrophins function along the HPG axis, which is a classical example of an endocrine regulatory circuit, with positive and negative feed-forward and feedback regulatory events (Fig. 3.1). Notably, the functional activity of the HPG axis varies considerably during sexual development. In the female, ovarian function is independent of gonadotrophins during the fetal period and, at least in rodents, the onset of gonadotrophin receptor expression and function occurs postnatally (Sokka et al., 1992; Zhang et al., 1994). Data on the developmental onset of gonadotrophin receptor expression in human ovary are not available. Infancy is quiescent in this respect since tonic inhibition of the hypothalamic–pituitary (HP) unit results in low circulating gonadotrophin levels. As puberty approaches, the

Paediatric and Adolescent Gynaecology, ed. Adam Balen et al. Published by Cambridge University Press.
© Cambridge University Press 2004.

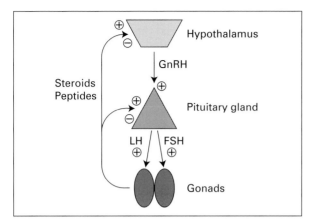

Fig. 3.1. Schematic presentation of the hypothalamic–pituitary–gonadal axis. LH, luteinizing hormone; FSH, follicle-stimulating hormone; GnRH, gonadotrophin-releasing hormone.

HPG axis is activated by enhanced central excitatory inputs. In addition, progressive desensitization of the HP unit to the feedback effects of inhibitory gonadal signals may participate in the onset of puberty. As a result, the increased circulating levels of gonadotrophins, and apparent appearance of gonadotrophin receptors in the ovary, induce complete sexual maturation and the attainment of reproductive capacity. This initiates the adult reproductive period, where the pulsatile cyclic secretion of gonadotrophins drives the cyclicity in ovarian function (i.e. follicular development and selection, ovulation, luteinization). Finally, reproductive senescence, with cessation of ovarian function owing to exhaustion of the follicular pool, takes place at menopause. In this period, high serum LH and FSH levels are detected as a consequence of the loss of negative feedback loops through impaired ovarian hormone secretion.

In the ovary, LHRs are expressed in theca, granulosa and luteal cells. In theca cells, LH elicits the production of aromatizable androgens (Hillier et al., 1994), whereas in granulosa cells it triggers ovulation by inducing rupture of the follicle wall, thereafter stimulating luteinization and progesterone production by the corpus luteum (Richards and Hedin, 1988). The ovarian FSHRs are solely expressed in granulosa cells. Consequently, FSH stimulates ovarian granulosa cell growth and activates the production of oestrogens by upregulating aromatase activity, thus initiating the normal menstrual cycle. In the absence of sufficient FSH, the follicles fail to develop beyond the early antral stage and ovulation does not occur. Although the earliest phases of follicular maturation may not be FSH dependent, this gonadotrophin is essential to support persistent follicular growth (Filicori and Cognigni, 2001). Overall, a large

body of evidence from studies in laboratory rodents as well as in primates and humans, clearly indicates that the initiation of follicular growth is gonadotrophin independent, but shortly thereafter it becomes responsive to FSH.

The maintenance of gonadotrophin secretion is critically dependent on pulsatile secretion of the hypothalamic gonadotrophin-releasing hormone (GnRH), at 1–2 hour intervals. GnRH is a decapeptide that acts upon gonadotroph cells of the anterior pituitary gland to elicit gonadotrophin synthesis and secretion. GnRH secretion is under positive and negative control by gonadal hormones (see below), but is also regulated by a number of central nervous system (CNS) neurotransmitters. The same GnRH peptide stimulates the release of both FSH and LH. A separate FSH-releasing peptide has also been proposed (Yu et al., 1997) but conclusive evidence for its existence has not been provided. GnRH effects are mediated through a G-protein-coupled receptor (GPCR), and its signal transduction entails activation of phospholipase C, generation of inositol trisphosphate (IP_3) and diacylglycerol (DAG) second messengers, increase of cytoplasmic free calcium and activation of protein kinase C (PKC). The major endocrine factors contributing to gonadotrophin secretion are gonadal steroid and peptide hormones. The steroid hormones, oestrogen and progesterone in the female, exert their negative feedback actions both on GnRH secretion at the hypothalamic level and directly on gonadotrophin gene expression in pituitary gonadotrophs. In addition, oestradiol has a positive feedback effect upon hypothalamic and pituitary levels of GnRH, resulting in the preovulatory surge of gonadotrophins that culminates in the ovulatory LH secretion peak. Of the ovarian peptide hormones, inhibin is a physiologically significant negative regulator of FSH secretion at the pituitary level (de Kretser and Phillips, 1998). The other peptide of this family, activin, and its binding protein, follistatin, exert regulatory effects on gonadotrophin secretion and action mainly in para/autocrine fashion within the anterior pituitary and gonads (de Kretser and Phillips, 1998). Notably, besides the endocrine regulation of the HPG axis, a complex network of paracrine and autocrine, intrapituitary and intragonadal regulatory mechanisms participate in the regulation of gonadotrophin secretion and action (Albertini et al., 2001; Hillier, 1999; Schwartz, 2000), yet the extent of their physiological role needs to be fully delineated.

It is noteworthy that the expression of the gene for LHR in nonclassical gonadotrophin target tissues, such as the placenta, brain and adrenal gland, has been independently reported by a number of groups (Kero et al., 2000; Rao, 1996; Ziecik et al., 2001), thus opening up the possibility of additional, as yet unknown, biological actions of LH

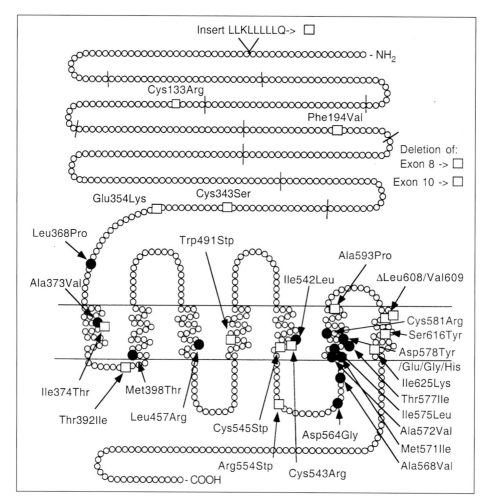

Fig. 3.2. The structure of the human luteinizing hormone receptor and the currently known activating (•) and inactivating (□) mutations. For details of original reports on the mutations, see Themmen and Huhtaniemi (2000).

in nongonadal tissues. Indeed, recent evidence indicates the presence of functional LHRs in the female mouse reproductive tract (Zheng et al., 2001). Analogous extragonadal expression of FSHRs has been reported in the bovine cervix (Mizrachi and Shemesh, 1999) and human myometrial smooth muscle (Kornyei et al., 1996). To date, the physiological relevance of such "ectopic" expression of LHR and FSHR has remained elusive.

Structure of gonadotrophin receptors

The gonadotrophin receptors belong to the large family of GPCRs, all having a domain of seven plasma membrane-traversing α-helices connected by three extracellular and three intracellular loops. The GPCRs are responsible for activation of the G-protein-mediated signal transduction

(Segaloff and Ascoli, 1993; Simoni et al., 1997; Themmen and Huhtaniemi, 2000) (Figs. 3.2 and 3.3). To date, the complementary DNAs (cDNA) encoding the LHR and FSHR have been cloned from several species (Themmen and Huhtaniemi, 2000). For the LHR, the nascent receptor is a 700 amino acid residue (aa) protein, where the first 26 aa comprise the signal peptide; the mature LHR protein has 674 aa and a molecular mass of 93 kDa (Segaloff and Ascoli, 1993). The immature FSHR contains 695 aa, where the first 17 aa function as signal peptide. Following cleavage of this fragment, the mature FSHR protein has 678 aa and a molecular mass of approximately 75 kDa (Minegishi et al., 1991).

Unlike most other GPCRs, the LHR and FSHR have a long extracellular domain that constitutes about 50% of the size of the receptor protein. The amino acid sequences and structural organization of the two gonadotrophin receptors

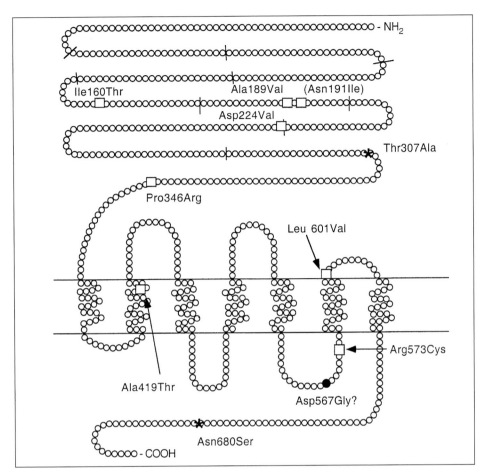

Fig. 3.3. The structure of the human follicle-stimulating hormone receptor with the currently known activating (•) and inactivating (□) mutations and functionally significant polymorphisms (∗). For details of original reports on the mutations, see Themmen and Huhtaniemi (2000).

are highly homologous, as is the case with their respective ligands (Segaloff and Ascoli, 1993; Simoni et al., 1997; Themmen and Huhtaniemi, 2000). The unusually large extracellular domain at the N-terminus of both receptors is responsible for specific high-affinity ligand binding. However, despite such selectivity in ligand binding, LH and human chorionic gonadotrophin (hCG) both bind to the same LHR, whereas FSH is the only ligand for FSHR. A similar large ligand-binding ectodomain is also present in the receptor for thyroid-stimulating hormone (TSH) receptor – TSHR – which is the third member of the subfamily of glycoprotein hormone receptors (Vassart and Dumont, 1992). Because of the structural similarity of ligands and receptors in this gene family, very high levels of hCG are able to bind to and activate to some extent the TSHR, and vice versa (Hosoi et al., 1999). In contrast, the structural organization of most other members of the GPCR family is defined by a fairly short extracellular domain, and their

ligand-binding site is a cleft in the transmembrane region (Jackson, 1991). The genes for LHR and FSHR comprise 11 and 10 exons, respectively, where the seven transmembrane segments and the G-protein-coupling domain are encoded by the last exon to encode the extracellular domain. In contrast, most of the shorter GPCRs have only one exon, homologous to the last exon of the glycoprotein hormone receptors. In humans, the genes *LHR* and *FSHR* are located on chromosome 2p21 and 2p21–16, respectively (Rousseau-Merck et al., 1993).

The extracellular domains of LHR and FSHR present a number of imperfect leucine-rich repeats (LRR), encoded by exons 2–9. These repeats with approximate lengths of 20–25 aa possess an amphiphilic β-sheet/α-helix structure that has been implicated in ligand–receptor binding (Segaloff and Ascoli, 1993). In fact, a number of glycoproteins with analogous structure have been identified where, despite the otherwise functional divergence, the presence of LRRs has been related to protein–protein interaction (Kobe and Deisenhofer, 1995). Concurrently, it has been theorized that the binding domain of the gonadotrophin receptors possesses a horseshoe-like structure, where the LRR direct their β-sheets to the inner face and their α-helices to the outer face of the U-shaped region (Moyle and Campbell, 1996). As the LRR motifs share 94% homology between LHR and FSHR, the question arises on their contribution to specific gonadotrophin binding. In this sense, variation in the location of the LRRs, presumed to determine the ligand specificity in LHR and FSHR, may be responsible for such a phenomenon (Song et al., 2001). The tertiary conformation of this binding domain depends, at least partly, on the presence of disulphide bonds between several cysteine residues in the extracellular region, essential for ligand binding and membrane insertion of the receptors (Dufau, 1996). Notably, in both receptors, the transit from the luminal side of the endoplasmic reticulum to the plasma membrane critically depends on the presence of a signal peptide, encoded by the 5′-terminal part of exon 1. Such a targeting process is also dependent on proper folding of the nascent protein, through interaction with the chaperone calnexin (Rozell et al., 1998).

The extracellular ligand-binding domain of the gonadotrophin receptors is connected by a cysteine-rich hinge region to the transmembrane signalling domain. The role of this connecting peptide has not been fully clarified, although convincing evidence indicates that it may serve functions other than merely acting as a spacer allowing correct location of the extracellular domain (Gromoll et al., 2000; Nakabayashi et al., 2000; Zhang et al., 1997, 1998). This hinge region is followed by the transmembrane domain with its seven membrane-spanning α-helices, connected by three exoloops and three cytoloops. This region is responsible for interaction and activation of the G-proteins, followed by signal transduction. However, the ligand binding *ectodomain* and signal transducing *endodomain* are intimately related in their functions. In this respect, the ectodomain of gonadotrophin receptors constrains the transmembrane region into a "resting" state under basal (unstimulated) ligand-free conditions. Overall, a molecular model for gonadotrophin receptor activation proposes that ligand binding to its receptor is a multistep process. Initially, ligand binding to a high-affinity site in the extracellular domain induces sensible modifications in receptor conformation, and eventually ligand interaction with a low-affinity site in the C-terminal part of the receptor triggers the signal transduction. Finally, the C-terminal part of the gonadotrophin receptor ends in a short cytoplasmic tail that contains several potential substrates for receptor phosphorylation, a phenomenon involved in the homologous

and heterologous modulation of receptor function. This involves the cessation of hormonal stimulation, by mediating the uncoupling of the receptor from its effector systems, as well as downregulation of the number of cell surface receptors (see below).

Function of gonadotrophin receptors

The gonadotrophin receptors appear as single-chain monomeric surface proteins and are fully capable of signal transduction. Nevertheless, recent reports indicate that functional LHR may be able to self-aggregate into dimers or oligomers, and that receptor functionality possibly involves receptor–receptor interaction (Roess et al., 2000). Transduction of the hormonal message and targeting to the biological actions of gonadotrophins to specific cells by gonadotrophin receptors involves different signalling systems. However, compelling evidence indicates that cAMP is the major second messenger for gonadotrophin action (Segaloff and Ascoli, 1993; Simoni et al., 1997). Indeed, LHR and FSHR are efficiently coupled with the G_s-protein, and ligand-induced receptor activation switches on the membrane-bound adenylyl cyclase to catalyse conversion of ATP into cAMP. In turn, increased intracellular cAMP levels induce activation of cAMP-dependent protein kinase A (PKA), which phosphorylates different cellular targets, including transcription factors such as the cAMP-responsive element binding protein (CREB), the cAMP-responsive element modulatory protein (CREM) and the inducible cAMP early repressor (ICER), which allow modulation of gene expression through interaction with consensus sequences (e.g. the cAMP-responsive element, CRE) located in promoters of gonadotrophin-regulated genes. In addition, coupling of the gonadotrophin receptors to the inhibitory G_i-proteins, decreasing cAMP levels, has been described. The ability of gonadotrophin receptors to interact with activators and repressors of the cAMP pathway has been implicated in the plasticity of gonadotrophic responses in target tissues (Arey et al., 1997).

In addition to cAMP, gonadotrophin receptor activation recruits other signalling systems. hCG, a "super-agonist" of LH, can stimulate phosphoinositide breakdown in ovarian cells, suggesting that inositol phosphates and DAG can operate as intracellular signals in biological actions of LH (Davis et al., 1984). In this pathway, receptor activation leads, through G_q-proteins or other members of the family, to stimulation of phospholipase C, which in turn catalyses the breakdown of phosphatidylinositol (IP) into DAG and IP_3. DAG activates PKC whereas IP_3 induces the release of calcium ions from intracellular stores. Conclusive evidence for the link between LHR and the IP–PKC pathway has been presented in humans and rodents (Gudermann et al., 1992). However, coupling of FSHR to the IP pathway appears to be species specific, being weak to absent in human FSHR (Hirsch et al., 1996; Tena-Sempere et al., 1999). In any case, the doses of LH or FSH required to elicit half-maximal responses of cAMP production are 10- to 50-fold lower than those needed for stimulation of IP_3. This emphasizes the major role of cAMP as the second messenger of gonadotrophin actions. In fact, gonadotrophin levels sufficient for IP_3 stimulation are observed only during the preovulatory surges and pregnancy (hCG) in females, thus suggesting that the physiological signalling role, if any, of the IP–PKC pathway is limited to those situations (Themmen and Huhtaniemi, 2000).

Besides the cAMP–PKA and IP–PKC pathways, other signals have been involved in the transduction and/or modulation of gonadotrophin actions in target cells. These include extracellular calcium, needed for the steroidogenic actions of LH; uptake of calcium ions has been shown in Leydig and Sertoli cells after LH and FSH stimulation, respectively (Grasso and Reichert, 1990; Manna et al., 1999). Similarly, autocrine or paracrine factor-mediated MAP (mitogen-activating protein) kinase signalling may participate in full granulosa cell responses to gonadotrophins (Johnson and Bridgham, 2001; Seger et al., 2001). Other intercellular signals may include other ions (e.g. chloride), arachidonic acid, leukotrienes and various free radicals (Cooke, 1996). From a functional stand-point, the concurrence of such a plethora of signalling systems might be linked to the differential signalling of specific gonadotrophin effects in target cells. In fact, intrinsic differences in signalling through LHR and FSHR have been recently described in granulosa cells, where, despite the use of the same second messenger (cAMP), LH and FSH provoke distinct biological actions (Bebia et al., 2001).

Physiological regulation of gonadotrophin receptor expression and function

The pivotal position of gonadotrophin receptors in the reproductive axis makes them a suitable target for tuning of gonadal function. The regulation of gonadotrophin receptor function can be conducted by homologous and heterologous signals: the former through alteration of the circulating gonadotrophin levels, the latter through action of other endocrine or para/autocrine factors. These modulatory effects can be stimulatory (*sensitization*) or inhibitory (*desensitization*), and they also include alteration of the number of cell surface receptors and expression of the receptor genes (*up-* and *downregulation*), as well as changes

in the functionality of receptor-mediated activation of signalling systems (*uncoupling*).

Concerning homologous regulation, physiological gonadotrophin levels are able to maintain or upregulate their cognate receptor levels, but supraphysiological levels, and especially prolonged elevation, result in receptor downregulation (e.g. LaPolt et al., 1992; Tilly et al., 1992), which is preceded by uncoupling of the signal transduction system. At least two mechanisms are involved in gonadotrophin receptor downregulation: increase in the rate of receptor internalization (Kishi and Ascoli, 2000; Lazari et al., 1999; Nakamura et al., 1991) and decrease in the level of receptor gene expression or mRNA half-life (LaPolt et al., 1992; Monaco et al., 1995; Themmen et al., 1991). The former apparently precedes the latter. The molecular mechanisms responsible for homologous desensitization of the LHR are thought to include phosphorylation of the cytoplasmic tail, through activation of G-protein-coupled receptor kinases (GRKs), and binding of nonvisual arrestins (e.g. β-arrestin and arrestin-3) to the third cytoplasmic loop, which have a role in uncoupling and internalization of the LHR (Mukherjee et al., 1999). A similar mechanism involving GRK-mediated receptor phosphorylation and arrestins seems to operate for the FSHR (Lazari et al., 1999; Troispoux et al., 1999). Several additional factors may modulate the rate of ligand-induced receptor desensitization, such as palmitoylation or self-aggregation of LHRs (Horvat et al., 2001; Munshi et al., 2001), and ADP ribosylation factor nucleotide exchange factor (ARNO)-induced β-arrestin release from the plasma membrane (Mukherjee et al., 2000a,b).

Besides homologous signals, a wide array of heterologous regulators of gonadotrophin receptor expression and function has been reported. For example, epidermal growth factor and phorbol ester can mimic the downregulation effect of LH on its receptor (Wang et al., 1991). Similarly, a number of factors have been shown to stimulate (transforming growth factors (TGF) α and β, activin, insulin-like growth factor 1 (IGF-1)) or inhibit (epidermal growth factor and retinoic acid) FSHR expression (Dunkel et al., 1994; Findlay and Drummond, 1999; Minegishi et al., 1999, 2000; Xiao et al., 1992). This heterologous regulation has many sexually dimorphic features. In the ovary, its functional cyclicity is associated with cyclic changes in the level of gonadotrophin receptor expression, and a number of heterologous signals are implicated in the regulation of ovarian gonadotrophin receptors. For instance, the induction of LHR expression in luteinizing granulosa cells occurs through synergistic action of FSH and oestradiol (Shi and Segaloff, 1995). Similarly, prolactin upregulates, together with LH, LHR expression in rodent corpora lutea (Segaloff

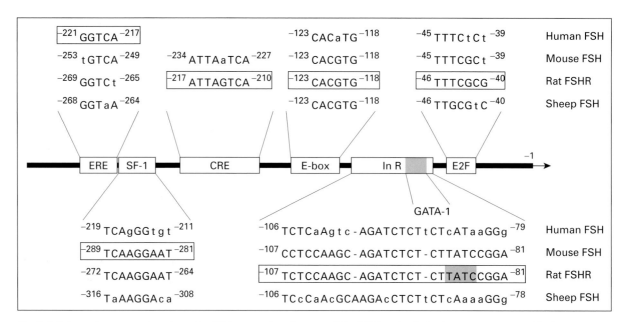

Fig. 3.4. Schematic presentation of putative DNA-responsive-elements of the follicle-stimulating hormone receptor 5′ flanking region. The nucleotides are numbered for respective species by allocating −1 to the first nucleotide above the translation initiation site. Each binding site sequence was compared with the sequence belonging to the species where the responsive element was first described (boxed). For references see text.

et al., 1990). Other heterologous factors playing roles in the regulation of gonadotrophin receptor expression are IGF-1, interleukin-6, activin, inhibin, follistatin, TGF-β_1, TGF-β_2, basic fibroblast growth factor, GnRH and TGF-α (e.g. Segaloff and Ascoli, 1993; Saez, 1994; Tamura et al., 2001; Themmen and Huhtaniemi, 2000). The physiological role of this complicated regulatory network remains to be explored, but it very likely operates in a redundant manner to ensure the optimal tuning of gonadotrophin receptor expression and, in turn, of gonadal function.

Unravelling the molecular mechanisms behind regulation of gonadotrophin receptor expression by homologous and heterologous signals has been made possible recently by the cloning and functional characterization of the promoter sequences of gonadotrophin receptor genes. Indeed, the 5′ flanking regions of the LHR and FSHR genes have been cloned from a variety of species, including the human (Atger et al., 1995; Gromoll et al., 1994; Heckert et al., 1992; Huhtaniemi et al., 1992; Tsai-Morris et al., 1991). Interestingly, analysis of the promoter areas revealed that all but the human LHR lack conventional TATA or CCAAT consensus sequences in the vicinity of the main transcription start sites. However, highly conserved crucial elements for positioning the RNA polymerase II complex have been located in the FSHR upstream region, overlapping the transcription start site. They include an initiator region (Inr) and an E box sequence able to bind the upstream regulatory

factors USF-1 and USF-2 (Heckert et al., 1998; Xing and Sairam, 2001). Another interesting feature of the LHR and FSHR promoters is their scattered pattern of transcription start sites, as well as the high CG content in the case of LHR: characteristics that apply also to the promoters of "housekeeping" genes. Notably, despite otherwise similar gene organization, no clear-cut structural relationship is found between the LHR and FSHR promoters. However, the promoter regions show high homology among different species for the same receptor. For instance, alignment of the proximal FSHR promoter regions of the human, mouse, rat and sheep genes (Fig. 3.4) showed that numerous positive regulatory elements, such as oestrogen receptor response elements (Gromoll et al., 1994), E2F and GATA elements (Kim and Griswold 2001), CRE (Monaco et al., 1995) and steroidogenic factor 1 (SF1)-binding sites (Heckert, 2001; Levallet et al., 2001), are roughly conserved between species.

Functional analyses have demonstrated that a large number of transcription factors do affect LHR and FSHR expression, thus revealing totally new information on these regulatory events. These studies have, for instance, demonstrated direct effects on LHR promoter function of thyroid hormones, progesterone, prolactin, IGF-1, FSH, nuclear orphan receptors and transcription factors Sp1, Sp2 and Ap2 and direct effects on the FSHR promoter of transcription factors SF1, USF-1 and USF-2 (Heckert et al.,

2000; Levallet et al., 2001; Manna et al., 2001; Nikula et al., 2001). Interestingly, the molecular basis for the conspicuous cAMP responsiveness of the LHR promoter, despite the absence of a classical CRE site, has been recently elucidated by the identification of two novel SAS (Sp1 adjacent site) in the rat promoter (Chen et al., 2000, 2001).

Finally, additional mechanisms are probably involved in the regulation of gonadotrophin receptor function. A recent suggestion is the regulation of gene expression by extensive DNA methylation at cytosine residues in the promoter and coding regions. In the rat FSHR promoter, seven specific CpG sites are methylated in cells that do not express the gene (Griswold and Kim, 2001). Moreover, demethylation treatment of the FSHR-negative Sertoli cell line MSC-1 reactivated transcription of the *FSHR* gene. To our knowledge, similar data have not been reported for the LHR.

An additional source of modulation of receptor function may derive from the generation of receptor isoforms through alternative splicing. Indeed, in all species tested so far, the expression of gonadotrophin receptor messages appears in a complex pattern of alternative splicing, which results in generation of mRNA transcripts of varying sizes. For instance, four major mRNA species of 7.0–6.8, 4.2, 2.6 and 1.8 kb have been described for the LRH, whereas FSHR mRNA transcripts of 2.5, 4.2, and 7.0 kb have been identified in Northern hybridization analyses (Segaloff and Ascoli, 1993; Tilly et al., 1992). However, the ability of those species to translate into functionally different receptor isoforms and, overall, the physiological significance of this phenomenon still remain unresolved (e.g. Tena-Sempere et al., 1999).

Structure–function relationships of gonadotrophin receptors

In recent years, detailed analyses of the structure–function relationships of gonadotrophin receptors have been carried out. Such studies have taken advantage of the characterization of several naturally occurring mutations in gonadotrophin receptor genes, as well as the development of potent molecular biological techniques. The latter has allowed selective modifications within the primary amino acid sequence of the receptors, construction of truncated and chimeric receptor molecules, as well as manipulation of the pattern of glycosylation of the nascent receptors. In this way, the function(s) of an expanding number of residues/portions of the functional receptors have been identified, as will be briefly summarized below.

The contribution of a number of structural features to folding and trafficking of the nascent protein, ligand binding, signal transduction and ligand-induced desensitization of LHR has been studied in detail. Studies using deleted and chimeric receptors have demonstrated that the binding region of gonadotrophin receptors presents both facilitatory binding determinants, responsible for high-affinity binding to the proper ligand (LRR 1–8 in LRR; LHR 1–11 in FSHR), and inhibitory binding determinants, responsible for blocking the binding of inappropriate ligands (exons 2–4 and 7–9 in LHR; exons 5–6 in FSHR) (Moyle and Campbell, 1996). Moreover, specific amino acid residues appear essential for proper ligand binding, as demonstrated by site-directed mutagenesis studies. For example, residues Glu132 and Asp135 of the rat LHR are absolutely required for hCG binding (Bhowmick et al., 1996). Mutational analyses have also identified several ionizable amino acid residues (i.e. Lys158, Lys183, Glu184, and Asp206) on the extracellular domain of LHR involved in ligand–receptor interaction (Bhowmick et al., 1999). Moreover, even amino acids located outside the N-terminal extracellular domain, such as Asp 383 of the LHR and His 407 of the FSHR, are likely involved in the ligand–receptor interaction (Ji and Ji, 1991, 1995).

The functional relevance of other structural characteristics of gonadotrophin receptors has also been a matter of analysis, for example the state of glycosylation. The extracellular domain of the LHR has six potential sites for N-linked glycosylation (Asn 99, 174, 195, 291, 299, and 313) whereas that of FSHR possesses four sites (Asn191, 199, 293, and 318, although the last site is not conserved among species) (Segaloff and Ascoli, 1993, Simoni et al., 1997). It is noteworthy that, although it has been demonstrated that the gonadotrophin receptors are glycosylated, the extent and importance of glycosylation in receptor function is not clear, and some apparently contradictory results have been presented. For example, chemical prevention of glycosylation of the rat LHR did not prevent correct receptor folding and trafficking, hormone binding and signal transduction (Davis et al., 1997). In contrast, mutational analysis in rats revealed a decrease or even complete loss of hormone-binding activity upon elimination of the potential glycosylation sites at Asn103, Asn178, and Asn199 (equivalent to Asn99, Asn174, and Asn195 in the human) (Zhang et al., 1991). An explanation for such a discrepancy is that disruption of the glycosylation sites by site-directed mutagenesis alters not only the glycosylation potential but also the conformation of the receptor. More detailed studies demonstrated that all potential consensus glycosylation sites were actually N-glycosylated. It was also shown that the deleterious effects of the mutated N-linked glycosylation sites on rat LHR function was a result of the amino acid substitutions per se and not the lack of glycosylation (Davis et al., 1997). Two of the three glycosylation sites

(Asn191 and Asn293) are glycosylated in the rat FSHR, and a carbohydrate at either residue is required for appropriate receptor folding during its synthesis (Davis et al., 1995).

Several cysteine residues located in the distal and middle region of the extracellular domain of the LHR, giving rise to disulphide bonds, have been proven essential for maintaining proper conformation of the binding domain and, thus, receptor function. Other cysteines located near, and in the transmembrane region, may play a role in insertion of the receptor into the cell membrane (Zhang et al., 1996). Detailed molecular analyses have indicated a role for specific amino acid residues or discrete domains within the primary sequence of gonadotrophin receptors in the processing/trafficking of the nascent receptor molecule. For example, a number of amino acid substitutions in the LHR and FSHR cause intracellular trapping of the mutant proteins, supporting a role for these residues in the proper folding and/or transport of the receptors to the cell surface (e.g. Rozell et al., 1995; Segaloff and Ascoli, 1993).

The structural requirements to activate signal transduction in the LHR have been assessed for specific amino acids and discrete areas. Several amino acid residues have been identified as essential to elicit cAMP responses after receptor activation. For example, mutation of residues Glu332 and Asp333 (close to the first transmembrane segment), Asp397 (in the first exoloop) and Lys583 (in exoloop 3) in the LHR resulted in blunted cAMP responses without altering ligand binding (Alvarez et al., 1999; Fernandez and Puett, 1996; Huang and Puett, 1995; Ji and Ji, 1993). Similarly, residues Asp405, Thr408 and Lys409 in the FSHR were found essential for signal transduction but not for ligand binding (Ji and Ji, 1995). Several amino acid substitutions, such as Ser277 and Asp578, were reported to induce constitutive activation (i.e. in the absence of ligand) of the LHR (Abell et al., 1998; Nakabayashi et al., 2000). Overall, it is apparent that specific areas within the receptor structure are critical for activation of the cAMP pathway. In fact, most of the activating mutations found to date in LHR and FSHR are located in a hot-spot comprising transmembrane segment 6 and cytoloop 3, thus suggesting that this area is highly relevant in G_s-protein coupling. In fact, this contention has been recently substantiated by the use of a synthetic peptide approach: a peptide designed to mimic the lower portion of transmembrane segment 6 of the LHR was able to activate adenylyl cyclase by interaction with G_s-proteins, whereas a peptide corresponding to an area in cytoloop 3 of FSHR was able to interact with G-protein and modulate signal transduction (Abell and Segaloff, 1997; Grasso et al., 1995).

As stated earlier, LHR and FSHR are also able to activate other signal transduction pathways, involving increased PI turnover and IP_3 production, elevated intracellular calcium ions and activation of MAP kinases. However, activation of these alternative intracellular pathways takes place in most cases at higher hormone concentrations than the cAMP pathway, likely restricting their physiological relevance to situations of elevated gonadotrophin levels such as the preovulatory surge and pregnancy (Themmen and Huhtaniemi, 2000). Interestingly, the ability of gonadotrophin receptors to activate different intracellular signals has been related to the plasticity of the biological actions of gonadotrophins. In this sense, it is tempting to speculate that the activation of different signals after receptor activation is carried out through different loci within the primary structure of the receptors. This seems to be the case with the LHR, where divergence of the cAMP and IP signalling pathways was detected at or near Lys583, located in exoloop 3. Mutations in this residue were incompatible with cAMP accumulation after receptor activation but permitted, at least in some cases, IP formation (Gilchrist et al., 1996). Similar divergence has been recently demonstrated for mutations in a highly conserved leucine residue (Leu457) located in transmembrane helix 3 of the human LHR (Shinozaki et al., 2001). It remains to be shown, however, whether LH can act at different sites of the binding domain of its receptor in order to activate cAMP and/or IP signals selectively. It would be intriguing if the different gonadotrophin isoforms would trigger a different array of second messenger responses, which could help to explain the pleomorphism of their actions according to the physiological state.

Finally, the structural determinants for ligand-induced gonadotrophin receptor desensitization (uncoupling *plus* internalization) have been thoroughly evaluated. Initial studies indicated that phosphorylation of certain serine/threonine residues in the cytoplasmic regions of LHR and FSHR were involved in receptor uncoupling. Agonist-induced phosphorylation of rat LHR was mapped to a locus of four serines (Ser635, 639, 649, 652) located in the C-terminus (Lazari et al., 1998). Concurrently, truncations of the cytoplasmic tail of the LHR were shown to prevent homologous uncoupling. More detailed analyses demonstrated that structural requirements for agonist-induced uncoupling and internalization are different (Lazari et al., 1998). In fact, mutational analyses in the second exoloop of human LHR emphasized the importance of receptor activation and de-emphasized the importance of receptor phosphorylation in ligand-induced internalization (Li et al., 2001). Several structural features of the LHR, including seven noncontiguous intracellular residues located in cytoloops 2 and 3 and the C-terminal tail (Nakamura et al., 2000), and a dileucine-based motif in the C-terminus (Nakamura and Ascoli, 1999), have been involved in ligand–receptor complex internalization, probably through their ability to modulate binding of the LHR to endogenous non-visual arrestins.

Clinical manifestations of gonadotrophin receptor mutations

Pathology linked to gonadotrophin receptor function of known aetiology is rare; most such pathologies are caused by constitutively activating or inactivating mutations of the receptor genes. Both activating and inactivating LHR mutations have been described, but the former seems to cause phenotype only in men. No clearly activating FSHR mutations have yet been characterized. In most sporadic cases with appropriate phenotype (e.g. hypergonadotrophic hypogonadism), no mutations are detected, and in these situations it is most likely that another gene involved in the cascade of gonadotrophin signal transduction harbours the mutation. Examples of such cases have not yet been identified, but it is likely that they will be detected in the future. A comprehensive list of gonadotrophin receptor mutations was published recently (Themmen and Huhtaniemi, 2000).

Mutations in luteinizing hormone receptors
Activating mutations
The first mutations detected in gonadotrophin receptors were those activating the LHR constitutively (Kremer et al., 1993; Shenker et al., 1993), apparently because of their striking phenotype. Interestingly, no female phenotype of these mutations has been described. It is a syndrome of male-limited gonadotrophin-independent precocious puberty, also called *testotoxicosis*. So far, a total of 12 activating mutations of the LHR gene have been described (Fig. 3.2). They all, understandably, are localized in the transmembrane region of the LHR, because this part of the receptor molecule plays a crucial role in the transduction of the LH signal. The mutations apparently change conformation of the transmembrane region of the receptor in such a fashion that it assumes, at least partially, activated conformation in the absence of ligand hormone. Functional consequences of gonadotrophin receptor mutations can be tested by transfecting the mutated receptor gene into cultured cells (Fig. 3.5). Second messenger (cAMP) response to increasing concentrations of the ligand hormone reveal whether the mutation has caused constitutive activation (elevated basal cAMP response) or inactivation (absent cAMP response to hormonal stimulation) of the receptor, or whether the mutation is neutral (no difference of cAMP response from control cells expressing wild-type receptor). Constitutively activating LHR mutations induce premature activation of Leydig cell testosterone production before the normal pubertal age of onset of LH secretion.

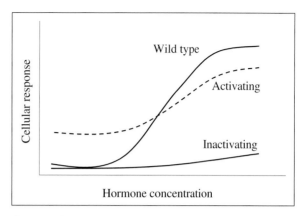

Fig. 3.5. Schematic presentation of hormone-stimulated response (e.g. cyclic adenosine monophosphate production) in cells transfected with complementary DNA encoding a wild-type receptor, and one carrying an activating and inactivating mutation. The elevated response in the absence of hormonal stimulation is typical of an activating mutation. In an inactivating mutation the response is almost or totally missing.

Despite the clear phenotype in males, no apparent phenotype is known in females with activating LHR mutations. One explanation is that the initiation of LH action in the ovary requires FSH priming and FSH-dependent paracrine factors (e.g. oestrogen) may be needed to induce the LHR responsiveness in theca cells. Since FSH secretion does not start in these women before the normal age of puberty, the necessary FSH induction cannot start prematurely. Another explanation is that, because prepubertal theca or granulosa cells do not express the LHR, it does not matter whether there is an activating mutation in the *LHR* gene. The developmental onset of ovarian *LHR* expression is an intriguing question, but it may remain unanswered since noninvasive methods to study *LHR* expression in the prepubertal ovary are not available. However, it remains curious why no hyperandrogenism is detected at any age in women expressing constitutively activated LHR: their theca cell androgen production should be elevated because of chronic LH stimulation.

Inactivating mutations
Today, close to 20 inactivating LHR mutations have been identified. They can be subdivided into two categories: partially or completely inactivating (Fig. 3.2; Themmen and Huhtaniemi, 2000). In the partially inactivating forms, some of the receptor activity remains and, therefore, the LH-dependent target cell functions are not totally absent. In men, LHR inactivation, depending on severity of the inactivation, causes a wide spectrum of phenotypes, ranging from complete lack of masculinization (46,XY

male pseudohermaphroditism) to mild undervirilization, in the form of micropenis or perineoscrotal hypospadias (Themmen and Huhtaniemi, 2000). Individuals with the complete form of mutation have female external genitalia, low testosterone and high LH levels, but normal FSH, total lack of responsiveness to LH/hCG challenge and no development of secondary male or female sex characteristics. There is a notable lack of breast development in the affected individuals at the age of puberty, which is the clearest phenotypic difference between this condition and complete androgen insensitivity syndrome (testicular feminization), caused by inactivating mutations in the androgen receptor gene. Because there is no testosterone secretion and action in the fetal period, the Wolffian duct-derived accessory sex organs (prostate, seminal vesicles) are totally absent. The uterus is also missing because the fetal Sertoli cells produce normal levels of anti-Müllerian hormone. It is, however, noteworthy that the individuals do have epididymides, which is a sign of minimal autonomous testosterone production and subsequent paracrine action on stabilization of the Wolffian ductal structures closest to the testis (Themmen and Huhtaniemi, 2000). As expected, the cryptorchid testes contain no mature Leydig cells upon histological examination, and spermatogenesis is totally arrested (Kremer et al., 1995; Latronico et al., 1996). In vitro studies of function of the mutated receptors have shown a clear correlation between the extent of receptor inactivation and severity of the symptoms (Martens et al., 1998; Themmen and Huhtaniemi, 2000).

Females with LHR inactivation have a milder phenotype than males, with normal puberty, primary or secondary amenorrhoea, hypo-oestrogenism, high LH but normal FSH (reviewed in Themmen & Huhtaniemi, 2000). Histological examination of ovarian biopsy samples reveals all stages of follicular development, including primordial follicles, preantral and antral follicles with a well-developed theca cell layer, but no preovulatory follicles or corpora lutea (Latronico et al., 1996). Nonovulated follicles may give rise to cysts. Upon clinical examination, the patients have a small uterus, normal-sized vagina with hyposecretory function and thin walls, as well as decreased bone mass, all indicative of low oestrogen levels. These observations strongly support the view that LH is essential for ovulation and sufficient oestrogen production, while follicular development is initially autonomous and at later stages dependent on intact FSH action. The normal feminization at puberty in those with inactivating LHR mutations indicates that this process in girls is mainly dependent on FSH.

In addition, there are several apparent polymorphisms in the *LHR* gene (Themmen and Huhtaniemi, 2000). Whether they are neutral polymorphisms, with no phenotypic expression, or whether they represent subtle alterations of receptor function with phenotypic effects, in particular when under the influence of specific modifier genes, remains to be explored.

Mutations in follicle-stimulating hormone receptors

Although FSH receptor mutations are rare compared with LHR mutations, they are very informative about the role of FSH in reproductive function. The relative paucity of FSH mutations (eight inactivating and one activating mutations; Table 3.1 and Fig. 3.3) compared with LHR mutations may indicate that the phenotypes caused by them are less evident and escape our attention. It is also possible that a selection mechanism operates against FSHR mutations, perhaps because of the infertility that is often associated with them. We describe below briefly the physiological and clinical consequences of FSHR mutations in female and male reproductive function.

Activating mutations

To date, a single activating mutation in the FSHR has been described (Fig. 3.3; Gromoll et al., 1996b): a hypophysectomized hypogonadotrophic patient treated with testosterone alone who fathered three children. The mutation was located at the C-terminal part of the third intracytoplasmic loop of exon 10, resulting in Asp567Gly transition. In transient transfection experiments, cells expressing the mutant receptor produced consistently higher (1.5-fold) concentrations of cAMP in the absence of FSH than did cells expressing wild-type receptor, while both receptor type reacted similarly to increasing concentrations of FSH.

Deletion mutations in the third intracellular loop of the TSH (Asp619) or LH (Asp564) receptor have been shown to cause constitutive receptor activation (Schultz et al., 1999). It was postulated with TSHR and LHR that there is interaction between the transmembrane domains (TM5/TM6 and TM6/TM7, respectively) to stabilize receptors in an inactive state, and gain-of–function mutations might destabilize these interhelical contacts (Schultz et al., 2000). However, deletion of Asp567 from FSHR exoloop 3 (corresponding to Asp564 in the LHR and Asp619 in the TSHR) did not alter function of the receptor (Schultz et al., 1999). Consequently, it may be that the Asp567Gly substitution is a nonfunctional polymorphism, and a different, as yet unidentified, mutation may cause the phenotype of the patient. Alternatively, the Asp567Gly mutation may cause a relatively small constitutive activation of the human FSHR that is difficult to observe in a reproducible manner. However, substitution of a highly conserved leucine residue in transmembrane helix 3 of the human FSHR with arginine caused a fivefold

Table 3.1. The currently known mutations in the human gene for the follicle-stimulating hormone receptor

Protein domain	Gene location	Base change	Amino acid change	Effect	Phenotype(s)	Reference
Extracellular	Exon 6	T479C	Ile160Thr	Inactivating	Compound heterozygous woman: with Arg573Cys mutation; secondary amenorrhoea, follicular development up to antral stage	Beau et al., 1998
	Exon 7	C566T	Ala189Val	Inactivating	Homozygous women: hypergonadotrophic ovarian failure. Homozygous males: normally masculinized, oligozoospermia	Aittomäki et al., 1995
	Exon 7	A572T	Asn191Ile	Inactivating	Heterozygous woman: healthy	Gromoll et al., 1996a Simoni et al., 1997
	Exon 9	A671T	Asp224Val	Inactivating	Compound heterozygote woman: with Leu601Val mutation; primary amenorrhoea, follicular development up to antral stage	Touraine et al., 1999
	Exon 10	C1118G	Pro346Arg	Inactivating	Homozygous woman: delayed puberty	Allen et al., 2000
Transmembrane 2	Exon 10	G1255A	Ala419Thr	Inactivating	Compound heterozygous woman: with Ala189Val mutation: delayed puberty	Docherty et al., 2001
Intracellular loop 3	Exon 10	A1700G	Asp567Gly	Activating	Heterozygous man: hypophysectomized, fertile under replacement therapy	Gromoll et al., 1996b
	Exon 10	C1717T	Arg573Cys	Inactivating	Compound heterozygote with Ile160Thr mutation	Beau et al., 1998
Transmembrane 6	Exon 10	C1801G	Leu601Val	Inactivating	Compound heterozygote with Asp224Val mutation	Touraine et al., 1999

increase in basal cAMP in transfected cells, while substitution with lysine, alanine or aspartate resulted in decreased FSH responsiveness (Tao et al., 2000). Only arginine caused constitutive activation, suggesting a role for Leu460 in FSH-stimulated cAMP production by the FSHR. Constitutive activation may arise by both disruption of Leu418 and introduction of a specific residue stabilizing the active receptor conformation. These data demonstrate that activating mutations in the FSHR are possible, but it is curious why clear-cut cases have not yet been demonstrated in humans. Maybe our "educated guesses" for their phenotypes have been incorrect. An animal model expressing a constitutively activated form of FSHR could elucidate the correct phenotype.

Inactivating mutations
A total of eight inactivating point mutations have so far been characterized in the human *FSHR* gene (Fig. 3.3

and Table 3.1). The first natural mutation reported in the human *FSHR* gene was found in a Finnish population of patients suffering from hypergonadotrophic ovarian dysgenesis or resistant ovary syndrome (Aittomäki, 1994). This syndrome is characterized by normal karyotype, normal female phenotype until puberty, variable development of secondary sex characteristics at puberty, highly elevated gonadotrophins, and streak gonads associated with primary amenorrhoea. Males homozygous for the same inactivating FSHR mutation had slightly or severely suppressed testicular size and spermatogenesis, but no azoospermia or absolute infertility (Tapanainen et al., 1997). Linkage analysis of the affected multiplex families located the affected gene to chromosome 2p, coinciding with the FSHR and LHR gene loci (Attomäki, 1994). Sequencing of the *FSHR* gene of the affected individuals revealed a homozygous cytosine/thymine to T transition at position 566, predicting an Ala189Val mutation in exon 6 encoding the extracellular receptor domain. The mutation segregated perfectly with the disease phenotype (Aittomäki et al., 1995). A cell line expressing the mutated FSHR showed near-total loss of FSH binding and FSH-evoked cAMP response, indicating the inactivating nature of this mutation. The majority of immunoreactive FSHR in cells transfected with mutated receptor cDNA seems to be sequestered intracellularly (A. Rannikko, P. Pakarinen, P. Manna, K. Aittomäki and I. Huhtaniemi, unpublished data).

The mutated Ala189 is the first of a stretch of five amino acids (AlaPheAsnGlyThr) that are perfectly conserved in all glycoprotein hormone receptors; this is, therefore, unlikely to be the site of ligand recognition and specificity. The conserved domain contains a consensus N-linked glycosylation signal, which was found to have functional importance for proper folding of the rat FSHR protein (Davis et al., 1995). Gromoll et al., (1996b) reported a heterozygous point mutation involving the same glycosylation site (Asn191Ile) in a healthy fertile woman. Functional studies of this FSHR mutant also demonstrated almost complete inactivation (Gromoll et al., 1996b; Simoni et al., 1997). These data suggest a critical role for this five residue domain. The presence of valine at position 189 may interfere with glycosylation, resulting in impaired receptor trafficking and folding, followed by defective transit of the receptor to the plasma membrane.

Two pairs of compound heterozygous FSHR mutations have been described from France in women with primary or secondary amenorrhoea, normal pubertal development and follicular development up to the antral stage (Table 3.1) (Beau et al., 1998; Touraine et al., 1999). Two of the mutations, Ile160Thr and Asp224Val, present in the extracellular domain of the receptor, caused almost complete loss of FSH binding. In accordance, cells expressing these receptor mutants showed absent or marginal cAMP response to FSH stimulation. The other two mutations, Arg573Cys and Leu601Val, caused less complete receptor inhibition, displaying clear ligand binding and residual cAMP responses to FSH (12–24% of wild-type control). More recent studies have identified two additional mutations, Ala419Thr in the second transmembrane loop of FSHR (Docherty et al., 2001) and Pro346Arg in the extracellular part of exon 10 (Allen et al., 2000). Both of these mutations abolished FSH signal transduction; in the former, this occurred in spite of normal FSH–receptor binding.

The FSHR mutants Ile160Thr and Asp224Val carry mannose-rich carbohydrates, suggesting that they have not reached the Golgi apparatus. This impairment of receptor cell trafficking may be caused by altered receptor conformation, which then further impedes the intracellular trafficking of the nascent protein (Touraine et al., 1999).

Alternatively, the intracellular accumulation may be caused by a failure of the mutated receptor to interact with a specific chaperone necessary for proper receptor folding (Rozell et al., 1998). Chaperone proteins are known to interact with a wide variety of glycosylated proteins and are thought to provide a quality control mechanism by binding and retaining misfolded proteins at the endoplasmic reticulum (Ruddon and Bedows, 1997). Similar intracellular retention of FSHR was also shown with the Ala189Val mutation (see above).

The Leu601Val and Arg573Cys substitutions were characterized by impairment in signal transduction, without any change in the FSH–receptor interaction. They thus highlight the role of the third extracellular loop and transmembrane domain in FSHR signal transduction. It seems likely that Leu601 may be involved in maintaining the proper conformation of exoloop 3 and of the adjacent transmembrane helices 6 and 7, as already suspected for the LHR (Fernandez and Puett, 1996). It appears that the degree of FSHR inactivation by mutations is largely determined by the degree of receptor sequestration inside the cell.

Besides mutations, there are also numerous polymorphisms in the gonadotrophin receptor genes. Although they may not cause clear-cut pathologies in gonadotrophin action, they may be responsible for borderline alteration in pituitary–gonadal function (e.g. subfertility) that might present especially in combination with additional polymorphisms with similar effect. In keeping with this, the first study has appeared on phenotypic effects of a common FSHR polymorphism (Perez Mayorga et al., 2000). In this study, the amount of FSH (number of ampoules) needed for ovarian stimulation in in vitro fertilization cycles was related to the two known allelic variants of the FSHR (Thr307/Asn680 and Ala307/Ser680; Fig. 3.3). The frequency of the two alleles was almost equal: Asn/Asn homozygotes 29%, heterozygotes 45%, Ser/Ser homozygotes 26%. Peak oestrogen levels, the number of preovulatory follicles and the number of retrieved oocytes were similar in the three groups. However, the basal FSH concentrations were significantly different between the three groups, being lowest in the Asn/Asn group and highest in the Ser/Ser group. The number of ampoules to induce similar ovarian stimulation was likewise 50% higher in the Ser/Ser group than in the Asn/Asn group. Hence, ovarian sensitivity to FSH seems to depend on the subtle structural difference of the FSHR brought about by the two polymorphic alterations in its amino acid sequence. This finding prompts more detailed studies of phenotypic effects of polymorphisms in the key genes regulating gonadal function.

Animal models for pathologies of gonadotrophin receptor function

Gene-modified mice provide a versatile approach to study further the molecular pathogenesis of human mutations. They are also useful in predicting the phenotype of a mutation that has not yet been detected in humans. Mouse knockout models exist now for the inactivating LHR and FSHR mutations, and they have partly corroborated the respective human phenotypes and partly elucidated novel features of gonadotrophin receptor function. Animal models for activating gonadotrophin receptor mutations have not yet been developed, but transgenic mice overexpressing LH/hCG or FSH can partly serve as models for these conditions and for prediction of the human phenotypes.

Luteinizing hormone receptor knockout mice

The phenotype of the LHR knockout mice has been reported by two laboratories (Lei et al., 2001; Zhang et al., 2001). As expected, no phenotype was found at birth in female homozygous (null) mice, in agreement with the concept in humans that female sex differentiation occurs independent of ovarian influences. In adults, the homozygous female knockout mice were infertile, as a result of poor oestrogen synthesis and lack of follicular maturation beyond the early antral stage. In this respect, the female knockout mouse is a full phenocopy of women with inactivating LHR mutations. The lack of progression of follicular growth from the antral to preovulatory stage in the knockout mice indicates that LH is important in the final stages of follicular maturation before ovulation, and not only for ovulation and maintenance of corpus luteum. A surprise was the normal-looking theca cell layer around the developing follicles, which showed that LH action is not needed at least for the morphological differentiation of the cells. In accordance, although the oestrogen levels of the null mutant mice were drastically suppressed, they were measurable, in keeping with LH-independent supply of androgen precursors from the theca cells for granulosa cell oestrogen synthesis.

The male LHR knockout mice were indistinguishable from controls at birth, displaying full intrauterine masculinization of their sex organs. This indicates that some nongonadotrophic factors are able to maintain fetal Leydig cell androgen production. In this respect, the mouse differs from man, where normal LHR function is vital for prenatal masculinization. However, the LHR knockout male mice totally lacked postnatal sexual development, which is known to be dependent on LH-stimulated testicular androgen synthesis.

The activity of the knockout mouse fetal testes in the absence of LHR is explained by an array of bioactive peptides that are able to stimulate rodent fetal Leydig cell steroidogenesis in paracrine fashion, thus providing a backup mechanism if gonadotrophin secretion fails (El-Gehani et al., 1998). In the human, hCG seems to provide this backup stimulus in the absence of pituitary LH. It is intriguing that the induction of male sexual differentiation is regulated so differently in the two mammalian species. The LHR knockout model will provide a model for further studies on the role of LH in gonadal function, in particular when these mutants are crossed with other knockout and transgenic models. It will also help to elucidate the elusive role of extragonadal gonadotrophin action.

Transgenic mice overexpressing luteinizing hormone

Although technically possible, no animal models have yet been developed for activating gonadotrophin receptor mutations. This would require production of a "knock-in" mutation in the endogenous LHR gene. The closest animal model so far produced for an activating LHR mutation is a mouse expressing the bovine LH β-subunit/hCG C-terminal peptide fusion gene under the bovine common α-subunit promoter (bLHβ–CTP) (Risma et al., 1995). The females of this model have very high levels of circulating LH and might, therefore, mimic constitutive LHR activation. The mice are infertile and the elevated LH levels appeared to prolong the lifespan of corpora lutea in pseudopregnancy-like fashion. The development of multiple cysts and increased LH/FSH and androgen/oestrogen ratios are akin to changes seen in human polycystic ovary syndrome. In addition, the mice develop granulosa cell tumours, nephropathy and become obese after puberty, for an unexpected reason. Upon LH overproduction, the mice started expressing LHR in their adrenal gland, which then stimulated high corticosterone production and a Cushing's syndrome-like phenotype (Kero et al., 2000). For this reason, the adrenal function of men with testotoxicosis, female carriers of the same mutations and postmenopausal women might be worth investigating, because all these groups are exposed to high LH levels or LHR activity for extended periods of time.

The ovarian tumorigenesis in bLHβ–CTP mice supports findings in some other transgenic models on tumour promoter effects of high gonadotrophin levels (Kananen et al., 1995, 1996; Kumar et al., 1999). On the one hand, this may be a consequence of the structural relationship of gonadotrophins with cystine-knot growth factors, including nerve growth factor, TGF-β and platelet-derived growth factor-α (Lapthorn et al., 1994) and could entail activation of signal transduction pathways other than that employing cAMP. This has been demonstrated with an activating LHR mutation detected in Leydig cell tumours; the IP$_3$ pathway was preferentially stimulated by the mutated LHR (Liu et al., 1999). On the other hand, chronically elevated cAMP levels may also provide a tumorigenic signal, as seems to be the case in the function of constitutively activated TSHR in toxic thyroid nodules (Vassart, 1998).

In males, the bLHβ–CTP transgene did not increase LH levels but, nevertheless, reduced for unknown reasons their fertility and testis size (Risma et al., 1995). It remains to be seen what phenotypic expression chronically elevated gonadotrophin levels would cause in the male. Our preliminary observations on an hCG-overexpressing transgenic mouse model suggests that the male phenotype in the presence of very high hCH levels is rather modest (S. Rulli, M. Poutanen and I. Huhtaniemi, unpublished observations). It remains unclear how well this type of transgenic animal with pharmacologically elevated gonadotrophin levels is able to simulate the human conditions of constitutive LHR activation, in particular since no clearcut phenotype has been related to this condition in women.

Knockout mice for follicle-stimulating hormone receptor

Two groups have developed targeted disruption (knockout) of the *FSHR* gene (Abel et al., 2000; Dierich et al., 1998). The female FSHR null mutant mice were infertile and had thin uteri, caused by low oestrogen production by the small ovaries, with blockade of follicular development at the pre-antral stage. No Graafian follicles or corpora lutea could be identified. The male FSHR knockout mice were fertile but had small testes and decreased testosterone levels. Semen analysis showed a decrease in the number and motility of sperm, and a relative increase in aberrant spermatozoa, such as bent tails and cytoplasmic droplets. The decrease in testis size appeared to be caused by a decrease in seminiferous tubule volume, although a decrease in tubule length, which would be caused by a decrease in Sertoli cell number, was not excluded. FSH levels were increased in both male (threefold) and female animals (15-fold), accompanied by a significant enlargement of the anterior lobe of the pituitary gland with a high number of FSH-producing cells.

In many respects, the FSHR null mutant mice of both sexes appear to be a complete phenocopy of human patients with inactivating FSHR mutations, as described above. The clearcut phenotypic features in females are infertility, as a result of blockade of follicular development,

but intact primordial follicular recruitment. In males, there is incomplete suppression of spermatogenesis, with increased proportion of aberrant spermatozoa, but persistent fertility. In contrast to the inactivating LHR mutations, those of FSHR seem to induce a more severe phenotype in females.

Mice overexpressing follicle-stimulating hormone

Kumar et al. (1992, 1999) have produced mice with both absent and enhanced FSH action and have studied their specific effects on mouse phenotype as well as explored their contribution to gonadal tumorigenesis of inhibin-deficient mice. The transgenic FSH-overexpressing females were infertile, with highly haemorrhagic and cystic ovaries, and elevated serum testosterone, oestradiol and progesterone. The last may have caused the kidney and urinary tract abnormalities observed in these animals, which, interestingly, were also found in LH-overproducing mice (Risma et al., 1995). No gonadal tumours were found in these mice, indicating that FSH alone is not oncogenic. The infertility resulted from disrupted folliculogenesis and development of ovarian cysts. Therefore, these mice ovaries mimicked the human ovaries observed in hyperstimulation and polycystic ovary syndrome. Likewise, women with elevated serum FSH levels, in conditions such as postmenopausal ovarian cancer (Cochrane and Regan, 1997), ovarian hyperstimulation syndrome (Agrawal et al., 1997) and with FSH-secreting pituitary adenomas (Djerassi et al., 1995), present with cystic and haemorrhagic ovaries. Interestingly, the female phenotypes of the FSH- and LH-overexpressing mice are very similar (see above). How well the FSH-overexpressing mouse simulates activating *FSHR* mutations in women remains open, since such causes have not yet been detected.

FSH-overexpressing male mice had normal testicular differentiation and spermatogenesis. Nevertheless, they were infertile, possibly as a result of some behavioural effects, functional incompetence of the sperm or abnormal secretory products of the enlarged seminal vesicles (Kumar et al., 1999). Interestingly, these mice presented with elevated testosterone production and enlarged seminal vesicles secondary to elevated androgens, demonstrating that supraphysiological FSH levels somehow stimulated Leydig cell function, possibly through a Sertoli cell paracrine factor (Saez, 1994). Whether a gain-of-function mutation of the *FSHR* gene would produce a similar phenotype in human males remains to be seen. With present knowledge, this seems unlikely, since men with pituitary adenomas secreting large amounts of FSH have no abnormal testicular phenotype (Galway et al., 1990).

Future perspectives

Today, both activating and inactivating mutations of gonadotrophin receptor genes are known. Likewise, animal models exist for most of these conditions, both in the form of gonadotrophin ligand and receptor knockouts and in forms overexpressing gonadotrophin genes. Of the possible permutations in the human, the largest number of cases have been reported for the activating and inactivating LHR mutations, and their phenotypic expression is now relatively well known. The finding that women with activating mutations of LHR seem to have no altered phenotype is puzzling, and animal models with activating LHR mutation could help in predicting the missing phenotypic changes.

Much less is known about the consequences of FSHR mutations. Females with inactivating *FSHR* mutations display the expected lack of follicular development; the findings are identical with the inactivating *FSHR* mutations and the FSH β-subunit (Kumar et al., 1997) and FSHR (Abel et al., 2000; Dierich et al., 1998) knockout mice and, therefore, the role of FSH in the female can be considered to be quite well explored. Since no undisputed activating mutations of the *FSHR* have yet been found, a mouse model would be useful in predicting the phenotype, which might turn out to be either nonexisting or unexpected.

Several polymorphisms have been detected in genes of gonadotrophin receptors. Their impact on pituitary–gonadal function is still largely unexplored. It will be intriguing to find out whether the polymorphisms that are known to exist in genes of the gonadotrophins and their receptors, in specific combinations with those of other genes involved in reproduction, could contribute to the larger individual variation of fertility. In the future, it may even become possible to construct a panel of polymorphisms in these genes to be used to predict the reproductive capacity of a couple and to select specific treatments for infertility.

The finding of activating TSHR mutations in thyroid adenomas suggested that similar mutations in LHR and FSHR might also have tumorigenic effects. Constitutive activation of the cAMP pathway by activating mutations in the gene for the G_s-protein α-subunit (Weinstein et al., 1991) has been found to be oncogenic in human ovarian stromal and testicular Leydig cell tumours (Fragoso et al., 1998), but no association has been indicated between activating LHR mutations and Leydig cell adenomas, suggesting that increased cAMP levels are not necessarily oncogenic. The activating LHR mutation (Asp578His) that was identified in Leydig cell adenomas (Liu et al., 1999) has the special characteristic that it causes, besides cAMP response, constitutive coupling to the IP_3 pathway, suggesting that this coupling by itself or through synergism with the cAMP pathway is essential for the tumorigenic activity of this mutation. By and large, it will be interesting to address the possible specific roles and interactions of the different signal transduction systems in the overall actions of gonadotrophins, including the mounting information on their oncogenic effects in specific conditions.

The discovery of gonadotrophin receptor expression in extragonadal tissues (Rao, 1996) still remains without explanation. All phenotypes observed with human gonadotrophin receptor mutations are related to specific gonadal expression, suggesting that extragonadal gonadotrophin effects are unlikely to be of major physiological significance. Possibly, extragonadal LHR expression is caused by illegitimate or "leaky" transcription, which is detected by the very sensitive polymerase chain reaction techniques that are often applied in these studies. The LHR knockout mouse would indicate that there is no major physiological role for the extragonadally expressed LHR (Lei et al., 2001; Zhang et al., 2001).

Structural studies of the LHR have been hampered by difficulties in expressing high-affinity receptors, but the recent development of a soluble hCG–LHR complex (Remy et al., 2001) suggests that a crystallization strategy may be within reach. Detailed understanding of the gonadotrophin receptor structure would have two benefits: improved understanding of the receptor structure–function relationships and the possibility that specific gonadotrophin agonists and antagonists could be developed. These would have tremendous clinical potential.

The physiology and pathophysiology of gonadotrophin receptor function has been characterized in great detail using classical physiological and biochemical research methods. Today, the novel information revealed by molecular approaches has elucidated totally new aspects of the role of gonadotrophin receptors in functions of the HPG axis.

REFERENCES

Abel M H, Wootton A N, Wilkins V, Huhtaniemi I, Knight P G, Charlton H M (2000). The effect of a null mutation in the follicle-stimulating hormone receptor gene on mouse reproduction. *Endocrinology* 141, 1795–1803.

Abell A N, Segaloff D L (1997). Evidence for the direct involvement of transmembrane region 6 of the lutropin/choriogonadotropin receptor in activating Gs. *J Biol Chem* 272, 14586–14591.

Abell A N, McCormick D J, Segaloff D L (1998). Certain activating mutations within helix 6 of the human luteinizing hormone receptor may be explained by alterations that allow transmembrane regions to activate Gs. *Mol Endocrinol* 12, 1857–1869.

Agrawal R, Chimusoro K, Payne N, van der Spuy Z, Jacobs H S (1997). Severe ovarian hyperstimulation syndrome: serum and ascitic fluid concentrations of vascular endothelial growth factor. *Curr Opin Obstet Gynecol* 9, 141–144.

Aittomäki K (1994). The genetics of XX gonadal dysgenesis. *Am J Hum Genet* 54, 844–851.

Aittomäki K, Dieguez Lucena J L, Pakarinen P et al. (1995). Mutation in the follicle-stimulating hormone receptor gene causes hereditary hypergonadotropic ovarian failure. *Cell* 82, 959–968.

Albertini D F, Combelles C M, Benecchi E, Carabatsos M J (2001). Cellular basis for paracrine regulation of ovarian follicle development. *Reproduction* 121, 647–653.

Allen L, Achermann J C, Kotlar T J, Jameson J L, Cheetham T D, Ball S G (2000). A novel loss of function mutation in exon 10 of the FSH-receptor gene causing hypergonadotropic hypogonadism: clinical and molecular characteristics. *Proceedings of the 82nd American Endocrine Society Annual Meeting*, Toronto, Canada. Abstract 2333.

Alvarez C A, Narayan P, Huang J, Puett D (1999). Characterization of a region of the lutropin receptor extracellular domain near the transmembrane helix 1 that is important in ligand-mediated signaling. *Endocrinology* 140, 1775–1782.

Arey B J, Stevis P E, Deecher D C et al. (1997). Induction of promiscuous G protein coupling of the follicle-stimulating hormone (FSH) receptor: a novel mechanism for transducing the pleiotropic actions of FSH isoforms. *Mol Endocrinol* 11, 517–526.

Atger M, Misrahi M, Sar S, Le Flem L, Dessen P, Milgrom E (1995). Structure of the human luteinizing hormone-choriogonadotropin receptor gene: unusual promoter and 5′ non-coding regions. *Mol Cell Endocrinol* 111, 113–123.

Beau I, Touraine P, Meduiri G et al. (1998). A novel phenotype related to partial loss of function mutations of the follicle stimulating hormone receptor. *J Clin Invest* 102, 1352–1359.

Bebia Z, Somers J P, Liu G, Ihrig L, Shenker A, Zeleznik A J (2001). Adenovirus-directed expression of functional luteinizing hormone (LH) receptors in undifferentiated rat granulosa cells: evidence for differential signaling through follicle-stimulating hormone and LH receptors. *Endocrinology* 142, 2252–2259.

Bhowmick N, Huang J, Puett D, Isaacs N W, Lapthorn A J (1996). Determination of residues important in hormone binding to the extracellular domain of the luteinizing/chorionic gonadotropin receptor by site-directed mutagenesis and modeling. *Mol Endocrinol* 10, 1147–1159.

Bhowmick N, Narayan P, Puett D (1999). Identification of ionizable residues on the extracellular domain of the lutropin receptor involved in ligand binding. *Endocrinology* 140, 4558–4563.

Chen S, Liu X, Segaloff D L (2000). A novel cyclic adenosine 3′,5′-monophosphate-responsive element involved in the transcriptional regulation of the lutropin receptor gene in granulosa cells. *Mol Endocrinol* 14, 1498–1508.

(2001). Identification of an SAS (Sp1c adjacent site)-like element in the distal 5′-flanking region of the rat lutropin receptor gene essential for cyclic adenosine 3′, 5′-monophosphate. *Endocrinology* 142, 2013–2021.

Cochrane R, Regan L (1997). Undetected gynaecological disorders in women with renal disease. *Hum Reprod* 12, 667–670.

Cooke B A (1996). Transduction of the luteinizing hormone signal within the Leydig cell. In *The Leydig Cell*, Payne A H, Hardy M P, Russell R D, eds., pp. 351–363. Cache River Press, Vienna, IL.

Davis D, Liu X, Segaloff D L (1995). Identification of the sites of N-linked glycosylation on the follicle-stimulating hormone (FSH) receptor and assessment of their role in FSH receptor function. *Mol Endocrinol* 9, 159–170.

Davis D P, Rozell T G, Liu X, Segaloff D L (1997). The six N-linked carbohydrates of the lutropin/choriogonadotropin receptor are not absolutely required for correct folding, cell surface expression, hormone binding or signal transduction. *Mol Endocrinol* 11, 550–562.

Davis J S, West L A, Farase R V (1984). Effects of luteinizing hormone on phosphoinositide metabolism in rat granulosa cells. *J Biol Chem* 259, 15028–15034.

de Kretser D M, Phillips D J (1998). Mechanisms of protein feedback on gonadotropin secretion. *J Reprod Immunol* 39, 1–12.

Dierich A, Sairam M R, Monaco L et al. (1998). Impairing follicle-stimulating hormone (FSH) signaling in vivo: targeted disruption of the FSH receptor leads to aberrant gametogenesis and hormonal imbalance. *Proc Nat Acad Sci USA* 95, 13612–13617.

Djerassi A, Coutifaris C, West V A et al. (1995). Gonadotroph adenoma in a premenopausal woman secreting follicle-stimulating hormone and causing ovarian hyperstimulation. *J Clin Endocrinol Metab* 80, 591–594.

Docherty E, Pakarinen P, Tiitinen A et al. (2002). A novel mutation in the follicle-stimulating hormone receptor inhibiting signal transduction and resulting in primary ovarian failure. *J Clin Endocrinol Metab* 57, 1151–1155.

Dufau M L (1996). The luteinizing hormone receptor. In *The Leydig Cell*, Payne A H, Hardy M P, Russell R D, eds., pp. 333–350. Cache River Press, Vienna, IL.

Dunkel L, Tilly J L, Shikone T, Nishimori K, Hsueh A J (1994). Follicle-stimulating hormone receptor expression in the rat ovary: increases during prepubertal development and regulation by the opposing actions of transforming growth factors beta and alpha. *Biol Reprod* 50, 940–948.

El-Gehani F, Zhang F P, Pakarinen P, Rannikko A, Huhtaniemi I (1998). Gonadotropin-independent regulation of steroidogenesis in the fetal rat testis. *Biol Reprod* 58, 116–123.

Fernandez L M, Puett D (1996). Lys^{583} in the third extracellular loop of the lutropin/choriogonadotropin receptor is critical for signaling. *J Biol Chem* 271, 925–930.

(1997). Evidence for an important functional role of intracellular loop II of the lutropin receptor. *Mol Cell Endocrinol*, 128, 161–169.

Filicori M, Cognigni G E (2001). Clinical review 126: roles and novel regimens of luteinizing hormone and follicle-stimulating hormone in ovulation induction. *J Clin Endocrinol Metab* 86, 1437–1441.

Findlay J K, Drummond A E (1999). Regulation of the FSH receptor in the ovary. *Trends Endocrinol Metab* 10, 183–188.

Fragoso M C, Latronico A C, Carvalho F M et al. (1998). Activating mutation of the stimulatory G protein (gsp) as a putative cause of ovarian and testicular human stromal Leydig cell tumors. *J Clin Endocrinol Metab* 83, 2074–2078.

Galway A B, Hsueh A J, Daneshdoost L, Zhou M H, Pavlou S N, Snyder P J (1990). Gonadotroph adenomas in men produce biologically active follicle-stimulating hormone. *Journal of Clinical Endocrinology and Metabolism* 71, 907–912.

Gilchrist R L, Ryu K-S, Ji I, Ji T H (1996). The luteinizing hormone/chorionic gonadotropin receptor has distinct transmembrane conductors for cAMP and inositol phosphate signals. *J Biol Chem* 271, 19283–19287.

Grasso P, Reichert L E, Jr (1990). Follicle-stimulating hormone receptor-mediated uptake of $^{45}Ca^{2+}$ by cultured Leydig cells does not require activation of cholera toxin- or pertussis toxin-sensitive guanine nucleotide binding proteins or adenylate cyclase. *Endocrinology* 127, 949–956.

Grasso P, Dexiel M R, Riechert L E, Jr (1995). Synthetic peptides corresponding to residues 551 to 555 and 650 to 653 of the rat testicular follicle-stimulating hormone (FSH) receptor are sufficient for post-receptor modulation of Sertoli cell responsiveness to FSH stimulation. *Regul Pept* 60, 177–183.

Griswold M D, Kim J S (2001). Site-specific methylation of the promoter alters deoxyribonucleic acid–protein interactions and prevents follicle-stimulating hormone receptor gene transcription. *Biol Reprod* 64, 602–610.

Gromoll J, Dankbar B, Gudermann T (1994). Characterization of the 5′ flanking region of the human follicle-stimulating hormone receptor gene. *Molecular and Cellular Endocrinology* 102, 93–102.

Gromoll J, Simoni M, Nordhoff V, Behre H M, de Geyter C, Nieschlag E (1996a). Functional and clinical consequences of mutations in the FSH receptor. *Mol Cell Endocrinol* 125, 177–182.

Gromoll J, Simoni M, Nieschlag E (1996b). An activating mutation of the follicle-stimulating hormone receptor autonomously sustains spermatogenesis in a hypophysectomized man. *J Clin Endocrinol Metab* 81, 1367–1370.

Gromoll J, Eiholzer U, Nieschlag E, Simoni M (2000). Male hypogonadism caused by homozygous deletion of exon 10 of the luteinizing hormone (LH) receptor: differential action between human chorionic gonadotropin and LH. *J Clin Endocrinol Metab* 85, 2281–2286.

Gudermann T, Birnbaumer M, Birnbaumer L (1992). Evidence for dual coupling of the murine luteinizing hormone receptor to adenylate cyclase and phosphoinositide breakdown and Ca^{2+} mobilization. *J Biol Chem* 267, 4479–4488.

Heckert L L (2001). Activation of the rat follicle-stimulating hormone receptor promoter by steroidogenic factor 1 is blocked by protein kinase A and requires upstream stimulatory factor binding to a proximal E box element. *Mol Endocrinol* 15, 704–715.

Heckert L L, Daley I J, Griswold M D (1992). Structural organization of the follicle-stimulating hormone receptor gene. *Mol Endocrinol* 6, 70–80.

Heckert L L, Daggett M A, Chen J (1998). Multiple promoter elements contribute to activity of the follicle-stimulating hormone receptor (FSHR) gene in testicular Sertoli cells. *Mol Endocrinol* 12, 1499–1512.

Heckert L L, Sawadogo M, Daggett M A, Chen J K (2000). The USF proteins regulate transcription of the follicle-stimulating hormone receptor but are insufficient for cell-specific expression. *Mol Endocrinol* 14, 1836–1848.

Hillier S G (1999). Intragonadal regulation of male and female reproduction. *Ann Endocrinol* 60, 111–117.

Hillier S G, Whitelaw P F, Smyth C D (1994). Follicular oestrogen synthesis: the 'two-cell, two-gonadotropin' model revisited. *Mol Cell Endocrinol* 100, 51–54.

Hirsch B, Kudo M, Naro F, Conti M, Hsueh A J W (1996). The C-terminal third of the human luteinizing hormone (LH) receptor is important for inositol phosphate release: analysis using chimeric human LH/follicle-stimulating hormone receptors. *Mol Endocrinol* 10, 1127–1137.

Horvat R D, Barisas B G, Roess D A (2001). Luteinizing hormone receptors are self-associated in slow diffusing complexes during receptor desensitization. *Mol Endocrinol* 15, 534–542.

Hosoi Y, Murakami M, Minegishi T et al. (1999). Stimulation of Chinese hamster ovary cells expressing human thyrotropin receptors by serum human chorionic gonadotropin of patients with hydatidiform mole. *Thyroid* 9, 1205–1210.

Huang J, Puett D (1995). Identification of two amino acid residues on the extracellular domain of the luteinizing hormone/choriogonadotropin receptor important for signaling. *J Biol Chem* 270, 30023–30028.

Huhtaniemi I T, Eskola V, Pakarinen P, Matikainen T, Sprengel R (1992). The murine luteinizing hormone and follicle-stimulating hormone receptor genes: transcription initiation sites, putative promoter sequences and promoter activity. *Mol Cell Endocrinol* 88, 55–66.

Jackson T (1991). Structure and function of G protein coupled receptors. *Pharmacol Ther* 50, 425–442.

Ji I H, Ji T H (1991). Asp^{383} in the second transmembrane domain of the lutropin receptor is important for high affinity hormone binding and cAMP production. *J Biol Chem* 266, 14953–14957.

(1993). Receptor activation is distinct from hormone binding in intact lutropin-choriogonadotropin receptors and Asp^{397} is important for receptor activation. *J Biol Chem* 268, 20851–20854.

(1995). Differential roles of exoloop 1 in the human follicle-stimulating hormone receptor in hormone binding and receptor activation. *J Biol Chem* 270, 15970–15973.

Johnson A L, Bridgham J T (2001). Regulation of steroidogenic acute regulatory protein and luteinizing hormone receptor messenger ribonucleic acid in hen granulosa cells. *Endocrinology* 142, 3116–3124.

Kananen K, Markkula M, Rainio E, Su J G, Hsueh A J, Huhtaniemi I T (1995). Gonadal tumorigenesis in transgenic mice bearing the mouse inhibin alpha-subunit promoter/simian virus T-antigen fusion gene: characterization of ovarian tumors and establishment of gonadotropin-responsive granulosa cell lines. *Mol Endocrinol* 9, 616–627.

Kananen K, Markkula M, El-Hefnawy T et al. (1996). The mouse inhibin alpha-subunit promoter directs SV40 T-antigen to Leydig cells in transgenic mice. *Mol Cell Endocrinol* 119, 135–146.

Kero J, Poutanen M, Zhang F P et al. (2000). Elevated luteinizing hormone induces expression of its receptor and promotes steroidogenesis in the adrenal cortex. *J Clin Invest* 105, 633–641.

Kim J S, Griswold M D (2001). E2F and GATA-1 are required for the Sertoli cell-specific promoter activity of the follicle-stimulating hormone receptor gene. *J Androl* 22, 629–639.

Kishi H, Ascoli M (2000). Multiple distant amino acid residues present in the serpentine region of the follitropin receptor modulate the rate of agonist-induced internalization. *J Biol Chem* 275, 31030–31037.

Kobe B, Deisenhofer J (1995). A structural basis of the interactions between leucine-rich repeats and protein ligands. *Nature* 374, 183–186.

Kornyei J L, Li X, Lei Z M, Rao C V (1996). Restoration of human chorionic gonadotropin response in human myometrial smooth muscle cells by treatment with follicle-stimulating hormone (FSH): evidence for the presence of FSH receptors in human myometrium. *Eur J Endocrinol* 134, 225–231.

Kremer H, Mariman E, Otten B J et al. (1993). Cosegregation of missense mutations of the luteinizing hormone receptor gene with familial male-limited precocious puberty. *Hum Mol Genet* 2, 1779–1783.

Kremer H, Kraaij R, Toledo S P et al. (1995). Male pseudohermaphroditism due to a homozygous missense mutation of the luteinizing hormone receptor gene. *Nat Genet* 9, 160–164.

Kumar T R, Fairchild-Huntress V, Low M J (1992). Gonadotrope-specific expression of the human follicle-stimulating hormone beta-subunit gene in pituitaries of transgenic mice. *Mol Endocrinol* 6, 81–90.

Kumar T R, Wang Y, Lu N, Matzuk M M (1997). Follicle stimulating hormone is required for ovarian follicle maturation but not male fertility. *Nat Genet* 15, 201–204.

Kumar T R, Palapattu G, Wang P et al. (1999). Transgenic models to study gonadotropin function: the role of follicle-stimulating hormone in gonadal growth and tumorigenesis. *Mol Endocrinol* 13, 851–865.

LaPolt P S, Tilly J L, Aihara T, Nishimori K, Hsueh A J (1992). Gonadotropin-induced up- and down-regulation of ovarian follicle-stimulating hormone (FSH) receptor gene expression in immature rats: effects of pregnant mare's serum gonadotropin, human chorionic gonadotropin, and recombinant FSH. *Endocrinology* 130, 1289–95.

Lapthorn A J, Harris D C, Littlejohn A et al. (1994). Crystal structure of human chorionic gonadotropin. *Nature* 369, 455–461.

Latronico A C, Anasti J, Arnhold I J P et al. (1996). Testicular and ovarian resistance to luteinizing hormone caused by inactivating mutations of the luteinizing hormone receptor gene. *N Engl J Med* 331, 507–512.

Lazari M F, Bertrand J E, Nakamura K et al. (1998). Mutation of individual serine residues in the C-terminal tail of the lutropin/choriogonadotropin receptor reveal distinct structural requirements for agonist-induced uncoupling and agonist-induced internalization. *J Biol Chem* 273, 18316–18324.

Lazari M F, Liu X, Nakamura K, Benovic J L, Ascoli M (1999). Role of G protein-coupled receptor kinases on the agonist-induced phosphorylation and internalization of the follitropin receptor. *Mol Endocrinol* 13, 866–878.

Lei Z M, Mishra S, Zou W et al. (2001). Targeted disruption of luteinizing hormone/human chorionic gonadotropin receptor gene. *Mol Endocrinol* 15, 184–200.

Levallet J, Koskimies P, Rahman N, Huhtaniemi I (2001). The promoter of murine follicle-stimulating hormone receptor: functional characterization and regulation by transcription factor steroidogenic factor 1. *Mol Endocrinol* 15, 80–92.

Li S, Liu X, Min L, Ascoli M (2001). Mutations on the second extracellular loop of the human lutropin receptor emphasize the importance of receptor activation and de-emphasize the importance of receptor phosphorylation in agonist-induced internalization. *J Biol Chem* 276, 7968–7973.

Liu G, Duranteau L, Carel J C, Monroe J, Doyle D A, Shenker A (1999). Leydig-cell tumors caused by an activating mutation of the gene encoding the luteinizing hormone receptor. *N Eng J Med* 341, 1731–1736.

Manna P R, Pakarinen P, El-Hefnawy T, Huhtaniemi I T (1999). Functional assessment of the calcium messenger system in cultured mouse Leydig tumor cells: regulation of human chorionic gonadotropin-induced expression of the steroidogenic acute regulatory protein. *Endocrinology* 140, 1739–1751.

Manna P R, Kero J, Tena-Sempere M, Pakarinen P, Stocco D M, Huhtaniemi I T (2001). Assessment of mechanisms of thyroid hormone action in mouse Leydig cells: regulation of steroidogenic acute regulatory protein, steroidogenesis, and luteinizing hormone receptor function. *Endocrinology* 142, 319–331.

Martens J W, Verhoef-Post M, Abelin N et al. (1998). A homozygous mutation in the luteinizing hormone receptor causes partial Leydig cell hypoplasia: correlation between receptor activity and phenotype. *Mol Endocrinol* 12, 775–784.

Minegishi T, Nakamura K, Takakura Y, Ibuki Y, Igarashi M, Minegishi T (1991). Cloning and sequencing of human FSH receptor cDNA. *Biochem Biophys Res Commun* 175, 1125–1130.

Minegishi T, Kishi H, Tano M, Kameda T, Hirakawa T, Miyamoto K (1999). Control of FSH receptor mRNA expression in rat granulosa cells by $3'$, $5'$-cyclic adenosine monophosphate, activin, and follistatin. *Mol Cell Endocrinol* 149, 71–77.

Minegishi T, Nakamura K, Takakura Y, Ibuki Y, Igarashi M, Minegishi T (2000). A role of insulin-like growth factor I for follicle-stimulating hormone receptor expression in rat granulosa cells. *Biology of Reproduction* 62, 325–33.

Mizrachi D, Shemesh M (1999). Follicle-stimulating hormone receptor and its messenger ribonucleic acid are present in the bovine cervix and can regulate cervical prostanoid synthesis. *Biol Reprod* 61, 776–784.

Monaco L, Foulkes N S, Sassone-Corsi P (1995). Pituitary follicle-stimulating hormone (FSH) induces CREM gene expression in Sertoli cells: involvement in long-term desensitization of the FSH receptor. *Proc Nat Acad Sci USA* 92, 10673–10677.

Moyle W R, Campbell R K (1996). Gonadotropins. In *Reproductive Endocrinology, Surgery, and Technology*, Adashi E Y, Rock J A, Rosenwaks Z, eds., pp. 683–724. Lippincott-Raven, Philadelphia, PA.

Mukherjee S, Palczewski K, Gurevich V, Benovic J L, Banga J P, Hunzicker-Dunn M (1999). A direct role for arrestins in desensitization of the luteinizing hormone/choriogonadotropin receptor in porcine ovarian follicular membranes. *Proc Nat Acad Sci USA* 96, 493–498.

Mukherjee S, Casanova J E, Hunzicker-Dunn M (2000a). Desensitization of the luteinizing hormone/choriogonadotropin receptor in ovarian follicular membranes is inhibited by catalytically inactive ARNO(+). *J Biol Chem* 276, 6524–6528.

Mukherjee S, Gurevich V V, Jones J C et al. (2000b). The ADP ribosylation factor nucleotide exchange factor ARNO promotes beta-arrestin release necessary for luteinizing hormone/choriogonadotropin receptor desensitization. *Proc Nat Acad Sci USA* 97, 5901–5906.

Munshi U M, Peegel H, Menon K M (2001). Palmitoylation of the luteinizing hormone/human chorionic gonadotropin receptor regulates receptor interaction with the arrestin-mediated internalization pathway. *Eur J Biochem* 268, 1631–1639.

Nakabayashi K, Kudo M, Kobila B, Hsueh A J (2000). Activation of the luteinizing hormone receptor following substitution of Ser-277 with selective hydrophobic residues in the ectodomain hinge region. *J Biol Chem* 275, 30264–30271.

Nakamura K, Ascoli M (1999). A dileucine-based motif in the C-terminal tail of the lutropin/choriogonadotropin receptor inhibits endocytosis of the agonist-receptor complex. *Mol Pharmacol* 56, 728–736.

Nakamura K, Minegishi T, Takakura Y et al. (1991). Hormonal regulation of gonadotropin receptor mRNA in rat ovary during follicular growth and luteinization. *Molecular and Cellular Endocrinology* 82, 259–263.

Nakamura K, Liu K, Ascoli M (2000). Seven non-contiguous intracellular residues of the lutropin/choriogonadotropin receptor dictate the rate of agonist-induced internalization and its sensitivity to non-visual arrestins. *J Biol Chem* 275, 241–247.

Nikula H, Koskimies P, El-Hefnawy T, Huhtaniemi I (2001). Functional characterization of the basal promoter of the murine LH receptor gene in immortalized mouse Leydig tumor cells. *J Mol Endocrinol* 26, 21–29.

Perez Mayorga M, Gromoll J, Behre H M, Gassner C, Nieschlag E, Simoni M (2000). Ovarian response to follicle-stimulating hormone (FSH) stimulation depends on the FSH receptor genotype. *J Clin Endocrinol Metab* 85, 3365–3369.

Rao C V (1996). The beginning of a new era in reproductive biology and medicine: expression of low levels of functional luteinizing hormone/chorionic gonadotropin receptor in non-gonadal tissues. *J Physiol Pharmacol* 47(Suppl. 1), 41–53.

Remy J-J, Nespoulous C, Grosclaude J et al. (2001). Purification and structural analysis of a soluble human choriono-gonadotropin hormone–receptor complex. *J Biol Chem* 276, 1681–1687.

Richards J S, Hedin L (1988). Molecular aspects of hormone action in ovarian follicular development, ovulation and luteinization. *Annu Rev Physiol* 50, 441–463.

Risma K A, Clay C M, Nett T M, Wagner T, Yun J, Nilson J H (1995). Targeted overexpression of luteinizing hormone in transgenic mice leads to infertility, polycystic ovaries, and ovarian tumors. *Proc Nat Acad Sci USA* 28, 1322–1236.

Roess D A, Horvat R D, Munnelly H, Barisas B G (2000). Luteinizing hormone receptors are self-associated in the plasma membrane. *Endocrinology* 141, 4518–4523.

Rousseau-Merck M F, Atger M, Loosfelt H, Milgrom E, Berger R (1993). The chromosomal localization of the human follicle-stimulating hormone receptor gene (FSHR) on 2p21-p16 is similar to that of the luteinizing hormone receptor gene. *Genomics* 15, 222–224.

Rozell T G, Wang H, Liu X, Segaloff D L (1995). Intracellular retention of mutant gonadotropin receptors results in loss of binding activity of the follitropin receptor but not the lutropin/choriogonadotropin receptor. *Mol Endocrinol* 9, 1727–1736.

Rozell T G, Davis D P, Chai Y, Segaloff D L (1998). Association of gonadotropin receptor precursors with the protein folding chaperone calnexin. *Endocrinology* 139, 1588–1593.

Ruddon R W, Bedows E (1997). Assisted protein folding. *J Biol Chem* 272, 3125–3128.

Saez J H (1994). Leydig cells: endocrine, paracrine and autocrine regulation. *Endocr Rev* 15, 574–626.

Schulz A, Schoneberg T, Paschke R, Schultz G, Gudermann T (1999). Role of the third intracellular loop for the activation of gonadotropin receptors. *Mol Endocrinol* 13, 181–190.

Schulz A, Bruns K, Henklein P et al. (2000). Requirement of specific intrahelical interactions for stabilizing the inactive conformation of glycoprotein hormone receptors. *J Biol Chem* 275, 37860–37869.

Schwartz J (2000). Intercellular communication in the anterior pituitary. *Endocr Rev* 21, 488–513.

Segaloff D L, Ascoli M (1993). The lutropin/choriogonadotropin receptor . . . 4 years later. *Endocr Rev* 14, 324–342.

Segaloff D L, Wang H, Richards J S (1990). Hormonal regulation of luteinizing hormone/chorionic gonadotropin receptor mRNA in rat ovarian cells during follicular development and luteinization. *Mol Endocrinol* 4, 1856–1865.

Seger R, Hanoch T, Rosenberg R et al. (2001). The ERK signaling cascade inhibits gonadotropin-stimulated steroidogenesis. *J Biol Chem* 276, 13957–13964.

Shenker A, Laue L, Kosugi S et al. (1993). A constitutively activating mutation of the luteinizing hormone receptor in familial male precocious puberty. *Nature* 36, 652–654.

Shi H, Segaloff D L (1995). A role for increased lutropin/choriogonadotropin (LHR) gene transcription in the follitropin stimulated gene transcription of the LHR in granulosa cells. *Mol Endocrinol* 9, 734–744.

Shinozaki H, Fanelli F, Liu X, Jaquette J, Nakamura K, Segaloff D L (2001). Pleiotropic effects of substitutions of a highly conserved leucine in transmembrane helix III of the human lutropin/choriogonadotropin receptor with respect to constitutive activation and hormone responsiveness. *Mol Endocrinol* 15, 972–984.

Simoni M, Gromoll J, Nieschlag E (1997). The follicle-stimulating hormone receptor: biochemistry, molecular biology, physiology, and pathophysiology. *Endocr Rev* 18, 739–773.

Sokka T, Hämäläinen T, Huhtaniemi I (1992). Functional LH receptor appears in the neonatal rat ovary after changes in the alternative splicing pattern of the LH receptor mRNA. *Endocrinology* 130, 1738–1740.

Song Y S, Ji I, Beauchamp J, Isaacs N W, Ji T H (2001). Hormone interactions to Leu-rich repeats in the gonadotropin receptors. I. Analysis of Leu-rich repeats of human luteinizing hormone/chorionic gonadotropin receptor and follicle-stimulating hormone receptor. *J Biol Chem* 276, 2426–2435.

Tamura K, Kawaguchi T, Kogo H (2001). Interleukin-6 inhibits the expression of luteinizing hormone receptor during maturation of cultured rat granulosa cells. *J Endocrinol* 170, 121–127.

Tao Y X, Abell A N, Liu X, Nakamura K, Segaloff D L (2000). Constitutive activation of G protein-coupled receptors as a result of selective substitution of a conserved leucine residue in transmembrane helix III. *Mol Endocrinol* 14, 1272–1282.

Tapanainen J S, Aittomäki K, Min J, Vaskivuo T, Huhtaniemi I T (1997). Men homozygous for an inactivating mutation of the follicle-stimulating hormone (FSH) receptor gene present variable suppression of spermatogenesis and fertility. *Nat Genet* 15, 205–206.

Tena-Sempere M, Manna P R, Huhtaniemi I (1999). Molecular cloning of mouse follicle-stimulating hormone receptor complementary deoxyribonucleic acid: functional expression of alternatively spliced variants and receptor inactivation by a C566T transition in exon 7 of the coding sequence. *Biol Reprod* 60, 1515–1527.

Themmen A P N, Huhtaniemi I T (2000). Mutations of gonadotropins and gonadotropin receptors: elucidating the physiology and pathophysiology of pituitary–gonadal function. *Endocr Rev* 21, 551–583.

Themmen A P, Blok L J, Post M et al. (1991). Follitropin receptor down-regulation involves a cAMP-dependent posttranscriptional decrease of receptor mRNA expression. *Mol Cell Endocrinol* 78, R7-R13.

Tilly J L, LaPolt P S, Hsueh A J (1992). Hormonal regulation of follicle-stimulating hormone receptor messenger ribonucleic acid levels in cultured rat granulosa cells. *Endocrinology* 130, 1296–1302.

Touraine P A, Beau I, Meduri G et al. (1999). New natural inactivating mutations of the follicle-stimulating hormone receptor:

correlations between receptor function and phenotype. *Mol Endocrinol* 13, 1844–1854.

Troispoux C, Guillou, F, Alalouf J M et al. (1999). Involvement of G protein-coupled receptor kinases and arrestins in desensitization to follicle-stimulating hormone action. *Mol Endocrinol* 13, 1599–1614.

Tsai-Morris C H, Buczko E, Wang W, Xie X, Dufau M L (1991). Structural organization of the rat luteinizing hormone (LH) receptor gene. *J Biol Chem* 266, 11355–11359.

Vassart G (1998). Hypo- and hyperthyroidism caused by mutations of the TSH receptor. In *Contemporary Endocrinology: G Proteins, Receptors, and Diseases*, Spiegel A M, eds., pp. 119–138. Humana Press, Totowa, NJ.

Vassart G, Dumont J E (1992). The thyrotropin receptor and the regulation of thyrocyte function and growth. *Endocr Rev* 13, 596–611.

Weinstein L S, Shenker A, Gejman P V, Merino M J, Friedman E, Spiegel A M (1991). Activating mutations of the stimulatory G protein in the McCune–Albright syndrome. *N Eng J Med* 325, 1688–1695.

Wang H, Segaloff D L, Ascoli M (1991). Epidermal growth factor and phorbol esters reduce the levels of the cognate mRNA for the LH/CG receptor. *Endocrinology* 128, 2651–2653.

Xiao S, Farnworth P G, Findlay J K (1992). Interaction between activin and follicle-stimulating hormone-suppressing protein/follistatin in the regulation of basal inhibin production by cultured rat granulosa cells. *Endocrinology* 131, 2365–2370.

Xing W, Sairam M R (2001). Characterization of regulatory elements of ovine follicle-stimulating hormone (FSH) receptor gene: the role of E-box in the regulation of ovine FSH receptor expression. *Biol Reprod* 64, 579–589.

Yu W H, Karanth S, Walczewska A, Sower S A, McCann S M (1997). A hypothalamic follicle-stimulating hormone-releasing decapeptide in the rat. *Proc Nat Acad Sci USA* 94, 9499–9503.

Zhang F P, Hämäläinen T, Kaipia A, Pakarinen P, Huhtaniemi I (1994). Ontogeny of luteinizing hormone receptor gene expression in the rat testis. *Endocrinology* 134, 2206–2213.

Zhang F P, Rannikko A S, Manna P R, Fraser H M, Huhtaniemi I T (1997). Cloning and functional expression of the luteinizing hormone receptor complementary deoxyribonucleic acid from the marmoset monkey testis: absence of sequences encoding exon 10 in other species. *Endocrinology* 138, 2481–2490.

Zhang F P, Kero J, Huhtaniemi I (1998). The unique exon 10 of the human luteinizing hormone receptor is necessary for expression of the receptor protein at the plasma membrane in the human luteinizing hormone receptor, but deleterious when inserted into the human follicle-stimulating hormone receptor. *Mol Cell Endocrinol* 142, 165–174.

Zhang F P, Poutanen M, Wilbertz J, Huhtaniemi I (2001). Normal prenatal but arrested postnatal development of luteinizing hormone receptor knockout (LuRKO) mice. *Mol Endocrinol* 15, 172–183.

Zhang R, Tsai-Morris C H, Kitamura M, Buczko E, Dufau M L (1991). Changes in binding activity of luteinizing hormone receptors by site directed mutagenesis of potential glycosylation sites. *Biochem Biophys Res Commun* 181, 804–808.

Zhang R, Buczko E, Dufau M L (1996). Requirement of cysteine residues in exons 1 to 6 of the extracellular domain of the luteinizing hormone receptor for gonadotropin binding. *J Biol Chem* 271, 5755–5760.

Zheng M, Shi H, Segaloff D L, van Voorhis B J (2001). Expression and localization of luteinizing hormone receptors in female mouse reproductive tract. *Biol Reprod* 64, 179–187.

Ziecik A J, Derecka K, Gawronska B, Stepien A, Bodek G (2001). Nongonadal LH/hCG receptors in pig: functional importance and parallels to human. *Semin Reprod Med* 19, 19–30.

4

Normal childhood, puberty and adolescence

Clementina La Rosa, Cristina Traggiai and Richard Stanhope

Department of Paediatric Endocrinology, Great Ormond Street Hospital for Children and The Middlesex Hospital, London, UK

Introduction

Sex determination, or genetic sex, is a process starting at conception by which the undifferentiated genitalia evolve into male or female reproductive organs. It depends on chromosomal complement and is influenced by endocrine events and by nongenetic and nonendocrine factors such as nutrition, toxins (fetal alcohol syndrome), intrauterine environment (altered uterine blood flow, placental function, local uterine circulation and placental and umbilical circulation).

Initially this cascade of events is dependent on chromosomal or genetic sex, and then appropriate development of the hypothalamic–pituitary–gonadal axis is necessary for sex steroid secretion as well as for oogenesis and ovulation in the female and spermatogenesis in the male.

Genotype and phenotype

Genetic sex directs the embryonic gonad to differentiate into either testis or ovary and is determined by the presence or the absence of the Y chromosome.

The sex-determining region of the Y chromosome (*SRY*) has been mapped to the tip of the Y chromosome (Parker et al., 1999) and has been shown to be necessary and sufficient to initiate the male differentiation pathway and acts as a genetic switch towards testis development. If it is absent (or delayed in expression), ovarian differentiation occurs. However, many other factors involved in sex differentiation have been identified and are located on autosomal genes. In the presence of "male differentiating signals", testosterone and Müllerian inhibiting factor (anti-Müllerian

hormone (AMH) or Müllerian inhibiting substance) are secreted by the fetal gonads. Testosterone is converted to dihydrotestosterone by the 5α-reductase enzyme in target tissues. These hormones control the differentiation of the reproductive tract and genitalia (Jost et al., 1953) and lead to male sexual differentiation. In the absence of androgens, the pathway of sexual differentiation is female.

For normal female differentiation of the reproductive tract, oestrogens are (probably) not required. At 8 weeks of gestation, the human ovary has the capacity to produce oestrogens from androgens but it secretes only small amounts of steroids. However, the presence of oestrogen receptors in the female external genitalia suggests that maternal oestrogen may influence development.

Hypothalamic–pituitary–gonadal axis

Luteinizing hormone (LH) and follicle-stimulating hormone (FSH) are hormones secreted by the anterior pituitary gland, and their secretion is stimulated by hypothalamic gonadotrophin-releasing hormone (GnRH or LHRH). FSH induces gametogenesis (Watkins et al., 1987), stimulating the Sertoli cells and the production of LH receptors in the male, and follicular development in the female. LH is primarily responsible for the regulation of gonadal steroid production by Leydig cells of the testis and by ovarian follicles through the LH receptor. GnRH is released in a pulsatile pattern in order to produce a pulsatile release of the pituitary gonadotrophins, especially LH. Secretion of LH and FSH is regulated both by feedback of gonadal steroids and peptides (as inhibin) and by the GnRH signal,

Paediatric and Adolescent Gynaecology, ed. Adam Balen et al. Published by Cambridge University Press.
© Cambridge University Press 2004.

which interacts with a membrane receptor to regulate their release.

There is a sex difference in fetal, infancy and pubertal gonadal function (Faiman and Winters, 1971; Takagi et al., 1977). The sequential development of the pituitary–gonadal axis before and after birth in terms of secretion of oestrogens and testosterone reflects GnRH and human chorionic gonadotrophin (hCG) secretion. The latter is produced by the placenta (Julier et al., 1984) and maintains the secretion of oestrogen and progesterone by the corpus luteum during pregnancy. It has been recognized that there are five different stages of activity of the hypothalamic–pituitary–gonadal axis: fetal, early infancy, childhood, late prepuberty and puberty (Grumbach and Kaplan, 1990; Kaplan and Grumbach, 1976).

Fetus

In the first 20 weeks of gestation, there is GnRH neuron activity with LH and FSH secretion and a peak of hCG secretion (12 weeks). In the male, the secretion of testosterone from the testes starts at 7 weeks and has a peak at 15–18 weeks. In the female, oestrogen secretion is low. From mid-gestation to birth, the negative feedback by steroid (Backer and Scrimgeour, 1980) produced by the fetoplacental unit and the control of inhibition by the central nervous system (CNS) causes a suppression of GnRH secretion. Thus, prematurely born infants have higher serum LH and FSH levels than full-term infants (Shinkawa et al., 1983).

In germ cell development in the female, three cell types can be distinguished: gonocytes, oogonia and oocytes. The primitive germ cells migrate into the ovary from the yolk sac endoderm during the first month of gestation. The oogonia then go through mitotic division; maximal mitotic activity in the oogonia occurs between the 11th and the 26th weeks. They then undergo oogenesis, entering the prophase of meiosis, to become primary oocytes. The onset of ovarian activity is in early fetal life (Rajpert-De Meyts et al., 1999). Human follicles begin their development during the fourth month of fetal life; a maximum of approximately 7 million germ cells are present around 20 weeks of gestational age. Thereafter, associated with meiosis, the pool of immature follicles begins to diminish, so that by menarche approximately 500 000 remain and by menopause the pool reduces to less than 100. When oocytes enter the diplotene stage of meiotic prophase, they must be furnished with granulosa cells to form a primordial follicle or they undergo atresia.

The maintenance of the oocyte population is clearly dependent on the presence of a normal X chromosome complement within the germ cells. In 45,XO Turner's syndrome, the unequal number of chromosomes leads to abnormal spindle formation at meiosis; although the initial increase in oocytes, associated with mitosis, is normal, there is a dramatic reduction in numbers associated with meiosis (Stanhope et al., 1993).

The main stages of follicular development are primordial follicle, primary follicle, secondary follicle, preantral follicle, early follicle, early antral follicle and small antral follicle. Follicular growth even before birth is gonadotrophin dependent. In anencephalic fetuses, there is no follicular development (Backer and Scrimgeour, 1980); no follicles reach the preovulatory size as they degenerate at various stages of their development. Therefore, it seems that the survival of gametes depends on secretion from the pituitary gland; certainly when follicles are > 2 mm diameter growth becomes increasingly dependent on gonadotrophin hormones.

Early infancy

At two weeks after birth and until six months of age in boys and 12 months in girls, the activity of GnRH causes an elevation of FSH and LH concentrations (de Zegher et al., 1992). These episodic discharges occur in association with both serum testosterone and oestrogen increases. These phenomena appear to be related to a lack of maturation of CNS inhibitory tracts and to insensitivity to sex hormone concentrations.

Serum FSH levels are higher in female infants than in males and significant amounts of oestradiol or its precursors are secreted from the infant ovary; however, this response is less uniform than testosterone production in male infants, and it may reflect the regression of ovarian follicles at this time. Serum concentration of FSH in girls remains elevated after birth, in some cases until as late as four years of age. This may result from relative ovarian resistance to gonadotrophin stimulation or it may represent a delay in the maturation of the feedback mechanism controlling gonadotrophin secretion.

Childhood

After six months of age, the negative feedback from gonadal steroids and the maturation of intrinsic CNS inhibition cause a progressive decline in LH and FSH levels. This inhibition is maximal at four years of age (Winter et al., 1975).

The number and the size of antral follicles increase after the age of six years, coinciding with the progressive increase in FSH output in childhood.

During childhood, there is a relationship between follicle growth, hormone response and hormone production.

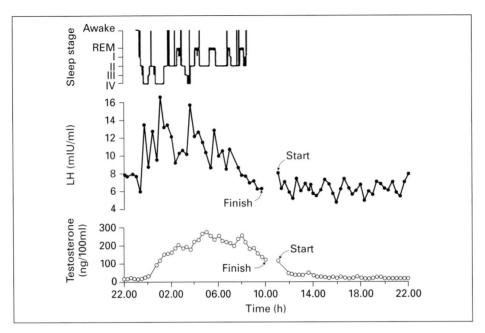

Fig. 4.1. Spontaneous serum luteinizing hormone (LH) and follicle-stimulating hormone (FSH) secretion for a normal boy in early puberty. An electroencephalogram emphasises the period of sleep. (From Boyar et al., 1974.)

Some chromosome abnormalities alter normal follicular development, with a reduction of the pool of available follicles, and inhibit follicular growth (Peters et al., 1976).

Late prepubertal period

In the late prepubertal period, these inhibitory influences decrease contemporaneously with the increasing of amplitude and frequency of GnRH pulses. The preparation for the onset of female puberty may begin in girls at five or six years of age. The diurnal rhythms of LH, FSH and sex steroid levels increase many years before the onset of phenotypic puberty; there is a time delay between LH and oestrogen time series, which decreases before the onset of puberty (Mitamura et al., 2000).

Puberty

Puberty is the stage of transition from childhood to adult life during which secondary sexual characteristics and growth acceleration appear; it results in the potential for fertility. Other physical features appearing in puberty are alteration in fat distribution, increase in muscle mass and deepening of the voice in boys. The aetiology of suppression (and desuppression) of the hypothalamus–pituitary–gonadal axis is unknown. The first endocrine events of puberty come several years earlier than phenotypic

puberty (breast development in girls and increase of testicular volume in boys); this event is an increase in the pulsatile secretion of LH from the pituitary gland in response to pulsatile GnRH secretion from the hypothalamus at night. LH release is a result both of gonadal hormone secretion and of increased pituitary sensitivity to GnRH, caused by prolonged unopposed oestrogen exposure of the gonadotrophin cells. The nocturnal rise in serum LH is sleep dependent (Boyar et al., 1974, 1976) (Figs. 4.1 and 4.2) and the amplitude increases until the early hours of the morning. As puberty progresses, there is an increase in the amplitude of nocturnal gonadotrophin pulses and a gradual change to the adult pattern of one pulse approximately every 90 minutes throughout the day and the night (Stanhope and Brook, 1988). In contrast to LH, no diurnal variation is found for FSH at any of the pubertal stages. For FSH, the mean levels increase progressively from prepuberty to mid-puberty, with a slight increase in the mean pulse amplitude at the onset of puberty, but no change in pulse frequency is found (Peters et al., 1978). LH is secreted in a pulsatile manner well before the onset of puberty; furthermore, the gonadotrophin secretory patterns characteristic of early puberty result from the amplification of an already existing circadian pattern.

The nocturnal pulsatile LH secretion is equally true for boys and girls; in boys, testosterone increases after the first nocturnal pulse of LH and reaches a peak in the early hours

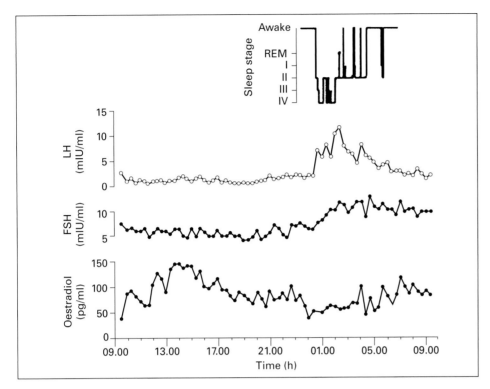

Fig. 4.2. Spontaneous serum luteinizing hormone (LH) and follicle-stimulating hormone (FSH) and oestradiol secretion for a normal girl in early puberty. The electroencephalogram emphasises the period of sleep. (From Boyar et al., 1976.)

of the morning. It then falls to low concentrations during the daytime (Fig. 4.1); this is why spontaneous erections occur in the early hours of the morning. For this reason, the measurement of LH, FSH and testosterone in boys in early puberty are of little use, unless the samples are taken in the middle of the night. Although boys enter puberty approximately six months later than girls, they are potentially fertile at an earlier age. Spermaturia (the appearance of sperm in the urine) occurs from a 6 ml testicular volume (Nilsen et al., 1986). In girls, high-amplitude pulsatile secretion of gonadotrophin does not commonly occur during the daytime until one or two years after menarche, when ovulatory cycles are established. Oestrogen concentrations rise much later at night in girls than testosterone does in boys, probably because of aromatase induction, and continue rising to achieve peak values by mid-morning (Fig. 4.2).

Age-related standards for the onset and progression of puberty are derived from longitudinal and cross-sectional surveys of normal children. The appearance of secondary sexual characteristics occurs in 95% of girls between 8.5 and 13 years, as evidenced by enlargement of the breasts, and in 95% of boys between 9.5 and 13.5 years as assessed by enlargement of the testes (Fig. 4.3). The average age at which the individual events of puberty occur in normal girls is variable. Usually the first event to be noticed is the appearance of the breast bud (breast-stage 2); this is an elevation of breast papilla with slight enlargement of the areola and occurs at the average age of 11.2 years. Pubic hair usually begins to appear six months later; however, in about one-third of all girls, pubic hair may appear before breast development. These two events are independent and each individual event of puberty is a reflection of different endocrine events (e.g. breast development reflects oestrogen secretion; pubic and axillary hair reflects adrenal androgen secretion; and increasing testicular volume reflects gonadotrophin secretion). Menarche occurs late in puberty, at the average age of 13 years, and it is independent from the other pubertal characteristics but correlates well with the waning of the growth spurt; girls start to menstruate when their height velocity is falling to approximately 4 cm/year. The adolescent growth spurt in girls occurs earlier than in boys; in girls the first event of puberty may be the growth spurt whereas in boys the onset of the growth spurt commences between genitalia stages 3 and 4 and it is never the first sign of puberty (Tanner, 1989).

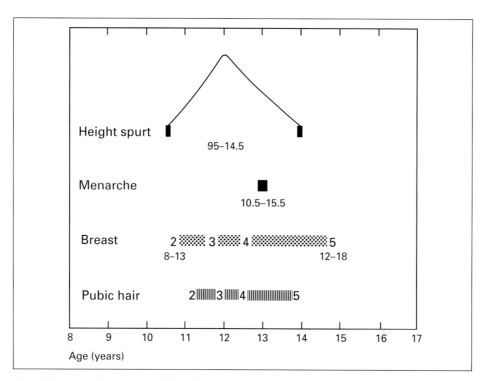

Fig. 4.3. Sequence of acquisition of signs of secondary sexual characteristics for normal girls in puberty. (From Tanner, 1989.)

The progressive physical changes during normal puberty (breast development, pubic hair distribution, and testicular and penile enlargement) are described in each category by "Tanner stages" (Tanner, 1962). Puberty is a slow process and it is important to mimic this time scale when puberty is induced. The fastest girls progress through puberty in 18 months although the slowest boys may take five years.

Bone age is not a useful guideline to identify the onset of puberty. Similarly, pelvic ultrasound is not precise but is a noninvasive method of assessing ovarian and uterine changes caused by the pulsatile release of gonadotrophins from the pituitary gland. Necropsy studies have shown that ovarian size increases gradually during childhood (Simbkins, 1932). Ovarian size increases from a mean of 1 cm^3 at two years of age to a mean of 2 cm^3 at seven years. Multicystic ovaries describes the morphological appearance characterized by more than six follicles greater than 4 mm in diameter (Stanhope et al., 1985). This multicystic appearance is the ovarian response to pulsatile gonadotrophin secretion. The ovaries of normal adolescents contain multiple follicular cysts (Polhemus, 1953), the development of which causes the rapid ovarian enlargement at puberty (Krants and Atkinson, 1967). Both ovarian and follicular size increase progressively from fetal life to puberty and there is histological evidence of a continued turnover of follicles throughout childhood (Peters et al., 1981). Ovaries containing multiple cysts have been shown by ultrasound in normal prepuberty (Cabrol et al., 1980) and single or multiple follicular cysts have been reported in girls with precocious puberty (Haller et al., 1983). A different pattern of ovarian morphology is polycystic ovaries; this occurs in approximately 20% of normal women. It has been documented that multicystic ovaries may change into a polycystic pattern but this change is probably irreversible. The multicystic ovary is the ovarian morphological response to nocturnal pulsatile secretion of gonadotrophins and can be used as a marker for this. However, in adolescence, the chronobiological pattern of pulsatility of LH and FSH with predominant pulsatility during the daytime rather than at night is associated with the presence of polycystic ovaries (Porcu et al., 1987). This reversal of the night-time predominance of gonadotrophin secretion is unexplained.

During puberty, the uterus undergoes a steady increase in size and the corpus gradually becomes larger than the cervix. Uterine length, ovarian volume, fundus: cervical ratio and hormones (serum oestradiol, FSH, LH) show a significant correlation with Tanner score but they cannot be considered as markers of pubertal stages (Orbak et al., 1998). Menarche occurs in girls during late puberty, when growth velocity is < 4 cm/year. Initial menstrual cycles are usually anovulatory and this is associated with irregular and often painful periods. After approximately one to two years, the capacity for oestrogen-positive feedback develops, culminating in a mid-cycle LH surge and ovulation. At this stage, the endocrine mechanism of potential fertility has been achieved (Stanhope, 1998).

Adolescence

The term adolescence is not synonymous with puberty. Adolescence incorporates the social adaptation to adult life and refers to a whole process of changing physically and psychologically, which takes a longer period of time than puberty. Puberty is the process associated with gonadal maturation and the development of fertility.

The correlation between psychological disturbances and mood swings in adolescence, and the secretion of sex hormones is well recognized. Adolescents are exposed to changing patterns and timing of oestrogen and testosterone secretion, which may influence behaviour. The association between emotional problems and sex hormone secretion is complex, but there are few data available on the subject. Adolescents need to become independent and to develop a sense of identity. During adolescence, the difference between individuals in attitude and physique becomes more evident than ever before. Some children grow up faster and earlier than others do. There may be numerous psychological difficulties when puberty occurs at the limits of the normal range. The timing of pubertal development may have profound importance for adolescence and affect physical strength and sporting prowess, social adaptation and relations with the opposite sex. Children whose pubertal development occurs earlier than average have an earlier growth spurt and are taller and stronger than their peers in the short term. This may allow them earlier independence.

Delayed puberty in normal adolescence causes a physical delay in maturation compared with peers, and it often leads to psychological difficulties. This phenomenon may lead to aggressive and antisocial behaviour. For these reasons, although children with delayed puberty may be endocrinologically normal, reassurance may not be sufficient. Such children may need some practical help with pubertal induction and advancement of the timing of their growth spurt. Surprisingly most boys with delayed puberty are more concerned about their short stature than their delay in acquiring secondary sexual characteristics (Krants and Atkinson, 1967). The diagnosis of constitutional delayed puberty is clinical, and such children require treatment rather than intensive investigation. Those who do not respond to sex steroid therapy in a predictable fashion require investigation.

Summary

Puberty and adolescence are two complex stages of life during which the potential of fertility and reproduction and the psychosocial adaptation to adult life occur. Puberty is the process of gonadal maturation, which is characterized by the appearance of secondary sexual characteristics and an associated growth spurt and results in the attainment of fertility. Adolescence encompasses more than just puberty; it takes a longer period of time than puberty and leads to the social adaptation to adult life.

These processes start at conception by the determination of genetic sex and the differentiation of genitalia into male or female reproductive organs. Through a cascade of endocrine events, controlled by the hypothalamic–pituitary–gonadal axis, physical and psychological changes occur, which mark the transition from childhood to adult life.

REFERENCES

Baker T G, Scrimgeour J B (1980). Development of the gonad in normal and anencephalic human foetuses. *J Reprod Fertil* 60, 193–199.

Boyar R M, Rosenfeld R S, Kapen S et al. (1974). Human puberty: simultaneous secretion of lutenizing hormone and testosterone during sleep. *J Clin Invest* 54, 609–614.

Boyar R M, Wu R H, Roffwarg H et al. (1976). Human puberty: 24-hour estradiol in pubertal girls. *J Clin Endocrinol Metab* 43, 1418–1421.

Cabrol S, Haseltine F P, Taylor K J, Viscomi G, Genel M (1980). Ultrasound examination of pubertal girls and of patients with gonadal dysgenesis. *J Adolesc Health Care* 1, 185–192.

de Zegher F, Devlieger H, Veldhuis J D (1992). Pulsatile and sexually dimorphic secretion of luteinizing hormone in the human infant on the day of birth. *Pediatr Res* 32, 605–607.

Faiman C, Winter J S (1971). Sex differences in gonadotropin concentrations in infancy. *Nature* 232, 130–131.

Grumbach M M, Kaplan S L (1990). The neuroendocrinology of human puberty: an ontogenic prospective. In *Control of the Onset of Puberty*, Grumbach M M, Sizonenko P C, Aubert M L, eds., pp. 1–62. Wilkins & Wilkins, Baltimore, MD.

Haller J O, Friedman A P, Schaffer R, Lebensart D P (1983). The normal and the abnormal ovary in childhood and adolescence. *Semin Ultrasound* 4, 206–225.

Jost A (1953). Problems of fetal endocrinology. The gonadal and hypophyseal hormones. *Rec Prog Horm Res* 8, 379–418.

Julier C, Weil D, Couillin P et al. (1984). The beta chorionic gonadotrophin-beta luteinizing gene cluster maps to human chromosome 19. *Hum Genet* 67, 174–177.

Kaplan S L, Grumbach M M (1976). The ontogenesis of human foetal hormones. II. Luteinizing hormone (LH) and follicle-stimulating hormone (FSH). *Acta Endocrinol* 81, 808–829.

Krants K E, Atkinson J P (1967). Paediatric and adolescent gynaecology: gross anatomy. *Ann N Y Acad Sci* 142, 551–571.

Mitamura R, Yano K, Suzuki N, Ito Y, Makita Y, Okuno A (2000). Diurnal rhythms of luteinizing hormone, follicle-stimulating hormone, testosterone and estradiol secretion before the onset of female puberty in short children. *J Clin Endocrinol Metab* 85, 1074–1080.

Nilsen C T, Skakkebaek N E, Richardson D W et al. (1986). Onset of the release of spermatozoa (spermarche) in boys in relation to age, testicular growth, pubic hair and height. *J Clin Endocrinol Metab* 62, 532–535.

Orbak Z, Sagsoz N, Alp H, Tan H, Yildirim H, Kaya D (1998). Pelvic ultrasound measurements in normal girls: relation to puberty and sex hormone concentration. *J Pediatr Endocrinol Metab* 11, 525–530.

Parker K L, Schedl A, Schimmer B P (1999). Gene interactions in gonadal development. *Annu Rev Physiol* 61, 417–433.

Peters H, Himelstein-Braw R, Faber M (1976). The normal development of the ovary in childhood. *Acta Endocrinol* 82, 617–630.

Peters H, Byskov A G, Grinsted J (1978). Follicular growth in fetal and prepubertal ovaries of humans and other primates. *J Clin Endocrinol Metab* 7, 469–485.

(1981). The development of the ovary during childhood in health and disease. In *Functional Morphology of the Human Ovary*, Coutts J R T, ed., pp. 26–34. MTP Press, Lancaster, UK.

Polhemus D W (1953). Ovarian maturation and cyst formation in children. *Pediatrics* 11, 588–594.

Porcu E, Venturoli S, Magrini O et al. (1987). Circadian variations of luteinizing hormone can have two different profiles in adolescence and ovulation. *J Clin Endocrinol Metab* 65, 488–493.

Rajpert-De Meyts E, Jorgensen N, Gram N et al. (1999). Expression of anti Müllerian hormone during normal and pathological gonadal development: association with differentiation of Sertoli and granulosa cells. *J Clin Endocrinol Metab* 84, 3836–3844.

Shinkawa O, Furuhashi N, Fukaya T, Suzuki M, Kono H, Tachibana Y (1983). Changes of serum gonadotrophin levels and sex differences in premature and mature infants during neonatal life. *J Clin Endocrinol Metab* 56, 1327–1331.

Simbkins C S (1932). Development of the human ovary from birth to sexual maturity. *Am J Anat* 51, 465–505.

Stanhope R (1998). Endocrinology. In *The Practice of Medicine in Adolescence*, Brook C G D, ed., pp. 120–133. Edward Arnold for Bioscientifica, London.

Stanhope R, Brook C G (1988). An evaluation of hormonal changes at puberty in man: a review. *J Endocrinol* 116, 306–305.

Stanhope R, Adams J, Jacobs H S, Brook C G D (1985). Ovarian ultrasound assessment in normal children, idiopathic precocious puberty, and during low dose pulsatile gonadotrophin releasing hormone treatment of hypogonadotrophic hypogonadism. *Arch Dis Child* 60, 116–119.

Stanhope R, Massarano A, Brook C G D (1993). The natural history of ovarian demise in Turner syndrome. In *Basic and Clinical Approach to Turner Syndrome*, Hibi I, Takano K, eds., pp. 91–99. Excerpta Medica, Japan.

Takagi S, Yoshida T, Tsubata K et al. (1977). Sex differences in fetal gonadotrophin and androgens. *J Steroid Biochem* 8, 609–620.

Tanner J M (1962). *Growth at Adolescence*. Blackwell, Oxford.

(1989). *Foetus into Man: Physical Growth from Conception to Maturity*, 2nd edn. Castlemead, Ware.

Watkins P C, Eddy R, Beck A K et al. (1987). DNA sequence and regional assignment of the human follicle-stimulating hormone beta-subunit gene to the short arm of human chromosome 11. *DNA* 6, 205–212.

Winter J S, Faiman C, Hobson W C, Prasad A V, Reyes F I (1975). Pituitary–gonadal relations in infancy. I. Patterns of serum gonadotrophin concentrations from birth to four years of age in man and chimpanzee. *J Clin Endocrinol Metab* 40, 545–551.

5

Control of the menstrual cycle and fertility

Gillian Lockwood

Midland Fertility Services, Aldridge, UK

Introduction

During her reproductive 'lifespan' of approximately 35 years, a woman who neither conceives nor uses hormonal contraception will experience over 400 menstrual bleeds. It is a remarkable feature of human ovulation that the sequence of events is so finely coordinated to ensure that there is maximum chance of achieving a pregnancy by synchronizing the release of a mature oocyte with the time of maximum receptivity of the endometrium and, in addition, if a pregnancy is not established that cycle, the entire sequence of events is repeated the next month (Fig. 5.1). Even more extraordinary perhaps, given the enormous hormonal and biochemical changes wrought by pregnancy, is the fact that, in the absence of lactation and breastfeeding, the whole sequence can start up again shortly after delivery.

From an evolutionary standpoint, it is clear that this is a wasteful and potentially hazardous situation. One must remember, however, that during the long eons of evolutionary time, women would not have entered puberty until they were much older than is the current case and pregnancies not only would have been "unavoidable" but would have been followed by a prolonged period of breastfeeding during which time ovulation, and hence menstruation, would have been suppressed. Our ancestors would probably have experienced only a fraction of the number of menstrual cycles that modern women have to endure. The present day "epidemic" of gynaecological diseases such as endometriosis, fibroids, endometrial and ovarian cancer can perhaps be accounted for by the fact that women's bodies are experiencing a hormonal environment that they did not encounter during evolutionary development. The apparent protective value of the combined oral contraceptive pill

against gynaecological disease can be explained by the fact that it suppresses ovulation and renders the hormonal milieu much closer to the state of "perpetual pregnancy or lactation" that was the fate of our female ancestors. We could also perhaps speculate that the "extended reproductive lifespan" in which a woman "outlives" her menopause is a relatively modern phenomenon.

Embryology: development of the ovary

At approximately four to five weeks of embryonic life, genital ridges (which are identical in the two sexes at this stage) are formed overlying the embryonic kidney. The primitive gonad is formed between five and seven weeks of embryonic life, at which time the undifferentiated germ cells migrate from the yolk sac to the genital ridges by amoeboid movement.

In the absence of male determinants, the cortical portions of the primitive gonad develop into ovaries. Granulosa cells derived from proliferating coelomic epithelium cells migrate and surround the germ cells, thus forming primordial follicles. Each primordial follicle consists of an oocyte within a single layer of granulosa cells. Theca cells, also derived from proliferating coelomic epithelium, form now and are separated from the layer of granulosa cells surrounding the follicles by a basal lamina.

The maximum number of primordial follicles is reached at approximately 20 weeks of gestation, by which time six to seven million are present. Atresia gradually reduces this number so that by birth only one to two million are present. This process, which is independent of hormonal changes, continues throughout childhood and by the onset

Paediatric and Adolescent Gynaecology, ed. Adam Balen et al. Published by Cambridge University Press.
© Cambridge University Press 2004.

51

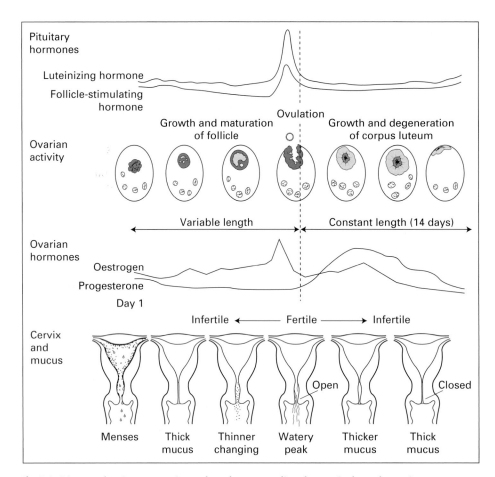

Fig. 5.1. Diagram showing one ovarian cycle and corresponding changes in the endometrium.

of puberty, 300 000–400 000 primordial follicles are present within the ovaries. Only 300–400 will be ovulated between menarche and menopause, while the remainder will undergo atresia. The oocyte of a primordial follicle is developmentally arrested at the prophase of its first meiotic division and remains in that state until it either regresses or re-enters the meiotic process shortly before ovulation. The relative infertility of older women, and the high incidence of miscarriage associated with aneuploidy in their embryos, thus reflects the fact that some oocytes may be arrested in this state of meiotic "suspended animation" for 45–50 years.

Puberty: the onset of the menarche

Puberty represents a transition between childhood and adulthood and it is vital to distinguish between the hormonal and reproductive attributes of this transition and the social and sociobiological consequences. Within a few centuries in the Western world, "childhood", as a state of

entitlement to nurturing and absence of responsibility, has been alternately advanced and delayed. In the seventeenth century, children were dressed as adults and expected to undertake adult work and responsibilities from their early teens. They could be married and held accountable for their actions at law. More recently, "childhood" has been idealized and extended, and children have been protected, restricted and arguably "infantilized" until they are 18 or even 21 years of age.

The endocrine and hormonal events that occur during puberty are designed to prepare the organs of reproduction for their procreative role, and it is perhaps unfortunate that the social and cultural support for this new role is neither as predictable nor as reliable as the series of hormonal phenomena that accompany them.

The hypothalamic–pituitary–ovarian axis begins to function during fetal life, but it does not usually become fully active until the second decade. Throughout childhood, serum gonadotrophin levels are very low and remain so until the onset of puberty. The hypothalamic and pituitary system for gonadotrophin release is exquisitely sensitive to the negative feedback effects of oestradiol, and during childhood serum levels of oestradiol remain at levels less than 10 pg/ml. The central nervous system of the prepubertal girl displays an increased sensitivity to even the small amounts of circulating oestrogens that are present. Its sensitivity to this negative feedback gradually decreases as puberty begins, allowing the release of gonadotrophin-releasing hormone (GnRH) and the gonadotrophins.

The onset of puberty occurs when a level of physical maturity is achieved. This level is most closely related to the skeletal age of the girl, with a secondary influence of body mass. Because the first menstrual period is a precise event, there are data covering many years and we find that the age at menarche has decreased significantly during the twentieth century. This is probably a result of improvements in nutrition and in environmental conditions; in Norway, where detailed records go back for over a century, there has been a progressive lowering of the mean age of menarche from the seventeenth to the thirteenth year. In the southern USA, where childhood obesity is recognized to be a major health and social problem, "precocious puberty" at 9 or 10 years is usually caused by a high calorific diet and sedentary lifestyle alone. The first changes to herald puberty are the occurrence of small nocturnal spikes of luteinizing hormone (LH) and follicle-stimulating hormone (FSH); these in turn, stimulate afternoon rises in oestradiol levels. FSH spikes are detected first, but the amplitude of LH rises is greater and, during this phase, nocturnal levels of LH may exceed those of adult women.

Menarche, the first menstrual period, occurs when sufficient ovarian oestrogens are synthesized to promote endometrial proliferation. Ovulation rarely occurs during the first few cycles, and less than half the cycles in the first two years are ovular. The discomfort, irregularity and unpredictability of these early anovular menstrual cycles unfortunately may encourage many young girls to seek, and their doctors to prescribe, the oral contraceptive pill to "regulate" the cycles. This may have a long-term deleterious effect of "re-setting" an immature endocrine "thermostat".

The endocrine basis for ovulation

Regular cyclic ovulation in women is achieved by an elegant and complex interaction of hormonal signals that prevent the "default to atresia" which is the fate of the majority of the primordial follicles that exist in the ovaries of the newborn infant. The female reproductive system functions within an integrated classical model with hypothalamic stimulation of the pituitary by a specific releasing hormone, GnRH,

resulting in pituitary secretion of LH and FSH. GnRH is produced and released from a group of connected neurons in the medial basal hypothalamus, primarily within the arcuate nucleus and in the preoptic area of the ventral hypothalamus. It is released by axonal transport in a pulsatile fashion into the complex capillary net of the portal system, and it binds to specific receptors in the plasma membrane of the anterior pituitary gonadotrophs, where it stimulates synthesis, storage and release of LH and FSH.

Physiological secretion of gonadotrophins from the pituitary requires intermittent, pulsatile GnRH secretion. The short half-life (< 3 minutes) of GnRH makes it impossible to measure GnRH secretion directly in human subjects, but animal studies suggest that the pulsatile pattern of LH secretion represents pulses of GnRH. Human females show a wide variation in GnRH pulse frequency, ranging from the shortest interpulse frequency of 70 minutes in the late follicular phase to 216 minutes in the late luteal phase. The quality of pulsatile gonadotrophin stimulation is critical in achieving ovulation, as even minor abnormalities in the frequency or amplitude of GnRH-induced LH pulses may interfere with ovulatory function. Paradoxically, continuous or high-frequency pulses of GnRH or its analogues results in desensitization of the pituitary gonadotrophs and blockade of gonadal function. The frequency and amplitude of GnRH stimulation regulate LH and FSH secretion and synthesis in a differential manner. In the absence of gonadal steroids and peptides, a decrease in GnRH pulse frequency is associated with a decrease in LH, but an increase in FSH. In the early follicular phase, the LH interpulse interval is approximately 90 minutes, and slowing of the GnRH pulse generator with sleep is a unique feature of this stage of the menstrual cycle. GnRH pulse frequency increases in the mid-follicular phase to every 60 minutes, with a marked diminution of pulse amplitude that is secondary to the negative feedback effect of oestradiol on LH. In the late follicular phase, GnRH pulse frequency remains at every 60 minutes while LH pulse amplitude begins a gradual increase concomitant with the rapid rise in oestradiol (Fig. 5.2). The mid-cycle LH surge in the human does not rely on an increase in the frequency or amount of GnRH secreted as it does in other mammals. The luteal phase is associated with a progressive decrease in the frequency of pulsatile GnRH secretion, with an interpulse interval of 100 minutes during the early luteal phase, widening to 4 hours in the late luteal phase. The decrease in GnRH pulse frequency is associated with an increase in LH pulse amplitude.

Preantral stages of follicular growth occur independently of gonadotrophic stimulation. However, antrum formation requires stimulation by FSH, acting via its receptor in the

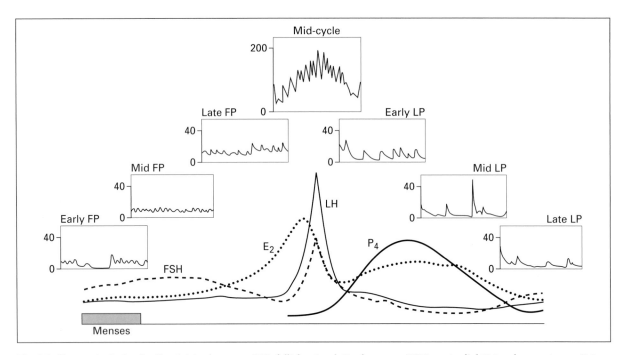

Fig. 5.2. Changes in the levels of luteinizing hormone (LH), follicle-stimulating hormone (FSH), oestradiol (E_2) and progesterone (P_4) during the normal menstrual cycle. The insert boxes show the changing pattern of pulsatile LH secretion measured during 24 hour frequent-sampling studies. FP, follicular phase; LP, luteal phase. (After Hall, 1997.)

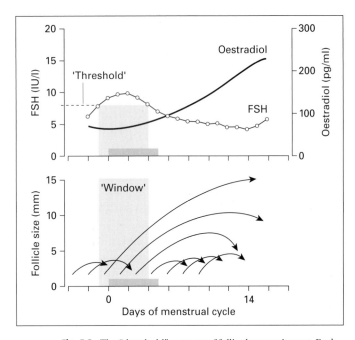

Fig. 5.3. The "threshold" concept of follicular recruitment. Each developing follicle has a "threshold" for stimulation by follicle-stimulating hormone (FSH); when the hormone exceeds that level, the follicle secretes oestradiol, which causes FSH levels to fall and other follicles to undergo atresia. (Adapted from Fauser et al., 1993.)

granulosa cell surface membrane. The increment in FSH that is required to initiate folliculogenesis is relatively small, and within the normal menstrual cycle it begins during the luteofollicular transition. The mechanisms for this increase in FSH include release from the negative feedback control of oestradiol, which occurs in conjunction with the demise of the corpus luteum since the FSH rise can be prevented by administration of mid-luteal phase levels of oestradiol. A contributory mechanism is found in inhibin A, which has a suppressive effect on FSH levels during the luteal phase and is significantly reduced with the demise of the corpus luteum. The luteofollicular rise in FSH occurs concomitantly with a dramatic increase in GnRH pulse frequency, suggesting that the dynamic modulation of GnRH pulse frequency which occurs between the luteal and follicular phases of the cycle may also play an important role in the luteofollicular rise in FSH.

From puberty, cyclic increases in pituitary FSH secretion rescue a cohort of follicles from atresia according to the "threshold" concept (Fig. 5.3). Although multiple follicles are recruited to begin preovulatory development, as the FSH concentration rises at the beginning of each cycle, usually only one survives to become dominant: the follicle with granulosa cells that are most responsive to FSH. During follicular growth, FSH acts via granulosa cell FSH receptors coupled to cyclic AMP-mediated postreceptor signalling to stimulate the formation of factors that locally modulate cell proliferation and differentiation. Autocrine factors that affect FSH-regulated granulosa cell proliferation include growth and differentiation factors such as activin and transforming growth factor β that activate serine/threonine kinase-mediated postreceptor signalling. Paracrine factors of thecal cell origin that influence FSH actions include the androgens. The granulosa cell androgen receptor that mediates paracrine androgen action is developmentally regulated by FSH. Development of the dominant follicle is characterized by the secretion of increasingly large amounts of oestradiol and inhibin into the circulation, and there is evidence to suggest that the maintenance of dominance is effected by intraovarian paracrine signalling, with inhibins and activins acting as important paracrine messengers. As follicular dominance develops, LH-stimulated thecal androgen is required as an oestrogen precursor in FSH-stimulated granulosa cells. In vitro studies on isolated granulosa and thecal cells and whole follicles have shown that FSH stimulates granulosa cells to produce factors that upregulate LH-stimulated thecal P450c17α mRNA expression and androgen synthesis during preovulatory follicular maturation. There is a role for inhibins (and insulin growth factors 1 and 2) as the functional growth and differentiation factors implicated in this positive feedback loop, especially as inhibin enhances LH-stimulated human thecal cell androgen production in vitro and is produced in a development-related manner by the ovary.

Inhibin B levels in peripheral serum rise from early in the follicular phase to reach a peak coincident with the onset of the mid-follicular phase decline in FSH levels. That temporal coincidence is strong evidence for an important role for inhibin B in ensuring mono-ovulation, as the maintenance of high FSH levels is truncated before more than one "dominant" follicle can be recruited. Inhibin B levels then decline during the luteal phase apart from a peri-ovular peak, which may represent release of follicular inhibin B from the rupturing follicle into the circulation (Groome et al., 1996) (Fig. 5.4). By contrast, inhibin A levels are low in the early follicular phase, show a small mid-follicular phase peak, rise rapidly with ovulation and are maximal during the mid-luteal phase.

During the luteal–follicular transition, inhibin B concentrations rise rapidly to their mid-follicular peak whereas inhibin A concentrations fall synchronously with oestradiol and progesterone to reach a nadir at the time of the intercycle FSH peak. In a study of the luteal–follicular transition in normal cycling women and GnRH-deficient women who were administered pulsatile exogenous GnRH, Welt et al. (1997) demonstrated that, in normal women, inhibin B levels rose in association with FSH at the time associated

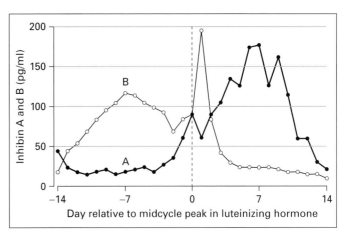

Fig. 5.4. Graph of inhibin A and B normalized to ovulation. (After Groome et al., 1996.)

with the increase in GnRH pulse frequency that occurs before menses. The different patterns of circulating inhibin A and B during the two phases of the ovarian cycle are strong evidence for their playing different physiological roles during follicular recruitment, maturation and ovulation (Groome et al., 1996).

Much experimental evidence has accrued concerning the role of activin (an ovarian product structurally related to inhibin but with the opposite effect of enhancing FSH release from the pituitary) in the female reproductive axis (Woodruff and Mather, 1995). Primate studies have shown that injection of recombinant human activin stimulates basal or GnRH-stimulated FSH synthesis and release (Stouffer et al., 1993) and activin also regulates a variety of pituitary and ovarian hormones. During the menstrual cycle, serum activin A levels vary in a biphasic manner with highest levels at mid-cycle during the luteofollicular transition at the specific times when FSH levels are highest, and nadirs occur in the mid-follicular and mid-luteal phases (Muttukrishna et al., 1996).

The mechanism of ovulation

The events leading to ovulation are initiated by the mid-cycle surge of LH and FSH. The surge initiates an increase in the concentration of plasminogen activator by a process mediated by oestradiol and progesterone. LH and FSH also stimulate the production of hyaluronic acid within the corona radiata cell mass and this weakens the cohesive bonds within the cumulus. Ovulation is essentially an inflammatory process (an assertion given enhanced credence by the finding that nonsteroidal anti-inflammatory

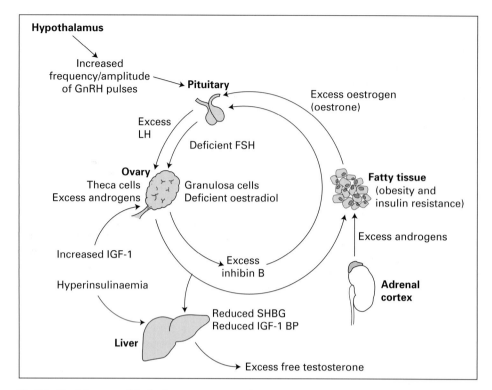

Fig. 5.5. The "viscous cycle" of polycystic ovarian syndrome. LH, luteinizing hormone; FSH, follicle-stimulating hormone; GnRH, gonadotrophin-releasing hormone; IGF-1, insulin-like growth factor 1; BP, binding protein; SHBG, sex hormone-binding globulin.

drugs and the newer cyclooxygenase 2 inhibitors can prevent ovulation). As ovulation approaches, there is an increased capillary permeability associated with follicular oedema and migration of inflammatory cells into the surrounding tissues. A variety of cytokines such as interleukin 1 and tumour necrosis factor are associated with ovulation, and enhanced blood flow through the ovary is promoted by vascular endothelial growth factor and nitric oxide (Norman and Brannstrom, 1996).

The formation of the corpus luteum

After ovulation, a separate and distinct endocrine organ, the corpus luteum, is formed. The corpus luteum produces progesterone and has a lifespan of approximately 14 days. The corpus luteum attains its maximum activity seven or eight days after the LH peak, and luteolysis begins two to three days before the onset of menses. The corpus luteum is dependent on continuing LH support for four or five days after ovulation, and at this point the corpus luteum is vulnerable to the luteolytic effect of GnRH

agonists or antagonists, which interfere with both LH pulse amplitude and pulse frequency and bring about an abrupt decrease in progesterone levels and a premature onset of menses. By contrast, the life of the corpus luteum can be prolonged when human chorionic gonadotrophin is administered at this point in the luteal phase. The close homology between human chorionic gonadotrophin and LH molecules means that the former can bind to the LH receptors of the luteal cells and maintain the function of the corpus luteum, just as chorionic gonadotrophin produced by the early embryo supersedes any luteolytic mechanism.

Dysovulation and anovulation

The exquisite fine tuning required for the hypothalamic–pituitary–ovarian axis to function correctly explains why ovulatory dysfunction remains one of the commoner causes of infertility. Many of the dysovular states will be described in detail in other chapters, but a brief overview is required here for completeness.

Polycystic ovarian syndrome (PCOS) is a heterogeneous clinical entity characterized by hyperandrogenism, oligomenorrhoea or amenorrhoea (Dunaif et al., 1992; see Ch. 27). The syndrome may be more broadly characterized by the presence in the ovary of multiple small circumferential antral follicles that have become arrested at a diameter of less than 10 mm. The ovaries are enlarged as a result of stromal and thecal hyperplasia and many women with PCOS are hyperinsulinaemic, suggesting that a metabolic disorder may be contributing to the syndrome (Morales et al., 1996).

In many patients with PCOS, the hyperinsulinaemia and insulin resistance is associated with obesity. Obesity is an important pathogenetic factor involved in the development of hyperandrogenism in women with PCOS and obese PCOS women have lower sex hormone-binding globulin levels than PCOS women who are not obese. The clinical and biochemical heterogeneity of PCOS is reflected in the range of neuroendocrine disturbances associated with the syndrome. An increased serum LH concentration is common and occurs primarily as a result of an increase in the amplitude of pulsatile LH.

There have been conflicting reports in the literature on inhibin levels in PCOS. Early reports using the "Monash" assay found that the levels of immunoreactive inhibin (inhibin pro-alpha C and alpha-containing dimers) in the serum of women with PCOS were similar to those found in ovular women in the early follicular phase of the cycle (Buckler et al., 1988; Reddi et al., 1989). Using a specific assay for dimeric inhibin A, Lambert-Messerlian et al. (1994) found that the concentration in the serum of women with PCOS was similar to that of ovular women. The use of enzyme-linked immunosorbent assays for dimeric inhibin B (Anderson et al., 1998) has confirmed the original report that inhibin B levels in anovular women with PCOS are significantly higher than those of normal women (Lockwood et al., 1996). The dysovular state of PCOS can, therefore, be explained as the consequence of a "vicious cycle" in which excess androgens, deranged GnRH release and elevated inhibin B levels conspire to suppress FSH levels below the level at which functional follicles can be recruited and progress towards ovulation (Fig. 5.5).

Hyperprolactinaemia and anovulation

That lactation causes amenorrhoea, and is hence contraceptive, is one of the most important aspects of reproductive endocrinology, and its evolutionary significance is obvious. Our baby ancestors simply could not have survived if

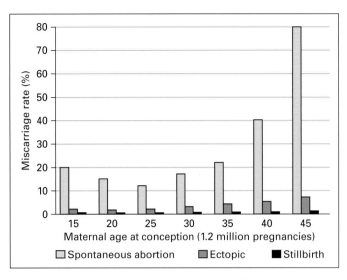

Fig. 5.6. Miscarriage rates by age. (From Anderson et al., 2000.)

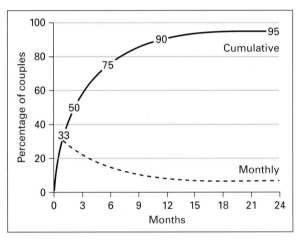

Fig. 5.7. Cumulative conception and monthly fecundity rates in a normal population of proven fertility during the first 2 years trying to conceive. Cumulative refers to the total conceiving at a particular length of time; monthly refers to the proportion conceiving in any particular month among those who have not already conceived.

their mothers had become pregnant again before they were ready to be weaned. Prolactin is unique among the anterior pituitary hormones in that its release is under tonic inhibition, principally by dopamine. There is clear diurnal variation in prolactin levels, with peak levels occurring at night, but there is no evidence of menstrual cyclicity. High levels of prolactin are inhibitory for ovulation because they reduce aromatase activity in developing follicles, block folliculogenesis and interfere with the luteal phase production of progesterone. Prolactin also has a direct effect on the hypothalamus leading to a reduction of both amplitude and frequency of GnRH pulses.

Normal fertility

Compared with other mammals, or even other primates, humans are not very fertile. Successful conception occurs only one time in three or four even when appropriately timed intercourse takes place. Unlike other mammals, which have a recognizable oestrus cycle, have distinct behavioural features indicating fecundity or are "reflex" ovulators, ovulation in women is concealed, and it is interesting to speculate on the evolutionary significance of this, and the behavioural adaptations it has engendered.

Natural fertility in women declines rapidly after the age of 32 and even more steeply from 38 years onwards. By the age of 40, 40% of recognized conceptions will end as miscarriages. It is estimated that 50% of all fertilized ova fail to implant successfully and the cause of this, and the relatively high miscarriage rate (which is 15–20% even for young women) is the high incidence of chromosomal abnormalities that arise at fertilization (Fig. 5.6).

Notwithstanding, about half of all normally fertile couples (where the woman is under 35 years) will have conceived within 3 months, two-thirds by 6 months and 90% within a year (Fig. 5.7).

REFERENCES

Anderson R A, Groome N P, Baird D T (1998). Inhibin A and inhibin B in women with polycystic ovarian syndrome during treatment with FSH to induce mono-ovulation. *Clin Endocrinol* 48, 577–584.

Dunaif A (1997). Insulin resistance and the PCOS: mechanism and implications for pathogenesis. *Endocr Rev* 18, 774–800.

Groome N P, Illingworth P J, O'Brien M et al. (1996). Measurement of dimeric inhibin-B throughout the human menstrual cycle. *J Clin Endocrinol Metab* 81, 1401–1405.

Lambert-Messerlian G M, Hall J E, Sluss P M et al. (1994). Relatively low levels of dimeric inhibin circulate in men and women with polycystic ovarian syndrome using a specific two-site ELISA. *J Clin Endocrinol Metab* 79, 45–50.

Lockwood G M, Muttukrishna S, Groome N P, Matthews D R, Ledger W L (1998). Mid-follicular phase pulses of inhibin B are absent in polycystic ovarian syndrome and are initiated by successful laparoscopic ovarian diathermy: a possible mechanism regulating emergence of the dominant follicle. *J Clin Endocrinol Metab* 83, 1730–1735.

Morales A J, Laughlin G A, Butzow T, Maheshwari H, Baumann G, Yen S S (1996). Insulin, somatotrophic, and luteinizing hormone axes in lean and obese women with polycystic ovary syndrome: common and distinct features. *J Clin Endocrinol Metab* 81, 2854–2864.

Muttukrishna S, George L, Fowler P A, Groome N P, Knight P G (1995). Serum concentrations of 'total' activin A during the human menstrual cycle and pregnancy. *J Reprod Fertil* 15, 226.

Reddi K, Wicking E J, Hillier S G, Baird D T (1989). Bioactive and FSH and inhibin concentrations during ovulation induction in patients with polycystic ovarian disease. *J Endocrinol* 123(Suppl.), 26.

Stouffer R, Woodruff T, Dahl K, Hess D, Mather J, Molkness T (1993). Human recombinant activin A alters pituitary LH and FSH secretion, follicular development and steroidogenesis during the menstrual cycle in rhesus monkeys. *J Clin Endocrinol Metab* 77, 241–248.

Welt C K, Martin K A, Taylor A E et al. (1997). Frequency modulation of follicle-stimulating hormone (FSH) during the luteal-follicular transition: evidence for FSH control of inhibin B in normal women. *J Clin Endocrinol Metab* 82, 2645–2652.

Woodruff T K, Mather J P (1995). Inhibin, activin and the female reproductive axis. *Annual Review of Physiology*, 57, 219–244.

6

Nutrition and reproductive function

Howard S. Jacobs

Royal Free and University College London School of Medicine, The Middlesex Hospital, London, UK

Introduction

Optimum fertility requires an adequate level of maternal nutrition. Women who conceive while underweight, usually it must be admitted through medical treatment, have a higher than normal risk of producing a premature child that is itself underweight (van der Spuy et al., 1988). Recent epidemiological studies have indicated that subnormal weight at birth is associated with an adverse pattern of health during adult life, particularly with respect to the development of metabolic and cardiovascular disorders (Barker, 1997). Clearly, then, risks to normal intrauterine development are greater during times of maternal starvation than when nutrition is normal. At the other end of the scale, obesity is associated with impaired health at all ages (Norman and Clark, 1998). Obesity impairs most aspects of fertility, causes insulin resistance and is a major determinant for the expression of polycystic ovary syndrome.

Role of leptin

We now understand that nutrition is regulated in large part by hormonal signals from fat cells interacting with the neuroendocrine system to control feeding and energy expenditure (Kalra et al., 1999). Leptin is a recently discovered cytokine, encoded by the *ob* gene, that is secreted by white fat cells in response to a number of influences (Mantzoros, 1999). Stimulation of hypothalamic leptin receptors suppresses neuropeptide Y production and thereby controls a variety of reproductive and vegetative functions. Much recent work has focused on factors determining circulating leptin concentrations in an attempt to understand better the influence of fat cell repletion, that is, of nutritional "status", on reproductive function.

Serum leptin concentrations correlate with fat mass (Mantzoros, 1999). Prolonged fasting decreases and overfeeding increases leptin concentrations, so the levels are also thought to reflect energy balance. Leptin production is higher in subcutaneous than in visceral fat. Several endocrine factors regulate leptin secretion. Prolonged infusion of insulin, supraphysiological insulin levels and administration of glucocorticoids increase leptin secretion, while isoprenaline (isoproterenol) and β_3-adrenergic receptor agonists reduce circulating leptin levels in humans. Women have higher levels of leptin than men, even after adjustment for fat mass, probably because of their different body fat distribution together with the stimulating effects of oestrogens and the suppressive effect of androgens on leptin secretion. Cigarette smoking is associated with decreased serum leptin concentrations, and several cytokines, such as tumour necrosis factor-α, interleukin-1 and interleukin-6, alter both leptin mRNA expression and its circulating levels.

Leptin is thought to signal attainment of the amount of fat necessary for initiation of puberty and for maintenance of menstrual cycles and reproductive ability (Bray, 1997). In contrast, individuals with inactivating mutations of the leptin receptor, who are hyperphagic and obese, remain prepubertal because of hypogonadotrophic hypogonadism (Clement et al., 1998). Although leptin has been considered mainly as an appetite-regulating antiobesity hormone, the leptin–neuropeptide Y (NPY) system also contributes to the body's adaptation to starvation. In this context, its main role is to conserve energy by decreasing thyroid hormone-induced thermogenesis and to mobilize energy stores by

Paediatric and Adolescent Gynaecology, ed. Adam Balen et al. Published by Cambridge University Press.
© Cambridge University Press 2004.

increasing the secretion of glucocorticoids. At the same time, suppression of gonadal function avoids the energy demands of pregnancy and lactation. NPY is itself an inhibitor of gonadotrophin-releasing hormone (GnRH) pulsatility and so, by suppressing NPY, leptin permits GnRH pulse activity and fertility.

Variations in serum leptin concentrations are related to minute-to-minute changes in adrenocorticotrophic hormone and cortisol levels in normal men (Licinio et al., 1997) and to luteinizing hormone (LH) and oestradiol levels in normal women (Licinio et al., 1998). Decreased leptin levels may, therefore, underlie the metabolic and neuroendocrine changes seen in patients with anorexia nervosa and which may accompany therapeutic dieting for obesity.

Serum leptin levels in patients with anorexia nervosa, bulimia and nonspecific eating disorders are similar to those of healthy people of comparable body mass index (BMI) (Grinspoon et al., 1996). In patients with anorexia nervosa, who in recovery preferentially gain fat mass, leptin concentrations in cerebrospinal fluid return to normal sooner than the body mass index does (Mantzoros et al., 1997) which may, therefore, contribute to the difficulty they have in regaining weight. Weight loss-related amenorrhoea is characterized by low leptin levels (Audi et al., 1998), consistent with the notion that the body senses its fat content through leptin and inhibits ovulation when nutritional reserve is depleted, as signalled by a critical leptin level. The recovery of LH secretion in response to refeeding closely mirrors the rise in serum leptin levels.

Subnormal nutrition and reproductive function

The neuroendocrine adaptations discussed above are designed to assist the individual's survival in times of famine. In clinical practice, they are commonly observed in patients with self-imposed starvation. The eating disorders to be considered are anorexia nervosa, bulimia nervosa and binge eating disorder. There are naturally milder forms of these conditions that do not meet the formal criteria for the above diagnoses but which have a similar if milder impact on the patient's metabolic and endocrine condition. Exercise-related amenorrhoea shares many features of these conditions. Correlation of the reproductive disturbance with the intensity of training is, however, variable and it is likely that women who develop exercise-related amenorrhoea are also underweight, at least with respect to their fat mass.

Becker et al. (1999) give an authoritative review of the formal diagnostic criteria and clinical psychiatric features

of these eating disorders. Here the points to be emphasized are the endocrine changes that develop as the patient loses weight. The characteristic endocrine pattern of mild-to-moderate weight loss-related amenorrhoea (roughly corresponding to a BMI of 17.5–$19.0\,kg/m^2$) is a marked reduction in the serum LH concentration (Boyar et al., 1974), associated with subnormal oestrogen levels. As the patient continues to lose weight, serum follicle-stimulating hormone (FSH) concentrations also fall into the range seen in women with hypogonadotrophic hypogonadism (see also Ch. 26). It is in subjects with more severe weight loss that the metabolism of thyroxine favours the production of the noncalorigenic reverse triiodothyronine (Moshang et al., 1975) and endocrine features of hypothalamic hypothyroidism develop. Plasma cortisol levels may be elevated throughout the day, although episodic and diurnal variation is maintained (Boyar et al., 1977). To some extent the increase in cortisol levels can be attributed to a reduction in metabolic clearance, but dexamethasone suppression may be incomplete, unbound cortisol levels raised and the corticotrophin response to corticotrophin-releasing hormone (CRH) impaired (Warren et al., 1996). Moreover production of CRH is increased, as suggested by the finding of increased CRH concentrations in cerebrospinal fluid (Hotta et al., 1986). Intravenous injection of CRH acutely reduces LH secretion (Warren et al., 1996), so activation of the hypothalamic–pituitary–adrenal axis may contribute to the impairment of gonadal function as well as mobilizing energy stores during starvation.

In women with weight loss-related amenorrhoea, the reduction in oestrogen levels may be very profound. The loss of follicular secretion of oestradiol is accompanied by a reduction in extra ovarian conversion of androstenedione to oestrone because of the loss of fat tissue. The marked suppression of LH secretion also results in subnormal testosterone secretion by theca cells, so reducing the amount of substrate available for aromatization. Significant numbers of women with anorexia nervosa are vegetarian. Since a vegetarian diet can alter the intestinal microflora, enterohepatic recirculation of oestrogens may be interupted, resulting in a faecal leak of oestrogen conjugates and reduced reabsorbtion of free oestrogens (Goldin et al., 1982). Finally, the metabolic fate of oestrogens is influenced by nutrition so that, in thin women, the pathway of metabolism favours formation of antioestrogenic catechol oestrogens rather than oestriol.

The combination of severe oestrogen deficiency with subnormal gonadotrophin secretion indicates a functional hypogonadotrophic hypogonadism. Characteristically there is a reduction of the amplitude of gonadotrophin pulsatility, initially during the daytime but, as weight continues to fall, nocturnal gonadotrophin secretion is also reduced. The ovarian ultrasound image of the woman with the milder degrees of weight loss shows an ovarian multifollicular pattern, similar to that seen in the early stages of normal puberty (Adams et al., 1985). This is in contrast to a "polycystic ovary", in which the follicles/cysts are usually smaller (2–8 mm compared with 6–12 mm in multifollicular ovaries); additionally, the ovarian stroma is more prominent in polycystic ovaries. With severe weight loss, the ovaries are small and show little follicular activity. Uterine dimensions are reduced and there is little endometrial thickening. These changes reverse when normal gonadotrophin secretion resumes with regain of weight.

A number of women with anorexia nervosa present to infertility clinics with anovulatory infertility. More commonly, women referred with the latter diagnosis are discovered to be underweight (BMI less than $19\,kg/m^2$), with the characteristic endocrine profile of low serum LH and oestradiol concentrations. On ultrasonography, they have multifollicular ovaries and a small uterus with little endometrial thickening. Bone densitometry usually reveals skeletal decalcification. In clinics drawing referrals from universities, such patients may represent as many as 20% of those referred with amenorrhoea.

In considering the optimum method for women with weight loss-related amenorrhoea to recover their fertility, two important issues need to be considered. The first relates to the experience of such patients as mothers, the second to more medical concerns, such as the obstetric outcome of pregnancies in underweight women. As mentioned earlier, the obstetric outcome of underweight women who conceive without treatment is impaired; for example, they have twice the rate of small-for-dates babies as do women of normal weight. When underweight women with amenorrhoea conceive as a result of induction of ovulation, the proportion of small-for-dates infants rises to 50% and there is a significant increase in the rate of obstetric interventions needed to protect the baby (van der Spuy et al., 1988). When these observations are coupled with the problems in parenting that may be experienced by women with anorexia nervosa (Russell et al., 1988) and the presumed adverse effects of impaired nutrition during pregnancy on patterns of childhood and adult health (Barker, 1997), the arguments against induction of ovulation by medical means become overwhelming. In the author's opinion, appropriate management is by weight increase, coupled with psychiatric support. Women with weight loss-related amenorrhoea can expect to resume ovulation when their BMI reaches 19–$19.5\,kg/m^2$. A point to remember, however, is that some 20% of all women have ultrasound-detected polycystic ovaries (Polson et al., 1988; see also Ch. 27), including those with amenorrhoea caused by weight loss. It has been known for some years that a similar proportion of women recovering from anorexia nervosa do not resume menstrual cycles when they reach their target weight (Crisp and Stonehill, 1971). It is appropriate therefore to monitor recovery with serial ultrasonography and offer induction of ovulation to those who achieve their target weight but do not resume regular and predictable ovulation cycles.

Osteoporosis in underweight women with amenorrhoea

Osteoporosis is an important problem in patients with anorexia nervosa (Miller and Klibanski, 1999; see also Ch. 39). It is common and associated with a serious risk of overt fracture. The precise mechanisms underlying its development are not clear and so not surprisingly current regimens of treatment, other than by weight gain, are not at all successful.

Most women with anorexia nervosa have evidence of bone loss and 50% have a bone mineral density (BMD) that is more than two standard deviations below that of age-matched controls. Peak bone mass is achieved by a woman's third decade and thereafter gradually falls at a rate of about 1% per decade, accelerating to 2% per decade after the menopause. One study reported that the BMD of 19 young anorectic patients was equivalent to that of postmenopausal women in the seventh or eighth decade (Biller et al., 1991). In a community-based retrospective cohort study of 208 women diagnosed with anorexia nervosa, long-term follow-up revealed that the relative risk of fracture was increased threefold (Lucas et al., 1999). This figure was remarkably consistent with predictions based on the average results of bone densitometry. Fractures occurred at all three sites (hip, radius and vertebrae) and, most worryingly, their peak incidence occurred some 30 years after diagnosis. Patients with anorexia nervosa are particularly vulnerable to fracture because, in addition to the reduction in bone mass, they lack the protective padding normally provided by fat tissue. Moreover, if the onset of the anorexia was during adolescence their bones are frequently quite slender and, if the oestrogen deficiency persists, their muscles may be relatively weak too.

While underweight women with anorexia nervosa are certainly very oestrogen deficient, the pattern of markers of bone formation is different from that seen in women with postmenopausal osteoporosis. In the latter condition, there is evidence of accelerated bone turnover, with a disproportionate increase of resorption compared with formation. In underweight anorectic women with osteoporosis, the markers that reflect resorption of bone (urinary excretion of deoxypyridinoline, serum concentrations of pyridinoline, deoxypyridinoline and N-telopeptide) are indeed increased but those that reflect formation (serum type 1 collagen C-terminal propeptide, osteocalcin) are low or normal whereas they are raised in postmenopausal osteoporosis (Stefanis et al., 1998). The observation that, in vitro, leptin enhances osteoblast differentiation in human marrow stromal cells (Thomas et al., 1999) is, therefore, intriguing and suggests yet another implication of the hypoleptinaemia of undernutrition. Clinically, the pattern of bone markers is actually more consistent with that seen in osteoporosis caused by glucocorticoids than that associated with oestrogen deficiency (Lems et al., 1998).

The response to treatment of osteoporosis in patients with anorexia nervosa emphasizes the relevance of these results. While BMD reliably improves when patients regain sufficient weight to resume menstrual cycles (Gulekli et al., 1994), little or no improvement is observed in persistently underweight women treated over an 18 month period with oestrogen-based hormone replacement (Klibanski et al., 1995). Several explanations suggest themselves. Diversion of oestrogen metabolism toward 2-hydroxylation, with the formation of the antioestrogenic catechol 2-hydroxyoestrone rather than oestriol (Fishman et al., 1975), might contribute to the ineffectiveness of oestrogen treatment, analogous to the way smoking diverts oestrogen metabolism (Michnovicz et al., 1988) and impairs the response to treatment (Jensen et al., 1985). As in patients with depression, elevation of plasma cortisol levels caused by activation of the hypothalamic–pituitary–adrenal axis may be contributory (Biller et al., 1989). Nutritional deficiency itself may be critical, either because of lack of specific nutrients or because of the consequent low circulating concentrations of insulin-like growth factor 1 (IGF-1). The latter mechanism would be consistent with the increase in the serum markers of bone formation in response to treatment with recombinant IGF-1 in osteoporotic women with anorexia nervosa (Grinspoon et al., 1995). Other factors to be considered are dietary deficiencies of calcium and vitamin D.

At the present time, management of osteoporosis in women with anorexia nervosa is focused on restoration of body weight and ovarian function together with calcium supplementation. The results of trials of IGF-1 and of bisphosphonates are awaited with interest, the former because of the potential enhancement of bone formation, the latter by analogy with their beneficial effect in steroid-induced osteoporosis (Eastell et al., 1998).

Overnutrition and reproduction: the effect of obesity

During the 1990s, there was increasing appreciation of the role of hypersecretion of insulin in the pathogenesis of the polycystic ovary syndrome (Dunaif, 1997, see also Ch. 27). This work has stressed the importance of extrasplanchnic resistance to the glucose-lowering actions of insulin, which results in compensatory hypersecretion of insulin. The insulin resistance is thought to spare the ovary. As insulin levels rise, ovarian function decompensates. Since obesity is an important cause of insulin resistance, it can be readily appreciated that its development is a frequent harbinger of reproductive dysfunction in women with polycystic ovaries (Poretsky et al., 1999).

The obesity that occurs in some 40% of women with polycystic ovary syndrome (Balen et al., 1995) is to a large extent central, that is to say, visceral. There is a considerable literature describing the pattern of leptin secretion in such women, as reviewed by Jacobs and Conway (1999). The central predominance of fat suggests that serum leptin concentrations are unlikely to reflect the BMI to the same magnitude as they do in "simple" obesity. Our own studies showed that, in women with polycystic ovary syndrome, for any BMI, leptin concentrations were some 25% lower than in the normal control group (Jacobs and Conway, 1999). Levels do, however, rise as the patient's weight increases. The resulting hyperleptinaemia may contribute further to insulin resistance and to the preservation of skeletal calcification despite the development of amenorrhoea (Davies et al., 1990). It has been shown in vitro that leptin impairs oestradiol production, both that stimulated by LH (Karlsson et al., 1997) and that stimulated by FSH (augmented with IGF-1) (Zachow and Magoffin, 1997). Perhaps the balance between the inhibitory effects of leptin and the stimulatory effects of insulin contribute to the otherwise surprisingly impaired response of the polycystic ovary to stimulation by gonadotrophins (White et al., 1996).

While the major impact of obesity on reproduction in women is to cause clinical expression of the polycystic ovary syndrome, there are other important adverse effects on fecundity (Norman and Clark, 1998): there is an increase of other forms of infertility, miscarriage rates are raised, and obstetric outcome impaired. The implications for clinical management are clear: medical treatments must be combined with efforts to control weight. With respect to polycystic ovary syndrome, a dietary-induced fall of body weight by as little as 5% may be associated with a return of ovulatory cycles (Kiddy et al., 1992), perhaps because of preferential loss of the metabolically active visceral fat. Norman and Clark (1998) emphasize the importance of modifications to lifestyle such as changing eating habits and increasing exercise, particularly important if long-term complications are to be avoided.

REFERENCES

Adams J, Franks S, Polson D W et al. (1985). Multifollicular ovaries: clinical and endocrine features and response to pulsatile gonadotropin releasing hormone. *Lancet* ii, 1375–1379.

Audi L, Mantzoros C S, Vidal-Puig A, Vargas D, Gussinye M, Carrascosa A (1998). Leptin in relation to resumption of menses in women with anorexia nervosa. *Mol Psychiatry* 3, 544–547.

Balen A H, Conway G S, Kaltsas G et al. (1995). Polycystic ovary syndrome: the spectrum of the disorder in 1741 patients. *Hum Reprod* 10, 2107–2111.

Barker D J (1997). Fetal nutrition and cardiovascular disease in later life. *Br Med Bull* 53, 96–108.

Becker A E, Grinspoon S K, Klibanski A, Herzog D B (1999). Eating disorders. *N Engl J Med* 340, 1092–1098.

Biller B M, Saxe V, Herzog D B, Rosenthal D I, Holzman S, Klibanski A (1989). Mechanisms of osteoporosis in adult and adolescent women with anorexia nervosa. *J Clin Endocrinol Metab* 68, 548–554.

Biller B M, Coughlin J F, Saxe V, Schoenfeld D, Spratt D I, Klibanski A (1991). Osteopenia in women with hypothalamic amenorrhea: a prospective study. *Obstet Gynecol* 78, 996–1001.

Boyar R M, Katz J, Finkelstein J W et al. (1974). Anorexia nervosa. Immaturity of the 24-hour luteinizing hormone secretory pattern. *N Engl J Med* 291, 861–865.

Boyar R M, Hellman L D, Roffwarg H et al. (1977). Cortisol secretion and metabolism in anorexia nervosa. *N Engl J Med* 296(4): 190–193.

Bray G A (1997). Obesity and reproduction. [Review; 41 refs] *Hum Reprod* 12(Suppl. 1), 26–32.

Clement K, Vaisse C, Lahlou N et al. (1998). A mutation in the human leptin receptor gene causes obesity and pituitary dysfunction. *Nature* 392, 398–401.

Crisp A H, Stonehill E (1971). Relation between aspects of nutritional disturbance and menstrual activity in primary anorexia nervosa. *Br Med J* 3, 149–151.

Davies M C, Hall M L, Jacobs H S (1990). Bone mineral loss in young women with amenorrhoea. *Br Med J* 301, 790–793.

Dunaif A (1997). Insulin resistance and the polycystic ovary syndrome: mechanism and implications for pathogenesis. [Review; 277 refs.] *Endocr Rev* 18, 774–800.

Eastell R, Reid D M, Compston J et al. (1998). A UK Consensus Group on management of glucocorticoid-induced osteoporosis: an update. *J Intern Med* 244, 271–292.

Fishman J, Boyar R M, Hellman L (1975). Influence of body weight on estradiol metabolism in young women. *J Clin Endocrinol Metab* 41, 989–991.

Goldin B R, Adlercreutz H, Gorbach S L, Warram J H, Dwyer J T, Swenson L, Woods M N (1982). Estrogen excretion patterns and plasma levels in vegetarian and omnivorous women. *N Engl J Med* 307, 1542–1547.

Grinspoon S K, Baum H B, Peterson S, Klibanski A (1995). Effects of rhIGF-I administration on bone turnover during short-term fasting. *J Clin Invest* 96, 900–906.

Grinspoon S, Gulick T, Askari H et al. (1996). Serum leptin levels in women with anorexia nervosa. *J Clin Endocrinol Metab* 81, 3861–3863.

Gulekli B, Davies M C, Jacobs H S (1994). Effect of treatment on established osteoporosis in young women with amenorrhoea. *Clin Endocrinol* 41, 275–281.

Hotta M, Shibasaki T, Masuda A et al. (1986). The responses of plasma adrenocorticotropin and cortisol to corticotropin-releasing hormone (CRH) and cerebrospinal fluid immunoreactive CRH in anorexia nervosa patients. *J Clin Endocrinol Metab* 62, 319–324.

Jacobs H S, Conway G S (1999). Leptin, polycystic ovaries and polycystic ovary syndrome. *Hum Reprod Update* 5, 166–171.

Jensen J, Christiansen C, Rodbro P (1985). Cigarette smoking, serum estrogens, and bone loss during hormone- replacement therapy early after menopause. *N Engl J Med* 313, 973–975.

Kalra S P, Dube M G, Pu S, Xu B, Horvath T L, Kalra P S (1999). Interacting appetite-regulating pathways in the hypothalamic regulation of body weight. *Endocr Rev* 20, 68–100.

Karlsson C, Lindell K, Svensson E et al. (1997). Expression of functional leptin receptors in the human ovary. *J Clin Endocrinol Metab* 82, 4144–4148.

Kiddy D S, Hamilton-Fairley D, Bush A et al. (1992). Improvement in endocrine and ovarian function during dietary treatment of obese women with polycystic ovary syndrome. *Clin Endocrinol* 36, 105–111.

Klibanski A, Biller B M, Schoenfeld D A, Herzog D B, Saxe V C (1995). The effects of estrogen administration on trabecular bone loss in young women with anorexia nervosa. *J Clin Endocrinol Metab* 80, 898–904.

Lems W F, van Veen G J, Gerrits M I et al. (1998). Effect of low-dose prednisone (with calcium and calcitriol supplementation) on calcium and bone metabolism in healthy volunteers. *Br J Rheumatol* 37, 27–33.

Licinio J, Mantzoros C, Negrao A B et al. (1997). Human leptin levels are pulsatile and inversely related to pituitary–adrenal function. *Nat Med* 3, 575–579.

Licinio J, Negrao A B, Mantzoros C et al. (1998). Synchronicity of frequently sampled, 24-h concentrations of circulating leptin, luteinizing hormone, and estradiol in healthy women. *Proc Natl Acad Sci USA* 95, 2541–2546.

Lucas A R, Melton III J L, Crowson C S, O'Fallon W M (1999). Long-term fracture risk among women with anorexia nervosa: a population-based cohort study. *Mayo Clin Proc* 74, 972–977.

Mantzoros C S (1999). The role of leptin in human obesity and disease: a review of current evidence. *Ann Intern Med* 130, 671–680.

Mantzoros C, Flier J S, Lesem M D, Brewerton T D, Jimerson D C (1997). Cerebrospinal fluid leptin in anorexia nervosa: correlation with nutritional status and potential role in resistance to weight gain. *J Clin Endocrinol Metab* 82, 1845–1851.

Michnovicz J J, Naganuma H, Hershcopf R J, Bradlow H L, Fishman J (1988). Increased urinary catechol estrogen excretion in female smokers. *Steroids* 52, 69–83.

Miller K K, Klibanski A (1999). Clinical review 106: amenorrheic bone loss. *J Clin Endocrinol Metab* 84, 1775–1783.

Moshang T J, Parks J S, Baker L et al. (1975). Low serum triiodothyronine in patients with anorexia nervosa. *J Clin Endocrinol Metab* 40, 470–3.

Norman R J, Clark A M (1998). Obesity and reproductive disorders: a review. *Reprod Fertil Dev* 10, 55–63.

Polson D W, Adams J, Wadsworth J, Franks S (1988). Polycystic ovaries – a common finding in normal women. *Lancet* i, 870–872.

Poretsky L, Cataldo N A, Rosenwaks Z, Giudice L C (1999). The insulin-related ovarian regulatory system in health and disease [in process citation]. *Endocr Rev* 20, 535–582.

Russell G F, Treasure J, Eisler I (1998). Mothers with anorexia nervosa who underfeed their children: their recognition and management. *Psychol Med* 28, 93–108.

Stefanis N, Mackintosh C, Abraha H D, Treasure J, Moniz C (1998). Dissociation of bone turnover in anorexia nervosa. *Ann Clin Biochem* 35, 709–716.

Thomas T, Gori F, Khosla S, Jensen M D, Burguera B, Riggs B L (1999). Leptin acts on human marrow stromal cells to enhance differentiation to osteoblasts and to inhibit differentiation to adipocytes. *Endocrinology* 140, 1630–1638.

van der Spuy Z M, Steer P J, McCusker M, Steele S J, Jacobs H S (1988). Outcome of pregnancy in underweight women after spontaneous and induced ovulation. *Br Med J Clin Res Ed* 296, 962–965.

Warren M P, Adashi E Y, Rock J A, Rosenwaks Z (eds.) (1996). *Reproductive Endocrinology, Surgery, and Technology,* Ch. 50, *Eating Disorders and the Reproductive Axis.* pp. 1039–1060. Lippincott-Raven, Philadelphia, PA.

White D M, Polson D W, Kiddy D et al. (1996). Induction of ovulation with low-dose gonadotropins in polycystic ovary syndrome: an analysis of 109 pregnancies in 225 women. *J Clin Endocrinol Metab* 81, 3821–3824.

Zachow R J, Magoffin D A (1997). Direct intraovarian effects of leptin: impairment of the synergistic action of insulin-like growth factor-I on follicle-stimulating hormone-dependent estradiol-17 beta production by rat ovarian granulosa cells. *Endocrinology* 138, 847–850.

7

Normal bladder control and function

Nikesh Thiruchelvam[1] and Peter M. Cuckow[2]

[1]The Institute of Child Health, London, UK
[2]Great Ormond Street Hospital for Children and the Institute of Urology, London, UK

Introduction

The bladder is an amazing organ with an ability to increase its volume dramatically with little increase in its internal pressure whilst maintaining a securely closed outlet. This enables the bladder to collect urine excreted by the kidneys and store it securely within the body. When the time is appropriate, contraction of the bladder muscular wall causes a rapid rise in its internal pressure and, together with simultaneous relaxation of its outlet, allows urine to be expelled via the urethra. The bladder empties to completion before its outlet closes and its walls relax again to start the next filling cycle.

We start this chapter with a discussion of the anatomy, innervation and control mechanisms of the normal bladder, followed with the evolution of its function from the fetus to the continent adult, the means by which we assess its function and, finally, what is currently known about the effect of sex steroids, the menstrual cycle and pregnancy on the female bladder.

Anatomy

The bladder is an abdominal organ in the fetus and infant that descends as the pelvis deepens towards puberty to become a truly pelvic organ in the mature female (Fig. 7.1). At its apex is the fibrous remnant of the urachus, which ascends in the midline to the umbilicus. Its posterosuperior surface is covered by peritoneum, which is continuous with that of the anterior abdominal wall. As it fills with urine, the bladder rises out of the pelvis between the anterior abdominal wall and its covering peritoneum. Posteriorly,

the peritoneum is reflected over the uterus to form the vesico-uterine pouch and then over the rectum to form the rectouterine pouch (Fig. 7.2, colour plate). The base of the bladder, the bladder neck and the urethra rest on the anterior vaginal wall. The vagina is attached to the levator ani muscle, the contraction of which will lift the bladder neck upwards and forwards. Below and lateral to the bladder lie the retropubic fat pads and pubic bone (anteriorly), and the obturator internus and levator ani posteriorly (Fig. 7.1). The ureters enter the lower part of the bladder and with the bladder outlet define a specialized triangular area of the bladder called the trigone. From the bladder outlet, where there is a functionally important region referred to as the bladder neck, the urethra extends along the distal third of the anterior vaginal wall to the external urinary meatus.

Histology

The bladder wall is made up of three distinct cell layers: the innermost urothelium, the intermediate muscular layer (also called the detrusor) and the outermost serosal (or peritoneal) layer (Fig. 7.3, colour plate).

The urothelium

The urothelium comprises the inner lining of transitional bladder epithelium, which is folded when the bladder is empty and smoothed when it distends with urine. Deep to this is the lamina propria: a relatively thick layer of fibroelastic connective tissue that allows the bladder to distend and is responsible for its viscoelastic properties. The urothelium of the trigone is thinner and smoother, as its dimensions do not change appreciably during filling and emptying of the bladder.

Paediatric and Adolescent Gynaecology, ed. Adam Balen et al. Published by Cambridge University Press.
© Cambridge University Press 2004.

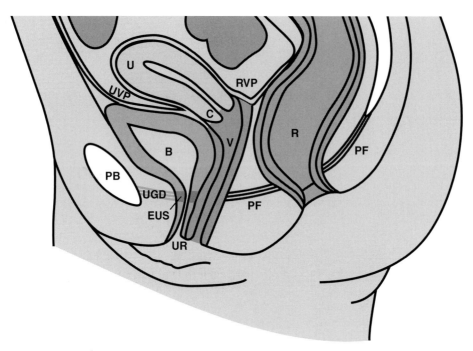

Fig. 7.1. Bladder relations. The bladder (B) lies in front of the anterior wall of the vagina (V), cervix (C) and uterus (U) but its position alters depending on the intravesical urine volume. The outflow from the bladder is via the urethra (UR), which, in part, is surrounded by the external urethral sphincter (EUS). The supporting urogenital diaphragm anteriorly (UGD) lies anterior to the EUS and this structure continues posteriorly as the pelvic floor (PF) or levator ani. The rectovaginal pouch (RVP) lies behind the vaginal fornix and, in part, covers the rectum (R). PB, pubic bone.

The intermediate muscle layer

The detrusor layer consists of smooth muscle fibres arranged into interlacing bundles, which are loosely organized into inner longitudinal, middle circular and outer longitudinal layers (Fig. 7.3, colour plate). This muscle layer of the bladder is adapted in the specialized areas of the organ. At the bladder neck, the smooth muscle fibres are smaller and finer and are morphologically and functionally different from the rest of the bladder. In females, the inner longitudinal fibres become continuous with the inner longitudinal layer of smooth muscle of the urethra. The outer two layers may also converge with this inner layer but this point is contentious (Gosling, 1985). Unlike the male bladder neck, the female bladder neck contains very little adrenergic (or sympathetic) innervation (see below) and contributes little to continence (Versi et al., 1986). The other specialized area is the trigone, where the muscle is supplied with adrenergic (or sympathetic) innervation. The ureteric muscle is incorporated into the area of the trigone and this helps to prevent retrograde flow of urine up the ureters during bladder emptying (otherwise known as vesico-ureteric reflux).

The urethral sphincter

The urethral sphincter is a cylindrical structure wrapped around the urethra, which is thicker anteriorly than posteriorly. Innermost is a smooth muscle layer that is continuous with the bladder neck smooth muscle (see above). Outside this is a layer of striated muscle that extends from the bladder neck to the mid-urethra. The anatomical maturation of this sphincter has been described (Kokoua et al., 1993) and variations and abnormalities of this process may contribute to the discrepancies observed in voiding that seem to occur in early infant life.

Bladder innervation

Micturition or voiding is the process of emptying the bladder. Micturition is a complex chain of events involving the detrusor muscle and the urethral sphincter, which are activated by autonomic and somatic nerves, respectively, and influenced by the central nervous system. As the bladder fills with urine, relaxation of its wall and the maintenance of tone in the sphincter (see below) allow it to

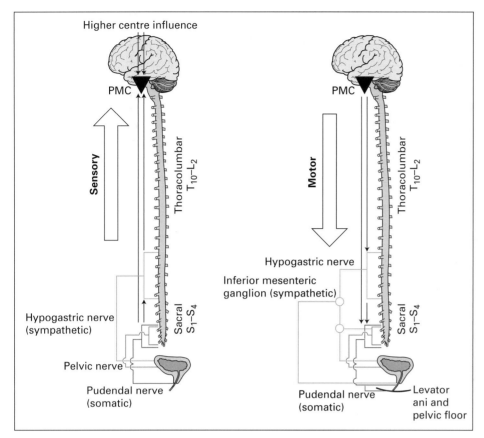

Fig. 7.4. Sensory and motor innervation of the bladder. To allow for bladder filling, the bladder relaxes its tone (by negative feedback of the sympathetic nervous system) and maintains bladder outflow closure by the somatic nerves. With further filling, impulses are carried up the pelvic nerve to enter into the sacral region of the spinal cord and eventually reach the pontine micturition centre (PMC) in the pons; this area may also be influenced by further higher cerebral control. Voiding is achieved by coordinated parasympathetic activation (impulses pass via the preganglionic parasympathetic nerves 1, the pelvic ganglion 2 to reach the bladder by the pelvic nerve 3), sympathetic activation (via the hypogastric nerve and the inferior mesenteric ganglion to cause bladder trigonal contraction) and somatic activation (to alter the tone of the levator ani and the pelvic floor).

contain the urine at low pressure. When it is distended, signals indicating a full bladder are transmitted to the spinal cord in sensory (afferent) nerves and ascend to the brain (Fig. 7.4).

Neurotransmitter release in the brain results in signals being sent back down the spinal cord to converge on the two main areas involved in spinal micturition control. These are the thoracolumbar region (thoracic nerves 10, 11 and 12 and lumbar nerves 1 and 2) and the sacral region (sacral nerves 2, 3 and 4). The autonomic parasympathetic and sympathetic nerves (otherwise known as preganglionic fibres) pass outside the spinal cord to synapse with the cell bodies of peripheral autonomic nerves in specialized areas

adjacent to the spinal cord known as ganglia (or plexuses). Neurotransmitter release here results in impulses leaving the ganglia in postganglionic nerves to reach the bladder muscle, bladder trigone or urethra. A further somatic outflow passes directly to supply the pelvic floor and urethral sphincter via the pudendal nerve.

Further neurotransmitter release from nerve endings adjacent to the bladder muscle cell results in receptor activation on its membrane and causes the release of numerous chemical messengers within the muscle cell, which result in its contraction. Similarly, the somatic supply to the sphincter modifies its tone and may effect relaxation and opening of the bladder outlet.

Central control

The pontine micturition centre is found in the dorsolateral region of the pons (Blok et al., 1998). This centre receives inputs from the peripheral nervous system, cerebral cortex, cerebellum, extrapyrimidal system and the brainstem (Valentino et al., 1999), indicating the extent to which conscious, psychological and emotional activity can influence micturition.

Peripheral control

From the inferomediolateral cell column of the second, third and fourth sacral spinal cord segments, preganglionic parasympathetic nerves are conveyed via the pelvic nerve to the pelvic and vesical plexuses, where they synapse before principally supplying the detrusor muscle, although a few fibres pass to the urethral smooth muscle. From the tenth thoracic to the second lumbar segments of the cord, sympathetic preganglionic fibres pass into the sympathetic chain and synapse in the inferior mesenteric ganglion. Postganglionic sympathetic fibres pass down the hypogastric nerve and through the pelvic plexus to supply principally the bladder neck and urethra (which both have an abundant adrenergic innervation) with a few fibres to the remainder of the bladder. Thus, the pelvic plexus acts as an autonomic focal point. Located anteriorly to the parasympathetic outflow, somatic motor neurons also arise from the lower three sacral segments (in a region known as Onuf's nucleus) and form the pudendal nerve, which mainly supplies the urethral sphincter and the pelvic floor.

Bladder storage reflexes

There are two reflexes involved in bladder storage function. The first of these is effected by the pudendal (somatic) nerve acting on the sphincter and causing it to be held closed (Buzelin, 1995). The second is negative feedback (via the sympathetic system) acting on the preganglionic parasympathetic input to the bladder to reduce its influence and cause a reduction of tone in the detrusor. Consequently, it is the communication between parasympathetic, sympathetic and somatic pathways in the spinal cord that permits increased urine accommodation.

Voiding reflexes

Bladder filling and subsequent distension is detected by mechanoreceptors in the bladder wall, which send afferent (sensory) impulses to the spinal cord. These signals pass via the pelvic nerve and enter the dorsal root of S2, S3 and S4 spinal cord segments. The majority ascend up the spinal cord to the pontine micturition centre, where other higher functions may influence micturition. Effector impulses descend down the long tracts of the spinal cord and leave by three routes. First, they enter the pelvic plexus in preganglionic fibres via the S2, S3 and S4 parasympathetic outflow. Postganglionic parasympathetic neurons pass from here to the detrusor smooth muscle and cause contraction. Second, and coordinated with the parasympathetic outflow, impulses pass down the pudendal (somatic) nerve to modify the tone of the sphincter muscle (to allow relaxation and cause micturition) and to control the tone of the levator ani and the pelvic floor (de Groat, 1993). In addition sympathetic outflow, via the hypogastric nerve, passes to the trigone.

The pharmacology of bladder detrusor muscle contraction

A multitude of chemicals are involved in the generation of a bladder contraction. These include the many described neurotransmitters and modulators that allow communication between the central, autonomic and peripheral nervous systems and the lower urinary tract. In addition, other chemicals, referred to as local trophic factors, influence the maintenance and growth of nerves that supply the bladder. The release of neurotransmitter at the detrusor level synapse initiates a whole series of events involving receptor activation, ionic movement through specialized membrane channels and activation of membrane-bound enzymes and second messengers, which finally result in detrusor muscle contraction.

The principal neurotransmitter is acetylcholine (ACh). This is released from preganglionic parasympathetic neurons to activate receptors in peripheral ganglions (termed nicotinic receptors because they may be directly stimulated by nicotine). This results in transmission of the impulse down the postganglionic neuron to the detrusor muscle cell. Here further ACh release results in excitatory activation of the cell via other receptors. These receptors are known as muscarinic receptors because they may be directly stimulated by muscarine; in the urinary tract these are further divided into M_2 and M_3 muscarinic receptors (Wang et al., 1995). Smooth muscle contraction follows a chain of membrane-bound reactions leading to the production of intracellular inositol trisphosphate. The latter results in release of intracellular calcium from the sarcoplasmic reticulum. This calcium complexes to calmodulin, a soluble protein, which then, by phosphorylation, activates a portion of the myosin molecule. Following this, with ATP consumption, interaction of actin and myosin protein contractile filaments results in filament, and thus muscle, contraction (Fry and Wu, 1998) (Fig. 7.5).

Noradrenergic (sympathetic) innervation to the detrusor is sparse but nerve terminals are present in the bladder base, urethra and trigone. Furthermore, the bladder and urethra have been shown to respond to adrenergic drugs (Gosling et al., 1999; Taki et al., 1999). Numerous other neurotransmitters have been described. These include ATP (acting via p_{2x} receptors; Elneil et al., 2001), neuropeptide Y, tachykinins, vasoactive intestinal peptide and calcitonin gene-related peptide (Dixon et al., 1998; Smet et al., 1996) and vasopressin (Holmquist et al., 1991). In addition, sex steroids may modulate bladder receptors and influence bladder growth (see below). Finally, nitric oxide has a role in neurologically mediated relaxation in the lower urinary tract, especially in the urethra (Andersson and Persson, 1995).

Neurotransmitters that act centrally on the brain include glutamate, dopamine, serotonin (5-hydroxytryptamine), noradrenaline, gamma-aminobutyric acid, neuropeptides, enkephalins and also ACh (de Groat, 1990).

Evolution of voiding and voiding control

The above discussion relates to the mature or adult type of micturition. However, there is a progressive evolution of this function from the fetus through the early years of childhood, prior to attaining full voluntary voiding control.

Our own studies in the fetal lamb (using urachal catheters) (Thiruchelvam and Cuckow, 1999) have demonstrated that filling and emptying of the bladder (cycling) is established by mid-gestation and continues through to term (Fig. 7.6). Others have demonstrated voiding in fetal lambs by the third trimester (Kogan et al., 1989; Wlodek et al., 1989), and bladder storage and voiding function in fetal pigs in the latter part of gestation, together with urethral sphincter activity (Olsen et al., 2001). Human fetal voiding data have been collected by ultrasound. Studies in the second half of gestation show that bladder cycling is established and strongly correlates with hourly urine output (Mitra, 1999). The fetal bladder volume increases linearly with time before it empties during micturition. The length of this cycle does not appear to change with gestation, as the mean bladder capacity increases to accommodate the

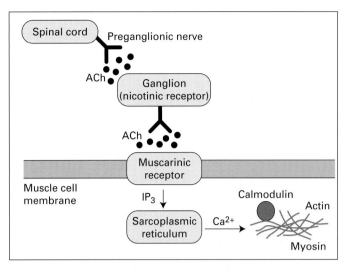

Fig. 7.5. Bladder pharmacology. At a molecular level, acetylcholine (ACh) is released from preganglionic nerves to activate nicotinic receptors on peripheral ganglia. This causes nerve stimulation and acetylcholine release at the bladder, which activates muscarinic receptors on the muscle cell membrane. This activates a chain of molecular reactions leading to inositol trisphosphate (IP_3) release. This subsequently results in calcium (Ca^{2+}) release from the sarcoplasmic reticulum; binds to calmodulin to form a calmodulin complex. The formation of this complex causes myosin and actin contractile proteins to interact, producing muscle cell contraction.

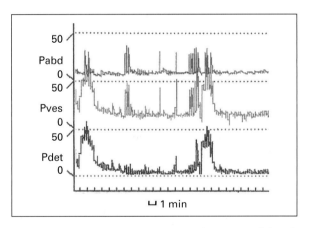

Fig. 7.6. Fetal urodynamics. Fetal abdominal pressure (Pabd) and fetal bladder (or vesical) pressure (Pves) are shown; the true bladder muscle (detrusor, Pdet) pressure is given by Pves – Pabd. These fetal urodynamic studies allow the characterisation of bladder function, as assessed by parameters such as bladder voiding pressure, duration of voiding and voiding interval. This figure clearly shows two fetal voids, as seen by two peaks in Pdet.

increase in fetal urine production (Nicolaides et al., 1988). During the last trimester, the bladder fills and empties approximately 30 times every 24 hours (Goellner et al., 1981). After birth, voiding is infrequent for the first few days and then increases rapidly to a peak of approximately once per hour by two to four weeks of age. At the end of the first year of life, voiding frequency has decreased to 10 to 15 times a day. By three years of age, a child voids between 8 and 10 times daily and the mean voided volume (and bladder capacity) has increased up to fourfold (Holmdahl et al., 1996; Yeung et al., 1995). By 12 years of age, the adult pattern of voiding four to six times a day is established.

Increasing bladder capacity accommodates both the increase in urine production and the decrease in voiding frequency with age, and there is no significant difference between boys and girls. The bladder capacity for young infants can be calculated (Holmdahl et al., 1996):

Bladder capacity (ml) $= 38 + (2.5 \times$ age in months)

After 1 to 2 years of age, a more simple formula for calculating bladder capacity can be applied (Hjalmas, 1988):

Bladder capacity (ml) $= 30 + (30 \times$ age in years)

Some children under 1 year of age have incomplete maturation of their voiding mechanism. The coordination between detrusor contraction and sphincter relaxation is lacking, so they void in an interrupted or staccato fashion. (Bachelard et al., 1999). This phenomenon tends to disappear by two years of age. Bladder pressures during micturition are much higher in boys than in girls, although infants of both sexes have significantly elevated pressures compared with adults. These progressively decrease to lower adult levels with age (Bachelard et al., 1998; Yeung et al., 1998).

It used to be thought that babies and young infants void automatically by spinal reflex when the bladder is full, and that there was no cortical influence. With time, the child learns to inhibit this micturition reflex and imposes voluntary control. More recent studies have shown, however, that fetuses and newborn babies do exhibit some higher control over micturition. Fetuses near to term only seem to micturate when awake (Ohel et al., 1995) or when stressed (Zimmer et al., 1993). Similarly, infants seem to be roused by a distended bladder to void when awake (Yeung et al., 1998). Potty training, or the attainment of the adult pattern of voluntary control and continence, occurs in most children by three to four years. This is a product of both lower urinary tract development (increasing bladder capacity and decreasing voiding pressures) and

adaptation of the reflex micturition by higher cognitive function.

Female continence

In addition to voluntary control of the reflex bladder activity outlined above, there are four distinct characteristics of the urethra that prevent urinary leakage and promote continence in females:
1 urethral support
2 the internal sphincter
3 the external or striated sphincter
4 intrinsic urethral mechanisms.

Urethral support
Dense bands of connective tissue, called the pubourethral ligaments, pass between the pubic bones and the paraurethral tissues. These supportive ligaments are continuous with the urogenital diaphragm (Milley and Nichols, 1971) (Fig. 7.1). In addition, the levator ani provides support to the bladder neck, with contraction lifting it upwards and forwards and maintaining the angle between the bladder and urethra. This angle is lost during relaxation of the levator muscle, which is able to maintain its tone because of its slow-twitch striated muscle fibre composition (Critchley et al., 1980). The urethra and the anterior vaginal wall are closely bound together and supported by the endopelvic fascia.

Increases in intra-abdominal pressure will tend to push the bladder backwards and downwards. This movement is prevented by the support mechanisms outlined above and urethral compression is the result. In addition, increased intra-abdominal pressure will be transmitted directly to the urethra via the anterior vaginal wall. Thus, increases in urethral pressure are observed during abdominal pressure rises and urethral closure is enhanced at times when leakage is most likely to occur (De Lancey, 1990).

Internal sphincter
The internal sphincter is a loop of detrusor muscle at the bladder neck (with regional adrenergic innervation, see above) and a more proximally placed ring of elastin and smooth muscle (Huisman, 1983). When levator ani contracts, this region is compressed against the endopelvic fascia anteriorly (the pubovesical ligament; Chou and De Lancey, 2001), an important factor in urethral closure.

External sphincter
In the outer layer of the urethra, circularly orientated slow-twitch striated muscle fibres are well suited to exert a

continuous resting pressure and sustain continence (Klevmark et al., 1991). Inside this striated muscle are layers of longitudinal and circular smooth muscle fibres. The functional significance of this smooth muscle is questioned, although its activity has been shown to alter urethral luminal pressure during anaesthesia (Kulseng-Hanssen, 1987).

Intrinsic mechanisms

The urethral wall has a well-developed vascular plexus, which may assist in forming a water-tight closure of the urethra (De Lancey, 1990). Rises in intra-abdominal pressure, for example those caused by coughing, will also cause engorgement of this vascular plexus, thereby helping to prevent urinary leakage. In addition, the female urethral epithelium is richly folded with a plentiful network of submucosal collagen and elastin fibres, which are able to promote a urethral seal effect.

Assessing bladder function

Various investigations are available to evaluate bladder function (and primarily dysfunction) in the clinical setting and may be collectively referred to as urodynamics. Taking a careful history and examining the patient should not be neglected in the initial assessment of patients. Simple measurements of the volume and frequency of voids and objective data about wetting can be collated by the parents and/or the patient. Noninvasive tests include bladder and urinary tract ultrasound, performed before and after voiding. If the patient can void into a simple flow rate machine, these data can be collected at the same time. Thus information about bladder anatomy, its capacity and emptying can be obtained.

Uroflowmetry

Voiding into a flowmeter generates a urinary flow curve and measures voided volume, from which the mean and maximum flow rates may be derived. Care must be taken in the interpretation of a single test as results may vary within an individual, so tests are best repeated to obtain a representative view. A normal test produces a bell-shaped curve (Fig. 7.7) and reflects detrusor contraction with urethral relaxation and absence of any mechanical obstruction to bladder outflow. Flow rates are higher in girls (Gutierrez, 1997), reflecting their short urethras. Bladder outlet obstruction is rare in females, although a characteristic staccato pattern may be seen in detrusor–sphincter

dyssynergia (Fig. 7.7). This investigation is more commonly applied to males.

Cystometry

Measurement of the pressure–volume relationships of the bladder involves a more invasive approach. Pressure inside the bladder is measured by a urethral (or suprapubic) catheter. A second catheter within the abdomen (in most cases placed in the rectum) allows the abdominal component of this to be measured separately and subtracted, to give the pressure that is produced by the bladder muscle alone: this is known as the detrusor pressure (Fig. 7.6). Abdominal pressure can also be measured using vaginal pressure transducers but this is rarely appropriate in children. The abdominal pressure methodology must be stated in urodynamics reports for proper interpretation of results (Wall et al., 1995).

The bladder may be allowed to fill naturally with urine (natural fill urodynamics), which is more physiological but will also take longer to perform. However, the bladder can be filled artificially with warm saline via a separate lumen in the catheter, enabling several filling and voiding cycles to be studied in a relatively short period. If X-ray contrast is used as the filling fluid, screening of the bladder during the test provides additional information about its anatomy, its emptying, its position relative to the pelvic floor and the presence or absence of vesico-ureteric reflux. During filling, the compliance (the change in volume of the bladder/change in pressure), sensation and capacity of the bladder or its storage function is assessed (videourodynamics). During normal filling, the pressure stays low (compliance is high) until the bladder is full, at which time it rises coincident with the sensation to void. The patient is then asked to micturate and the characteristics of their voiding – including detrusor pressures, urine flow and completeness of emptying – are assessed.

Cystometry can be combined with perineal electromyographic skin electrodes, which can record pelvic floor activity during the micturition cycle for more detailed investigation.

Miscellaneous investigations

The intraluminal pressure of the urethra at rest can be measured by pulling a pressure-recording catheter along it. This urethral pressure profile reflects sphincteric tone, urethral support and closure (see above), but this is an uncomfortable procedure that is largely confined to adult urology. With the development of compact recording equipment

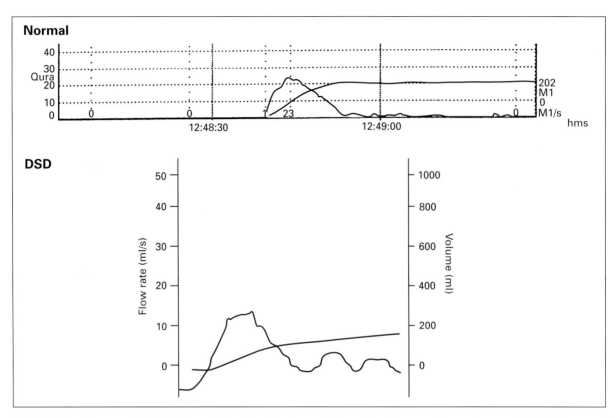

Fig. 7.7. Urinary flow rates. This simple investigation identifies abnormalities such as detrusor–sphincter dyssynergia (DSD). The normal flow rate shows increasing urine volume (to a plateau) with a smooth, bell-shaped flow rate. In DSD, there are intermittent flow rates (usually with normal urine volume) because of abnormal bladder–sphincter coordination.

and the use of longer-term catheters, for 12 or 24 hours, ambulatory urodynamics studies can also be performed (Fig. 7.8). Similar to natural fill urodynamics, ambulatory urodynamics studies are more physiological and may be particularly useful in the diagnosis of bladder instability (where the bladder is hyperactive during urine filling and storage) or detrusor–sphincter dyssynergia (where the bladder attempts to empty against an inappropriately closed urethral sphincter).

Sex steroids and the bladder

Oestrogen

Receptors for oestrogen have been demonstrated in parts of the brain involved with micturition, including the cerebral cortex, cerebellum and the pontine micturition centre (Maggi and Perez, 1985). They are also present in the bladder and urethra (Urner et al., 1983). The highest

receptor concentration is thought to occur in the urethra, compared with the trigone and the remainder of the bladder (Iosif et al., 1981). Studies show inconsistent expression of oestrogen receptors throughout the lower urinary tract. Blakeman et al. (2000) have reported finding oestrogen receptors in the urothelial layer of the female bladder, and then only in the epithelium of the trigone and proximal urethra that had undergone squamous metaplasia.

Oestrogen administration has been shown to potentiate the muscle contractility produced by muscarinic stimulation. (Levin et al., 1981). This effect may be the result of oestrogen increasing the density of muscarinic receptors on the muscle cell membrane (Batra and Andersson, 1989). Oestrogen also enhances the adrenergic responses of the detrusor (Levin et al., 1980) and the urethra (Callahan and Creed, 1985). This effect is mediated by a trophic effect on adrenergic nerves (increasing their number; Levin et al., 1981), altering electrolyte shift across smooth muscle cell membranes (Callahan and Creed, 1985), and

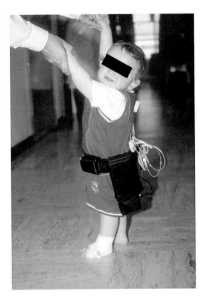

Fig. 7.8. Ambulatory urodymanics. Bladder pressure can be recorded with bladder and rectal catheters in situ for 12–24 hours to enable physiological urodynamics parameters to be measured with minimal disturbance to the child. This equipment will allow the child to wander freely as the bladder fills naturally rather than by the conventional method of artificially filling the bladder, which may produce some artefact.

by increasing adrenergic receptor density (Levin et al., 1980).

As mentioned above, nitric oxide is a possible modulator of smooth muscle activity in the urinary bladder. Oestrogen has been shown to induce calcium-dependent nitric oxide synthase activity and influence the bladder neck and urethral relaxation during micturition (Weiner et al., 1994). By improving the efficiency of the pelvic floor (Hilton and Stanton, 1983) and improving local blood flow (Versi and Cardozo, 1986), oestrogen improves transmission of abdominal pressure to the proximal urethra and increases urethral closure pressure (Rud, 1980).

In summary, oestrogen will tend to increase bladder muscle tone, enhance the urethral continence mechanism and improve voiding function, with an overall positive influence on urinary tract function.

Progesterone

Less is known of progesterone receptors. They are also expressed inconsistently in the lower urinary tract and have been found in the suburothelial region of the bladder dome,

trigone (Blakeman et al., 2000) and the urethra (Batra and Iosif, 1987). Progesterone is generally thought to antagonize oestrogen, and in the urinary tract may either act by reducing the influence of oestrogen (Batra et al., 1985) or by the direct stimulation of progesterone receptors (Blakeman et al., 2000).

In addition, separate studies have suggested that progesterone alters bladder responsiveness to certain neurotransmitters, although this is not a consistent finding. Ekstrom et al. (1993) showed that progesterone increased the sensitivity of the detrusor and the contractile response of the urethra to bethanecol (an ACh analogue). Conversely, Tong et al. (1995) showed that progesterone produced a reduction in maximal detrusor response secondary to acetylcholine stimulation.

Progesterone would appear to decrease detrusor tone and urethral resistance and negatively influence lower urinary tract function.

The menstrual cycle

During the menstrual cycle, bladder muscle tone is increased during the follicular phase and relatively decreased during the secretory phase of the cycle (Gitsch and Brandstetter, 1954). Urethral pressure, length and closure all increase in the follicular phase (Schreiter et al., 1976) and decrease before menstruation. These effects corroborate with the clinical observation that urinary symptoms are increased just prior to menstruation (Hextall et al., 1999). Interestingly, urodynamic indices do not appear to alter during the menstrual cycle of mature women (Visco et al., 2000) but it is possible that this assessment is too crude to detect the more subtle changes observed in bladder tone and contractility.

Oral contraceptive pill and pregnancy

Women taking an oral contraceptive pill with a high progesterone content have an increased incidence of urinary symptoms (Zahran et al., 1976). Similarly, the higher incidence of symptoms during pregnancy (especially stress and urge incontinence) may be contributed to by the progesterone effect (Stanton et al., 1980), although it is difficult to separate this from the more obvious mechanical factors (secondary to uterine enlargement and ligamentous laxity). At a cellular level, the reduction during pregnancy of receptors in the bladder to respond to cholinergic stimulation (Levin et al., 1991; Tong et al., 1995) and in the bladder neck and urethra to respond to adrenergic stimulation is probably progesterone mediated (Tong et al., 1995).

In women who remain continent throughout pregnancy, the urethra appears to adapt to the challenge by an increase in its length, maximum pressure and closure pressure (Iosif et al., 1980), although these findings have not been consistent (van Geelen et al., 1982). A study of pregnant women with stress incontinence demonstrated decreased maximum urethral closure pressure (Meyer et al., 1998). Cystometry has shown a rise in resting bladder pressure (Clow, 1995) and a decrease in bladder capacity, peak and mean urinary flow rates in pregnancy (Nel et al., 2001). Bladder instability during the filling phase increases in incidence towards term, leading to urge incontinence.

REFERENCES

Andersson K E, Persson K (1995). Nitric oxide synthase, the lower urinary tract: possible implications for physiology and pathophysiology. *Scand J Urol Nephrol* 175(Suppl.), 43–53.

Bachelard M, Sillen U, Hansson S, Hermansson G, Jodal U, Jacobsson B (1999). Urodynamic pattern in asymptomatic infants: siblings of children with vesicoureteral reflux. *J Urol* 162, 1733–1737.

Batra S, Andersson K E (1989). Oestrogen-induced changes in muscarinic receptor density and contractile responses in the female rabbit urinary bladder. *Acta Physiol Scand* 137, 135–141.

Batra S, Iosif C S (1987). Progesterone receptors in the female lower urinary tract. *J Urol* 138, 1301–1304.

Batra S, Bjellin L, Iosif S, Martensson L, Sjogren C (1985). Effect of oestrogen and progesterone on the blood flow in the lower urinary tract of the rabbit. *Acta Physiol Scand* 123, 191–194.

Blakeman P J, Hilton P, Bulmer J N (2000). Oestrogen and progesterone receptor expression in the female lower urinary tract with reference to oestrogen status. *Br J Urol Int* 86, 32–38.

Blok B F, Sturms L M, Holstege G (1998). Brain activation during micturition in women. *Brain* 121, 2033–2042.

Buzelin J M (1995). [Physiology of continence, micturition.] *Rev Prat* 45, 286–291.

Callahan S M, Creed K E (1985). The effects of oestrogens on spontaneous activity, responses to phenylephrine of the mammalian urethra. *J Physiol* 358, 35–46.

Chou Q, De Lancey J O (2001). A structured system to evaluate urethral support anatomy in magnetic resonance images. *Am J Obstet Gynecol* 185, 44–50.

Clow W M (1975). Effect of posture on bladder, urethral function in normal pregnancy: a preliminary report. *Urol Int* 30, 9–15.

Critchley H O, Dixon J S, Gosling J A (1980). Comparative study of the periurethral, perianal parts of the human levator ani muscle. *Urol Int* 35, 226–232.

de Groat W C (1990). Central neural control of the lower urinary tract. *Ciba Found Symp* 151, 27–44.

(1993). Anatomy and physiology of the lower urinary tract. *Urol Clin North Am* 20, 383–401.

De Lancey J O (1990). Anatomy and physiology of urinary continence. *Clin Obstet Gynecol* 33, 298–307.

Dixon J S, Jen P Y, Gosling J A (1998). Immunohistochemical characteristics of human paraganglion cells and sensory corpuscles associated with the urinary bladder. A developmental study in the male fetus neonate and infant. *J Anat* 192, 407–415.

Ekstrom J, Iosif C S, Malmberg L (1993). Effects of long-term treatment with estrogen and progesterone on in vitro muscle responses of the female rabbit urinary bladder and urethra to autonomic drugs and nerve stimulation. *J Urol* 150, 1284–1288.

Elneil S, Skepper J N, Kidd E J, Williamson J G, Ferguson D R (2001). Distribution of p2x(1), p2x(3) receptors in the rat and human urinary bladder. *Pharmacology* 63, 120–128.

Fry C H, Wu C (1998). The cellular basis of bladder instability. *Br J Urol* 81, 1–8.

Gitsch E, Brandstetter F (1954). Phasen-sphinctero-cystometrie. *Z Gynakol* 76, 1746–1754.

Goellner M H, Ziegler E E, Fomon S J (1981). Urination during the first three years of life. *Nephron* 28, 174–178.

Gosling J A (1985). The structure of the female lower urinary tract and pelvic floor. *Urol Clin North Am* 12, 207–214.

Gosling J A, Dixon J S, Jen P Y (1999). The distribution of noradrenergic nerves in the human lower urinary tract: a review. *Eur Urol* 36(Suppl. 1), 23–30.

Gutierrez S C (1997). Urine flow in childhood: a study of flow chart parameters based on 1361 uroflowmetry tests. *J Urol* 157, 1426–1428.

Hextall A, Bidmead J, Cardozo L D, Hooper R (1999). Hormonal influences on the female lower urinary tract: a prospective evaluation of the effects of the menstrual cycle on symptomatology and the results of urodynamic investigation. *Neurourol Urodyn* 18, 363–364.

Hilton P, Stanton S L (1983). The use of intravaginal oestrogen cream in genuine stress incontinence. *Br J Obstet Gynaecol* 90, 940–944.

Hjalmas K (1988). Urodynamics in normal infants and children. *Scand J Urol Nephrol* 114(Suppl.), 20–27.

Holmdahl G, Hanson E, Hanson M, Hellstrom A L, Hjalmas K, Sillen U (1996). Four-hour voiding observation in healthy infants. *J Urol* 156, 1809–1812.

Holmquist F, Lundin S, Larsson B, Hedlund H, Andersson K E (1991). Studies on binding sites contents and effects of AVP in isolated bladder and urethra from rabbits and humans. *Am J Physiol* 261, R865–R874.

Huisman A B (1983). Aspects on the anatomy of the female urethra with special relation to urinary continence. *Contrib Gynecol Obstet* 10, 1–31.

Iosif C S, Batra S, Ek A, Astedt B (1981). Estrogen receptors in the human female lower urinary tract. *Am J Obstet Gynecol* 141, 817–820.

Iosif S, Ingemarsson I, Ulmsten U (1980). Urodynamic studies in normal pregnancy, in puerperium. *Am J Obstet Gynecol* 137, 696–700.

Klevmark B, Kulseng-Hanssen S (1991). Continence mechanism in the female. *Scand J Urol Nephrol* 138(Suppl.), 35–40.

Kogan B A, Iwamoto H S (1989). Lower urinary tract function in the sheep fetus: studies of autonomic control and pharmacologic responses of the fetal bladder. *J Urol* 141, 1019–1024.

Kokoua A, Homsy Y, Lavigne J F et al. (1993). Maturation of the external urinary sphincter: a comparative histotopographic study in humans. *J Urol* 150, 617–622.

Kulseng-Hanssen S (1987). Urethral pressure variations in women with neurourological symptoms. II Relationship to urethral smooth muscle. *Neurourol Urodyn* 6, 79–85.

Levin R M, Shofer F S, Wein A J (1980). Estrogen-induced alterations in the autonomic responses of the rabbit urinary bladder. *J Pharmacol Exp Ther* 215, 614–618.

Levin R M, Jacobowitz D, Wein A J (1981). Autonomic innervation of rabbit urinary bladder following estrogen administration. *Urology* 17, 449–453.

Levin R M, Zderic S A, Ewalt D H, Duckett J W, Wein A J (1991). Effects of pregnancy on muscarinic receptor density and function in the rabbit urinary bladder. *Pharmacology* 43, 69–77.

Maggi A, Perez J (1985). Role of female gonadal hormones in the CNS: clinical and experimental aspects. *Life Sci* 37, 893–906.

Meyer S, Bachelard O, de Grandi P (1998). Do bladder neck mobility and urethral sphincter function differ during pregnancy compared with during the non-pregnant state? *Int Urogynecol J Pelvic Floor Dysfunct* 9, 397–404.

Milley P S, Nichols D H (1971). The relationship between the pubourethral ligaments and the urogenital diaphragm in the human female. *Anat Rec* 170, 281–283.

Mitra S C (1999). Effect of cocaine on fetal kidney and bladder function. *J Matern Fetal Med* 8, 262–269.

Nel J T, Diedericks A, Joubert G, Arndt K (2001). A prospective clinical and urodynamic study of bladder function during and after pregnancy. *Int Urogynecol J Pelvic Floor Dysfunct* 12, 21–26.

Nicolaides K H, Rosen D, Rabinowitz R, Campbell S (1988). Urine production and bladder function in fetuses with open spina bifida. *Fetal Ther* 3, 135–140.

Ohel G, Haddad S, Samueloff A (1995). Fetal urine production, micturition and fetal behavioral state. *Am J Perinatol* 12, 91–92.

Olsen L H, Dalmose A L, Swindle M M, Jorgensen T M, Djurhuus J C (2001). Male fetal pig lower urinary tract function in mid second and early third trimester of gestation. *J Urol* 165, 2331–2334.

Rud T (1980). The effects of estrogens and gestagens on the urethral pressure profile in urinary continent and stress incontinent women. *Acta Obstet Gynecol Scand* 59, 265–270.

Schreiter F, Fuchs P, Stockamp K (1976). Estrogenic sensitivity of alpha-receptors in the urethra musculature. *Urol Int* 31, 13–19.

Smet P J, Edyvane K A, Jonavicius J, Marshall V R (1996). Neuropeptides and neurotransmitter-synthesizing enzymes in intrinsic neurons of the human urinary bladder. *J Neurocytol* 25, 112–124.

Stanton S L, Kerr-Wilson R, Harris V G (1980). The incidence of urological symptoms in normal pregnancy. *Br J Obstet Gynaecol* 87, 897–900.

Taki N, Taniguchi T, Okada K, Moriyama N, Muramatsu I (1999). Evidence for predominant mediation of alpha1-adrenoceptor in the tonus of entire urethra of women. *J Urol* 162, 1829–1832.

Thiruchelvam N, Cuckow P M (1999). Fetal urodynamics: report of preliminary findings. In *Proceedings of the International Feto-Maternal Medicine Society Annual Meeting*, Newcastle 1999.

Tong Y C, Hung Y C, Lin J S, Hsu C T, Cheng J T (1995). Effects of pregnancy and progesterone on autonomic function in the rat urinary bladder. *Pharmacology* 50, 192–200.

Urner F, Weil A, Herrmann W L (1983). Estradiol receptors in the urethra and the bladder of the female rabbit. *Gynecol Obstet Invest* 16, 307–313.

Valentino R J, Miselis R R, Pavcovich L A (1999). Pontine regulation of pelvic viscera: pharmacological target for pelvic visceral dysfunctions. *Trends Pharmacol Sci* 20, 253–260.

van Geelen J M, Lemmens W A, Eskes T K, Martin C B Jr (1982). The urethral pressure profile in pregnancy, after delivery in healthy nulliparous women. *Am J Obstet Gynecol* 144, 636–649.

Versi E, Cardozo L D (1986). Urethral instability: diagnosis based on variations in the maximum urethral pressure in normal climacteric women. *Neurourol Urodyn* 5, 535–541.

Versi E, Cardozo L D, Studd J W, Brincat M, O'Dowd T M, Cooper D J (1986). Internal urinary sphincter in maintenance of female continence. *Br Med J (Clin Res Ed)* 292, 166–167.

Visco A G, Cholhan H J, O'Toole L, Guzick D S (2000). Effects of menstrual cycle and urinary tract instrumentation on uroflowmetry. *Neurourol Urodyn* 19, 147–152.

Wall L L, Hewitt J K, Helms M J (1995). Are vaginal and rectal pressures equivalent approximations of one another for the purpose of performing subtracted cystometry? *Obstet Gynecol* 85, 488–493.

Wang P, Luthin G R, Ruggieri M R (1995). Muscarinic acetylcholine receptor subtypes mediating urinary bladder contractility and coupling to GTP binding proteins. *J Pharmacol Exp Ther* 273, 959–966.

Weiner C P, Lizasoain I, Baylis S A, Knowles R G, Charles I G, Moncada S (1994). Induction of calcium-dependent nitric oxide synthases by sex hormones. *Proc Natl Acad Sci USA* 91, 5212–5216.

Wlodek M E, Thorburn G D, Harding R (1989). Bladder contractions and micturition in fetal sheep: their relation to behavioral states. *Am J Physiol* 257, R1526–R1532.

Yeung C K, Godley M L, Ho C K et al. (1995). Some new insights into bladder function in infancy. *Br J Urol* 76, 235–240.

Yeung C K, Godley M L, Dhillon H K, Duffy P G, Ransley P G (1998). Urodynamic patterns in infants with normal lower urinary tracts or primary vesico-ureteric reflux. *Br J Urol* 81, 461–467.

Zahran M M, Osman M I, Kamel M, Fayad M, Mooro H, Youssef A F (1976). Effects of contraceptive pills and intrauterine devices on urinary bladder. *Urology* 8, 567–574.

Zimmer E Z, Chao C R, Guy G P, Marks F, Fifer W P (1993). Vibro-acoustic stimulation evokes human fetal micturition. *Obstet Gynecol* 81, 178–180.

8

Development of sexuality: psychological perspectives

Lih Mei Liao

University College Hospital, London

In biomedicine, there are morphological and biochemical characteristics that can be measured with varying degrees of accuracy, rendering it more possible to describe variations in physical development and to define typical ranges. Sexuality dimensions, by comparison, afford no such luxury. "Normal" sexuality is contentious – in psychology and in society – and is destined to remain so.

What do psychologists have to say about human sexuality and its development? Why do some psychologists test children for "gender-appropriate" toy preferences, while others "un-define sex differences"? The simple answer is that they subscribe to different theoretical viewpoints, ask different questions and use different research methods to address their questions. The aim of this chapter is to describe and discuss key psychological perspectives in sexuality development. It is not possible to be a neutral presenter of rival positions, so I should make explicit my own biases. While I have come from a positivist framework and still apply that knowledge in selective projects, I have found that this framework alone is not adequate for examining and addressing sexuality events that are presented to me in clinical settings. My current view is that individual sexuality events cannot be understood without reference to cultural representations of such events. I hope it becomes clear why many psychologists now find it important to integrate discursive analysis in sexuality studies.

In this chapter, multiple facets of sexuality are discussed including gender identity (subjective identification with being a man or a woman), sexual partner choice and sexual activity, each set of events representing a complex interplay of thoughts, emotions, sensations, behaviours and our own subjective interpretation of them. All of these are encapsulated by our culture-specific linguistic framework. As any

one aspect of sexuality development is already a vast area, it is not possible to offer a detailed exposition of all the key areas. Rather, I aim to offer an abridged discussion of the main theoretical frameworks that health professionals are likely to come across in paediatric and adolescent gynaecology. As I do so I will describe some research to anchor the discussion. This chapter considers, in turn, the naturist position, social learning, sex of rearing, biopsychosocial framework, psychoanalysis and social constructionism. It ends with proposing a more integrated analysis of the sexual subject within a material-discursive framework, with special reference to psychological research and practice relating to conditions associated with nonnormative physicosexual development.

Nature

In the natural sciences, sex is conceptualized as biologically given. It is taken for granted that there can only be two mutually exclusive and oppositional sexual categories: male and female. The development of attributes such as "masculine" or "feminine" gender identity, sexual behaviour and partner orientation is assumed to be congruent with either male or female sex chromosomes, hormonal profile, brain, physique and reproductive capacity. Psychologists who study sexual development within this framework focus their research upon the correlational relationships between physiological variables and observable behaviour.

Naturist sex research has several characteristics. There is the tradition of animal research: mostly experimentation in laboratory conditions but sometimes observations of animals in their natural habitat. Experimental manipulations

Paediatric and Adolescent Gynaecology, ed. Adam Balen et al. Published by Cambridge University Press.
© Cambridge University Press 2004.

such as hormonal injections or lesions along hypothesized neuroendocrine pathways enable the researcher to assess corresponding variations in reproductive markers (e.g. sperm production in the male, lactation in the female) and mating behaviour (e.g. *intromission*, *lordosis*, homosexual approaches and receptivity). Animals provide an acceptable compromise for looking at biological factors in sexual behaviour, since procedures such as castration and anaesthesia of the genitalia present ethical and technical problems in human research. Of all the laboratory animals, the sexual behaviour of rats is undoubtedly the most thoroughly researched.

The extent to which animal data can be extrapolated to humans has been debated for a century in psychology and remains a moot point. It is worth noting that human sexuality is more varied than copulation and considerably more diverse even when compared with that in primates. Take genital intercourse alone, it is not just the male partner who performs pelvic thrusting, the female partner also commonly performs pelvic movement leading to ejaculation. Likewise, ejaculation without intromission is common for men. It would be even more difficult for biological theories to account for phenomena such as fetishes or sadomasochism.

In research with humans, a range of observational and survey techniques and psychometric tests are used to measure "sex differences". Sex differences research is essentially an elaboration of the naturist position and in general has focused mostly on the cognitive and performance capacities of boys and girls, men and women, with sexuality studies occupying only a relatively small corner of this research platform. A concise review of the vast area of sex differences research can be found in Collaer and Hines (1995).

One of the observational techniques used to examine the relationship between anatomical sex and gendered behaviour in humans is to identify "masculine" and "feminine" preferences and behaviours in boys and girls. Experiments are set up so that children choose between various toys and play activities, playmates, clothing and potential future occupation. Both children and parents may be asked questions about preferences. In the general population, differential preferences between boys and girls have been described. For example, boys seem to prefer cars, guns and trains while girls seem to prefer dolls and dressing up (Alexander and Hines, 1994). Studies using such techniques indicate that boys as young as three years of age show a preference for masculine toys and games. In kindergarten, girls are more likely to show a preference for masculine toys than boys do for feminine toys. With increasing age, both girls and boys make increasingly more sex-stereotyped choices,

but boys consistently make more of them than girls do. Researchers are careful to point out that within-sex variations can be as wide as between-sex variations (Hines and Kaufman, 1994). Consequently, when it comes to defining "normal" ranges of gender attributes, complications arise.

In mainly animal and some human sexual research, studies have concentrated on the role of prenatal androgens in gender differentiation. Other studies have examined the activation potential of the sex hormones, especially testosterone, on current sexual desire, activity and partner orientation in men and women.

It is often said that, without androgens, nature makes a female, and that it is the presence of prenatal androgens at *critical periods* that result in masculine sexual differentiation. The search for the hormonal role of gender differentiation has, therefore, broadly targeted the effects of fetal androgens. Again, animals provide the first opportunities, and critical periods have been determined for a number of species. However, ambiguous genital–sexual differentiation and development has also fascinated psychologists precisely because of their potential for elucidating the relative contributions of nature and nurture to human sexuality.

Ehrhardt et al. (1968) reported that girls with congenital adrenal hyperplasia (CAH) who have been exposed to high levels of fetal androgens at critical times exhibit "tomboyism". By this, the authors meant a preference for outdoor active play over indoor and less active play. It is important to bear in mind that behavioural observations had come from parents and teachers who knew of the girls' condition. More recent studies directly comparing girls who have been exposed to fetal androgens and those who have not also suggested that the former can have a greater predisposition towards stereotypically masculine behaviour. They are more likely to report that they prefer masculine toys, engage in rough and tumble play, choose outdoor activities, have more male playmates, and so on. As described by Ehrhardt et al. (1968), these girls are also more likely to describe themselves as tomboys (see Collaer and Hines, 1995). Interestingly, men with 46,XY who have been exposed to prenatal "feminizing" hormones do not appear to be predisposed towards stereotypically female behaviours. This discrepancy is explained in terms of the stronger pressure for boys to conform to stereotypically masculine behavioural patterns than for girls to conform to feminine stereotypes (Hines and Kaufman, 1994).

Biological theories of differential gender attributes so far do not explain why some girls who have not been exposed to fetal androgens also describe themselves as tomboy and/or express stereotypically masculine preferences and/or describe themselves as homosexual or bisexual. Furthermore, the idea that there is greater social pressure on boys to exhibit masculinity, and that this could potentially override the influence of feminizing hormones, is an important acknowledgement of cultural determinants in gendered development.

Different rates of self-reported homosexuality and bisexuality have been found for women with CAH. These range from 5% (Mulaikal et al., 1987) to 11% (May et al., 1996), 22% (Dittman et al., 1992), 29% (Money and Schwatz, 1977) and 37% (Money and Ehrhardt, 1972). Different findings in research studies probably reflect methodological differences such as age of participants, timing of "feminizing" treatments, severity of illness and so on. How homosexuality is defined would also influence results. For example, Dittman et al. (1992) included homosexual desire in their definition of homosexual orientation, while some studies include multiple experiences of homosexual acts as a criterion.

Meyer-Bahlburg et al. (1984) investigated women who had been exposed to prenatal diethylstilbestrol (DES, known to "masculinize" female rats). Compared with a so-called control group with a higher proportion of Roman Catholic married women, this mainly single, student, DES-exposed sample was more likely to describe themselves as lesbian or bisexual. The authors found "no consistent group differences in other domains of gender–role behaviour" including parental reporting of childhood rough and tumble play, age of first boyfriend and first sexual intercourse, expressed preference between motherhood and career. The fact that the two samples differed in important dimensions – not least because DES-exposed women were more at risk of certain reproductive cancers – did not seem to concern the authors about accepting this research as evidence for the relationship between adult sexual orientation and prenatal hormones. Studies of this kind raise the important and vexing question of what constitutes a suitable control group (see *Biopsychosocial framework* below).

Asking the question in another way, is there evidence that different social groups such as homosexuals, sex offenders and "normals" differ biologically? It would seem that this area of investigation has also not produced reliable evidence (Bancroft, 1989). For example, a study comparing homosexual and heterosexual women failed to find significant differences in serum testosterone, androstenedione or cortisol (Downey et al., 1987). Various brain regions have also been investigated with mixed results, but so far no known researcher has linked any human anatomical brain difference to any hormonal event in the womb (Vine, 1993). Moreover it is possible that lived experiences can

affect brain development. Theoretical coherence in this area has yet to be developed. Be that as it may, the more recent tragedy of deaths from acquired immunodeficiency syndrome (AIDS) has produced opportunities for new research to identify differences between gay and straight brains. A detailed exposition of this research and a critical analysis can be found in Le Vay (1996) and Hegarty (1997), respectively. As well as other methodological problems in these postmortem studies, Ussher (1997) points out that if partner choice was indeed a tight and stable category, "the men were all dead when they were recruited for the study and therefore could not give any report".

If scientists have yet to prove that the brain, hardwired by sex steroids while in utero, predicts future gender attributes, or that current hormonal profile varies meaningfully between social groups, what about the activation potential of sex steroids on sexual behaviour? Dabbs and Mohammad (1992) examined the short-term effects of testosterone on the sexual behaviour of healthy heterosexual adults. They reported that levels of early evening testosterone measured in saliva did not predict sexual activity that night for sexual partners who were living together. Testosterone levels were raised after sexual activity. A study of heterosexual college students failed to find any relationship between the women's testosterone levels and sexual activities, or their satisfaction with their male partners (Alexander et al., 1990). Interestingly, low testosterone levels in hypogonadal men do not appear to affect erectile responses to erotic stimulation or fantasies (Bancroft, 1988). It is possible that the level of testosterone necessary to fuel sexual desire is low and levels above this have no measurable effect (Bancroft, 1989).

Despite a vast volume of research of which only a few examples are given here, it remains equivocal as to how closely adult human sexuality relates to the hormonal environment during fetal life. In general, the explanatory and predictive power of naturist hypotheses is greater in relation to the courtship and mating behaviour of animals, though even then data do not reliably generalize from one species of rodent to another. When it comes to human studies, results are at their most equivocal. It is possible that, in controlled conditions when other factors can be screened out, "pure" hormonal effects are more salient. The question is, how influential are hormonal effects where competing influences such as fatigue, shyness, distraction, perceived attractiveness of partner, opportunity, religious sanctions and socialization processes have also to be negotiated? Hormonal influences are probably important, but we do not yet know how important, for what aspects of sexuality, for whom and in what situations.

Social learning

Each culture prescribes approved standards for the behaviour of boys, girls, men and women. Let us call these gender stereotypes for that culture. Definitions of masculine and feminine behaviour have changed considerably across historical periods within the same culture, so some of what is acceptable today differs radically from what used to be tolerated. Take education in this country for example; it was once regarded as a male domain and higher education was believed to be too arduous for the delicate female mind and might even damage women's fertility. If this is history, again take contemporary Western societies, which supposedly enjoy a greater degree of gender equity; it is obvious that relatively few women are employed as taxi drivers or brain surgeons, few men work as secretaries or speech therapists, and few children are cared for by men. The debate has never been on the existence of gender differences. Differences – whatever their form and content – are observable in most cultures in any historical period, but are these biological destiny or are they largely shaped by family, peer groups and institutions tied to the survival or political economy of that culture?

It has been shown that from birth the responses of adults are influenced by the expectations held for the presumed sex of the baby (Condry and Condry, 1976; Frisch, 1977). In a study by Smith and Lloyd (1978), six-month-old babies were stereotypically dressed as either a boy or a girl and named accordingly, and mothers of similar aged infants were invited to play with them. Mothers' verbal behaviour and responses to the physical actions of the baby differed according to the presumed sex of the infant. In particular, they responded to the baby boys with more physical action and to the baby girls with more comforting and soothing behaviour. These early differences are said to continue throughout childhood (Rebelsky and Hanks, 1971). Fathers have been found to be particularly more boisterous in their play but especially with sons, with whom they are more likely to initiate rough-and-tumble activities (Lamb, 1981). By the time the infant is 12 months of age, parents are found to be encouraging their sons and daughters to play with sex-typed toys and to avoid playful activities that are considered more appropriate for children of the opposite sex (Snow et al., 1983).

Gender socialization continues throughout childhood aided by direct and indirect, intended and unintended, messages from teachers, peers and families. As it continues into adulthood, it would be strange if there were no clear differences in behaviour, expectations and social roles between men and women. Nurturists believe that gender

characteristics are socially shaped rather than biologically determined. The very notion that men and women are fundamentally different organizes social structures and interactions between people in that society (Bem, 1993). Imagine if gender rigidity–permissiveness in parents had been the subject of investigation instead of the children's toy preferences, scales might have been developed questioning child carers as to how likely they were to gift-wrap a train engine as a birthday present for a two-year-old girl or a tutu for a little boy. In a society that judged gender-rigid rearing style rather than juvenile play that does not conform to gender stereotypes, parents who reported insufficient permissiveness might be offered interventions to help them to become less rigid. In such a culture, one might speculate a somewhat different scenario in the playrooms of boys and girls.

It is generally accepted that attitudes expressed by significant adults towards one another and towards the child are a major influence on the child's interpretation of masculine and feminine roles. However, like its naturist counterpart, social learning research is limited mainly to the study of gendered social behaviour, but these may not be connected to sexual fantasies and acts or to gender identity. Social learning offers only a limited framework for sexuality development, but some of the psychological differences found for people with intersex conditions could be interpreted within this model.

When it comes to the rearing of children born with ambiguous genitalia, it is possible that parental and medical doubts about the sex of the neonate may result in ambiguous expectations about appropriate behaviour. Unclear expectations about appropriate behaviour may encourage the development of some behaviour perceived by society as more appropriate for the other gender. Social learning takes place not only in the home but also in public institutions such as schools and, of course, hospitals. An individual's experience of the healthcare system itself could be a profoundly important learning process and can partly explain future adjustment. Problematic interactions and encounters with significant adults, including health professionals, are well documented in lay accounts by people who have grown up with an intersex condition (see Ch. 17). These are corroborated by professional accounts (May, 1998; Liao, 2003). In particular, many of the adults appear to have had few role models to help them to manage feeling different and to learn to communicate with greater confidence in intimate relationships. By comparison, the opportunities for learning about negative aspects of themselves appear to have been abundant. Through silence and secrecy, individuals may grow up with the notion that aspects of themselves are too catastrophic to be mentioned. Through lack of control over their medical care they may learn to be passive and helpless. Through intrusive gazing of their genitalia they may learn to associate it with deviance and shame rather than sensual and sexual pleasure. The sexuality differences of intersex people could be the result of their differential treatment by others rather than any intrinsic biological difference.

A detailed project (May, 1998) compared adult women with CAH and adult women with diabetes – a research design superior to that comparing people with CAH with those without any chronic medical condition at all. Participants from both adult samples had been treated at the same hospital as children. Results indicated that the two groups of women had similar social and sexual aspirations, but the CAH group was less socially and sexually experienced. When relationships failed, the women with CAH were more likely to blame themselves, fulfilling expectations of their inadequacies, expectations that have been fuelled by messages about their sexual inadequacies. When people with stigmatizing conditions do not do sexuality in the way we expect them to, there may be many reasons for this. To tie these differences back to their biological condition when there are other possible explanations is scientifically unsound, if nothing else.

Sex of rearing

The sex of rearing approach developed by John Money and coworkers is discussed separately because it is not congruent with any of the other theoretical perspectives. According to Money and Ehrhardt (1972), all infants are gender-neutral at birth. They are said to remain malleable until about two and a half years old. Sex has to be fixed by then so genital congruence must be achieved in this period. Once sex is assigned, the parents must be left in no doubt that their child is of the given sex. If surgical modification has taken place in childhood to achieve genital congruence, gender is further consolidated with appropriate hormonal management at puberty. If these strategies were in place, children are thought to develop subsequently into well-adjusted men or women.

Such an approach is probably more appropriately thought of as a case-management protocol for genital ambiguity rather than as a theory of sexuality development. Proponents of the sex of rearing approach have been cited as champions of the nurture end of the sexuality debate; I think mistakenly so. Although Money believes that gender is developed through being reared as boy or girl, implicit in

his recommendations are several fundamentally naturist assumptions: sexual dimorphism, the normality of genital and gender congruence and heterosexual partner choice, and critical periods for imprinting. Sex of rearing is a hybrid approach strangely combining aspects of biological, social learning and psychoanalytic theories of sexual maturation; it also reflects cultural conflation of penis size and masculinity. I will first summarize the biological concepts within the sex of rearing approach.

Interest in the study of instinct (innate behaviour) by evolutionary psychologists declined in the early part of the last century because it did not prove very helpful in understanding human behaviour. However, it was temporarily revived in the 1950s by a group of European psychologists and zoologists who called themselves ethologists. A key concept introduced by ethologists was *imprinting*, which refers to a type of early learning that forms the basis for the young animal's attachment to its parents. The Austrian zoologist Konrad Lorenz famously demonstrated how young ducklings followed him instead of the mother duck because he was the first moving object that they saw after hatching and were repeatedly exposed to him within the first two days of life: the *critical period* for ducklings to imprint. Imprinting within a critical period has also been described for other species (e.g. wild dogs are said to be most predisposed to taming in the first seven weeks of life). Ethological studies have also shown that, in certain circumstances, say following the death of a parent, animals can imprint onto another species and later attempt to mate with a member of this other species. Such ethological concepts were extrapolated onto human gender development by sex of rearing proponents. As well as that, the sex of rearing approach was also clearly influenced by Freudian ideas (see *Psychoanalysis* below).

Like Freud, Money and coworkers also assumed that the presence or absence of the penis was of prime importance in psychosexual differentiation. Gender must be fixed before entry into the Freudian phallic stage, because now children are supposedly very preoccupied with their genitalia and would notice penis presence or absence. However, unlike Freud, who did not specify actual penis size as the main determinant of masculine development, Money and colleagues assumed it best to avoid the (as yet undocumented) worse problems of having a small penis in adulthood by assigning children with current or anticipated small penis to the female gender (Money et al., 1981). Such an approach reflects a conflation of penis size and masculinity, and a conflation of masculinity and men's well-being. It is as if a small penis is hardly worth having, and in the case of a very small penis, a man might as well be a woman. The recommendation of the morphology of the penis as the best criterion for separating the genders has had its critics from early on (e.g. Diamond, 1965). In fact one of the children cited as a major source of evidence for Money's approach has reassigned himself back to his genetic sex. The discrediting accounts of John/Joan's problematic life are now published in a best seller (Colapinto, 2000). It is a story of a twin baby boy who lost a section of his penis through a botched circumcision and was subsequently assigned female. The success of this case was hailed as scientific evidence for the sex of rearing approach. After not inconsiderable personal suffering, this person has in fact reassigned himself as male and apparently lives a happier life with his wife and stepchildren.

As well as being epistemologically confused, the sex of rearing approach is built on unsubstantiated assumptions. For example, there is no evidence to suggest that gender assignment mitigates parental doubt of the sex of the child (Wilson and Reiner, 1998) and prevents ambiguous rearing. Indeed Money and Ehrhardt (1972) described parents who still had doubts about the sex of the child and tended to monitor their child's behaviour "looking vainly for signs to resolve their doubt". Parental vigilance and zealousness in promoting gender stereotyped behaviour could potentially lead the child to adopt oppositional behaviour patterns.

Sex of rearing did not account for cogent philosophical argument, neither did the proponents produce convincing empirical evidence for the predicted long-term social, emotional and sexuality trajectory of sex assignment, yet critics had little impact. Interestingly, Van Seters and Slob (1988) and Reilly and Woodhouse (1989) briefly described a few men with micropenis who reported a mutually satisfying sex life with their heterosexual partners, albeit the authors had not sought partner corroboration. The men were said to be able to de-emphasize the importance of genital intercourse and to have found alternative ways for themselves and their partners to reach orgasm. Likewise, in a recent study with men who have experienced prepubertal onset hypogonadism, measures of sexual experiences and aspects of psychological well-being were similar to the general population. Self-perceived penis size was no more significant than other secondary sexual characteristics in the experience of delayed puberty (Chadwick et al., 2002). A number of recent studies using a mixture of methodologies contradicted the claim that sex of rearing results in uncomplicated psychosexual outcome for intersex women (May et al., 1996; Minto et al., 2003a,b).

With support from only a handful of frequently cited cases (Kessler, 1998) and limited conceptual richness, it is astonishing how sex of rearing could have received so much scientific credibility. Its wide adoption in the management of genital ambiguity has been something akin to an uncontrolled social experiment. One interpretation is that sex of rearing owes its impact to its face validity, to technical expedience because it was easier to remove than to build an appendage and to the rising opposition to biological theories of gender determination. Most of all, the protocolized management of ambiguous sexual differentiation resonated with contemporary attitudes to sex.

Perhaps the greatest theoretical challenge for both sex of rearing and the naturist position comes from transsexuals. These individuals have chromosomal pattern, anatomical characteristics and parental rearing that are congruent with one sex, yet they have difficulties in developing a congruent gender identity. As early as 1978, Kessler and McKenna produced a detailed exposition of gender construction based on their work with transsexuals. However, this work has been largely invisible in the scientific community, with only two references to it between 1978 and 1995 in the *Science Citation Index* (Diamond, 2000).

Biopsychosocial framework

Within psychology, the biopsychosocial framework (see Sarafino, 2001) is most centrally endorsed by the subspecialism *health psychology*. The development of health psychology parallels the shift in emphasis in medicine from the elimination of infectious diseases to the management of chronic illness and disability. Engel (1977) introduced the biopsychosocial model as a framework for integrating knowledge about the biological, psychological and social aspects of health problems. Much of health psychology research examines the relationship between variables such as health and illness perceptions (e.g. perceived control of health and illness, expectancy of health outcome) and psychological well-being (e.g. mood, quality of life). This type of research is being carried out in an increasing number of disease contexts. These measures are sometimes hypothesized to predict health-enhancing behaviour or lifestyle change (e.g. adherence to medical regimen, smoking cessation). They are also thought to influence outcome variables of medical treatment (e.g. diabetes control, postsurgery recovery time). This framework of inquiry has several points of relevance for this chapter. First, a literature of the psychology of chronic illness and medical management has amassed and should not be ignored by researchers who want to assess long-term outcome – sexual or nonsexual – of people who present any chronic condition affecting sexual development. Second, a biopsychosocial framework has been the predominant psychological model of adolescent development, and the formulation of psychological difficulties arising from atypical physicosexual development falls within this framework. Third, theories and treatment of sexual difficulties tend to be conceptualized within a biopsychosocial framework.

The section *Nature* (above) discussed the question as to what constitutes a suitable control group when examining the social and sexual outcome of medical conditions that could disrupt physicosexual development. A biopsychosocial framework can help in considering this question. Individuals with such medical diagnoses differ from other groups on important counts. Compared with "healthy normals" (e.g. relatives), they differ in having a chronic medication condition. Compared with other medical populations, they differ in bodily presentation and attendant experiences, including intrusive gazing and not being given adequate information. Compared with most people, they may differ in the experience of ambiguous rearing. I will first discuss the psychology of living with a chronic condition requiring continuing contact with medical services.

Chronic conditions affect the psychological development of children. In a meta-analysis involving 82 peer-reviewed studies examining the psychosocial aspects of chronic childhood conditions, Nolan and Pless (1986) concluded that "the presence of a birth defect or chronic disorder significantly increases the risk of emotional problems in children". Cassileth et al. (1984) studied across different disease categories, including cancer, arthritis and renal disease, and found that the emotional impact appeared to be fairly uniform across diseases. Absences from school, visits to hospitals, surgery, treatment regimens, parental anxiety, invasion of personal privacy, pain or physical discomfort, early or late physical development may all lead to feelings of being "different" from one's peers. Any differences in social and sexual dimensions found for these children would need to be explained within a theoretical model that could take account of the transactions with the social systems of hospital, school, family, friendship network, the type of condition and treatment demands and the communication effectiveness of the treatment team responsible for managing the condition. Children are not passive recipients of these influences but can themselves affect the course of their illness by their behaviour.

Since medicalization of children can have a profound impact on their psychological development, Slijper (1984) was careful not to compare the test results of children with CAH with "normal" children but rather with another group with a chronic condition (diabetes). She argued that both had suffered chronic illness and hospitalization and both had rebelled against the intrusion of medical authority into their lives. She found no group differences in their gender ideas and preferences. May (1998) found some support for the view that feelings of alienation become particularly salient in adolescence. In her detailed analyses of women with CAH and diabetes treated at the same children's hospital, she found CAH women to be less sexually experienced than diabetic women, for example fewer of the former group had masturbated or had intercourse. However, those medical condition factors described above were also different for the two groups. For example, the diabetic women knew where to get information, had people to discuss their problems with and had not been advised to keep their condition secret. So it is not clear whether any sexuality differences between those with CAH and other female patients result from prenatal hormones, other factors or both. As intersex activist Cheryl Chase said in an interview, "The whole family is distorted and unusual, so there's no way you're gonna tease out "nature" and "nurture" without over-looking all of the trauma that intersexed children and their families experience" (Hegarty, 2000). Researchers will need to examine further the comparability of children (and adults) whose sexual development is compromised and those who have other health problems or who do not have any significant health problem.

The biopsychosocial framework is currently also the dominant model of adolescent development (Adelson, 1980). Within this model, pre-eminence is given to pubertal changes in adolescence, but it is also recognized that biological changes occur in a context of broader, reciprocal changes in intellectual, emotional and social capacities. Pubertal changes are said to provide the substrate upon which psychological and social influences act. For example, changes in the physical body generate new social opportunities; these could lead to changes in that individual's emotional repertoire, which, in turn, could generate expectations of new social roles, and so on (Petersen and Taylor, 1980). The degree to which the body conforms to a male or female stereotype is thought to determine the degree to which typically male and female psychological characteristics are attributed to that child's personality. These attributions, in turn, organize the social interactions between the child and the social environment and, over time, become reflected in stable, typically male or female personality configurations. This theorizing appears to state nothing beyond the idea that typically male bodily characteristics result in a typically male adult personality, as for female.

Because development is multifaceted, the influence of variations in the rate and timing of specific bodily developments on psychosexual outcome cannot be easily established. Where pubertal development is nonnormative (e.g. delayed or early), negative outcome is generally assumed, though little is understood about the social, emotional and sexual consequences (Rekers, 1992). For boys and men, conclusions of negative outcome are based upon a few descriptive studies using unreliable methodology of questionable validity and focusing on the relationship between psychosexual outcome and undersized penis at the expense of other concurrent developmental factors (Money and Clopper, 1975; Money et al., 1980, 1985). These studies conclude that concerns about small penis size were central to the experience of psychological distress. However, for most of the men described by Money et al. (1980, 1985), having a smaller than average penis was not their only difference. A recent study examining sexual experiences, psychological well-being and quality of life suggested that, where puberty is delayed, appearance factors such as absent facial hair, unchanged musculature, non-deepened voice and gynaecomastia were the important factors that organized social interaction in adolescence, not penis size (Chadwick et al., 2002). Such appearance factors prevented the young men from being able to "pass" in their social world.

Interestingly, Milton Diamond's latently expressed ideas relating to intersex would also place him within a bio-psychosocial framework, even though he has often been put in the naturist camp because of his opposition to Money. In a recent summary of his position, Diamond (2000) proposes: "One is born with a biological psychosexual predisposition that is fixed by the genetic–endocrine heritage and with it a propensity for certain sexual and gender patterns to be expressed". Which pattern gets expressed apparently depends on the level of tolerance that "cultural mores" allow. Diamond further proposed that we have an inner "sexual identity" that is prenatally organized and an outer "gender identity" that comes with self-evaluation against social norms. Sexual identity is forged by some "brain template" and/or "early engrams" and will override subsequent rearing-activated ones.

Diamond sees transsexuals as "intersex" in that their body is one sex and their brain is another, but that their "mind" takes precedence such that they eventually change their body to fit with their mind. He cites the famous John/Joan to support his view and states: "John, and other males sex-reassigned as females, "knew" that they were not girls". There are many possible reasons why this troubled individual had reassigned himself back to a male gender rather than those that Diamond cited. The fact that this same life has been used to support two rival theoretical positions offers a glimpse of the speculative nature of the science of gender development. Implied in Diamond's theorizing are some very contentious ideas, for example

that somehow one's engrams (whatever they are and wherever they are located) cause one to "know" one's (real) sexual identity. Our current understanding of neuroscience does not enable us to speculate about these ideas. In a bizarre way, Diamond aligned some of his thinking to Kessler and McKenna's (1978) theory that gender is a social construction (see *Social constructionism* below), failing to note that it is ideas such as true sex that are being deconstructed. The mistake is easily made, because discursive and essentialist theorists both advocate against early sex assignment, but on an entirely different theoretical basis. This difference matters.

The rise of *discursive* theory and methods in psychology has led some critics to question the adequacy of the biopsychosocial framework for understanding and researching experiences of health, illness and their management (Yardley, 1999). Of particular relevance here is the criticism levied at mainstream psychological conceptualization of sexuality events, with the majority of researchers and clinicians still clinging on to *realist* assumptions, failing to question the influence of their own subjectivity or ideological standpoint on the theories or therapies that they develop, or the role of discourses in social regulation (Ussher, 1997a). This critique applies to most psychological therapies for "sexual dysfunction" (e.g. vaginismus, low libido).

Within a biopsychosocial formulation of sexual difficulties, bodily pathology (e.g. hormonal deficiencies, side effects of drugs, ill-health) is seen to "interact" with the individual's psychological diatheses (e.g. low self-esteem, health anxiety). Psychological diatheses may have psychological origins (e.g. marital discord, parental attitude towards sexual matters) or they may be events external to the person (e.g. unemployment, an accident). The social part of the formulation may be conceptualized as environmental stress, religious prohibition and so on. This is inadequate. The process of diagnosis and treatment itself operates from unspoken cultural ideologies and itself requires interrogation. Boyle (1993) draws our attention to the unquestioned acceptance of the centrality of genital intercourse in the assessment and treatment of sexual difficulties. Other sexual activities are consigned to the secondary status of "foreplay" – something dispensable except as means to the real thing. Boyle points out that, almost 50 years ago, Kinsey and coworkers had already reported a greater frequency with which women appeared to experience orgasm in homosexual encounters. She quotes Hite, who points out that most women do not have difficulty having orgasms but that society has difficulty coming to terms with the way they have them. In marginalizing other sexual activities, female pleasure is subordinated. Failure to question the centrality of genital intercourse communicates something of its sacredness in our culture.

However, phallocentric assumptions also disadvantage some men, whose "premature" ejaculation must be extended. Acceptance of derogatory labels such as "impotence" and "frigidity" are often prerequisite for getting support, but this professional terminology could itself undermine greater acceptance of the diversity of human sexuality and define for the rest of society "normal" and inadequate sex.

Psychoanalysis

Freud was the first person to build a sustained psychosexual theory. Since then, psychoanalytic theory has branched off in many directions but as a whole, its treatise of human sexuality has remained influential. Common to all psychoanalytic theories is the notion that consciousness is only a partial picture of mental life, that the dynamic unconscious shades into the conscious, and that the unconscious is knowable only through decoding of the conscious. Freud developed the notion of the three-pronged psyche: the *id* (a sea of impulses and strivings for gratification, gradually repressed as development progresses but continuing to influence even the adult), the *superego* (parental authority internalized) and the *ego* (the conscious self-striving for balance as the id and superego push forward).

Psychosexual development is said to begin in infancy and experience of this is said to structure the adult personality. The psychosexual stages are: *oral* (characterized by gratification through stimulation of the lips and mouth region), *anal* (characterized by gratification through withholding and expelling faeces), *phallic* (characterized by gratification through fondling the genitalia), *latent* (in which sexual interests are no longer active so children of elementary school age turn their interests to the enviroment) and finally *genital* (at which point normal heterosexual interests arise). Both constitutional factors (e.g. each of the erotogenic zones is differentially capable of excitation for each person) and environmental factors (e.g. the duration and nature of the weaning process) are important determinants of the child's experience of each stage. Excessive indulgence in feeding or excessive frustration through rapid and early weaning, for example, means that the individual is loath to renounce oral eroticism. This refusal to renounce the pleasure from a particular erotogenic zone is known as *fixation*. Freud states that "The permanent character traits are either unchanging perpetuations of the original impulse, sublimations of them or reaction-formations against them" (quoted in Kline, 1972). For instance,

character traits such as impatience, envy and ambition are thought to be part of the *oral personality*, and obstinacy, parsimony and orderliness are attributed to the *anal personality*.

But how do gender differences develop? How do newborn babies, who can have no psychological representation of their genitalia and who, according to Freud, have a bisexual psychological potential, develop a masculine or feminine gender identity? Freud asserts that in the first three or so years of life there is little, if any, difference between boys and girls in the expression of their infantile sexuality. He begins to differentiate their sexual development at the age of three or four (phallic stage). He theorizes with certainty about boys, but with hesitancy and many afterthoughts about girls, admitting on several occasions that he was baffled by the psychology of women (Jahoda, 1977).

The boy enters the period of the *Oedipus complex*, characterized by passionate but aimless sensual attachment to the mother and jealousy of the father or a sibling in intimate bodily contact with the mother, and *phantasizes* about the disappearance of the rival. Having derived pleasure from fondling his penis, the boy notices that his much loved mother is without one. If the penis can be removed from his mother (and other females), his own may also be in danger. This fear of loss of the penis is termed *castration complex*. The mother who has lost her penis is now seen as not quite as strong and powerful as father. The boy turns to father for protection and wants to be like father. The Oedipus complex is dissolved, and jealousy and hatred of the father is replaced by identification with him. This identification encourages the internalization of parental standards and establishes the foundation of the superego.

The girl's path to feminine identity is not quite so neat in Freudian theory. She is just as passionately attached to mother. Her new source of sensual pleasure is clitoral masturbation but, on discovering that boys have a bigger pleasure object, she feels underprivileged and envious. She must identify with the mother, who is inferior like her, and convert her *penis envy* into love for those who have a penis. Unlike the boy whose oedipal attachment to mother precedes the castration complex, the girl's passionate oedipal attachment follows the discovery of her castration and the accompanying feelings of envy and of resentment against her fate as female. In the end, if things go well, envy changes into the wish to have a baby.

Freud's ideas make gender development crudely derivative of anatomical sexual difference. His conceptualizing of feminine development as thwarted masculine development was soon to be challenged by Horney (1932). Horney developed the idea that it is mother and not father who is agentic in masculine gender differentiation, that the growing boy's deep-seated fear of being overwhelmed by mother is more important and more energetically repressed than his fear of the castrating father. In that sense, adult masculinity is founded on reactions against femininity. Horney interpreted men's tendency to choose as love objects women with less social power than themselves in terms of the men's need to support an "ever precarious self-respect of the "average man"". Her reformulation saw the beginning of feminism in psychoanalysis. In *The Second Sex*, de Beauvoir (1949) applied *existential psychoanalysis* directly to the feminine gender. She wrote about different types of femininity and theorized that different gender forms are negotiated ways of contemporary life and not fixed character types. Her treatise allows gender to be seen as an evolving engagement with situations and social structures. On the whole, however, the development of feminist psychoanalytic theories did not take off for another two decades.

The public tends to associate psychology with psychoanalysis. However, mainstream psychology in the UK (and USA) has had a very ambivalent relationship with psychoanalysis. Psychology has been bent on becoming a behavioural and natural science and psychoanalysis did not fit easily within a framework of positivist science. Consequently, the teaching of psychoanalysis within psychology is extremely variable. In clinical psychology, some practitioners work exclusively within a psychoanalytic framework while others ignore it completely.

Freud first became a physician before he turned to psychology. This coincidental link of psychoanalysis with medicine through its founder has meant a loss of some of its original radical potential (Connell, 1995) and alienation by some practitioners of psychology. Mainstream psychoanalysis is criticized for first pathologizing the individual then normalizing them by way of orientating them towards culturally prescribed norms through "therapy". Mainstream practice is still characterized by orthodox interpretation of sexuality theories and no longer emphasizes the contradictory nature of gender or the clash between individual desire and social order.

Freud was clear about the continuum between pathologized events (*neuroses*) and nonpathologized events such as jokes, slips of the tongue, dreams, choice of occupation or partner, the significance of which, if decoded, would turn out to be sexual. Freud also asserted that all human beings – not just those identified as patients – have a bisexual potential. Classical Freudian theory emphasizes the precarious rather than fixed nature of sexuality, development of which is characterized by conflict. Sexuality develops through hazardous relational processes and remains

fragile. Although in any given individual one sexual character will prevail, Freud hypothesized that it never enjoys monopoly and that masculine and feminine currents coexist in all of us. According to Connell (1995), in *Civilisation and its Discontents*, Freud's treatise of the superego – internalized prohibitions from the parents (and presumably culture) – suggested the beginning of a sociological dimension. However, he did not complete the hypothesizing of the superego as the means by which culture overcomes individual desire, or the relationship between parental and cultural authority.

Psychoanalytic ideas have been heavily criticized for different reasons and by different groups (including psychoanalysts) since their inception. However, in recent decades, some of the original radical notions that were lost have been reinterpreted and integrated with postmodernist analyses of sexuality. Revisionist psychoanalytic theories, which continue to develop, have been possible partly because, as Goldner (1991) stated, the generic analytic stance "fosters scepticism about the knower and the known by illuminating the motivational structures underlying ideas, actions, and systems of knowledge (including itself). Moreover, the analytic method of inquiry and interpretation defines itself in terms of the elaboration of multiply-layered meanings, as opposed to a 'final truth'." Goldner questions the taken for granted concept of stable gender identity itself. She quotes May, who argued that "The very notion of identity can imply a sense of self too final, smooth and conflict-free to do justice to our clinical (or personal) experience". Goldner quotes Rubin who went further: "Far from being an expression of natural differences, exclusive gender identity is *suppression of natural similarities*".

Social constructionism

To the question "Is a culture-free psychology possible? Can man acquire any knowledge uncontaminated by the social and historical conditions of the knower?" (Jahoda, 1977), the social constructivists' answer would be a definitive "no". Social constructionism has developed outside psychology by postmodernist theorists. It provides a framework for challenging traditional knowledge claims, offers a more coherent analysis of body and culture, and enables the development of research methods that examine subjective accounts of bodily events.

If knowledge is accepted reality, and reality is constructed through social discourses, then dominant discourses define reality for that culture. How reality is defined is conceptualized as a product of power relationships between social groups and as such is never neutral but always acting in the interests of certain groups. Social constructivist research is principally concerned with explaining the processes by which people come to describe, explain and account for the world in which they live. Developments within "psychological science" have themselves been treated as events for social analyses. Psychological research is not accepted as a neutral activity that objectively deciphers facts about people but as social practice both reflecting and fulfilling cultural ideologies. Likewise, psychological constructs are not accepted as truth but as social constructions. Psychological science is systematically *deconstructed*; few psychologists are prepared for such "wrenching, conceptual dislocation" (Gergen, 1985).

Within mainstream psychology, subjective experiences are investigated mainly from a *realist* perspective, taking for granted that psychological events are not only real and quantifiable but can be sorted into exclusive categories. Sexuality events have been reduced to hormonal variations, penile and vaginal swelling, intercourse frequency and duration, reports on questionnaires. Likewise "low libido" or "frigidity" are diagnosed and seen as real disorders that belong to the individual and which can be uncovered and treated. It is as if sexuality events mainly take place on one's own in a private chamber screened of all information and cultural influence. A recent interview study examining male partner's construction of intersex women demonstrated the relational nature of sexuality (Doyle, 2002). The positioning of the woman as doubtless feminine enabled the male partner to position himself as doubtless masculine. The positioning of the woman as doubtful casts a shadow on the male partner's own sexuality. People's positioning is often renegotiated in the context of new relationships. And negotiations take place in our wider culture.

Many social theorists analyse exclusively the *discursive* – communicative and symbolic – aspects of bodily experiences. The sexual body is treated as an object constructed within sociocultural discourses and practices; that is to say, in the impossible absence of discourses, the body means nothing. This is a difficult idea to grasp. Consider tribal rituals such as those involving piercing and cutting into body parts or walking on burning rocks. To the nonacculturated, these acts could be excruciating. Yet "pain" may never enter into the subjectivity of the tribesman, because "pain" is not available in the linguistic and symbolic representations of such rituals within his culture. Here in this oversimplified example, we have one material event but two subjective experiences informed by two different sets of social and historical conditions. According to some discursive theorists, bodily experiences are only as real as our

constructions of them, and our constructions are specific to our language and culture. This is why they argue that, in order to study bodily experiences, the focus should not be on the material body but on discourse, because bodily experiences cannot be understood without discourses of such experiences.

Constructivist treatise of body regulation in contemporary culture is relevant for our understanding of human sexuality. Anthropologists have argued that the human body has a role as a cultural text. For example, just as "primitive" rituals of body inscriptions by means of scarification define a sexual or courageous body, rituals and commodities such as hairstyles, cosmetics and body conditioning define a sexual and "civilized" body (Grosz, 1992). In addition, the body has been theorized as a locus of social control, principally through the work of Michel Foucault. Foucault introduced the concept of *disciplinary power*. Whereas judicial or legal power is authoritarian and orchestrated, disciplinary power works "from below" to produce and normalize bodies to serve prevailing relations of dominance and subordination. Disciplinary power maintains prevailing forms of selfhood (gender amongst them) via individual surveillance and correction of self to produce the "docile body", so-called because it is regulated by cultural norms (Bordo, 1993). Implied in this are also notions of plasticity or malleability of the human body (including its genital anatomy).

In modern times, disciplinary power operates through preoccupation with bodily appearance, especially for women. Feminist theorists have argued that, within our gender hierarchy, the current preoccupation with bodily appearance affects women more powerfully than men. Self-surveillance for cultural acceptability goes hand in hand with exhausting self-corrective regimens such as dieting, depilation, body building, dressing, cosmetic and, more recently, surgical alterations. According to recent bank surveys, 20% of personal bank loans to women in the UK in recent years were for cosmetic surgery. Appearance industries contribute substantially to our consumerist economy, but unachievable social norms such as "a body that is absolutely tight, contained, bolted down and firm" (Bordo, 1993) render many women psychologically vulnerable, feeling that they are "never good enough". Women's vulnerability increases as societal prescriptions gather pressure. This is thought to represent a backlash against the narrowing of gender power discrepancy in recent times. Women's vulnerability helps to reassert gender configurations against attempts to transform gender hierarchy. One might speculate that masculine and feminine body types will become even more extreme as other gender attributes become more diffuse – a return to the days of Ken and Barbie – as a way of restoring masculine–feminine differential and maintaining distinct the social categories and their attendant power relationship.

Social constructionism represents a paradigm shift in its analysis of normal and deviant sexualities in contemporary society and has much to say about the management of genital ambiguity. Constructivists are critical of mainstream psychology, with many of its theories failing to question in the first place the notion that there is a tidy divide between the two biologically given sexual categories. It is as if there can only be two kinds of person in the natural world, one with female reproductive and sexual capacity, feminine behaviour and a sexual orientation towards men, the other with male reproductive and sexual capacity, masculine behaviour and a sexual orientation towards women. All the attributes – chromosomes, brain, physique, social identity and sexuality – must be congruent and united in being either male or female (Vine, 1993). Most psychologists also tend to hypothesize about the individual psyche and fail to take account of the relationship between body and culture. Rather than look to the brain, childhood experience, or self-esteem in explaining presenting sexuality problems, discursive psychologists are more likely to ask what are the cultural notions of sex that make certain sexuality events taken for granted and others a subject of scrutiny and treatment. The insistence on two sexes has "calamitous personal consequences" for those who present sexual anatomy that fails to be easily distinguished as one biological sex or the other (Chase, 1998). Within a social constructivist framework, experiences of people whose genitalia are not typical of those of their biological sex would not be attributable to their body but to cultural allowances for only certain bodies and sexualities. Within this framework, individual problems and dilemmas are not conceptualized in terms of bodily inadequacies in need of alterations, it is the fact that individuals have to suffer material alterations in order to do "proper" sexuality that will come under scrutiny. Previous psychological studies are criticized for failing to pay attention to the personal meanings of genital ambiguity, the experience of living with it, and how meanings and experiences are produced by dominant discourses of body and sex.

In recent years, John Money has attempted to deconstruct paedophilia (even though he had previously neglected to apply a constructivist framework in the management of genital ambiguity). Since "age of consent" to sexual intimacy can also be said to be a contemporary cultural construction, it too can be deconstructed and with that the concept of "abuse" of the children involved. Ussher (1997b) argues that "such libertarian deconstructions simply do not wash" because there is a power discrepancy in paedophilic practices, that "the majority of adults who engage in such acts use threats or coercion, often leaving the child in a state of shame and self-blame". This argument is strong on moral ground but weak on theoretical ground, because power discrepancy can also be deconstructed, so can shame. As a philosophical framework detached from a humanitarian context, social constructionism can be potentially problematic as well as liberating for the underprivileged.

Social constructionism has been criticized for marginalizing individual corporeality (see *Material–discursive psychology* below). It does not address the dilemmas of clinicians, who are faced with often desperate requests from individuals and families to intervene. Solutions for the individual and for his or her society are conspicuous by their absence in the myriad of books and papers written by constructivist theorists. The less than obvious utility may partly explain why constructivist treatise on gender has remained largely invisible in the scientific community. It is also marginalized in psychology. Gender theorists find this perplexing but fail to ask how they could enable the target community (often clinical disciplines) to take their painstaking analyses more seriously.

Social analysis of the sexual body in contemporary culture is important. But subjective experiences do not reflect body and culture transactions only. They are also interpreted according to the developmental trajectory of the individual within a family system. Without integration with psychological theories, constructivist analysis itself cannot account for the wide variations between the ways in which people in similar social groups drawing from similar discourses might construct similar bodily events differently. In particular, many people are able to resist, challenge and deconstruct cultural ideals while others succumb and remain vulnerable to distress mediated by dominant culture. Finally, social constructivists' own *gazing* and critiquing of mainstream theory and practice relating to sexuality is itself a social practice unique to our culture. Who should analyse this?

Material–discursive psychology

According to discursive analysis, in the process of becoming man or woman, we follow the various scripts of manhood and womanhood that proliferate in our culture, in the form of myths, images, texts, advertisements, conversations. Having to negotiate between the many contradictory representations may render most of us vulnerable towards feelings of a compromised sexuality in certain situations.

At such moments, the usual desire is to repair the damage in order to pass as normal by adopting strategies, not to invite discreditation. The relationship between successful maintenance of "normal" facade and psychological functioning for the individual should not be underestimated. It is corroborated by a recent study of "hirsute" women (Keegan et al., 2003). While the experience of gender incongruence, "freakishness" and shame was salient for all the interviewees, successful concealment of hair growth through depilatory practices enabled the women to pass socially and accounted for the near normative levels of well-being despite a secret sense of shame.

Unlike artists, philosophers or social activists, clinicians have a duty to consider not just symbolic and representational aspects of sexuality events but also the most optimal solution for the individual. Psychological practitioners are presented with subjective feelings of distress that people relate to their corporeality, not just social discourse. The tension between alteration of the material body to pass and deconstruction of the discourses that necessitate such alteration occurs in many areas of clinical practice, and nowhere clearer than in intersex management. Like most individuals, intersex people aspire to be acceptable to society rather than to challenge it, even if it involves taking on medical procedures to achieve corporeal "passing". This is a legitimate desire. However, currently medical practice is not able to deliver "normality" and no technique can reverse intersex or remove the need to give explanations about difference. Can psychology also be part of the solution?

It would seem that a *material–discursive* healthcare psychology may have the potential to offer something useful to individuals and their families as well as to the healthcare system. Whereas medical practice tends to be positioned at the material, reflexive psychological practice must shuffle between material, subjectivity and discourse, to enrich our formulation of individual and systemic events and to maximize opportunities for solutions. Such a framework can help psychologists to be more sceptical of traditional realist theories and practice and to question the legitimacy of expert intervention (our own and by others). It will offer wider scope for creative case-by-case problem solving within our healthcare context. In deconstructing the "deviant" body, problems are externalized and, for many, deconstruction of their deviance can be liberating and material "passing in society" might become less salient. For others, however, the strong desire to continue to hide their difference and to "pass" will not diminish. In order to "normalize" their body to survive in the current – albeit constructed – reality, men and women, boys and girls or their guardians may choose techniques that currently have a limited evidence base. These decisions are legitimate. Sound practice

of healthcare psychology (see *Biopsychosocial framework* above) can facilitate optimal multidisciplinary care for the individual from decision making about treatment through to posttreatment and evaluation.

Materiality of the body is important; it both affords and delimits our interaction with the world and as such goes some way towards shaping our destiny and our identity. In marginalizing the materiality of clients' problems, we risk alienating them. So the scope for social activism in clinical practice remains unclear. Practitioners are not licensed to replace one set of cultural scripts with another, and individuals do not passively follow scripts, they also resist them. Past and new experiences are continuously reinterpreted, by our clients as well as ourselves. This is how discursive psychology arose in the first place. Cocreation of optimal individual solutions will only occur in the context of our commitment to reconcile our critical analyses with a full acknowledgement of the materiality of sexuality events.

Summary

The isolation of the "sex hormones" in the 1920s and 1930s brought with it the optimism that nature was about to reveal its secrets in sex differences. To date psychological research in sex differences has unfolded more questions than answers. Be that as it may, the political implications of naturist research can be significant; misrepresentation and misunderstanding of such research could perpetuate social injustice. For example, men's testosterone-driven, uncontrollable sexual urges have been used to justify rape, and women's inferior share of the economy has been explained on the basis of their innate tendency to domesticity. The argument for naturist research is sometimes based on the optimism that identification of culprit genes and hormones will remove blame from people considered sexual anomalies in society. This naive assumption reflects a failure to appreciate the force of dominant culture. For instance, how likely is it that the discovery of gay genes and brains will make homosexuality more socially acceptable? It is activism that has led to institutional changes relating to homosexuality, not science. A further lesson can be learned from intersex, where biological causes are crystal clear, but stigma remains and legislation to endorse this truly natural variation may be many years away.

Psychologists must evaluate whether a science of sex differences is worth continuing. The argument that certain behaviours are intrinsically masculine or feminine, and that these somehow provide independent criteria for some biological reality known as "masculinity" or "femininity", is tautological. When the criteria of normal masculine and feminine attributes are difficult to define, and the potential of sex hormones to change sexuality events is not well understood, it seems somewhat absurd to diagnose "abnormal" sexuality for men and women, to account for it and to treat it. It reflects a blurring of scientific practice and social convention. The constructs of masculinity and femininity are relational, neither has meaning without the other. Since understanding of masculinity and femininity arises out of understanding of gender relations, psychologists should arguably be more preoccupied with understanding gender relations.

Psychologists within a social learning framework have been quick to expose weaknesses in biological sexual research and to gather counterevidence supporting social causation of gender differences. This type of research is also limited. If masculine and feminine social behaviour is shaped through learning what is allowed and disallowed, encouraged and discouraged, are these behaviours the same thing as sexual partner choice, sexual fantasies and sexual acts? To date, social learning theory has not contributed greatly to our understanding of more complex sexuality events.

Psychological development does not end with the attainment of physical maturity, so sexuality development continues throughout life. Revisionist psychoanalytic theories, detached from the delimiting orthodoxy and preoccupation with "pathologies", have contributed to interesting accounts of the precarious sexual subject. However, most psychological theories have failed to question the imperatives of sex. In order to do so, some psychologists have moved beyond the individual focus. Instead they analyse what experts do.

Research and treatment of sexuality events is an act unique to our culture, we may well ask why some questions are asked and resources are given to answer them but not others, or why modify the person instead of educating the public towards greater tolerance? Other questions that arise are how would such actions change or maintain the social status quo and which social groups would benefit the most or the least from biological or cultural evidence for sexuality development. We have known for some time about the common initial developmental pathways of all individuals and the anatomical continuities between male and female external and internal sex organs; it is interesting that researchers have focused on resultant sexuality differences rather than similarities. The psychology of sex of rearing has been used to support phallocentric infant sex assignment, but it would seem that this practice is continuing, even though its supporting psychology is now in disrepute.

In our capacity as researchers, we need to be careful not to pander to cultural mandates that might disadvantage certain social groups. In formulating our research questions and clinical practice relating to atypical physicosexual development, we need to be mindful of heterosexist imperatives. It is heterosexist ideology within our culture that requires two oppositional sexual categories, their certification through acceptable frequency and duration of genital intercourse, and the capacity for procreation, preferably in the context of a state-registered union. In the absence of such imperatives, concepts such as male, female, intersexuality, lesbianism, fertility and marriage are less important. It is these powerful social scripts that produce distress in persons with nonnormative physicosexual development, not their body per se.

The separation of masculinity from femininity, homosexuality from heterosexuality, normal from abnormal have not been fruitful in psychology, neither has it been neutral, objective and value-free as claimed. Sexuality is not static but changes throughout our lifespan against a cultural context, so perhaps events are not so stable and discrete as imagined. They are also not understandable without relating to social discourse. The value of future psychological research will depend on our capacity to highlight some of these processes, to induct diverse and dynamic subjectivities, rather than deduct from preconceived, static, "objective" categories. The relevance of any new psychological knowledge of sexuality will rest with our success in cocreating with our informants interpretative rather than universal sexualities.

Box 8.1 Key points

1. It remains equivocal to what extent sexuality has its origins in the brain hardwired by the hormonal environment during fetal life. The transitory effects of the "sex hormones" for activating sexual events also appear to be variable in the research literature.
2. Family attitude and behaviour, influenced by the wider culture, are a major factor in the child's interpretation of masculine and feminine roles and on their gender development. But this alone cannot fully address the more complex and dynamic aspects of sexuality.
3. Psychology has been criticised for its inadequate conceptualisation of cultural factors. The neglect of cultural analysis is clear in the sex of rearing approach, which owes its impact not so much to empirical evidence but to its resonance with discourses of sexual dimorphism and with cultural conflation of penis size and masculinity.

4. It was Freud who first made gender development crudely derivative of penis presence and absence. But Freud was also clear that all human beings have a bisexual potential and emphasised the precarious rather than fixed nature of sexuality, development of which is characterised by conflict.

5. The majority of researchers and clinicians do not examine how their own ideological standpoint might have influenced the theories or therapies that they develop, how they might have been inadvertently engaged in the social regulation and control of the body without awareness of the dominant discourses that influence their thinking and action. Social constructionism, developed outside psychology by postmodernist philosophers, provides a framework for challenging traditional knowledge claims. The framework enables the development of research methods that examine subjective accounts of sexuality. Future development of sexuality theories will benefit from our capacity to deal with diverse and subjective accounts constructed within a cultural context; psychological know-how in stewing complex phenomena down to a minimum number of static categories will not be enough.

3. Our understanding of masculinity and femininity arises out of our understanding of gender relations, so perhaps it is gender relations that form a more strategic focus for psychological research and practice.

4. Sexuality development does not end with maturation of our sexual anatomy but continues through our lifespan. Rather than developing static categories to capture people's experiences, clinicians and researchers may need to be more reflexive in the formulation of research questions, clinical problems and solutions.

5. Sexuality is not understandable without relating to discourse, but discursive theories have few practical solutions to offer individuals. These debates create considerable tension between traditional medical practice of altering the material body to fit with dominant culture, and deconstruction of the discourses that necessitate such action. A material-discursive health care psychology may offer broader based knowledge and skills to co-create with colleagues and patients richer formulations of "clinical" problems and optimal individual solutions.

Box 8.2 Points for practice

1. There is always an ideology underlying research and practice. In investigating and treating aspects of sexuality, we especially need to be conscious of the ways in which our thinking and action are mediated by dominant discourses of sex and gender which privilege some groups and disadvantage others. We need to be aware of how our actions might change or maintain the social status quo, what things might we be perpetuating and which sections of society will gain or lose as a result.

2. In scrutinising the sexuality of people with non-normative physico-sexual development, we may have to pay more attention to the way in which our own practice such as the treatment choices we offer, the language we use and our silence might themselves lead to some of the negative effects we observe in patients with stigmatising diagnoses. The way in which we "contaminate" our own observations may render any observed difference un-interpretable.

REFERENCES

*Indicates key references.

Adelson J (1980). *Handbook of Adolescent Psychology*. Wiley, New York.

Alexander G A, Hines M (1994). Gender labels and play styles: their relative contributions to children's selection of playmates. *Child Dev* 65, 869–879.

Alexander G A, Sherwin B B, Bancroft J, Davidson D (1990). Testosterone and sexual behaviour in oral contraceptive users and non-users. *Horm Behav* 24, 388–402.

Baill C, Money J (1980). Physiological aspects of Female Sexual Development. In. *Women's Sexual Development*, Kirkpatrick M ed., pp. 45–59. Plenum Press, New York.

Bancroft J (1988). Sexual desire and the brain. *Sex Marital Ther* 3, 11–27.

   (1989). *Human Sexuality and its Problems*, 2nd edn. Churchill Livingstone, London.

Bem S L (1993). *The Lenses of Gender*. Yale University Press, London.

Bordo S (1993). *Unbearable Weight: Feminism, Western Culture and the Body*, p. 190. University of California Press, London.

Boyle M (1993). Sexual dysfunction or heterosexual dysfunction? *Feminism Psychol* 3, 73–88.

Cassileth B R, Lusk K E J, Strouse T B et al. (1984). Psychological status in chronic illness. *N Engl J Med* 311, 506–511.

Chadwick P M, Liao L M, Boyle M, Conway G S (2002). Size matters: fallacies about men presenting atypical genito-sexual development. *Proceedings of the British Psychological Society Division of Health Psychology Annual Conference*, Sheffield, UK.

Chase C (1998). Hermaphrodites with attitude: mapping the emergence of intersex political activism. *GLQ: J Lesbian Gay Studies*, 4, 189–211.

Colapinto J (2000). *As Nature Made Him: The Boy Who was Raised as a Girl*. Quartet Books, London.

*Collaer M L, Hines M (1995). Human behavioural sex differences: a role for gonadal hormones during early development. *Psychol Bull* 118, 55–107.

Condry J, Condry S (1976). Sex differences: a study of the eye of the beholder. *Child Dev* 47, 812–819.

Connell R W (1995). *Masculinities*, pp. 8, 10. Polity Press, London.

Dabbs J M, Mohammad S (1992). Male and female salivary testosterone concentrations before and after sexual activity. *Physiol Behav* 52, 195–197.

de Beauvoir S (1949; reprinted 1972). *The Second Sex*. Penguin, Harmondsworth, UK.

Diamond M (1965). A critical evaluation of the ontogeny of human sexual behaviour. *Q Rev Biol* 10, 147–175.

(2000). Sex and gender: same or different? *Femin Psychol* 10, 46–54.

Dittman R W, Kappes M E, Kappes M H (1992). Sexual behaviour in adolescent and adult females with congenital adrenal hyperplasia. *Psychoneuroendocrinology* 17, 153–170.

Downey J, Ehrhardt A A, Schiffman I, Dyrenfurth I, Becher J (1987). Sex hormones in lesbian and heterosexual women. *Horm Behav* 21, 347–357.

Doyle J (2002). Intersex women: male partner's perspective. PhD Thesis, University of East London.

Ehrhardt A A, Evers K, Money J (1968). Influence of androgen and some aspects of sexually dimorphic behaviour in women with the late treated adrenogenital syndrome. *Johns Hopkins Med J* 123, 115–122.

Engel G L (1977). The need for a new medical model: a challenge for biomedicine. *Science*, 196, 129–136.

Frisch H L (1977). Sex stereotypes in adult–infant play. *Child Dev* 48, 1671–1675.

Gergen K J (1985). The social constructionist movement in modern society. *Am Psychol* 40, 266–275.

Goldner V (1991). Toward a critical relational theory of gender. *Psychoanal Dialogue* 1, 249–272.

Grosz E (1992). Inscriptions and body maps: representations on the corporeal. In *Feminine/Masculine and Representation*, Threadgold T, Cranny-Francis A, eds., pp. 62–74. Allen and Unwin, Sydney, Australia.

Hegarty P (1997). Materializing the hypothalamus: a performative account of the 'gay brain'. *Femin Psychol* 7, 355–372.

(2000). Intersex activism, feminism and psychology: opening a dialogue on theory, research and clinical practice. *Femin Psychol* 10, 117–132.

Hines M, Kaufman F R (1994). Androgens and the development of sex-typical behaviour: rough-and-tumble play and sex of preferred playmates in children with congenital adrenal hyperplasia. *Child Dev* 65, 1042–1053.

Horney K (1932). The dread of woman: observations on a specific difference in the dread felt by men and by women respectively for the opposite sex. *Int J Psychoanal*, 13, 348–360.

Jahoda M (1977). *Freud and the Dilemmas of Psychology*, pp. 73–75. Hogarth Press, London.

Keegan A, Liao L M, Boyle M (2003). Hirsutism: a psychological analysis. *J Health Psychol*, 8, 311–329.

*Kessler S J (1998). *Lessons from the Intersexed*, p. 15. Rutgers University Press, New Brunswick, NJ.

Kessler S J, McKenna W (1978). *Gender: An Ethnomethodological Approach*. Wiley, New York.

Kline P (1972). *Fact and Fantasy in Freudian Theory*, p. 6. Methuen, London.

Lamb M E (1981). *The Role of the Father in Child Development*. Wiley, New York.

Le Vay S (1996). *Queer Science: The Use and Abuse of Research into Homosexuality*. MIT Press, Cambridge, MA.

Liao L M (2003). Learning to assist women born with atypical genitalia: journey through ignorance, taboo and dilemmas. *J Reprod Infant Psychol Special Issue*, 21, 226–236.

May B (1998). *Psychosocial outcome in women with congenital adrenal hyperplasia*. PhD Thesis, University of London.

May B, Boyle M, Grant D (1996). A comparative study of sexual experiences: women with diabetes and women with congenital adrenal hyperplasia due to 21-hydroxylase deficiency. *J Health Psychol* 1, 479–492.

Meyer-Bahlburg H, Ehrhardt A A, Rosen L et al. (1984). Psychosexual milestones in women prenatally exposed to diethylstilbestrol. *Horm Behav* 18, 359–366.

Minto C L, Liao L M, Conway G S, Creighton S M (2003a). Complete androgen insensitivity syndrome and sexual function. *Fertil Steril*, 80, 157–164.

Minto C L, Liao L M, Woodhouse C R, Ransley P, Creighton S (2003b). Adult outcomes of childhood clitoral surgery for ambiguous genitalia. *Lancet*, 361, 1252–1257.

Money J, Clopper R R (1975). Post-pubertal psychosexual function in post-surgical male hypopituitarism. *J Sex Res* 11, 22–38.

Money J, Ehrhardt A A (1972). *Man and Woman, Boy and Girl: The Differentiation and Dimorphism of Gender Identity from Conception to Maturity*, p. 153. Johns Hopkins University Press, Baltimore, MD.

Money J, Schwatz M (1977). Dating, romantic and non-romantic friendships and sexuality in 17 early-treated adrenogenital females aged 16–25. In *Congenital Adrenal Hyperplasia*, Leep P A, Plotnick L P, Kowarsi A A, Migeon C J, eds., pp. 419–431. University Park Press, London.

Money J, Hampson J G, Hampson J L (1957). Imprinting and the establishment of gender role. *Arch Neurol Psychiatry* 77, 333–336.

Money J, Clopper R R, Menefee J (1980). Psychosexual development in post-pubertal males with idiopathic panhypopituitarism. *J Sex Res* 16, 212–225.

Money J, Mazur T, Abrams C, Norman B F (1981). Micropenis, family mental health, and neonatal management: a report on 14 patients reared as girls. *J Prevent Psychiatry* 1, 17–27.

Money J, Lehne G K, Pierre-Jerome F (1985). Micropenis: gender, erotosexual coping strategy and behavioural health in nine paediatric cases followed to adulthood. *Compr Psychiatry* 26, 29–42.

Mulaikal R M, Migeon C J, Rock J A (1987). Fertility rates in female patients with congenital adrenal hyperplasia due to 21-hydroxylase deficiency. *N Engl J Med* 316, 178–182.

Nolan T, Pless I B (1986). Emotional correlates and consequences of birth defects. *J Paediatr* 109, 201–216.

Petersen A C, Taylor B (1980). The biological approach to adolescence: biological change and psychological adaptation. In *Handbook of Adolescent Psychology*, Adelson J, ed., pp. 286–290. Wiley, New York.

Rebelsky F, Hanks C (1971). Fathers' verbal interaction with infants in the first three months of life. *Child Dev* 42, 63–68.

Reilly J M, Woodhouse C R (1989). Small penis and the male sex role. *J Urol* 142, 569–571.

Rekers G A (1992). Development of problems of puberty and sex roles in adolescence. In *Handbook of Clinical Child Psychology*, 2nd edn, Walker C E, Roberts M C, eds., pp. 607–622. Wiley, New York.

*Sarafino E P (2001). *Health Psychology: Biopsychosocial Interactions*, 3rd edn. Wiley, New York.

Slijper F (1984). Androgens and gender role behaviour in girls with congenital adrenal hyperplasia (CAH). In *Progress in Brain Research*, Vol. 61, de Vries G J, de Bruin J P C, eds., pp. 417–433. Elsevier, Amsterdam.

Smith C, Lloyd B B (1978). Maternal behaviour and perceived sex of infant. *Child Dev* 49, 1263–1265.

Snow M E, Jacklin C N, Maccoby E E (1983). Sex-of-child differences in father interaction at one year of age. *Child Dev* 54, 227–232.

Ussher J M (1997a). Framing the sexual 'other': the regulation of lesbian and gay sexuality. In *Body Talk: The Material and Discursive Regulation of Sexuality, Madness and Reproduction*, Ussher J M, ed., pp. 131–138. Routledge, London.

*Ussher J M (ed.) (1997b). *Body Talk: The Material and Discursive Regulation of Sexuality, Madness and Reproduction*, p. 6. Routledge, London.

Ussher J M (1997c). Introduction: towards a material-discursive analysis of madness, sexuality and reproduction. In *Body Talk: The Material and Discursive Regulation of Sexuality, Madness and Reproduction*, Ussher JM ed., p. 142. Routledge, London.

Van Seters A P, Slob A K (1988). Mutually gratifying heterosexual relationship with micropenis of husband. *J Sex Marital Ther* 14, 98–107.

Vine G (1993). *Raging Hormones: Do They Rule Our Lives?* p. 95. Virago Press, London.

Wilson B E, Reiner W G (1998). Management of intersex: a shifting paradigm. *J Clin Ethics*, 9, 360–369.

*Yardley L (1999). Introducing material-discursive approaches to health and illness. In *Material Discourses of Health and Illness*, Yardley L, ed., pp. 1–24. Routledge, London.

Part II

Management of developmental abnormalities of the genital tract

9

Management of ambiguous genitalia at birth

Gary L. Warne

Royal Children's Hospital, Parkville, Victoria, Australia

About 1 in every 4000 infants is born with ambiguous genitalia (Hamerton et al., 1975). This event creates tremendous anxiety for the parents. Any health professionals involved in caring for them and the baby at the delivery will be immediately placed under great pressure to sort things out quickly. Under these circumstances, decision making is stressful, particularly for staff who are unprepared and inexperienced, and stress can increase the risk of mistakes. This chapter is intended to provide health professionals with clear guidelines on how best to proceed. The management of ambiguous genitalia at birth involves management of the medical condition in the infant and also management of the distressed parents, who become patients themselves. A team approach is required to provide the range of professional skills needed (medical, surgical, nursing and mental health) and the best team members for this situation are those with very good communication skills as well as clinical acumen.

Genitalia are "ambiguous" when they have an atypical appearance and no one in the room can decide if the baby is male or female. The phallus looks too small to be a penis and too large to be a clitoris. The urethra is malpositioned in relation to the size of the phallus, being usually on the shaft of the phallus or in the perineum. If there is a vagina, it may open into a urogenital sinus, so that there is only a single orifice. The extent of fusion between the genital folds may be intermediate between what is expected for a girl and what is expected for a boy. The skin of the genital folds may be rather rugose. Gonads may or may not be palpable in the genital folds.

"Ambiguous genitalia" or "hypospadias"?

There is a certain amount of subjectivity in saying whether or not genitalia are ambiguous. In any particular case, one doctor might declare that a baby is a boy with hypospadias (implying that gender is clear, no investigation is necessary and surgery will completely overcome all difficulties in due course), while another may say that the sex is unclear because the genitalia are ambiguous. In the latter, the parents would be made more anxious, referral to a specialist team would be more likely to be made and many costly investigations would be recommended. There would be discussions about what the sex should be. So why is the distinction between hypospadias and ambiguous genitalia important? It is important because of the serious nature of the underlying medical conditions that can cause genitalia to be ambiguous. These conditions include many that can cause significant morbidity and even death. They can cause acute metabolic derangement (salt-wasting forms of congenital adrenal hyperplasia (CAH)), gonadal cancer (as in XY gonadal dysgenesis), arterial hypertension (as in some adrenal enzyme defects), disordered skeletal growth (CAH) and infertility. There may be genetic implications for the extended family and future offspring. Accurate diagnosis is, therefore, very important.

If an infant has an ectopic urethral orifice (hypospadias), there are a number of *additional* features that should prompt referral to an endocrinologist for further investigation. They are:

Paediatric and Adolescent Gynaecology, ed. Adam Balen et al. Published by Cambridge University Press.
© Cambridge University Press 2004.

97

- perineal hypospadias (more likely to be part of a wider developmental defect)
- a dysmorphic facial appearance (suggesting a possible chromosomal anomaly)
- hypoplasia of the phallus
- one or more undescended testes
- growth retardation (either intrauterine or postnatal)
- other congenital malformations.

Causes of ambiguous genitalia

The following classification of causes of ambiguous genitalia is based on knowing the sex chromosome karyotype. In this classification, the author has deliberately avoided the use of older terms such as male pseudohermaphrodite and female pseudohermaphrodite because these terms are unacceptable to parents. Simple descriptive terms are preferred.

46,XX karyotype

Within the normal female karyotype:
- virilizing forms of CAH
  - 21-hydroxylase deficiency
  - 11β-hydroxylase deficiency
  - 3β-hydroxysteroid dehydrogenase deficiency
- a virilizing condition in the mother or side effect of a maternally ingested drug
- placental aromatase deficiency
- true hermaphroditism.

46,XY karyotype

Within the normal male karyotype:
- partial gonadal dysgenesis, including true hermaphroditism
  - single gene mutations: *SRY, WT1, SF1, SOX9, XH2*
  - duplication of *DAX1*
  - chromosomal deletion (9p, 10q)
- a defect in testosterone biosynthesis
  - 17β-hydroxysteroid dehydrogenase deficiency
  - 3β-hydroxysteroid dehydrogenase deficiency
  - 17α-hydroxylase deficiency
  - lipoid adrenal hyperplasia
- androgen insensitivity
  - androgen receptor gene mutation (complete or partial androgen insensitivity syndrome [CAIS or PAIS, respectively])
  - 5α-reductase deficiency
- Leydig cell hypoplasia caused by a mutation in the gene for the luteinizing hormone receptor or by congenital hypopituitarism.

Abnormal karyotype

Abnormal karyotype includes mosaicism and aneuploidy:
- partial gonadal dysgenesis, including true hermaphroditism.

Clinical assessment of the infant

Full examination

Usually the ambiguity of the genitalia is noticed as soon as the baby is born, but more subtle anatomical variations may go unnoticed for some time. In resource-poor countries, the birth may occur at home or in a village health station with no doctor or nurse in attendance. In such cases, the significance of atypical genitalia may be overlooked for weeks or months and the underlying condition causing the ambiguity may run a longer course than would be the case in another medical setting. By the time the baby is brought for assessment, its general health may have deteriorated severely. Therefore, before the genital appearance becomes the complete focus of the examination, the baby should be given a full examination looking for signs of illness and for associated congenital abnormalities. The following features need to be carefully considered:
- illness: poor feeding, vomiting, poor tone, dehydration, low blood pressure (all suggestive of adrenal insufficiency and salt-wasting)
- signs of hypoglycaemia associated with adrenal insufficiency (jitteriness, seizures, coma)
- hyperpigmentation of the skin induced by adrenocorticotrophic hormone, associated with adrenal insufficiency
- facial and other features of Turner's syndrome associated with a chromosomal abnormality (downturned angles of the mouth, webbing of the neck, high-arched palate, deformities of the external ear, epicanthic folds, strabismus, heart murmur, absent femoral pulses, hypoplasia of nails, peripheral oedema)
- skeletal anomalies associated with a dysmorphic syndrome such as campomelic dysplasia (short, bowed tibiae and other long bones).

Inspection of the genitalia

Inspection of the genitalia should include:
- The genital folds
  - symmetrical or asymmetrical (presence of a gonad on one side will make for asymmetry)
  - colour of the skin: daylight is best for determining the presence or absence of subtle hyperpigmentation, looking for evidence of CAH

Table 9.1. Clinical features of causes of ambiguous genitalia

Clinical feature	XY gonadal dysgenesis	Congenital adrenal hyperplasia (21-hydroxylase deficiency)	Androgen insensitivity	Defect in testosterone biosynthesis (17β-hydroxysteroid dehydrogenase deficiency)
Pattern of inheritance	Usually sporadic	Autosomal recessive	X-linked	Autosomal recessive
Dysmorphic	+/−	−	−	−
Gonad(s) palpable	+	−	+	+
Systemic illness	−	+/−	−	−
Hyperpigmentation	−	+	−	−
Genital asymmetry	+	−	−	−
Uterus present	+ (75%)	+	−	−

- —skin texture: rugosity suggests exposure to androgens
- —is there posterior fusion: fusion of the genital folds is also an androgen effect
- the phallus
  - —the length and breadth of the phallus should be measured and recorded
  - —erectile tissue should be detected by palpation
- position of all orifices should be determined and recorded on a diagram: pulling the genital folds towards the examiner allows a single perineal orifice to be converted into a funnel and it may be possible to see that there are two passages opening into a urogenital sinus
- the gonads should be palpated carefully along the inguinal region starting from the anterior superior iliac spine to assess
  - —the number that can be palpated
  - —the size, shape, consistency (normal, hard, soft, homogeneous or formed from more than one component)
  - —the position (record on a diagram)
- the presence or absence of a uterus should be determined by
  - —rectal examination (only in a term infant and if the examiner's fifth finger is slender enough): the uterus can readily be palpated in the midline behind the pubis
  - —pelvic ultrasound
  - —pelvic magnetic resonance imaging.

History

Essential information from the history would include:
- any family history
  - —CAH is autosomal recessive
  - —PAIS is X-linked
  - —XY gonadal dysgenesis is usually sporadic
- medications the mother took during the pregnancy
  - —babies with ambiguous genitalia have been born to mothers treated with progestins for threatened abortion

- —antiandrogens such as cyproterone or spironolactone may prevent complete masculinization in a male fetus
  - —cytotoxic drugs
- any changes experienced by the mother during pregnancy suggesting virilization (deepening of the voice, temporal hair loss, acne, enlargement of the clitoris)
  - —placental aromatase deficiency allows fetal adrenal androgens to cross the placenta and virilize both mother and fetus
  - —mothers with poorly controlled CAH.

Collation and interpretation of the clinical information

Table 9.1 lists the clinical features associated with some causes of ambiguous genitalia.

Investigation strategy

The following investigations should be made.
1. Urgent serum 17-hydroxyprogesterone measurement *in patients with clinical features suggestive of CAH.* This investigation is not needed if a gonad can be palpated because 21-hydroxylase deficiency only virilizes genetic females and they do not have palpable gonads.
2. Urine collection (preferably 24 hour but a shorter period (4–6 hours) may provide a useful result) for steroid analysis to detect an enzyme defect.
3. Urgent DNA analysis by fluorescent in situ hybridization (FISH) to detect Y chromosome sequences.
4. Karyotyping.
5. Pelvic ultrasound to define
   - presence of uterus
   - presence and location of gonads.
6. Further studies to define anatomy
   - urogenital sinugram
   - cystoscopy performed by a paediatric urologist
   - in selected cases, laparoscopy and gonadal biopsy.

7. Serial urine tests for albumin over the first 3 months in patients with XY gonadal dysgenesis. Where there is a mutation in *WT1*, there is a risk of associated glomerulosclerosis, Wilms' tumour, or both (Denys–Drash syndrome) (McTaggart et al., 2001).

Medical management

Any infant with ambiguous genitalia should be assumed to have salt-wasting CAH until proven otherwise.

Overall, approximately 40–50% of infants with ambiguous genitalia have CAH (most of the rest have gonadal dysgenesis). The clinician who makes this assumption will be on the lookout for signs of impending adrenal crisis or other metabolic disturbance such as hypoglycaemia. Vomiting and dehydration owing to salt wasting are not usually evident until the second week of life or later, although lack of interest in feeding may appear in week 1. Hypoglycaemia, however, may occur in the first hours or days of life in infants with CAH. Monitoring of blood glucose is important in these infants and intravenous glucose can be given to control hypoglycaemia pending the results of investigations to establish the diagnosis. Serum electrolytes start to become abnormal (as indicated by a rising potassium level) towards the end of the first week, by which time the diagnosis of CAH will usually have been made. Once a firm diagnosis of CAH has been made, oral hydrocortisone (15–20 mg/m² per day) combined with fludrocortisone 0.1 mg/day is appropriate in the absence of vomiting. For a vomiting infant, intravenous glucose, saline and hydrocortisone should be given.

Infants with ambiguous genitalia and palpable gonad(s) usually prove to have a positive FISH test for Y chromosome sequences. The chances of the infants becoming acutely ill are much smaller than in the XX group, in that the enzyme defects that may be responsible are rare and only three of these rare defects are associated with adrenal impairment.

Psychological support for the parents

A group of parents was interviewed by two social workers (Elizabeth Loughlin and Margaret Sahhar, unpublished) in the author's clinic in the mid-1980s. The parents were asked to recall what had been said to them following the birth of their baby with ambiguous genitalia, and by whom. What parents found most difficult to cope with was:

- being given conflicting information about the baby's sex and the prognosis by different staff members
- staff who were clearly unprepared to deal with the situation and who could not control their own emotions
- poor communication from staff about what was happening in the first few hours (one mother thought her baby had died because the baby was taken away and no one said anything for hours)
- lack of specific counselling on how to deal with friends and relatives: it is difficult if they feel the need to keep certain facts a secret from loved ones
- the strong emotions they were feeling at the time: more help in dealing with these would have been appreciated.

Parents need to be told that the baby appears healthy but that there is a problem deciding about the gender. Showing the baby to the parents will give them the chance to see this for themselves and they will be more accepting. Both parents should be counselled together. They will be grateful to hear that there are other babies with the same condition and that there are a number of well-known and *treatable* medical conditions that can cause genitalia to look atypical. They should be told that an expert in such conditions will be called in without delay and should be given reassurance that a good outcome can be anticipated. They will want to know how long the process of investigation will take and who will be involved. A clinical pathway prepared for them, giving appointment times and names of people who will be seeing them, will be helpful. They may need to be told the same things several times before they fully absorb what is being said. They should ideally be referred to an experienced mental health professional (social worker or psychologist) whose role will be to assist them to understand and work through their intense emotions. These emotions may include guilt, shame, grief for the loss of the "normal" child, anxiety about other people's reactions, and anger. Where appropriate, they can be offered the chance to meet other parents who have been through the same experience. They will be glad to know that support groups exist to help people like them. They may be worried about the future sexual identity and sexual orientation of their child and may be glad to talk about these fears. They will want support when it comes to facing their own friends and relatives. Should they tell other people or keep the nature of the baby's condition a secret? Some people find it easy to be open while others do not. Either way, they need to talk about which words they can use and to feel that there is someone they can talk to along the way as the week progresses.

Gender assignment

Gender assignment is a profoundly difficult area because, sooner or later, it is likely that the patient will require surgery to make the genitalia look either male or female. An intense debate about the timing of surgery is taking place, with some patient advocacy organizations and clinicians opposing early surgery (Diamond and Sigmundson, 1997). The former patients who oppose early surgery do so because they are unhappy with their own outcome following surgery. Some are unhappy in the gender assigned to them when they were infants, and many also claim to derive little or no enjoyment from their sexual relationships. Many doctors, however, remain unconvinced that children would benefit from having their genital surgery delayed. The following observations are relevant to the debate.

- With few exceptions, genetic females with 21-hydroxylase deficiency CAH grow up content with their female gender identity (van der Kamp and Slijper, 1996).
- Women with 21-hydroxylase deficiency CAH have ovaries and a uterus and are fertile, provided they take their hormone replacement therapy and have regular monitoring.
- There are medical benefits from early surgery for patients who have a urine-storing vagina and recurrent urinary tract infections. Division of fused labia in these patients allows the free passage of urine onto the perineum and further urinary infections are prevented (De Jong and Boemers, 1995).
- Although there are some isolated reports of a successful psychosexual outcome in people who have grown to adulthood with ambiguous genitalia, their numbers are unclear, their case histories have not been well documented, and the medical profession remains unconvinced that it is reasonable, let alone best, to ask a child to grow up with ambiguous genitalia and make a decision about surgery for him/herself. Observations made by the author in India and Vietnam (unpublished) suggest that most children who grow up with ambiguous genitalia because surgery was not available are miserable and that they suffer discrimination and abuse on a daily basis.
- Long-term follow-up studies of patients with XY gonadal dysgenesis and PAIS show that most are satisfied with their assigned gender, whether male or female (Wisniewski et al., 2001). This is not to deny their psychosexual difficulties and their need for help in dealing with them. Many factors influence the psychological outcome in people whose parents were perhaps traumatized and inadequately counselled, and whose endocrine management may not have been optimal.
- There are objective reasons why patients being treated with genital surgery now should expect a better outcome than patients treated 20–30 years ago. Clitoral surgery has clearly improved. (Removal was the norm

until the mid-1960s. Later operations often led to severe pain, intra-operative haemorrhage, and an avascular glans. Better operations were developed in the late 1970s.) In addition, better criteria for evaluation of outcomes have been developed, and counselling methods have improved.

For all of these reasons, the author advocates continuation of the practice of early surgery, particularly for girls with CAH in view of their fertility. Gender assignment is more problematic when the patient has no chance of fertility. This is the case for almost all conditions that cause ambiguous genitalia except CAH and a few cases of true hermaphroditism. In patients who cannot possibly be fertile, gender is usually assigned according to the appearance of the external genitalia. If the phallus looks like a penis, the child will most likely be raised male, especially if a palpable gonad is present and there is no uterus. If the child has a uterus, no testes and a small phallus looking more like a clitoris, the female gender will usually be selected. However, it is essential that all major centres should carry out long-term follow-up studies on their patient populations, preferably in collaboration with patient advocacy organizations, so that their concerns can be taken into account. Parents do have the legal right to decide about genital surgery if in their opinion and in the opinion of the responsible medical practitioner the benefits of operating outweigh the risks, and they have been fully informed about these risks.

Gonadectomy for prevention of cancer

In patients with gonadal dysgenesis, ambiguous genitalia and Y chromosome sequences, the risk of seminoma is high. On the basis of that, it has been accepted dogma that dysgenetic gonads should be excised during childhood. Parents are often reluctant to allow this to be carried out when they have elected to raise the child as a boy. In these boys, the gonads, although dysgenetic, may produce enough testosterone to make hormone replacement therapy unnecessary. It is a significant benefit not to require testosterone injections or implants for life, and the cost saving is also considerable.

What are the facts?

In dysgenetic gonads, seminoma is preceded by a premalignant condition, gonadoblastoma. Gonadoblastoma occurs in 55% of gonads in partial XY gonadal dysgenesis and in 30–66% of gonads of females with complete XY gonadal dysgenesis (Gourlay et al., 1994; Sultana et al., 1995). All gonadoblastomas are believed to progress eventually to seminoma, but the age at which this occurs is unclear. The actual risk of cancer during childhood and adolescence has not been accurately defined. Seminoma has a 95% 5-year survival with current modes of treatment (Power et al., 2001). If a patient at risk of seminoma was under appropriate medical surveillance (meaning palpation of the gonads by an experienced practitioner every 6–12 months), the treatment for a seminoma that did develop would be surgery alone. Based on this, a case can be made for *not* excising the gonads, provided that the patient is compliant and under optimal long-term surveillance. Where these are not present, gonadectomy and hormone replacement therapy should be advised.

If dysgenetic gonads are not excised, they should always be biopsied. Gonads containing gonadoblastoma should be excised and others left until puberty, when a second biopsy should be done. It is important to understand that, when one gonad is clearly dysgenetic and the other is not, the risk of cancer applies equally to the better-differentiated gonad. A well-differentiated testis does not develop gonadoblastoma; instead, it may develop carcinoma in situ (Ramani et al., 1993). The risk of cancer in other conditions, such as PAIS, testicular enzyme defects and 5α-reductase deficiency, is much lower than the risk in XY gonadal dysgenesis and is probably negligible before adulthood. In true hermaphroditism, the risk of gonadal cancer is low in the 75% who are 46,XX and higher in the testes of those who have a Y chromosome.

Gonadectomy to remove source of testosterone

Often the reason for wanting to remove gonads has less to do with the risk of cancer and more to do with the risk that the gonads will secrete an unwanted hormone, testosterone. Testosterone will definitely be unwanted once the decision has been made to raise the child as a girl. If the gonads are left in and testosterone levels are outside the normal female range, virilization of the genitalia and other parts of the body will progress. However, surgery is not the only way of preventing testosterone secretion: treatment with a gonadotrophin-releasing hormone analogue could achieve the same result.

Informed consent for genital surgery and gonadectomy

Parents are entitled to be informed about the material risks faced by their child if surgery is carried out. These risks,

which are additional to the usual risks of surgery and anaesthesia, are:
- a risk (considered to be very small) that the child will one day want to be the opposite sex to that assigned, because of hormonal effects on the developing brain
- the risk that the person having the surgery might be dissatisfied in adult life with the sexual function and sensitivity of the genitalia
- the risk that removing the only source of testosterone could be regretted, if the child subsequently wanted to be a boy rather than a girl.

The parents should be informed that some patients who are now adult are advocating postponement of surgery, even if the local medical team does not agree with this policy. Furthermore, parents should be advised that they may defer the decision about surgery if they so desire and that their child can continue to receive the best care available regardless of the parents' choice. Doctors should stop advising parents that the need to remove gonads is urgent and that there is an imminent risk of cancer, when this is not the case. Parents can be allowed time to think. Similarly, an honest and ethical approach demands that doctors should tell parents what the real indication for removing gonads is; if the real reason is to prevent testosterone secretion rather than to prevent cancer, then that should be made very clear.

None of the above is intended to discourage clinicians from advising gonadectomy when it is clearly needed. It is simply arguing for a more honest and ethical approach to the process of obtaining informed consent.

REFERENCES

De Jong T P V M, Boemers M L (1995). Neonatal management of female intersex by clitorovaginoplasty. *J Urol* 154, 830–832.

Diamond M, Sigmundson H K (1997). Management of intersexuality. Guidelines for dealing with persons with ambiguous genitalia. *Arch Pediatr Adol Med* 151, 1046–1050.

Gourlay W A, Johnson H W, Pantzar J T M, McGillivray B, Crawford R, Nielson W R (1994). Gonadal tumors in disorders of sexual differentiation. *Urology* 43, 537–540.

Hamerton J L, Canning N, Ray M, Smith S (1975). A cytogenetic survey of 14 069 newborn infants. I. Incidence of chromosome abnormalities. *Clini Genet* 8, 223–243.

McTaggart S J, Algar E, Chow C W, Powell H R, Jones C L (2001). Clinical spectrum of Denys–Drash and Frasier syndrome. *Pediatr Nephrol* 16, 335–339.

Power D A, Brown R S D, Brock C S, Payne H A, Majeed A, Babb P (2001). Trends in testicular carcinoma in England and Wales, 1971–99. *Br J Urol Int* 87, 361–365.

Sultana R, Myerson D, Disteche CM (1995). In situ hybridization analysis of the Y chromosome in gonadoblastoma. *Genes Chromosome Cancer* 13, 257–262.

Ramani P, Yeung CK, Habeebu SS (1993). Testicular intratubular germ cell neoplasia in children and adults with intersex. *Am J Surg Pathol* 17, 1124–1133.

van der Kamp HJ, Slijper FME (1996). The quality of life in adult female patients with congenital adrenal hyperplasia: a comprehensive study of the impact of genital malformations and chronic disease on female patients life. *Eur J Pediatr* 155, 620–621.

Wisniewski AB, Migeon CJ, Gearhart JP, Meyer-Bahlburg HFL, Berkovitz GD, Rock JA (2001). Partial androgen insensitivity syndrome (PAIS) and partial gonadal dysgenesis: long-term medical, surgical and psychological outcome of patients reared male or female. *Pediatr Res* 49 (Part 3), 51A.

10

Imaging of the female pelvis in the evaluation of developmental anomalies

Christopher Schelvan[1], Margaret A. Hall-Craggs[1] and Rose de Bruyn[2]

[1]UCH Hospital Trusts, London
[2]Great Ormond Street Hospital for Children, London

Introduction

The use of imaging for the evaluation of developmental anomalies of the female pelvis has rapidly expanded since the 1980s mainly because of the development and availability of imaging technology, particularly high-resolution ultrasound with Doppler, spiral computed tomography (CT) and magnetic resonance imaging (MRI). Imaging is now used in virtually every case to confirm diagnosis or to show the anatomy of the structural abnormalities of the genital tract and other related disorders. Imaging is used extensively for planning the surgical management of the primary condition and any associated complications.

The most commonly used imaging modalities are fluoroscopy (usually with contrast agents), ultrasound and MRI. Each technique has particular advantages and disadvantages, and knowledge of these is important for the appropriate choice of imaging technique. A major consideration when imaging children is the use and dose of ionizing radiation, particularly as many patients are likely to need multiple investigations during the course of their lifetime.

Imaging modalities

Fluoroscopy

Genitograms and micturating cystourethrography are the traditional fluoroscopic methods for evaluating children with disorders of sexual differentiation. All perineal orifices are examined with the catheter inserted only a short distance into the orifice. Contrast is injected gently under direct fluoroscopic screening to allow visualization of the morphology of the urogenital sinus. The important features that are noted include the presence or absence of a vagina, its relationship to the urethra and the level of the external sphincter (which has important surgical implications), and the recognition of a male or female type urethral configuration (Aaronson, 1992). Occasionally the uterus and Fallopian tubes will be demonstrated.

Hysterosalpingography involves cannulating the cervix and then injecting contrast into the uterus under fluoroscopy. This will demonstrate the patency of the cervical canal, show the internal uterine contour and demonstrate any tubal occlusion (Yoder and Hall, 1991; Zanetti et al., 1978). (Fig. 10.1).

The disadvantages of this technique include the radiation and contrast exposure of the patient, and the potential discomfort of the examination itself. Hysterosalpingograms are inappropriate investigations in the young or sexually inactive, and they cannot be carried out in patients with vaginal agenesis or nonpatent genital tracts. Equally, while the study gives accurate information on the luminal characteristics of the genital tract, there is no information on the external uterine contour and surrounding structures. It will miss noncommunicating uterine horns and double cervices, for example.

Ultrasound

Ultrasound provides a quick and generally noninvasive method for assessing the abdomen and pelvis without the use of ionizing radiation. Excellent image resolution can be achieved using a small footprint, high-frequency

Paediatric and Adolescent Gynaecology, ed. Adam Balen et al. Published by Cambridge University Press.
© Cambridge University Press 2004.

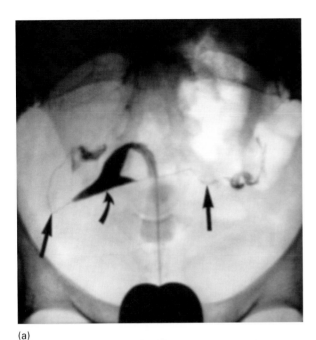

(a)

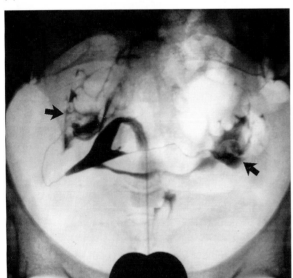

(b)

Fig. 10.1. Normal hysterosalpingogram. The cervix has been canulated and contrast has been slowly injected into the uterus. The normal intrauterine contour (a: curved black arrow) and the normal Fallopian tubes (a: straight black arrows) are demonstrated. There is normal spill of contrast into the peritoneal cavity indicating tubal patency (b: straight small black arrows).

transducer (operating at or above 7.5 mHz) with variable focus to allow visualization of the deeper structures (de Bruyn, 1997). Ultrasound may be performed using a transabdominal or transvaginal approach. For transab-

dominal imaging, a full bladder is necessary to provide an acoustic window when imaging the pelvis. Transvaginal ultrasound yields images of higher resolution and accuracy (Lyons et al., 1992) but can only be employed in older girls who are sexually active. Its use in paediatric gynaecology is, therefore, limited, although it provides good views of the uterine shape and configuration and an accurate measure of the endometrial thickness.

Ultrasound can be used to identify the absence or presence of gonadal and Müllerian structures, primarily the uterus and ovaries (Cohen et al., 1993; Horowitz and Glassberg, 1992; Kutteh et al., 1995; Siegel, 1991). It may be used to measure the ovarian follicles and endometrial thickness. Renal and adrenal examination form an integral part of the assessment because of the close embryological development of the renal tract, and because adrenal hyperplasia may be associated with ambiguous genitalia (females with virilizing congenital adrenal hyperplasia (CAH)). Ultrasound may be used to detect the complications of Müllerian duct abnormalities such as hydrocolpos and hydrometrocolpos (Nussbaum Blask et al., 1991).

A disadvantage of transabdominal pelvic ultrasound is that it depends on the bladder being full to provide a suitable transonic window. This cannot always be achieved in babies and young children, particularly those with associated urological and abdominal wall abnormalities and those who have undergone extensive surgery. The technique is extremely operator dependent and great expertise is required to achieve a full evaluation of patients with complex anomalies. Even in the best hands, there may be insufficient information because of inadequate views.

Magnetic resonance imaging

MRI is a further nonionizing imaging modality that may be used to assess the paediatric abdomen and pelvis. The best images are obtained with relatively high field systems (1 Tesla or above) and using appropriate surface coils. The majority of coils are designed to fit adults and to be loaded by adult weight and volume. Consequently, some ingenuity may be required to image small babies, such as examining the whole child in a "head and neck" coil and using bags of saline to obtain adequate loading of the coils. The amount of radiofrequency energy that can be deposited during a scan sequence is related to weight as it results in tissue heating, and this can limit the examination in very small babies and infants.

The main advantages of MR are that it produces multiplanar images and generates high tissue contrast without the use of radiation. The disadvantages are that it is very susceptible to movement (physiological and patient movement) and is relatively slow, with a detailed pelvic and abdominal assessment taking between 20 and 60 minutes. Physiological motion artefact can be minimized by the use of buscopan or glucagon to reduce bowel movement, specific sequences to reduce breathing artefact and saturation bands to reduce blood-flow artefact. Patient movement can be reduced by feeding and sedating babies or by using general anaesthesia. Older children can be helped by counselling before the study, using music and by having a familiar person with them in the scanner during the examination.

MRI studies generally consist of a combination of T_1- and T_2-weighted images acquired in several planes (often oblique). Intravenous contrast agents may be useful for confirming the position of the gonads and for showing the vagina. The structure of the uterus is much easier to define in a postpubertal patient as the organ enlarges and the layered structure becomes apparent (see below). Consequently, even where a prepubertal study has been relatively unrewarding, repeating the examination after menarche may be helpful.

MRI can provide detailed anatomical information about Müllerian and Wolffian structures and the position of the gonads (Gambino et al., 1992; Secaf et al., 1994). These advantages are particularly relevant to the female genital tract as the uterus, Fallopian tubes and ovaries can have a very variable position. MRI will also demonstrate the internal architecture of the uterus, allowing greater anatomical classification of the Müllerian duct anomalies (Carrington et al., 1990; Doyle, 1992; Pellerito et al., 1992).

MRI remains the best noninvasive imaging modality to show the uterine and parauterine anatomy (Togashi et al., 2001). While this is less important if the clinical question is merely to identify the gonads, it is vital for detailed assessment of Müllerian duct anomalies with a view to surgical intervention. MRI may also provide supplementary information in the assessment of congenital anomalies in that it may identify abnormal pelvic bones and musculature (Minto et al., 2001). As with ultrasound, the study can be extended to cover the upper abdomen to examine the kidneys and adrenal glands.

The normal Fallopian tubes are often difficult to see and separate from adjacent bowel loops (Outwater and Mitchell, 1996). Unless they are clearly obstructed, tubal patency cannot be assessed without the use of intraluminal contrast. The technique of MR hysterosalpingography has been developed as an alternative to fluoroscopic hysterosalpingography to avoid the use of ionizing radiation (Rouanet de Lavit et al., 2000; Tello et al., 1997; Wiesner et al., 2001).

Normal development and appearances

The appearance of the female genital tract varies through childhood owing to variation in hormonal activity. The configuration of the uterus and ovaries changes with age as a result of hormonal influences (Salardi et al., 1985). The neonatal uterus and ovaries are enlarged as a result of the physiological effects of maternal hormones and this makes them more prominent. Consequently, the optimum time to assess the paediatric pelvis is in the newborn period. After this, the examination becomes more difficult as the uterus and ovaries reduce in size.

Uterine development

In the neonate, maternal hormones cause the uterus to have a more "adult" type configuration, with a prominent corpus and endometrium. After 1 month, the uterus starts to regress, and it assumes a normal prepubertal configuration with prominence of the cervix, with a cervix to corpus ratio of 2:1. This appearance remains until the onset of adrenarche (about 9 years) (Salardi et al., 1985).

The uterus grows during adrenarche and assumes a tubular shape (with equal growth of the corpus and cervix). With the onset of puberty and mature ovarian follicular development, the uterus attains an adult pear-shaped configuration with fundal (corpus) dominance (Garel et al., 2001) (Fig. 10.2).

On ultrasound, the endometrium can be clearly seen as an echogenic midline echo. On MRI, the configuration of the uterus changes with age as described above. With the onset of puberty, the uterus develops the normal adult "zonal" appearance. The uterine corpus consists of three zones on T_2-weighted images (Hricak et al., 1983; Lee et al., 1985). Centrally is the high-signal endometrium, then the low-signal junctional zone with the myometrium peripherally being of intermediate to high signal. The junctional zone was initially considered to be the MR equivalent of the subendometrial hypoechoic layer seen on ultrasound, but no histological equivalent has been defined. More recently, ultrafast sequential MRI has shown that the junctional zone of the uterus varies in thickness and signal return with time (Togashi et al., 2001). It is, therefore, likely that it represents the summation of ceaseless uterine peristalsis and is not a discrete anatomical structure per se.

The appearance of the uterus changes in response to physiological effects such as the menstrual cycle and the contraceptive pill (McCarthy et al., 1986). The endometrium gradually thickens during the proliferative phase of the menstral cycle, to reach around 7–14 mm during the secretory phase. The zonal appearance of the corpus

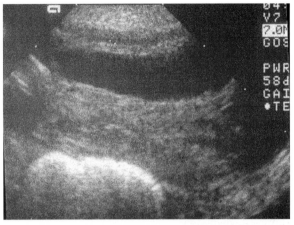

(a)

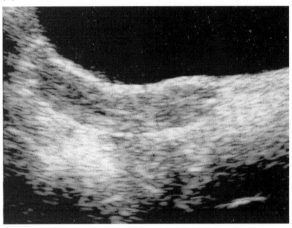

(b)

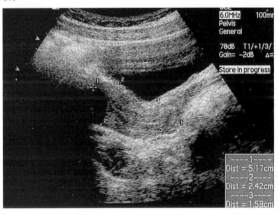

(c)

Fig. 10.2. Longitudinal ultrasound appearances of normal uterine development. (a) A neonatal uterus with a prominent corpus (fundus) and endometrium. (b) A tubular uterus (with equal growth of the corpus and the cervix) usually seen in adrenarche. The prepubertal uterus usually shows cervical dominance. (c) shows a postpubertal uterus, with a pear-shaped configuration and fundal dominance.

becomes much less distinct during menstruation in some girls/women (Demas et al., 1986; Haynor et al., 1986; McCarthy et al., 1986).

The cervix may have a two- or three-layered appearance on T_2-weighted images. The central layer is constant and represents the high-signal endocervix. Peripheral to this is the cervical stroma; this is predominantly low signal because of the presence of fibrous connective tissue. Peripheral to this is the inconstant intermediate outer layer, which is of higher signal return (Hricak et al., 1983; Lee et al., 1985).

Ovarian development

There is continuous growth and activity of the ovaries throughout childhood, with two periods of accelerated growth (Peters et al., 1976). The first of these occurs at around eight years and coincides with the rise in androgen secretion from the adrenal cortex. The second spurt occurs just before and during puberty. The ovarian volume changes from 0.8 ml in the first three months, to 1 ml at two years and 2 ml by the age of 12 years (Cohen et al., 1990).

In addition to changes in volume, there is follicular development and this can be seen with ultrasound. In the neonate, follicles of varying size are apparent and result from maternal hormonal influences. The number and size of follicles increases during childhood and at approximately eight or nine years of age the ovaries become multi-follicular in appearance (Adams et al., 1985), that is containing six or more follicles of 6–14 mm in size. During puberty the follicles continue to increase in size.

Other structures

The extensive paracervical and periuterine venous complexes can be well seen on MRI using angiographic sequences. Many supporting muscles and ligaments may be visualized, including the pelvic floor muscles and the anal sphincters; this is particularly useful in patients with complex developmental anomalies (Togashi et al., 2001).

Congenital abnormalities

There is a wide range of developmental anomalies that potentially can affect the female genital tract because of the complex embryological development of the urogenital tract. These can range from ambiguous genitalia and intersex conditions to complex developmental anomalies.

Assessment of ambiguous genitalia and intersex conditions

The role of the radiologist in the assessment of ambiguous genitalia and the intersex conditions is to demonstrate accurately the anatomy of the genitourinary tract and the effects of the condition on other organs (Faure and Garel, 1981). This may be a complex task as there is marked diversity between these conditions and often a variable expression, leading to a wide range of anatomical variability. The appropriate assignment of gender is fundamental to the physical and psychological development of the child, as well as for parental bonding (Izquierdo and Glassberg, 1993). Defining the anatomy plays an integral role in the multidisciplinary management of the child. It is important to remember that the appropriate assignment of gender may not be concordant with the genetic sex of the child.

There are several clinical manifestations of the disorders of sexual differentiation. These may be children with ambiguous genitalia, male phenotypes with bilateral/unilateral impalpable testes and hypospadias, and female phenotypes with clitoral hypertrophy and fused labia, or with a gonad present in a hernial sac (Aaronson, 1992).

Classification of sexual differentiation disorders can be based around gonadal histology: female and male pseudohermaphroditism, true hermaphroditism and conditions of dysgenetic gonads (Aaronson, 1992; Page, 1994). Making a definitive diagnosis requires correlation of the clinical findings with biochemical, cytological and radiological evaluation. Imaging strategies aim to identify the presence or absence of the gonadal (ovary/testis) and Müllerian (usually the uterus) structures. Ultrasound provides an easy noninvasive method in the first instance (Horowitz and Glassberg, 1992; Kutteh et al., 1995; Siegel, 1991). With increasingly complex anatomy, MRI may prove a useful adjunct to image ectopic gonadal tissue (Gambino et al., 1992; Secaf et al., 1994). If there is ambiguous genitalia with an associated hydrometrocolopos, with only two perineal orifices visible, then fluoroscopic investigation may provide useful information about the anatomy of the urogenital sinus.

The intersex conditions are a heterogeneous group of disorders with a variable expression. In the normal female child, the Müllerian structures (from which the Fallopian tubes, uterus, cervix and upper vagina are derived) are fully developed. In the male child, the Müllerian structures regress (under the influence of anti-Müllerian hormone (AMH), which is produced by the Sertoli cells of the fetal testis). The Wolffian structures (from which the vas deferens, epididymis and seminal vesicles are derived) develop under the influence of testosterone from the Leydig cells of the fetal testis (McGillivray, 1992; Page, 1994). Therefore, a normal testis will prevent Müllerian structures forming on the ipsilateral side. Any disruption of this hormonal cycle (either by a poorly functioning/dysgenetic testis or the absence/insensitivity to androgenic (testosterone) stimulation) will allow the simultaneous development of both male and female structures, or failure of development of the male structures in a genetically male fetus.

Female pseudohermaphroditism

Most children with ambiguous genitalia will have female pseudohermaphroditism. This is a result of excessive androgenic exposure of genetic females 46,XX in utero. The majority are secondary to virilizing CAH. The excessive production of androgens caused by an enzyme deficiency in the corticosteroid/mineralocorticoid pathway leads to virilization of a female fetus: with clitoromegaly and ambiguous genitalia.

Ultrasound should be performed in the newborn period to confirm the presence of normal female internal genitalia, and to assess the size of the adrenal glands. There may be a hydrocolopos present if there is a urogenital sinus malformation present. If there is a urogenital sinus malformation present, this can be demonstrated fluoroscopically (Josso et al., 1969) (Fig. 10.3).

Virilized females have ovaries and a uterus in the presence of a normal female karyotype (46,XX). However, if there is nonvisualization of gonadal tissue either unilaterally or bilaterally, then further imaging is required to confirm or exclude the presence of ectopic testicular tissue or an ovatestis. This can be achieved by ultrasound assessment of the inguinal and perineal areas (Wright et al., 1995). If these are present, the diagnosis of female pseudohermaphroditism is excluded. If these are absent, then the diagnosis of female hermaphroditism is probably still correct, as identification of only one or neither ovary can occur in a significant number of normal infants (> 40%) (Cohen et al., 1993).

Male pseudohermaphroditism

The presence of ambiguous genitalia with absent Müllerian structures (uterus, Fallopian tubes and upper third of the vagina) suggests male pseudohermaphroditism.

Male pseudohermaphroditism is most commonly a result of a complete or partial androgen insensitivity syndrome (C/PAIS) in genetic males 46,XY (Page, 1994; Williams et al., 1993). A combination of human chorionic gonadotrophin stimulation test, evaluation of the testosterone and dihydrotestosterone levels and an assay of androgen-binding activity in skin fibroblasts makes the

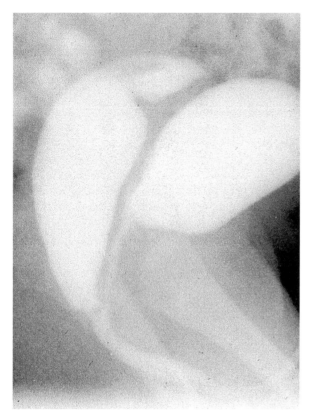

Fig. 10.3. Genitogram demonstrating a urogenital sinus. The female infant has ambiguous genitalia secondary to congenital adrenal hyperplasia, and a single perineal orifice. The genitogram shows an elongated urethra and a urogenital sinus communicating with the vagina (there is a hydrocolpos present).

definitive diagnosis (Berkovitz et al., 1984). PAIS usually presents with ambiguous genitalia, but there can be wide anatomical variability in the imaging findings. CAIS (formerly known as testicular feminization) presents in late adolescence with primary amenorrhoea, when the pelvic ultrasound fails to demonstrate any normal female organs. The testicular tissue must be sort out because of the risk of malignant transformation; this can be achieved with ultrasound initially for inguinal gonads, but MRI will yield more positive results for pelvic gonads (Fritzsche et al., 1987; Gambino et al., 1992; Secaf et al., 1994) (Fig. 10.4). If a genitogram is performed, this will show a short blind-ending vagina, with no cervical impression.

True hermaphroditism

True hermaphroditism is a rare cause of intersexuality but is the most common intersex state after virilizing CAH in a 46,XX child. It is characterized by the presence of ovarian and testicular tissue, either as a single tissue type or an

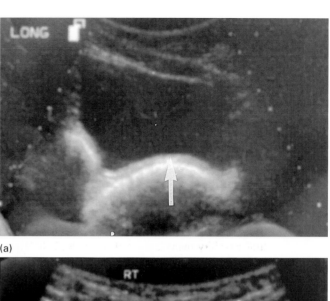
(a)

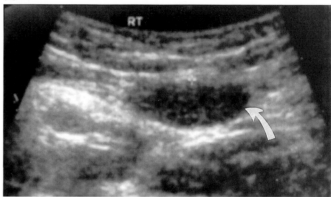
(b)

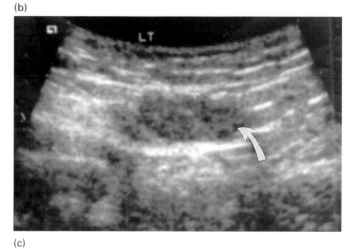
(c)

Fig. 10.4. Ultrasound scans in complete androgen insensitivity syndrome, demonstrating an absent uterus and bilateral ectopic testes within the inguinal canals. This 16-year-old girl presented with primary amenorrhoea. (a) The uterus is absent on transabdominal ultrasound scanning: the posterior wall of the bladder is in direct contact with the anterior wall of the gas-filled rectum, with no intervening viscus (straight white arrow). (b,c) Scans of the inguinal regions demonstrate intermediate echogenicity soft tissue masses typical of ectopic testes (curved white arrows). (Courtesy of A. Patel.)

ovatestis. Usually this is in the form of bilateral ovatestes or a combination of ovary–ovatestis (Hadjiathanasiou et al., 1994). The uniform echogenicity of the normal testis is replaced by a heterogeneous appearance because of the presence of multiple ovarian follicles.

If the gonads cannot be visualized unilaterally or bilaterally by pelvic ultrasound in a 46,XX child with ambiguous genitalia, a search of testicular tissue is warranted. The testis or ovatestes may been seen on perineal or inguinal ultrasound.

The presence of both testicular and ovarian tissue can lead to a wide range of anatomical features: these children may have a normal or hypoplastic uterus and unilateral or bilateral Fallopian tube development, depending on the relative local levels of androgens, oestrogens and AMH production (Yordam et al., 2001).

Precise anatomical evaluation is best achieved with a combination of fluoroscopy and MRI. Genitograms will demonstrate the exact anatomical relationships of the urogenital sinus which is needed for surgical planning. The demonstration of the level at which the vagina opens into the urogenital sinus and its relationship to the external sphincter have important surgical implications (Aaronson, 1992).

MRI can provide detailed anatomical information about Müllerian and Wolffian structures, and position of gonads. T_1-weighted scans are useful for anatomical clarity, while T_2-weighted scans will show ectopic gonads (testes or ovaries) as high signal.

Complex Müllerian duct anomalies

The Müllerian ducts develop within the first six weeks of fetal life. Abnormal development may result from genetic errors or from teratogenic events, and it is estimated that the prevalence of Müllerian abnormalities may be 0.5% in the female population (Nahum, 1998). Congenital abnormalities of the Müllerian system can occur in isolation or in association with other developmental disorders involving the cloaca, urogenital sinus and anorectal areas (Levitt et al., 1998). With simple anomalies, the majority of women (up to 75%) will be asymptomatic (Golan et al., 1989) and the remainder will present in a variety of ways depending on the particular abnormality. The most common clinical manifestations range from haematometrocolpos and haematosalpinx (in an obstructed genital tract) to premature labour, obstetric complications and recurrent miscarriages. In contrast, patients with complex congenital abnormalities often present earlier because of associated abnormalities and may require neonatal surgical intervention to deal with the urinary and gastrointestinal aspects

of the condition. With improved neonatal care and surgical techniques during the 1990s, many of these girls are now surviving into adolescence. It is at this stage of their development that evaluation of the female genital tract becomes important, to address issues around menstruation, sexual function and fertility.

With simple anomalies, imaging is infrequently performed in childhood unless there are gynaecological complications such as haematometrocolpos that require surgical intervention (Fig. 10.5). In the complex anomalies, surgery to the bladder, abdominal wall, anus, rectum and perineum is frequently necessary in the neonatal period and during childhood and this will require appropriate imaging of the urinary and gastrointestinal tracts. In later childhood, adolescence and in early adulthood, imaging of genital tract structures becomes necessary to aid diagnosis and to allow for appropriate surgical planning to deal with either the complications of the anomaly or to perform corrective surgery. Detailed understanding of the abnormality is also extremely valuable for counselling patients as to the likely outcome in terms of fertility and sexual function. In the past, Müllerian anomalies have been imaged with a combination of clinical examination, examination under anaesthetic, ultrasound, hysterosalpingography and laparoscopy. More recently, MRI has been used and there is now some evidence to suggest that MRI is a valuable alternative/adjunct to these techniques in both simple anomalies (Carrington et al., 1990; Pellerito et al., 1992) and the more complex conditions (Minto et al., 2001) (Figs. 10.6–10.10). MRI can also provide additional information on coexisting abnormalities of the pelvic bones and musculature, which may influence surgical planning (Fig. 10.11).

Where surgical intervention is contemplated, accurate knowledge of the surgical anatomy is necessary. The surgeon should ideally know whether there is a uterus present with the potential for menstruation or pregnancy (i.e. uterine type, dimensions and presence of an endometrium, and also whether the cervix is of normal patency and configuration), and whether any complication (e.g. haematosalpinx/hydrosalpinx) has arisen. Planning of vaginal surgery is enhanced with measurements of vaginal dimensions and septae. Where partial vaginal agenesis has occurred, measurements of the size of the aplastic segment and its distance from the perineum and the cervix allow accurate choice of vaginoplasty technique (Figs. 10.12–10.14) Differentiation of the types of Müllerian anomaly is needed to decide if surgery is appropriate and to plan the surgical approach (Hurst and Schlaff, 1993). Vaginal and uterine septae can be removed hysteroscopically. An abdominal approach is required for metroplasty in bicornuate uteri (although this operation is rarely performed nowadays).

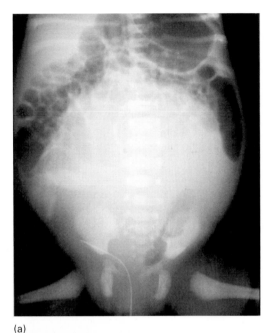

(a)

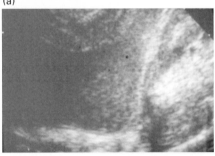

(b)

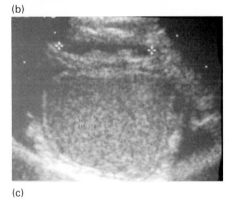

(c)

Fig. 10.5. Hydrometrocolpos presenting as a neonatal pelvic mass. This girl presented in the neonatal period with a pelvic mass. (a) The plain abdominal radiograph shows a large mass arising out of the pelvis, which is displacing the bowel loops superiorly and laterally within the abdomen. (b,c) The longitudinal and transverse ultrasound images, respectively, show a pelvic mass lying behind the empty bladder, which contains multiple echoes. These are the typical appearances of a hydrometrocolpos.

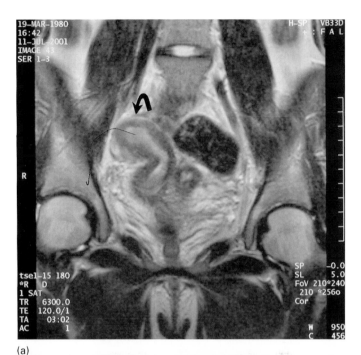

(a)

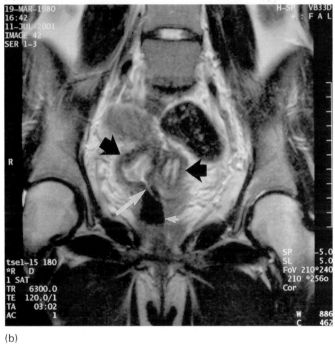

(b)

Fig. 10.6. Uterus didelphys, bicollis with unilateral partial obstruction. Coronal T_2-weighted scans from posterior to anterior. The scans show two distinct and separate uteri (a,c: curved arrows), each with a normally developed cervix (b: large arrow). The left cervix communicates normally with the vagina. The right cervix communicates with the vagina through a pinhole tract (b: large white arrow). The vagina is seen as low signal (b: small arrow) on this scan as a result of an air-filled tampon.

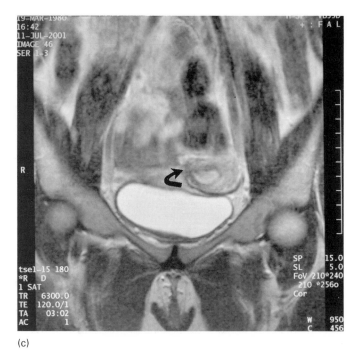

(c)

Fig. 10.6. *(Cont.)*

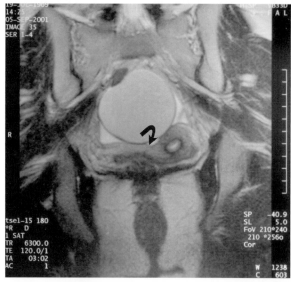

(b)

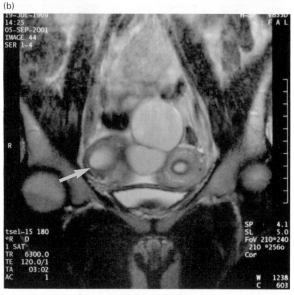

(c)

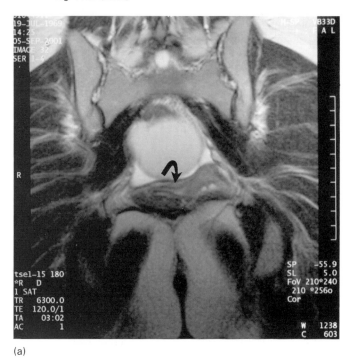

(a)

Fig. 10.7. Complex Müllerian anomaly with unicornuate cavitatary left uterus and an obstructed fused right uterus. Magnetic resonance T_2-weighted images: (a–d) coronal posterior to anterior; (e,f) sagittal; (g) transverse. There is a well-developed cavitatary left unicornuate uterus (f). The right unicornuate uterus is fused to the left uterus (a,b: curved arrows) and is obstructed. The uterine cavity is distended with blood (c: small white arrow), and there is a gross right haematosalpinx (d,e: straight arrows). There are two normally sited ovaries that show multiple follicles (g: large white arrows).

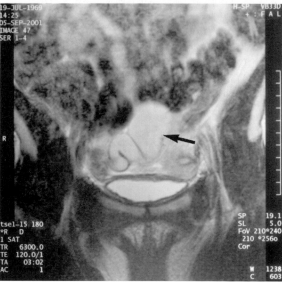

(d)

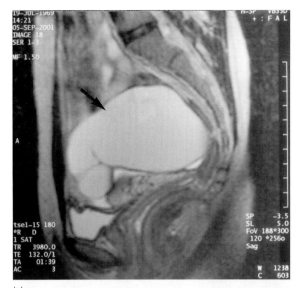

(e)

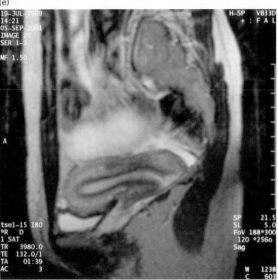

(f)

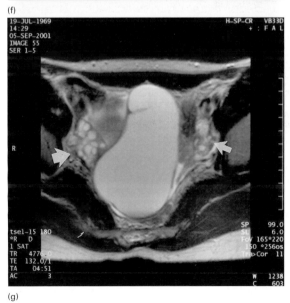

(g)

Fig. 10.7. *(Cont.)*

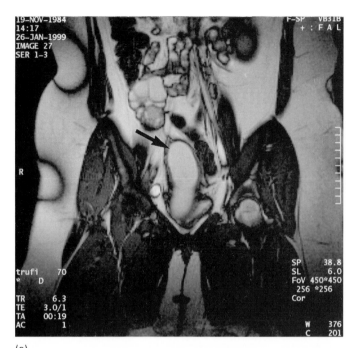

(a)

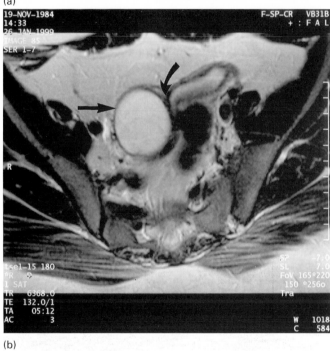

(b)

Fig. 10.8. Complex Müllerian anomaly with a unicornuate left uterus and an obstructed right fused horn. Magnetic resonance images: (a) coronal T_2-weighted; (b) transverse T_2-weighted: transverse T_1-weighted; (d) transverse T_2-weighted; (a–c) pelvis; (d) lower abdomen. There is a distended right uterine horn (a–c: straight arrows). The horn is fused to the left unicornuate uterus (b: curved arrow) and is obstructed at the level of the external cervical os (a). The distended cervix is partially obstructing the left uterus, which is slightly dilated. The right horn contains fluid, which is bright on both T_1 and T_2-weighted images; these are the imaging characteristics of blood. There is also a cystic structure in the lower right abdomen (d: open arrow), which is the remnant of a malformed right kidney.

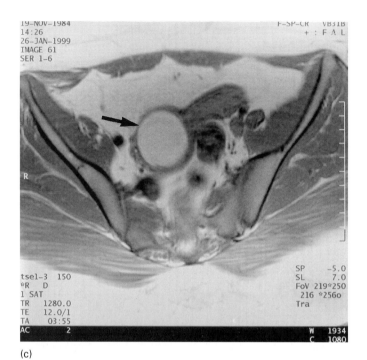

(c)

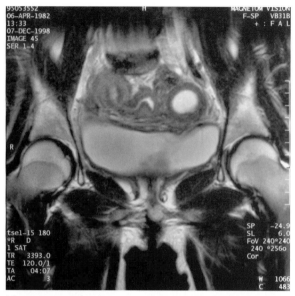

(a)

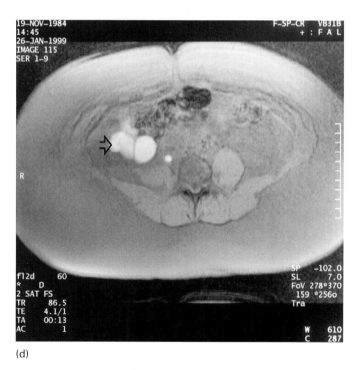

(d)

Fig. 10.8. (*Cont.*)

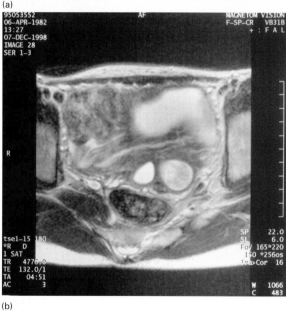

(b)

Fig. 10.9. Complex Müllerian anomaly with haematuria in adolescence. Magnetic resonance T_2-weighted scan in the coronal (a), transverse (b,d) and sagittal (c) planes. A pelvic surgical procedure had been performed in infancy and the girl presented in her mid-teens with haematuria. The scans show a uterus didelphys bicollis. Both uteri (a) and cervices (b) are partially obstructed and distended with blood. The cervices communicate directly with the posterior wall of the bladder through a fistulous tract (c,d: straight arrows). There is patchy mucosal thickening of the bladder wall (d: curved arrow).

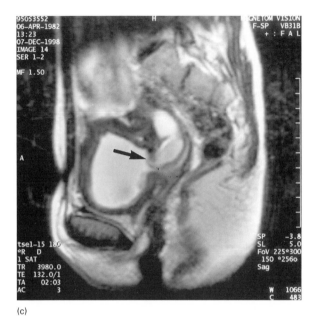

(c)

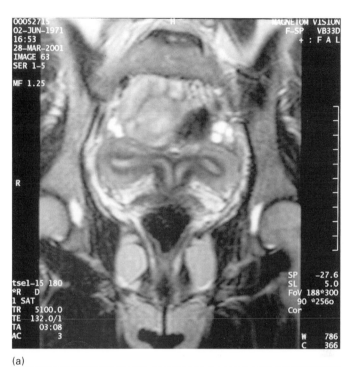

(a)

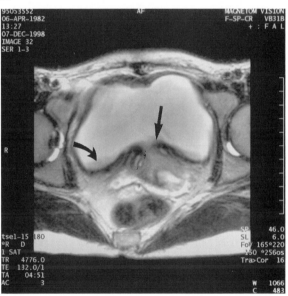

(d)

Fig. 10.9. (*Cont.*)

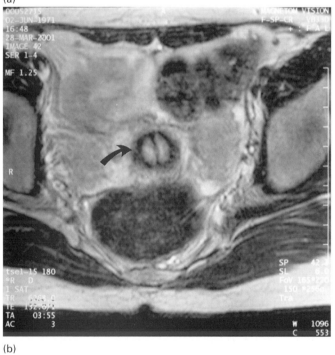

(b)

Fig. 10.10. Uterus didelphys bicollis with a partial vagina. Magnetic resonance T_2-weighted coronal (a) and transverse (b,c) scans. There are two separate uteri (a) with clearly defined double cervices (b: curved arrow). There are two separate vaginas, which are fused in the midline. The vaginal vaults can be seen (c: straight arrows).

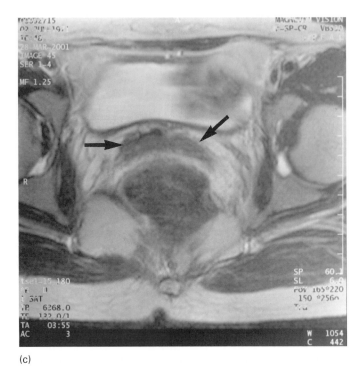

(c)

Fig. 10.10. (*Cont.*)

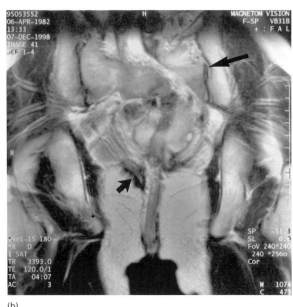

(b)

Fig. 10.11. (*Cont.*)

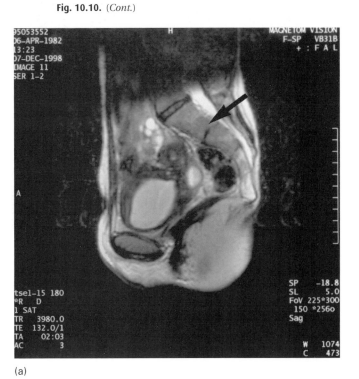

(a)

Fig. 10.11. Bony and pelvic floor anomalies. Sagittal (a) and coronal (b) T_2-weighted magnetic resonance scans. The sacrum and coccyx are abnormally formed (a,b: large arrows). The right levator ani is abnormal (b: small arrow) while the left levator ani is absent.

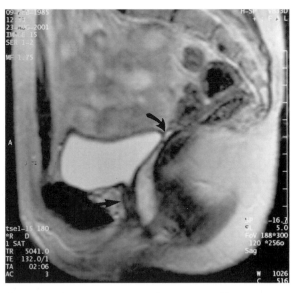

Fig. 10.12. Absent vagina as part of a complex Müllerian anomaly. The sagittal T_2-weighted image shows a fluid-filled bladder and urethra (straight arrow). The rectum contains gas and lies posterior to the bladder. The dome of the bladder is immediately opposed to the rectum (curved arrow) as there is no normally sited uterus and cervix. The space between the bladder base and the rectum is filled with fat as there is no vagina.

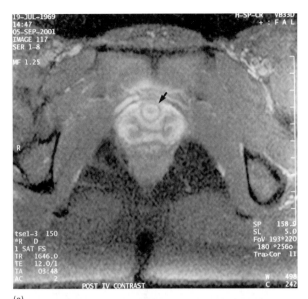

(a)

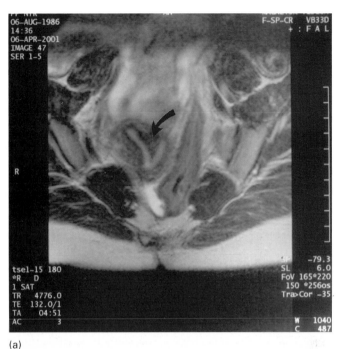

(a)

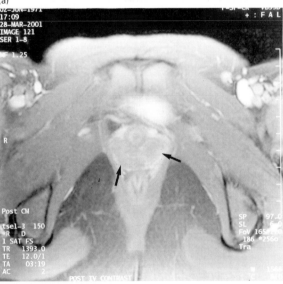

(b)

Fig. 10.13. Single and double vagina. Transverse contrast-enhanced and fat-suppressed magnetic resonance scans through the vagina and the urethra at the level of the pubic symphysis. (a) The structure of a normal single vagina. The vaginal stroma shows diffuse enhancement with a central H-shaped submucosal region of nonenhancement. The urethra (small arrow) lies immediately anterior to the vagina. (b) A double vagina (large arrows). The H-shape is not visualized and the vaginas are fused in the midline.

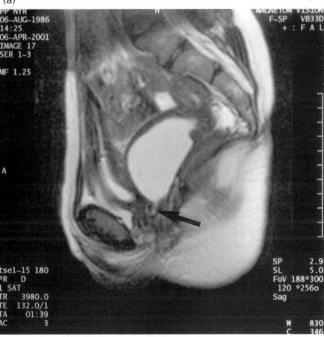

(b)

Fig. 10.14. Bicornuate uterus with partial vaginal agenesis. T_2-weighted transverse (a) and sagittal (b) magnetic resonance scans. This adolescent girl presented with primary amenorrhoea, and a perineal dimple in place of a vaginal orifice. (a) A bicornuate uterus (curved arrow) can be seen. (b) The proximal vagina is distended with blood and terminates in a blind-ending nipple (straight arrow), which lies 1.5 cm proximal to the perineal dimple.

Partial vaginal agenesis may be effectively reconstructed via a perineal approach and didelphic uteri without vaginal septae require no surgery.

Although corrective surgery is being attempted in patients with complex anomalies, there are no prospective studies yet available reporting the long-term outcome of these procedures. Consequently, the imaging features predictive of a successful surgical outcome have not yet been determined.

Summary

The developmental anomalies of the female genital tract show marked anatomical variability. Imaging is now an essential component in the assessment of each patient. Its role may be twofold: either to confirm the diagnosis or to provide a detailed demonstration of the anatomy of the genital tract and associated abnormalities. This is particularly useful if surgical intervention is being considered. Ultrasound and fluoroscopy have been the traditional imaging modalities used, but MRI is probably the most useful imaging technique in the assessment of complex anomalies.

REFERENCES

Aaronson I A (1992). Sexual differentiation, intersexuality. In *Clinical Pediatric Urology*, 3rd edn, Kelalis P P, King L R, Belman A B, eds., pp. 977–1014. Saunders, Philadelphia, PA.

Adams J, Polson D W, Abulwahid N et al. (1985). Multifollicular ovaries: clinical, endocrine features and response to pulsatile gonadatrophin releasing hormone. *Lancet* ii, 1375–1379.

Berkovitz G D, Lee P A, Brown T R, Migeon C J (1984). Etiological evaluation of male pseudohermaphroditism in infancy and childhood. *Am J Dis Child* 138, 755–759.

Carrington B, Hricak H, Nuruddin R N et al. (1990). Mullerian duct anomalies: MR imaging evaluation. *Radiology* 176, 715–720.

Cohen H L, Ticc H M, Mandel F S (1990). Ovarian volumes measures by ultrasound: bigger than we think. *Radiology* 177, 18.

Cohen H L, Shapiro M A, Mandel F S, Shapiro M L (1993). Normal ovaries in neonates and infants; A sonographic study of 77 patients from 1 day to 24 months old. *Am J Roentgenol* 160, 583–586.

de Bruyn R (1997). Ultrasonagraphy of the normal female pelvis in childhood and adolescence. *Imaging* 8, 1–9.

Demas B E, Hricak H, Jaffe R B (1986). Uterine MR imaging: effects of hormonal stimulation. *Radiology* 159, 123–126.

Doyle M B (1992). Magnetic resonance imaging in mullerian fusion defects. *J Reprod Med* 37, 33–38.

Faure C, Garel L (1981). Radiology in intersex states. In *Pediatric and Adolescent Endocrinology*, Vol. 8, *The Intersex Child*, Josso N, ed., pp. 40–50. Karger, Basel.

Fritzsche P J, Hricak H, Kogan B A, Winkler M L, Tanagho E A (1987). Undescended testis: value of MR imaging. *Radiology* 164, 169–173.

Gambino J, Caldwell B, Dietrich R, Walot I, Kangarloo H (1992). Congenital disorders of sexual differentiation: MR findings. *Am J Roentgenol* 158, 363–367.

Garel L, Dubois J, Grignon A, Filiatrault D, van Vliet G (2001). US of the pediatric female pelvis: a clinical perspective. *Radiographics* 21, 1393–1407.

Golan A, Langer R, Bukovsky I, Capsi E (1989). Congenital anomalies of the Mullerian system. *Fertil Steril* 51, 747–755.

Hadjiathanasiou C G, Brauner R, Lortat-Jacob B et al. (1994). True hermaphroditism: genetic variants, clinical management. *J Pediatr* 125, 738–744.

Haynor D R, Mack L A, Soules M R, Shuman W P, Montana M A, Moss A A (1986). Changing appearance of the normal uterus during the menstrual cycle: MR studies. *Radiology* 161, 459–462.

Horowitz H, Glassberg K I (1992). Ambiguous genitalia: diagnosis evaluation and treatment. *Urol Radiology* 14, 306–318.

Hricak H, Alpers C, Crooks L E, Sheldon P E (1983). Magnetic resonance imaging of the female pelvis: initial experience. *Am J Roentgenol* 141, 1119–1128.

Hurst B S, Schlaff W D (1993). Congenital anomalies of the uterus and their treatment. In *Congenital Malformations of the Female Reproductive Tract*, Verkauf B S, ed., pp. 91–115. Appleton & Lange, Norwalk, CT.

Izquierdo G, Glassberg K I (1993). Gender assignment and gender identity in patients with ambiguous genitalia. *Urology* 42, 232–242.

Josso N, Fortier Beaulieu M, Faure C (1969). Genitography in intersexual states. *Acta Endocrinol* 165–180.

Kutteh W H, Santos-Ramos R, Ermel L D (1995). Accuracy of ultrasonic detection of the uterus in normal newborn infants: implications for infants with ambiguous genitalia. *Ultrasound Obstet Gynecol* 5, 109–113.

Lee J K, Gersell D J, Balfe D M, Worthington J L, Picus D, Gapp G (1985). The uterus: in vitro MR anatomic correlation of normal and abnormal specimens. *Radiology* 157, 175–179.

Levitt M A, Stein D M, Peña A (1998). Gynaecological concerns in the treatment of teenagers with cloaca. *J Pediatr Surg* 33, 188–193.

Lyons E A, Gratton D, Harrington C (1992). Transvaginal sonography of normal pelvic anatomy. *Radiol Clin North Am* 30, 663–675.

McCarthy S, Tauber C, Gore J (1986). Female pelvic anatomy: MR assessment of variations during the menstrual cycle, with use of oral contraceptives. *Radiology* 160, 119–123.

McGillivray B C (1992). Genetic aspects of ambiguous genitalia. *Paediatr Clin North Am* 39, 307–317.

Minto C L, Hollings N, Hall-Craggs M A, Creighton S (2001). Magnetic resonance imaging of complex Mullerian anomalies. *Br J Obstet Gynaecol* 108, 791–797.

Nahum G G (1998). Uterine anomalies: how common are they and what is the distribution amongs subtypes? *J Reprod Med* 43, 877–887.

Nussbaum Blask A R, Saunders R C, Gearhart J P (1991). Obstructed uterovaginal anomalies: demonstration with sonography. Part 1 Neonates and infants. *Radiology* 179, 79–83.

Outwater E K, Mitchell D G (1996). Normal ovaries and functional cysts: MR appearance. *Radiology* 201, 751–755.

Page J (1994). The newborn with ambiguous genitalia. *Neonat Netw* 13, 15–21.

Pellerito J S, McCarthy S M, Doyle M B, Glickman M G, de Cherney A H (1992). Diagnosis of uterine anomalies: relative accuracy of MR imaging endovaginal sonography and hysterosalpingography. *Radiology* 183, 795–800.

Peters H, Himelstein-Braw R, Faber M (1976). The normal development of the ovary in childhood. *Acta Endocrinol* 82, 617–630.

Rouanet de Lavit J P, Maubon A J, Thurmond A S (2000). MR hysterography performed with saline injection and fluid attenuated inversion recovery sequences: initial experience. *Am J Roentgenol* 175, 774–776.

Salardi S, Forsini L, Cacciari E et al. (1985). Pelvic ultrasonography in premenarchal girls: relation to puberty and sex hormone concentrations. *Arch Dis Child* 60, 120–125.

Secaf E, Hricak H, Gooding C A et al. (1994). Role of MRI in the evaluation of ambiguous genitalia. *Pediatr Radiol* 24, 231–235.

Seigel M J (1991). Paediatric gynaecological sonography. *Radiology* 179, 593–600.

Tello R, Tempany C M, Chai J, Ainslie M, Adams D F (1997). MR hysterography using axial long TR imaging with three-dimensional projections of the uterus. *Comput Med Imaging Graph* 21, 117–123.

Togashi K, Nakai A, Sugimura K (2001). Anatomy and physiology of the female pelvis: MR imaging revisited. *J Magn Reson Med* 13, 842–849.

Wiesner W, Ruehm S G, Bongartz G, Kaim A, Reese E, de Geyter C (2001). Three-dimensional dynamic MR hysterosalpingography: a preliminary report. *Eur Radiol* 11, 1439–44.

Williams D M, Patterson M N, Hughes I A (1993). Androgen insensitivity syndrome. *Arch Dis Child* 68, 343–344.

Wright N, Smith C, Rickwood A M K, Carty H M L (1995). Imaging children with ambiguous genitalia and intersex states. *Clin Radio* 50, 823–829.

Yoder I C, Hall D A (1991). Hysterosalpingography in the 1990s. *Am J Roentgenol* 157, 675–683.

Yordam N, Alikasifoglu A, Kandemir N, Caglar M, Balci S (2001). True hermaphroditism: clinical features, genetic variants and gonadal histology. *J Pediatr Endocrinol Metab* 14, 421–427.

Zanetti E, Ferrari L R, Rossi G (1978). Classification and radiographic features of uterine malformations: hysterosalpingographic study. *Br J Radiol* 51, 161–170.

11

Surgical correction of vaginal and other anomalies

Jane MacDougall[1] and Sarah Creighton[2]

[1] Addenbrooke's Hospital, Cambridge, UK
[2] Elizabeth Garrett Anderson and Obstetric Hospital, University College Hospitals, London, UK

Historical perspective

The surgical correction of vaginal anomalies dates from the early 1800s. Surgery on the clitoris is a more recent practice and has evolved over the last 50 years or so. The existence of uterine anomalies was first noted in 1681 by Dionis, who described simultaneous pregnancies in each side of a hemi-uterus (Letterie, 1998). Their impact on reproduction was recognized but the first systematic review was not until 1922 (Miller, 1992). The first metroplasty was described in 1884 by Ruge.

Correction of vaginal anomalies

Many different techniques to create or reconstruct a vagina have been described by a variety of different authors, which suggests that there continues to be controversy over the optimal form of surgery. The evidence base on which to select a particular technique is limited to, at best, a series of case reports with short-term follow-up. This is, in part, inevitable because of the rarity of these conditions, but it does not help decision making. It is useful to look at how and what prompted the development of these various techniques (Schober et al., 1998).

Dupuytren described the first vaginoplasty in 1817 (Judin, 1927). This involved creating a perineal pouch between bladder and rectum. Wharton (1938) and Counsellor (1948) subsequently refined this technique by using a mould to hold the pouch open, which allowed spontaneous epithelialization to take place. This procedure fell into disrepute when it was found to have a 46% failure rate (Cali and Pratt, 1968) and also when it was realized that the mould had to be used for several hours every day, sometimes

indefinitely. Just under 30 years later this method was resurrected (Jackson and Rosenblatt, 1994) using an absorbable adhesion barrier wrapped around the mould.

Abbe (1898) was the first surgeon to use skin over a mould to create a vagina. Subsequently, McIndoe and Bannister (1938) used split-thickness skin grafts over a mould to create a vagina. This again involved dissection to create a space between the bladder and rectum. However, there were problems with fistula formation secondary to the use of the mould and the need for lubrication as the skin graft tended to be rather dry. Newer softer moulds reduced the incidence of the former complication. A subsequent problem was long-term scarring with stenosis of the created vagina, particularly at its distal end.

Skin flap vaginoplasty was first described in 1921 when Graves used labia minoral tissue as a pedunculated flap. Subsequently, Sheares (1960) described a flap based posteriorly, which was used to line the posterior vagina, and Fortunoff (1964) utilized a U-shaped skin flap. Williams (1964) used labial tissue to line a pouch formed by a U-shaped perineal incision. This technique was refined by Passerini-Glazel (1989), who used skin flaps brought down from a reduced phallic shaft to form labia majora and minora. Other flaps used include rotated buttock flaps (Hendren and Donahoe, 1980), pudendal thigh fasciocutaneous flaps and rectus abdominis flaps. All can suffer from scarring at the donor site, plus lack of lubrication and hair growth within the neovagina, which can become stenosed.

Apart from skin, surgeons have used a variety of other tissues to line new vaginas. These include bowel, amnion, peritoneum and bladder mucosa. Amnion was first used by Ashworth et al. (1986), who lined a perineal space with

Paediatric and Adolescent Gynaecology, ed. Adam Balen et al. Published by Cambridge University Press.
© Cambridge University Press 2004.

sterile amnion that was held in place by a mould. Again, subsequent contracture may be a problem and the technique seems to have fallen from favour, in part because of concern about the transmission of human immunodeficiency virus.

The use of other tissues involves more complex procedures that may necessitate a combined abdominoperineal approach. The use of bladder mucosa (Claret et al., 1988) involves opening the bladder and harvesting tissue, which is then used over a mould to line a perineal space. Little is known about complications. The use of bowel dates back to the beginning of the twentieth century when Baldwin (1904) sutured an open end of a segment of ileum to the vaginal introitus. The other end was closed and care was taken to retain the blood supply to the ileum by rotating the segment on its vascular pedicle. However, there were complications, including deaths, and the procedure was largely abandoned until 1961, when Pratt described the use of a sigmoid loop. This method tends to overcome the problem of lack of lubrication and distal vaginal stenosis but outlet stenosis and prolapse can occur and vaginal discharge may be offensive.

Pelvic peritoneum has been used in a combined abdomino perineal approach. Davydov and Zhvitiashvili (1974) described dissection of a cylinder of peritoneum within the abdomen that was then brought down into a newly dissected vaginal space. The upper end was closed and the lower end sutured to the introitus.

It is very occasionally necessary to create a vagina using full-thickness skin flaps that are rotated on a vascular pedicle to create a cylindrical tube. A vagina may be created in this way using skin from the inner thigh (trying to avoid using skin that is too hairy) or by taking skin from the surface of the rectus abdominis and rotating it into the pelvic cavity. Alternatively, a full-thickness free flap can be taken, for example from the scapular region, and a microsurgical vascular anastomosis performed. These complex plastic surgical procedures are rarely required but may be of benefit to patients who have undergone extensive surgery for cloacal anomalies and so may have no suitable skin in the genital region.

Nonsurgical methods were first described by Frank in 1938, who used pressure generated by frequent use of dilators to create a vagina that was, therefore, lined with skin stretched from the perineum (see Ch. 13).

Surgery on the clitoris

The history of clitoral surgery is shorter but also characterized by a variety of techniques (Schober, 1999) mostly aimed at reducing clitoral size. Development of surgical techniques has also been influenced by concepts of clitoral and sexual function, an area that is explored in Chapters 8, 14 and 37. Many surgeons in the 1950s considered that the clitoris was unnecessary for normal sexual function and, therefore, clitorectomy could be performed. However, increasingly it was recognized that the clitoris might be important and subsequent surgery attempted to retain its function.

Ombredanne (1939) was the first to describe what was effectively clitoral reduction; this was achieved by overlapping the untouched clitoris with skin flaps to give a cosmetically smaller clitoris. Subsequently, several other techniques that involved burying the mostly intact glans and corpora gave way to attempts to reduce the size without loss of function or tissue. However, this was found to cause bowstringing of erectile tissue and surgery focused on removal of appropriate tissue. Schmid (1961) removed the corpora retaining the glans and its neurovascular pedicle. Various authors since have described variations on this technique (Kumar et al., 1974; Passerini-Glazel, 1989). Some have also described suturing the remaining glans to the pubic bone (Sagehashi, 1993; Spence and Allen, 1973). It is still unclear which technique, if any, is optimal.

Correction of uterine anomalies

There are so many different types of uterine anomaly that one might expect many different surgical techniques. In fact, there is rather less variation in technique than might be expected. Controversy in this area has largely centred on the indications for surgery. Surgery itself can be broadly subdivided into transcervical and transabdominal techniques. The first metroplasty was actually performed transcervically with excision of a uterine septum in a woman who had a history of two pregnancy losses (Ruge, 1884). She subsequently delivered a baby at term. Strassman and later his son advocated uterine unification operations (Rock, 1997), which necessitated an abdominal approach. The first of these was reported in 1907. Subsequently, Jones and Jones (1954) reported a series of abdominal metroplasties dating from 1936. The other surgeon closely associated with the abdominal approach to metroplasty is Tompkins, who described his technique in 1962.

More recently, surgeons have readvocated the transcervical approach, particularly with the development of hysteroscopic techniques that allow direct visualization of uterine septa (Chervenak and Neuwirth, 1981; Daly et al., 1983; De Cherney et al., 1986; Israel and March, 1981). The advantages of this approach will be discussed below.

General principles of current practice

Underlying concepts

It is important before embarking on surgery aimed at correcting vaginal or uterine anomalies to bear certain general principles in mind. Careful preoperative workup is essential so that an accurate diagnosis is made prior to surgery. This then allows a full discussion with the patient and/or parents in advance.

A multidisciplinary approach to care both preoperatively and postoperatively has many advantages. This may include liaison with specialist nurse counsellors and psychologists before and after surgery. Medically, we have found enormous benefit at the planning stage from joint patient consultations in clinics attended by paediatric surgeons, endocrinologists and gynaecologists. Clinical decisions may also be informed by input from geneticists.

Joint operating lists with paediatric surgeons and gynaecologists provide an opportunity to discuss the management of individual cases both in the long and short term based on findings at examination under anaesthesia (EUA). These cases are often complex and may not follow the textbook descriptions. In such situations, two or several heads are generally better than one in deciding optimal management and the transition of care from paediatric to adult surgeon is streamlined. As far as the definitive operation is concerned there are also advantages in some situations in a joint approach; other surgeons that may need to be involved include plastic surgeons, urologists and bowel surgeons. As far as specific gynaecological care is concerned, the authors believe it wise, indeed vital, to involve gynaecological oncologists in the management preoperatively, intraoperatively and postoperatively of young girls with ovarian tumours. Depending on their individual skills, paediatric and adolescent gynaecologists may choose to involve laparoscopic and hysteroscopic surgeons in management of specific patients. The underlying principle to all this is the importance of assembling the optimal surgical expertise to manage a particular patient.

Other advantages of the multidisciplinary approach are discussed in Chapter 17 and include for the patient, and/or parents, less visits to clinics, better long-term healthcare planning, an easier transition from paediatric to adult care and better decision making from several experts rather than one. As far as healthcare professionals are concerned, there are advantages as well. The opportunity to discuss difficult cases with colleagues is enormously educational. For doctors in training, such clinics and theatre lists provide them with a chance to see a number of related cases in a session, which in normal circumstances might take them

several years to see. The educational benefits to them are obvious.

There is currently considerable controversy, discussed elsewhere in this book, over the choice of surgery particularly in regard to vaginal and clitoral anomalies (see Ch. 17). There is much to be gained from a more conservative approach. This is perhaps best exemplified by the current management of patients presenting with complete androgen insensitivity syndrome where the use of Frank's dilators has superceded surgery as first-line treatment (see Ch. 13).

Preservation of fertility should always be considered. The knowledge of what can be achieved using assisted conception techniques is important when making management decisions. A crystal ball that could show us what might be possible in 10–20 years time would also be helpful, but in the absence of this it seems wise to avoid removing tissue without good reason. As far as uterine anomalies are concerned, surgery should be chosen with subsequent reproductive performance in mind.

The problem of urinary incontinence tends to be underestimated in patients with Müllerian tract abnormalities (Caione et al., 1995). The psychological problems associated with incontinence, particularly in this age group, can be almost insuperable and it is, therefore, important to consider this both pre- and intraoperatively when selecting an operative procedure.

The timing of surgery is another controversial area (Hall et al., 1985). Is it better to operate early or late? Can surgery be postponed until after the menarche or will this cause additional medical complications? Should gonads be removed prepubertally to avoid any risk of malignant change or should they be retained until after puberty so that the patient can benefit from the physiological output of hormones? At the moment, there seem to be more questions than answers. What is becoming increasingly clear is that each patient should be considered individually and the management discussed on its own merits. Further discussion takes place in the following chapters on individual conditions.

Preoperative decision making

As discussed above, this should be team based with parents and child. It is important to assemble as much information as possible preoperatively so that there is a clear diagnosis. This may have involved endocrinological and genetic evaluation as well as ultrasound, magnetic resonance imaging (MRI) and examination under anaesthetic. It is important to have an unhurried consultation with both parents and child or adolescent so that all know what to expect.

This is also an opportunity to sign the relevant consent forms.

Several studies have suggested that it is beneficial to prepare children and adolescents for surgery and that this reduces the psychological upset resulting from hospitalization (Emans et al., 1998). Educating the patient and parents before an operation can help to reduce anxiety; booklets, films, artwork, puppet shows and tours of operating suites and recovery rooms can be used. In order to do this successfully, it is important for doctors and other staff involved to understand the different stages of child development, from the limited reasoning of the curious toddler to the adolescent who is capable of abstract thought and is able to consider hypotheses. It is important to provide appropriate advice, pitched at the right level and delivered in the right way (see Ch. 17).

Surgical correction of a vaginal anomaly does not correct the patient's self-image. It is important to address the psychological and sexual issues, as well as the reproductive ones, if possible before embarking on surgery (Spence, 1998). It is sensible to involve the psychologist preoperatively. Patients should be given information about support groups relevant to their condition. If operations require significant input from the patient postoperatively, for example the use of dilators, it is important to ensure preoperatively that the patient is happy and ready to do this. It is becoming increasingly clear that one of the most important factors determining the success of operations such as vaginoplasty is the psychosocial adjustment of the patient preoperatively (Rock, 1997).

There is increasing evidence that parents should be encouraged to stay with the child while they are in hospital, both to provide support and to help with their care (Emans et al., 1998). Most children taken into hospital, which is after all an unfamiliar environment, are frightened and, if separated from their parents as well, may focus on this separation. Parents now are encouraged to accompany children undergoing operations to theatre and to be present in the recovery room afterwards. They will obviously need preparation for such a role as well.

If care is taken to address the social, psychological and developmental needs of patients undergoing gynaecological procedures, the outcome is likely to be better than if attention is solely paid to the abnormality with which they present.

Type of surgery

The different types of reconstructive surgery are described in the relevant chapters and will not be discussed in detail here.

Uterine anomalies

Incidence

The true prevalence of Müllerian duct abnormalities in the general population is not clearly established, with estimates of between 0.001 and 10% (Buttram, 1983; Hamilton et al., 1998; Manesci et al., 1995; Raga et al., 1997; Sharara, 1998; Stampe-Sorenson, 1988). Most authors have estimated prevalence in infertile or fertile women. One such study identified rates of 0.17% in fertile women and 3.5% in infertile women, a difference that was statistically significant (Nahum, 1998). If hysterosalpingography (HSG) is used, up to 16% of infertile women may have a uterine anomaly (Makino et al., 1992a). In contrast, only 1.9% of women undergoing sterilization had a uterine anomaly on HSG. Up to 10–15% of women with recurrent pregnancy loss have a uterine anomaly (Bacsko, 1997; Makino et al., 1992b).

Attempts to assess prevalence in the general population have proved more difficult. Nahum (1998) reported a prevalence of 0.5%. Jurkovic et al. (1997) found major anomalies in 2.3% of women attending for gynaecological ultrasound scans. Byrne et al. (2000) attempted to estimate prevalence in girls and women who had ultrasound scans for reasons unrelated to the presence of uterine anomalies and found a rate of 3.9 per 1000 (0.4%). However, both of these studies are not estimating prevalence in the general population, but rather in a population with some, albeit apparently unrelated, gynaecological problem. Of course, such estimates also depend on how uterine anomalies are defined and the detection methods used.

Definitions

Several classifications have been used for upper tract anomalies but that adopted by the American Society of Reproductive Medicine (ASRM; previously known as the American Fertility Society (AFS)) is probably the most useful. This was adapted from a classification proposed by Buttram and Gibbons in 1979, which was based on the degree of failure of normal development of the Müllerian tract (Letterie, 1998). Abnormalities are divided into groups with similar clinical presentations, treatments and prognosis. The classification was updated by the ASRM in 1988 (AFS, 1988) and divides abnormalities into seven groups: type I hypoplasia and agenesis (vagina, cervix, uterus, tubes); type II unicornuate uterus (both patent and obstructed); type III uterine didelphys; type IV bicornuate uterus (partial and complete); type V septate uterus (partial and complete); type VI arcuate; type VII exposure to

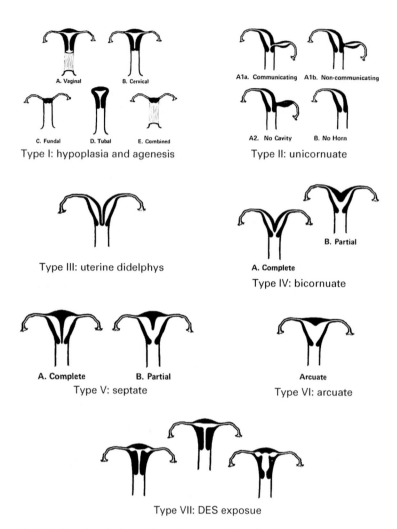

Type I: hypoplasia and agenesis

A. Vaginal   B. Cervical   C. Fundal   D. Tubal   E. Combined

Type II: unicornuate

A1a. Communicating   A1b. Non-communicating   A2. No Cavity   B. No Horn

Type III: uterine didelphys

Type IV: bicornuate

A. Complete   B. Partial

Type V: septate

A. Complete   B. Partial

Type VI: arcuate

Arcuate

Type VII: DES exposue

Fig. 11.1. American Society of Reproductive Medicine classification of Müllerian anomalies. DES, diethylstilbestrol.

diethylstilboestrol (DES) (Fig. 11.1). Subsequently, further classification of communicating uteri (types III and IV) has been recommended to help the management of these often complex anomalies (Edmonds, 1994; Fedele et al., 1988; Toaff et al., 1984). It is important also to clarify the anatomy of the renal tract in such patients as there are often associated anomalies (Golan et al., 1989). This can be recorded on the ASRM classification forms.

Use of a classification scheme such as that recommended by the ASRM helps the clinician to clarify the diagnosis, counsel the patient and select appropriate management, be that surgical or conservative.

Importance

Uterine anomalies have been associated with an increased incidence of urinary tract anomalies and an in-creased likelihood of infertility, early pregnancy loss, mid-trimester loss, antepartum bleeding, premature rupture of membranes, preterm labour, malpresentation, postpartum haemorrhage and retained placenta (Bacsko, 1997; Ben Rafael et al., 1991; Gemer and Segal, 1994; Musich and Behrman, 1978; Rock and Schlaff, 1985; Sharara, 1998; Tulandi et al., 1980). They will tend, therefore, to have a high caesarean section rate. Rarely, pregnancy can occur in noncommunicating rudimentary uterine horn with subsequent rupture (Hickey et al., 1998). Uterine anomalies have also been associated with endometriosis and pelvic pain (Keltz et al., 1994; San Filippo, 1986) and menstrual dysfunction (Ansbacher, 1983; Emans et al., 1998). The incidence of such problems is dependent on the type of anomaly.

There is some debate over the link between uterine anomalies and infertility (Ashton et al., 1988). Several authors conclude that uterine anomalies are rarely the cause of infertility (Heinonen and Pystynen, 1983; Musich and Behrman, 1978; Papp et al., 1986; Wiersma et al., 1976).

Indications for operation

If uterine anomalies are rarely the cause of infertility and many women with such anomalies are fertile, then operations to restore normal anatomy should only be used as a last resort (Musich and Behrman, 1978). It is important to identify other causes of infertility first and also to be aware of the long-term effects of such operations on reproductive behaviour.

Currently, many women undergoing in vitro fertilization treatment who are found to have a septate uterus are advised to have surgery as it is believed that this increases implantation rates (Lavergne et al., 1996). The evidence on which to base this decision is, however, somewhat limited.

Patients with a past obstetric history of recurrent miscarriage, mid-trimester loss, premature delivery or malpresentation who also have a uterine anomaly may benefit from surgery (Golan et al., 1989; Heinonen, 1982; Ludmir et al., 1990; Makino et al., 1992a). Heinonen et al. (1982) noted that obstetric outcome improved from 10% successful pregnancies to 88% after metroplasty. However, some recent studies have questioned this (Kirk et al., 1993; Manesci et al., 1993). The type of anomaly may also be important; Musich and Behrman (1978) noted that patients with septate and bicornuate uteri were more likely to be poor obstetric performers than those with didelphic uteri. Metroplasty seems to prevent breech delivery and to reduce the caesarean section rate, which are potential benefits although not necessarily an indication for surgery (Heinonen, 1997).

Several authors have recommended cervical cerclage in patients with symmetric uterine anomalies in association with premature labour and recommended that this should be tried first before embarking on more radical surgery (Abramovici, 1983; Golan et al., 1989). It is important that any decision to proceed with surgery is only taken after careful evaluation of the individual patient and their reproductive history. Other causes of reproductive loss must be excluded first.

Most women with a longitudinal vaginal septum and double vagina will be asymptomatic. A few will report difficulty with inserting tampons or dyspareunia, in which case surgical excision of the septum may be indicated (Heinonen, 1982). Occasionally, patients present with a double uterus and unilateral haematocolpos secondary to an obstructed hemivagina. Such patients characteristically have ipsilateral renal agenesis. In this situation, excision of the vaginal septum is the preferred surgical option (Rock, 1997).

A rudimentary uterine horn can present with dysmenorrhoea in the adolescent if there is functioning endometrium present (Emans et al., 1998). These patients are at increased risk of endometriosis. This tends to regress after surgery (San Filippo et al., 1986). Spontaneous pregnancies have also been reported in obstructed uterine horns. These are unlikely to progress to viability and may rupture, causing intra-abdominal haemorrage (Hickey et al., 1998). On balance, therefore, it may be sensible to excise rudimentary horns with functioning endometrium.

Preoperative workup

As discussed earlier in this chapter, careful preoperative workup is important. An accurate preoperative diagnosis allows a planned and efficient surgical approach (Keltz et al., 1994). Genital tract aberrations are very variable and do not always fall into a specific category. They may also be associated with renal anomalies and urinary difficulty, for instance incontinence (Caione et al., 1995). It is, therefore, vital to evaluate all patients thoroughly (Spence, 1998).

MRI is particularly valuable in this group of patients and may obviate the need for an EUA prior to definitive surgery (Doyle, 1992; Lang et al., 1999; Olson et al., 1992; Pellerito et al., 1992; Wagner and Woodward, 1994; Woodward et al., 1995). Its usefulness was first recognized in the late 1980s (McCarthy, 1990; Mintz et al., 1987); it is particularly helpful in determining the site of obstruction in obstructive uterovaginal anomalies (haematometros, haematocolpos). Other investigations may include ultrasonography (Jurkovic et al., 1995) and HSG (Damario and Rock, 2000). Wu et al. (1997) argue that three-dimensional ultrasound can give similar information to an HSG while being less invasive. Saline hysterosonography has also been recommended by some authors as an acceptable first-line screening procedure (Alatas et al., 1997; Hamilton et al., 1998). EUA plus vaginoscopy, hysteroscopy and laparoscopy may be necessary to clarify the diagnosis in the more complex cases. Laparoscopy may be contraindicated in some patients, for example after multiple complex surgical procedures for cloacal anomalies, in which case MRI is the investigation of choice (Minto et al., 2001).

Surgical techniques

Some papers have been published evaluating the various surgical techniques (Ansbacher, 1983; Spence, 1998) but they are probably more comprehensively described in textbooks of gynaecological surgery (Edmonds, 1994; Jones, 1992; Rock, 1997).

Rudimentary uterine horn

A rudimentary uterine horn, if functioning and causing dysmenorrhoea, may need removal. This can be performed as an open technique or laparoscopically.

Bicornuate and septate uteri: metroplasty

Metroplasty is the surgical treatment of bicornuate and septate uteri. Traditionally this procedure was performed abdominally via a pfannenstiel approach. However, there are advantages to the hysteroscopic approach. Both will be described here.

Hysteroscopy can be used to visualize the uterine cavity and also to resect uterine septae. Preoperative treatment with a gonadotrophin-releasing hormone analogue for one to two months is recommended to thin the endometrium. The septum can either be divided using hysteroscopic scissors (Assaf et al., 1990) or be excised using a resectoscope with a cutting blade (De Cherney et al., 1986; Taylor and Gordon, 1993; Valle, 1999). Whichever is used, a continuous flow system to wash out debris is advised. The septum is divided in the midline in order to avoid blood vessels close to the uterine wall. Concurrent laparoscopy is recommended; this allows observation of transillumination of the hysteroscopic light through the uterine wall and reduces the risk of perforation. Laparoscopy can also be used to assess the rest of the pelvis and helps to differentiate the bicornuate uterus from the septate one. When the uterine septum is fully divided, this light becomes uniform across the whole uterus and both tubal ostia can be seen clearly when moving the hysteroscope from side to side. Bleeding will tend to occur when healthy myometrium is excised at the top of the septum; dissection can then be halted. Finally, the intrauterine pressure can be reduced and bleeding vessels selectively cauterized (if electrocautery is used it is important to use a nonelectrolyte distending medium, e.g. glycine, sorbitol, mannitol). For wider septae, a resectoscope can be used or a Nd:Yag (neodymium/yttrium–aluminium–garnet) laser. Septae that extend to the cervix may require fenestration prior to their removal (Valle, 1999).

Complications include uterine perforation, fluid overload and bleeding. The advantages over laparotomy are less postoperative morbidity, shorter inpatient stay and quicker recovery. Patients can also have a subsequent vaginal delivery. As a result, hysteroscopic resection has now largely replaced the abdominal approach for septate uteri (Heinonen, 1997).

Open metroplasty (the Jones or Tompkin technique) can be used when the uterine septum is broad and not easily incised with the resectoscope. The Strassman procedure is used to unify a bicornuate uterus (Rock, 1997).

In the Jones metroplasty, a wedge of uterine tissue is excised to include the uterine septum. It is important that the incisions at the top of the uterine fundus are not too close to the insertion of the Fallopian tubes (certainly no closer than 1 cm). If the incisions are then directed to the apex of the wedge, transection of the interstitial portion of the tubes should be avoided. The uterus is then closed in layers with interrupted sutures. Rock (1997) describes a modified Jones metroplasty that advocates using either tourniquets around the uterine and ovarian arteries or injections of vasopressin into the uterus to reduce the bleeding.

The Tompkins metroplasty involves a longitudinal incision in the midline extending anteriorly and posteriorly from the uterine fundus until the operator enters the uterine cavity and has effectively bivalved the uterus. Each lateral septal half is then incised to within 1 cm of the tubes until the septum has been excised. The single uterine cavity is repaired in a similar way to the Jones' metroplasty.

Strassmans' operation for unifying a bicornuate uterus involves a transverse incision across the uterine fundus from cornua to cornua, avoiding the uterotubal junctions, which exposes both uterine cavities. The septum is then divided. The transverse incision is converted into a vertical one using layers of interrupted sutures and the two uterine cavities can be united (Letterie, 1998). If present, a rectovesical ligament extending over and attached between the two uterine corpora may need to be excised prior to making the incision on the uterus. As in the hysteroscopic procedure, no attempt should be made to unify a double or septate cervix, as this can result in cervical incompetence (Rock, 1997).

Postoperative care after metroplasty

Most authors suggest that there is no need to insert an intrauterine device postoperatively to prevent intrauterine adhesion formation. Some recommend high-dose oestrogen (e.g. 2.5 mg conjugated oestrogen twice daily for 30 days) followed by a progestogen challenge (e.g. medroxyprogesterone 10 mg for 10 days) (Letterie, 1998).

Follow-up evaluation with an hysteroscopy or HSG is advised to confirm that the procedure was adequate and that there are no postoperative intrauterine adhesions.

As far as advice is concerned, Rock (1997) advises that patients wait four to six months after an open metroplasty before trying to conceive. Elective caesarean section is recommended after an open procedure whereas patients who have had hysteroscopic removal of a septum can have a vaginal delivery (Bacsko, 1997).

Longitudinal vaginal septae

Longitudinal septae may be asymptomatic or may present with dyspareunia or difficulty with tampon insertion. Less commonly, one side of the vagina may be obstructed. Surgical incision is relatively straightforward although the vagina is very vascular and care must be taken with haemostasis. The increasing availability of the hand-held harmonic scalpel may simplify this. Care must be taken not to incise too close to the vaginal mucosa to prevent causing a defect or stricture to the vagina.

Transverse vaginal septae

Transverse septae are much more complex to manage. They are most commonly found at the junction of the middle and upper vagina and usually present with haematocolpos, which may be complicated by haematometra, bilateral haematosalpinges and pelvic endometriosis. It is essential to identify the amount of vagina above and below the septum and this is best done with MRI (Minto et al., 2001).

If the septum is thin and low within the vagina it may be possible to remove it from below. Once the septum is removed, the upper and lower vagina can be reanastomosed. It is essential to ensure the whole septum is removed otherwise contracture may occur. If the septum is thick, then a combined abdominal and perineal approach may be required. It is usually possible to reanastomose the upper and lower vagina, provided that adequate mobilization can be achieved. In some cases, however, the distance to be bridged is too great and an interposition skin or intestinal graft may be required. Postoperatively, it is usually necessary to use vaginal dilators for a period of time to preserve patency and prevent stricture. Fertility may be affected if significant endometriosis resulted from retrograde menstruation.

Improvements in outcomes after surgery

A number of authors have attempted to evaluate the benefits of surgery in patients with uterine anomalies. It is worth remembering that outcomes in reproductive medicine tend in general to improve with successive pregnancies and this can make assessment of outcome after surgery difficult. Outcome studies that compare pregnancies before and after surgery may, therefore, be difficult to interpret.

A number of studies have demonstrated an improvement in reproductive performance after surgery (Ayhan et al., 1992; Gray et al., 1984; Hannoun et al., 1989; Khalil et al., 1995; Makino et al., 1992a; Spiritos et al., 1987; Zorlu et al., 1996). However, many of these report small numbers, are retrospective and some patients may have had other reasons for their infertility that were treated at the same time (Kirk et al., 1993).

A few studies have compared patients with similar conditions who have or have not had surgery. In one study, the percentage of patients with living children after the diagnosis of septate or bicornuate uteri was 73% for those who had undergone metroplasty and 67% for those who did not have surgery, which was not statistically significant (Kirk et al., 1993). Fetal salvage rates did improve after surgery but obstetric outcome was similar to that of the control group after the diagnosis was made and surgery deferred. In another study that compared reproductive outcomes after abdominal metroplasty for bicornuate uterus, cumulative pregnancy rates were 88% after two years compared with 95% in patients with no surgical correction (Manesci et al., 1993). These studies, therefore, question the value of metroplasty in the treatment of multiple pregnancy loss in association with uterine anomalies and support the need for a randomized prospective study to investigate the efficacy of metroplasty. However, the debate continues, as Makino et al. (1992a) have reported significant improvements in maintaining pregnancy after metroplasty (84%) compared with a randomly selected group that did not have surgery and where 94% of pregnancies terminated spontaneously before 12 weeks of gestation.

Most women with a uterine anomaly will successfully achieve a pregnancy without intervention, although the likelihood of early pregnancy loss, malpresentation and caesarean section is increased (Matts et al., 2000). There is no clear evidence that metroplasty is of benefit in recurrent pregnancy loss or infertility but it may help in women with a history of second-trimester loss or preterm labour.

Summary

Box 11.1 outlines the key points for reconstructive surgery of the genital tract. Preoperative planning and psychological preparation of the patient is the key to a successful outcome. Most of the conditions described are rare and should be managed in specialist centres with not only surgical expertise but also access to multidisciplinary and wide-ranging clinical support services.

Box 11.1 Key points

- The aim of reconstructive surgery of the genital tract is to facilitate menstruation, allow comfortable and enjoyable sexual intercourse, maximize fertility prospects and ensure a good cosmetic outcome.
- A multidisciplinary approach pre- and postoperatively is advantageous using optimal surgical expertise to manage a particular case; this may involve gynaecologists, paediatric surgeons, urologists and plastic surgeons.
- The patient's psychological, sexual, reproductive and developmental needs should be addressed before embarking on surgery. Such preoperative planning is essential and includes full discussion with the patient and her parents.
- The evidence base for choosing the surgical method is limited and the timing of surgery is controversial: hence care should be individualised.

REFERENCES

Abbe R (1898). A new method of creating a vagina in a case of congenital absence. *Med Rec* 54, 836–838.

Abramovici H, Faktor J H, Pascal B (1983). Congenital uterine malformations as indication for cervical suture (cerclage) in habitual abortion and premature delivery. *Int J Fertil* 28, 161–164.

Alatas C, Aksoy E, Akarsu C, Yaakin K, Aksoy S, Hayran M (1997). Evaluation of intrauterine abnormalities in infertile patients by sonohysterography. *Hum Reprod* 12, 487–490.

American Fertility Society (1988). The American Fertility Society classifications of adnexal adhesions, distal tubal occlusion, tubal occlusion secondary to tubal ligation, tubal pregnancies, mullerian abnormalities and intrauterine adhesions. *Fertil Steril* 49, 1944–1955.

Ansbacher R (1983). Uterine anomalies and future pregnancies. *Clin Perinatol* 10, 295–304.

Ashton D, Amin H K, Richart R M, Neuwirth R S (1988). The incidence of asymptomatic uterine anomalies in women undergoing transcervical tubal sterilization. *Obstet Gynecol* 72, 28–30.

Ashworth M F, Morton K E, Dewhurst J, Lilford R J, Bates R G (1986). Vaginoplasty using amnion. *Obstet Gynecol* 67, 443–446.

Assaf A, Serour G, Ackady A, El-Agizy H (1990). Endoscopic management of the intrauterine septum. *Int J Gynaecol Obstet* 32, 43–51.

Ayhan A, Yucel I, Tunrer Z S, Kisnisci H A (1992). Reproductive performance after conventional metroplasty: an evaluation of 102 cases. *Fertil Steril* 57, 1194–1196.

Bacsko G (1997). Uterine surgery by operative hysteroscopy. *Eur J Obstet Gynaecol Reprod Biol* 71, 219–222.

Baldwin J F (1904). The formation of an artificial vagina by intestinal transplantation. *Ann Surg* 40, 398.

Ben Rafael Z, Seidman D S, Recabi K, Bider D, Mashiach S (1991). Uterine anomalies: a retrospective matched control study. *J Reprod Med* 36, 723–727.

Buttram V C (1983). Mullerian anomalies and their management. *Fertil Steril* 40, 159–161.

Buttram V C Jr, Gibbons W E (1979). Mullerian anomalies: a proposed classification (an analysis of 144 cases). *Fertil Steril* 32, 40–46.

Byrne J, Nussbaum-Blask A, Taylor W S et al. (2000). Prevalence of mullerian duct anomalies detected at ultrasound. *Am J Med Genet* 94, 9–12.

Caione P, Silveri M, Capitanucci M L, Capozia N, De Gennaro M (1995). Urinary incontinence in mullerian duct anomalies. *Pamminerva Med* 37, 14–17.

Cali R W, Pratt J H (1968). Congenital absence of the vagina: long term results of vaginal reconstruction in 175 cases. *Am J Obstet Gynecol* 100, 752–763.

Chervenak F A, Neuwirth R S (1981). Hysteroscopic resection of the uterine septum. *Am J Obstet Gynecol* 141, 351.

Claret I, Castanon M, Rodo J et al. (1988). Neovagina con injerto libre do mucosa vesical (technical original de Claret). *Libro de Actas del XXVIII Congreso de la Sociedad Espanola de Chirugia Pediatrica*, Lloret de Mar, Spain.

Counsellor V S (1948). Congenital absence of the vagina. *J Am Med Assoc* 136, 861.

Daly D C, Walters C A, Soto-Albors et al. (1983). Hysteroscopic metroplasty: surgical technique and obstetrical outcome. *Fertil Steril* 39, 623.

Damario M A, Rock J A (2000). Uterovaginal anomalies. In *Paediatric and Adolescent Gynaecology*, 2nd edn, Koehler Carpenter S E, Rock J A, eds, pp. 332–353. Lippincourt Williams & Wilkins, Philadelphia, PA.

de Cherney A, Russell J B, Graebe R A (1986). Resectoscopic management of mullerian fusion defects. *Fertil Steril* 45, 726.

Davydov S N, Zhvitiashvili O D (1974). Formation of vagina (colpopoiesis) from peritoneum of Douglas pouch. *Acta Chir Plast* 16, 35–41.

Doyle M B (1992). Magnetic resonance imaging in mullerian fusion defects. *J Reprod Med* 37, 33–38.

Edmonds D K (1994). Sexual development anomalies and their reconstruction: upper and lower tracts. In *Pediatric and Adolescent Gynecology*, Sanfillipo J, Muram D, Lee P, Dewhurst J, eds., pp. 535–566. Saunders, Philadelphia, PA.

Emans S J, Laufer M R, Goldstein D P (1998). *Paediatric and Adolescent Gynaecology*. Lippincourt Williams & Wilkins, Philadelphia, PA.

Fedele L, Vercellini P, Marchini M et al. (1988). Communication uteri: description and classification of a new type. *Int J Fertil* 33, 168.

Fortunoff S, Lattimer J K, Edson M (1964). Vaginoplasty technique for female pseudohermaphrodites. *Surg Gynecol Obstet* 118 545–548.

Frank R T (1938). The formation of an artificial vagina without operation. *Am J Obstet Gynecol* 35, 1053–1055.

Gemer O, Segal S (1994). Incidence and contribution of predisposing factors to transverse lie presentation. *Int J Gynaecol Obstet* 44, 219–221.

Golan A, Ranger R, Burkousky I, Caspi E (1989). Congenital anomalies of the mullerian system. *Fertil Steril* 1989 51, 747–755.

Gray S E, Roberts D K, Franklin R R (1984). Fertility after metroplasty of the septate uterus. *J Reprod Med* 29, 185–188.

Hamilton J A, Larson A J, Lower A M, Hasnain S, Grudzinskas J G (1998). Routine use of saline hysterosonography in 500 consecutive unselected infertile women. *Hum Reprod* 13, 2463–2473.

Hall R, Fleming S, Gysrer M, McCorie G (1985). The genital tract in female children with an imperforate anus. *Am J Obstet Gynecol* 151, 169–171.

Hannoun A, Khalil A, Karan K (1989). Uterine unification procedure: postoperative obstetrical outcome. *Int J Gynaecol Obstet* 30, 161–164.

Heinonen P K (1982). Longitudinal vaginal septum. *Eur J Obstet Gynaecol Reprod Biol* 13, 253–258.

(1997). Reproductive performance of women with uterine anomalies after abdominal or hysteroscopic metroplasty or no surgical treatment. *J Am Assoc Gynecol Laparosc* 4, 311–317.

Heinonen P K, Pystynen P P (1983). Primary infertility and uterine anomalies. *Fertil Steril* 40, 311–316.

Heinonen P K, Saarikoski S, Pystynen P (1982). Reproductive performance of women with uterine anomalies: an evaluation of 182 cases. *Acta Obstet Gynecol Scand* 61, 157.

Hendren W H, Donahue P K (1980). Correction of congenital abnormalities of vagina and perineum. *J Pediatr Surg* 15, 751–763.

Hickey K, Cairns A, Balen A H (1998). Rupture of a rudimentary uterine horn at 19 weeks' gestation. *J Obstet Gynecol* 18, 394.

Israel R, March C M (1981). Hysteroscopic incision of the septate uterus. *Am J Obstet Gynecol* 140, 867.

Jackson N D, Rosenblatt P L (1994). Use of Interceed absorbable adhesion barrier for vaginoplasty. *Obstet Gynecol* 84, 1048–1050.

Jones H W Jr (1992). Reconstruction of congenital uterovaginal anomalies. In *Female Reproductive Surgery*, Rock J, Murphy A, Jones H W, eds. Williams & Wilkins, Baltimore, MD.

Jones H W Jr, Jones G E S (1954). The gynaecological aspects of adrenal hyperplasia and allied disorders. *Am J Obstet Gynecol* 68, 1330.

Judin S (1927). *Surg Gynecol Obstet* 44, 530.

Jurkovic D, Geipel A, Grboeck K, Jauniaux E, Natucci M, Campbell S (1995). Three dimensional ultrasound for the assessment of uterine anatomy, detection of congenital anomalies: a comparison with hysterosalpingography and two dimensional sonography. *Ultrasound Obstet Gynecol* 5, 233–237.

Jurkovic D, Gruboeck K, Tailor A, Nicolaides K H (1997). Ultrasound screening for congenital uterine anomalies. *Br J Obstet Gynaecol* 104, 1320–1321.

Keltz M D, Berger S B, Comite F, Olive D I (1994). Duplicate cervix and vagina associated with infertility, endometriosis and chronic pelvic pain. *Obstet Gynecol* 84, 701–703.

Khalil A M, Azar G B, Hannoun A B, Sawaya J T, Abumasa A A (1995). Reproductive outcome following abdominal metroplasty. *Int J Gynaecol Obstet* 49, 157–160.

Kirk E P, Chyong J, Coulam C B, Williams T J (1993). Pregnancy after metroplasty for uterine anomalies. *Fertil Steril* 59, 1164–1168.

Kumar H, Kiefer I E, Rosenthal I E, Clark S S (1974). Clitoroplasty: experience during a 19 year period. *J Urol* 111, 81–84.

Lang I M, Babyn P, Oliver G D (1999). MR imaging of paediatric uterovaginal anomalies. *Pediatr Radiol* 29, 163–170.

Lavergne N, Aristizabal J, Zarka V, Erny R, Hedon B (1996). Uterine anomalies and in vitro fertilization: what are the results? *Eur J Obstet Gynaecol Reprod Biol* 68, 29–34.

Letterie G S (1998). *Structural Abnormalities and Reproductive Failure.* Blackwell Science, Oxford.

Ludmir J, Samuels P, Brooks S, Mennuti M T (1990). Pregnancy outcome of patients with uncorrected uterine anomalies managed in a high risk obstetric setting. *Obstet Gynecol* 75, 906–910.

McCarthy S (1990). Gynecological applications of MRI. *Crit Rev Diagn Imaging* 31, 263–281.

Makino T, Umeuchi M, Nakada K, Nozawa S, Iizuka R (1992a). Incidence of congenital uterine anomalies in repeated reproductive wastage and prognosis for pregnancy after metroplasty. *Int J Fertil* 37, 167–170.

Makino T, Hara T, Oka C et al. (1992b). Survey of 1120 Japanese women with a history of recurrent spontaneous abortions. *Eur J Obstet Gynaecol Reprod Biol* 44, 123–130.

Manesci F, Marana R, Muzii L, Manusco S (1993). Reproductive performance in women with bicornuate uterus. *Acta Eur Fertil* 24, 117–120.

Maneschi F, Zupi E, Marconi D, Valli E, Romanini C, Mancuso S (1995). Hysteroscopically detected asymptomatic mullerian anomalies: prevalence and reproductive implications. *J Reprod Med* 40, 684–688.

McIndoe A H, Bannister J B (1938). An operation for the cure of congenital absence of the vagina. *J Obstet Gynaecol Br Emp* 45, 490–494.

Matts S J, Clark T J, Khan K S, Gupta J K (2000). Surgical correction of congenital uterine anomalies. *Hosp Med* 61, 246–249.

Miller N F (1992). Clinical aspects of uterus didelphys. *Am J Obstet Gynecol* 4, 398–408.

Minto C L, Hollings N, Hall-Craggs M, Creighton S (2001). Magnetic resonance imaging in the assessment of complex Mullerian anomalies. *Br J Obstet Gynaecol* 108, 791–797.

Mintz M C, Thickman D I, Gussman D, Kressel H Y (1987). MR evaluation of uterine anomalies. *Am J Roentgenol* 148, 287–290.

Musich J R, Behrman S J (1978). Obstetric outcome before and after metroplasty in women with uterine anomalies. *Obstet Gynecol* 52, 63–66.

Nahum G G (1998). Uterine anomalies. How common are they and what is their distribution among subtypes? *J Reprod Med* 43, 877–887.

Olson M C, Posniak H V, Tempany C M, Dudiak C M (1992). MR imaging of the female pelvic region. *Radiographics* 12, 445–465.

Papp Z, Toth Z, Csecsei K (1986). Ultrasound surveillance of pregnancies after metroplasty for septate uteri. *Z Gynakol* 108, 1307–1311.

Passerini-Glazel G (1989). A new I stage procedure for clitorovaginoplasty in severely masculinised female pseudohermaphrodites. *J Urol* 142, 562–568.

Pellerito J S, McCarthy S M, Doyle M B, Glickman M G, de Cherney A H (1992). Diagnosis of uterine anomalies: relative accuracy of MR imaging, endovaginal sonography and hysterosalpingography. *Radiology* 183, 795–800.

Raga F, Bauset C, Remohi J, Bonilla-Musoles F, Simon C, Pellicer A (1997). Reproductive impact of congenital Mullerian anomalies. *Hum Reprod* 12, 2277–2281.

Rock J A (1997). Surgery for anomalies of the Mullerian ducts. In *Te Linde's Operative Gynaecology*, 8th edn, Rock J A, Thompson J D, eds., pp. 687–729. Lippincott-Raven, Philadelphia, PA.

Rock J A, Schlaff W D (1985). The obstetric consequences of uterovaginal anomalies. *Fertil Steril* 43, 681–692.

Ruge P (1884). Fall von schwangerschaft bei uterus septus. *Z Gebutshilfe Gynakol* 10, 141–143.

Sagehashi N (1993). Clitoroplasty for cliteromegaly due to adrenogenital syndrome without loss of sensitivity. *Plast Reconst Surg* 91, 950–955.

Sanfilippo J S, Wakin N G, Schikler K N, Yussman M A (1986). Endometriosis in association with uterine anomalies. *Am J Obstet Gynaecol* 154, 39–43.

Schmid M A (1961). *Arch Klin Chic* 298, 977.

Schober J (1999). Feminising genitoplasty for intersex. *Br J Urol Int* 83, 39–50.

Sharara F I (1998). Complete uterine septum with cervical duplication, longitudinal vaginal septum and duplication of a renal collecting system. A case report. *J Reprod Med* 43, 1055–1059.

Sheares B H (1960). Congenital atresia of the vagina: a new technique for tunneling the space between the bladder and rectum and construction of a new vagina by a modified Wharton technique. *J Obstet Gynaecol Br Emp* 67, 24–31.

Spence J E (1998). Vaginal and uterine anomalies in the pediatric and adolescent patient. *J Pediatr Adolesc Gynecol* 11, 3–11.

Spence J M, Allen T D (1973). Genital reconstruction in the female with the adrenogenital syndrome. *Br J Urol* 45, 126–130.

Spiritos N J, Evans T N, Magyar D M, Moghissi K S (1987). The reproductive performance of women before and after metroplasty. *Int J Fertil* 32, 46–49.

Stampe-Sorenson S (1988). Estimated prevalence of mullerian anomalies. *Acta Obstet Gynecol Scand* 67, 441–445.

Taylor P J, Gordon A G (1993). *Practical Hysteroscopy*. Blackwell Scientific, Oxford.

Toaff M E, Lev-Toaff A S, Toaff R (1984). Communicating uteri: review, classification with introduction of two previously unreported types. *Fertil Steril* 41, 661.

Tompkins P (1962). Comments on the bicornuate uterus and twinning. *Surg Clin North Am* 42, 1049.

Tulandi T, Arronet G H, McInnes R A (1980). Arcuate and bicornuate uterine anomalies and infertility. *Fertil Steril* 34, 362–364.

Valle R F (1999). Hysteroscopic resection of uterine septum. In *Atlas of Laparoscopic and Hysteroscopic Techniques for Gynecologists*, Tulandi T W B, ed., pp. 239–246. Saunders, London.

Wagner B J, Woodward P J (1994). Magnetic resonance evaluation of congenital uterine anomalies. *Semin Ultrasound CT MR* 15, 4–17.

Wharton L R (1938). A simplified method of constructing a vagina. *Ann Surg* 107, 842.

Wiersma A F, Peterson L F, Justema E J (1976). Uterine anomalies associated with unilateral renal agenesis. *Obstet Gynecol* 47, 654–657.

Williams E A (1964). Congenital absence of the vagina: a simple operation for its relief. *Br J Obstet Gynaecol* 4, 511–512.

Woodward P J, Sohaey R, Wagner B J (1995). Congenital uterine malformations. *Curr Probl Diagn Radiol* 24, 178–197.

Wu M H, Hsu C C, Huang K E (1997). Detection of congenital mullerian duct anomalies using 3 dimensional ultrasound. *J Clin Ultrasound* 25, 487–492.

Zorlu C G, Yalcin H, Ugur M, Ozden S, Kara-Soysal S, Gokmen O (1996). Reproductive outcome after metroplasty. *Int J Gynaecol Obstet* 55, 45–48.

12

Laparoscopic techniques

Azad S. Najmaldin[1] and Alfred Cutner[2]

[1]St James University Hospital, Leeds, UK
[2]Elizabeth Garrett Anderson Hospital, London, UK

Introduction

The first gynaecological reports for laparoscopy came from Hope in 1937 (Hope, 1937) on the diagnosis of extrauterine pregnancy but it was not until the 1970s that laparoscopic surgery started to become established (Semm, 1970). The introduction of good-resolution camera systems and the development of new surgical instruments have enabled the advancement of laparoscopic surgery. In addition, advances in technology have increased the safety parameters and enabled surgery to be performed more efficiently. These technological developments include the expansion of bipolar technology and the introduction of laser modalities, the harmonic scalpel and haemostatic stapling devices.

Originally laparoscopic surgery was referred to as minimally invasive surgery but it soon became apparent that the surgery was highly invasive but performed through small incisions, and hence the term minimal access surgery was coined. Minimal access surgery can be considered as an alternative procedure to the traditional operation; it aims to achieve the same end result as the traditional operation but is performed through small incisions. In hysteroscopic surgery, most laparoscopic procedures should aim to emulate the open operation, the only difference being the size of the incision. However, there may be modifications in the minimal access route as a result of the improved vision that it affords or the difficulty in emulating the open procedure. The perceived disadvantages of the laparoscopic route over the open route are the potential complications, the time to perform the operation and the cost. The length of operations and safety have improved with increased sophistication of equipment and increased surgical expertise. Without doubt, the laparoscope gives better vision and is also a useful teaching aid. In addition, hospital stay and recovery once home are reduced (Cutner and Rymer, 1998; Vermesh et al., 1989). Laparoscopy was developed more slowly.

The first part of this chapter will deal with applications in paediatric surgery and gynaecology. The second part will discuss the technique in more detail and its application in adolescents and adults.

Paediatric gynaecology

AZAD S. NAJMALDIN

The application of laparoscopy in children as a safe diagnostic measure was recognized in the early 1970s (Gans and Berci, 1971). Throughout the 1970s and 1980s, the technique was used by a few paediatric surgeons to aid in the diagnosis of impalpable testes, abdominal pain, hepatobiliary disease, intersex anomalies, ascites and abdominal trauma (Gans and Berci, 1973). The introduction of multipuncture laparoscopic cholecystectomy heralded the development of laparoscopic/minimal access techniques in all surgical specialities including paediatric surgery.

Initially, paediatric surgeons did not embrace the new method with the fervour witnessed in adult surgery and gynaecology. This is because some surgeons argued that infants and children recover from conventional open operations quickly, while others felt that there is no single organ, such as the gall bladder in adult surgery or reproductive system in gynaecology, that frequently becomes diseased and

Paediatric and Adolescent Gynaecology, ed. Adam Balen et al. Published by Cambridge University Press.
© Cambridge University Press 2004.

would benefit from laparoscopic surgery. The development of paediatric laparoscopic surgery was further impeded by the slow development of miniaturized and specialized instruments.

Children do suffer the consequences of trauma from open surgery as do adult patients. The benefit of diminished postoperative pain, shorter hospital stay, low incidence of scarring and better cosmesis should be considered as important for children, if not more important, as they are for adults. In recent years, however, the practice of laparoscopy has mushroomed across the various paediatric surgical specialities and increasing numbers of surgeons are applying the new technique in their routine daily clinical practice.

This first part of the chapter highlights some of the applications of laparoscopic gynaecology in infants and children.

Operative considerations

Preoperative investigations, and preparation of the patient prior to laparoscopy should be identical to that of conventional surgery. The patients and parents/carers are fully informed and consent is obtained for both laparoscopy and the open technique in case of emergency and/or conversion. As for most surgical procedures in children, laparoscopy is performed under general anaesthesia with endotracheal intubation and full muscle relaxation (Najmaldin and Grousseau, 1999). A preliminary inspection and palpation of the abdomen for previous scars and enlarged intra-abdominal organs or masses are important. This helps towards further understanding the pathology, deciding whether laparoscopy is likely to succeed and optimizing access by changing the routine position of cannulae. It is important that the urinary bladder is empty before inserting the cannula during the lower abdominal and pelvic procedures. Catheterization is required only if the bladder is palpable, for monitoring renal function and in prolonged lower abdominal/pelvic procedures. In children, a palpable bladder can be adequately emptied by expression. The use of a nasogastric tube to drain the stomach is required only for considerations of anaesthesia. A routine preoperative enema is not necessary.

The patient must be properly and securely positioned to facilitate safe insertion of the cannulae, optimize exposure and allow for the comfort of the operator. The surgeon, assistant and nurse may stand on either side of the patient depending on the type of the procedure to be executed and surgeon's preference, with the monitors placed towards the end of the table. In infants and small children, and for bilat-

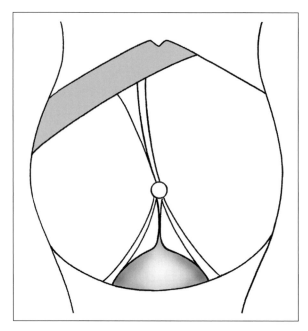

Fig. 12.1. Anatomy in infants and small children. The surface area for access is small and the abdominal wall is thin. The liver margin is below the rib cage, the bladder is an intra-abdominal structure and the obliterated structures are relatively prominent.

eral procedures, the surgeon may find it more comfortable to operate standing at the head of the table. A degree of Trendelenburg position and/or lateral tilt often improves exposure.

In paediatric patients, the whole abdomen is usually prepared and draped. This is because the sites of cannulae insertion are often away from the operative field, and additional cannulae may be necessary for retraction or manipulation, or wide access may be necessary for conversion or emergency open surgery.

It is important to recognize that in children, particularly infants, the surface area for laparoscopic access is small, the abdominal wall is thin and highly compliant, the liver margin is often below the rib cage, the bladder is largely an intra-abdominal structure, the viscera are close to the anterior abdominal wall and the peritoneal cavity is small (Fig. 12.1). In small infants, an established pneumoperitoneum may only require 400 ml carbon dioxide. The so-called obliterated structures, umbilical vessels and urachus, remain relatively large and partially patent in infants. These anatomical characteristics make access and manipulation in children more difficult and complicated compared with adults. However, children have well-defined anatomical landmarks owing to lack of excess fat, making recognition and dissection of structures a relatively easy exercise (Najmaldin and Grousseau, 1999).

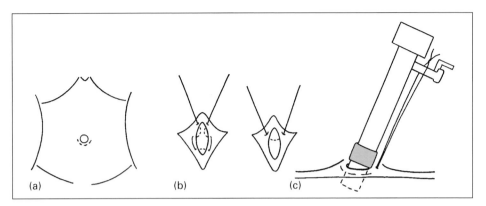

Fig. 12.2. Open technique laparoscopy. (a) A peri-umbilical incision includes the peritoneum. (b) A purse string or single suture includes the fascia/muscle and peritoneum. (c) The cannula is shown in position with the suture tied first at the level of wound using a single throw and then at the gas port using multiple throws, leaving 1–2 cm of the cannula inside the peritoneal cavity. Note: a cuff of rubber tube may be used to prevent the cannula from falling inside.

Open-technique laparoscopy (Fig. 12.2) is the preferred method for insertion of the primary cannula and creation of a pneumoperitoneum in children (Humphrey and Najmaldin, 1994). In an unscarred abdomen and for bilateral procedures, an incision to fit the size of the primary cannula is usually made at the umbilical region (infants and small children at upper margin or above; older children and adolescents through upper or lower margins depending on the shape of the umbilicus and thickness of fat in the periumbilical region). Alternatively, and in unilateral procedures or a scarred abdomen, the primary cannula can be placed anywhere in the abdomen, usually along the para-rectal lines (Najmaldin and Guillou, 1998). The incision is then carried through the fascia and peritoneum and a 2/0 vicryl, simple or purse-string suture in inserted. Care is taken to include both the fascia and peritoneum with each bite (otherwise the insufflation gas may dissect through the extraperitoneal plain). An ordinary "primary" cannula is pushed off its trocar into the abdominal cavity and secured with a single throw of suture, thus allowing snug opposition of the peritoneum and fascia to the cannula during the procedure, thereby preventing a gas leak. The suture is then secured around the gas port of the cannula, allowing 1 cm of the cannula to remain inside the abdominal cavity (side holes near the tip of cannula must be placed beyond the peritoneal layer). This suture prevents the cannula from falling out; if desired, a preadjusted rubber tube on the cannula may be used to prevent the cannula from falling in (Najmaldin and Grousseau, 1999). Alternatively, a cannula with Hasson's configurations may be used.

An insufflation pressure of 6–8 mmHg in infants and small children and 8–10 mmHg in older children and adolescents with a carbon dioxide flow of 0.2 to 1 l/min are adequate parameters for all laparoscopic procedures. The number, size, length and site of working "secondary" cannulae are modified according to the size of the patient, type of surgical procedure, size of available instruments for use, individual anatomy and surgeon's preference (Fig. 12.3). In general, short and light in weight cannulae are preferred. A purpose built-in thread, or a cuff of preadjusted rubber tube on any ordinary cannula with a stitch through the abdominal wall (Fig. 12.4), prevents the cannulae from falling in and out of the abdominal cavity. This is particularly important in infants and small children because of their thin abdominal wall and in prolonged surgical procedures.

At the end of the procedure, fascial incisions greater than 4 mm are closed with 3/0 absorbable sutures; local infiltration of anaesthetic agents is helpful. Some surgeons prefer local infiltration of long-acting anaesthetic agents at the time of cannula insertion.

Equipment and instruments
In addition to the basic equipment (camera, light, monitor, insufflator, suction, energy apparatus (e.g. diathermy)) and a set of laparotomy instruments for emergency use or conversion to an open technique, the following instruments are adequate for most if not all laparoscopic gynaecological procedures in children.
- One to four 2.5–12 mm cannulae/trocar. In general 3.5–5 mm short cannulae are utilized for most procedures. However, longer cannulae may be required for older and/or fat children and adolescents.
- A 5 mm telescope preferably angled (30–45°) serves all purposes. However 2.5–3.5 mm scopes may be adequate

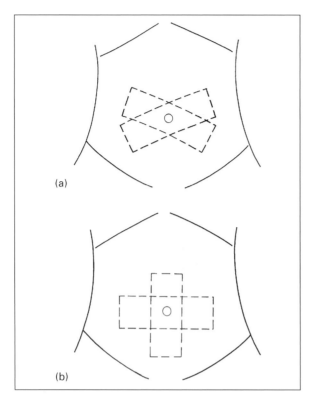

Fig. 12.3. The position of the cannula for pelvic/ovarian surgery. (a) The site is shown for the primary and secondary cannulae for unilateral left or right surgery. (b) Two different sites "vertical" or "transverse" are shown for the primary and secondary cannulae in bilateral pelvic procedures.

but only for diagnostic and very minor surgical procedures. A 10 mm scope is readily available in all departments and may prove useful for long and complicated procedures.

- Two 3.5–5 mm atraumatic, preferably curved, grasping forceps without ratchet. One additional grasper with ratchet.
- One 3.5–5 mm double jaw action curved scissors with a diathermy point and preferably the insulation sleeve extending to the blades.
- Unipolar fine hook and/or needle diathermy probe and a bipolar forceps (3.5–5 mm).
- One 5 mm clip applicator and appropriate sized clips. Alternatively, ordinary suture materials and/or pretied suture loops may be used.
- One 3.5–5 mm needle holder and one suction irrigation probe may occasionally prove useful.

In general, normal length instruments are good to use, but short instruments may be more appropriate for very small children and infants.

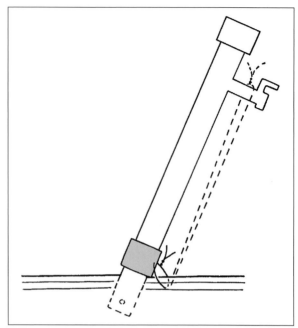

Fig. 12.4. Fixation of the secondary cannulae in position. A single suture including skin and fascia/muscle is fixed either through a cuff of rubber tube or around the gas port leaving 1 or 2 cm of the cannula inside.

Management of ovarian cysts in the newborn

Small benign cysts of less than 2 cm in diameter are common findings in the prenatal and early postnatal period (Desa, 1997). Large cysts are rare, and malignant tumours are an exceedingly rare phenomenon in the newborn. The majority of benign cysts, particularly those smaller than 5 cm in diameter, tend to regress spontaneously either prenatally or soon after birth (Bagolau et al., 1992; Luzzatto et al., 2000). Small cysts are considered less liable to torsion than large cysts (more than 5 cm in diameter) (Bagolau et al., 1992). Torsion of the ovarian cyst mostly occurs prenatally (Grapin et al., 1987; Mohammed et al., 1998) (Fig. 12.5, colour plate) and can mimic a solid mass on the ultrasound scan.

The differential diagnosis includes hydrometrocolpos and uterine duplication; bladder, ureter and renal anomalies; mesenteric or enteric cysts; liver, pancreas or choledochal cysts; pelvic component of sacrococcygeal teratoma; or anterior meningomyelocele. Clinical examination, laboratory tests and repeat ultrasound scan should exclude malignancy in the majority of cases. The treatment strategy depends on consideration of the exact nature of the cyst and the chance of either regression or complications. The aim for treatment is to avoid torsion and to preserve as much functioning tissue as possible. All small, benign (less than 5 cm in diameter) cysts and large cysts that are

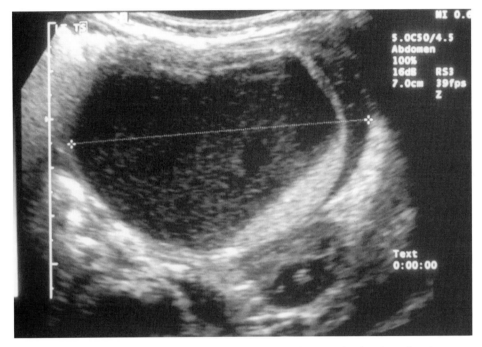

Fig. 12.6. Antenatally diagnosed ovarian cyst larger than 5 cm in diameter showing signs of torsion on ultrasound scan in the first few weeks of life. Generalized echogenicity within the cyst indicates torsion.

showing signs of spontaneous regression may be treated conservatively and followed up by ultrasound scan to ensure a return to normality. Indications for early surgery include cysts larger than 5 cm in diameter and showing no signs of spontaneous regression and acute or chronic torsion (Fig. 12.6). Laparoscopy allows visual assessment of the lesion and definitive treatment of the nonmalignant cysts (Esposito et al., 1998; Mohammed et al., 1998; Waldschmidt and Schier, 1992) as well as assessment of the contralateral ovary.

With possible malignancy having been certainly excluded by investigations and imaging, ultrasound-guided or a laparoscopically guided needle aspiration may provide valuable information and prevent unnecessary surgery for large ovarian cysts (Doligin, 2000). However, recurrence after simple aspiration is common (Bagolau et al., 1992; Sapin et al., 1994).

Techniques (salpingo-oophorectomy, cystectomy)

The open technique for laparoscopy is mandatory in the newborn. The exact site of the primary cannula is determined by the size of the patient, the size and site of the ovarian mass and whether the cyst is thought to have ruptured. After a preliminary exploration, the site, number and size of one or more working cannulae are selected depending on the position of the primary cannula and the nature of the procedure to be executed. In large benign cysts and/or

difficult assessment, a percutaneous needle aspiration (Fig. 12.7, colour plate) improves exposure and facilitates safe insertion and appropriate positioning of the working cannulae.

In inexperienced hands, misdiagnosis is not uncommon. Therefore, before committing to any definitive surgical procedure, careful examination of the ipsilateral ovary, cyst, tube and pedicles is mandatory. This assessment may necessitate adhesiolysis for pericystic adhesions. The contralateral ovary must also be examined.

With malignancy having been excluded, the surgical manoeuvre depends on the state of the ovary and the Fallopian tube, and the discovery of acute or chronic torsion and pericystic adhesions. A detorsion with or without a preliminary puncture should be attempted in all acute cases without clear signs of gangrene (Doligin, 2000). The place of prophylactic oophoropexy remains uncertain (Grunewald et al., 1993). The discovery of torsion associated with gangrene (acute) or necrosis (chronic) demands surgical resection, often in the form of salpingo-oophorectomy (Fig. 12.8, colour plate).

The procedure is carried out by first securing the proximal and distal main blood supply using suture ligature, clips or bipolar electrocoagulation, followed by a clip or suture ligation and division of the proximal part of the tube very close to the uterus. Finally, the specimen is freed using diathermy scissors or probes and removed through an extended cannula site. Care must be taken to identify and preserve iliac vessels, ureter and uterus. A linear stapler is not required in children, and the procedure should be bloodless.

Alternatively, salpingo-oophorectomy may be executed via a laparoscopic-assisted technique. Here the cyst is decompressed first through a percutaneously inserted needle and then the intact diseased organs are delivered outside the abdominal wall through a small suprapubic or inguinal incision for resection using conventional instruments (Fig. 12.9, colour plate).

The treatment of large cysts without signs of ischaemia remains controversial, although an increasing number of surgeons advocate oophorectomy or excision of cyst with maximum preservation of compressed parenchyma (Esposito et al., 1998). As for salpingo-oophorectomy, both oophorectomy and ovarian cystectomy may be accomplished outside the abdominal wall (by a laparoscopic-assisted technique). In laparoscopic oophorectomy, the proximal and distal blood supplies of the ovary are secured, and the remaining attachments are divided by needle or hook monopolar diathermy or scissors. In infants and small children, preservation of the associated healthy tube, especially the fimbriated end, can be difficult because of the close proximity of the two structures.

Laparoscopic resection of the cyst is carried out by enucleating the cyst through an adequate antimesenteric incision. The ovarian tissue is stripped from the cyst using a combination of sharp and blunt dissection. Haemostasis is achieved by diathermy, suturing the edges or even biological glue. The resulting cavity may either be left open or obliterated by absorbable sutures. Care must be taken to minimize damage to the very thinned-out normal functioning residual ovarian tissue during diathermy dissection, haemostasis and suturing. The previously aspirated cyst/ovary is usually easy to extract through a small cannula or the site of the cannula insertion. The efficacy and long-term results of simple de-roofing of benign ovarian cysts is uncertain.

Laparoscopy and intersex

Paediatric surgeons have long known that the laparoscope provides an opportunity to view deep cavities such as the pelvis with magnification and illumination (Gans and Berci, 1971). The indications for its use in intersex disorders are:

- diagnostic evaluation and biopsy as part of investigation for sex assignment (Fig. 12.10, colour plate)
- diagnostic evaluation and relocation of testes in assigned males with intra-abdominal testes

- the removal of normal gonads with or without ductal structures that are contrary to the assigned gender: when the diagnosis of true hermaphroditism is made, gender assignment depends largely on the karyotype and anatomic findings and gonads and internal duct structures that are contradictory to the assigned sex should be removed
- removal of dysgenetic gonads that present a potential for malignancy.

The possibility of malignant changes in gonads is diagnosis and age related. The risk of tumour formation in patients with mixed gonadal dysgenesis is approximately 30–50% (Rosenfield et al., 1980; Shellhas, 1974). The risk of malignancy in patients with true hermaphroditism and prepubertal androgen insensitivity syndrome (AIS), while reported, are low (Van Niekerk, 1976). Gonadectomy is often delayed until after puberty as the testes secrete androgen, which is converted to oestrogen and allows more natural development of the breasts than can be achieved with oestrogen therapy. Patients with AIS are expected to receive close and lifelong follow-up and female hormones after the age of 11 years or so.

The gonads in phenotypic males are infertile and have a high risk of developing tumours. Therefore, all streak gonads and intra-abdominal testes that cannot be relocated in the scrotum and/or associated with ipsilateral Müllerian duct structures should be removed.

Bilateral gonadectomy in Turner's syndrome

The risk of gonadal malignancy, especially gonadoblastoma, in patients with mosaicism involving the Y chromosome sharply increases after puberty (Krasna et al., 1992; Olsen et al., 1988) (Fig. 12.11, colour plate) and the incidence may reach as high as 80% in the fourth decade of life (Shellhas, 1974). Consequently streak gonads should be removed in any adolescent or young adult with evidence of virilization or a Y-containing cell line.

Laparoscopy provides excellent visualization and allows a relatively easy bilateral gonadectomy. However, special attention must be paid to the rather unusual and ill-defined nature of the gonads (Fig. 12.12, colour plate). Streak gonads extend close to the body of uterus medially, run adjacent to the Fallopian tubes, with a narrow mesentery in between the two structures, and are almost inseparable from the fimbriated end of the tubes. These anatomical characteristics, and the fact that preserving the tubes is unnecessary, makes laparoscopic bilateral salpingo-oophorectomy the technique of choice in patients with Turner's syndrome who require gonadectomy.

Three 3.5–5 mm preferably short cannulae provide adequate access. An angled (30–45°) 5 mm telescope allows good visualization and versatility. In prepubertal girls, the specimens are usually extractable through a 5 or possibly a 3.5 mm cannula. Dissection first proceeds towards the medial aspects of the gonad and Fallopian tube. A window is created through the mesentery above and below the ovarian ligament using a pair of fine scissors and fine curved or angled grasping forceps. The isthmus, ovarian ligament and their respective branches of the uterine vessels are secured using either clips or ligatures. The proximal ovarian vessels are then secured and divided in between ligatures, clips or even bipolar diathermy. The entire gonad and its related tube are mobilized using either scissors or a monopolar diathermy hook/needle. Care must be taken not to leave any gonadal tissue behind, and the close proximity of structures such as iliac vessels, ureter, uterus and even bowel must be respected throughout the procedure.

Laparoscopic transposition of the ovaries

In children, the therapeutic protocol for treating pelvic malignancies (soft tissue, bony or lymphatic) may include radiotherapy. The doses of radiation used usually lead to ovarian failure (Shalet et al., 1976). The minimal radiation dose that can produce ovarian failure is age related: 20 Gy in children and young adults, and 6 Gy if over 40 years of age (Lushbaugh and Casarett, 1976). The ovarian irradiation and the risks of ovarian failure can be reduced significantly by surgical transposition of one or both ovaries (Baker et al., 1972; Thibaud et al., 1992).

The risk of transposing a metastatic ovary, recurrent malignancy on the retained but relocated ovary, reduced ovarian blood supply, ovarian dystrophy and failure to protect ovaries against radiation have all been reported in adult patients (Anderson et al., 1993; Tabata et al., 1987). Information about the effectiveness and long-term outcome of ovarian transposition in children is scarce. Sporadic reports indicate that ovarian transposition performed during childhood or adolescence preserves ovarian function and that short-term complications are uncommon (Thibaud et al., 1992). In addition to avoiding the trauma of any open surgical procedure, especially in immuno compromised cancer patients, the minimally invasive technique allows radiotherapy and chemotherapy to be commenced almost immediately after surgery without concerns for the healing of a larger wound after open surgery.

Positioning of the ovarian tissue can be customized to the radiation plan required. In children, because of their small size, median transposition provides inadequate protection. Therefore, lateral or high lateral transposition, depending on the exact field of radiation, are the preferred methods. Moving the ovary and an intact Fallopian tube as a single unit, which may allow the patient to conceive in the future, must be considered in all children.

In paediatric patients, since pelvic radiation may be administered almost immediately after laparoscopic transposition, absorbable sutures (PDS) provide adequate fixation. In some patients, the use of absorbable sutures may allow the ovaries to migrate back to their original position in the pelvis without the need for further surgery (Gugliemi et al., 1980).

Lateral ovariopexy

The position of three cannulae for standard bilateral ovariopexies is demonstrated in Fig. 12.3. This, however, can be modified as necessary in unilateral procedures or in the presence of a pelvic lesion such as pelvic sarcoma.

A satisfactory, but limited, degree of lateral transpositioning may be achieved without dividing either the ovarian ligaments or the peritoneum. The ovary is picked up with an atraumatic grasper and stretched over and beyond the iliac vessels. A single 5/0 or 4/0 PDS suture on a round needle is used to fix the inferior part of the ovary to the peritoneum and the underlying muscle as high and lateral as possible (Fig. 12.13, colour plate). Care must be taken not to damage the ovary, ureter or the iliac vessels.

A desired level of lateral transposition without transecting the Fallopian tube (maintaining the natural relationship between the ovary and the fimbriated end of the tube) can be achieved by one or more of the following procedures in sequence.

1. Division of the ovarian ligament between clips or by bipolar or unipolar diathermy. Care must be taken not to damage the isthmus and its accompanying vessels.
2. Division of the mesovarium in between the tubal and the ovarian arcades of vessels using diathermy scissors or needle as close to the fimbriated end of the tube as safely possible. Care must be taken not to damage the blood vessels or tube and its fimbriated end.
3. A releasing incision through the peritoneum inferior to the ovary. Care must be taken not to damage the ureter or iliac vessels.

If necessary, a very high and lateral transposition can be accomplished by total mobilization of the ovary on its proximal ovarian vessel. Here care must be taken not to damage the ovarian vessels and to avoid twisting the vascular pedicle.

A metal clip is applied to either the inferior pole of the ovary (mobilization without dissection) or the detached ovarian ligament adjacent to the lower pole of the ovary (mobilization with dissection), in order to mark the location on pelvic X-ray.

Oophorectomy for cryopreservation

Most children and adolescents treated for cancer can now expect to be cured. However, their disease and aggressive chemotherapy may cause infertility in a significant minority. Immature germ cell harvesting, storage and in vitro maturation is an evolving but challenging procedure (see Ch. 33). Despite its experimental nature and ethical issues gonadal cryopreservation provides the only chance to conserve the fertility of young cancer patients (Rutherford et al., 1999).

A laparoscopic ovarian wedge resection or cortical tissue biopsy are effective methods for collecting ovarian tissue for cryopreservation in adult patients (Meirow et al., 1999). In children, the size of ovary is such that a total removal of one ovary is usually required.

Careful planning and appropriate consent and liaison with responsible laboratory personnel are essential preoperative requisites. The technique requires three cannulae, one of which has to be large enough (usually 5 or 10 mm depending on the age) to allow the harvested ovary to be delivered outside the body without undue damage to the ovarian tissue. The ovarian vascular pedicles are secured and divided in between clips, bipolar diathermy or monopolar needle/hook diathermy. The ovary is then mobilized using scissors and/or diathermy. Care must be taken not to cause thermal damage to the ovary. In children, the fimbriated end of the Fallopian tube is almost inseparable from the ovary. However, preservation of the tube is not essential for future in vitro fertilization.

Laparoscopy for acute and chronic abdominal pain

Missed preoperative diagnoses, which lead to delayed surgery for important conditions such as appendicitis or unnecessary surgery for a benign gynaecological condition, are not uncommon encounters in prepubertal girls. An early and accurate diagnosis would, therefore, undoubtedly lead to less morbidity for the patients and a considerable saving in resources (Rahejo et al., 1980). The ovarian cyst rarely causes acute abdominal pain. However, haemorrhage into the cyst and torsion can present with acute pain. Occasionally ovulation-induced intraperitoneal haemorrhage may cause abdominal pain and localized peritonitis (Fig. 12.14, colour plate). Recurrent or chronic abdominal pain in girls may be caused by an ovarian cyst, endometriosis (see below), pelvic inflammatory disease and dysmenorrhoea. The limitations of preoperative evaluation,

including computer-aided diagnosis (Adams et al., 1986), ultrasonography and spinal computed tomography, and the need to proceed with emergency surgery in acute or even recurrent situations prompt the use of laparoscopy (Decadt et al., 1999; Salky, 1988). Laparoscopy allows for exploration of the entire abdominal cavity and execution of most definitive general surgical or/and gynaecological procedures, making unnecessary open surgery a thing of the past.

An angled telescope via the first, usually periumbilical, cannula allows adequate preliminary exploration in most cases. A degree of Trendelenburg and/or side tilt often improves access. However, in the minority of cases, additional one or two "working" cannulae are required to manipulate organs, and/or to allow suction irrigation or even adhesiolysis before the diagnosis is reached. Most definitive surgical procedures can be accomplished using a total of three cannulae. In difficult or suspected malignant cases, conversion to an open technique or referral to an appropriate paediatric surgical oncologist, respectively, must be considered promptly.

Adolescent gynaecology

ALFRED CUTNER

This section of the chapter will examine first the principles of laparoscopy before considering the management of the various developmental abnormalities in adolescents and adults. Finally, the laparoscopic management of endometriosis will be reviewed, as this is a common complication of congenital abnormalities that result in menstrual outflow obstruction.

Principles of laparoscopy

Laparoscopic surgery has four components each with its own concerns:
1. obtaining the pneumoperitoneum
2. insertion of additional ports
3. the specifics of the planned procedure
4. the removal and closure of ports.

Gynaecological surgical training in laparoscopic surgery has been formalized in the UK by the Royal College of Obstetricians and Gynaecologists (RCOG). Different grades of operation are categorized according to their complexity. Level 1 refers to diagnostic and very simple procedures. Level 2 refers to moderate operative procedures and level 3 to complex operative procedures. Most paediatric laparoscopic surgery for congenital abnormalities has not been classified.

Obtaining a pneumoperitoneum

Although obtaining a pneumoperitoneum is straightforward in the majority of patients, it is not without risk. The RCOG confidential enquiry in 1978 reported a 0.1 per 1000 death rate for diagnostic and sterilization procedures (Chapron et al., 1998). There are four methods used to obtain a pneumoperitoneum. The first utilizes a Verres needle, the second direct insertion of the first trocar in a blind manner (Copeland et al., 1983; Jarrett, 1990), the third a direct method using an optical port (Hallfeldt et al., 1999; String et al., 2001) and the fourth a surgical approach to entry with insertion of a blunt trocar. The Verres needle and the direct surgical approach are the commonly used methods; the Verres needle is described below; the direct surgical approach was discussed in the first part of this chapter.

Verres needle

The Verres needle is traditionally inserted at the umbilicus. An incision is made in the umbilical region, as it is at this point that the layers of the rectus sheath and peritoneum are fused. The patient is initially catheterized to empty the bladder as this removes the risk of perforating a distended bladder. The patient is placed supine with no tilt and the needle is first directed towards the sacral promontory; when the characteristic clicks of passing through the layers is felt, the needle is then directed towards the pelvis. A water test should be used to confirm entry into the correct space and the abdomen is insufflated. Insufflation is ceased when flow ceases as the pre-set pressure is reached (10 mm in children, 20 mm in adults). The main trocar, either 5 mm or 10 mm (depending on the size of the patient and the planned procedure) is then placed, through the umbilical region (Anon, 1999).

Where there is difficulty in obtaining a pneumoperitoneum, other sites may be considered. These include the pouch of Douglas (Neely et al., 1975), transuterine (Wolfe and Pasic, 1990) and suprapubic insertion. However none of these are suitable where there is a risk of pelvic adhesions or if there is a large abdominal mass. A common alternative site now used in high-risk cases is Palmer's point (Cilders et al., 1993; Pasic et al., 1999) (the left subcostal area in the mid-clavicular line). The spleen should be detected by palpation prior to insertion of the Verres needle and a nasogastric tube should be considered to reduce the chance of perforating an inflated stomach.

Additional ports

The placement of additional ports is important. All additional ports must be placed under direct vision in order to avoid injury to viscera or vessels. Ports should either be placed very lateral or medial so as to avoid the inferior epi-gastric vessels (Balzer et al., 1999; Hurd et al., 1994). They should be placed so that adequate dexterity can be achieved during the operation.

Another consideration is large ports. All 10 mm lateral ports should be formally closed to reduce the incidence of incisional hernias (Coda et al., 1999; Montz et al., 1994). Because even umbilical ports can result in subsequent hernia formation (Montz et al., 1994), it is probably advisable to close central ports when operating on children.

Laparoscopy for diagnosis

After insertion of the ports, the abdomen should be examined in a systematic manner. The liver and appendix should be visualized and the pelvic organs assessed (Fig. 12.15, colour plate). Their mobility and structure should be noted, as should any adhesions or endometriosis. The pouch of Douglas should be viewed, as should the course of the ureters. Even in a young child, the Fallopian tubes should be adequately visualized as this may give information with regards to future fertility.

Congenital abnormalities

The first part of this chapter also discussed congenital abnormalities in paediatric laparoscopy.

Uterine abnormalities

Where a uterine abnormality exists, the minimum preoperative workup should include an intravenous urograph and hysteroscopy. The incidence of renal tract abnormalities ranges from 31 to 100% (Buttram and Gibbons, 1979; Silber et al., 1990) and this will have major implications for the surgical approach (Kadir et al., 1996), as the number and course of the ureters needs to be known prior to surgery.

Hysteroscopy will enable determination of whether or not the uterine horn is communicating with the other uterus or the vagina (Heinonen, 1997) (Fig. 12.16, colour plate). Also when the uterine horn is to be removed, considerations as to whether the remaining uterus is of adequate size to contain a pregnancy needs to be considered, as otherwise a meteroplasty should be undertaken (Creighton et al., 2000).

Where there is a uterine horn that *communicates* with the main uterine body (Fig. 12.17a, colour plate) but is not adequate for pregnancy, then removing the Fallopian tube has been suggested as a more straightforward procedure than removing the rudimentary horn itself, which may jeopardize the integrity of the wall of the uterus. This may prevent pregnancy within the horn (Corleta et al., 2001; Handa et al., 1999; Heinonen, 1997; Pasini et al., 2001), which is important as there is a high incidence of uterine rupture during pregnancy, which carries a significant maternal mortality. Also the chance of a successful outcome of pregnancy is exceedingly rare in a rudimentary horn (Buttram and Gibbons, 1979; Chang et al., 1994; Kriplani et al., 1995) although it has been reported (McCarthy, 1999; Nahum, 1997). Laparoscopic salpingectomy is a straightforward operation. Either an endoloop can be placed around the tube and it can then be excised or the mesosalpinx is coagulated and the tube is then excised.

If the horn is *noncommunicating*, surgery would normally entail removal of the horn because of problems with haematometra, pain and endometriosis (Ansbacher, 1983; Chang et al., 1994; Falcone et al., 1997; Heinonen, 1983; Olive and Henderson, 1987; Rock and Schlaff, 1985). A simple approach to this problem has been reported (Corleta et al., 2001) where a vaginal connection was made to the uterine horn and then an endometrial ablation was performed on the noncommunicating horn. This was combined with a salpingectomy on the ipsilateral side. This is a simplified approach but it may be that there will not be long-term relief as it is known that endometrial resection only has a 20–50% amenorrhoea rate (O'Connor and Magos, 1996).

Laparoscopic removal of an accessory uterine horn was first reported by Nezhat et al. in 1994, and there have been numerous case reports subsequently. To remove the horn, the ureter needs to be identified and the ovarian ligament coagulated and divided. The uterovesical fold is then incised and the bladder reflected. The space between the two uteri is then incised and the accessory uterus excised. The raw aspect of the remaining uterus may then be sutured to prevent adhesions. Some authors advocate the use of diathermy (Kadir et al., 1996), while others prefer the use of endoscopic stapling devices (Canis et al., 1990; Yahata et al., 1998). However, we have found that the hormonic scalpel is a useful tool in such surgery making it relatively bloodless and decreasing the operating time (Creighton et al., 2000) (Fig. 12.17, colour plate).

The accessory uterus can then be morcellated to remove it from the abdomen. This technique results in minimal scarring and quick patient recovery (Creighton et al., 2000). It is advisable to remove the Fallopian tube on the ipsilateral side as this would remove the chance of an ectopic pregnancy on that side.

Some authors have preferred posterior colpotomy (Kadir et al., 1996) to remove the accessory uterus from the abdomen, but the morcellator is quick and removes the need to incise the vagina. When a morcellator is not available, the specimen can be cut up in the abdomen laparoscopically so that it can be removed through one of the ports

(Giatras et al., 1998). This will, however, add additional operating time to the surgery. Some authors have made a small suprapubic abdominal incision to remove the specimen (Chapron et al., 1995) but this will increase morbidity.

The variation in anatomy needs to be considered when performing this surgery. An abnormal urinary system will influence surgery. Indeed, if there is not a kidney on the side of the rudimentary horn, then surgery will be easier as there is no requirement to dissect the course of the ureter (Kadir et al., 1996). Some authors have suggested that concomitant hysteroscopy should be performed at the time of laparoscopic surgery because of the variation in connection between the two horns (Corleta et al., 2001; Falcone et al., 1997; Perrotin et al., 1999) to prevent damage to the remaining uterus (Kadir et al., 1996; Nezhat et al., 1994).

Consideration should be given to the use of gonadotrophin-releasing hormone (GnRH) analogues preoperatively to reduce vascularity and make surgery easier, especially when there is severe endometriosis (Canis et al., 1990; Nezhat et al., 1994; Nezhat and Smith, 1999). Removal of a pregnant uterine horn has been reported (Dulemba et al., 1996; Yahata et al., 1998; Yoo et al., 1999) and the principles of surgery are much the same. However the pedicles are larger and more vascular. One report has suggested the use of a stapling device to facilitate surgery in such cases. In early pregnancy, consideration should be given to initial treatment with methotrexate (if early) or fetocide and a delayed operation for excision of the accessory horn. This will give the advantage that GnRH analogues can be given preoperatively, which will decrease the blood supply and aid in the treatment of concomitant endometriosis. The downside is the time delay as it may take several months for the pregnancy to resorb. The same principles to removing an accessory uterine horn can be applied to the excision of a small rudimentary uterus (Connell et al., 2000). This may present with symptoms of pain where there is no connection with the vagina. It will also predispose to the development of endometriosis.

Vaginal agenesis

Vaginal agenesis may occur in isolation or in association with absence of the cervix and uterus. The initial treatment will normally be conservative with the use of vaginal dilators. Surgery is, however, indicated when there is a functioning uterus, as this will result in a haematometra, pelvic pain and the development of endometriosis. There are four main surgical approaches using an open or vaginal approach. These can be classified as the use of bowel for reconstruction (Ruge procedure), the use of a skin graft (McIndoe procedure), the use of pelvic peritoneum (Davydov procedure) and the use of a pressure device

(Vecchietti procedure). All of these have been reported using either a complete laparoscopic approach or a laparoscopically assisted approach. There are reports of other less-commonly used techniques in the literature but these have been largely replaced by the above approaches.

The use of bowel for reconstruction (Ruge procedure)
The Ruge procedure was described in 1914 (Ruge and Ersatz, 1914) and involves the formation of a neovagina using a sigmoid colon graft. Advantages of this approach are less scarring and stenosis of the neovagina. However, the two main disadvantages are the morbidity of the operation itself and the problems with chronic mucus discharge.

Ota et al. (2000) reported a laparoscopically assisted Ruge procedure. Preoperatively angiography of the inferior mesenteric artery was performed to visualize the feeding arteries of the sigmoid colon. A three port technique was used to mobilize a section of the bowel and an endoscopic stapler was used to sever the connection between the colon and rectum. A 3 to 5 cm abdominal incision was then made to apply the stapling device to reconnect the rectum and upper colon and to suture the opening of the colonic stump. The abdominal incision was then closed. The vaginal opening was then developed caudally and the colonic stump guided laparoscopically into the created cavity. This was then sutured to the vaginal entrance and the serosa of the colonic stump sutured to the pelvic peritoneum laparoscopically. This is the only report in the literature of this technique, where essentially a traditional operation has used laparoscopic assistance to reduce a midline incision to a small transverse incision. This should result in faster patient recovery but all the advantages and disadvantages of using bowel for the neovagina remain the same (see also Ch. 11).

The use of a skin graft (McIndoe procedure)
The McIndoe procedure is a vaginal operation whereby a false tract is created between the urethra and rectum and this is then lined with a full-thickness skin graft (McIndoe, 1950).

There is one report in the literature of using a laparoscopically assisted approach (Lee et al., 1999). The indication for the use of the laparoscope was that the patient had a uterus and the aim was to preserve the uterus and enable a connection between the uterus and the neovagina. A routine McIndoe procedure was performed and laparoscopic guidance was used to confirm that the direction of the created canal was correct. A probe was passed into the uterus to create a cervical canal. The graft was then applied to the vagina and sutured to the created cervix. A Foley catheter was used to maintain the cervical canal and a pack to maintain the vaginal canal. The authors merely used a laparoscope to guide the vaginal surgery and also to treat coexisting pelvic pathology, such as endometriosis, at the time of surgery. Essentially, the operation did not differ from that originally described by McIndoe.

The use of pelvic peritoneum (Davydov procedure)
The Davydov procedure consists of making a vaginal passage between the urethra and rectum and then via an abdominal incision passing pelvic peritoneum into the vagina and suturing it to the vaginal opening. The top end is then closed with a purse string to create the top of the vagina (Davydov, 1969). The potential advantages of creating a neovagina lined by peritoneum is that it may be oestrogen sensitive and does not have the problems associated with bowel. In addition, the additional morbidity of taking a skin graft from another site is avoided.

There are several reports in the literature of using a modified laparoscopic approach (Adamyan, 1995; Soong et al., 1994, 1996; Templeman et al., 2000). The first report did not contain follow-up (Soong et al., 1994) and the authors later reported a large series (18 patients) with a follow-up of 8 to 40 months (Soong et al., 1996). There were no intraoperative complications and they reported an 85% sexual satisfaction rate. They did, however, have one late rectovaginal fistula, which they felt was not a consequence of the operation itself. The technique they used was a three port approach. Initially, they merely passed the peritoneum down to the created vaginal opening. The later approach involved releasing incisions to free the peritoneum further and create a greater vaginal length. In all cases, a rudimentary uterus was excised if present. This is in contrast to the report by Templeman et al. (2000), who left the rudimentary horn as it was felt that by incorporating it into the purse string at the top of the vagina there would be greater vaginal support. The report by Adamyan (1995) compared a completely vaginal route with a laparoscopically assisted route. He found that the laparoscopically assisted approach resulted in a shorter operating time and a lower intraoperative complication rate. There was a similar functional result in the two groups.

It would appear that the laparoscopically assisted Davydov procedure does not subtract from the original operation. It does, however, improve visualization and reduce morbidity.

The use of a pressure device (Vecchietti procedure)
The Vecchietti procedure was first described in 1965 (Vecchietti, 1965). It has been likened to the Frank's method of vaginal dilators to create a functioning vagina (Frank,

1938). The difference is that Frank's method involves a prolonged period of self-dilator use and marked patient motivation whereas the Vecchietti bypasses the need for self-application with a surgical approach. This method has become the standard surgical option in Europe (Fedele et al., 2000) although it has yet to be reported as being carried out in the UK.

The operation entails the placement of an acrylic olive in the vaginal dimple (see Fig. 13.2, p. 148). Traction sutures are passed from the olive to the anterior abdominal wall. Abdominal traction from above creates a cavity in the vesicorectal space. This results in the creation of a neovagina over several days. The original procedure entailed a laparotomy to pass the traction sutures and this resulted in morbidity especially as there would be pressure over the site of the recent laparotomy.

The first description of a laparoscopically modified Vecchietti procedure was in 1992 (Gauwerky et al., 1992). There have been many subsequent reports in the literature since then. The variations in technique depend on whether the sutures are passed transabdominally (Giacalone et al., 1999) in the peritoneal cavity or tunnelled extraperitoneally (Fedele et al., 2000). The other variations include whether the sutures are passed from above down (Fedele et al., 1994, 2000) or below up (Giacalone et al., 1999; Veronikis et al., 1997) and the degree of dissection that is carried out at the time of surgery (Chatwani et al., 1999; Fedele et al., 2000; Gauwerky et al., 1992). In addition, some authors have used ultrasound guidance to confirm that the needles have not penetrated the bladder (Busacca et al., 1996; Giacalone et al., 1999) while others have used concomitant cystoscopy to achieve the same aim (Fedele et al., 1994, 2000; Veronikis et al., 1997). The final variation is whether one or two passes of the needle are made (Fedele et al., 2000).

The largest case series in the literature is from Fedele et al. (2000). They had no significant complications. The follow-up, however, was short (6 to 64 months) but initial results demonstrated a good vaginal length with 94.2% having a satisfactory sexual relationship after the operation and an 80.8% reported rate of orgasm. The different laparoscopic methods of creating a neovagina have been described but a true comparison of outcome is not possible. This would require a randomized study. However, at the very least, detailed sexual questionnaires are required. Most reports in the literature include only small numbers and follow-up is inadequate. It would appear, however, from the number of cases in the literature that the laparoscopic Vecchietti procedure is gaining the most popularity and the time has come to apply standardized questionnaires so that real outcome measures can be compared.

Endometriosis

Endometriosis is defined as the finding of tissue outside the uterus that is histologically similar to the endometrium. It is the presence of ectopic endometrium and the associated damage that gives rise to symptoms. Although it was described 140 years ago (Von Rokitansky, 1860), it still remains a poorly understood condition. The three main theories are retrograde menstruation and implantation, lymphatic spread, and haematogenous spread and transformation of coelomic epithelium (van der Linden, 1996). In addition, there is thought to be a genetic and racial influence and some workers have suggested autoimmune and immunological factors. The retrograde menstruation theory appears to be pertinent to developmental abnormalities.

Superficial endometriotic lesions may be red, white or black and show varying degrees of cellular activity (Vernon et al., 1986). Deep endometriosis is also associated with cellular activity and may be hidden. The most common areas affected by endometriosis are the ovaries, especially endometriomas on the affected side, the pelvic sidewall and the pouch of Douglas (Fig. 12.18, colour plate).

Infiltration may result in anatomical distortion and, in the extreme case, complete obliteration of the pouch of Douglas. Many women have incidental findings of surface endometriosis and are asymptomatic (Moen, 1995). Even in symptomatic patients, spontaneous regression of implants have been noted, with only some patients going on to have progressive disease (Mahmood and Templeton, 1990). These observations make management difficult.

The definitive diagnosis is made at laparoscopy. The whole pelvis should be systematically assessed. Treatment must be individualized to the patient, taking into account the age, reproductive wishes, symptoms, severity of the disease and expectations of the patient. In addition, if the underlying predisposing factor such has imperforate hymen has been removed, there is the theoretical chance of spontaneous resolution. Medical treatments have greater success with superficial endometriosis whereas surgery is the preferred option for deep disease. Combination therapy affords the best outcome.

Objectives of surgical treatment are the removal or ablation of endometrial implants, restoration of normal anatomy and the prevention or delay of disease progression. Laparoscopic surgery offers better visualization, less tissue handling and trauma and possibly less adhesion formation than laparotomy (Koh and Janik, 1999).

For the management of endometriomas, either the cyst can be ruptured and the capsule ablated or the cyst wall excised. With the latter, there is a lower recurrence rate but there is debate as to which method results in fewer adhesions (Jones and Sutton, 2002).

The treatment of rectovaginal disease is in its infancy. The principles are to excise all endometriotic tissue. The ureter needs to be dissected laterally, often after stenting, and the bowel dissected off the vagina so that the nodule can be excised safely. Initially, the ovaries are freed from the pelvic sidewall. Temporary suturing of the ovaries to the obliterated umbilical ligament will aid surgical exposure. The ureters are then dissected to lateralize them from the nodule. The dissection should start at an area of normal tissue, usually at the pelvic brim. A probe inserted in the rectum will aid opening of the pararectal and rectovaginal space. The nodule can then be safely excised (Fig. 12.19, colour plate). The need for bowel excision is currently controversial.

This radical surgery is high-risk major surgery and requires significant laparoscopic skills. However, improvements in quality-of-life scores have been demonstrated although there are only short-term follow-up data in the literature (Garry et al., 2000; Jacobson et al., 2001; Redwine, 1991). The need for such radical excision in young girls should be limited, as normally the disease will not be severe. However, where there is extensive disease resulting in marked debilitation and loss of quality of life, then such surgery may be considered.

Many reports in the literature for treatment of noncommunicating uteruses describe the treatment of coexisting severe endometriosis. However, whether or not the condition will undergo some resolution once the underlying cause has been treated is not known.

Conclusions

This chapter has highlighted the principles of laparoscopic surgery for congenital uterine and vaginal abnormalities (Box 12.1). The basic principles of open surgery are adhered to in the laparoscopic technique but the improved visualization may enable more exact surgery to be carried out. In some areas, such as the treatment of endometriosis, laparoscopic techniques have resulted in more complete surgery and the end results appear superior. So far in the field of surgery for congenital anomalies, most of the papers are case series of patients with the emphasis on surgical technique. More data on outcome measures such as improvement in quality of life and sexual function are required.

Box 12.1 Key points

- At initial laparoscopy the whole pelvis should be visualized.
- In communicating uterine horn, the Fallopian tube on the side of the communicating uterine horn should be removed to remove the risk of ectopic pregnancy.
- In an accessory horn, the size of the remaining uterus should be considered prior to surgery to remove the accessory horn.
- The renal tract should be assessed prior to surgery in patients with congenital tract abnormalities.
- The standard laparoscopic surgical treatment for vaginal agenesis is probably the laparosiopic Vecchietti procedure.
- When treating vaginal agenesis, sexual function needs to be assessed in greater detail than is currently reported.

REFERENCES

* Indicates key references.

Adams I D, Chan M, Clifford P C et al. (1986). Computer aided diagnosis of acute abdominal pain: a multi-centre study. *Br Med J* 293, 800–804.

Adamyan L V (1995). Laparoscopic management of vaginal aplasia with or without functioning noncommunicating rudimentary uterus. In *Principles of Laparoscopic Surgery*, Arrequi M E, Fitzgibbons R J, Katkhouda N, McKernan J B, Reich H eds., pp. 646–651. Springer-Verlag, New York.

Anderson B, La Polla J, Turner D, Chapman G, Buller R (1993). Ovarian transposition in cervical cancer. *Gynecol Oncol* 49, 206–214.

*Anon. (1999). A consensus document concerning laparoscopic entry techniques: Middlesbrough, March 19–20 1999. *Gynecolog Endosc* 8, 403–406.

Ansbacher R (1993). Uterine anomalies and future pregnancies. *Clin Perinatol* 10, 295–304.

Bagolau P, Rivosecchi M, Giorlandino C (1992). Prenatal diagnosis and clinical outcome of ovarian cyst. *J Pediatr Surg* 27, 879–881.

Baker J W, Morgan R C, Peckham M J, Smithers D W (1972). Presentation of ovarian function in patients requiring radiotherapy for paraortic and pelvic Hodgkin's disease. *Lancet* i, 1307–1308.

Balzer K M, Witte H, Recknagel S, Kozianka J, Waleczek H (1999). Anatomic guidelines for the prevention of abdominal wall hematoma induced by trocar placement. *Surg Radiol Anat* 21, 87–89.

Busacca M, Perino A, Venezia R (1996). Laparoscopic–ultrasonographic combined technique for the creation of a neovagina in Mayer–Rokitansky–Kuster–Hauser syndrome. *Fertil Steril* 66, 1039–1041.

*Buttram VC, Gibbons WE (1979). Mullerian anomalies: a proposed classification (an analysis of 144 cases). *Fertil Steril* 32, 40–46.

Canis M, Wattiez A, Pouly JL et al. (1990). Laparoscopic management of unicornuate uterus with rudimentary horn and unilateral extensive endometriosis: case report. *Hum Reprod* 5, 819–820.

Chang WF, Lin HH, Ho HN et al. (1994). Ultrasound diagnosis of rudimentary uterine horn pregnancy at fourteen weeks of gestation: a case report. *Asia-Oceania J Obstet Gynecol* 20, 279–282.

Chapron C, Morice P, Dupre La Tour M, Chavet, X, Dubuisson J-B (1995). Laparoscopic management of assymetric Mayer–Rokitansky–Kuster–Hauser syndrome. *Hum Reprod* 10, 369–371.

Chapron C, Querleu D, Bruhat MA et al. (1998). Surgical complications of diagnostic and operative gynaecological laparoscopy: a series of 29 966 cases. *Hum Reprod* 13, 867–872.

Chatwani A, Nyirjesy P, Harmanli OH, Grody MH (1999). Creation of neovagina by laparoscopic Vecchietti operation. *J Laparoendosc Adv Surg Tech A* 9, 425–427.

Childers JM, Brzechffa PR, Surwit EA (1993). Laparoscopy using the left upper quadrant as the primary trocar site. *Gynecol Oncol* 50, 221–225.

Coda A, Bossotti M, Ferri F et al. (1999). Incisional hernia and fascial defect following laparoscopic surgery. *Surg Laparosc Endosc Percutan Tech* 9, 348–352.

Connell R, Cutner A, Creighton S (2000). Laparoscopic removal of an ectopic uterus in a patient with Mayer–Rokitansky–Kuster–Hauser syndrome. *J Obstet Gynecol* 20, 97.

Copeland C, Wing R, Hulka JF (1983). Direct trocar insertion at laparoscopy: an evaluation. *Obstet Gynecol* 62, 655–659.

Creighton S, Minto CL, Cutner A (2000). Use of the ultrasonically activated scalpel in laparoscopic resection of a non-communicating rudimentary horn. *Gynecol Endosc* 9, 327–329.

Cutner A, Rymer, J (1998). Patient recovery after laparoscopic colposuspension. *Gynecol Endosc* 7, 307–308.

Davydov SN (1969). Colpopoiesis from the peritoneum of the ueterorectal space. *Obstet Gynecol* (Moscow) 12, 255–257.

Decadt B, Sussman L, Lewis MPN et al. (1999). Randomised clinical trial of early laparoscopy in the management of acute nonspecific abdominal pain. *Br J Surg* 86, 1383–1386.

Desa DJ (1975). Follicular ovarian cysts in stillbirth and neonates. *Arch Dis Child* 50, 45–50.

Doligin SE (2000). Ovarian masses in newborn. *Semin Pediatr Surg* 9, 121–127.

Dulemba J, Midgett W, Freeman M (1996). Laparoscopic management of a rudimentary horn pregnancy. *Am Assoc Gynecol Laparosc* 3, 627–630.

Esposito C, Garipoli V, Di Matteo G, De Pasquale M (1998). Laparoscopic management of ovarian cysts in newborns. *Surg Endosc* 12, 1152–1154.

Falcone T, Gidwani G, Paraiso M, Beverly C, Goldberg J (1997). Anatomical variation in the rudimentary horns of a unicornu-

ate uterus: implications for laparoscopic surgery. *Hum Reprod* 12, 263–265.

Fedele L, Busacca M, Candiani M, Vignali M (1994). Laparoscopic creation of a neovagina in Mayer–Rokitansky–Kuster–Hauser syndrome by modification of Vecchietti's operation. *Am J Obstet Gynecol* 171, 268–269.

*Fedele L, Bianchi S, Zanconato G, Raffaelli R (2000). Laparoscopic creation of a neovagina in patients with Rokitansky syndrome: analysis of 52 cases. *Fertil Steril* 74, 384–389.

Frank RT (1938). The formation of an artificial vagina without operation. *Am J Obstet Gynecol* 35, 1053–1055.

Gans SL, Berci G (1971). Advances in endoscopy of infants and children. *J Pediatr Surg* 6, 199–223.

(1973). Peritoneoscopy in infants and children. *J Pediatr Surg* 8, 399–405.

Garry R, Clayton R, Hawe J (2000). The effect of endometriosis and its radical laparoscopic excision on quality of life indicators. *Br J Obstet Gynaecol* 107, 44–54.

Gauwerky JFH, Wallwiener D, Bastert G (1992). An endoscopically assisted technique for construction of a neovagina. *Arch Gynecol Obstet* 252, 59–63.

Giacalone PL, Laffargue F, Faure JM, Deschamps F (1999). Ultrasound-assisted laparoscopic creation of a neovagina by modification of Vecchietti's operation. *Obstet Gynecol* 93, 446–448.

Giatras K, Licciardi F, Grifo JA (1998). Laparoscopy for pelvic pain in the Mayer–Rokitansky–Kuster–Hauser syndrome. *J Reprod Med* 43, 203–205.

Grapin C, Montague JP, Sirinelli D et al. (1987). Diagnosis of ovarian cysts in the perinatal period and therapeutic implications (20 cases). *Ann Radiol* 30, 497–502.

Grunewald B, Keating J, Brown S (1993). Asynchronous ovarian torsion. The case for prophylactic oopheropexy. *Postgrad Med J* 69, 318–319.

Gugliemi R, Galzavena F, Pizzi GB et al. (1980). Ovarian function after pelvic lymphnode irradiation. *Eur J Gynecol Oncol* 2, 99–107.

Hallfeldt KK, Trupka A, Kalteis T, Stuetzle H (1999). Safe creation of pneumoperitoneum using an optical trocar. *Surg Endosc* 13, 306–307.

Handa Y, Hoshi N, Yamada H et al. (1999). Tubal pregnancy in a unicornuate uterus with rudimentary horn: a case report. *Fertil Steril* 72, 354–356.

Heinonen PK (1983). Clinical implications of the unicornuate uterus with rudimentary horn. *Int J Gynaecol Obstet* 21, 145–150.

(1997). Unicornuate and rudimentary horn. *Fertil Steril* 68, 224–230.

Hope R (1937). The differential diagnosis of ectopic gestation by peritoneoscopy. *Surg Gynaecol Obstet* 64, 229.

Humphrey G, Najmaldin A (1994). Modification of Hasson's technique in paediatric laparoscopy. *Br J Surg* 81, 1319.

Hurd WW, Bude RO, De Lancey JO, Newman JS (1994). The location of abdominal wall blood vessels in relationship to abdominal landmarks apparent at laparoscopy. *Am J Obstet Gynecol* 171, 642–646.

Jacobson T Z, Barlow D H, Garry R, Koninckx P (2001). Laparoscopic surgery for pelvic pain associated with endometriosis (Cochrane Review). *Cochrane Database Syst Rev* 4, CD001300.

Jarrett J C II (1990). Laparoscopy: direct trocar insertion without pneumoperitoneum *Obstet Gynecol* 75, 725–727.

Jones K D, Sutton C J (2002). The ovarian endometrioma: why is it so poorly managed? Indicators from an anonymous survey. *Hum Reprod* 17, 845–849.

Kadir R A, Hart J, Nagele F, O'Connor H, Magos A L (1996). Laparoscopic excision of a noncommunicating rudimentary uterine horn. *Br J Obstet Gynaecol* 103, 371–372.

Koh C H, Janik G M (1999). Laparoscopic microsurgery: current and future status. *Curr Opin Obstet Gynecol* 11, 401–407.

Krasna I H, Lee M I, Smilour P, Sciorra L, Eirman L (1992). Risk of malignancy in bilateral streak gonads: The role of the Y-chromosome. *J Pediatr Surg* 27, 1376–1380.

Kriplani A, Relan S, Mittal S, Buckslee K (1995). Pre-rupture diagnosis and management of rudimentary horn pregnancy in the first trimester. *Eur J Obstet Gynaecol Reprod Biol* 58, 203–205.

Lee C-L, Wang C-J, Liu Y-H, Yen C-F, Lai Y-L, Soong Y K (1999). Laparoscopically assisted full thickness graft for reconstruction in congenital agenesis of vagina and uterine cervix. *Hum Reprod* 14, 928–930.

Lushbaugh C C, Casarett G W (1976). The effects of gonadal irradiation in clinical radiation therapy: a review. *Cancer* 37, 1111–1120.

Luzzatto C, Midrio P, Toffolutti T, Suma V (2000). Neonatal ovarian cysts: management and follow up. *Paediatr Surg Int* 16, 56–59.

Mahmood T A, Templeton A (1990). The impact of treatment on the natural history of endometriosis. *Hum Reprod* 5, 965–970.

McCarthy E (1999). A case report and review of pregnancies in rudimentary noncommunicating uterine horns. *Aust N Z J Obstet Gynecol* 39, 188–190.

McIndoe A (1950). The treatment of congenital absence and obliterative condition of vagina. *Br J Plast Surg* 2, 254–267.

Meirow D, Fasouliotis S J, Nugent D, Schenker J G, Gosdon R G, Rutherford A J (1999). A laparoscopic technique for obtaining ovarian cortical biopsy specimens for fertility conservation in patients with cancer. *Fertil Steril* 71, 948–951.

Moen M H (1995). Why do women develop endometriosis and why is it diagnosed? *Hum Reprod* 10, 8–11.

Mohammed A, Jibril A, Youngson G (1998). Laparoscopic management of a large ovarian cyst in the neonate. *Surg Endosc* 12, 1272–1274.

Montz F J, Holschneider C H, Munro M G (1994). Incisional hernia following laparoscopy: a survey of the American Association of Gynecologists and Laparosiopists. *Obstet Gynecol* 84, 881–884.

Nahum G G (1997). Rudimentary uterine horn pregnancy. A case report on surviving twins delivered eight days apart. *J Reprod Med* 42, 525–532.

Najmaldin A, Grousseau D (1999). Basic Technique. In *Endoscopic Surgery in Children*, Bax N M A, Georgeson K E, Najmaldin A S, Valla J S, eds., pp. 14–34. Springer Verlag, Berlin.

Najmaldin A, Guillou P (1998). *A Guide to Laparoscopic Surgery.* Najmaldin A, Guillou P, eds. Blackwell Science, London.

Neely M R, McWilliams R, Makhlouf H A (1975). Laparoscopy: routine pneumoperitoneum via the posterior fornix. *Obstet Gynecol* 45, 459–460.

Nezhat C R and Smith K S (1999). Laparoscopic management of unicornuate uterus with two cavitated, non-communicating rudimentary horns. *Hum Reprod* 14, 1965–1968.

Nezhat F, Nezhat C, Bess O, Nezhat C H (1994). Laparoscopic amputation of a noncommunicating rudimentary horn after a hysteroscopic diagnosis: a case study. *Surg Laparosc Endosc* 2, 155–156.

O'Connor H, Magos A (1996). Endometrial resection for the treatment of menorrhagia. *N Engl J Med* 335, 151–156.

Olive D L, Henderson D Y (1987). Endometriosis and Mullerian abnormalities. *Obstet Gynecol* 69, 412–415.

Olsen M M, Caldamore A A, Jackson C L et al. (1988). Gonadoblastoma in infancy: indications for early gonadectomy in 46XY gonadal dysgenesis. *J Pediatr Surg* 23, 270–271.

Ota H, Tanaka J-I, Murakami M et al. (2000). Laparoscopy-assisted Ruge procedure for the creation of a neo-vagina in a patient with Mayer–Rokitanski–Kuster–Hauser syndrome. *Fertil Steril* 73, 641–644.

Pasic R, Levine R L, Wolf W M Jr (1999). Laparoscopy in morbidly obese patients. *J Am Assoc Gynecol Laparosc* 6, 307–312.

Pasini A, Alfieri L, Belloni C (2001). Spontaneous ectopic contralateral pregnancy with unicornuate uterus. A case report. *Minerva Ginecol* 53, 215–218.

Perrotin F, Betrand J, Body G (1999). Laparoscopic surgery of unicornuate uterus with rudimentary horn. *Hum Reprod* 14, 931–933.

*Redwine D B (1991). Conservative laparoscopic excision of endometriosis by sharp dissection: life table analysis of reoperation and persistent or recurrent disease. *Fertil Steril* 56, 628–634.

Raheja S K, McDonald P J, Taylor I (1990). Nonspecific abdominal pain: an expensive mystery. *J Roy Soc Med* 88, 10–11.

Rock J A, Schlaff W D (1985). The obstetric consequences of uterovaginal anomalies. *Fertil Steril* 43, 681–691.

Rosenfield R L, Lucky A W, Allen T D (1980). The diagnosis and management of intersex. *Curr Probl Pediatr* 10, 1–66.

Ruge E (1914). Ersatz der vagina durch die flexur mittels laparotomie. *Dtsch Med Wochenschr* 40, 120–122.

Rutherford A J, Gosdon R G (1999). Ovarian tissue cryopreservation: a practical option? *Acta Paediatr Suppl* 88, 13–18.

Salky B A (1988). The role of laparoscopy in the diagnosis and treatment of abdominal pain syndrome. *Surg Endosc* 12, 911–914.

Sapin E, Bargy F, Lewin F et al. (1994). Management of ovarian cyst detected by prenatal ultrasounds. *Eur J Pediatr Surg* 4, 137–140.

Semm K (1970). Weitere Entwicklungen in der gynäkologischen Laparoskopie-Gynäkologische Pelviskopie. *Klin Frauenheilk Geburt* 1, 326–329.

Shalet S M, Beardwell C G, Morris-Jones P H, Pearson D, Orrell D H (1976). Ovarian failure following abdominal irradiation in childhood. *Br J Cancer* 33, 655–658.

Shellhas H F (1974). Malignant potential of dysgenetic gonad. *Obstet Gynecol* 44, 298–309.

Silber C G, Magness R L, Farber M (1990). Duplication of the uterus with a noncommunicating functioning uterine horn. *Mt Sinai J Med* 57, 374–377.

Soong Y K, Chang F H, Lee C L, Lai Y M (1994). Vaginal agenesis treated by laparoscopically assisted neovaginoplasty. *Gynecol Endosc* 3, 217–220.

*Soong Y K, Chang F H, Lai Y M, Lee C L, Chou H H (1996). Results of modified laparoscopically assisted neovaginoplasty in 18 patients with congenital absence of vagina. *Hum Reprod* 11, 200–203.

String A, Berber E, Foroutani A, Macho J R, Pearl J M, Siperstein A E (2001). Use of the optical access trocar for safe and rapid entry in various laparoscopic procedures. *Surg Endosc* 15, 570–573.

Tabata M, Ichineok, Sakuragi N, Shina Y, Yamaguchi T, Mabuchi Y (1987). Incidence of ovarian metastasis in patients with cancer of the uterine cervix. *Gynecol Oncol* 28, 255–261.

Templeman C L, Hertweck S P, Levine R L, Reich H (2000). Use of laparoscopically mobilised peritoneum in the creation of a neovagina. *Fertil Steril* 74, 589–592.

Thibaud E, Ramirez M, Brauner R et al. (1992). Presentation of ovarian function by ovarian transposition performed before pelvic irradiation during childhood. *J Pediatr* 121, 880–885.

van der Linden P J (1996). Theories on the pathogenesis of endometriosis. *Hum Reprod* 11(Suppl 3), 53–65.

Van Niekerk W A (1976). True hermaphroditism: an analytic review with a report of 3 new cases. *Am J Obstet Gynecol* 126, 890–907.

Vecchietti G (1965). Neovagina nella sindrome di Rokitansky–Kuster–Hauser. *Attual Obstet Ginecol* 11, 131–147.

Vermesh M, Silva P D, Rosen G F, Stein A L, Fossum G T, Sauer M V (1989). Management of unruptured ectopic gestation by linear salpingostomy: a prospective, randomized clinical trial of laparoscopy versus laparotomy. *Obstet Gynecol* 73, 400–404.

Vernon M W, Beard J S, Graves K, Wilson E A (1986). Classification of endometriotic implants by morphologic appearance and capacity to synthesize prostaglandin F. *Fertil Steril* 46, 801–806.

Veronikis D K, McClure G B, Nichols D H (1997). The Vecchietti operation for constructing a neovagina, indications, instrumentation, and techniques. *Obstet Gynecol* 90, 301–304.

von Eye Corleta H, Villodre L C, Reis R, Capp E (2001). Conservative treatment for a noncommunicating rudimentary uterine horn. *Acta Obstet Gynecol Scand* 80, 668.

Von Rokitansky C (1860). Ueber uterusdrusenneubildung in Uterus and Ovarilsarcomen. *Z Gesellschaft Aerzte Wien* (van der Linden PJ) 37, 577–593.

Waldschmidt J, Schier F (1992). Laparoscopical surgery in neonates and infants. *Eur J Pediatr Surg* 1: 145–150

Wolfe W M, Pasic R (1990). Transuterine insertion of Veress needle in laparoscopy. *Obstet Gynecol* 75, 456–457.

Yahata T, Kurabayashi T, Ueda H, Kodama S, Chihara T, Tanaka K (1998). Laparoscopic management of rudimentary horn pregnancy: a case report. *J Reprod Med* 43, 223–226.

Yoo E H, Chun S H, Woo B H (1999). Laparoscopic resection of a rudimentary horn pregnancy. *Acta Obstet Gynecol Scand* 78, 167–168.

13

A nonsurgical approach to the treatment of vaginal agenesis

Julie Alderson[1] and Julie Glanville[2]

[1]Department of Adolescent Psychology, St James Hospital, Leeds, UK
[2]Department of Reproductive Medicine, Leeds General Infirmary, Leeds, UK

Introduction

Vaginal dilator pressure treatment is a nonsurgical treatment method to extend or create a vagina for patients with vaginal agenesis. In this chapter, the term dilation is used to describe the extension of width and length of the vaginal pit (dilatation). The dilator is a cylindrical instrument of moulded plastic, which is repeatedly applied with pressure. Treatment to develop a short or absent vagina is offered to women who desire the capacity for sexual activity that includes sexual intercourse or other vaginal penetration. Dilation treatment relies upon patient adherence and, therefore, requires a scrupulous patient-centred approach by the multidisciplinary team.

History of dilation

Since the first descriptions of congenital absence of the vagina, physicians have described and performed various techniques for the creation of a neovagina in order that women can achieve sexual function including vaginal penetration. Frank was the first to describe treating young women with vaginal agenesis using a vaginal pressure dilation technique (Frank, 1938). He reported the treatment of six patients using vaginal dilators. Dilation treatment occurred two to three times per day and dilators were placed in the vagina throughout the night. Frank reported that five of his patients achieved a vaginal length of 6.5–7 cm within six to eight weeks of treatment and three of the women had sexual intercourse after treatment.

Since Frank detailed his method, there have been variations of his pressure dilation technique. Ingram (1981) described a bicycle stool method whereby patients were instructed to sit on a bicycle seat-shaped stool for short periods with a vaginal dilator held in position in or at the vaginal opening to stretch the vaginal tissue. This was thought to supersede the Frank method by virtue of the fact that the patient was not required to maintain direct pressure by hand, a process that can be uncomfortable and tiring.

Variations of dilators have been developed in recent years and many are commercially available. Most are produced in sets in a range of sizes. They can, however, be expensive and difficult to source. As a result, some centres including our own, have produced their own sets of dilators (Fig. 13.1), often based on the needs of individual patients. Dilator design continues to be influenced by Frank and Ingram, who both emphasized the need for a range of dilator width as well as length. They describe the importance of first creating a narrow vaginal canal and only then progressing to using wider dilators. This method prevents dilatation of the urethral meatus or dorsal angulation of the urethra, leading to urethrocele.

A surgical development of Frank's pressure dilation by Vecchietti (1979) has received much interest in Europe and Australia. Vecchietti describes a surgically inserted tension mechanism used to stretch a neovagina. The Vecchietti procedure uses the same principles as Frank but, by developing a surgical method of applying regular pressure, aims to decrease the length of the treatment time and to circumvent the significant challenge of patient adherence to a home regimen for dilator use (Fig. 13.2). Some modified versions of this technique have been suggested. One example minimizes the surgical component and further reduces the treatment time to an average of 8 days (Fedele et al., 2000; Keckstein et al., 1995). A central argument for the

Paediatric and Adolescent Gynaecology, ed. Adam Balen et al. Published by Cambridge University Press.
© Cambridge University Press 2004.

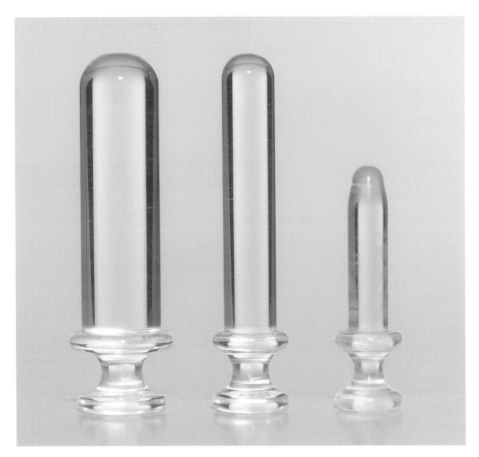

Fig. 13.1. Dilators.

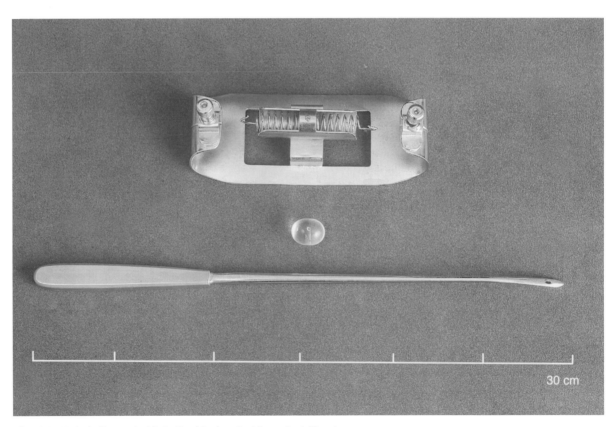

30 cm

Fig. 13.2. Vaginal olive used with the Vecchietti method for vaginal dilatation.

development of surgical stretch techniques such as these is that, while manual stretch-based treatments can be effective, the level of committed adherence required for treatment success is too great.

Timing of treatment

The timing of any treatment of vaginal agenesis must be acutely sensitive to the psychological and social development of the girl or young woman. Not only must she undergo what may feel like invasive procedures, she must be extremely active in her treatment and must remain active in the process over a period of months. She must be able to commit to an initial training period, regular monitoring, follow-up appointments and regular use of the dilators at home. There has been debate regarding whether any treatment for vaginal agenesis, including pressure dilation, should take place before a young woman is sexually active or once she has established a personal (potentially sexual) relationship (Mobus et al., 1993). Shah et al. (1992) recommended that surgical treatment for vaginal agenesis should occur when the patient has decided to become sexually active. Garden (1998), however, believed that it is obvious that girls should have a functioning vagina before they start a sexual relationship, adding that having intercourse will increase the length of the vagina. This suggests that confidence to begin intercourse may be established during the treatment process and in a sense may form part of the treatment. Harkins et al. (1981), writing about surgery, said that treatment for vaginal agenesis should take place when the patient is physically and emotionally mature enough. Foley and Morley (1992) echoed this and guarded against the use of dilators for younger patients long before the start of sexual activity. It is not a prerequisite that a patient be in a heterosexual relationship prior to the commencement of vaginal dilation. Rather, decisions about timing of treatment must be based primarily on an assessment of the individual patient's desire and ability to undertake the treatment procedures. This individual-based approach needs skilful evaluation and negotiation with the patient and in some cases her parents or partner. For many girls and perhaps sexually immature women, the desire to progress with treatment and develop a functioning vagina will be countered by anxiety about the need to penetrate the introitus with the dilator. For others, specific psychological or practical barriers may complicate the use of dilators. If these problems can be identified and countered before the start of treatment, then the likelihood of a positive outcome will be increased. An appropriate timing of treatment should help to prevent fear of failure, limited adherence,

treatment drop out and consequent loss of confidence in the dilation process.

Consent and decision making

To ensure that a patient is able to consent to the treatment with a clear understanding of its demands, it is necessary to help her to gain a thorough appreciation of the dilation process (for full discussion of competency to consent and decision making see Ch. 17). This is a task for each of the clinicians involved and begins when the possibility of vaginal dilation is introduced. It is important to present the benefits of pressure dilation without minimizing the challenges of the process. At this point, it is useful for the specialist nurse to show the patient examples of dilators, give written information about their use and answer initial questions. Dilation should be presented to the patient as a treatment process that includes joint decision making and regular contact with the team of clinicians. Deciding whether to go ahead with treatment, careful consideration of the timing of the start of treatment, training in the use of dilators, regular monitoring examinations, and recognition of a treatment end point and follow-up are all necessary elements of the nonsurgical vaginal dilation process. In this manner, patients must be made aware that dilation is a lengthy process, and that poor adherence will limit success. They may then be able to appreciate that it is necessary to undertake dilation at the optimal time, considering both practical and psychological aspects of their situation.

Psychological preparation and support

After dilation is proposed, the patient can be given a separate appointment for a more detailed discussion of the procedures. It is useful if this appointment occurs at least one week after the initial clinic appointment and presentation of the dilator and written information, leaving time for the patient (and parents) to have considered her initial thoughts and also to have identified concerns and preliminary questions.

The aims of the initial preparation appointment are:
- to ensure that the patient understands that the decision to take up the offered dilation treatment is her own; treatment is neither compulsory nor life saving, but elective
- to ensure that the patient is aware of the treatment process including consent, the initial training, the self-administered regimen and the monitoring appointments
- to anticipate the demands of the dilation process and if possible to begin to consider ways of meeting those demands

- to consider the woman's desires and expectations of treatment and outcome
- to assess any psychological contraindications to commencing dilator use
- to identify any psychological intervention needed prior to dilator use
- to think psychologically and practically about the optimum timing of the start of the treatment process
- to offer and discuss support group or other voluntary agency information.

Depending on the staffing or referral pathways of the service, this consultation might be conducted by a clinical psychologist, counselling psychologist, a heath psychologist, counsellor, psychotherapist or member of a liaison psychiatry team. However, in some services, the specialist gynaecology or endocrinology nurse will be trained and supervised to perform this task. Often the aims of the initial preparation appointment can be met within one extended appointment, usually lasting 50–90 minutes. When working with girls or adolescents, additional liaison with parents will be necessary and will extend the duration of the initial preparation consultation.

When offered treatment for vaginal agenesis, patients and their parents are likely to reconsider the advice they have been given by other health workers prior to referral to the current service. It can be helpful to begin with a review of their journey since initial presentation. In our experience, we often find that patients have been given conflicting advice, for example about the likelihood or timing of surgery; they may have established certain expectations and perhaps made consequent adaptations such as limiting social contacts or withdrawing from personal relationships. Dilation or dilators may have been mentioned by previous clinicians, perhaps in relation to surgery or may have been used in the past. A review of any existing feelings and beliefs about dilators will assist in the assessment of possible hurdles to adherence. This detailed history approach leads on to a discussion of the previous clinic appointment, what was understood, the patient's initial thoughts and her concerns since. Once any misunderstandings have been corrected, the patient's response to the prospect of dilation should be discussed in detail. Throughout this discussion, the clinical psychologist or equivalent will focus on trying to understand the patient's experiences, both of the past and of the present task of talking about the issue of adaptation to and treatment of vaginal agenesis. The listener's genuine struggle for empathic understanding will mean that this consultation might not only be informative but also psychologically therapeutic in relation to distress associated with the matters discussed.

Patients' attitudes to dilator treatment

There is a range of frequent responses to the offer of dilator treatment. Some women, girls and parents express relief when offered an alternative to surgery. Some see dilation as an easier option while others are disappointed that they have not been offered an operation that in their perception would "get it all over with". Patients with a very short vagina may have difficulty accepting that dilation can be effective. It is common for younger women or teenagers to be quite appalled by the idea of inserting an instrument into the vulval region. It may be that, despite concerns about amenorrhoea, the girl has not explored her genitalia or may even have developed a phobic response to her genital area. It is necessary to explore the nature and extent of these fears, to offer information or reassurance wherever possible and to estimate the impact of remaining anxiety on adherence to therapy. It is common to have fear of pain, concern about hospitalization and repeat appointments. It is important at this stage to help the patient to accept these concerns as appropriate and useful considerations for discussion. It is only by becoming aware of anxieties that adequate preparation and well-founded decisions about treatment can be made. A brief explanation and demonstration of the use of dilators is likely to be insufficient. Some patients recall being given dilators as embarrassing, confusing and painful, and they confess to disposing of the dilators after very little use. Others have recalled how they had found the idea of using dilators abhorrent or frightening and had failed to use their dilators on more than the rare occasion (Alderson, 2000). Had these patients been able to talk openly about their concerns with the clinicians providing their care, they may have been helped to make better use of the dilators and the process may have been much less distressing.

When the clinician presents the dilation procedure in detail, he or she invites the patient to imagine her own experience of the process at each stage. By this mechanism, anxieties and possible barriers can be anticipated. For example, the practicalities such as hospitalization and home administration may raise the issue of the degree of disclosure and openness regarding the underlying condition, or the importance of regular privacy and time to use the dilators at home. In some cases, this careful consideration will reveal specific psychological problems that may need addressing before dilator use can take place, may require onward referral or may effect the expected outcome of dilation. These can include trauma responses to child sexual abuse, hospital anxiety or procedural distress, body dysmorphia or psychosexual problems.

A decision to go ahead with dilation treatment is made when the girl or woman fully understands and consents to the proposed procedure, the demands it places upon her and the range of possible outcomes. Further preparation may include additional appointments or telephone discussions with the nurse specialist to discuss treatment and sessions of psychological intervention such as cognitive behavioural therapy to ameliorate specific anxieties for the reduction of procedural distress. Dilation treatment may be delayed by the presence of psychological disorder such as depression, which would be likely to mitigate against adherence and, therefore, treatment outcome. Treatment could then be commenced after psychotherapeutic or pharmacological treatment.

Additional psychological support may be beneficial as the dilation process begins. It is sometimes helpful for the patient to be seen by the psychologist immediately before the initial dilation demonstration by the specialist nurse. Anxiety management techniques can be revised, and as treatment begins the psychologist can help the patient to maximize her motivation gained from its initial impact. Robinson et al. (1999) recommended the provision of psychological support for younger women during dilator treatment. Following a randomized control trial of a psychoeducational group, they concluded that most women, particularly younger women, are unlikely to follow the recommendation to use a dilator unless they are given assistance in overcoming their fears and are taught behavioural skills.

Vaginal dilator treatment

It is essential that patients undergoing dilator therapy are properly instructed, supervised and supported by a trained and skilled nurse or doctor. A specialist nurse can often best combine the role of trainer and supporter of the patient and family. The nurse specialist provides continuity of care via frequent contact with the patient while liasing with other members of the multidisciplinary team and making onward referrals when appropriate.

A philosophy of care that emphasizes the necessary partnership between patient and nurse is essential in the practice of dilation treatment. A useful nursing model that may be applied throughout the treatment process is that of Orem (1995). Orem describes three types of nursing system where the responsibility for patient care is differently apportioned to the nurse and the patient depending on the needs of the patient at a particular time or situation. Dilator treatment exemplifies Orem's supportive–educative

system, where the patient, having learned to perform the needed self-care from the nurse, is then competent in that care but still requires periodic guidance. This approach is in line with the Nursing and Midwifery Council Code of Professional Conduct (2002): "You must recognize and respect the role of patients and clients as partners in their care and the contribution they make to it. This involves identifying their preferences regarding care and respecting these within the limits of professional practice, existing legislation, resources and the goals of the therapeutic relationship." Information leaflets with diagrams, anatomical models and example dilators can all be used to inform patients fully about the treatment process. Such explanation forms part of the preparation and consent processes but should be reviewed at the start of treatment. As it is common for patients to feel able to express anxieties and discuss sensitive subjects with a nurse, by remaining accessible the nurse can encourage the patient to seek nursing, psychological or medical advice at the earliest stage. Box 13.1 summarizes the recommendations for dilator treatment.

Box 13.1 Recommendations for practice

- Dilation treatment of vaginal agenesis should be undertaken within a multidisciplinary context.
- Informed consent and psychological preparation processes must take place before treatment begins.
- The clinician should be aware of individual patient factors (including cultural beliefs and values) that may influence adherence.
- Dilation training and ongoing review should be provided by a named clinician with the support of other team members.
- Psychological approaches to the promotion of adherence should be considered.
- Evaluation of multidisciplinary outcome should be undertaken and disseminated.

Inpatient training

Instruction and training in the use of vaginal dilators is aimed at establishing effective independent use by the patient. Some UK centres have found that this process is more effective when the patient is admitted to hospital to undertake intensive training over a period of two to four days. Admission enables supervised trials three times a day and ensures that the patient has adequate privacy to practise locating the vaginal pit and using the dilators. The initial progress achieved within the first few days of intensive treatment can be a strong motivating factor that promotes future adherence. Extended training periods with feedback on the patient's own performance can develop confidence in her ability to use the dilators correctly. This is likely to increase confidence and establish habitual use once at home. Inpatient training is also useful when the patient must travel a considerable distance to the treatment centre and attendance at frequent appointments is difficult.

Initial instruction

The dilation training session should begin with a relaxed discussion of the patient's expectations and the aims of the treatment. The specialist nurse can encourage the patient to express her anxieties and ask questions. The patient is advised to be in a semirecumbent position (on the bed or chair) and is shown how to locate her vaginal dimple or introitus using a mirror. The nurse demonstrates the placing of the dilator, including its angle; the pressure to be applied; and the use of local anaesthetic gel and lubricants as required. The rounded end of the dilator is inserted parallel to the normal axis of the vagina and intermittent pressure is applied for 10 to 15 minutes, gradually stretching the vaginal tissue. Some patients may prefer the bicycle seat method, which eliminates the hand fatigue that can occur during this exercise. The patient starts using the smallest dilator dependent upon the start size of the vaginal pit. The dilators increase in size in 5 mm width sizes until approximately 30 mm width and 100 mm length can be used with comfort (or until the patient is happy with the size of dilator used). At initial sessions, the patient may require oral analgesia prior to the procedure, as the dilation process can be painful. Pain or discomfort appears to occur less frequently and usually resolves as the dilation therapy progresses. Relaxation exercises may be taught in addition or in place of analgesia as required, and used throughout the subsequent dilation. The training process includes supervised trials by the patient and the patient's independent practice. During and after practice, the patient can ask any questions and check that she has used the dilator correctly. Common questions concern the correct amount of pressure to be applied and enquiries about the nature and commonality of the physical sensations experienced during therapy. Whether inpatient or outpatient based, the training process should develop the patient's confident independent use of the dilators.

Ongoing use of dilators

On discharge, the patient is advised to establish a habitual routine of dilation at home and the nurse and patient agree the periodicity of further reviews. Frank (1938)

recommended use for 30 minutes per session and nighttime use while Ingram recommended that patients sit on the bicycle seat with the dilator in place for at least 2 hours per day. The frequency and duration of dilation must be planned with the patient, based on a detailed discussion of her daily schedule. Our practice is to recommend routine use three times daily for 15 minutes per session. The initial estimation of the most appropriate and convenient times to use the dilators can be revised during later discussions in clinic. It is vital for adequate adherence that the patient and the specialist nurse continue to review the most convenient times for home dilation and to counter any difficulties as they arise. The same specialist nurse should review the patient's progress at an outpatient nurse-led clinic. In this clinic, the patient would be seen by the specialist nurse only, unless the nurse and patient have requested the presence of an additional member of the multidisciplinary team. Loftus and Weston (2001) suggest that there is evidence that a positive impact on the quality of outpatient care can occur when a service is led by a specialist nurse. Their conclusion that nurse-led clinics are "developed to meet unmet patient need, solve actual or potential patient problems and improve the quality of a service" concords with the rationale for the development of dilation treatment services. Initial reviews should occur approximately every two weeks and then more or less frequently, depending on progress, the level of support needed, and the patient's travelling distance, school or work commitments, etc. Patients are encouraged to contact the nurse between appointments to ask questions, seek advice or reassurance or to arrange the most convenient review appointment times.

Assessment of progress is made by vaginal examination and by measuring the width and length of the dilator that can be inserted by the patient at each stage. Measurements are recorded on the nursing assessment sheet at each visit. The patient can be asked to contribute to the monitoring process by charting the frequency of home dilation. Such a diary chart may aid adherence by serving as a reminder to the patient, and patchy completion might highlight patterns of adherence. Central to the nursing follow-up is a discussion of the patient's assessment of her progress. Both objective and subjective progress form the basis of the goals for the next stage of treatment, the amount of time before return to clinic and the inclusion of telephone contact with the nurse or additional support from any other member of the team.

Counselling

Both during the inpatient-training phase and during outpatient reviews, the nurse specialist needs significant

Table 13.1. Summary of the nurse specialist role

Activity	Components
Nursing process	Assessment, planning, implementation and evaluation
Assessment of individual needs	Flexible appointment times fitted around college or work commitments; awareness of social situation and support; choice of dilation method and instruments
Self-care planning	Promotion of active participation by patient in own care planning (e.g. start of treatment, frequency of dilation, frequency of review appointments); patient information, education and supervision
Continuity of care	Named nurse leads the team involvement throughout the treatment process
Access	Telephone contact for appointments or counselling; long-term follow up; treatment breaks
Support	Patient support and encouragement; support for other family members and partners
Liaison	With other members of multidisciplinary team; with appropriate support groups
Evaluation and dissemination	Monitor and audit treatment process and outcomes; professional links with other centres (benchmarking); share clinical experience

counselling skills to instruct, motivate and support the patient. The nurse specialist role includes maintaining the therapeutic relationship, monitoring behavioural programmes for adherence and referring on to the clinical psychologist or other psychological staff when appropriate (Table 13.1). Telephone counselling skills as well as face-to-face counselling skills may be needed. Supervision of this counselling role can be provided by a clinical psychologist or by a nursing clinical supervisor with training and expertise in counselling relationships. Reasons for psychological referral might include continued poor adherence, increased anxiety, awareness of previously undetected psychosexual problems or the patient's desire to talk in depth about her feelings and thoughts regarding adjustment to the underlying condition promoted by the treatment process. The specialist nurse should be able to assess the need for onward referral and be able to discuss this with the patient. Liaison with the wider clinical team allows the nurse to answer many of the patient's questions regarding treatment and promotes continuity of care when other team members are directly involved (Table 13.1).

When the desired vaginal length and width has been achieved a review appointment in the main clinic can mark success for the patient and allows the whole team, including the consultant, to be involved in the review. This permits discussion of each patient's treatment process and outcome, which then informs future practise.

In an ongoing review of dilator treatment in our unit, over three years (February 1998 to February 2002), 19 women used dilators as a nonsurgical approach to the treatment of vaginal agenesis. The women were aged between 15 years 6 months and 50 years 3 months (average age 20 years 1 month). Of those 19, two were still ongoing with the process at the time of writing and one woman had dropped out.

Table 13.2. Changes in patient's vaginal lengths and widths achieved by dilator treatment

	Pretreatment mean (range)	Posttreatment mean (range)	Change achieved mean (range)[a]
Length (mm)	36 (25–60)	83 (25–100)	68 (20–75)
width (mm)	20 (10–25)	28 (25–35)	10 (0–20)

[a]Results from 16 of the 19 women treated; one woman dropped out of the study and two were still undergoing treatment.

Sixteen women (84%) had completed treatment to their satisfaction. The women used the dilators over an average period (from first examination to last) of 8.9 months. Those who had completed treatment did so within an average period of 7.4 months. Table 13.2 shows the patient's vaginal lengths and widths pre- and posttreatment and the changes they achieved.

None of the women was able to experience penetrative sex at the start of treatment, whereas by posttreatment follow-up (approximately three months after last examination) 62% of those who completed dilation were sexually active (i.e. 11 (57%) of the original 19).

Adherence

The non-surgical creation of a vagina via pressure dilation techniques is largely dependent upon the patient's correct and conscientious use of the dilation instruments. The woman must be active in the training process and negotiate aspects of the process with the specialist nurse. The term adherence refers to the extent to which the negotiated health-related behaviours (such as repeating an exercise-taking medication) is undertaken towards achievement of an agreed therapeutic goal. This conceptualization of adherence implies more than a passive compliance to a given treatment regimen and emphasizes the patient's active involvement. It is, of course, very difficult for women and adolescents to sustain the use of vaginal dilators and the high level of commitment needed for success. It is vital that, with the introduction of vaginal pressure dilation treatment, the whole team is aware that they are not merely *applying* a treatment but are working to maximize the patient's commitment and promote her continued adherence. Because adherence underpins the effectiveness and efficiency of vaginal dilation, it is extremely influential in clinical decision making, as in other areas of healthcare (Rapoff, 2001). Poor adherence to the demands of nonsurgical vaginal dilation have significantly contributed to the development of surgical stretch methods for the creation of a neovagina (Fedele et al., 2000; Keckstein et al., 1995; Vecchietti, 1979).

Of course the development of the vagina via pressure dilation is not a single event but is extended over a period of months during which adherence is likely to reduce (La Greca and Schuman, 1995; Rapoff and Barnard, 1991). In a study of cancer patients undergoing vaginal dilation, Bruner found that patients reported a rapid decline in adherence even after receiving counselling (Bruner et al., 1993; Flay and Matthews, 1995; Schover, 1989). Another follow-up study of oncology patients found that 57% of the group still used the dilator at 6 months but only 14% reported adherence to the recommended frequency of three times per week (Robinson et al., 1999). The demands of home dilation can be compared to those of physiotherapy regimens. A study of compliance to prescribed physiotherapy noted that up to two-thirds of adult patients were compliant during supervised treatment, but there was a fall in self-reported compliance from 64% to only 23% once supervision ended (Sluijs and Kuiper, 1990). Robinson et al. (1999), therefore, recommended that close follow-up is needed to maintain compliance. Another physiotherapy study concluded that a lack of multidisciplinary support contributed to a reduction in adherence to a prescribed exercise regimen.

The personal nature of vaginal dilation is likely to compound the adherence challenge, along with other factors such as the speed of change and invisible consequences of less than optimal adherence. In addition, measurement of the level of adherence can be made only by means of self-report, clinical judgement and clinical outcome. Patient account is considered the most unreliable and is believed to grossly overestimate adherence (Gordis et al., 1969; Sheiner et al., 1974). Even the reliability of clin-

ical outcome as a measure of adherence is said to vary depending upon the individual, the underlying condition and the clinical acumen of the clinician. However, while outcome may be considered to be of limited value as a stand-alone measure of compliance to health behaviour advice (McGavoc, 1996), it is perhaps the best measure of the appropriate use of vaginal dilators. This distinction highlights both the difference between compliance and adherence and the emphasis of collaborative working with the patient. It is more important that the patient uses her vaginal dilators in the way that produces the best clinical outcome in her case (adherence to working towards a negotiated clinical goal) than it is for her to follow the nurse specialist's advice to the letter (compliance to a given regimen).

Adherence by adolescents

While recognized as a challenge to all patient groups, it has been suggested that adherence further reduces in adolescence (Koocher et al., 1990), when dilation is likely to commence. Central to child or adolescent adherence is that treatment must be recognized as a family issue (Lemanek, 2001). Health- and treatment-related behaviours take place in the family home, are prompted by a parent and are timed around the family schedule. In many cases, even the older child will in practical terms be adhering to the advice of both parent and clinician. At times, the patient, parents and physician may have subtly different goals for treatment, such as achieving normalcy, the capacity to use tampons or the capacity for sexual intercourse (Bryon, 1998; Gordis et al., 1969; Reid and Appleton, 1991). It is important, therefore, to work with parents to promote their understanding and beliefs in the efficacy of treatment, to reduce any ambivalence and to improve their motivation to provide proper support for their daughter's motivation.

A review of 27 studies of the efficacy of interventions to promote adherence in paediatric care found that only three showed clear improvements in disease outcomes (Rapoff and Barnard, 1999). In general, the studies supported behavioural strategies. Glasgow and Anderson (1995), Johnson et al. (1986) and La Greca and Schuman (1995) each recommend focusing adherence interventions on individual family needs. With either an individual or family approach it is necessary to consider the family or parent/adolescent barriers to adherence. Aspects as varied as a shared room or dilation as a focus for opposition or control within a parent–child relationship may form barriers to adherence (Rapoff and Barnard, 2001).

Overcoming adherence problems

If a patient has actively consented to the dilation treatment yet appears unable to use her dilators at home, then it is necessary to try to identify and attempt to remove her barriers to adherence. The psychological perspective on adherence has been to take a patient-centred approach, using the patient's insights as the most valuable way of understanding the mechanisms of poor adherence, and then work to alter these mechanisms. All advice following is informed by the patient's knowledge, beliefs and attitudes, which influence her decision making. Therefore, to understand adherence is to understand behaviour, its antecedents and consequences, its context, the patient's beliefs and the attitudes that underpin those beliefs. The patient's rationality might not follow medical authodoxy but if her idiosyncratic understanding and thinking can be accessed by the psychologist or other clinician then intervention can be based on discussion and explanation rather than superficially challenging the patient's behaviour. Using similar processes, qualitative studies based on patients' accounts of their beliefs and experiences have developed models of patient adherence and have advanced knowledge in this area. Some of the findings from adherence studies can shed light on adherence to vaginal dilation (concepts from research are shown in italics).

The extent of *positive attitude* towards the treatment, the clinical team and the likelihood of success is thought to be influential upon adherence. Indeed, the *perceived efficacy* (her beliefs about how likely the dilation is to work) will be central to her motivation to repeat the exercises regularly. Because efficacy can be defined in different ways, it is necessary to discuss what rate of treatment effect is desirable clinically and what the patient feels is necessary for her to feel satisfied (Arluke, 1980; Falsberg, 1991). In addition, the views of others will impact on the patient's prospective judgement about the likelihood of dilation to be effective. *Lay views* of significant people such as parents and partners and any *past experience* of efficacy, either the patient's own or that of others known to her, are likely to affect her perception of the efficacy of dilation and, in turn, her adherence. The *mode of production* has been highlighted in adherence research. This often pertains to the patient's views of the unnaturalness of medicines. Similarly, some patients contemplating vaginal dilation might require help to overcome a sense that it is not right or not natural to touch her genitals or to insert a foreign body into her vagina. As with certain medicines, it may help to present dilation as a natural and gradual mode of treatment. Although professionals might see vaginal dilation as a benign treatment, patients may still feel that they are *balancing risks or benefits* when going ahead. Such concerns are most likely when dilation follows previous surgical intervention to the genital region and the patient suspects that they may be applying pressure to a vulnerable site. Even without prior surgery, a patient might still worry about harming delicate tissue. In addition, if clear beneficial effects are not observed then treatment may be stopped prematurely, especially when balanced against side effects such as pain.

A perhaps rare but significant side effect could occur in relation to previous traumatic experiences. Beginning dilation could trigger flashbacks to sexual abuse, assault or unsuccessful attempts at intercourse. Other traumatic memories might include painful medical procedures, embarrassing examinations or the diagnosis itself. If the patient experiences any of these associations, she is likely to balance them against the desired therapeutic outcome. *Social context* of any treatment is said to influence adherence. This includes the possible unorthodox meaning of the treatment within the patient's social context. For many, vaginal dilation will mean an introduction to a sexual life; for others it might mean the conclusion of an episode of medical involvement. In some cultures or subcultures, the creation or opening of the vagina when fertility is not affected might signal the desire for sexual activity aside from reproduction. If this is not openly acceptable within her culture, it will be more difficult for the patient to adhere to the demands of the treatment despite her desire or intention. Commonly, the patient's social context may include practical variables such as the amount of privacy available or the amount of family support for the patient.

Practical approaches to improving adherence

While characteristics of a certain disease are said not to determine the level of adherence, characteristics of the treatment certainly do. Efforts can be made to alter a dilation treatment regimen to promote patient's treatment-related behaviours and, therefore, the treatment outcome. A good clinician–patient relationship prevents adherence problems remaining undisclosed, but there are additional, serviced-based strategies that can be used to maximize the effectiveness of nonsurgical dilation treatments for vaginal agenesis (Table 13.3).

Summary

Nonsurgical vaginal dilation is neither an easy option for the treatment of vaginal agenesis nor is it an unachievable

Table 13.3. Practical approaches to improving adherence

Approach	Features
Individualize care	Provide choices regarding date time of admission and of ward environment (side room); option for parent to be resident or partner to be involved in treatment
Be sensitive to cultural differences in need	Needs of minority groups or people of different cultures may vary
Provide written information	Written information can influence adherence, correct misunderstanding and alter attitude to treatment; a well-designed and relevant leaflet can increase satisfaction with care; written information (in the patient's first language) should be supplemented by discussion
Utilize peer support opportunities	Groups for women undertaking dilation, and paired admission during training can be offered; introductions to national support groups
Recommend monitoring	Patient monitoring of dilator use and treatment progress can aid patient motivation by showing patterns of activity and progress
Use behavioural interventions	Negotiate a programme of rewards with use of dilators or treatment progress

task for many adolescents and women (Box 13.2). All professionals involved should understand the process required to maximize the patient's adherence and the outcome of this procedure.

Box 13.2 Key points

- Dilation treatment of vaginal agenesis is a genuine alternative to surgery.
- Adherence is the foundation of dilation treatment of vaginal agenesis.
- Timing of treatment must be sensitive to the psychosocial development of the patient.
- All decisions regarding treatment must be made jointly by the patient, parents and clinicians.
- An experienced nurse specialist is the most appropriate lead clinician for this treatment.

REFERENCES

*Indicates key references.

Alderson J (2000). XY women with androgen insensitivity syndrome (AIS): a qualitative study. Unpublished Thesis, University of Leeds.

Arluke A (1980). Judging drugs: patients' conceptions of therapeutic efficacy in the treatment of arthritis. *Hum Organization* 39, 84–88.

Bruner D, Lanciano R, Keegan M, Corn B, Martin E, Hanks G (1993). Vaginal stenosis and sexual function following intracavitary radiation for the treatment of cervical and endometrial carcinoma. *Int J Radiat Oncol Biol Phys* 27, 825–830.

Bryon M (1998). Adherence to treatment in children. In *Adherence Treatment to Medical Conditions*, Myers L B, Midence K, eds., pp. 161–190. Harwood, Amsterdam.

Falsberg M (1991). Reflections on medicines and medication; a qualitative analysis among people on long-term drug regimens. Studies in Education Dissertation 31, Linkoping University, Linkoping, Sweden.

Fedele L, Bianchi S, Zanconato G, Raffaelli R (2000). Laparoscopic creation of a neovagina in patients with Rokitansky syndrome: analysis of 52 cases. *Fertil Steril* 74, 384–389.

Flay L, Matthews J (1995). The effects of radiotherapy and surgery on the sexual function of women treated for cervical cancer. *Int J Radiat Oncol Biol Phys* 31, 399–404.

Foley S, Morley G W (1992). Care and counselling of the patient with vaginal agenesis. *Female Patient* 17, 73–80.

*Frank R T (1938). The formation of an artificial vagina without operation. *Am J Obstet Gynecol* 35, 1053–1055.

Garden A S (1998). Problems with menstruation. In *Paediatric and Adolescent Gynaecology*, Garden A S, ed., pp. 127–154. Arnold, London.

Glasgow R E, Anderson B J (1995). Future directions for research on pediatric chronic management: lessons from diabetes. *J Pediatr Psychol* 20, 389–402.

Gordis L, Markowitz M, Lilienfeld A M (1969). The inaccuracy in using interviews to estimate patient reliability in taking medications at home. *Med Care* 7, 49–54.

Harkins J L, Gysler M, Cowell C A (1981). Anatomical amenorrhea: the problems of congenital vaginal agenesis, its correction. *Paediatr Clin North Am* 28, 345–354.

Ingram J M (1981). The bicycle seat stool in the treatment of vaginal agenesis and stenosis: a preliminary report. *Am J Obstet Gynecol* 140, 867.

Johnson S B, Silverstein J, Rosenbloom A, Carter R, Cunninham W (1986). Assessing daily management in childhood diabetes. *Health Psychol* 9, 606–631.

Keckstein J, Buck G, Sasse V, Tuttlies F, Ulrich U (1995). Laprascopic creation of a neovagina: modified Vecchitti method. *Endosc Surg* 3, 93–95.

Koocher G P, McGrath M L, Gudas L J (1990). Typologies of non-adherence in cystic fibrosis. *Dev Behav Pediatr* 11, 353–358.

La Greca A M, Schuman W B (1995). Adherence to prescribed medical regimens. In *Handbook of Pediatric Psychology*, 2nd edn, Roberts M C, ed., pp. 55–83. Guilford, New York.

*Lemanek K (2001). Adherence issues in the middle management of asthma. *J Pediatr Psychol* 15, 437–458.

Loftus L A, Weston V (2001). The development of nurse-led clinics in cancer care. *J Clin Nurs* 10, 215–220.

McGavoc H (1996). *A Review of the Literature on Drug Adherence: Taking Medicines to Best Effect*. Royal Pharmaceutical Society of Great Britain, London.

Mobus V, Sachweh K, Knapstein P G, Kreienberg R (1993). Women after surgically corrected vaginal aplasia: a follow up of psychosexual rehabilitation. *Geburtsh Frauenh* 53, 125–131.

*Nursing and Midwifery Council (2002). *Code of Professional Conduct*, 2.1 p. 3. Nursing and Midwifery Council, London.

*Orem D E (1995). *Nursing: Concepts of Practice*, 5th edn. Mosby, St Louis, MO.

Rapoff M J (2001). Commentary: pushing the envelope. Furthering research on improving adherence to chronic pediatric disease regimens. *J Pediatric Psychol* 26, 277–278.

Rapoff M A, Barnard M U (1991). Compliance with pediatric medical regimens. In *Patient Compliance in Medical Practice and Clinical Trials*, Cramer J A, Spiker B, eds., pp. 73–98. Raven, New York.

Reid P, Appleton P (1991). Insulin dependent diabetes mellitus: regimen adherence in children, young people. *Irish J Dev Behav Pediatr* 10, 307–312.

*Robinson J W, Faris P D, Scott C B (1999). Psychoeducational group increases vaginal dilation for younger women and reduces sexual fears for women of all ages with gynaecological carcinoma treated with radiotherapy. *Int J Radiat Oncol Biol Phys* 44, 497–506.

Schover L, Fife M, Gershenson D (1989). Sexual dysfunction and treatment for early stage cervical cancer. *Cancer* 63, 204–212.

Shah R, Wooley M M, Costin G (1992). Testicular feminisation: the androgen insensitivity syndrome. *J Pediatr Surg* 27, 757–760.

Sheiner L B, Rosenberg B, Marathe V V, Peck C (1974). Differences in serum digoxin concentrations between outpatients and inpatients: an effect of compliance? *Clin Pharmacol Ther* 15, 239–246.

Sluijs E M, Kuiper E B (1990). Problemen die Fysiotherapeuten ervaren bij het geven van voorlichting aan Patienten: een Inventarisatie. [Problems physical therapists encounter in educating patients.] *Ned Tijdschr Fysiother* 100, 128–132.

Vecchietti G (1979). Le neo-vagin dans le syndrome de Rokitanski–Kuster–Hauser. *Rev Med Suisse Romande* 99, 593–601.

14

Psychological care in disorders of sexual differentiation and determination

Polly Carmichael[1] and Julie Alderson[2]

[1] Department of Psychological Medicine, Great Ormond St Hospital for Children, London, UK
[2] Department of Adolescent Psychology, St James Hospital, Leeds, UK

Psychosocial functioning and quality of life are of increasing emphasis in consideration of outcome for people with chronic health conditions. The World Health Organization's assessment of quality of life has six domains, three of which refer to psychosocial outcomes (WHOQOL group, 1995). While few will experience clinically significant psychopathology, children with chronic illness are more likely to have psychosocial problems and a child's illness can impact on the whole family (Drotar and Crawford 1985; Eiser, 1990; Wallander et al., 1989).

Healthcare services for children and adolescents with disorders of sexual differentiation and determination (DSDD) are in part aimed at the prevention of psychopathological responses to diagnosis and treatment. Medical and nursing staff aim to provide healthcare that is designed to be sensitive to patients' psychological needs, but it is acknowledged that specialist psychosocial care should also be available and integrated with the medical care. A clinical psychologist or other applied psychologist in a health setting with experience of DSDD generally provides this service.

The psychologist has a dual role of supporting the family and working with the wider team to ensure that individual child or family needs are incorporated into treatment from the outset. Recognition of the psychological components of healthcare does not represent a presumption of psychological disorder, rather an acknowledgement of the possible impact on the child's psychological development and the wider family adaptation. Although families can feel wary of the notion that they require psychological support, this is a key element of routine care based upon the significant emphasis on psychological outcome in DSDD. Familiarity with the team psychologist should reduce suspicion and enable families to discuss their concerns about their child at an early stage. Seeking a balance between remaining accessible to families and not overloading the child with hospital appointments and interventions, psychological care provision is focused on the prevention of difficulties throughout medical care.

Psychologists may be involved in decision making regarding sex of rearing either at birth or, in cases of later diagnosis, via assessment of a child's psychosexual development. They can work with a child or family to promote fully informed consent to surgical or medical interventions. They frequently focus on talking to parents and children about the condition and play a significant role in transition to adolescent or adult services. Some children may require individual therapeutic work in response to specific difficulties including adaptation to diagnosis, nonadherence, problems of body image, gender identity or family functioning.

Despite the increasing anecdotal and clinical knowledge concerning the psychological demands of DSDD, there remains little evidence on which to base psychosocial services. However, increasing interest in the psychological sequelae, the prevention of psychopathology and the role of psychological or psychosocial care for this patient group is fuelling current research activity.

Theories of psychosexual development

The optimum management for children born with DSDD is currently the subject of controversial debate. Divergent theories of psychosexual development underpin this debate and continue to inform the medical, surgical and psychosocial care of children.

Paediatric and Adolescent Gynaecology, ed. Adam Balen et al. Published by Cambridge University Press.
© Cambridge University Press 2004.

John Money and his colleagues in the 1950s and 1960s proposed and developed the dominant theory of psychosexual development used to guide treatment of children born with ambiguous genitalia (Money et al., 1955, 1957; see also Ch. 8). Money suggested that socialization exerts a decisive role in the development of gender identity. He proposed that in the sex assignment or reassignment of babies there is latitude of choice in gender as psychosexual identity is as yet undifferentiated. This meant that sex assignment and subsequent rearing could direct the course of differentiation. This paradigm gives precedence to the role of nurture over nature in the development of a gender identity as it is suggested that "genetic, hormonal or other prenatal determinates do not exercise a gross, inevitable predisposing effect" (Money, 1975).

The recommendation that followed was that, when a child was assigned a sex following presentation with ambiguous genitalia, parents should unequivocally adhere to the assigned sex. It was said that the child would then develop a gender identity in line with this sex of rearing. In order to protect the child and parents from any ambiguity regarding gender, early surgery aimed to make the external genitalia congruent with the assigned sex of rearing. Fears about the negative impact on gender development of any delay in sex assignment have led to the recommendation that children born with ambiguous genitalia should be treated as a medical emergency. In order to make decisions about sex assignment, Money proposed that a fundamental rule, irrespective of the chromosomal karyotype and gonadal sex, was never to assign a baby to be reared as male unless the phallus in the neonatal period was the same as that of same aged males with a "small–average" phallus (Money 1975).

This model of psychosocial and medical management for children with a DSDD has been termed the "optimal gender policy". The policy aimed to facilitate the best prognosis across a range of variables. These included a stable gender identity, psychosocial well-being, gender-appropriate appearance, good sexual function, fertility where possible and minimal medical procedures (Meyer-Bahlberg, 1999).

For many years, the success of the optimal gender policy was illustrated with the now infamous case of monozygotic twins, one of whom had a circumcision that resulted in the loss of his penis. At the age of 17 months, he was reassigned female and underwent gonadectomy and genital reconstruction. He reportedly developed a female gender identity and the case was cited as evidence for the role of nurture over nature in the development of gender identity (Money and Ehrhardt, 1972). This case has since become the cornerstone of recent challenges to Money's conceptualization of the development of gender identity. Diamond and Sigmundson (1997a) reported that at the age of 14 years the child rejected the female gender and began to live as a male. In adulthood, he married a woman. This example of the "failure" of sex reassignment has been used to argue that socialization factors are secondary to biological factors in the development of gender identity and sexual orientation (e.g., Diamond, 1997).

In what has been termed the "true-brain sex policy" it is posited that gender-identity development in babies with ambiguous genitalia is not a malleable process and cannot be predicted in infancy (Kipnis and Diamond, 1998). On this basis, it is recommended that no feminizing surgery should take place before the child or adolescent is able to give consent.

The optimal gender and true-brain sex models represent polar positions in the conceptualization of the aetiology of gender development. This leads to divergent recommendations for the criteria used to inform gender assignment decisions and subsequent clinical interventions. However, both propose that a male or female sex assignment should be made. Social constructionist critiques of the medical model (Dreger, 1998; Fausto-Sterling, 1993, 2000; Kessler, 1998), with its focus on sex assignment in terms of male and female, have prompted exploration of the possibility of a "third sex".

Secrecy in medical care

The medical and psychological management of DSDD have long been interrelated. Medical interventions have attempted to establish individuals as one sex or the other and to promote successful psychological adjustment to the established sex and corresponding gender. The psychosexual theory that the chosen course for gender-identity development would be disturbed by ambiguity regarding the assigned gender demanded secrecy regarding aspects of medical management. However, over time, this practice became distanced from its theoretical origins and changed in nature. The imposition of secrecy has been employed without critical scrutiny of its value in each case. Its use appears to have reinforced feelings of stigma and shame for those affected by DSDD. It can be argued that the perceived need for secrecy has protected health practitioners from addressing some difficult aspects of care. This has effectively precluded the opportunity for individuals to explore any concerns they may have about their condition. It has also limited the development of thinking and practise in the medical and psychological care of children with DSDD. Secrecy became a doctrine rather than a considered way of promoting psychological well-being.

The negative effects of secrecy are becoming more widely known but medical practices based on the optimal gender policy are well established. For example, in a 1989 text doctors talking to new parents of a child with ambiguous genitalia were advised to say, "Your child has been born with an abnormality of the external genitalia, which make it impossible for us to be sure at this stage whether the child is a boy or a girl. We are quite sure that your child will prove to be one or the other and not something in between." A caveat was added: "This is not strictly true, but it should be said to relieve fear" (Edmonds, 1989). The desire to reduce the possibility of gender-ambiguous rearing by protecting parents, as well as their child, from information that may be difficult to reconcile is evident. "It is more satisfactory to give confident advice to the parents even though this means misleading them to some extent, and to avoid disclosing the male karyotype". In line with optimal gender policy, Edmonds also recommended continued psychological support for the child and suggested that parents' distress should be correctly managed in the early stages, and "the sex [chromosomal pattern] at birth, should never be communicated to the child". Regarding management of the older child or adolescent, the same author advised: "The need for removal [of the gonads] must be carefully broached with the patient along lines similar to those discussed previously".

Preves (1998) was direct in her assertion that the very approach that was adopted to prevent psychological maladjustment to DSDD had in fact, been the cause of the high levels of psychological distress reported. She describes a phenomenon of "medicalization", as a result of which people suffer through "living with bodies that have been classified as deviant" (Preves, 1998). She suggested that well-intended medical treatment (e.g. hormone therapy and surgery) to reinforce a single sex in people with intersex conditions is experienced by the patients as degrading and shaming. Preves recommended further psychosocial research and dialogue between doctors and adults with intersex about how to improve the future treatment of children.

Preves' suggestions are echoed in the findings of one of the authors (JA), who conducted an in-depth qualitative study of women with partial or complete androgen insensitivity syndrome (PAIS and CAIS, respectively) (Alderson et al., 2003). This suggested that an approach to the medical management of AIS that includes the withholding of information about diagnosis and treatment to competent children, adolescents and their parents can actually foster the development of a negative psychological response. The struggle to make sense of the signs of disorder or early treatment in an environment of secrecy appeared to contribute to the affected person's sense of herself. The findings of Preves and Alderson counter the proposition that with-holding medical information promotes psychological well-being in a person with a DSDD. Rather, it suggests that confusion and fear about the truth concerning one's body and health is central to the psychological distress experienced by this group. Coupled with the confusion associated with lack of information is a sense of the duplicity of doctors, healthcare staff, and sometimes parents, which was felt by many of the research participants.

It is apparent that the "clinical management of disorders of physical sex differentiation – intersexuality – is in a state of great flux, debate, and controversy" (Zucker, 2002). Advances in medical knowledge and understanding of psychosexual development, together with an increased emphasis on the rights of the individual and changing attitudes towards gender, have all contributed to debate about the role and efficacy of medical intervention. Clinical practice that has developed to promote psychological health is the subject of current critical review.

There is no consensus on how we should proceed. Research on medical and psychological outcomes is ongoing and it is difficult to interpret preliminary or inconsistent findings. There is a danger that the strength of opinion expressed by clinicians, patients and patient groups could result in overly defensive healthcare practice. Alternatively, an opportunity is presented to develop a model of healthcare that is flexible and incorporates evidence as it emerges. A multidisciplinary team approach provides a forum for discussion from different perspectives and promotes the development of individual-based care that is informed in a dynamic and thoughtful way by outcome data. There must be ongoing assessment of outcome across medical and psychological domains to give us a better understanding of the factors that support psychological adjustment and coping across the lifespan.

Gender schema

A diagnosis of a DSDD in a child or adolescent will inevitably raise questions for parents about some aspect of their child's gender development. These may relate to physical appearance, fertility, behaviour, sexual orientation or gender identity. Questions and concerns may arise at predictable times, such as time of diagnosis, or in relation to aspects of their child's behaviour. At the time of diagnosis, parents are often trying to come to terms with their own reactions while facing difficult decisions regarding their child's medical management. Many parents find it difficult to comprehend information that simply does not fit into their existing perceptions of gender. If they then observe aspects of their child's behaviour that they associate with the other sex, this can confuse or perturb parents. In the case of children where a decision about sex of rearing was made in infancy, cross-gender behaviour can trigger doubts about the original decision. Parents can also interpret this behaviour as an indication of adult sexual orientation.

It is important to address parents' concerns promptly. As healthcare provision has moved towards patient-led models of care with an emphasis on collaboration and patient consent, it is important that parents have a full understanding of their child's medical diagnosis if they are to be in a position to make informed decisions. If parents feel unable to cope with aspects of their child's diagnosis, their anxiety may have an adverse psychological effect both on themselves and their child. Slijper et al. (1998) found that parents of girls with PAIS had considerable difficulty coping with their child's ambiguous external genitalia and XY karyotype. It was hypothesized that parental inability to cope with the diagnosis may have been one of the causes of the psychopathology found in a number of the children in the study.

It is crucial that parents are given appropriate help to enable them to come to terms with their child's diagnosis. Gender schema theory has been used to describe how concepts of gender are developed and organized. One basic way we use concepts is to judge whether something belongs to a category. For example, an individual is judged to be female if she has certain characteristic features or attributes. Concepts of male and female derived from physical and biological features tend to be based on mutually exclusive differences. Hence, we may hypothesize that difficulties are created when we receive information that describes an individual in terms of attributes that are located in both female and male schema. Schema must change before this seemingly incongruent information can be accommodated (Carmichael and Ransley, 2002). The concept of gender schema suggests that if parents are able to develop a less rigid understanding of the differences between male and female they will be more able to integrate previously incongruent information.

Aspects of gender development

It is important for professionals working with families to have a good understanding of psychobiological theories of gender. Helping parents to understand the relationships between the various aspects of gender – behaviour, gender identity and sexual orientation – and to gain an awareness of what is known about how they develop places them in a much better position from which to discuss their concerns and make decisions.

Psychosexual differentiation is often conceptualized as having four components. The aetiology of the development of and association between these elements remains the topic of debate.

- *Sex role* behaviour or *gender role behaviour* refers to behaviours, attitudes and personality traits that are typically associated with masculine and feminine. What is considered appropriate for male and female role behaviour may vary across different societies and cultures and may change over time.
- *Sexual orientation* refers to an individual's responsiveness to sexual stimuli. Thus sexual orientation is defined by the sex of the person to whom one is attracted to sexually in relation to one's own sex. In our culture this may be homosexual, lesbian, bisexual or heterosexual.
- *Gender identity* refers to a child's developing sense of themselves as belonging to one sex or the other and developing a core concept of him- or herself as male or female (Stoller, 1964).
- *Sexual identity* is differentiated from sexual orientation by Zucker (2002). He notes that there may be differences between what an individual is aroused by and how they view themselves. For example, an individual may be aroused by same-sex stimuli and yet view themselves as heterosexual.

In the general population, gender identity is usually consistent with genetic and phenotypic sex. Gender identity is most often linked to gender role, but gender role cannot be predicted from sexual orientation. Discordance between biological sex and gender identity is seen as a problem and is termed gender identity dysphoria.

Sex role behaviour

A number of human behaviours show reliable sex differences. Sex differences are defined as average differences between groups of girls and boys or men and women. In terms of gender role behaviour, activity preferences (e.g. rough and tumble play; DiPietro, 1981), childhood toy preferences (e.g. boys preferring cars and girls preferring dolls; Liss, 1981), physical aggression and certain cognitive abilities all show sex differences (for a comprehensive review see Collaer and Hines (1995)). Evidence suggests that, in part, preferences are developed through social factors such as copying and differential reinforcement of behaviour. However, because gonadal hormones influence behaviours that show sex differences in behaviour and the brain of other species, it is hypothesized that they influence human behaviours in a similar way (Hines, 1998).

Research findings support the suggestion that early hormone exposure affects the development of sex-typed behaviour in humans. It has been suggested that high levels of androgen during sensitive periods of human development produce masculine-typical behaviour. Conversely, very low levels of androgens during these periods are said to result in female-typical behaviour.

Girls with congenital adrenal hyperplasia (CAH), who have been exposed to high levels of antenatal androgens have been studied extensively. This group of children provide an opportunity to consider the differential effects of hormones and environment on sex-typed behaviour. For example, behaviours that are associated in typical girls may be disassociated in CAH girls if the social environment predominantly influences one of the behaviours and early hormones predominantly influence the other. Toy choice, activity level and activity and playmate preference, which show sex differences in the general population, have been assessed in a number of ways including interview and direct observation of behaviour.

There is robust evidence to suggest that early exposure to male sex hormones in females with a XX karyotype has a masculinizing effect on sex-typed toy preferences and activities (Berenbaum and Hines, 1992; Berenbaum and Snyder, 1995). The activity preferences found in girls with CAH, while similar to those of boys, tend not to be as extreme. It is generally agreed that these differences are caused by the influence of sex hormones and not social or illness factors. Although findings are consistent with an androgen influence on sex-typed toy choices, the way in which hormones influence behaviour is not certain. There may be a direct effect on brain structures linked to specific behaviours or an indirect effect, for example an influence on activity levels, motor skills or temperament (Berenbaum and Hines, 1992).

Some behaviours, such as activity preference, are thought to show meaningful within-sex variation whereas others such as the tendency to associate with same sex peers reflect social factors common to all members of the sex (Maccoby, 1988; Maccoby and Jacklin, 1987). This suggests that there is independence between sex-typed behaviours and that they have different aetiologies. In girls with CAH, early exposure to androgens seems to have a major effect on childhood activity preferences but only a weak influence on playmate preferences. This suggests that the two are only minimally related and have different aetiologies.

It has been found that individuals with salt-wasting CAH show more masculinization of gender-related behaviour than do those with the milder simple virilizing form of CAH (Dittman et al., 1990). However, a number of studies have found that behavioural masculinization in women and children with CAH does not relate to degree of virilization (Berenbaum and Hines, 1992; Slijper et al., 1992). Slijper et al. (1998) suggested that this supports the view that parental acceptance of gender affects the way the child

is treated and, in turn, the gender behaviours of the child. This suggests that we need to consider the influence of socialization in combination with pre- and postnatal androgens.

The research evidence to date requires cautious interpretation. The relationship between prenatal hormone environment and sex-typical behaviours is not uniform. It is likely that there are critical periods in which hormones have an influence on behaviour and that social and cultural factors need to be taken into account. It is also likely that hormonal effects on behaviour are a reflection of a number of factors, such as timing, duration, dose, type of hormone, individual variations in sensitivity to hormones and different sensitive periods for different aspects of behaviour (Berenbaum, 1998). The effects are complex and reflect the multidimensional nature of sex-typed behaviour (Berenbaum and Snyder, 1995).

In order to answer parents' questions, further research is needed to elucidate the way in which early gonadal hormones influence behaviour and if early sex-typed toy choice and/or activity preferences may predict later behaviour, in particular sexual orientation.

Sexual orientation

There has been considerable interest in the idea that sex-typed behaviours are predictive of adult sexual orientation. It is hypothesized that gonadal hormones play a key role in the development of sexual orientation as well as sex-role behaviour (Berenbaum and Snyder, 1995). However, the relationship between hormones, childhood sex-typed behaviour and sexual orientation is complex and as yet remains unclear. It is likely that the development of sexual orientation is influenced by a number of factors, both biological and environmental. The finding in some studies that women with CAH are more likely than controls to have bisexual or homosexual interests would suggest that prenatal hormone environment influences sexual orientation (Dittman et al., 1992; Money et al., 1984). However, others have found that both homosexual and heterosexual interests were reduced in women with CAH compared with a control group (Zucker et al., 1996). Several suggestions have been made to explain these inconsistent findings (Hines, 1998). It may be that sexual interest requires appropriate hormonal activation in adulthood and as such is not expressed in adult women with CAH as high levels of androgens are not present. Alternatively, the variable initial hormonal exposure to androgens of women with CAH might account for the differences in sexual orientation.

Gender identity

Money et al. (1957) suggested that children are psychosexually neutral until about the age of two years. This is seen as a "sensitive" or "optimal" period of time in which gender identity can develop as male or female, under the influence of socialization. After this period, gender identity is said to be established and, therefore, difficult to change. This hypothesis led to the recommendation that sex assignment should be made no later than 18–24 months, otherwise the child may be vulnerable to what Money termed "psychologic unhealthiness". This corresponds with consensus amongst developmental psychologists that the emergence of gender identity differentiation can be seen from around two years of age.

There is, however, evidence that appears to contradict both the decisive role of socialization and a sensitive period of gender identity formation. There are reports of successful reversal in gender identity in later years, for example the reversal of gender identity associated with spontaneous pubertal change in 5 α-reductase deficiency (Imperato-McGinley et al., 1979). In addition, there are a number of case reports of individuals who in their teenage and adult years have rejected an assigned sex (e.g. Diamond and Sigmundson, 1997a; Gooren et al., 1991; Meyer-Bahlburg et al., 1996; Phornphutkul et al., 2000; Reiner, 1996). These cases are cited as evidence for the biological basis of the development of gender identity. There have been associated cogent critiques of the theoretical underpinnings of the optimal gender policy and recommendations for changes in practice (Kipnis and Diamond, 1998). It is argued that the brain is not psychosexually neutral at birth and that hormone exposure in utero acts on the brain to predispose an individual to behave in male-typical or female-typical ways (Diamond and Sigmundson, 1997a). In this paradigm it is recommended that sex assignment should be based on the underlying diagnosis, taking into account what is known about the causes and prognosis of the specific disorder. Implicit in this recommendation is that genetic and hormonal events will dictate eventual gender identity (Kipnis and Diamond, 1998) and that gender identity cannot be predicted or irreversibly decided upon at birth on the basis of physical attributes. Therefore, it is proposed that surgery should be delayed until the child's emerging gender identity can be taken into account (Diamond and Sigmundson, 1997b; Phornphutkul et al., 2000).

Unfortunately, the evidence supporting the relative salience of socialization and biological factors in the development of gender identity is equivocal. While there are individual case reports that appear to support a biological basis for gender identity development, this is not yet a well-established finding as little is known about the timing of hormone exposure on the developing brain (Phornphutkul et al., 2000).

The adoption of a particular theoretical stance or philosophical position has profound practical implications for the psychological and medical management of some individuals with a DSDD. The ramifications of the recommendation not to perform surgery until a child is able to consent must be considered. A number of researchers indicate that the appearance of genitalia may have an influence on gender identity development (Donahue, 1987; Meyer-Bahlberg, 1994). Slijper et al. (2000) suggested that surgery to correct virilization immediately after birth aims to avoid cross-gender identification in the child as well as the parent. It is thought that genital ambiguity can lead to uncertainty regarding gender for both the parents and the child, which they suggest can lead to problems in the gender identification process.

It is unclear to what extent children rely on the appearance of the external genitalia in making judgements about gender. Some research suggests that initially children pay more attention to hair and clothing style as the features that define sex than they do to the genitalia (Thompson and Bentler, 1971). It is not until around the age of seven years that children use the external genitalia in correct gender labelling of self and others (McConaghy, 1979). It is critical to assess further the role, if any, of the appearance of external genitalia on the development of gender identity.

It seems most likely then that postnatal "rearing environment" may interact with biological predisposition (Zucker, 2002) but the relative contributions of and interactions between these factors require further exploration. For example, a number of studies have looked at adult gender identity in individuals with CAH reared as girls, a small proportion of whom have later been found to be living as male (Meyer-Bahlberg et al., 1996; Zucker et al., 1996). The majority of girls with CAH, however, have sex-atypical activity preferences together with a female gender identity. It has been argued that, while androgen exposure may have shaped gender role behaviour, the exposure has not been sufficient to create a male gender identity. Environmental influences (i.e. being raised unambiguously as a girl) are likely to contribute further to shape a female gender identity (Berenbaum and Hines, 1992).

Appraisal of the available studies indicates that gender identity development is a complex interaction between pre- and postnatal biological and psychological processes. The relative contribution and the relationship between these factors in gender identification are not yet fully understood. Meanwhile, cautious interpretation of the evidence can be used to inform future research and clinical decisions on a case-by-case basis, taking into account the individual, family and wider social and cultural context.

Psychological disorder in children with disorders of sexual differentiation

Few studies have looked at psychological or psychiatric disorder associated with DSDD. However, available evidence is a cause for concern. One study evaluated psychological outcome for 59 patients, 54 of whom were female. The group included individuals with a diverse range of conditions (Slijper et al., 1998) but 39% of the girls met diagnostic criteria (DSM-IV; American Psychological Association, 1994) for at least one psychiatric disorder and 15% had more than one, with a mean age of onset of 9.8 years. Depression, anxiety, sexual problems, oppositional defiant disorder, attention-deficit hyperactivity and conduct disorders were reported, although there were no significant associations found between specific medical diagnoses and psychopathology. In contrast to the level of psychological disturbance seen in this study, an abstract report of a UK questionnaire survey of adults with AIS concluded that neither CAIS nor PAIS need necessarily be associated with a reduced psychological well-being (Hines et al., 1998).

Gender identity disorder

Problems of gender identity occurring in the general population are classified as a psychiatric disorder under the heading gender identity disorder (GID) as in the *Diagnostic and Statistical Manual of Mental Disorders* (American Psychiatric Association, 1994) and the *International Classification of Diseases* (World Health Organization, 1992). However, there is debate about how problems with gender identity in children and adolescents with DSDD should be conceptualized: specifically whether they should be diagnosed by the same criteria as generally used with biologically typical children (Meyer-Bahlberg, 1994). Following a review of the literature, Meyer-Bahlberg concluded that the prevalence of spontaneous gender change (i.e. in 5α-reductase deficiency) and gender change requests in patients with DSDD (termed intersex in his study) is considerably higher than in the general population. Furthermore, that intersex patients with a significant gender identity problem differ from non-intersex patients with GID in prevalence, age of onset, presentation and in sex ratio. While he acknowledged the shortcomings of the existing literature, Meyer-Bahlberg concluded that gender identity problems in intersex and non-intersex patients are unlikely to be the same disorder. Slijper et al. (1998) agreed noting that the younger group of

children thought to have some level of GID do not show the "obsessive preoccupation" associated with this diagnosis. This is taken as an indication that the type of psychopathology described differed from that found in biologically typical boys and girls with GID.

It is difficult to interpret questions regarding gender as indicating psychological disturbance when they are raised by a child with a DSDD. When a person's karyotype or antenatal hormonal environment is unusual in relation to their gender, defining a sex of reference against which a GID is measured can be problematic. Children and adolescents may be aware of differences in their behaviour or their physical appearance and feel that these do not fully accord with their assigned role. This may create uncertainty and prompt questions without a desire to change gender, and as such is perhaps better described as gender confusion rather than as GID (or the American term "gender dysphoria") (Meyer-Bahlberg, 1994).

Psychological assessment and intervention

Assessment of gender

Formal assessment of gender can be used to monitor a child's psychological well-being or to inform decisions about gender assignment. However, there is a need for validated measures for use by researchers and clinicians in different centres as current lack of consistency in the assessment techniques makes comparison of results difficult.

It is necessary to assess aspects of gender separately because while they are interrelated it is possible that they vary independently. An example of this is that a given gender identity can accommodate a wide range of gender role behaviours. Two standardized measures have been developed to obtain information from parents about children's gender-related behaviour: the Child Game Participation Questionnaire (Meyer-Bahlberg et al., 1994b) and the Child Behaviour and Attitude Questionnaire (Meyer-Bahlberg et al., 1994a). It is also helpful to observe a child's play. Meyer-Bahlberg (2002) suggested using gender typical toys and dressing-up clothes and scoring the percentage of time spent in gender-stereotypic activities. Assessment of a child's gender identity can be facilitated with the Gender Identity Interview developed by Zucker et al. (1993). This is a semistructured interview designed to elicit a child's disclosure of any cross-gender wishes or ambivalence.

Assessment requires a long-term perspective as problems with gender and sexuality are more common in adolescence. Meyer-Bahlberg (2002) suggested that assessment of gender in adolescents should include occupational and hobby preferences, retrospective recall of gender role behaviour and activities, gender identity and an assessment of sexual orientation.

Methods of gender assessment have been criticized as being too narrow in focus and unable to reflect either the dynamic and complex nature of gender or the individual and family reactions to difference (Kessler, 2002). However, standardized measures are useful in conjunction with a broader assessment and must be interpreted carefully with reference to the child's specific diagnosis, personal history and social context.

There are particular problems related to the assessment of young children who are unaware of their diagnosis. Parents can fear that assessment alone may trigger doubt or confusion about gender identity in their child. It may be that the process of assessment allows a child to share doubts about their gender identity that have not been previously mentioned. This ultimately may be beneficial for the child. The purpose and value of assessment should be explored and parental consent given. As is always the case in psychological assessment of children, the individual child's perception and understanding of the assessment process should be considered prior to seeking their agreement to take part in each activity. This is particularly important when assessing gender identity as we do not yet know whether assessment or ongoing monitoring of children with DSDD contributes in any way to the development of psychological difficulties or distress.

Assessment of quality of life

Assessment of psychosexual development alone is not sufficient to monitor outcome for children with DSDD. Methods for the assessment of health-related quality of life (HrQoL) need to be developed to extend the range of outcomes of interest. Available measures of HrQoL do not assess aspects of health and psychological functioning that are particular to this group of children (Gerharz, 1997). In fact, very few studies have attempted to address HrQoL in children with DSDD (Schober, 1999; Schober et al., 2002). Meyer-Bahlberg (1999) proposed that assessment of HrQoL for DSDD should incorporate a number of factors relevant to this group of children. In addition to "generic broad-band" assessment, he suggested assessment of gender role/identity and sexuality and "syndrome-specific" factors, for example medication or specific techniques of genital surgery. When beginning to collect quality-of-life data in a new patient group Kind and Rosser (1997) suggested that the use of five-point clinical global impression scales (with grading from excellent to poor) will generate important and useful information.

Psychological intervention

A small number of studies have investigated the effectiveness of psychological intervention for children with DSDD and have found that it is associated with improved outcome for children and their families. Slijper et al. (1998) assessed children with a variety of diagnosis including AIS and CAH and found that psychological problems were twice as prevalent among children who did not receive psychological support and help from diagnosis onwards. They conclude that early counselling has a preventative effect.

There are some guidelines available for psychological counselling (Meyer-Bahlberg, 1993; Money, 1994) but, most often, mention of psychologically therapeutic intervention is made in passing. The content, frequency or rationale for interventions is rarely described. In general, it seems that therapeutic input with children believed to be experiencing gender identity difficulties has been aimed at reinforcing and supporting the originally assigned gender. An exception is the study of Slijper et al. (1998), who gave some detail of the psychological approach used with children presenting with features of GID. It is apparent that their aim was to reinforce and support children in their assigned gender by "make[ing] the patient aware of the conflict between the fantasy of being a boy and the reality of having the female gender" (Slijper et al., 1998). Associated work with parents sought to reinforce that they had made the right decision in gender assignment. This approach was based on the hypothesis that parents' doubts may be expressed via their child in the form of "gender fantasies". In this case, it is clear that the aim of psychological therapy is informed by Money's theory of psychosexual development. It is important that the aims and methods of psychological therapy are made overt to allow for a comparison of effectiveness. Different theoretical conceptualization will suggest a specific therapeutic approach. These may differ greatly and yield different results.

Future directions in psychological assessment and intervention

Considerable emphasis has been placed on identifying psychopathological responses in children with a diagnosis of DSDD. While it is important to assess psychopathology, broader assessment that does not "pathologize" the individual in relation to their medical condition is required to inform the development of appropriate interventions.

There is a need to develop more imaginative ways of exploring gender and difference in a therapeutic context with young children. Therapeutic approaches that explore the child's understanding of gender within her individual and contextual experience are essential.

The use of therapeutic stories is one suggestion and has been instigated by Warne (1992). Carefully constructed stories, personalized for individual children, may be a useful way of introducing complex concepts at an early stage. Stories allow open exploration of the views of a child and family about different aspects of the child's medical diagnosis and treatment, and they provide a framework for making sense of perceived difficulties. Discussion of a story can initiate more personally related discussion of the child's experience.

Psychological therapy and intervention should be integrated into the overall care of the child and their family. It should be sensitive to the varied needs of children at different stages of development and medical intervention. It is essential that effectiveness of therapeutic intervention is evaluated both for child and adult outcomes. Family and individual factors, psychological and medical intervention and psychological outcome are intimately related. Careful assessment of the relationship between these elements will help to ensure that both psychological and medical interventions are appropriately re-evaluated and can remain flexible in relation to individual needs.

The family context of psychological care

The task of a clinical psychologist or other applied psychologist in a medical setting is to elicit the unique experience of the patient or family and gather the emotional and subjective information that might not otherwise be included in a medical understanding of their healthcare needs. Within a multidisciplinary healthcare team, psychologists will then promote recognition of the interactions between the biological, interpersonal, familial and cultural factors of patients and families, alongside the concerns and practices of the medical and nursing staff. In this way, psychological care of children with DSDD is aimed at shaping the healthcare process to minimize psychological problems and promote psychological well-being.

The psychological task for families where there is a child with a DSDD is to adjust or adapt to the condition and its consequences. Optimal adaptation would ultimately be for a child to develop into an autonomous, healthy, and well-functioning adult – both socially and occupationally – as defined by their cultural and social context. Behaviour during childhood would be age appropriate and adaptive in terms of the demands and circumstances of their condition and other aspects of life.

Adaptation and coping in children

Psychological understanding of children's coping and adjustment to health conditions emphasizes the influential role of stress, referring to a demand on mental energy or an amount of psychological distress (Thompson et al., 1992; Wallander et al., 1989). Environmental factors (such as changing school), individual factors (such as temperament) and relationship factors (such as the adaptation of parents) can all contribute to an individual child's stress during the management of their health condition. Illness is seen as an additional stress to which the individual child needs to adjust. The models of children's adaptation to health conditions put forward by both Thompson et al. (1992) and Wallander et al. (1989) suggest that psychological processes are more influential than biomedical factors in mediating adjustment and coping. Thompson's model particularly emphasised the impact of parental adaptation on the adaptation of children. Both models illustrated how the promotion of adaptation and coping should not focus solely on symptom reduction or surgical outcome. Rather, these models suggest that psychosocial factors in a child's life are likely to be more powerful than medical treatment outcome on overall adaptation.

In order to promote good adaptation to a health condition, it may be necessary to intervene to minimize other stresses in the child's life and to maximize coping resources. Psychological help to minimize a child's distress and promote adaptation may be directed at the individual child, her parent or her family. While psychologists working within the healthcare team will contribute to this process in matters relating to the actual condition, in cases where there are comorbid psychological difficulties it will be necessary to refer patients and their families to community-based child and adolescent mental health services. In contrast to disorder-focused intervention, psychological health literature suggests that other factors such as individual coping styles and family functioning can mediate positive adaptation to diagnosis and treatment.

DSDD brings particular challenges to adaptation. These can include concerns about physical appearance (e.g. appearance of genitalia, hirsutism), demanding treatment regimens (e.g. dilation, frequent medication) and involvement with a complex medical system (e.g. travelling to specialist services and multidisciplinary care). While adapting to these stresses, children must also negotiate typical childhood tasks such as the development of autonomy, identity formation, establishment of peer relationships and transitions through secondary school, college and work.

Proactive psychological support

With increased awareness of diagnosis, prognosis and experiences of individuals and families where there is a child with DSDD, psychologists in the healthcare setting are able to offer proactive intervention aimed at prevention of psychological problems as well as reactive intervention aimed at the amelioration of distress.

Drotar et al. (1984) suggested that prevention of psychological difficulties in children with health conditions should focus on:

- reduction of anxiety and fears related to the illness and compliance with treatment regimens
- promotion of developmentally appropriate understanding
- the integration of the illness into family life
- the adaptation to important systems

They point out that these protective processes are most likely to occur within an ongoing therapeutic relationship with care staff (Drotar et al., 1984). They recommended that psychosocial care staff be proactive in their interventions to these ends, using an approach they termed *anticipatory guidance*. By gaining a thorough knowledge of the illness process, psychosocial aspects of the illness for child and family, child development and the individual child and family's coping resources, psychologists can time and focus their interventions around anticipated illness transitions or developmental tasks. This individual approach to each family must also be sensitive to that family's cultural values. The approach emphasized the clinician's anticipation of hurdles for the child and family and aimed to prevent problems by offering in advance the kind of help they might need. For example, because adherence appears to pose a particular challenge to adolescents (Koocher et al., 1990), it may be appropriate to offer additional support at the beginning of hormone therapy. Using the foci of prevention described by Drotar et al. (1984), an assessment of a patient's fears about taking hormone therapy might reveal, for example, that she is worried that her friends will think that she has begun to take the contraceptive pill without telling them (*reduction of anxiety and fears related to the illness and compliance with treatment regimens*). Emphasis on effects of more immediate interest (e.g. breast development) rather than long-term effects such as bone density might help her to appreciate the need for hormone therapy (*promotion of developmentally appropriate understanding*). Thoughtful discussion and review with a psychologist might enable the girl to counter practical barriers to taking her medication, or for her to negotiate an acceptable level of parental involvement, for example by receiving prompts or reminders to take tablets (*the integration of the illness into family life*). Finally, additional support by a trusted psychologist or specialist nurse might enable the child to report effectively her response to the medication to the consultant during clinic visits (*adaptation to important systems*).

Parents' reactions to diagnosis

It is acknowledged that a child's diagnosis of a DSDD can be a traumatic experience for parents (Slijper et al., 1998). Two studies have looked at the experiences of parents of children with AIS (Le Maréchal, 2001; Slijper et al., 2000). Both of these studies found that the reaction of most parents to a diagnosis of AIS was one of shock. Le Maréchal found that parents commonly reported devastation, disbelief, denial and confusion and likened their feelings to those experienced during bereavement.

At the time of diagnosis, parents are often concerned about the potential fertility and future sexual expression of their baby. It can be helpful for parents to have the opportunity to discuss their fears about their child's condition, care and future. In Le Maréchal's (2001) study, almost all participants talked about their grief, which was most often directly related to the discovery that their child was infertile and the consequent loss of future grandchildren. Their sense of grief and loss also related to their child's future as they identified fears that their child may not have satisfactory relationships or sexual intimacy as a result of her DSDD. Mothers, in particular, experienced feelings of guilt and self-blame, feeling that they passed on the condition to their child, either genetically or because of something they may have done during pregnancy.

Parents often express concerns about what to tell friends and family. When their child's genitalia appear unusual, parents may have worries about leaving their child with others. It can be useful for parents to think through the implications of sharing information about their child's condition with close friends and family and to identify explanations they feel are appropriate. Parents often request written information about their child's condition and future treatment, and some parents express a wish to meet other parents of children with a similar diagnosis. Support groups can be extremely helpful in both regards.

Although there are some commonly observed experiences of parents of a child with DSDD, it is necessary to explore with patients the idiosyncratic meaning of information for the individuals and the family. Families have different experiences and histories in relation to the circumstances of a diagnosis, which can impact on later adjustment and concerns.

Le Maréchal (2001) found that for many parents their recollections of what they were told at the time of diagnosis were limited to a few words or phrases. It seems likely that the powerful emotions experienced at the time of diagnosis affect the ability to take in and retain information, and parents were rarely able to give an accurate description of the condition. Slijper et al. (2000) suggested that receiving full information at the time of the clinical diagnosis was one of the most important factors in determining positive parental coping. To this end, parents need to be given a full explanation; however, to enable them to appreciate such complex and emotionally challenging information it should be presented on more than one occasion. In practice, giving information is a process of exploration rather than a simple exchange. Parents often have difficulties adjusting to the information that their child's chromosome pattern is not congruent with their gender. This is not surprising as information that challenges our fundamental understanding of a concept creates anxiety and confusion. It can be helpful to present the usual process of sexual differentiation, divided into a series of components – chromosomal, gonadal, phenotype and hormonal – together with the evidence base for distinctions between gender identity, sex role behaviour and sexual orientation (Carmichael and Ransley, 2002). This explanation, which, challenges existing concepts of gender, helps parents to appreciate that physical sex is multidimensional and that one parameter does not hold precedence over another. The aim is to help parents to integrate information and to evaluate the implications of particular aspects of the diagnosis for their child. Parents' understanding of their child's diagnosis and future is the basis of family adaptation and acceptance. Children develop in the context of their families, and parental understanding and acceptance is fundamental to the long-term psychological adjustment of the child. It also enables parents to be active in decision making and equips them to give their child information in the future. An awareness of the experiences of parents is important in order to develop appropriate support with which to address their needs and concerns.

Families have different styles of coping and in some cases families and individuals do not want detailed information. However, in the period following diagnosis, a parent's rejection of further information can result from feeling overwhelmed and unable to process more information. The pace of information giving should be governed by individual family needs.

Parents' decision making

In the past, the diagnosis of a child with ambiguous genitalia has been treated as a medical and psychological emergency, with the emphasis on making decisions as quickly as possible to reduce distress and uncertainty. However, the importance of giving parents adequate time to come to terms with and fully appreciate the implications of their child's diagnosis cannot be overemphasized.

Parents are increasingly involved in decision making with regard to their child's care. This is particularly so with regard to elective procedures, as in some aspects of the medical care of children with DSDD. Appraisal of possible outcomes can be particularly difficult for parents for many of the reasons already outlined.

Following diagnosis, parents are encouraged to contribute to decisions about their child's future at a time when they may be experiencing overwhelming and difficult emotions. Faced with this situation, parents will need both information and time to think about what they believe will be in the best interests of their child as well as their own reactions. Parents' considerations take place within an environment of family values and cultural beliefs that will affect what the diagnosis means for themselves and their view of their child's future. Parents may need to come to terms with the potential "loss" of a healthy child or the possibility of grandchildren. In this situation, parents can experience high levels of anxiety and may show signs of psychological disturbance. While this is a necessary and valued process, it can be exceedingly challenging.

In Le Maréchal's (2001) study of parents of girls with AIS, participants said that they believed that they made little contribution to decisions regarding their daughters' treatment and were without the relevant knowledge or status to be in a position to take more of an active role. Parents can often feel disempowered by the medical system and defer to the views of doctors. Moreover, in many cases, parents ask doctors to make decisions on their behalf or do as they would with their own child. This can be challenging for staff who may believe that parents can never fully relinquish responsibility and may not be afforded impunity by their child in years to come. Provision of effective support and adequate information are essential to enable parents to be involved in the decision-making process. Parents often express their strong desire to make the right decision. It is useful to emphasize that they can only do what they perceive to be best for their child on the basis of the evidence available at the time. Clear documentation of parental decisions, perhaps in the form of a letter to the child that could remain in the medical records, can aid later review by the older child.

Parental decisions about early surgery

The debate that questions the value of irreversible treatment of ambiguous genitalia in childhood (e.g. Diamond and Sigmundson, 1997b; Schober, 1998) is based not only on the functional outcome of genital surgery performed in childhood but also on the intrinsic reliance on parental consent only, with decisions made by parents based on their view of their child's best interests.

Some authors have viewed parents' decisions in favour of surgery as reflecting their own needs rather than those of their child. Schober (1998) commented that "the surgery of early genitoplasty only addresses the way the infant appears to parents and others", emphasizing parents' desire for cosmetic normalcy. She argued that if surgery is warranted at all it can only be considered when the individual child is competent to consent and that parental consent is not a viable alternative (Diamond, 1999; Schober, 1998). These arguments are persuasive but tend to focus on the adult gender identity. The impact on child development is rarely discussed. However, parental views about surgery are important, as early childhood emotional development is predominantly dependent on secure relationships with primary caregivers. If parents are likely to have difficulty accepting their child or if they lack confidence in rearing their child with ambiguous genitalia, then psychological work to maximize attachment relationships and family acceptance must accompany a no-surgery option. It is essential to evaluate outcome of this treatment path on a range of developmental and psychological measures, both in the short and long term.

The suggestion of deferring decisions regarding surgery until children are old enough to make their own decisions has raised questions about the management of possible teasing and bullying regarding ambiguous genitalia (Melton, 2001). Some suggest that the benefits of not having surgery outweigh the possibility that a child will be bullied despite the evidence that bullying in childhood is associated with low self-esteem and can cause both short-term and long-term mental health problems (Hawker and Boulton, 2000; Salmon et al., 1998). The promotion of a child's coping strategies for dealing with bullying depends to a large extent on parents' and school's ability to support the child. However, concern has been expressed that children with genital ambiguity may be stigmatized by their family or peers (Money et al., 1986), which in turn may limit the support available to them.

Because children develop in the context of families and social groups, the feelings of parents, siblings and peers are directly relevant to the psychological well-being of the child. Guidelines from the British Association of Paediatric Surgeons (2001) suggested that there are so many specific issues related to the different diagnostic groups that a policy of no cosmetic surgical intervention in childhood would be too prescriptive. However, they do suggest that fully informed consent requires parents to be aware of the option of nonoperative management with ongoing psychological support for the child and family. We would add that availability of psychological support must be guaranteed before such offers can be made.

Parental uncertainties following gender assignment

Retrospective research regarding long-term outcomes of families affected by CAH and CAIS found that, while parents continued to be concerned about the gender or chromosome pattern of their daughter, most were able to accept the incongruities (Slijper et al., 1998). However, the same study suggested that parents are more likely to experience continued concerns following a female gender assignment in the case of children born with ambiguous genitalia when there was uncertainty about the most appropriate sex assignment, for example children with PAIS. The number of participants in the study was small and, consequently, interpretation must be tentative, but we can speculate as to some of the reasons why this might occur. In clinical practice, discussions subsequent to a decision about female sex of rearing often reveal continued parental fear that their child may develop male secondary sexual characteristics at puberty. We can hypothesize that if this fear is not addressed it will influence parental ability to accept fully the assigned gender and thus confound one of the primary rationales for early surgery (unambiguous sex of rearing). This indicates that it is important to discuss physical development at puberty with parents at the time of sex assignment.

Parents of girls with a DSDD are often confused and perturbed by behaviour that they perceive as boyish. There is some evidence that parents anticipate male-typical behaviour in patients where the karyotype is incongruent with the sex of rearing. This occurs even in the case of parents of children with CAIS where XY girls would not be expected to display cross-gender behaviour on the basis of androgen synthesis. Le Maréchal's (2001) study found that parents were aware of heightened sensitivity towards any boyish behaviour shown by their daughter. They reported difficulty resisting an assumption that this behaviour brought into question the child's adaptation to her female gender. This finding reinforces the need to help parents to understand psychosexual conceptualizations of gender and the evidence that suggests that sex role behaviour is independent from gender identity.

Parents' views on disclosure to children

A detailed study of 20 parents of children with a diagnosis of CAIS or PAIS identified distinct reservations with regard to giving children information about their condition (Le Maréchal, 2001). The participants' overarching desire was to protect their child from harm. Their main dilemma was whether withholding or giving information would cause more harm. Parents felt stuck in a double bind. They felt their child was "normal" and that by not giving them information they were perpetuating the view that AIS was "abnormal". However, they expressed a wide range of feelings and fears associated with the thought of giving full information to their children. They feared that their child would blame them for their condition or would be angry with previous decisions made about treatment. They were particularly concerned about how their child might react to the diagnosis. The intensity of these concerns ranged from a worry that their child would be upset to a fear that she would be thrown into a state of extreme psychological distress and experience a complete personality change. Such feelings are not unique to parents of this patient group and can be compared to those of parents of children with human immunodeficiency virus, who also try to protect their child from depressive or fearful reactions to diagnosis (Funck-Brentano et al., 1997). However, specific fears that information about their condition may trigger a gender identity crisis in the child are likely to be particular to the parents of children with CAIS or PAIS.

Notably, none of the parents in Le Maréchal's (2001) study were able to give a full or accurate account of their child's diagnosis. A number said that while they wanted to give their child information they did not know how to begin. This is, of course, an argument for improvements in communication with parents and the provision of additional support to aid disclosure to children.

Telling children about their condition

It is generally agreed that patients should be fully informed about their diagnosis and medical history. Many paediatricians treating children with DSDD now routinely advise parents that their child should be given full information. This represents a phenomenal shift in practice. Until recently nondisclosure, particularly in childhood, was upheld as essential. The emphasis on the key role of unequivocal sex of rearing provided a rationale for not telling children about their diagnosis of a DSDD. In practice, when patients received information in adulthood they have often felt angry and betrayed. These feelings can be directed at parents and can affect family relationships, or can hamper future relationships with doctors (Alderson, 2000).

It is important for paediatric services to offer parents the encouragement, guidance and support they require to enable them to give their daughters full information about their condition as early as possible. Some parents prefer a professional to give information to their child. Prior to any information giving, it is important to have a discussion with the parents about what will be discussed. When talking

to younger children, parents should be present and be involved in the process as far as possible. This promotes an atmosphere of openness and acceptance and prevents any suggestion to the child that the information is secret. Older children or adolescents may elect to discuss their condition without their parents present. Nevertheless, it can be useful to hold summary sessions with both parties to promote more open discussion at home.

Timing of information for children

Effective communication with children regarding DSDD remains a challenge both to parents and to professionals. Some believe that children will ask questions about their underlying condition or medical treatment at a time when they are ready to receive information. However, a medical setting of clinic appointments and examinations will not always be conducive to a child feeling comfortable or confident enough to ask difficult questions. What is more, in the context of limited information, it may be difficult for children to know what questions to ask. Children are often aware that there are "secrets" concerning their body or their health and may interpret this as an indication that something unspeakably grave is wrong. They may then seek to protect themselves and their parents from discomfort by not asking questions.

Debate regarding the "right" time to give information is ongoing. The tension revolves around the age at which information can be meaningfully understood, balanced against the impact of the "delivery of painful information during the very vulnerable teenage years" (Goodall, 1991). Warne (1989) suggested that it is important for children to know about their condition before adolescence, when a child's desire to minimize difference and conform to a group is amplified. From the age of 12 years onwards it is suggested that children develop the ability to think in conceptual terms and only then will a child be able to understand a discussion about the complex nature of her condition.

In the sparse published guidance, the process of giving information to children regarding DSDD is loosely based on cognitive models of child development. Goodall (1991) advocated that information should be given in a staged or step-by-step way: "matching simple statements to the child's conceptual growth until the personal implications are finally realised as part of a maturing process". Similarly Slijper et al. (2000) propose a three-step process starting, "at an early age", with education about the biological and psychological aspects of normal sexual differentiation. At 11 years, they suggest that the child should have a full explanation of AIS, with the exception of the XY karyotype. The final disclosure of the chromosomal pattern is given last when the child reaches the age of 16 or 17 years. While published recommendations generally agree that chromosomal information should be given last, we must question whether, in fact, this reflects the salience adults attach to a chromosomal pattern that is incongruent with gender of rearing. It may be that giving chromosomal information earlier would allow a child to integrate this into their developing constructs of male and female and hence their self-concept, rather than having to accommodate the information later when their constructs are more fixed.

Approaches to talking to children about disorders of sexual differentiation

Parents often provide general information to their daughter before linking it to her own experience. For example by introducing the idea that some people are unable to conceive or carry a child but are able to become parents by other means. This strategy uses what may be called "buffers", the purpose of which is to provide a less-distressing framework into which personal information can be fitted.

Throughout childhood, children are constantly constructing their own understanding of what it means to be female or male (Golombok and Fivush, 1994). When new information is given, it should be considered in the light of the ideas or constructs children already have about gender. If new information does not fit into these constructs, it is likely to cause confusion and distress. Girls with DSDD often ask if information they have been given means they are male. This can be extremely upsetting for parents who are not prepared and do not know how to respond. A common response of parents and perhaps poorly prepared health professionals is to foreclose discussion with firm reassurances. It may be more helpful to see the child's question as her way of exploring the personal implication of the information and not necessarily a prelude to gender identity problems.

Research with adult patients and parents of children with DSDD has found that specific phrases that caused distress are still remembered many years after they were first said and continue to cause discomfort (Alderson, 2000; Le Maréchal, 2001). This finding reminds us that the words or phrases used to explain an underlying condition must be carefully considered.

Resources for children

There are a small number of resources available to facilitate parents talking to their child about CAH and AIS, each written by Warne (1989, 1992, 1997). Stories or fairytales can be used with children of all ages as a nonthreatening and engaging way to give information. In psychological therapies,

metaphor is often used to present complex concepts and explore difficult feelings. As a method of teaching and giving information, the use of symbolic language is centuries old (Mills and Cowley, 1986). In this tradition, Warne (1992) has written a fairytale as a medium through which parents can introduce the matter of ambiguous genitalia to a child or their sibling aged between four and seven years. However, the content reflects how quickly practice has changed and may need revision. It is written with the aim of preventing fear in children but in doing so could be misleading for parents. Surgical intervention is assumed via a definitive treatment plan, without mention of the elective nature of genital surgery. Furthermore, surgical procedures are minimized ("a small operation to complete the parts that nature had not quite finished") and expectations of excellent surgical outcome are implied ("after that no-one would be able to tell that there had been anything different at all").

Prior planning of the stages or steps in giving information allows parents to review their own information and understanding. Role play can be a useful way to help parents to prepare what to say to the child.

Children's disclosure to others

Parents often have valid concerns about the ability of children to appreciate the possible consequences of being open about their condition with their friends. We recommend that parents avoid talking about aspects of their child's condition as secrets. There is a danger that the idea of having secrets can make a child feel worried or ashamed. If parents want to advise their child against discussion with others, it may be better to refer to the information as "special" or "private" (Lipson, 1994). Clinical evidence suggests that children have often talked to a close friend about aspects of their diagnosis or medical care. It is, therefore, helpful to think with children about what they might say to people who ask them questions. This helps them to think about how much they want others to know and helps them to find the words they would like to use.

Older children sometimes find it difficult to discuss their concerns in the company of their parents. This reflects a normal developmental stage in adolescence in which children move away from their parents and tend to identify more closely with their peers. Adolescence is also associated with a need to conform to peer group standards, and feeling different can result in isolation; both factors can make disclosure to friends more difficult. It should be recognized that an offer of surgery might inadvertently introduce the idea of difference to an adolescent. A desire to conform can increase pressure for surgery from adolescents or their parents, seeking to eradicate difference as soon as possible.

Professional practice

Cultural and contextual considerations

The distinction between male and female serves as a basic organizing principle for most cultures. However, what it means to be male and female and the status afforded to men and women, can vary greatly. Families have different beliefs and values and these need to be taken into account when considering the impact and meaning of information. For example, cultural or individual values attached to fertility may be of particular importance for some when faced with decisions about sex assignment.

Consent and capacity

Outside of medical emergencies and in the circumstances described in the Mental Health Act (Department of Health, 1983, 1999), accepted UK healthcare practice upholds consent as a necessary prerequisite for the treatment of any young person (Shaw, 2001). Children's contribution to medical decision making was highlighted when the Children Act for England and Wales (Department of Health, 1989) stated (Part V, Section 43(8)): "if the child is of sufficient understanding to make informed decisions he may refuse to submit to medical or psychiatric examination or other assessment". However, in English law, competent children aged 16–17 can consent to treatment but a parent or the court can overrule their refusal. This tension makes crucial the careful consideration of a child's capacity to make competent decisions and the recognition of parents' responsibility for proxy consent.

Understanding competence

Children's competence to consent in healthcare has been heavily influenced by the Gillick decision (*Gillick* v. *West Norfolk and Wisbech Area Health Authority*, 1986). This case law defined competence as the ability to understand considerable information about the proposed treatment, including its purpose, nature, likely effects and risks, the probability of success and the availability of alternatives to that proposed. Because this definition of understanding is affected by an ability to consider a risk–benefit ratio, simple low-risk procedures (such as abdominal ultrasound) require a lesser degree of competence than do those when outcomes are speculative and have a potential cost (such as cosmetic genital surgery). It is worth noting, however, that judging a child's competence can be further complicated by the possibility that a health professional's preference for one treatment or another may inadvertently influence their perception of the level of competence needed. Where dif-

ficulty is anticipated, a team approach to the assessment of competence may be needed. Pearce (1994) argued that a more stringent test of competence must be applied when a child refuses consent, as this is potentially more dangerous to her (physical or psychological) health. This position presumes that those offering treatments have a full appreciation of what is best for that child. Pearce cautioned that the ability to overrule a child in her best interests must not replace good communication about the benefits and risks of treatment. Consideration of "best interest" is relevant in all patients aged 17 years or less, even those deemed competent, but becomes irrelevant at the age of 18. A competent 17 year old (or younger) who withholds consent can still be overruled by a court or person with parental responsibility. According to the Children Act (Department of Health, 1989), adults making decisions for children must have regard in particular to the "ascertainable wishes and feelings of the child concerned" (Section 1 (1)(b)). While competency to consent must be judged on an individual basis, taking into account the type of decision and the particular circumstances of that decision, care must be taken not to set a higher standard of competence for consent than would be expected of adults. The British Medical Association and the Law Society offer succinct guidance for the assessment of a child's competence (Box 14.1).

Box 14.1 Recommendations on competence

Assessments of competence should assess a young person's:
- ability to understand that there is a choice and that choices have consequences
- willingness and ability to make a choice (including the option of choosing that someone else makes treatment decisions)
- understanding the nature and purpose of the procedure
- understanding the procedures risks and side effects
- understanding of the alternatives to the procedure and the risks attached to them, and the consequences of no treatment
- freedom from pressure.

From British Medical Association and the Law Society (1995).

Describing consent in general terms, Prescilla Alderson (1993) wrote "It is about deciding one's own best interests and preferences". There is no universally acceptable level nor simple measure of competence according to Rutter (1999). He argued that a child's competence can only be estimated "in a particular context, for a particular type of decision, given particular circumstances".

Consent in practice

In practice, the consent process is embedded in the overall care of a child and family. The focus is to foster the child's understanding, cooperation and involvement in her healthcare. A child should be given information along with help to make sense of that information, its impact and ramifications. Once the child has achieved an understanding of her condition, she can move on to consider treatment options, what to expect during treatment and possible outcomes, before she is able to consent. Although it can be very difficult for a child to appreciate the range of long-term implications of treatment, she should be helped to appreciate as far as possible the risks and benefits. If this is achieved, her expectations should be realistic, thus preventing her later disappointment or resentment. When long-term outcome data are limited, clinicians must be open about the limits of their knowledge or evidence base.

A child's consent to assessment procedures should not be overlooked. For example, sensitive preparation for clinical photography is essential to prevent the potentially traumatic and shaming effect of this process experienced in the past (Creighton et al., 2002).

Although children should not be treated against their will, other than when they are likely to suffer significant harm without treatment (Shaw, 2001), there may be rare occasions when parents and the healthcare team will consider overruling a young child. For example, if gonadectomy is recommended for an eight-year-old girl with mixed gonadal dysgenesis and an unambiguous female gender, her agreement to her parent's consent would be sought. If the child did not agree, according to the Children Act her wishes would be paramount in decision making. However, in current English law she would not be able to refuse surgery that has been decided upon by her parents and doctors. In such circumstances, it would be important to delay surgery and attempt to reach an agreement between the child, the parents and the healthcare team. In some cases, specific concerns can be met and overcome by offering the child as much control over the process as possible, such as the timing of the operation. The child should be given help to understand their treatment and make a significant contribution to the decision. Equally the healthcare team and parents should be helped to understand the child. In Table 14.1, Shaw (2001) captures the complexity of what is required.

Putting children at the centre of decisions about their medical treatment can be challenging to staff, parents and children themselves. Although some research has indicated that there is little to distinguish the decision-making ability of older adolescents (14–18) from young adults (18 and over) (Weithorn and Campbell, 1982), it remains important to avoid placing too much responsibility on a child. Although the age of majority is 16 years it is considered good practice that additional agreement of a person with parental responsibility is sought when a competent person under the age of 18 gives consent.

Consent to treat the abused child

Gaining formal or informal consent for treatment from children or young people who have been abused may be particularly challenging as the child has experience of their trust being exploited. A girl who has experienced sexual abuse may be additionally anxious about genital examination. Parental authority may be inappropriate in these circumstances and management discussion with psychological care team members becomes essential. In some cases, involvement of medical social work or a court application may be necessary. For a thorough account of the emotional aspects of child sexual abuse see Warner (1998).

Transition to adult services

It is a widespread concern that outpatient services offered to adolescents can be ill-fitting. The needs of adolescents can rest between a paediatric service with a family-centred developmental paradigm and an adult service that assumes individualism and autonomy but may neglect family concerns (Royal College of Paediatrics and Child Health, 2002). Transition from paediatric to adult services is defined by the Society for Adolescent Medicine (USA) as "the purposeful, planned movement of adolescents and young adults with chronic physical and medical conditions from child-centred to adult orientated health care systems" (Blum et al., 1993). The UK government has emphasized the importance of transitional care in the *Diabetes National Service Framework* (Department of Health, 2001).

Where numbers of patients are great enough, an adolescent or transition service would ideally allow an extended period of attendance at a clinic that encompasses the range of developmental needs of adolescents within an adult-like model of medical and nursing care. When fewer patients are cared for in one centre, many clinicians have opted for hand-over appointments, where the paediatric and adult specialist attend and discuss care together with the patient and family. It is important when either of these approaches are taken that transition must not be viewed as a one-appointment event but rather a process where patients and their parents are prepared gradually and learn what to expect before each aspect of the transition process occurs. Patients and their parents should be helped to understand

Table 14.1. Conditions that encourage young people to be competent and contribute to decision making

The presence of	Free from	Understanding	Able to
A supportive and affectionate parent–child relationship	Pressure	That there is a decision to make	Retain an understanding
Trust and confidence in the doctor–patient relationship	Panic	That decisions have consequences	Appreciate its importance
Adequate information presented in an appropriate way	Pain	The nature of the recommended intervention and alternatives	See how it applies to them
	Other "temporary factors" that could impair judgement	Risks and benefits of interventions or no intervention	Weight the issue in the balance
		Longer-term consequences of each option	

Note: Adapted from Shaw (2001).

how aspects of their care might change, such as the care team's expectations of the patient's role and responsibility for their health. The transition process should reflect the multidisciplinary nature of both services and include psychological support during adaptation to the changes. The *Intercollegiate Working Party on Adolescent Health* (Royal College of Paediatrics and Child Health, 2002) recommends the following for good practice in outpatient care and transition:

- clear protocols of good practice for the management of young people's health during adolescent transfer to adult care should be developed
- young people should not be transferred fully to adult services until they have the necessary skills to function in adult services
- an identified person within the paediatric and adult teams must be responsible for transition arrangements, e.g. nurse specialists
- evaluation of transition must be undertaken
- a planned review by a clinical geneticist should be considered
- every paediatric general and speciality clinic should have a specific transition policy
- for adults with mental health problems, specific services should be available for those in the 16 to 19 years age group linking with adult teams.

Working with parents at transition

Transition from paediatric to adult services usually occurs towards the end of adolescence when processes of individuation are near or at completion. However, parents and the family system often retain great influence and this may be amplified in some cases if the development of the adolescent's autonomy has been delayed because of the effects of managing a lifelong health condition. During transition, families of children with DSDD may need to be handled with extraordinary sensitivity. The historical management of such conditions, followed by recent changes in practices of care, may create a mismatch between the style of care families were given when their child was in infancy and that presently offered at adolescence. The changes to an open management style, following a general shift away from paternalism, may be amplified by healthcare staff's respect for the autonomy of the adolescent child. Furthermore, a review of an adolescent patient's history may revive in her parents memories of traumatic events during their child's early years. Review of past care and preparation for future assessment or intervention will often include discussion of previous decision-making processes that occurred before the patient was involved in discussions of treatment. Because responsibility for consent now shifts from parent to child, the adolescent patient must be made fully aware of their medical condition and all aspects of ongoing or planned treatment. However, placing sole focus on the named patient at this stage can be divisive and lead to misunderstanding and conflict between parent, grown-up child and medical care team. Parents of adolescent patients will often need psychological support to enable them to speak openly about aspects of their child's past care, especially if they have previously been advised to keep this information secret. Without the parent's involvement it can be difficult to help the patient to gain a full understanding of her medical care during childhood. The transition period is a valuable opportunity for parents to provide additional information about aspects of the adolescent's health or family history. For example, in assessing any psychological distress or disorder in the adolescent patient, it is most helpful if a parent can provide information about other family members' adjustment to the patient's diagnosis or treatments.

The process of transition between age-based services, or indeed any services, should improve in future years as moves towards openness mean that parents and children understand more about their healthcare than they have in the past. The ability for different members of staff or teams to continue a lifespan process of care can be aided by careful documentation in contemporaneous medical records. When different professional groupings within multidisciplinary teams keep their own notes, it is particularly important that they also use a central, accessible record to document the process of information given and decisions reached. This will allow future workers to help families and children to continue care, aiding a seamless transition between services.

Summary

The debates regarding the appropriate medical management of children with DSDD are welcome. The psychological aspects of DSDD are complex and relate to the condition and associated treatment. When working with individual children and their families, it is important to maintain an open approach that is flexible in line with families' differing needs (Box 14.2). Real collaboration in decisions about gender assignment, surgery and other aspects of treatment is reliant upon effective communication of appropriate information regarding the treatment options and outcome evidence. This process requires time. Meanwhile, uncertainty can often create anxiety, which must be addressed. Time is needed for the family of a child with a DSDD to adapt or come to terms with the demands of understanding and managing the child's condition and its consequences. If we are not to succumb to making changes in management without good quality evidence, we need to establish collaborative research, long-term clinical follow-up and robust methods of communication between healthcare specialisms, age-based services and geographically based services (Box 14.3). In the future, this patient group will include individuals who have chosen not to undergo surgery, along with those who have opted for any of the range of surgical interventions available. Over time, changes in healthcare technologies and hopefully societal tolerance of difference will alter the specific pressures upon children and their families. Genuine flexibility in treatment and service adap-

tations to changes in information derived from emergent research evidence places great demands on children and families, healthcare workers and the structures and systems within which treatment is provided. It must be recognized that all parties need time and encouragement to consider their role and contribution when dealing with the inherent uncertainty involved in achieving optimal care. Certain factors are vital to achieving successful managemen (Box 14.3).

Box 14.2 Recommendations for practice

- Psychological support for children and parents should parallel all key stages of medical intervention and psychological assessment should inform decisions about gender assignment in infancy and later.
- Parents are required to be partners in treatment decisions and need information and support as part of this process.
- Children should be given information about their condition from the earliest stage: parental understanding is essential to achieve this.
- Children's involvement in decision making is central to collaborative family-based care and a team member should be responsible for coordinating family transition.
- A team approach should be used when assessment of a child's competence to consent is challenging.

Box 14.3 Key points

- A multidisciplinary team approach is essential, integrating different aspects of a child's life and health, with effective communication between healthcare staff and services.
- Psychological and psychosexual theory underpins many current medical practices in the care of those with DSDD.
- Children's adaptation is based on psychological and family factors in addition to treatment outcome factors.
- A philosophy of openness and flexibility in treatment options should be the starting point of care.
- Robust assessment must evaluate both medical and psychological interventions and outcomes and use standardized assessment tools that are sensitive to the needs of the group. Multicentre collaboration in data sharing and analysis is necessary.

REFERENCES

*Indicates key references.

Alderson J (2000). XY women with androgen insensitivity syndrome (AIS): a qualitative study. Thesis University of Leeds.

Alderson J, Madill A, Balen A (2003). Fear of devaluation: understanding the experience of intersexed women with androgen insensitivity syndrome. *Br J Health Psychol* in press.

Alderson P (1993). *Children's Consent to Surgery*, p. 35. Open University Press Buckingham, UK.

American Psychiatric Association (1994). *Diagnostic and Statistical Manual of Mental Disorders*, 4th edn revised. American Psychiatric Association, Washington DC.

*Berenbaum S (1998). How hormones affect behavioral and neural development: introduction to the special issue on gonadal hormones and sex differences in behavior. *Dev Neuropsychol* 14, 175–196.

Berenbaum S, Hines M (1992). Early androgens are related to childhood sex-typed toy preferences. *Psychol Sci* 3, 203–206.

Berenbaum S, Snyder E (1995). Early hormonal influences on childhood sex-typed activity and playmate preferences: implications for the development of sexual orientation. *Dev Psychol* 31, 31–42.

Blum R, Garell D, Hodgman C (1993). Transition from child-centred to adult health-care systems for adolescents with chronic conditions. A position paper of the Society for Adolescent Medicine. *J Adolesc Health* 14, 570–576.

British Association of Paediatric Surgeons (2001). *Intersex Surgical Guidelines: Statement of the British Association of Paediatric Surgeons Working Party on the Surgical Management of Children Born with Ambiguous Genitalia.* British Association of Paediatric Surgeons, London.

British Medical Association and the Law Society (1995). Assessment of mental capacity: guidance for doctors and lawyers. BMA, London.

*Carmichael P A, Ransley P G R (2002). Telling children about a physical intersex condition. *Dialog Pediatr Urol* 25, 7–8.

Collaer M L, Hines M (1995). Human behavioral sex differences: a role for gonadal hormones during early development? *Psychol Bull* 118, 55–107.

Creighton S, Alderson J, Brown P, Minto C (2002). Medical photography: ethics consent and the intersex patient. *Br J Urol Int* 89, 67–72.

Department of Health (1983). Mental Health Act. The Stationary Office, London.

(1989). Children Act Section 1(1)(b). The Stationary Office, London.

(1999). Mental Health Act 1983 Revised Code of Practice. The Stationary Office, London.

(2001). *National Service Framework for Diabetes: Standards.* UK Department of Health, London.

Diamond M (1997). Sexual identity and sexual orientation in children born with traumatised or ambiguous genitalia. *J Sex Res* 34, 199–211.

(1999). Paediatric management of ambiguous and traumatized genitalia. *J Urol* 162,1021–1028.

Diamond M, Sigmundson H K (1997a). Sex reassignment at birth. Long-term review and clinical implications. *Arch Pediatr Adolesc Med* 151, 298–304.

*Diamond M, Sigmundson H K (1997b). Management of intersexuality guidelines for dealing with persons with ambiguous genitalia. *Arch Pediatr Adolesc Med* 151, 1046–1050.

DiPietro J A (1981). Rough and tumble play: a function of gender. *Dev Psychol* 17, 50–58.

Dittman R W, Kappes M H, Kappes M E et al. (1990). Congenital adrenal hyperplasia II: gender-related behavior and attitudes in female salt-wasting and simple-virilizing patients. *Psychoneuroendocrinology* 15, 421–434.

Dittman R W, Kappes M E, Kappes M H (1992). Sexual behavior in adolescent and adult females with congenital adrenal hyperplasia. *Psychoneuroendocrinology* 17, 153–170.

Donahue P K (1987). The diagnosis and treatment of infants with intersex abnormalities. *Paediatr Clin North Am* 34, 1333–1348.

Dreger A (1998). *Hermaphrodites and the Medical Intervention of Sex.* Harvard University Press, Cambridge MA.

Drotar D, Crawford P (1985). Psychological adaptation of siblings of chronically ill children: research and practice implications. *J Dev Behav Pediatr* 6, 355–362.

Drotar D, Crawford P, Ganofsky M A (1984). Prevention with chronically ill children. In *Prevention of Problems in Childhood: Psychological Research and Applications*, Roberts M C, Peterson L, eds., pp. 233–265. Wiley, New York.

Edmonds D K (1989). Intersexuality. In *Dewhurst's Practical Paediatric and Adolescent Gynaecology*, Edmonds D K, ed., pp. 6–26. Butterworths, London.

Eiser C (1990). *Chronic Childhood Disease: An Introduction to Psychological Theory and Research.* Cambridge University Press, Cambridge.

Fausto-Sterling A (1993). The five sexes. *The Sciences* 33, 20–25.

(2000). *Sexing the Body: Gender Politics and the Construction of Sexuality.* Basic Books, New York.

Funck-Brentano I, Costagliola D, Seibel N et al. (1997). Patterns of disclosure and perceptions of the human immunodeficiency virus in infected elementary school age children. *Arch Pediatr Adolesc Med* 151, 978–985.

*Gerharz W (ed.) (1997). Quality of life research in children: Fashion or future? *Dialog Pediatr Urol* 20, 2–8.

Gillick v. West Norfolk and Wisbech Area Health Authority (1986). AC 112.

Golombok S, Fivush R (1994). *Gender Development.* Cambridge University Press, Cambridge, UK.

Goodall J (1991). Helping a child to understand her own testicular feminisation. *Lancet* 337, 33–35.

Gooren M D, Cohen-Kettenis P T (1991). Development of male gender identity/role and a sexual orientation towards women in a 46 XY subject with an incomplete form of the androgen insensitivity syndrome. *Arch Sex Behav* 20, 459–470.

Hawker D S J, Boulton M J (2000). Twenty years' research on peer victimization and psychosocial maladjustment: a meta-analytic review of cross sectional studies. *J Child Psychol Psychiatry* 44, 441–455.

Hines M (1998). Abnormal sexual development and psychosexual issues. *Baillières Clin Endocrinol Metab* 12, 173–189.

Hines M, Ahmed S F, Fane B A, Hughes I A (1998). Gender development and psychological well being in patients with androgen insensitivity syndrome (AIS). *Horm Res* 50, 116.

Imperato-McGinley J, Peterson R E, Gautier T, Sturla E (1979). Androgens and the evolution of male-gender identity among male pseudohermaphrodites with 5-reductase deficiency. *N Engl J Med* 300, 1233–1237.

Kessler S J (1998). *Lessons from the Intersexed*. Rutgers University Press, New Brunswick.

(2002). Questioning assumptions about gender assignment in cases of intersexuality. *Dialog Pediatr Urol* 25, 3–4.

Kind P, Rosser R (1997). Quality of life research: clinical relevance and practical value. *Dialog Pediatr Urol* 20, 2–3.

Kipnis K, Diamond M (1998). Pediatric ethics and the surgical assignment of sex. *J Clin Ethics* 9, 398–410.

Koocher G P, McGrath M L, Gudas L J (1990). Typologies of nonadherence in cystic fibrosis. *J Dev Behav Pediatr* 11, 353–358.

Le Maréchal K (2001). Bringing up an XY girl: parents' experience of having a child with androgen insensitivity syndrome. Thesis, University College London.

Lipson M (1994). Disclosure of diagnosis to children with human immunodeficieny virus or acquired immunodeficiency syndrome. *J Dev Behav Pediatr* 15(Suppl.), S61–S65.

Liss M B (1981). Patterns of toy play: an analysis of sex differences. *Sex Roles* 7, 1143–1150.

McConaghy M (1979). Gender permanence and the genital basis of gender: stages in the development of constancy of gender identity. *Child Dev* 50, 1223–1226.

Maccoby E E (1988). Gender as a social category. *Dev Psychol* 24, 755–765.

Maccoby E E, Jacklin C N (1987). Gender segregation in childhood. In *Advances in Child Development and Behaviour*, Vol. 20, Reese H W, ed., pp 239–287. Academic Press, New York.

Melton L (2001). New perspectives on the management of intersex. *Lancet* 357, 2110.

*Meyer-Bahlberg H F (1993). Gender identity development in intersex patients. *Child Adolesc Psychiatr Clin North Am* 2, 501–512.

(1994). Intersexuality and the diagnosis of gender identity disorder. *Arch Sex Behav* 23, 21–40.

(1999). Health related quality of life in intersexuality. *Acta Paediatr Suppl* 428, 114–115.

(2002). Gender: aspects and assessment. *Dialog Pediatr Urol* 25, 2–3.

Meyer-Bahlberg H F, Sandberg D E, Yager T J, Dolezal C L, Ehrhardt A A (1994a). Questionnaire scales for the assessment of atypical gender development in girls and boys. *J Psychol Hum Sex* 6, 19–39.

Meyer-Bahlburg H F, Sandberg D E, Dolezal C L, Yager T J (1994b). Gender-related assessment of childhood play. *J Abnorm Child Psychol* 22, 643–660.

Meyer-Bahlberg H F, Gruen R S, New M I (1996). Gender change from female to male in classical adrenal hyperplasia. *Horm Behav* 30, 319–332.

Mills J, Cowley R (1986). *Therapeutic Metaphors for Children*. Brunner/Mazel, New York.

Money J (1975). Psychologic counseling: hermaphroditism. In *Endocrine and Genetic Diseases of Childhood and Adolescence*, 2nd edn, Gardner L I, ed., pp. 609–610. Saunders, Philadelphia, PA.

(1994). *Sex Errors of the Body and Related Syndromes: A Guide to Counselling Children, Adolescents and their Families*, 2nd edn. Brookes, Baltimore, MD.

Money J, Ehrhardt A A (1972). *Rearing of a Sex-reassigned Normal Male Infant after Traumatic Loss of the Penis: Man and Woman/Boy and Girl*. pp. 44–51. John Hopkins University Press. Baltimore MD.

Money J, Hampson J G, Hampson J L (1955). Hermaphroditism: recommendations concerning assignment of sex, change of sex and psychologic management. *Bull Johns Hopkins Hosp* 97, 284–300.

Money J, Hampson J G, Hampson J L (1957). Imprinting and the establishment of gender role. *Arch Neurol Psychiatry* 77, 333–336.

Money J, Schwartz M, Lewis V G (1984). Adult erotosexual status and fetal hormonal masculinization and demasculinization: 46 XX congenital virilizing adrenal hyperplasia and 46 XY androgen-insensitivity syndrome compared. *Psychoneuroendocrinology* 9, 405–414.

Money J, Devore H, Norman B F (1986). Gender identity and gender transposition: longitudinal outcome of study of 32 male hermaphrodites assigned as girls. *J Sex Marital Ther* 12, 165–181.

Pearce J (1994). Consent to treatment during childhood. The assessment of competence and avoidance conflict. *Br J Psychiatry* 165, 713–716.

Phornphutkul C, Fausto-Sterling A, Gruppuso P A (2000). Gender self-reassignment in an XY adolescent female born with ambiguous genitalia. *Paediatrics* 106, 135–136.

Preves S E (1998). For the sake of the children: destigmatizing intersexuality. *J Clin Ethics* 9, 411–420.

Reiner W G (1996). Case study: sex reassignment in a teenage girl. *J Am Acad Child Adolesc Psychiatry* 35, 799–803.

Royal College of Paediatrics and Child Health (2002). *Intercollegiate Adolescent Working Party*, March 2002. Royal College of Paediatrics and Child Health, London.

Rutter M (1999). Research and the family justice system: what has been the role of research and what should it be? *Newslett Natl Council Fam Proc* 15, 2–6.

Salmon G, James A, Smith D M (1998). Bullying in schools: self-reported anxiety depression and self-esteem in secondary school children. *Br Med J* 317, 924–925.

Schober J M (1998). Early feminizing genitoplasty or watchful waiting. *J Pediatr Adolesc Gynecol* 11, 157–159.

(1999). Quality-of-life studies in patients with ambiguous genitalia. *World J Urol* 17, 249–252.

Schober J M, Carmichael P A, Hines M, Ransley P G (2002). The ultimate challenge of cloacal exstrophy. *J Urol* 167, 300–304.

Shaw M (2001). Competence and consent to treatment in children and adolescents. *Adv Psychiatr Treat* 7, 50–159.

Slijper F M, van der Kamp H J, Brandenburg H, Muinck Keizer-Schrama S M, Drop S L, Molenaar J C (1992). Evaluation of psychosexual development of young women with congenital adrenal hyperplasia: a pilot study. *J Sex Educ Ther* 18, 200–207.

Slijper F M E, Drop S L S, Molenaar J C, de Muinck Keizer-Schrama S M P F (1998). Long-term psychological evaluation of intersex children. *Arch Sex Behav* 27, 125–144.

Slijper F M E, Frets P G, Boehman A L M, Drop S L S, Niermeijer M F (2000). Androgen insensitivity syndrome (AIS): emotional reactions of parents and adult patients to the clinical diagnosis of AIS and its confirmation by androgen receptor gene mutation analysis. *Horm Res* 53, 9–15.

Stoller R (1964). The hermaphroditic identity of hermaphrodites. *J Nerv Mental Dis* 139, 453.

Thompson S K, Bentler P M (1971). The priority of cues in sex discrimination by children and adults. *Develop Psychol* 5, 181–185.

Thompson R J Jr, Gustafson K E, Hamlett K, Spock A (1992). Psychological adjustment of children with cystic fibrosis: the role of child cognitive processes and maternal adjustment. *J Pediatr Psychol* 17, 741–755.

Wallander J L, Varni J W, Babani L, Banis H, Wilcox K (1989). Family resources as resistance factors for psychological maladjustment in chronically ill and handicapped children. *J Pediatr Psychol* 14, 157–173.

Warne G L (1989). *Your Child with Congenital Adrenal Hyperplasia.* Royal Children's Hospital, Australia.

Warne G L (1992). The baby who was different. A fairy tale. *Matern Child Health* 159–160.

(1997). *Complete Androgen Insensitivity Syndrome.* Royal Children's Hospital, Australia.

Warner S (1998). Psychological aspects. In *Paediatric and Adolescent Gynaecology*, Garden A S, ed., pp 190–214. Arnold, London.

Weithorn L A, Campbell S B (1982). The competency of children and adolescents to make informed treatment decisions. *Child Dev* 53, 1589–1598.

World Health Organization (1992). *International Classification of Diseases and Health Related Problems, 10th revision (ICD-10).* World Health Organization, Geneva.

WHOQOL Group (1995). The World Health Organization Quality of Life Assessment (WHOQOL). (Position paper from the World Health Organization.) *Soc Sci Med* 41, 1403–1409.

Zucker K (2002). Intersexuality and gender identity differentiation. *J Pediatr Adolesc Gynecol* 15, 3–13.

Zucker K, Bradley S, Lowry Sullivan C, Kuksis M, Birkenfield-Adams A, Mitchell J N (1993). A gender identity interview for children. *J Personality Assess* 61, 443–456.

Zucker K, Bradley S, Oliver G, Blake J, Fleming S, Hood J (1996). Psychosexual development of women with congenital adrenal hyperplasia. *Horm Behav* 30, 300–318.

15

The needs of the adolescent patient and her parents in the clinic

Jane MacDougall

Addenbrooke's Hospital, Cambridge, UK

Introduction

Adolescence is a time of transition – of a child becoming an adult. Are adolescents different from children and adults and do they, therefore, have different needs? We would argue that they do. Patients' needs should dictate how the service is run and, therefore, an understanding of these is important. The consultation is pivotal in the doctor–patient relationship, and the way in which this is conducted will influence how patients perceive their illness. Parents are often involved, which adds an extra dimension to the consultation with the adolescent. They may have a different agenda to their offspring. Both can benefit from the opportunity the clinic presents for health education.

In this chapter, the needs of children and adolescents as users of healthcare are discussed. Wider issues include the more political questions such as "Who speaks for adolescents" and "Why bother?" This is followed by a discussion of their needs when they present with gynaecological problems. Parents have needs too and these are outlined. Issues such as consent and confidentiality are important. The way in which such needs can be used to develop a clinical service follows. The consultation itself is discussed in detail.

Definitions

First some definitions. Adolescence is characterized by physiological, psychological, sexual, social and educational change. The physiological changes have been ably described in Chapter 4 and include rapid growth, weight gain and maturation of the reproductive system. Cognitive and psychological changes occur: the child changes into an independent, problem-solving adult. Children tend to be "concrete" thinkers and find abstract concepts difficult. In adolescence, they develop the ability to think more abstractly, employ logic, consider hypothetical situations and view issues from different angles (Coupey, 2000; Yordan, 2000). Interestingly, one of the most recognized adolescent specialities in the UK is adolescent mental health. Psychiatrists have realised for some time that adolescents are different and present particular challenges. Add to this changing parent–child relationships, the increasing influence of the peer group plus a developing sexuality and it is hardly surprising that adolescence can be a difficult time even for the fit teenager. For those with medical problems, the difficulties just seem to multiply.

Age definitions vary; adolescence has been described as between 11 and 25 years. The lower age varies from 11 to 13 years, whereas the upper end can be anywhere from 16 to 25 years. For the purpose of this chapter, it will be restricted to 11 to 19 years, which appears to be the most generally used range. Pragmatically, adolescent gynaecology clinics are run in conjunction with paediatric gynaecology clinics and, therefore, the latter will also be discussed.

Adolescents' needs

The central theme here is how we organize or should organize our adolescent clinics; this should depend on the needs of the attending patients. So what are adolescents' needs? Are they so different from the needs of other patients, from adults or from children? What makes the adolescent special? We would like to argue that adolescents with gynaecological problems have specific needs, both in

Paediatric and Adolescent Gynaecology, ed. Adam Balen et al. Published by Cambridge University Press.
© Cambridge University Press 2004.

relation to their age and in relation to their specific gynaecological condition.

Asking adolescents for their views

One way to identify such needs is to ask the adolescents themselves. This has been done in several studies (Burack, 2000; Donovan et al., 1997; Jacobson et al., 2000) mostly based in primary care or abroad (primarily the USA). Many of the issues are not specific to gynaecology and consequently it is also worthwhile looking at studies from other areas of adolescent medicine (Hodgson et al., 1986; Quadrel and Lau, 1990).

Burack (2000) devised a questionnaire for teenagers aged 13–15 years that sought their opinions and attitudes towards general practitioner (GP)-based sexual healthcare services. Most were aware of the sexual health services offered by GPs and were positive about being given helpful advice at the consultation. However, many believed that they had to be over 16 years to access these services and had concerns over confidentiality. The author concluded that work was needed to improve teenagers access to and use of primary care sexual health services and in particular to improve their awareness of services as well as encouraging GPs to alter their approach to teenagers.

The Adolescent Working Group at the Royal College of General Practitioners (RCGP) also addressed teenagers' views (Jacobson et al., 2000) particularly in respect to the consultation and concluded that most were satisfied with services available in primary care. They also tried to identify the most common teenage health concerns and discovered that many teenagers did not seek help for their own individual concerns. The group recommended the provision of a more sensitive primary care service that would encourage teenagers to attend when they perceived a health problem. The same group looked in more detail at the provision of contraceptive services to teenagers and identified several factors that inhibited consultation with GPs. These included lack of trust in confidentiality, lack of staff friendliness and delays in appointment. Removing such blocks might well improve services (Donovan et al., 1997).

The issue of confidentiality and need for privacy during consultations is key to all patients, but particularly so in adolescents (Court, 1993; Donovan et al., 1997), who also appreciate some degree of informality and optimal waiting room conditions (Court, 1993). In the patient with long-term health problems, continuity of care by the same physician, who the adolescent trusts, is valued (Court, 1993). Court's study, which looked at adolescents with insulin-dependent diabetes, also suggested that transfer of care to adult services should take place after the age of 17 years (Court, 1993). The author recommended that transition services for young people with a chronic illness should be developed at those children's and adult's hospitals that provide specialist help for them. As far as adolescent gynaecology is concerned, this could easily apply to intersex conditions and premature ovarian failure following treatment for childhood malignancy.

Similarly, a questionnaire study of adolescents (Hodgson et al., 1986) identified delays in appointments as a common concern. These adolescents emphasized the importance of the personal characteristics of the doctor. They also discovered that adolescents with health concerns such as nervous/emotional problems, obesity and birth control often did not consult health professionals. There may be answers to this. A study describing an Adolescent Health Service in Israel (Halevy et al., 1995), which comprised a multidisciplinary school-linked community-based adolescent health clinic, found that students did attend and that most of their visits related to psychosocial and nutritional issues. This clinic applied a comprehensive approach to the biopsychosocial needs of adolescents, which was not addressed at other health services – and it proved popular.

Rather unsurprisingly, it has been suggested that adolescents' orientations toward physician use are associated with those of their parents and that this link is generally stronger and more specific during late adolescence (Quadrel and Lau, 1990). So it would be wise for anyone trying to optimize medical services for teenagers to look also at parents' views.

Asking parents for their views

There have been few studies examining parents' views. Gulati and Minty (1998) explored parental health attitudes in association with childhood illness in the context of paediatric neurology. They found that maternal attitudes were particularly important; mothers with children referred with headaches were more likely to report illness themselves and previous illness in the family, to express concern about serious disease in themselves, to be reluctant to accept medical reassurance, to express feelings of loneliness and were more likely to have lost their mothers through death than a comparison group presenting with epilepsy (a recognized structural pathology).

Asking doctors for their views

How about the medical profession? Their input is vital for service development to take place. Again studies are limited. Klitsner et al. (1992) surveyed practitioners of paediatrics, internal medicine, obstetrics and gynaecology, family practice and adolescent medicine in a large multispeciality prepaid group practice in the USA. Adolescent medicine physicians expressed the highest perceived knowledge and competence, with family practitioners rated second. Physicians in all specialities reported a need for a teen health centre for both consultation and education.

In an editorial, Bennett and Bauman (2000) stressed the importance of taking a "psychosocial biopsy" at each encounter with a young person and that it is important to focus on concerns, feelings and behaviours, whatever the presenting complaint. Although this was written mainly in the context of mental health, discussing its relationship with risky sexual behaviour, their conclusion is that young people need healthcare that covers psychological, sexual and social areas. There is no doubt that this is also applicable to patients attending with gynaecological problems.

Balen et al. (2002) sent a postal questionnaire to all 248 departments of obstetrics and gynaecology in the UK and 64 of the 137 units that responded felt that adolescents in this area had special needs. As far as service provision was concerned, family planning, teenage pregnancy and drug/alcohol abuse were the most often quoted. This study concluded that there was no consensus on who actually constituted the adolescent population and there was a marked lack of data on the numbers of patients presenting with obstetric and gynaecological problems.

What is different about the adolescent?

The identification of adolescent needs will depend on an understanding of the differences between adult, child and adolescent. So what are these differences? Psychiatrists have long recognized the differences in cognitive and psychological behaviour. We know that adolescence is a time when the reproductive system matures. The adolescent needs time to adapt to a changing sexual body. Many adolescents find it difficult to talk about gynaecological problems. In some cultures, such discussions are considered taboo (Balen et al., 2002). Patients with disorders of sexual development have particular difficulties; not only are they changing into adults, but they are also having to come to terms with a diagnosis of anomalous sexual development, which may be associated with a reduction of normal sexual function and fertility. It is important that those caring for these individuals are able to give them the support they need to understand their condition.

Adolescence is also a time of identity development and of changes in relationships (Renteria and Narring, 2000). The different stages of adolescent development depend on biological and environmental factors, which either favour resilience or weaken the individual if there has been lack of affection or the occurrence of an abusive relationship. Certain adolescents whose families have social problems, such as divorce, may be at increased risk of physiological and psychological disturbance (Thompson, 1998).

The parent–child relationship does of course change; young teenagers, as part of normal psychological development, are developing an identity that is separate from their parents (Coupey, 2000). This can cause conflict, which can spill over into other areas including healthcare.

In addition, adolescents have specific nonmedical needs (Hofman and Gaman, 1971; Uribe, 1986). These include social, emotional, educational and recreational needs as well as a need for privacy. Adolescents with chronic long-term illnesses can miss large portions of schooling. Some units address this by providing tutors for long-stay patients. Little such provision is available to the frequent outpatient attender.

There is major concern over the impact of teenage pregnancy on the teenage mother's subsequent educational performance and achievement and her long-term socio-economic contribution. One study suggested that pregnant and parenting teens wanted to remain in school despite the struggles they encountered (Weinman et al., 1999). School-based programmes aimed at increasing the use of health services and facilitation of attendance without students missing school may help. The key elements that enable teenagers to receive targeted services are communication and cooperation between programme staff and school nurses (Weinman et al., 1999).

Adolescents presenting with gynaecological problems, therefore, have two sets of needs: general (social, emotional and educational) and medical (specific to the illness and generic to the ill teenager). Clinic organization should take all these needs into account.

The adolescent clinic

The consultation

The patient–doctor consultation is central to all healthcare encounters. At its core is the need to make a diagnosis and decide a plan of management. However, there are other essential elements without which the whole process may fail. These include building rapport with patients, explaining and reassuring, discussing alternative treatment strategies and providing health education. It is important to listen to and subsequently address the patient's concerns.

Healthcare is more effective and better in quality in the adolescent or paediatric gynaecology patient if various principles are followed. There must be an understanding of the complexities of adolescent development: biological, social and psychological (Hirsch, 1978 and earlier chapters). It is vital that the clinician is conversant with the "normal" adolescent female – normal physiology and anatomy – and understands the developmental processes of sexual determination and puberty. The developmental stage of the patient should dictate clinical practice. Confidentiality is vital when caring for adolescents. Providing autonomy in medical choices leads to patients taking responsibility for their own health (Craighill, 1998).

The medical consultation for a gynaecological problem, questions on puberty and development or on contraception, provide an opportunity for gynaecologists to address sexual issues naturally and to anticipate questions as well as contraceptive needs. The consultation can also be used to screen for behaviour associated with lack of information. Of course this extension to the conventional view of a consultation needs time.

The setting

The clinic should be quiet, comfortable and be able to provide privacy. Appropriate toys, books and magazines and relevant medical information should be placed in the waiting area. Staff should be used to communicating with children and adolescents. Work on paediatric patients suggests that services need to be child friendly with trained paediatric nurses and play areas with play leaders. Ideally, adolescents should be seen in separate clinics at times to suit them.

It is important to provide privacy as well as ensuring confidentiality. In a teaching hospital with trainee doctors and medical students, this can be difficult. Patients should always be asked if they mind the presence of others in the consultation room – and their wishes should be respected.

The beginning: communication skills

Doctors sometimes find it difficult to communicate with adolescents (as do parents) while adolescents are often anxious and reluctant to visit a doctor (Sanci and Young, 1995). The young female adolescent poses particular problems; she is often reluctant to volunteer any information and is usually accompanied by her mother, who tends to dominate the situation. It may take several visits to develop the necessary rapport to facilitate communication and to extract all the relevant information. This is often easier in primary care than it is in the hospital situation. The gynaecologist specializing with adolescents needs to develop strategies to develop rapport with new patients quickly but should recognize that this may take more time. It is very gratifying to observe a young girl with a long-term gynaecological health problem (for example one of the intersex disorders) become increasingly independent of parents and able to take on responsibility for her own healthcare. Easing this transition is one of the physician's tasks.

Some physicians running adolescent clinics find it helpful to send parents of patients attending their clinics an introductory letter or leaflet in advance of their first appointment (Coupey, 2000). This might include a description of the visit and include information on confidentiality and the examination. It can be helpful to suggest that adolescence is a time when young people need to learn to start taking responsibility for their own healthcare. If confidentiality is also mentioned, it may well be easier for the physician to have a discussion with the girl on her own.

Consideration of ethnic and cultural differences is important; often the only member of the family that speaks English is the father and this can cause difficulty. Interpreters may need to be arranged. Alternatively, a close female friend or relative who does speak English can be encouraged to attend.

The approach to history taking will tend to vary according to the age of the child or adolescent (Coupey, 2000; Yordan, 1996). In line with cognitive development, the younger girl thinks in concrete terms and these should be used during the interview. She also tends to be shy and anxious about the appearance of her body. The older adolescent is beginning to think in a more abstract way and, therefore, a more "adult" approach can be used. The older adolescent is more preoccupied with exploring her identity and discovering what kind of adult she will become; other concerns include body image and sexual health. She may also, although often not willing to admit it, be anxious about future fertility. This obviously has implications for the way in which the interview is conducted.

There are various approaches that can help to start the therapeutic relationship in a positive manner (Lucas et al., 1986). Different physicians will use different methods to build rapport early. In secondary and tertiary care, where contact may be limited to a single encounter, this can be more difficult. It is worthwhile initiating physical contact with a patient during the interview and prior to the examination (shaking or touching a hand for instance) (Yordan, 1996).

Little is, in fact, known regarding teenage health. One study looked at time spent on consultations and found that there was a statistically significant mean shortfall of nearly two minutes in consultations with adolescents when compared with other age groups (Jacobson et al., 1994). This may imply a difficulty with communication.

The history

Most adolescents, and certainly those who are younger and are attending for their first visit, will be accompanied by one or both parents. The clinician should begin by speaking to the patient and parent(s) together. Questions should be directed to the adolescent (without alienating the parent). With the dominant mother and quiet teenager, this can at times prove difficult but it is important to make the adolescent central to the consultation. As well as providing the history, this is an opportunity to assess the parent–child relationship. Use of questionnaires may aid data gathering (Silber and Rosenthal, 1986). Occasionally it may be necessary to see the parents separately. It may be possible to address any sensitive issues while their daughter is changing for the examination in another room. I often ask birth history at this point and finish with the question "is there anything else you are worried about?"

In addition to the history of the presenting complaint, it is important to ask specific questions about puberty, past history, related systems, birth history, developmental milestones and the family. It may be easier to use a specific history sheet such as that shown in Box 15.1. While taking the history, it is important to make some sort of assessment of general adolescent well-being; are there psychological problems here that may be impacting on the physical symptoms? One way to do this is to ask questions that explore family and peer relationships (Is there conflict within the family? Do they have many friends?), school performance (Is it below expectations?), hobbies (Do they have any?) and evidence of unusual behaviour (Any truancy, drug abuse?) (Blotchky, 1997). The psychosocial history is often very important and can impact on perceptions of illness (Coupey, 2000).

Ideally, the gynaecologist should find time to talk to the girl on her own. Initially, this conversation is often one-sided, but most young girls will eventually open up and talk, although this may take several visits. It is important, in keeping with their cognitive development, to use concrete rather than abstract terms. Once they start talking it is important to listen and show that you are doing so. Signposting and summarizing are useful communication techniques as in adult consultations (Kurtz et al., 1998).

Box 15.1 An adolescent gynaecology patient sheet

Date
Age
Main Complaint(s)

HPC [history of presenting complaint]

Birth History: Gestation
                     Mode of Delivery

Milestones/School History

Pubarche   Thelarche   Menarche
Cycle

Sexually active   Y/N   If Y – smear

PMH [past medical history]

Drugs   Allergies   Smoke

FH [family history] parents   Siblings

Examination

Height   Weight   BMI [body mass index]

Tanner Staging
    Breasts   Public/Axillary Hair

Abdomen

Pelvic Examination
    External Genitalia
    Vaginal Examination/Speculum

Provisional Diagnosis

Plan
• Investigations
• Advice Given
• Treatment
• Follow Up

This may be the adolescent's first contact with the hospital health system and it will influence that particular girl's attitude toward medical care and other healthcare professionals that she will meet in the future. There is evidence that adolescents, in particular, place emphasis on the personal characteristics of the doctor when asked about their healthcare preferences (Hodgson et al., 1986). It is important to get it right the first time. Gynaecologists should be nonjudgemental (particularly in regard to sexual issues), supportive, sympathetic and interested. One strategy that has been employed successfully in the clinic is to postpone this one-to-one conversation until after the examination.

It can then be combined with reassurance about the examination findings. Parents are subsequently brought back from the waiting room and the final conversation and summing up can then involve them. Alternatively, the parent can be asked to sit in the waiting room just before the examination, allowing time for specific questions to the adolescent.

It is important to obtain a sexual history. Asking the adolescent, particularly those under 16 years, about sexual activity in front of their mothers may not yield the correct information. It is vital that this particular question takes place away from the parent. This can be asked either during the one-to-one conversation or just before the examination. It is very important that the gynaecologist respects the adolescent's confidentiality over this, especially if the mother is not aware that her daughter is sexually active. Conversations about contraception and sexually transmitted disease in the sexually active adolescent who has not told her parents are very important but should obviously take place during the one-to-one part of the consultation prior to including the parent in any discussion.

One case illustrates this well. A 16-year-old girl who had previously had chemotherapy and total body irradiation plus pelvic irradiation for a childhood malignancy and had subsequently developed premature ovarian failure was referred to the adolescent gynaecology clinic by the paediatric oncologists. They had two main concerns: her hormone replacement and the effect of the irradiation on her pelvis. Would she be able to achieve pregnancy by oocyte donation and would she have problems with intercourse because of narrowing of the vagina? During the course of the one-to-one conversation, it transpired that she had a boyfriend, had had intercourse and had no problems with this. However, her mother did not know and the daughter was not keen to tell her. Great care was taken to only speak to the mother subsequently *in front of her daughter*. It is important that the girl is sure that you have not told her parents anything that she told you in confidence. Going off to speak to the parents separately will immediately raise the adolescent's suspicions that you have told them this confidential information. In this case, by the follow-up visit 6 months later, she had told her mother anyway and all was in the open. Meanwhile her trust in us as physicians who respected her confidentiality was retained.

The hospitalized adolescent presents different challenges. Gathering information can be a problem. A systems questionnaire may help (Silber and Rosenthal, 1986) and can enhance communication between patients and physicians: 82 of the 100 patients completing a standard questionnaire (The Mile Square Youth Clinic Questionnaire)

presented new information that resulted in a better understanding of the individual patient's needs.

The examination

After the history has been taken, it is important to give the adolescent a clear unambiguous explanation of why an examination is necessary and what form the examination will take (RCOG, 1997). Verbal consent should always be sought and obtained prior to examination, both from the adolescent and from the parent if present. The techniques involved should be explained. They must be aware that they can ask to stop the examination at any stage; you are giving them control over the situation. A commitment should be made to avoid discomfort. Some adolescents and children will decline any or part of the examination. It is vital not to force the issue. They need to build confidence and trust in their doctor; this may take several visits.

It is important to ensure the comfort and privacy of the patient. Adolescents should be left to undress alone. They do not need to remove all their clothing and most prefer not to. A chaperone should always be present during the examination, whether or not a parent is present; this protects both the doctor and the patient. Drapes can be used to cover the lower body. After the examination, the patient should be left to redress and brought back into the consultation room for the "summing up". There should be a rule preventing any discussion with a patient (of whatever age) while that individual is undressed or partially clothed: the patient is immediately put at a disadvantage. At the very least, the discussion should be kept relevant and personal comments avoided (GMC, 1996).

General examination should include measurement of the body mass index (BMI), blood pressure, thyroid status, congenital abnormalities and breast examination as well as assessment of pubic and axillary hair. Tanner staging of secondary sexual development can then be recorded. Abdominal examination is then performed prior to moving on to pelvic examination. This should include palpation of the groins for lymphadenopathy and herniae.

If the patient is not sexually active, vaginal examination is inappropriate, particularly in the younger child. The perineum and external genitalia can be inspected and an ultrasound scan of the pelvis organized. There is, in fact, little extra that can be gleaned from a bimanual examination if the above has been arranged. If a foreign body is suspected or if investigation is required for bleeding or recurrent vaginal discharge, then an examination under anaesthetic (EUA) should be arranged. If the adolescent is postpubertal and using tampons it may be feasible to do a one finger

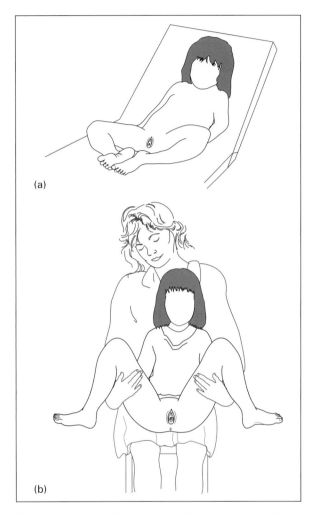

Fig. 15.1. Inspection of external genitalia. (a) Frog-leg position; (b) seated on mother's lap.

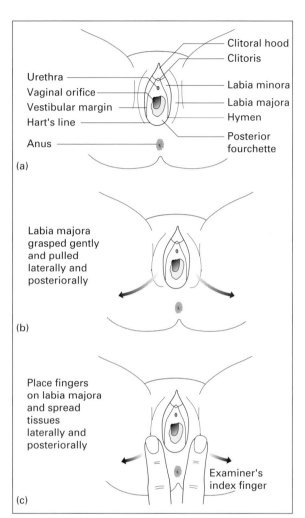

Fig. 15.2. The external genitalia. (a) Normal anatomy; (b) lateral traction method; (c) lateral spread method.

vaginal examination. If the adolescent is sexually active, a vaginal examination can be performed with or without a speculum examination (using a small Huffman or Pedersen speculum). This may be the patient's first such examination and it is important to be slow and very gentle. The patient should feel in control and able to stop the examination at any point if it is uncomfortable. It is important to explain this in advance and to reassure the patient. If the examination is incomplete an ultrasound scan can be arranged. (Goldforb, 1998). The optimal position is probably the "frog-legged" position with the patient lying supine but propped up with the hips flexed and soles of feet together (Fig. 15.1). Girls under three can sit on their mother's lap. Some authors have advocated the lithotomy position, but this should not be necessary. The use of hand-held mirrors has also been advocated to give the child more control.

Children may like to see what is going on; in the main, adolescents prefer not to. Some children may prefer to spread the labia themselves. Some gynaecologists use a nurse as "their hands" (Yordan, 1996) to provide lateral labial spread or traction while the doctor visualizes the vulva, vestibule and vagina.

Various techniques have been described for inspection of the external genitalia (Emans et al., 1998). These include alternative positioning, the lateral spread and lateral traction methods and "extinction of stimuli" method (Fig. 15.2). The lateral spread method involves pressure posterolaterally on the perineum, which causes the labia to spread. Alternatively, the labia can be gently gripped and pulled towards the examiner and slightly posterolaterally (lateral traction method). If the child takes a deep breath, the vestibular tissues, vagina and hymen can be visualized.

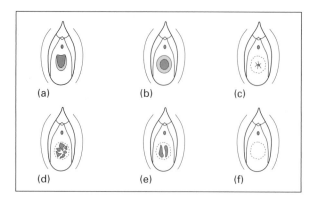

Fig. 15.3. Variations is appearance of normal hymen. (a) crescentic; (b) annular; (c) fimbriated; (d) microperforated (cribiform); (e) septate; (f) intact.

An otoscope or colposcope can be used to provide magnification. Another position is the prone knee-chest position with the back relaxed, which is advocated by several authors (Pokorny, 1994). This allows a better inspection of the vaginal canal and hymen than the frog-legged position. However, some children do find this frightening (Huffman et al., 1981) and it should only be used in the cooperative relaxed child. The "extinction of stimuli" phenomenon has been described in relation to the first speculum examination (Pokorny, 1994). A primary distracting stimulus is used to lessen, defuse and extinguish the intensity of a second stimulus. The non-examining finger is pressed into the patient's perineum before the introitus is touched with the examining finger.

The external genitalia should be inspected for the presence of pubic hair, clitoral size, configuration of the hymen, relationship of the anus to the vagina and urethral orifice to the hymen. The degree of oestrogenization and perineal hygiene should also be assessed. The appearance of the hymen can be variable (Fig. 15.3) and is not addressed here in detail. Normal types described include annular (circumferential), crescentic (posterior rim) and fimbriated (denticular) (Pokorny, 1994). Other variations include the microperforated and septate hymen. Glaister rods (glass rods or bulbs) can be used to demonstrate the edge of the hymen. The size of the hymenal opening varies according to position and relaxation and measurement is unhelpful (Robson, 1998). The adolescent and paediatric gynaecologist needs to be aware of this variability and should be cautious in interpreting any "abnormal" appearance and especially in attributing this to sexual abuse. The clitoris should be no larger than the average adult clitoris (5.4 mm $\times$ 4.4 mm) (Carson, 2000).

Some older textbooks advocate rectal examination in this age group as an alternative to vaginal examination. Most

children and adolescents find this upsetting and we would not recommend it. With the advent of reliable ultrasound scanning it has no indication. Occasionally EUA may be necessary and involve the use of a vaginoscope (or hysteroscope) and cystoscope. A nasal speculum with light source can be helpful for direct visualization of vagina and cervix.

Documentation of findings is important: a labelled sketch of the external genitalia is useful. Photographs may be helpful, after appropriate written consent. Records need to be clear, legible and contemporaneous (Robson, 1998). The vulva should be staged according to Tanner's classification.

Many women in their twenties and older attribute their fear and dislike of vaginal examinations to an unpleasant experience as a young woman or adolescent: "the doctor was rough". It is important to get it right the first time; remember that it will affect that patient's future attitude to gynaecological healthcare. Therefore, be gentle, take time, stop if there is discomfort and allow the patient to remain in control. The basic principles of respect, privacy, explanation and consent should always apply (RCOG, 1997). Most examinations can be completed by being gentle, caring and at every level empowering the girl to participate in the examination (Yordan, 1996). This will leave them with a positive experience that should inform their attitude to future gynaecological care.

The summing up

The discussion after the examination should include a summary of the findings and proposed management. The importance of doing this in front of the patient has already been discussed. Reassurance is important, both to patient and parents. It is helpful to ask the patient for her permission to discuss the findings with the parent and then invite the latter back into the room in order to do this. It is important to explain what is normal, what can be expected and how things may change. Box 15.2 summarizes the recommendations for practice.

Box 15.2 Recommendations for practice in the clinic

- Make the adolescent central to the consultation.
- Respect privacy and maintain confidentiality.
- Take great care over examination; always obtain consent.
- Provide clear explanations.
- Be aware of parents' concerns and address if possible.
- Help adolescents to take responsibility for own health.

The consultation is also an opportunity for health education. One area is weight reduction; up to 25% of adolescent girls are obese. Weight is a particularly sensitive area for many adolescent girls – even more so than for adults. Although it may be important in some cases to advise weight loss, the sensible gynaecologist treads very gently; it is easy to antagonize the adolescent and undo all the previous hard work in developing rapport. It is often easier to include such advice in a general conversation about diet. Other areas include advice on smoking, contraception and sexually transmitted disease. Literature should be available, in different languages, to supplement verbal advice.

Parents' needs in the clinic

There is no doubt that the presence of parents who may have a different agenda to their daughters can make the consultation process more complex. The interaction between child and parent may throw light on the child's illness. So far, the emphasis has been on the adolescent's or child's needs. It is important also to understand and be aware of parents' concerns. There are several issues: consent, confidentiality and the need to keep parents informed.

As far as consent is concerned, in this country a parent or guardian needs to sign consent forms for operative procedures if the adolescent is under 16 years. There are occasions when this can be waived. For example, a girl of 14 years may be pregnant and requesting a termination of pregnancy yet not wish to involve her parents. She should be encouraged to do so. However, if she refuses and two doctors consider that she is "Gillick competent" then she can sign her own consent form (Department of Health, 2001). The concept of "Gillick competency" arose from the case of "Gillick" where the courts held that children who had sufficient understanding and intelligence to enable them to fully understand what was involved in a proposed intervention would be able to consent to that intervention (*Gillick* v. *West Norfolk and Wisbech Area Health Authority*, 1986). Between the ages of 16 and 17 years, adolescents can consent to their own medical treatment. However, unlike adults, refusal of a competent person aged 16–17 years may, in certain circumstances, be overridden by either a person with parental responsibility or by a court (Department of Health, 2001).

Parents should be included as much as possible in important medical decisions but the adolescent's needs for medical privacy and confidentiality should be respected. Parents may need help to communicate more effectively with their adolescent. It is important to explain to the parents the extent of confidentiality and why this is important. In a survey of high school students, Cheng et al. (1993) found that 25% of adolescents would forgo healthcare in some situations if their parents found out and only 57% would go to their regular physicians for questions about pregnancy. The parents of older adolescents need to be educated by the clinician about the need to provide private confidential care for their daughter; however, they should also be reassured that they will be informed if a major health problem is uncovered (Coupey, 2000).

Parents may, understandably, feel protective of their daughters, particularly when they are ill. It is common for the mother to dominate the consultation and this situation is not always easy to deal with. The mother–daughter relationship tends to be particularly fraught when the daughter is between the ages of 14 and 17 years. Daughters may feel a need to reject the values and opinions of their mothers in an effort to differentiate themselves from them. Some mothers experience grief and sadness over the loss of their close relationship with their daughter and may react by being "controlling". The mother may need extra support and parenting advice at this time (Coupey, 2000). She should be encouraged to keep lines of communication open.

The wider view

It is important to identify the health needs of adolescents; it is also important to use such knowledge to improve adolescent healthcare services. Concern has been expressed that adolescents' health needs are not being recognized at policy level (Aynsley-Green et al., 2000; Royal College of Paediatrics and Child Health, 2002). Demographic changes are resulting in an increasingly ageing society and it seems likely that the needs of the elderly population may, in future, drain resources from children's services (Hall, 1999). Children and young people are a nation's most valuable resource, yet compared with other groups they do not have a vocal patient group. This is particularly true of adolescents, especially those estranged from their parents. It is perhaps not surprising that improving the health of children in the UK is not really a key government target (Aynsley-Green et al., 2000). These authors argue that a strategy needs to be developed for children and young people and that there must be recognition and protection of children's fundamental human rights.

These and other issues are discussed in more detail in Chapter 40, but will of necessity have an impact on funding of service development. A perception of the different needs of adolescents compared with children and adults is important in encouraging developments to take place.

Organization of the clinic

So what does all this mean for the organization of the clinic? Several studies have examined different aspects of this (Chavasse et al., 1995; Cohen et al., 1975; Court 1993; Fakeyke and Adegoke, 1994). School-based clinics have some advantages (Chavasse et al., 1995) and may overcome barriers such as access, cost and confidentiality. Fakeyke and Adegoke (1994) argued for the establishment of a multidisciplinary school health-counselling programme within Nigeria aimed at menstrual dysfunction. Others have argued for similar provision in the UK (Williams et al., 1994), primarily for general adolescent health advice.

Cohen et al. (1975) stressed the importance of tailoring a service to the current health needs of youth by using a variety of settings including an inpatient unit, outpatient service, primary care service within teenage detention and prison facilities, addictive disease diagnostic and treatment programmes, and school health programmes. These authors underlined the importance of using each unit as a "clinical laboratory and classroom" so that training and research activities were integral parts of each service area. They also described the organization as flexible and evolving to meet new demands from patients and staff. Another study evaluating linked services demonstrated that teenage pregnancy could be reduced by linking contraceptive services to school-based education, while increasing the access to young person's sexual health services and gaining the support of local community and youth organizations (Centre for Review and Dissemination, 1997). It is important that patients with gynaecological problems such as abnormal bleeding can be referred to a gynaecologist who has experience of adolescents (Anderson et al., 1986), particularly if paediatricians are not comfortable in dealing with such conditions. Continuity of care is also important (Court, 1993).

Viner (2001) argued for the provision of specific adolescent facilities within hospitals. This is based on bed occupancy by adolescents and refers predominantly to inpatient facilities. Even where numbers do not justify a separate ward for adolescents, a multidisciplinary approach from health professionals with interest and expertise in adolescent health is still possible in every hospital (MacFarlane and Blum, 2001). One way of ensuring that this happens is to develop guidelines for managing adolescents in hospital. These authors also stressed the importance of educating involved professionals so that they can provide optimal healthcare for this age group.

We, and others, have been running multispeciality, multidisciplinary clinics with consultant colleagues and other healthcare professionals. Such joint clinics, which cross directorate boundaries, may include paediatric and adult endocrinologists, paediatric surgeons, geneticists, plastic surgeons, psychiatrists, psychologists, nurse specialists and counsellors as well as gynaecologists. Links with radiologists and chemical pathologists are also helpful. There are several advantages for patients. These include a reduction in the number of visits to outpatient clinics as they can see a variety of clinicians in a single visit, consultant-based care, the opportunity to see experts in each area who understand adolescent needs and improved standards of care. There are some disadvantages however; there tends to be less flexibility for appointments as such clinics tend to be held on an infrequent basis. Fewer patients can be seen per clinic and some patients may find groups of doctors intimidating – particularly if trainees and medical students are also present.

As far as clinicians are concerned, joint clinics can be very valuable; they allow the discussion of difficult complex cases and also provide an opportunity for discussion of more general patient management issues. If confined to a particular area (e.g. intersex), it is possible to bring together a critical mass of patients with similar conditions, which provides a brilliant training resource. There is also an opportunity for coordinated research on rare conditions so that an evidence base can be developed. Such clinics also spawn the development of management guidelines. The main disadvantages for clinicians are organizational, and good administrative backup is essential. The present funding arrangements, which tend to be speciality based within a hospital, make funding across speciality boundaries problematic. Clinically, the main difficulty seems to be the limited scope for individual confidential discussions with patients and parents. This can be overcome by the use of video links. (As in the Great Ormond Street Intersex Clinic, where the patients and parents are seen by one or two clinicians in a separate room that has a video link to a room with other clinicians. Permission is of course sought from parents and patients in this situation.) Alternatively, the patient can just be taken into a separate clinic room by an individual clinician.

Novel strategies

There have been a number of descriptions of "novel" strategies of service organization. Many of these are aimed at improving accessibility of services and some make use of the technology that the adolescent age group is particularly familiar with. The *TeleHealth* project is a model telecommunications programme that provides health education and consultation to adolescents on the Internet (Cox, 1998). Set up by a health education centre in the USA in collaboration with East Carolina University, this involves interactive distance learning and is aimed at ninth grade students plus educators and health professionals. *Teen line* is a peer telephone listening service for adolescents that provides information on general issues as well as health-related problems (Boehm et al., 1991).

Many of the strategies have been developed in an attempt to reduce teenage pregnancy; most of these have come out of North America, where this is seen as a major health issue. Such strategies may, however, be extendable to other areas of adolescent health and, in particular, to adolescent gynaecology, and they are, therefore, worthy of examination. Direct targeting of "at risk" individuals may be helpful. Tiezzi et al. (1997) described a school-based pregnancy prevention programme that used an intensive risk-identification and case-management approach; it successfully reduced pregnancy rates among teenagers younger than 15 years by 34% over 4 years. Badger et al. (1976) described an innovative service programme designed to help adolescent mothers become more effective parents. Peer-led programmes may be particularly helpful. For example, the Nike programme in the USA enlists teenage mothers to advise their pregnant teenage peers.

Outreach clinics have been used with some success; Reuler (1991) described a clinic organized by a voluntary health agency and based at a drop-in centre for street youth. Respiratory, dermatological and gynaecological problems accounted for 56% of all diagnoses, while pregnancy tests accounted for 38% of all procedures. Location, opening hours and ability to perform a few simple laboratory procedures, along with an on-site pharmacy, were thought to be important features.

How to increase the uptake of healthcare and what adolescents get out of a clinic

Adolescents will tend to return for follow-up appointments if they feel that a healthcare consultation went well; so it is important to look at what they can get out of such a contact. The consultation is also a valuable opportunity for health education. Are such messages getting across?

There is a high consultation rate during childhood and infancy, which then decreases rapidly at 10 years of age, only to increase again at 16 years (Settertobulte and Kolip, 1997). The consultation rate does not appear to be gender specific nor is it influenced by social status, stress at school

or the quality of the parent–child relationship. However, the rate does depend on satisfaction with the previous medical consultation and concern over health.

There has undoubtedly been an increase in the range of health problems in adolescents (Sanci et al., 2000). Unmet health needs tend to lead to an underutilization of adolescent healthcare services. (Taylor et al., 1991). There appears to be a need to increase accessibility and quality of health services for young people (Sanci et al., 2000). Adolescents are more likely to use primary care services when an appointment is not needed, opening times are convenient, the location easy to access, provision of advice on any health problem possible and where staff are friendly, preferably female and informal, but nevertheless confidentiality is ensured (Peckham, 1997). There is evidence that attendance for follow-up appointments improves when adolescents are given autonomy and ownership of their condition.

One way of increasing the quality of healthcare in any arena is by improving the quality of medical education. In a randomized controlled trial, Sanci et al. (2000) evaluated the effectiveness of an educational programme in adolescent health designed for GPs in Australia. They demonstrated an improvement in knowledge, skill and self-perceived competency on the part of the GPs. The programme was also well received by the participants and confirmed a need for professional development in adolescent health.

Opportunity for health education

Attempts to impart health information at consultations is likely to be worthwhile, although there are limited studies to support this. Walker et al. (2000) evaluated the effectiveness of inviting teenagers to UK GP consultations that contained health behaviour advice. Around half reported some change in health-related behaviour at one month. In the context of sexual health, the messages may be more difficult to get across, although this is an area that is particularly important (Creatsas, 1997; Williams et al., 1994). Young people advised to attend genitourinary medicine clinics for sexually transmitted infection screening from community-based advisory centres rarely do so (Vanhegan and Wedgwood, 1999). However, a consultation for emergency contraception may present an opportunity to discuss more reliable and acceptable methods of contraception (Seamark and Pereira-Gray, 1997). We certainly have a responsibility to provide adolescents seeking advice on sexual matters with accurate advice as well as free family planning services in a setting where they can be counselled on the prevention of unwanted pregnancy and sexually transmitted diseases (Creatsas, 1997). Promoting the importance of a healthy sexual and reproductive life to adolescents requires openness and better sex education, together with support if things go wrong (Williams et al., 1994). There is also a need for sexually related education targeted at healthcare providers, especially doctors (Whatley et al., 1989).

Research

Research in this area is important but often difficult. Riesch et al. (1999) identified three strategies that can help in the recruitment and retention of adolescents and their families: community involvement, adherence to principles of adolescent development and ease of participation for school personnel and families. Fisher et al. (1996) discuss the impact of adolescent perspectives on research ethics. The conflict between confidentiality and legality with the need for exposure can at times be difficult. This is an area in which educationalists undertaking research into the education of children and adolescents are well versed (Cohen et al., 2000). Some of the lessons learned in the field of educational research can be usefully applied to medical research in this age group, particularly in regard to ethics and confidentiality.

Summary

As anyone who has adolescent children knows, adolescence is a time of change. Children are dependent on their parents whereas adults on the whole are not. Adolescence is the transition between the two states; adolescents are learning to take responsibility for their own healthcare. Our role as professionals is to help them through this process.

Adolescents with gynaecological problems present additional problems to those of teenagers utilizing medical care. Important issues are taking a sexual history and the examination of the external genitalia and pelvis and sensible involvement of parents. Reassurance is important. As can be seen from many of the chapters in this book, some conditions are rare. There is a need for appropriate management, which requires a certain level of expertise. It is important to "get it right" the first time: teenagers are quick to spot inconsistencies and failures in approach and will vote with their feet – they will not return to clinics. This is a specific group of patients with specific needs (Box 15.3).

Box 15.3 Key points

- Adolescents needs can be divided into four areas: learning to take responsibility for their own healthcare, the need to be listened to, the need to have medical problems clearly explained and to have educational and psychological issues addressed.
- Adolescents with gynaecological problems have general and medical needs. Healthcare professionals should consider social, educational, sexual and psychological needs in addition to medical needs specific to the illness and generic to the ill teenager.
- The foundations of a successful consultation include an understanding of the normal, good history taking, appropriate examination, and sensible involvement of parents.
- Parents may have different agenda and needs to adolescents.
- Multispeciality and multidisciplinary clinics have many advantages. Clinics should be organized according to patients' needs.
- The consultation is an opportunity for health education.

REFERENCES

Anderson M M, Irwin C E, Snyder D L (1986). Abnormal vaginal bleeding in adolescents. *Paediatr Ann* 15, 697–701, 704–707.

Aynsley-Green A, Barker M, Burr S et al. (2000). Who is speaking for children and adolescents and for their health at the policy level? *Br Med J* 321, 229–232.

Badger E, Burns D, Rhoads B (1976). Education for adolescent mothers in a hospital setting. *Am J Public Health* 66, 469–472.

Balen A H, Fleming C, Robinson A (2002). Health needs of adolescents in secondary gynaecological care: results of a questionnaire survey and a review of current issues. *Hum Fertil* 5, 127–132.

Bennett D L, Bauman A (2000). Adolescent mental health and risky sexual behaviour. *Br Med J* 321, 251–252.

Blotchky M J (1977). Adolescence. When isn't it just a phase? *J Am Med Assoc* 237, 2232–2233.

Boehm K, Chessare J B, Valko T R, Sager M S (1991). Teen line: a descriptive analysis of a peer telephone listening service. *Adolescence* 26, 643–648.

Burack R (2000). Young teenagers attitudes towards general practitioners and their provision of sexual health care. *Br J Gen Pract* 50, 550–554.

Carson S A (2000). Gynecological examination of the adolescent. In *Pediatric and Adolescent Gynecology*, Carpenter S E K, Rock J A, eds., pp. 69–77. Lippincott, Williams & Wilkins, Philadelphia, PA.

Centre for Review and Dissemination (1997). *Effective Health Care 3 (1), Preventing and Reducing the Adverse Effects of Unintended Teenage Pregnancies.* NHS Centre for Review and Dissemination, University of York, York, UK.

Chavasse M, North D, McAvoy B (1995). Adolescent health: a descriptive study of a school doctor clinic. *N Z Med J* 108, 271–273.

Cheng T L, Savageau J A, Sattler A L et al. (1993). Confidentiality in health care: a survey of knowledge, perceptions and attitude among high school students. *J Am Med Assoc* 269, 1404.

Cohen L, Manion L, Morrison K (2000). The ethics of educational and social research. In *Research Methods in Education*, 5th edn, Cohen L, Manion L, Morrison K, eds, pp. 49–72. Routledge-Falmer, New York.

Cohen M I, Litt R F, Schonberg S K, Sheehy A J, Daum F, Hein K (1975). Perspectives on adolescent medicine: concepts and program design. *Acta Paediatr Scand* 256(Suppl.), 9–16.

Coupey S M (2000). The middle adolescent girl: ages 14–17 years. In *Primary Care of Adolescent Girls*, Coupey S M, ed., pp. 17–26. Hanley & Belfus, Philadelphia, PA.

Court J M (1993). Issues of transition to adult care. *J Paediatr Child Health* 29(Suppl. 1), S53–S55.

Cox C G (1998). Highway to health: on line health education. *J Sch Nurs* 14, 48–51.

Craighill M C (1998). Paediatric and adolescent gynaecology for the primary care paediatrician. *Pediatr Clin North Am* 45, 1659–1688.

Creatsas G (1997). Improving adolescent sexual behaviour: a tool for better fertility outcome and safe motherhood. *Int J Gynaecol Obstet* 58, 85–92.

Department of Health (2001). *Reference Guide to Consent for Examination or Treatment.* Department of Health, London.

Donovan C, Mellanby A R, Jacobson L D, Taylor B, Tripp J H (1997). Teenagers' views on the general practice consultation and provision of contraception. The Adolescent working Group. *Br J Gen Pract* 47, 715–718.

Emans S J, Laufer M R, Goldstein D P (eds.) (1998). *Pediatric and Adolescent Gynecology.* Lippincott, Williams & Wilkins, Philadelphia, PA.

Fakeye O, Adegoke A (1994). The characteristics of the menstrual cycle in Nigerian schoolgirls and the implications for school health programmes. *Afr J Med Med Sci* 23, 13–17.

Fisher C B, Higgins D'Alessandro A, Rau J M, Kuther T L, Belanger S (1996). Referring and reporting research participants at risk: views from urban adolescents. *Child Dev* 67, 2086–2100.

Gillick v. *West Norfolk and Wisbech Area Health Authority* (1986). AC 112.

GMC (General Medical Council) (1996). *Intimate Examinations.* GMC, London.

Goldfarb A F (1998). *Atlas of Clinical Gynecology*, Vol. 1, *Pediatric and Adolescent Gynecology*, Steichever M A, ed. Current Medicine, Philadelphia, PA.

Gulati A, Minty B (1998). Parental health attitudes, illnesses and supports and the referral of children to medical specialists. *Child Care Health Dev* 24, 295–313.

Halevy A, Hardoff D, Knishkowy B, Palti H (1995). A school linked health service for adolescents in Jerusalem. *J Sch Health* 65, 416–419.

Hall D M B (1999). Children in an ageing society. *Br Med J* 319, 1356–1358.

Hirsch J G (1978). Understanding the adolescent patient. *Major Probl Clin Paediatr* 19, 28–38.

Hodgson C, Feldman, Corber S, Quinn A (1986). Adolescent health needs. II: Utilisation of health care by adolescents. *Adolescence* 21, 383–390.

Hofman A D, Gaman M (1971). The adolescent outpatient: medical, social and emotional needs. *Postgrad Med* 13, 764–783.

Huffman J W, Dewhurst C J, Capraro V J (1981). *The Gynecology of Childhood and Adolescence*, pp. 85–87. Saunders, Philadelphia, PA.

Jacobson L D, Wilkinson C, Owen P A (1994). Is the potential of teenage consultations being missed? A study of consultation times in primary care. *Fam Pract* 11, 296–299.

Jacobson L D, Mellanby A R, Donovan C, Taylor B, Tripp J H (2000). Teenagers' views on general practice consultations and other medical advice. The Adolescent Working Group, RCGP. *Fam Pract* 17, 156–158.

Klitsner I N, Borok G M, Neinstein L, Mackenzie R (1992). Adolescent health care in a large multispeciality prepaid group practice. Who provides it and how well are they doing? *West J Med* 156, 628–632.

Kurtz S, Silverman J Draper J (1998). *Teaching and Learning Communication Skills in Medicine*, pp. 186–191. Radcliffe Medical Press, Abingdon, UK.

Lucas S E, Spear B, Daniel W A (1986). Interviewing the adolescent. *Paediatr Ann* 15, 811–814.

MacFarlane A, Blum R W (2001). Do we need specialist adolescent units in hospital? *Br Med J* 322, 941–942.

Peckham (1997). Preventing teenage pregnancies: delivering effective services for young people. *Health Educ* 3, 103–109.

Pokorny S F (1994). Genital examination of prepubertal and peripubertal females. In *Pediatric and Adolescent Gynecology*, Sanfillipo J S, Muram D, Lee P A, Dewhurst J, eds., pp. 170–186. Saunders, Philadelphia, PA.

Quadrel M J, Lau R R (1990). A multivariate analysis of adolescents' orientations toward physician use. *Health Psychol* 9, 750–773.

RCOG (Royal College of Obstetricians and Gynaecologists) (1997). *Intimate Examinations: Report of a Working Party.* RCOG Press, London.

Renteria S C, Narring F (2000). Adolescent sexuality: epidemiology, clinical approach and preventive measures. [French] *Schweiz Rundsch Med Prax* 89, 5–16.

Reuler J B (1991). Outreach services for street youth. *J Adolesc Health* 12, 561–566.

Riesch S K, Tosi C B, Thurston C A (1999). Accessing young adolescents and their families for research. *Image J Nurs Sch* 31, 323–326.

Robson W J (1998). Gynaecological examination in childhood and adolescence. In *Paediatric and Adolescent Gynaecology.* Garden A S, ed., pp. 33–45. Arnold, London.

Royal College of Paediatrics and Child Health (2002). *Intercollegiate Adolescent Working Party*, March 2002. Royal College of Paediatrics and Child Health, London.

Sanci L A, Young D (1995). Engaging the adolescent patient. *Aust Fam Physician* 24, 2027–2031.

Sanci L A, Coffey C M M, Veit F C M et al. (2000). Evaluation of the effectiveness of an educational intervention for general practitioners in adolescent health care: randomised controlled trial. *Br Med J* 320, 224–329.

Seamark C J, Pereira-Gray D J (1997). Teenagers use of emergency contraception in a general practice. *J Roy Soc Med* 90, 443–444.

Settertobulte W, Kolip P (1997). Gender specific factors in the utilization of medical services during adolescence. *J Adolesc* 20, 121–132.

Silber T J, Rosenthal J L (1986). Usefulness of a review of systems questionnaire in the assessment of the hospitalized adolescent. *J Adolesc Health Care* 7, 49–52.

Taylor D K, Miller S S, Moltz K A (1991). Adolescent health care: an assessment of referral activities. *Adolescence* 26, 717–725.

Thompson P (1998). Adolescents from families of divorce: vulnerability to physiological and psychological disturbances. *J Psychosoc Nurs Ment Health Serv* 36, 34–39.

Tiezzi L, Lipshutz J, Wrobleski N, Vaughan R D, McCarthy J F (1997). Pregnancy prevention among urban adolescents younger than 15, results of the 'In your face' program. *Fam Plann Perspect* 29, 173–176, 197.

Uribe V M (1986). Adolescents: their special physical, social and metapsychologic needs. *Adolescence* 21, 667–673.

Vanhegan G, Wedgwood A (1999). Do young people attend genito urinary medicine clinics when referred by a community based Brook Advisory Centre? *Br J Fam Planning* 25, 23–24.

Viner R M (2001). National survey of use of hospital beds by adolescents aged 12–19 in the United Kingdom. *Br Med J* 322, 957–958.

Walker Z A, Oakley L L, Townsend J L (2000). Evaluating the impact of primary care consultations on teenage lifestyles: a pilot study. *Meth Infertil Med* 39, 260–266.

Weinman M L, Solomon C, Glass M B (1999). Opportunities for pregnant and parenting teenagers: a school based and school linked program. *J Sch Nurs* 15, 11–18.

Whately J, Thin N, Reynolds B, Blackwell A (1989). Problems of adolescents' sexuality. *J Roy Soc Med* 82, 732–734.

Williams E C, Kirkman R J, Elstein M (1994). Profile of young people's advice clinic in reproductive health, 1988–93. *Br Med J* 309, 786–788.

Yordan E E (1996). Tips, tricks and tests for the gynecological examination of young females. In *Clinical Problems in Pediatric and Adolescent Gynecology*, Goldfarb A F, ed., pp. 3–18. Chapman & Hall, New York.

(2000). The early adolescent girl: ages 10–13 years. In *Primary Care of Adolescent Girls*, Coupey, S M, ed., pp. 1–16. Nanley & Belfus, Philadelpia, PA.

16

Communicating a diagnosis

Gillian Lockwood[1], Alan Cooklin[2] and Sandra Ramsden[2]

[1]Midland Fertility Services, Aldridge, UK
[2]Department of Child and Adolescent Psychiatric Services, The Middlesex Hospital, London, UK

The right to know one's diagnosis

GILLIAN LOCKWOOD

As physicians we set great store by diagnosis. We feel that *making* the diagnosis is possibly the most important aspect of the consultation or medical interaction. And we feel that patients *need* a diagnosis, not only to ensure that they can be treated but also that the possession of a diagnosis somehow empowers them to face the medical establishment. As if, armed with their diagnosis, the patient can be viewed as an ally of the doctor, with the condition a common enemy that they can fight together. But it is not always so. Some diagnoses are bleak, incurable and unmanageable, and some do not reflect pathology at all, but just an alternative way of being. The timing of the diagnosis and even the way in which it is made, and by whom, can be as important as the diagnosis itself.

Giving a diagnosis

The following story from my early days as a gynaecology SHO may help to illustrate the importance of timing and how a diagnosis is given.

Baby Jane's mum

I met the mother of Baby Jane during my elective as a neonatal SHO on the Special Care Baby Unit. She was 39, had been pregnant before and had three teenage boys. She was surprised, but not distressed, to be pregnant again and if this pregnancy seemed "different" from the others she assumed that it was because she was so much older.

She was offered antenatal diagnosis but it seemed "a bit expensive" (the triple test) or "scary" (amniocentesis) and anyway she was too busy looking after her widowed mum who was not well.

She went into spontaneous labour at 41 weeks. The baby girl was floppy at birth (I was there because of meconium staining of the liquor) but pinked up nicely on oxygen. Baby Jane had bilateral single palmar creases and a heart murmur: the diagnosis was Down's syndrome. I was there when the Consultant gave her the diagnosis. "I wish I'd known" "I don't know what I would have done, but I wish I'd known" was all she said.

Baby Jane's granny

I finished the elective and returned to gynaecology where I met Baby Jane's grandmother. She was admitted with abdominal swelling, weakness and change of bowel habit. She was 60 and keen to tell everyone about her new little granddaughter. Exploratory laparotomy was "open and close" with a diagnosis of advanced ovarian carcinoma with metastases. Again I was with the consultant when the diagnosis and prognosis was told to her. She nodded and seemed to understand, but I was not surprised to be called back later and asked "If they had found anything wrong?"

Again I explained and later saw my registrar having the same conversation. Even the medical student and then the nurses were buttonholed in turn and again they gently explained. For three days she just cried and stopped eating, staring at the photos of her grandchildren on the bedside cabinet. The next day I was astonished to see her sitting up in bed tucking into breakfast. The lady that brought the tea and swept the floor had given her the only diagnosis that she wanted to hear, that "Doctors today were very clever and she was sure that she'd be alright!" She was enthusiastically

Paediatric and Adolescent Gynaecology, ed. Adam Balen et al. Published by Cambridge University Press.
© Cambridge University Press 2004.

looking forward to her daughter's visit as she was bringing little Jane!

Problems created by withholding a diagnosis

Androgen insensitivity syndrome (AIS) is a source of some of the most complex dilemmas in diagnosis making *and* telling. Diagnoses in children, which may require irreversible decisions to be made on their behalf by their parents, can inevitably lead to both regrets and secrets. A patient with AIS called Rosemary posted her story on the Support Group Website and her account of her slow and painful realisation of not only her diagnosis but also the way in which it had been kept from her makes for poignant reading. I reproduce a little of "Rosemary's Story" below.

I was about 14 when I concluded, with the aid of a hand mirror, that I was neither male nor female, but more female than male. In those days there was a social taboo about knowing about one's body so I kept this knowledge to myself and it was not until I was 17 that medical examination and subsequent surgery took place. My parents were told that my internal organs had not developed properly and that two hernias had been discovered and removed.

Thirty years later, a married woman in her late forties, Rosemary discovered the true nature of her condition and asked to see a copy of her medical records. She read:

It is felt that this person is really genetically and sexually a normal male ... in view of the fact that he has been brought up as a female since birth for 18 years.... it was decided to perform castration. The patient and her parents have been told that she will never menstruate and never conceive but that if she wishes to get married, an artificial vagina could be created. Neither the patient nor her parents have been told of the wrong diagnosis of sex; they still think that he is a female and we have done our best in our attitude to the patient not to alter their views about this.

There is no doubt that the series of doctors who looked after Rosemary for years without ever revealing the truth (even when she ran into severe complications from the medication she was prescribed) all felt that they were acting in her best interests. She commented: "... throughout my adult life I might well have taken different decisions had I been party to the true nature of my condition". Times have changed and it is unlikely that this extreme form of medical paternalism would occur today, but there is a generation of patients who were not considered to have the right to know their diagnosis and whose care we are now assuming.

A truthful diagnosis

When we make a diagnosis we are adamant that it must represent the truth and certain that it must be conveyed to the patient. The comfortable diagnoses of former times, full of false reassurances, that were easy for the doctor to make and easy for the patient to accept are rightly condemned nowadays. Truth is a very important value in our lives since we do not want to be deceived and we usually find it difficult to deceive others. In medicine, there are several approaches to the issue of truth-telling and we will return to some of these below. Briefly, defenders of rule or theory-based medical ethics hold that the decision whether or not to tell the truth can be made by applying various principles, especially the principle of respect for autonomy and the principle of beneficence to each individual patient. An alternative approach is based upon a therapeutic perspective whereby truth-telling is claimed to be crucial because it helps the patient to make sense of their world and to orientate themselves within it, with appropriate aims and goals. Perhaps we need to address first the more fundamental question, which relates to why this issue is of more than pragmatic importance in modern medicine.

A sense of personhood

There is something special about human beings – something tied-up with our ability to recognize that we exist – which distinguishes us, in morally relevant ways, from other animals. The great seventeenth century philosopher John Locke used the term *personhood* in referring to this specialness. A *person*, according to Locke (1694), is "a thinking intelligent being, that has reason and reflection, and can consider itself as itself, the same thinking thing, in different times and places". Persons, in this sense, have a highly articulated concept of self and of themselves as persisting over time. As rational beings, they are not mere slaves to their urges and passions. They can shape their behaviour according to plans that encompass more than the immediate future and act in ways that are rooted in values and goals that transcend mere animal instinct. Admittedly, *elements* of personhood, thus characterized, are to be found in other nonhuman animals. Nevertheless, there is a huge gulf between a normal human being beyond earliest infancy and even such sophisticated mammals as chimpanzees and dolphins. Though these animals possess their own complex signalling devices, what they have in the way of language – and what we could conceivably teach them – falls far short of our own linguistic capacities. Much of the richness of a normal human life derives directly or indirectly from language, not merely because of the depth that conversation lends to our relationships with others but also because it liberates the imagination and is a precondition of abstract thought. Perhaps the most significant abstract thoughts that we can have concern our view of ourselves and our recognition of who and what we are within the context of our family, our society, our environment.

When considering the question of "who we are", it seems obvious that we are the sum total of all the physical and psychological aspects of our bodily and mental selves. Our height, weight, build, physical prowess, talents, capabilities, strengths and weaknesses added to all our memories and experiences literally "make us who we are". As we develop and mature, our growing knowledge about all these features of ourselves is the source of our insight into our own personhood.

We may begin by asking whether we are essentially *persons*, in Locke's sense. In other words, could we have failed to be or could we at some point cease to be persons? Perceived from one angle, if the newborn baby that was me had died in early infancy, it would still be true that I had briefly existed, in spite of never achieving personhood. Likewise, if in old age I develop severe dementia it is possible that my mental faculties will eventually deteriorate to the point of loss of personhood. But it would still be me.

The Oxford philosopher and ethicist Michael Lockwood (2001) gave an example that highlights this vital difference between "persons" and "human beings".

Suppose you were suffering from severe heart disease, so severe as to be life threatening. In such circumstances, you would be delighted if, at the eleventh hour, a compatible heart became available for transplanting into your body. Now suppose, instead, that you were suffering from an inoperable brain tumour. Once again, your days appear to be numbered. But at the eleventh hour you are told that a new breakthrough in surgical technique has made it possible to remove your brain and replace it with another; and that a suitable brain has just become available in consequence of a tragic road accident. What then would be your reaction? Scarcely, I suggest, one of great delight or relief. For you would view such an operation not as saving *your* life but as saving that of the donor. It wouldn't even *be* a case of *you* getting a brain transplant. It would be a case of the donor getting a body transplant!

This response ties in well with the fact that death is now considered, in law, to mean brain death. This is why the continuation of biological life (with or without artificial aid) is insufficient for the continued existence of a human being. At a certain point, when a grieving relative objects to the doctors' proposal to withdraw life support, it is appropriate – given certain brain injuries – for the doctor to suggest that the patient is just "not there" anymore in any sense that conveys human value. This, of course, does not justify us treating "what's left" with anything less than dignity and respect, or merely as a source of potentially useful "spare parts", but the *person* has departed. What ceases to exist at brain death is what we recognize as a *human being*. And this is what we are *essentially*. The essential me

is the *mental* me, which resides in the brain; the rest of the body is merely a support system, toolbox, power pack and vehicle for getting about. What is central to our being are the brain structures that are directly implicated in consciousness. We cease to *be* when these structures become irreparably damaged in such a way that the brain can never again sustain any form of conscious mentality. And we literally *are* everything about us that consciousness supports and permits.

Consequently, if knowledge, insight and awareness are central to our concept of personhood, then it must follow that aspects of ourselves such as knowledge of the diagnosis and prognosis of conditions from which we suffer are similarly an inherent part of what it *is* to be *us*. As a parallel example, consider the very real distress and anguish of people who discover by accident in adulthood that they were adopted at birth, or that the man they have always known as dad is not their biological father. "What you don't know can't hurt you" is an inappropriate response to people who feel that their own sense of identity, their "concept of self" is bound up with the genetic as well as the social influences that have moulded them from the outset of their lives.

So if being a person ("*his own person*" as we say) is the most significant thing about being, what duties do we as persons have to other persons? As we have seen, responding to persons and respecting them is not identical with meeting their needs. It is possible to meet their needs (or our perception of their needs) without responding to them as persons. The distinction between persons and roles is also necessary: to respect persons is to refrain from reducing them to roles and functions and to refrain from seeing them from certain limited points of view. Bernard Williams (1967) stresses the distinction between "regarding a man's life, actions or character from an aesthetic or technical point of view", and "regarding them from a point of view which is concerned primarily with what it is for *him* to live that life and take those actions in that character". This would imply that a sick person is never to be regarded merely as the holder of the sick role, as the "owner" of the diagnosis. We may encounter people *through* roles: patient, relative, junior . . . . They are still persons and must be respected as such. We must try to see the world through their eyes and from their point of view. This is to show respect for their *autonomy* as persons.

The concept of autonomy is central to modern medical ethics and respect for an individual's or patient's autonomy can enhance and simplify the doctor–patient relationship in matters of truth-telling and information sharing. According to Beauchamp and Childress (1983), "Autonomy is a form of personal liberty where an individual determines his own course of action in accordance with a plan chosen by himself . . . A person's autonomy is his independence, self reliance and self-contained ability to decide."

We can recognize three types of autonomy: autonomy of thought, of will and of action. Autonomy of thought is literally thinking for oneself. But to be able to think for oneself one must have information about all the salient facts. Imagine the situation of a deaf child growing up in a signing household that conspired to maintain the fiction that there was no such thing as sound.

The brainwashed, addicted or severely depressed are all easy examples of individuals who lack autonomy of will. However, consider a little girl with AIS kept in ignorance of her diagnosis, but who plays with dolls and dreams one day of having babies of her own: her autonomy of will is just as compromised.

Autonomy of action implies the ability to move and to do in accordance with one's self-directing plan. A recent tragic court case provided an example of the unjustifiable thwarting of a patient's autonomy of action by well-meaning but misguided doctors. A young woman became paralysed from the neck down following a bleed from a vertebral vessel. Her autonomy of will and thought was intact but she was kept alive, ventilated and tube-fed, despite her repeated lucid and rational requests to be allowed to die. As you read the transcript of her bitter and angry rebuke of the doctors she felt were taking advantage of her helplessness to impose their will on her, it is hard to imagine a crueller fate.

Respect for an individual's autonomy would, therefore, seem to provide overwhelming justification for the right to know one's own diagnosis. After all, "Whose diagnosis is it anyway?" The doctor may *make* the diagnosis (and the Secretary of State for Health apparently owns the physical medical record), but the patient may be entitled to access the knowledge about themselves (particularly where that knowledge could be highly relevant to their decision making in fundamental life choices). "Knowledge is power" wrote Francis Bacon in the seventeenth century, and knowledge is certainly empowering for patients if it allows them to discuss their diagnosis with their doctor on near equal terms.

However, paternalism is not so easily dismissed. Many would agree with Ingelfinger (1980), who wrote: "If you would agree that the physician's primary duty is to make the patient feel better, a certain amount of authoritarianism, paternalism and domination are the essence of the physician's effectiveness". Likewise, the Hippocratic Oath states "I will follow that system or regimen which, according to my ability and judgement, I consider for the benefit of my patients". It says nothing about doing what they want, not deceiving them, explaining the consequences,

describing alternative courses of action, enhancing their autonomy, etc.

Real patients are scared, in pain, confused, undecided, in denial. Should we add to their distress by making them face harsh realities or make difficult choices for which we may have no evidence base to advise them? Deceit, evasions, half-truths and downright lies do not help; if doctors honestly believe that they should deceive the patient for "his own good", what about the relatives, the carers, the dependants? Advocates of strong paternalism may argue that patients "can't understand" or "can't assess what is in their own best interests" or may genuinely believe that doctors should "shoulder the burden", but the appropriate response is to educate, inform and support patients, not infantilize them.

Are we left with any cogent reasons for overriding a person's express wish for nondisclosure about an illness? This is clearly a different situation from those in which individuals are not even aware that they suffer from some pathology and are not consciously seeking medical help. Such is the situation when individuals with undiagnosed intersex disorders present to infertility clinics. They are expecting one kind of diagnosis (i.e. a probably treatable fertility problem) and they are confronted by another, that they have been living in their nongenetic gender.

It could actually be paternalistic to "force" information on unwilling patients on the grounds that it would be "best to know", so that they could "order their affairs" or prepare their families or even "reconcile themselves to God". Robert Veatch (1976) suggested that "Even in the extreme case, where the patient has freely chosen to avoid knowledge of his condition and no one else will suffer directly from his refusal, there may still be a moral duty to know one's self and one's fate". These "end of life" situations, in which Veatch seems to suggest that autonomy and dignity are goals to be promoted above all others, are clearly different from situations at the beginning of life where knowledge of a diagnosis, however painful, may be built on constructively and incorporated into a life plan. It may well be the case, as T. S. Eliot puts it, that "human kind cannot bear very much reality", but a reality that doctors have to bear, and bear bravely, is their patients' right to know their own diagnosis.

The child's need and right to understand

ALAN COOKLIN AND SANDRA RAMSDEN

Accessing the child's perspective

Some might see a need to access a child's perspective as quite a tall order. In fact, many doctors have continued to be uncertain about, or have been frankly antagonistic to, such a need with investigations and treatments that they wish to pursue.

Example

One young girl admitted for a gonadectomy had received what might be considered optimal preparation. In this case all the staff – endocrine, gynaecological, psychological, as well as others – had taken great care in her preparation for both the procedure and the adjustment issues with which she would be likely to require later help. Truly informed consent seemed to have been achieved. When this young person then suddenly refused treatment, after being informed of the possible need for a postoperative catheter by an unfamiliar admitting doctor, there was surprise and consternation.

So what happened here? In many ways the preparation was exemplary, and both the child and her parents participated actively in the decision process. Three factors were missed, however.

First, what the unfamiliar doctor explained could have had a quite different meaning for the girl from the previous explanations that had developed in a context she had begun to trust. Therefore, the fact that, from her perspective, she had not been warned about something which had a particular meaning for her – the catheter – could mean to her:

- that she was in "alien" territory and that people she did not know or feel connected to were going to do something unpredictable to her
- that if she was not warned about *this* then all her other preparations could be suspect
- that she was now in the care (and power) of someone who did *not* understand her feelings about the operation – in contrast with those who had prepared her and who she felt had understood.

Second, what has a particular meaning for a child may not be what the adults – professionals or parents – predict. The professional needs to include many of what they may have assumed are trivial details in the preparation and to seek regular and explicit confirmation from the child about how these have been understood.

Third, a particular aspect of a procedure may impinge other aspects of the child's life about which the doctor is unaware, unless he or she asks. So a child's key preoccupation may be her helplessness in being unable to influence events, such as a high level of conflict between her parents, actual divorce, illness or any other factor that she may fear could undermine the stability of the family or lead to a breakdown in her parents' capacity to function. Even a very small addition – as in this case the possible catheter – may be a trigger. This final burden may be linked to the

things that she feels are out of her control and may lead to a breakdown in her capacity to engage with a treatment process. Conversely, even a small area or issue over which she feels she has some choice may alleviate this sense of helplessness (see below).

Why talk to children about their condition and its treatment?

A meaningful answer to this question requires that one define one's model of a child and of childhood. Article 12 of the United Nations Convention on the Rights of the Child (Article 12) states:

... parties shall assure to the child who is capable of forming his or her own views the right to express those views freely in all matters affecting the child, the views of the child being given due weight in accordance with the age and maturity of the child ...

For this purpose, the child shall in particular be provided the opportunity to be heard in any judicial and administrative proceedings affecting the child, either directly, or through a representative or an appropriate body, in a manner consistent with the procedural rules of national law.

What is included in the term "administrative" is not defined but could include medical treatments. It is also not clear how a child should, or may, be represented. However, the UN convention does imply a model of a child as a potentially autonomous being with a capacity for thought and volition of his/her own, and rights that are independent of his/her parents or guardians. Although this model of childhood is implied in the legislature of some – but not all (the USA for example has not ratified the convention) – Western democracies, and is the philosophy underpinning the UK 1989 Children Act, the actual attitudes and behaviours of adults in authority towards the children for whom they are responsible may lag far behind. The implementation of adult behaviours that show respect for children's rights, and which may require new ways of eliciting a child's thought and opinions, may be much more difficult than writing legislation. Furthermore, such attitudes may be antithetic to the culture and beliefs of many cultures, particularly those based on fundamentalist religious dogma. In traditional oriental thinking, a child would not be seen as distinct from the other views and pressures of the family. In the UK, or at least in England and Wales, we have now officially abandoned the concept of parental rights, which are now replaced by "parental responsibilities". Case law is increasingly recognizing that the concepts of human rights, as represented in both the UK act and the UN convention, should be met for all UK residents regardless of race and culture.

Parental wishes

In a multicultural society, such as that in the UK, potential conflict of values between the prevailing legal framework and families own religiously or culturally determined value system may appear in many contexts such as child-care or education. In paediatric gynaecological practice, these conflicts seem predisposed to arise in cases where gender assignment and in cases where fertility may be compromised. Cultural sensitivity will be at a premium and may require the use not only of appropriate translation services and psychological services but also at times some "cultural consultation". "Same culture" medical staff may be invaluable; families may particularly appreciate a choice in sex of the examining doctor. It will be extremely important *not* to use or overuse the child patient as an interpreter where questions of consent are involved. Although this may be a familiar role for the child in many immigrant families for example, if the child does function as interpreter it may be impossible for the child to articulate their own view when consent is being considered. The concept that parents' wishes cannot take precedence over "the best interests of the child" is enshrined in the Children Act and assumes access to some dispassionate view of what is in the best interests of the child.

Example

A 15-year-old girl from a Muslim fundamentalist background and country was being treated for an abdominal tumour. Her father was heard to say she is "of no use if she cannot have children" when faced with the option of a treatment that might render her infertile. In such a case, the father's wishes cannot take precedence over "the best interests of the child".

The rights of the child

Where there is conflict beween the views of parents, medical staff and children, the right of the child to be heard is protected. In situations of dispute, at least concerning public law, a "dispassionate view" is sought from the appointment of a Guardian ad Litem (now renamed Children's Guardian) by the court. The Guardian is required take the child's point of view into account when formulating his/her own views of what is in the child's best interests but does not have to agree with or support the child's wishes. If a Guardian disagrees with a child, s/he is required to give cogent reasons why he or she has not followed the child's expressed wishes.

Children as young as 10 may sometimes be able to instruct their own lawyers, if they are in serious conflict with the views of their guardian, and it is the responsibility of the guardian's legal advisor to inform the child of his or her rights in such a case. However, the courts have also recognized a child's right to participate positively in decisions about his/her treatment, when the child is accepted as "Gillick competent" (*Gillick* v. *West Norfolk and Wisbech Area Health Authority*, 1986). This concept has no clear definition but is defined by the child's ability to understand the consequences of a decision about treatment; consequently, the age of "Gillick competence" will vary depending on the "maturity" of the child as well as the nature of the "consequences" that the child is required to understand. Furthermore, "Gillick competence" allows a child to accept treatment, independent of parental wishes, but does not allow a child under 16 years to refuse treatment that is deemed necessary by parents, guardians or doctors.

Example

AC was called urgently to the paediatric ward some years ago. He was already late for a meeting and could, therefore, only spare 20–30 minutes. There was an atmosphere of tension and anxiety in the staff when he arrived. A 15-year-old girl had been admitted for a gonadectomy as well as another abdominal procedure the following day. She was reported by her parents to have a learning disability, and her father in particular insisted on talking for her. He said she had agreed, and he thought had understood, about the gonadectomy, while adding "though she won't understand all the ins and out of it". He said he had told her about the intended additional abdominal operation the previous day ". . . and she hadn't said anything". When AC arrived on the ward, the girl had insisted to the staff that she would not have either operation. The nursing and junior medical staff were in a quandary about what to do. The father was enraged that they were listening to his daughter, rather than only to himself. There was also considerable anxiety about informing the surgeon, who had agreed to make special arrangements to carry out the operation. AC was asked what they should do.

The father's level of anger was if anything increased when AC insisted on talking to the girl on her own. After talking to her for 5–10 minutes, he concluded that she was herself angry at feeling "pushed around". He learnt that although she had some understanding about the significance of both operations, there were many aspects about which she was unclear, and she appeared not to have been able to articulate her various confusions about the nature and causes of her disorders, the goals of the operations and what she could actually expect to experience in terms of pain and discomfort, as well as long-term benefits. She herself attributed this in part to her father's tendency to decide things for her – without question – together with a complaint that the ward staff had not asked her what she knew and what she wanted to know. After they had been talking for about 15 minutes, AC further concluded that she was Gillick competent to consider the import of these procedures.

He, therefore, told her that he sympathized with her complaints and agreed that she should not agree to either of the operations without fully understanding what was involved. If it was then still her decision not to have the operations, he told her that he would fully support her decision, and she could go home. In the mean time, he said he would ask the ward doctor to arrange for the relevant doctors to come and answer any of her questions.

The girl seemed rather suspicious of this response. She was at first silent, then said she thought her father would not like it. AC said he understood this, but that in a girl of her age the doctors would not want to, and should not, operate on her unless she could understand and accept the operations. She thought for a few moments, and then when AC asked her if she would talk to the different doctors if he sent them to see her, she smiled and wished him goodbye quite cheerfully. As he was leaving the ward, AC had time to explain only briefly to her father what he had arranged. This did not appear to increase the father's equanimity. However, the nursing staff warned the surgical team about what had happened and asked for a consultant or SPR to visit to talk to the girl. The gynaecologist had already arrived. The girl decided later that day to go through with both operations. Perhaps being provided with an arena (for her unfamiliar) in which she could decide something about herself allowed her to think more objectively about and eventually decide positively about her operations (as described above).

The value of consulting the patient

In medicine there is an additional reason for ensuring that one has accessed a child's views about his/her condition and its treatment. There is now reasonable evidence that when patients in general, and children in particular, have "agency", or an element of active participation in decisions about their treatment, then their adjustment to treatment and its consequences is usually improved (Cooklin, 1989, 1993; Peterson, 1989). To achieve "agency", it is not enough to be given a "good explanation". This explanation also needs to be related to how the child currently thinks about, and perceives, his/her body, so that the "explanation" can then lead to a collaborative discussion between clinician and patient.

Overruling the child's opinion

It is important to note here that in some circumstances a child's refusal of treatment may be overridden by a person with parental responsibility for that child or by the court. Section 8 of the Family Law Reform Act 1969 entitles people of 16 or 17 years to consent to their own medical treatment, and to ancillary procedures attaching to that treatment. The 1986 Gillick judgement (*Gillick* v. *West Norfolk and Wisbech Area Health Authority*, 1986) determined that children under 16 years with sufficient understanding and intelligence to understand fully the nature of a proposed intervention will have the capacity to consent to that intervention. This is often known as "Gillick competence" and it is particularly important to note that this competence is *intervention specific*.

Decisions to overrule must, however, be based on the principle that the welfare of the child is paramount, a concept that includes the psychological well-being of that child. In the earlier example, the gynaecologist did not proceed with a procedure that was clearly necessary but in relation to which the child's consent was withdrawn. In this case, the patient was clearly *psychologically* not ready for the procedure. There is, however, no definitive guidance on when it is appropriate to overrule a competent child or young person's refusal. It should occur rarely, in individual cases and where the risk is of "grave and irreversible mental or physical harm" (Department of Health, 2001).

When to talk to children, and what to do with what they say

As already noted, the concept of competence is not codified and does not offer a set of ages or even stages when particular children can be expected to be competent to make particular decisions. Some clinicians have sought schema from the kinds of developmental stage defined by "traditional" developmental psychologists such as Piaget (1924, 1957, 1972) and Kohlberg (1981). However, the assumptions on which these are often based have been heavily criticized by Gilligan (1982), who has challenged the artificial hierarchy of "stages", which they took as read, and more significantly by Alderson (1993), who has produced one of the most "in depth" series of data on children's perceptions of their "consent" (or the lack of it) to surgery. She pointed out that the ability of quite young children to understand the complexities of relationships and events in such television programmes as *Neighbours* or *EastEnders* belies the misfit of many "standardized" tests based on the Piagetian model. In addition, changes in our different cultures, and child-rearing practices, which may actually require children to think more for themselves, may also lead to a change in children's capacity to process the information that can then be the basis of decisions. Alderson's (1993) book offered a compelling description of how different children, often as young as five years of age, can be helped to understand and positively participate in decisions about their treatment. It also demonstrated that children sometimes have a clearer technical understanding of their disorder and its treatment than their doctors realise (and sometimes more than their parents), and that they often endure considerable distress, which may not have been communicated to any adult and which may be intensified by their lack of access to direct discussion with an understanding doctor.

Reder and Fitzpatrick (1998) considered the advocacy of "a presumption of competence" of the child in the realm of consent to medical and surgical interventions, with the onus on adults to show where a child may be incompetent. These authors indicated an important omission in this approach, the vulnerability of children to personal or interpersonal conflict. Valid consent must be given voluntarily and children may be particularly influenced by parents, carers, peers, sexual partners or others. Consideration of these influences may be a complex clinical task.

Example

Andrew was aged 13 years and suffered from non-Hodgkins lymphoma. If asked if he knew of any disadvantages that might result from the treatment he was receiving, he would say, "No, only from missing some school and that . . . but my school have been really good and have helped me keep up".

The following conversation illustrates how an "active" conversation can enable a doctor to elicit more information regarding the level of understanding of their child patient.

DOCTOR And no-one has mentioned any other possible effects of the treatment?

ANDREW No . . . tho' my mum did tell me about fertility and that. She's seen a programme on the TV about it.

DOCTOR What did that tell you then?

ANDREW Well that as a result of the chemo, I might not be able to have a kid.

DOCTOR Had any of the doctors told you about that?

ANDREW No . . . and my Mum only told me after she saw the programme on Wednesday.

DOCTOR Do you think you would mind – trying to imagine now what you might think in say 10 years time – do you think you would mind if you could not – or at least [both laugh] if a woman could not – have a kid with you?

ANDREW Well not if the kid was anything like the way my brothers treat my Mum [both laugh].

The doctor establishes that Andrew is fully conversant with normal reproduction.

DOCTOR Well I realise that you do not yet know whether or not the treatment you have been given is likely to have that effect on your ball's ability to make sperm . . . and we can check on that with Dr Morton in a minute . . . but if it did have that effect in the future, do you know if there is any other way you could . . .

ANDREW Oh, you mean like sperm banking and that. Well, I don't know if I could because nobody's told me anything about it.

DOCTOR Right, something else we can check in a minute. So how do you think they get the sperm to put in the bank?

Andrew grins and makes a motion simulating masturbation.

Andrew had not been offered sperm-banking as it was assumed that he was too young, but no-one had elicited the fact that he had had wet dreams. It was assumed that he did not know about it, or how to *do* it. However, he did know (from his mother who had seen it on a TV programme). However, he did *not* know whether or not the treatment he had received was toxic to his germ cells, and he had not asked – and no-one knew that!

Engaging a child in an "active" conversation about his/her illness and treatment

There seems, then, to be no alternative for the doctor but to engage in a discussion with each child about what he/she already understands about his/her illness and treatment, what he/she needs and wants to know, how much he or she can balance the fears (for example of needles) against the need to treat the illness, and how much he or she wants to participate actively in any relevant clinical decisions. Lansdown (1998) has offered a thumbnail schema to help doctors in this task. This is based on a number of principles.

1 That children should be both listened to and taken seriously, regardless of whether or not the final decision is based on their expressed wishes.

2 That real consent is part of a process, involving continued discussion, rather than a "one off" talk. During that process, the child's competence to participate in the decision will not only become clearer but may itself be enhanced.

3 That all children, who can communicate, can take some decisions. The developmental stage of a child may only define the "weight" of decision that a particular child may be able to take on board.

4 That, although one needs to be alert to the danger that treatment may be "treating" principally the parent or even the doctor, rather than the child, the degree to which the clinical decision will affect other people should be a factor that is taken into consideration. Lansdown included the adult the child may become as one of those people.

All of the above assumes that doctors, Guardians or others who need to access children's perspectives are able to engage in a conversation with a child that will elicit that child's actual thinking and opinions, rather than those sought and/or expected by the professional. For many children, a concept of "consent" may have unexpected, or sometimes minimal, meaning, particularly when the child has no actual knowledge of what pain or other effects are involved. Among other factors, the child's view of the concept may be influenced by:

1 The age and maturity of the child.
2 The nature of, and the degree of anxiety associated with, and previous experience of the illness, and therefore the degree to which a child may expect and/or wish to hand over control to his or her parents.
3 The cultural traditions of the family, and the degree to which the child would expect to participate in any decisions about his or her own body.

The last of these is likely to determine the child's previous experience of being, or not being, invited to participate in giving consent about matters relating to him- or herself. Most children in all the different cultures with which we are likely to have contact will have had the experience of adults who expect them to "agree" with, or at least to acquiesce to, the "wisdom" of those adults. The child is, therefore, likely to perceive any attempt at "discussion" by a doctor as a demand for compliance.

It is particularly important not to mistake compliance for consent. It is also essential to review consent over time and if any significant changes occur, in the condition itself, in its treatment, in the child's coping strategies or in the wider family context. Consent will have in itself an evolving, changing state that is influenced by many factors including the treatment and the perceived responses to treatment in the patient by the patient and significant others (GMC, 1998). To elicit a child's active participation, a doctor will have to find ways to combat the child's expectation that he or she should comply with adults in general, and with doctors in particular. "Informed" consent requires not only that a child has been adequately helped to understand the issues pertinent to the decisions about treatment, but also that that child has been "informed" that his or her opinion matters. The question is how is a child, particularly one who is not used to having his or her opinions even considered or heard, going to be "informed" that this is a different situation and that this doctor genuinely wants to know how he or she is thinking about the treatment, and that this will have relevance for how the treatment will actually be conducted. This is not going to come about as a result of a simple "declaration" and explanation by a doctor on a "one off" basis. It requires that the doctor demonstrates that a different kind of conversation is both possible and sought after. This, in turn, can only be demonstrated through the kind of conversation that the doctor engages in with the child, which somehow conveys the message that "compliance" of opinion is not required and that the doctor will welcome hearing a different point of view from the child as a basis of their discussions.

Traditional forms of discussion between adults and children could often be defined as *didactic*. The ultimate goal never strays from that of ensuring that the child acknowledges the adult's wisdom. The worst examples can even include rhetorical questions masquerading as invitations to the child to express a point of view: "So what did I say when you said you were scared?" (To which the child is required to explain why he/she was afraid.) "I said you can tell me why." (So that the child's perspective can be demolished.) A *dialectic* conversation, by comparison, invites expression of real difference. (The *Shorter Oxford Dictionary* (1973) definition of dialectical is "The process of thought by which such contradictions are seen to merge themselves in a higher truth that comprehends them".) In a dialectical relationship, differences are juxtaposed as a valid subject for comment, debate and argument. It may, of course, lead to an argument or debate, but the essential ingredient of a dialectic relationship is that differences can be juxtaposed and considered. The problem for a doctor is less likely to be the intelligence or maturity of the child, although these are important factors, but whether the child's "thinking participation" is "switched on" or not. The level of the child's anxiety may be a further impediment acting against this "switching on".

Facilitating discussion

What will facilitate dialectic discussion? First, the doctor needs to establish a shared habit of discussion and banter with the child. This does not mean asking each child what his or her favourite football star is – particularly if the child detests football! It may mean finding out what this child enjoys, is good at, and his/her opinions about some aspects of his or her life. It will require that a doctor finds out in detail how this child understands his or her illness and its treatment, how he or she learnt what he/she "knows", and from whom. It may need the doctor to ask which aspects of the illness or the treatment the child would like to understand more about. The doctor may have to put considerable effort into distinguishing what is known from what is believed and/or hoped for, and to help the child to organize this into a form that fits both his or her developmental stage as well as the metaphors commonly used by the child. So a child who enjoys jigsaws may be able to understand antibodies easily in terms of pieces that do or do not fit.

Most children and young people will need to gain some visual image of what is being explained – of cells or of tumour cells as like "weeds" for example – in order for them to gain sufficient mastery over the idea for them to be able to consider options.

Some principles of a dialectical approach can be summarized.

1 Avoid "problem-focused" talk. To achieve any level of trust, a child needs to experience the adult as genuinely interested in his or her positive attributes and life, not only as sources of worry or anxiety. So rather than saying "You must have been very worried about all these treatments", it might be preferable to say "How did you find a way to manage all these treatments so well?"

2 Presume nothing: be "behind" rather than "ahead" of the child. Resist a common professional tendency to try and guess at, or even "suggest", what the child is thinking or feeling. It is preferable to ask a child to explain, and if necessary to acknowledge that one does not understand something a child is trying to express, and then to ask him or her to help you. So, rather than saying "You must have been very sad to see your Mum looking so low?", it might be preferable to say "So when you saw Mum like that what was it like?" If the child says "I don't know...", or "Nothing really", a question that is "easier to answer than to not answer" may be useful, such as "Well was it the sort of thing that might make a daughter more cross, more sad, or more worried?" (See below.)

3 Ask questions that are easier to answer than not to answer. A child who is anxious or frightened may respond to "open" questions by trying to, or fearing a failure to, find the answer the adult is "seeking". A child can often respond to binary or multiple-choice questions more freely, because he or she can select one of the choices, reject all of them or make a different point. So a "multiple-choice" question may be easier to answer, and more difficult to avoid, than an open question, as also may be the case if the question is not forcibly personalized. So rather than saying "You must feel very responsible for your Mum's upset", it may be preferable to say "Did you know that many kids in this situation seem to feel as though they are responsible for caring for their parents, rather than the other way round – its strange isn't it?"

4 Make no interpretations or presumptions about a child's experience... but ask! The importance of not playing "guessing games" with children and young people has already been highlighted. Given time, patience and a demonstration that the professional is prepared to wait for the child to think and speak, rather than "thinking for" him or her, children of all ages will attempt to articulate even their most complex ideas. Professionals who "suggest" the meaning of what the child is trying to say may "kill" the child's own attempts to clarify his or her own thoughts. However, if a child consistently talks with, or draws, some repetitive images that he or she seems stuck with, one might suggest to the child that these images have given a "funny" idea, and ask if he or she wants to hear about it. Occasionally a child will say firmly "No", in which case this should be respected. If the child says "Yes", then one might say: "You keep asking me about whether doctors learn to sew, and there's all those pictures you drew of people that didn't heal up. Do you think you could be worried about whether the doctors will be able to heal you up properly after the operation?" If the child says "Yes", one may need to say "OK lets think together about how they do it, now". If the child says "No! I just drew them because...", one should probably say "Oh...right...", but one may wish to add later "...by the way do you know how they do it?"

5 Challenge the child's expectation of compliance to adults. This is the most difficult part of a dialectical approach, because it goes against not only all adult habits of thinking about children's ideas, but also children's expectations of how they will be expected to behave. It requires not only a change of tone in the conversation with a child but often a change in one's expectations and the whole way of thinking about children and their ideas. One of the most useful ways to approach this is seriously to encourage a child to tell one about some area of expertise about which he or she is more competent than oneself, and then both question and respectfully debate his or her point of view. It could be something as simple as how some girls think boys are a disruptive influence in the class. One can then discuss why this might be: does she think she will never want boys in the same class and has she noticed how some girls seem to change their opinion about this when they get older.

6 Allow a language of contest (but not combat) and talk that may appear as "silly" and playful at the same time as being serious, but avoid insincere "forced" jocularity.

7 The *goal* is to help the child think, not to elicit feelings. Children will show what they feel as and when they choose.

Many doctors commonly do avoid such statements as "You must be very sad that... or very worried that...". These are often the currency of mental health professionals and this type of statement may err at the other extreme by not allowing a child a chance to describe any of his or her experience. However, it is generally better to focus on what the child has achieved or to frame questions in terms of possible achievements, such as: "...So if you were worried about that, how did you stop that worry from taking over your life/mind/thoughts etc.".

The goal is to help the young person to find his or her voice, and to articulate this voice. In situations of high stress, a child may be struggling with multiple, inconsistent or ambiguous voices inside him or herself. Reconciling these internal different voices makes it difficult for all children and young people to respond to key dilemmas that they may face in the course of treatment, but this is exacerbated if there are significantly different voices within the family, such as between the parents. In these situations, children and young people may often protect themselves by sticking steadfastly to one particular story, even though they may, in fact, often feel invaded by the multiplicity of the pressures from adults. In these situations, the child's mind is almost literally "switched off" – a form of language that is quite familiar to many children. If one asks, for example, if he or she will show you "where the switch is", they will often point with good humour to the back of the mastoid, the occiput or some other "location". When a child is in such a state, it is relatively futile to try to engage him or her in a conversation that requires participation in an important decision. The doctor or other professional then needs to try to influence the factors which might allow the child to become "switched on". There are some ways in which doctors may be able to increase the possibility of a child being "switched on" to think actively with them rather than just responding passively:

- the child's degree of anxiety needs to be at a level that he or she can manage
- the child needs information on which to base a choice
- information needs to be understandable and "imaginable"
- the professional needs to ensure that the child's "image" of the "words" is close enough to that being used professionally
- the relationship with the professional, and his/her way of defining questions and giving information, needs to challenge the expectation of compliance
- the child needs help to construct a "pros" and "cons" list.

The last of these can be particularly helpful. Not only does it allow the child to distance him- or herself from the painful nature of the decision to be taken, but it also provides a nonthreatening avenue through which the doctor can offer advise by suggesting factors for one or other side of the list.

Example

In the following conversation with Ginny, a 14-year-old girl, it can be seen that, in some ways, she has not understood some key points. Ginny was being offered oophoropexy prior to radiotherapy as a treatment for Hodgkin's disease. The interview lasted about 40 minutes. Four or five minutes were spent discussing her school, and the degree to which she had so far "beaten" her illness by nearly keeping up with her peers.

DOCTOR So how does your illness work then...what does it do?

GINNY I think the lymph cells keep growing...and they can like take over.

DOCTOR The lymph cells...so what are they exactly?

GINNY Well I'm not sure exactly...they're something to do with the blood, but not exactly blood, and they fight infection I think.

DOCTOR That's pretty good as a description...so why's it a problem do you think?

GINNY Well...I don't know exactly...I think if they take over they can harm the rest of the body.

DOCTOR So how do you think this treatment works then?

GINNY Can't remember...Oh yes, I think the radiation stops them from overgrowing.

DOCTOR Hmm...but then any idea how it would do that?

Ginny is pensive, then

GINNY I don't know...I suppose it kills them...or some of them.

DOCTOR So do you think there could be any disadvantages to this treatment?

GINNY Do you mean if it didn't work?

DOCTOR Well, no not exactly, because I believe there's a very good chance it would work in killing the excess overgrowth...but any other disadvantage you've been told about?

Ginny looks puzzled and a bit uncomfortable.

DOCTOR OK, let's draw it

He draws an "open" abdomen and highlights enlarged lymph glands in the lower abdomen, then turns to Ginny.

DOCTOR So now you've been shown what a radiation machine looks like. Let's direct a ray at those big glands.

Ginny looks tentatively at the drawing then draws a yellow beam (which is straight and parallel).

DOCTOR So, now let's put in all the other bits that are around there...do you know of any of them?

Ginny thinks for a few moments then hesitantly.

GINNY Well there's the bladder and (with slight embarrassment) the womb...

DOCTOR Yeah...do you know what an embryo is?

GINNY Yes, the beginnings of a baby.

DOCTOR Right, so where's it going to come from?

GINNY The eggs got to be fertilized.

DOCTOR Yes, I agree about that, but where's the egg going to come from?

GINNY Isn't it the ovaries?

DOCTOR Yes, could you draw them in, or would you like me to?

Ginny then draws a quite respectable diagram of ovaries next to, but not overlapping, the tumour.

DOCTOR The thing about the cells in the ovaries is that they are very sensitive and can be easily damaged by anything like radiation, so can you see a possible problem?

GINNY You mean like I might not be able to have babies?

Although this is said calmly, she in fact looks extremely anxious as she says it.

DOCTOR Well yes, unless there was a way to protect the ovaries.

The operation of oophoropexy was then explained to Ginny. It transpired that she had, in fact, known that there was an alternative treatment for Hodgkin's disease. She had not actually been offered a choice, but she was very relieved that she would not lose her hair, about which she had been very worried after a visit to the young people's cancer ward. She did, however, assume, although not explicitly informed of this, that the operation would be an almost automatic success. She became quite tearful when it was necessary to tell her that it was about a 1 in 2 chance that it would work. However she was then helped to build a "pro" and "cons" about the operation, and eventually opted for it.

Summary

This chapter has discussed various aspects of helping patients and their families to understand and participate in decisions about their treatment. This is particularly hard with children or those with learning difficulties. Talking to children is clearly advocated. The problem of the doctor's sense of competence or relative incompetence, or even his or her possible lack of knowledge about children's development, has not been addressed. Rather the chapter has intended to present doctors with the need and challenge of

communicating with their patients. This is, in the authors' view, a great opportunity. Some children may not appear to "want" (or have the habit of exercising) choice over their bodies, but they still need to be given the opportunity, which they may then chose to delegate back to their parents or carers.

REFERENCES

Alderson P (1993). *Children's Consent to Surgery*. Open University Press: Buckingham.

Beauchamp T, Childress J (1983). *Principles of Biomedical Ethics*. Oxford University Press, Oxford.

Cooklin A I (1989). Tenderness and toughness in the face of distress. *Palliative Med* 3, 89–95.

(1993). Psychological changes in adolescence. In *The Practice of Medicine in Adolescence*, Brook C, ed. Edward Arnold, London.

Department of Health (2001). *Reference Guide to Consent for Examination or Treatment*. Department of Health, London.

Family Law Reform Act (1969). HMSO, London.

GMC (General Medical Council) (1998). *Seeking Patients' Consent: The Ethical Considerations*. GMC, London.

Gillick v. *West Norfolk and Wisbech Area Health Authority* (1986). AC 112.

Gilligan C (1982). *In a Different Voice*. Harvard University Press, Cambridge, MA.

Ingelfinger F J (1980). Arrogance. *N Engl J Med* 303, 1507–1511.

Kohlberg L (1981). *The Philosophy of Moral Development*. Harper & Row, New York.

Lansdown R (1998). Ignoring the wishes and needs of an ill child cannot be right. *J Roy Soc Med* 91, 9.

Locke J (1694). *An Essay Concerning Human Understanding*, 2nd edn, II, xxvii. Oxford University Press, Oxford.

Lockwood M (2001). The moral status of the human embryo. *Hum Fertil* 4, 267–269.

Peterson L (1989). Coping by children undergoing stressful medical procedures: some conceptual, methodological, and therapeutic issues. *J Consult Clin Psychol* 57, 331–332.

Piaget J (1924). *The Language and Thought of the Child*. Routledge, London.

(1957). *Logic and Psychology*. Basic Books, New York.

(1972). *The Moral Judgement of the Child*. Routledge, London.

Reder P, Fitzpatrick G (1998). What is sufficient understanding? Clin Child Psychol Psychiatry, 3, 103–113.

Shorter Oxford Dictionary (1973). Oxford University Press, Oxford.

The Children Act (1989). HMSO, London.

Veatch R (1976). *Death, Dying and the Biological Revolution*. Yale University Press, Princeton, NJ.

Williams B (1967). The idea of equality. In *Philosophy, Politics and Society*, Laslett P, Runciman W G, pp. 116–117. Basil Blackwell, Oxford.

17

Patients and parents in decision making and management

Margaret Simmonds

Androgen Insensitivity Syndrome Support Group (AISSG),
www.medhelp.org/www/ais

So now, where should they begin? How should they co-ordinate their slow crawl back from the desert? What should they say? What could they tell people? Who was entitled to the whole story and who could be kept at a distance with a half-truth?

Anna's parents knew the facts – knew the possibilities, that is – but then settled for not talking about them. They pretended that they were sparing their daughter's feelings, but really they were sparing their own. Nothing in their lives had prepared them for catastrophe.

Hilary Mantel, 1995

Patients and parents whose lives are affected by intersex conditions such as androgen insensitivity syndrome (AIS) have chances to influence decision making and management both in the clinical setting and in the family. The prime qualifications for this are a knowledge-base and confidence to articulate concerns and information to doctors, family, partners and friends. This chapter explores some of the psychology of being a patient or a parent under these circumstances so that clinicians can better understand their needs and idosyncrasies in relation to some medical conditions that have been subject to a great deal of ignorance, secrecy, shame and taboo.

We shall examine chronologically, from birth to adulthood, the issues that affect decision making, bringing in parental issues. The basic assumptions are (i) that the doctors have truthfully disclosed the full diagnosis, at least to the parents, (ii) that we are considering decisions made not only in the clinical setting but also in the outside life of the parents/adults concerned, (iii) that the observations relate mainly to AIS and similar conditions, and (iv) that we are considering patients at the female end of the male–female continuum since that is the main area of experience/expertise of the AIS Support Group (AISSG) and since this is a gynaecology textbook.

For most of the 50 years since Morris first reported the phenomenon of "testicular feminization" in the medical literature (Morris, 1953), the main tenet of the doctor–patient relationship has been actively to discourage open and informed discussion about such topics, both within and outside of the clinical setting, and in the outside world. Since the early 1990s, this has started to change, helped by societal and technological changes. The advent of the acquired immunodeficiency syndrome (AIDS) gave the general public a vocabulary for talking about sex. The rise of Internet communications/publishing has provided an ideal medium for isolated "sufferers" to make contact with each other and discuss their situation (with a high degree of privacy or even anonymity) and for the patient support/advocacy groups that emerged in the early–mid 1990s to establish a worldwide presence.

For the 50% of AIS patients diagnosed in infancy/childhood, possibly as a result of inguinal herniae, it is probably the attitude of their parents that will be the most pervasive in their adjustment to their situation as they grow up. However, the parents themselves will be hugely influenced by the behaviour of the clinicians who care for their child, as will the older child to some extent through how she is treated during early clinic visits. For those patients diagnosed in adolescence as a result of primary amenorrhoea, their introduction to the subject is likely to be by direct interface with a diagnosing clinician, but with parents and family influencing the degree of openness and acceptance thereafter. Most patients in this category say that their interaction with the clinician who diagnosed them is hard-etched into their memory and has an enormous impact on the way they see their condition, and themselves in the years that follow. In either situation, it is the way in

Paediatric and Adolescent Gynaecology, ed. Adam Balen et al. Published by Cambridge University Press.
© Cambridge University Press 2004.

which the clinician handles the clinic interaction that is of supreme importance in setting the scene, with the parents playing a vital secondary role.

Of course it is the *patient* who *has* the condition and will have to deal with it on a practical level throughout her life, and yet so much of clinical practice over the years seems to have been aimed, not necessarily intentionally, at making the parents and even the doctors feel better about the situation, at the expense of the patient's long-term well-being.

Dr David Sandberg (1995/6), a health care professional (psychologist) and adult intersexual from Buffalo Children's Hospital's Psychoendocrinology Department wrote:

The program for treating intersexed children is actually geared towards the parents, not the child. When the child grows to adulthood, and is no longer the parents' child and charge, s/he is invariably "lost to follow-up". The problem disappears – for family and medical professionals – but *we* are left alone in our agony, isolated from peers and any emotional support, left to contemplate, alone, "what is wrong with me".

Doctors may say 'One might wish the world to be different [that parents should accept, and not feel compelled to "normalize", their intersexed child] but that's the way it is'. I was born intersexed, and my parents were horrified and ashamed. I was 'treated', and lied to, and I was made to feel like a freak and a monster *anyway*. And *that's* the way it is.

Surgery is not at the top of my personal list of grievances; that place is reserved for the cruelty of silence and the restriction of choice. I want to see parents and clinicians have as much information as possible – especially the stories and feelings of intersexed adults – as they make decisions about the care of intersexed infants and children.

With or without surgery, if the parents see their child as a 'freak', the prognosis is poor. Families need to receive counseling at all stages in the child's development. The child also needs age-appropriate information, with the goal of full [truth] disclosure. I cannot imagine anything worse than such an individual learning from a total stranger at some point in adulthood that all they had been told were lies or half-truths.

Neonatal/childhood treatment

Feminizing genitoplasty

There are essentially two related but somewhat separated situations here. First, there is the baby who has genitals that are "ambiguous" (i.e. not typical of either of the two currently recognized sexes) such that questions arise about the appropriate sex of rearing and about whether surgery should be employed to reinforce the chosen gender. Second, there is the child who is clearly at the female end of

the male/female continuum of genital appearance but has a larger than average clitoris so that surgery perhaps has a higher "cosmetic" component to it.

In a pioneering article, social psychologist Suzanne Kessler (1990) analysed interviews with six specialists in paediatric intersexuality concerning the medical decision-making process and described how *cultural* assumptions about sexuality in effect supersede objective criteria for gender assignment. In doing so she made three key statements:

There are no published studies on how these [intersexed] adolescents experience their condition and their treatment by doctors.

There is no reported data on how much emphasis the intersexed person himself, or herself, places upon genital appearance and functioning.

Most doctors claimed that the parents were equal partners in the whole process but they gave no instances of parental participation prior to the gender assignment.

Paediatric urologist Justine Schober (1998) wrote:

Success in psychosocial adjustment is the true goal of sexual assignment and genitoplasty. The psychosocial long-term outcomes represent the most necessary information to determine if we are successful in treating intersexual patients. However, in conditions other than CAH [congenital adrenal hyperplasia], outcomes are generally unavailable ... Surgery makes parents and doctors more comfortable but counseling makes people comfortable too, and is not irreversible. Patients wonder if thinking that surgery will improve the psychological outcome for the intersexual child is a mistake. They question if surgery could mean impairment of sexual function in adulthood. It may be illusory, but patients believe that the ability to choose for oneself may favourably affect the results of surgery. Surgery must be based on truthful disclosure and support, and permit decision-making by parents and patient.

The intelligent and articulate mother of a 15-month-old infant with partial AIS (PAIS) and ambiguous genitalia wrote a long letter to the UK AISSG in mid 1999 (Anon., 2001a). The infant had been whisked away following a caesarean birth and undergone feminizing genitoplasty on the recommendation of an endocrinologist, a surgeon and two paediatricians. The parents had been afforded very little say in the matter having been given no information to enable them to contribute to the decision. The mother said that she had later obtained a few copies of the group's newsletter, *ALIAS*, and that "It was a huge relief to finally get some in-depth and honest information, which as a concerned parent I was totally desperate for". She said that her endocrinologist had "told her to be wary of support group information and seemed to think the education he provided would be sufficient". "How very wrong he was!" she said.

She described the tumultuous emotions she went through after the birth and how she would sneak out of the bedroom at night to cry uncontrollably. She and her husband decided they needed more information but said that "pestering our endocrinologist and surgeon was of very little help as they had only scant answers where we needed in-depth discussions" and that "attempts to encourage our endocrinologist to help us make contact with other families affected by AIS [. . .] were met with rather weak excuses, e.g. [that] after the first year or so of diagnosis most families have come to terms with AIS and don't want to network but prefer to get on with life."

Their endocrinologist eventually sent them a copy of Dr Gary Warne's patient/parent booklet on complete AIS (CAIS) (Warne, 1997). Through him, and the support group, the mother made contact with other parents and affected adults. She said she "spent many hours on the phone [to these people] and began to have a sense of empowerment that knowledge brings . . . ". She expressed much gratitude for the support group's newsletter. However, she also said that reading in *ALIAS* about the growing debate concerning childhood genital surgery *after* her child had undergone this procedure had filled her with doubts and remorse that she had "allowed" this to happen. She wondered whether the support group was unhealthily biased against such surgery. Her anger and emotional turmoil were partly based on a fear that the wrong decision could have been made and her child's future compromised, but also on a feeling that her desire for information and her right to be involved in the decision making had been ignored, overridden or obstructed.

In 1995, at a time when adult intersexuals were just starting to question the wisdom of childhood genital surgery, and intersex support/advocacy groups were becoming established, the following was included in the *ALIAS* newsletter (Anon., 1995a).

In a recent TV documentary, made by a Jewish father, and bravely questioning the ethical basis of religious circumcision, a psychotherapist said: 'At one time the prospect of not sacrificing live animals to the Gods would have seemed unimaginable in our society. But once people start to question the accepted view and say "I'm going to do things differently", that gradually becomes "the way things are".'

However, it was difficult to imagine the bravery of those first few parents who went against the established practice with respect to genital surgery. Yet by 2000, not only had several intersex taskforces/working parties been set up to evaluate the issues (e.g. in North America, the North American Task Force on Intersex (NATFI); in the UK, the British Association of Paediatric Surgeons Working Party on the Problems of Children Born with Ambiguous Genitalia; in Australia, the

Murdoch Children's Research Institute (MCRI) Sex Study Group), with some of them involving support group representatives as well as clinicians, but some parents were doing their own research and rejecting surgery on their children.

The mother of a child aged three and a half years with 5α-reductase deficiency emailed from the USA in late 2000 (Anon., 2001b). She related how, about a year earlier, on the basis of tests that suggested 5α-reductase deficiency (and not the PAIS that was originally diagnosed), she and her husband had reassigned their child from girl to boy and did not plan any surgery unless the child requests it when older. She said:

Of course, if the doctors had had their way, his penis and testes would have been taken out *way* before results of the tests were available. As it was, the doctor waited 4 *months* to tell us that the initial diagnosis was incorrect. I was *so* angry. Research has shown that there is brain masculinization in utero for these children [with 5α-reductase deficiency] and that these children will continue to masculinize normally at puberty (although his penis and genital differences will never change). And these children do form a strong male gender identity.

The mother of an infant diagnosed with 46,XY mixed gonadal dysgenesis described whether or not to allow clitoral reduction surgery (Anon., 2000a). In November 2000, when the child was aged 18 months, she explaining how she and her husband had arrived at their decision not to allow the surgery (Anon., 2001b):

A mix of emotions surfaced for us [when problem was discovered at birth]; sadness, frustration and confusion. The surgeons attempted to console us by recommending cosmetic surgery, including a clitoral recession to 'normalize' the size of her 'moderately enlarged' clitoris . . . . The endocrinologist was not much help either, saying only to do "whatever the surgeons recommend".

Without any tangible education or support, we set out on our own . . . . We found helpful information on various websites including AISSG, ISNA and ISGI. We met with Cheryl Chase of ISNA who provided numerous articles and put us in touch with several parents. We spoke to Deborah Brown of ISGI at length on the telephone . . . . We met with Bruce Wilson, M.D., an Endocrinologist at Devos Children's Hospital in Grand Rapids, MI and spoke to his colleague William G. Reiner, M.D., a Psychiatrist at Johns Hopkins University. Some of the articles we read included *Management of Intersex: A Shifting Paradigm* by Bruce E. Wilson and William G. Reiner [1999]; *Rethinking Treatment for Ambiguous Genitalia* by Cheryl Chase [1999]; and *Care and Counseling of the Patient with Vaginal Agenesis* by Sallie Foley, ACSW and George W. Morley, M.D. [1992].

Some parents are also taking things into their own hands in areas such as diagnostic tests. A 38-year-old group member with CAIS emailed from Continental Europe (April 2001):

My sister is pregnant $5^{1}/_{2}$ months now and they do not know if she is a carrier. But they do know she will have a XY child, from a amniocentesis earlier in the pregnancy (the carrier tests did not have result yet, and the pregnancy came 'suddenly'). Last Friday they had a ultrasound to look at the baby's sex. The doctors whispered a lot, looked for almost an hour, but did not want to tell the results. The doctors wanted a team discussion – about the ultrasound video they made of it – after the weekend and told her they would let her obstetrician know. They left the parents in despair. This weekend they could not wait anymore, and they went to a commercial ultrasound office whom they did not tell the reason, but the lady there confirmed it was a baby girl, so an AIS child!

Gonadectomy/childhood hormone replacement therapy

Clinicians do not seem to have a consensus view on whether puberty in AIS is "better" or "more natural" via oestrogens from intact testes or from oestrogen from hormone replacement therapy (HRT) following early gonadectomy. On the cancer front, the risk in AIS seems so low before adulthood that early gonadectomy is not justified on these grounds alone (Anon., 1996a).

There is also the ethical issue of removing organs from a child without their informed consent and the question of whether early gonadectomy paves the way for the adults to gloss over the child's condition, and indulge in secrecy and subterfuge, in the teenage years. It has been suggested at a medical conference on AIS that childhood gonadectomy is more often practised for the convenience of the doctors/parents than because of any proven/documented benefit to the patient.

The mother of an infant with CAIS complained in 2001 that a paediatric endocrinologist's first words to her were "OK, so when's she coming in to have those gonads taken out?" and that she felt very pressured to agree to the surgery without any real discussion about it. The rapid advances in reproductive technology may mean that, when today's infants reach adulthood, the primitive spermatic material from intact AIS testes might be used to fertilize an egg donated perhaps by an XX relative? This is a good enough reason for not having them removed prematurely unless absolutely necessary.

At a UK AISSG meeting, one well-informed family said that they were not going to make the decision regarding gonadectomy on behalf of their nine-year-old AIS daughter and that the child's CAIS aunt still had her testes at age 32. Some parents are becoming aware of the high incidence of osteopenia and osteoporosis in adult women with AIS (Anon., 1996b) and are questioning whether early gonadectomy could contribute to this.

It seems also that XX girls start producing oestrogen earlier than previously thought, some years before any outward signs of puberty (Anon., 1997a) and produce more oestrogen from their ovaries than XY girls do from their testes. One of our UK medical advisors (Dr Richard Stanhope, Paediatric Endocrinologist, Institute of Child Health and Great Ormond St Children's Hospital, London) is, therefore, recommending that girls with AIS should be started on low-dose oestrogen HRT while still in childhood in order to help them to lay down healthy bone tissue, even if they still have their testes (Anon., 1996b). Some parents are starting to ask about this.

Tissue samples and informed consent

At a UK AISSG meeting, some parents of young children with AIS had many questions about diagnostic and carrier status testing. Concern was expressed about the time taken to gain the results of the latter. The practice of taking genital skin samples from the clitoris or labia of young children seemed to be a source of particular anxiety. Several parents expressed confusion as to the purpose of such samples; they questioned whether informed consent by parents was being observed, and they related how long-term physical discomfort and psychological trauma in their child had resulted from this practice.

They asked whether such procedures were needed in order to make a diagnosis. The combined wisdom of those at the meeting with medical knowledge suggested that a diagnosis of AIS could be reached by doing relatively simple tests on a blood sample (genetic karotyping, examination of the response to injected hormones, etc.) – tests which could be carried out by their own regional hospital. Any tests requiring a genital skin sample would be to research the exact mechanism of the inability of the body cells to respond to androgens, genital skin being chosen because of its high concentration of androgen receptors.

In some cases, parents were being told in vague terms that such tests "would help doctors understand more about AIS" but they were not receiving any feedback on what the tests had revealed and said they felt that the information flow was often one-way only: from the family to the doctors. One mother angrily told how, the day before a gonadectomy on her 8-year-old child (diagnosed as an infant), she received a phone call from a researcher at another, distant hospital asking her permission for a genital skin sample to be taken during the surgery, indicating that details of her child's condition had been passed on to a clinician who was not responsible for her care.

The mother of a 23 year old with AIS described how she had recently arranged to have carrier-status tests done on various family members by a specialist AIS research department in a hospital outside her health area and with whom her family had had no previous contact. While chasing the results by phone, she was shocked to be told that the department had known about her and her family in relation to AIS for many years.

Parental attitudes

Opportunities and problems

At a UK AISSG meeting, the AIS adults were asked by the parents how traumatic they thought the revelation of XY chromosomes and testes would be to a teenager (assuming a female gender identity). The adults thought it depended largely on how solidly the youngster had been able to build a positive sense of self and gender up to that point and, very importantly, how good her future prospects of fulfilling a role in relationships seemed to her.

The adults offered an analysis based on their observations of young women who had attended all the support group meetings to date. The worst outcome appeared to be where there had been a long-term awareness in the family of "a problem" (and possibly a diagnosis) but with secrecy and/or a lack of openness and discussion about it, or where there had been childhood hernias with mysterious unexplained operations and/or a discovery of vaginal hypoplasia. The best scenario appeared to be (i) where the first hint of a problem was the failure to menstruate in teenage years and (ii) where there was no severe vaginal hypoplasia. Paradoxically, the first situation gives the parents the most time to come to terms with things and plan how to help their daughter in an open and progressive way, and yet this so often *does not* happen. The second scenario is "a-bolt-out-of-the-blue," but since parents and teenager are learning the facts together there is less chance of an atmosphere of secrecy and shame developing; and, of course, the parents have already seen that their daughter has not grown up to be a freak, even if that is how *she* sees herself.

It is vital that parents of young children should meet affected adults and observe reality rather than living with their imaginations and fears. Parents need to "open the box", take everything out, have a really good look at it and maybe repack it in a different configuration so that they are swept along neither by clinicians' exhortations about how "normal" and "female" their daughter is, or will be, nor by their own irrational fears of unusual sexual development and "how terribly it could all work out". They need to steer a middle path, via *information, discussion* and *analysis*, not rhetoric and imaginings.

The parents of an infant/child newly diagnosed with an intersex condition have a very steep learning curve ahead of them. They need to grasp some complex genetic and embryological concepts, possibly with no prior education in biological subjects. There is a huge tendency for them to be overwhelmed, and to shut off and retreat into the safe territory of an overemphasis on the "normality" of their child (including the so-called "heterosexual imperative"), and the comforting notion of "my/our little girl". The "mirage of normality" and the resulting denial and secrecy become more important than acknowledging their child's need for emotional support and full medical care.

Parents may find it hard to consider their child as a future adult who will need to function emotionally and sexually; consequently, they may continue to try and protect them from the pain of knowing about the condition. This denial only hinders their youngster's healthy development (Anon., 1997b).

Willingness to learn

There are enormous benefits to be gained by parents and patients in dealing with any unusual condition from meeting other affected people, expanding their horizons and appreciating the wide variety of (often positive) responses to what one might have seen as a death sentence. At a UK AISSG meeting, one family attending with their 9-year-old AIS daughter described how their reaction, when told of their daughter's XY chromosomes, was "Wow – how interesting! She's really special! Let's see what we can find out about this". A 30 year old with AIS said that she felt like some kind of angel when she found out the truth of her condition (quite a common reaction). Parents attending the meeting might also have heard the words of a 33 year old with AIS, who had been fed the usual half-truths as a teenager about "underdeveloped ovaries" and had overheard nurses discussing her and saying "but she seems so female!".

When I was 21, I was travelling in India and came across a newspaper article in the Indian issue of *The Times* [Aug or Sept 1981?] about Joan of Arc and which speculated that the historical figure might have had a condition called AIS (TFS). There seemed to be similarities between my own symptoms and those described in the article. I rushed back to England and asked my consultant if I had this syndrome. I experienced a feeling of joy and relief on receiving confirmation of this, because there was a definite reassurance in knowing that my unusual condition was after all a 'known quantity', that it had a name, was documented in the literature, that there were other sufferers and that I was not just a one-off 'freak of nature' after all.

A woman with PAIS in her late thirties wrote:

Once they had finished all their tests, I was informed that a bikini cut from hip to hip would have to be done to carry out an internal examination. They didn't say what they were looking for and I didn't dare ask. I had just turned 14. The operation took place in the radiology theatre – I saw the sign on the door as they wheeled me in. The secret murmurings of my flustered parents and doctors convinced me of the fact that I had cancer and no-one was telling me. I thought they were going to give me radiotherapy during the operation. When I came round, the doctor told me that they had had to remove my ovaries and that I wouldn't be able to have children. That was a terrible shock....

...Having reached the youthful age of 35, I decided that the time had come for me to look things in the face.... My consultant had died, my medical notes had supposedly been destroyed. However, the endocrinologist was still alive and he put me in touch with Professor Ieuan Hughes in Cambridge. ...he spent a great deal of time examining me and patiently answering all the questions I had always wanted to ask. He explained that because my cells had been hardly able to absorb the male hormones in my body, the Y chromosome could not take effect and make me into a boy. Thus I had been born a girl. Afterwards I hopped on to my bike and drove back into town, filled with a deep sense of relief. I remember thinking, "I can live with THIS!"

Although the negative experiences should not be overemphasized, it is vital that today's parents and doctors should hear about the bad experiences of adults who have grown up with conditions like AIS and know what the adults are discussing, so that they learn about the issues that will be occupying their daughter's mind as she reaches maturity, and so that history does not repeat itself.

In the early–mid 1990s, when the AISSG list consisted merely of a few parents, the group was rather wary of the feminist-inspired discourses from some quarters, rallying opposition against patriarchal attitudes in intersex treatment such as the feminizing of male infants whose genitals do not make the grade (Anon., 1996c). However, this changed when we read more of the writings on psychosocial aspects of intersex (such as those mentioned under "AIS in Books and Articles" on the AISSG website) such as Suzanne Kessler (1990a,b), Anne Fausto-Sterling (1993), Morgan Holmes (1994), Cheryl Chase (1995) and Alice Dreger (1998, 1999). Further interest in these ideas came when increasing numbers of *adults* with AIS contacted us, told us their stories and started to discuss these aspects of AIS amongst themselves. We began to feel that these issues were, in fact, very important in explaining the attitudes of medicine to intersex (including the neglect of vaginal hypoplasia by paediatric specialists in their published material on AIS). This was even though questions of genital ambiguity were not of direct personal relevance to many of our members (who predominantly have CAIS or high-grade PAIS). Consequently, these issues began to be covered in *ALIAS*.

Many parents may find such sociological concepts/discussions difficult to handle; however, we believe our role is not to "cotton-wool" parents but to provide information and encourage openness and enquiry. We want to try and provide a balanced offering of support, information and "rocket fuel". We do feel parents should be prepared to consider some tough social, ethical and philosophical questions, even if the impact on their own situation is indirect. If parents read, think and talk (within the family, and with counsellors and other parents/patients) about these matters as much as possible – almost until they are saturated to the point of tedium – they will then get a sense of what all the angles and the outermost reaches of current discussion/knowledge are. Then, the less threatening the demons will become, the fewer murky, menacing corners there will be, and the better they will be equipped to put their own situation in perspective and to *manage* the situation in their child's best interests.

There *are* parents who are willing to get to grips with things but who, like the mother of the baby with PAIS mentioned above, are thwarted in their endeavours by the clinicians in their path. A mother related (in 1996) how she learnt about her 16-year-old daughter's CAIS (Anon., 1997c).

The gynaecologist told us that Sally had been born with no womb and that her ovaries were in a strange place, in her groin.... I phoned the gynaecologist a few weeks later and asked to see her (she had made the next appointment for Christmas time and I thought "You can't just tell someone they have no womb and to come back in four months").... The following week I took Sally to see her. She told Sally she could never have a child, that her vagina might need to be stretched and that her ovaries would have to be taken out. In my ignorance, I asked if they could leave the ovaries in place so that perhaps in the future her younger sister might act as a surrogate mother. But she was adamant that the ovaries had to go.

A couple of days later I told my GP the news. Meanwhile the gynaecologist had written to him to tell him everything. When I told the GP that the ovaries "had to go", it was then that he told me they were not ovaries, but testes. How I got home I'll never know. I couldn't say anything to Sally when she came in from school. My husband told me not to be so stupid, "How could she possibly have testes when she is a girl". I phoned the gynaecologist the next morning and told her what the GP had said. She asked my husband and I to go in the following day. She told us they were 'gonads', not testes. I asked if these 'gonads' would make her look any different than she looked already, and she answered no. That was all I wanted, gonads, testes, ovaries, or whatever – as long as she looked the same.

Then, on 17 November, Sally and I went for the final consultation with the gynaecologist. She asked to see Sally first; I sat outside. After an hour or so I was getting nervous. She then called me into her office, and with Sally sitting there she told me Sally had XY chromosomes. This meant nothing to me. I looked at Sally and she was pure white; she knew what it meant. The gynaecologist gave me the address and phone number of a lady at the 'AIS Support Group' in case I wanted to talk to anyone about it. The term 'AIS' meant nothing to me either.

The next day I called in to tell my GP the news. When he asked me how much I knew, I replied "Everything". He then said "Well you know you have a boy then. XY equals boy". I said that she couldn't be a boy as they weren't testes, they were gonads. He thought I was in denial, when I kept on saying that she couldn't be a boy. He was saying over and over again, "Mother, you have a boy. XY equals boy". I walked out of his surgery vowing never to enter it again. He should not have told me anything anyway since Sally was over 16 years of age.

I got straight onto a bus to town and looked up 'AIS' in the medical department of a large book shop near the university. It was then that I found out the truth. There I was, reading about my beautiful daughter, on my own, finding out exactly what 'AIS' meant. I was shaking all over. I was nearly fainting, at the clinical photographs etc., with the eyes blacked out, thinking this could have been Sally. I felt sick. Somehow I managed to get home, and I phoned the support group. The lady calmed me down and explained everything and the following day the group's factsheet was in the post.

On 4 January 95 Sally had her ovaries/testes/gonads removed. She started her HRT in the February, and in the March my husband and I went to the very first [UK] AIS Support Group meeting.... It all happened so quickly. If the lady I first phoned and the rest of you hadn't been there for us I can't think what might have happened.

I wanted to make a complaint about the GP at the time but there was Sally to consider, I would have had to mention her name etc. I changed to another GP in a different practice. I told him everything about AIS, and about the other GP, and he agreed to take on the whole family. I gave copies of every issue of ALIAS to both the new GP and the gynaecologist. Yet when I recently visited the new GP and told him I had written to a London gynaecologist about the possibility of Sally having a vaginoplasty, his reply was. "Why are you doing all this? It might never be used. After all she is neither woman nor man. She is an 'in-between' sex". I couldn't believe what he was saying and he even repeated it later on in the conversation. This was only a couple of days before the 4th support group meeting in Sept 96.

Whilst I feel so mad, and I want to complain, I do not want Sally to be involved. I have not told her what the new GP said about her. I've written to the gynaecologist and told her, and await her reply.

Support group members often encounter doctors like this who are not all singing to the same hymn sheet, as well as a great deal of ignorance amongst GPs. We have also been surprised to find that even paediatric specialists do not seem to be aware of the recent discourses on the psychosocial aspects of intersex. We feel that specialists who are making irreversible decisions (sometimes involving surgery) affecting how youngsters will function as social and sexual beings

really owe it to their patients to be conversant with these issues. How can they encourage parents to read around the subject if they have not done so themselves?

Guilt, denial and taboo

There are many excellent parents who cope well with their intersexed child, but there are significant problems in some cases. There is often a problem with maternal guilt/denial, with some parents projecting AIS as only a fertility problem, a notion often inherited from the clinician/s. There is commonly a fear of genetic and intersex aspects of the condition. It seems that mothers are particularly fearful of these matters and it is perhaps an unnecessary but understandable guilt that plays a large part in this, once they learn of the X-linked recessive nature of inheritance in AIS. We have observed that many fathers seem to cope better and appear to handle things more objectively, at least as judged by some very supportive yet rational fathers who have attended our meetings with their AIS daughters. Maybe there is less guilt at having brought what is seen as a defective baby into the world.

At a UK AISSG meeting, two adults with CAIS related how a childhood hernia and hints of a "reproductive problem" had led to fear and secrecy within their families and a delayed diagnosis; how in their teens they had resorted to medical libraries in order to find out their diagnoses (accurately in both cases) and how they had lived absolutely alone with the knowledge, and with no therapeutic intervention, for many years thereafter. The 47 year old was the first person with AIS that the 36 year old had become aware of (and only the previous week) and the 47 year old had made her first contact (with a 17 year old with AIS) only 2 years before. Neither of them had ever had a chance to articulate their anxieties about their condition to *anyone* until that point. They both expressed anger towards their otherwise very caring mothers for their complete lack of backbone and initiative when it came to facing reality, trying to overcome their taboos and seeking information/treatment for their child, and for not talking with them about their problem, albeit in a society much less open than that of today.

The two adults with AIS said that the idea of *blaming* their parents for their condition never had, and never would, enter their heads, since they had always accepted it as their own problem and a fact of nature, albeit a very stigmatizing one because of the censorial attitudes of doctors, parents and society. However, they did feel angry that their parents had defaulted in their duty to *manage* the situation. They felt that, instead, the child had been forced to "become the adult" and manage it by seeking information in secret. Both the adult women with AIS were adamant that the effects of the secrecy were far more damaging than the truth itself and that the enormous amount of energy invested by both parents and child in keeping their respective secrets would be much better spent in being open and seeking early medical and psychological guidance. Both women thought that parents were protecting themselves rather than their child by being secretive and withholding information.

Strange notions and "fixing" things

Some parents develop very strange notions about their youngster's condition/treatment and doctors should not underestimate the level of medical misunderstanding in parents. One mother in the support group believed that her daughter with CAIS might develop a hairy chest at puberty and understood vaginoplasty surgery to be the insertion of a plastic tube to serve as a vagina.

The mother of a 3-year-old girl with PAIS received our factsheet in response to a phone enquiry in late 1996 but she did not subscribe to the group. She had not responded to any of our subsequent communications encouraging her to get more involved in the group. In 1999, we heard through a third party that the mother felt antagonistic towards us because "the woman on the helpline would not accept that her (the mother's) brother had the *complete* form of AIS. OK, it's very rare; he might be the only recorded case, but ... ", the mother had explained. We told the go-between that if the mother had joined the group back in 1996, had obtained our newsletter, had come to meetings and heard guest clinicians speak, had talked with other group members and so on, she would not still, three years on, be failing to grasp the very basic medical facts (e.g. that it is almost impossible for her brother to have CAIS because he would almost certainly be her sister) and denying herself other vital support/information as a consequence.

A mother who has received *ALIAS* over a number of years was adamant that she preferred the term "testicular feminization syndrome" to the newer "androgen insensitivity syndrome" because Morris had coined the former term (and others later used the term "classical testicular feminization syndrome") to refer to patients with the *complete* form of the condition (before it was discovered that there was also an incomplete form, later known as partial AIS). She felt that the term AIS was "too general" and "covered other situations". The implication was that she could not face the fact that AIS is a spectrum that includes women with PAIS and with a larger than average clitoris, and even (heaven forbid) men with mild PAIS. Most adult women with AIS hate the older term, regarding it as very stigmatiz-

ing and inappropriate to their social status as females. We are not party to her daughter's view since it appears she has still not been told anything about her condition by parents or doctors even though she is now in her early twenties.

There is a natural desire amongst many parents to want to "fix" things for the future. There is general and pressing anxiety in parents of young children, even infants, over "what will happen at puberty". We usually recommend that, having asked a few relevant questions of their medical specialists, they do not overconcern themselves with this and devote more energy to reading about and understanding the psychosocial aspects. The mother of an infant with PAIS assigned as a girl had a piece of her own ovary frozen for possible future use by her child. Members of an AIS adults' email discussion circle could not agree on whether this was a caring self-sacrifice or an overanxious and unnecessary attempt to further "normalize" the infant's life experience (the child had already had extensive genital reconstruction surgery). Interestingly, the mother declined our offer to send her a newly published intersex issue of the *Journal of Clinical Ethics* (Dreger, 1999), which would have brought her right up to date on the very latest insights, from both affected adults and psychologists/doctors, on the psychosocial aspects of intersex treatment.

Parental control/censorship

There is a significant problem with some mothers making it into *their* problem. Some mothers seem focused on a relentless quest to turn themselves into AIS experts, seemingly without intention of ever sharing the information with their AIS daughters in their late teens, who still do not know the truth. They keep requesting information on AIS, and on truth disclosure, and yet seem embarked on a long-term academic exercise to try and justify *not* talking about things, appearing to have no plan to give their daughter her autonomy ever and allow her to deal with it herself like an adult.

Sometimes an extremely anxious mother of a daughter with AIS in, say, her mid/late teens will have attended group meetings for a number years without her daughter's knowledge. We do not know if these young women will ever be told the truth about their condition or will ever be told about the support group so that they can meet others and escape from their mother's well-meaning but unhelpful overprotection. How can they not know that "something is going on".

Some mothers are very controlling in the domestic setting, seeking to influence who *knows* what, and who *says* what about AIS within the family. A number of support group members have described how they had plans to hold a family meeting, to educate their parents and close relatives fully about their AIS and to give them literature, but this had been expressly forbidden by their mothers (Anon., 2000b).

Keeping it in the family

Some parents, like many clinicians, are inclined to believe they can handle everything without outside help (from counsellors, from the support group) and that they hold all the answers. Virtually all the glowing "fan letters" sent to the support group, saying how useful our literature/meetings have been, how it has changed their lives, etc., are from adults with the condition – not from parents of young children. Nearly all the personal stories submitted to our website are from affected adults rather than parents, and parents do not seem willing to take part in reputable media initiatives, in order to raise awareness, in the way that the adults are.

The long letter mentioned earlier from the parent whose baby had undergone genital surgery was really the first time that the parent of an infant/child had written to us at any length about their experience. We do very occasionally hear from parents of older children. The mother of a 13 year old with PAIS wrote (Anon., 1998a):

I am one of those guilty parents who have not given you any feedback, but you summed up the reasons why in your article "Parent Problems" [Anon., 1997b]. I could not have expressed it more articulately and it shows what a brilliant listener you have been. My daughter___ is now 13 (PAIS) and I'm still kind of shell-shocked, although now much more in control, thanks to the education through ALIAS and the one group meeting I attended in March '97. I was firmly of the opinion my daughter would not be told the full facts (i.e. that she was XY) until that meeting where I met___ and her three daughters. Her youngest girl, of 17, had the biggest impact when she said she would have liked full disclosure at an earlier age. There stood a bright, pretty girl and, although emotional during the meeting, she was in control.

We mothers wish to protect our children from every hurt, as we inflicted these XY chromosomes on our daughters through something beyond our control. [Not strictly true. The X comes from the mother, the Y from the father. However, the genetic fault that causes AIS is carried on the X.] I personally have been so afraid that my daughter could be so emotionally damaged by being told the full facts that she would no longer be able to cope with life. It has only been through ALIAS, and meeting with other mothers and affected adults, that I have changed my opinion. This parent/child emotional support, which has so far been missing, is the key to getting things right in the future.

But this sort of letter, in fact any communication, from a parent is very rare.

Although a significant proportion of the UK AISSG's subscribers are parents (44% in 1999/2000), most of the meeting attendees are adult women with AIS and similar conditions. There are notable exceptions. An overseas family have brought their PAIS daughter with them to several UK meetings since she was 9 years of age. There, the youngster herself, who speaks English, hears adult women talking freely about all the things that many parents might consider taboo. So she, like the adults at the meeting, sees how these can become just topics of normal dialogue. She may see some of the women cry but she also hears them laughing uncontrollably over dinner and late into the evening.

Parents, on the whole, seem to prefer to deal with AIS within the family. We perceive that while most parents are happy to receive newsletters, many may be too ashamed to attend meetings and confront the fact, and admit to others, that they have an intersexed child. It is our impression that more parents of young children used to attend in the early days when the meetings were smaller and more informal. Now that the adults have become stronger and more confident, maybe this has deterred the parents from attending because they feel intimidated (even though we provide a private parents' discussion group on the second day of our weekend meetings). Maybe this is a failing of our group, but no parents of young children have answered our calls for them to get involved and to help to plan and run our services.

Out of 35 parents only three with known email addresses even *acknowledged* an invitation in 2000 to join a parents' private email discussion circle we were offering to set up for them. Meanwhile the affected adults are all networking like crazy. Has the Internet revolution passed parents by? It is very important that clinicians should make parents (and patients) aware of the fact that increasing numbers of affected adults are every day discussing every angle and nuance of being intersexed (in meetings, in *ALIAS*, by private email and in online discussion groups and chatrooms tailored to every possible "flavour" of intersex (i.e. male, female, intergendered/androgynous etc.)) and that sections of society are becoming much more open and interactive on this subject. The UK AISSG recently helped a social anthropology student with her MA thesis on how intersexed people, and groups, talk about themselves on the Internet (Nahman, 2000).

Maybe parents do not have the concept of a *community* of peers in the way that the affected adults do. Parents sometimes want the impossible (one-to-one contact with a family with the *same* condition, with *same* aged child, in *same* geographical area) but that is usually difficult to arrange (these conditions are rare) and is not always the best option. We feel that they would benefit more by coming to meetings and hearing a variety of experiences/viewpoints.

The affected adults gain enormous benefit from their association with the support group, and by bonding and networking with others, but we have a problem on the whole in getting parents of young children actively involved, and this is where we need the help of the medical profession, specifically clinical psychologists, in trying to help parents *at the point of diagnosis* to realise the benefits of expanding their field of view beyond the family.

Counselling/psychotherapy

For parents

Parents of youngsters with AIS need a lot of help themselves before they can really understand and help their children. It is important that parents are encouraged to deal first with their own feelings/fears so that they will be better equipped to help their children through the learning/adapting process.

Doctors should *not* emphasize to parents that "It's very rare" or say "It's not something you'd really want to discuss with anyone". Rather, they need to encourage them to talk openly with a trained counsellor and to seek information on the options (what and when to tell their child, sources of ongoing psychological support, information about treating vaginal hypoplasia when the time comes, the timing of gonadectomy and HRT, etc.). Otherwise parents can become imprisoned by their own negative feelings, leading to isolation and inaction. It will be regarded as a lost cause, or something too terrible even to mention in the family, let alone to outside people who otherwise might have helped the child to realise her potential.

During a discussion on truth disclosure (Anon., 1998b) a 49 year old with CAIS said:

I agree [that parents often cannot be trusted to do the job on their own] and I think that AIS is so complicated biologically and psychologically that it is too risky to leave it to parents to explain things on their own. My parents just never grasped the biological facts or sought to inform themselves, never mind thought about them, or reached any sort of understanding or digest (beyond the concept of 'a normal girl with a fertility problem') that would have enabled them to help me (and I was far too stigmatized by my own independent discoveries and, above all, by their silence on the matter, and the obvious discomfort of the medics, to ask *any* questions *at all*).

I feel that at the time of diagnosis, the health care professionals must fully educate parents (and daughter, unless an infant/young child at the time), and provide professional psychological counseling, so that if the parents can't or won't get to grips with

it – scientifically/medically *and* emotionally – then at least the girl can be rescued from this nightmare situation, and be given a space in which to explore things with a professional, because if her doctors/parents don't explain it all to her in detail (and they all talk about it until they're blue in the face), she is going to find out all the biological facts anyway (or worse still, bits and pieces, and strange, stigmatizing terms) from sources like medical libraries, and will be completely on her own with it. In my view, parents should, with the help of counsellors, be forced (as it were) to overcome their hangups about discussing things openly, for the sake of their child's mental health.

For children

The following is the major part of a letter that first appeared in the newsletter of the Intersex Society of North America (ISNA), by a certified marriage, family and child counsellor (Slocum, 1995) who herself has PAIS.

Most of my life (I am 46 at present) I have endeavored to feel female. Most of my childhood my parents, especially my mother, labored to instill in me a female identity. These efforts have had some effect. I present myself as a woman, have many womanly attributes and am treated by and large as a female. Unfortunately, this struggle has almost exhausted me. All this time I have labored to prove something which is in some sense not true and at best a terrible simplification of a rather complex state of body and mind.

I'm not exaggerating when I say this process had for a while almost spent me. For much of my young adult life, for at least the years between the ages of 15 and 35, I remember having the experience almost daily of being in the midst of some positive experience (for example, a compliment being paid me, an exciting encounter, feelings of physical pleasure) when into my mind would intrude the thought that something was not quite right. I remember that almost daily experience as one of a lack of genuineness, an illegitimacy, a fear that I would be found out and ridiculed. From a very early age I felt my personal history was out of the norm, that I looked a bit different, felt a bit different and was treated differently than most females. This was never acknowledged. My doctors said only trivial things to me, my parents avoided any mention (and probably any thought) of my difference. My culture dealt with the only gender ambiguity that seemed speakable – transsexualism – with a snicker. I internalized the apparent taboo and lived with a great fear of myself. Another person I know with AIS has had to live in the same way and describes the anguish as her having, in her own words, "to every day slay the dragon".

I fear that parents in their attempts to give their children normal lives, will rob them of the chance to come to terms with their own difference. I suppose there is a great need to feel that the right thing has been done in choosing early surgical intervention. There might be a need to feel that everything has been fixed, or nearly fixed and that their child's acceptance of their difference will be as decisive as their surgery. Whether or not this type of surgery can ever be viewed as decisive is another critically serious topic. It would be nice if a young person didn't have to wrestle with puzzling terms like 'intersexed' and did not have to contemplate what existed before surgery. But that is not the fate of those of us born like this [just as it is not the fate of someone rendered paraplegic in an automobile accident to walk away from the scene (author's words paraphrased for publication in ALIAS)].

I don't wish to appear unkind or unfeeling to parents. I have so much empathy for these families, just as I have loved my family through our experience. What is important to emphasize, I believe, is that healing and a kind of wholeness and equanimity are possible. All children may not grow up to identify as intersexuals but there is a very good chance they will perceive of themselves as different to a greater or lesser degree. To not prepare such children for this self-confrontation is to do them a terrible disservice. These children will run the risk of never being comfortable in their own bodies and never at ease with the world around them.

I realize that the prospect of a lengthy course of [psycho]therapy may seem daunting to parents who have already suffered considerable trauma, but I can't imagine a substitute process. It would be hoped that these children can benefit from expert, informed counseling and be availed of the opportunity to join a group of others like themselves to facilitate self-exploration and gain support. I imagine the participation of loving, accepting parents in the early stages of this therapeutic process would be integral to success. Their child will become very special, someone who knows themself very well and someone who will very probably be capable of great courage and sensitivity to adversity.

But counselling has to be *appropriate* counselling. A father at a UK AISSG meeting told how he and his wife had been recommended to take their 9-year-old CAIS child to the Tavistock Centre in London (a family psychiatry centre with a unit specializing in gender dysphoria problems in children) for "gender counselling". However, he was concerned that "it [AIS] might be seen as being a gender dysphoria (transsexual) issue, which it is not, and that this might just create more problems in the mind of a child of that age". This is a valid concern and underlies the need for more psychological counselling tailored to biologically determined sexual anomalies.

John Money may be the bête noir of the moment because of his influence on the practice of genital surgery but he had some sound things to say concerning psychosocial matters, even before these issues became more prominently debated in the early–mid 1990s. In several of his papers/books, Money identified a need for counsellors who identify themselves as paediatric sexologists, specializing in the sexual problems of children (Money, 1987), an important qualification being an in-depth medical knowledge of intersex conditions. He referred to this "talking doctor" as a psychologist or psychiatrist with training in sexual medicine and psychoneuroendocrinology, whose services should be available throughout childhood and early adulthood. Unfortunately such professionals are very rare.

A discussion amongst some women with AIS (Anon., 1997d–f) covered the terminology and advice given in medical textbooks and its relevance to counselling and psychosocial well-being. One textbook had recommended "counselling and support for the parents, the individual and partners in later life". One of the women commented:

It must be really nice to have a physician who is so helpful and deeply involved in one's life that he'll take care of explaining things to your boyfriend! My impression is that, in real life, they don't even have the time to explain anything properly to parents, or to patients themselves. Anyway, by the time someone is old enough to have romantic partners she should long since have been provided with the words she can use to handle these situations herself. Instead, most of these books advise keeping the patient in at least partial ignorance, which makes her dependent on the "counseling and support" they recommend, but which few doctors are actually ready to supply.

From the patient's point of view, the best option is not to have a life so messed up that one needs support in order to face one's "special situation". I feel that such "supportive" counseling is a waste of time, and that counseling should be businesslike and oriented towards providing information, not "hand-holding". What I believe in is for a counselor to promote the patient's self-reliance and ability to cope with whatever situations he or she will encounter. They can do this best by providing accurate and complete *information* about his or her condition and treatment options, and about *sex* in general. Unfortunately, most counseling professionals are not geared to do this. Child clinical psychologists with specialized knowledge of AIS and related conditions, and of sex problems and their treatment, are very rare.

Also, there is a taboo on talking about sex with children, and people rationalize keeping them in ignorance as being necessary for their emotional well-being, when, in fact, it is more likely to be harmful. Counselors are unlikely to get into talking about erotic arousal, and sensation or orgasm with a child. They might fear getting into trouble with the parents or hospital authorities, or even being prosecuted under laws intended to protect children from pedophiles. Even when I saw counselors as a young adult (aged 21–22), I perceived an attitude of prudish avoidance of these topics on the counselors' part. It seemed this way to me even though I was shy and puritanical myself.

The current approach seems to be to avoid dealing with sexual problems until the person becomes an adult, even if the problem has by then become more complicated. One could call this protecting children from what they are not yet ready for, but one could also call it shrugging off a responsibility so that someone else can deal with it later. I think I've mentioned before that some of the overemphasis on gender identity in such conditions possibly stems from prudish avoidance of the real issue – *sexuality* – in dealing with a child . . .

... what I'm saying here is that by making gender identity the justification for whatever management/treatment is applied to a child, doctors can talk in terms of the existence of, or the achievement of cosmetic normality – whether the child looks, or can be made to *"look normal, like other boys (or girls)"* – rather than having to talk in terms of ability to have sexual intercourse.

Teamwork

In order for parents (and patients) to play a greater role in decision making there needs to be a shift in responsibility in the doctor/parent relationship, with parents and patients doing more thinking for themselves and not taking on board "hook, line and sinker" everything the doctor tells them. Doctors, in turn, need to relinquish some of their control over the situation and (funding of services permitting) delegate some responsibility to their clinical psychology colleagues.

There are, on the one hand, well-established, objective facts concerning the biological situation in AIS. On the other hand, any considerations of gender identity and orientation have an inherent degree of subjectivity, haziness, and unpredictability. However, it seems that clinicians sometimes offer fuzzy information, half-truths or straightforward untruths concerning the biological facts then issue dogmatic pronouncements and reassurances, as if from on high, concerning the more nebulous issues of sexual identity. It is time doctors stopped feeling that they have to issue edicts on such personal and mutable matters as gender identity and sexual orientation and arranged for counsellors or psychotherapists to help people to explore these and the many other psychological issues for themselves.

The parents are unlikely to seek counselling or contacts for their child if they have only one "script" running continuously in their heads: "Well the consultant kept on assuring us, over and over again, that she is a normal female, in spite of her XY chromosomes and testes, so that's all we need to keep telling ourselves for everything to be absolutely fine". They become fearful and intolerant of any discussion or intervention, or any contact with other people that might remotely question the truth of this Delphic proclamation. The script becomes a kind of life-raft that parents desperately cling to, trying to convince themselves that it was all a dream and the shipwreck never happened. I think this approach will be seen by the *patient* for what it is – a damage-limitation exercise.

Why do doctors think they have to hold all the answers? They are not trained in psychosocial or psychosexual aspects; and intersex conditions are not usually medical emergencies. It could even be argued that ex-perienced counsellors, and not doctors, should actually disclose the basic diagnostic information in such cases or that the case management around the time of diagnosis/treatment should be overseen by a psychology professional to ensure that the management plan will facilitate normal psychosexual development and enable the patient to anticipate personal relationships.

In 1996, a paediatrician commented to ISNA concerning some of their literature, saying that although it had been "remarkably illuminating" he felt that the medical profession came in for quite a "hammering". He thought it rather unfair to describe a urologist as merely a plumber whose role is to repair and lengthen pipes in infants to make them male. He said that he had always worked very closely with paediatric urologists in the management of infants with ambiguous genitalia and that their input went far beyond the pragmatic surgical management.

Cheryl Chase of ISNA replied to him (our italics):

It is very gratifying to hear that some of the information we are providing has been thought-provoking. In that light, I would like to open a dialog on several points from your letter with you. First, you say that the input of pediatric urologists goes far beyond the pragmatic surgical management. Indeed, as we see it, that *is a large part of the problem*. Pediatric urologists are not specialists in emotional issues. They do not generally have extensive training or experience in psychotherapy nor in sex therapy and sexological theory. We believe that the team which guides the treatment of these infants and children should be headed by such a mental health specialist.

The above recommendation has been strongly endorsed by the AIS Support Group (Anon., 1995b,c, 1996d).

At a symposium on intersex management held in London on 28 January 2002 (jointly organized by clinicians and AISSG), there was a general air of anxiety amongst paediatric clinicians. Several were getting quite agitated and saying things like: "Well, I have the parents in front of me..." or "I'm in the hot seat..." "...and they are asking me what I advise, so I *have* to tell them *something*... so what *do* I tell them (e.g. about early/late gonadectomy)?". Support group participants in the audience answered:

Well... you tell them that the risk of gonadal cancer, in AIS at least, is *very* low before puberty/early adulthood... you put them in touch with a clinical psychologist if possible, and you put them in touch with other parents via the support group... so they can discuss things at length, and in their own time, and can explore *all* the angles. There is no hurry to do surgery unless it's a life-threatening situation.

Intersex is largely a psychosocial phenomenon and not a medical emergency, and doctors should not feel they have to be the only people to advise parents.

Late childhood/adolescence

What/when to tell

At a UK AISSG meeting, there was discussion about the best time for truth disclosure and it emerged that there were probably no hard and fast rules because of differing family backgrounds, medical histories, character strengths/weaknesses in the youngster, etc. However, the adults with AIS advised that the sooner one is able to deal with the full psychological impact of the condition (by knowing that all the cards are on the table) the sooner one can get the immediate trauma over, and the sooner one can get on with one's life. The meeting heard of the experience of two young women with AIS: a 19 year old present at the meeting and a 23 year old (mother present without daughter). Both had experienced emotional difficulties until such time as they had been given the final pieces of the jigsaw, after which they were able, quite suddenly and dramatically, to get on with their lives in a positive way. After many years of anger, depression, low self-esteem, the 19 year old now had a steady boyfriend and the 23 year old had been recently married.

Suddenly to drop a bombshell on a teenager might well cause a degree of acute distress and might well mean that their school work suffers for a year, but life is not a bed of roses, and it is unlikely that a teenager with CAIS will not have been wondering exactly *why* she has not menstruated or developed pubic or underarm hair, or possibly *why* her vagina is very short. It is far better to be able to face reality and have a chance to talk about fears early on than to spend one's whole life under a stone because you are so stigmatized by an awareness that even those who brought you into the world cannot accept what you are.

All this seemed to give hope to some of the parents of young children, that there could be light at the end of the tunnel, in the face of their dread of having to talk truthfully to their daughter at some point. One set of parents announced that they were going to go home and start talking to their 8 year old. When it came to revealing information to a child diagnosed in infancy/childhood, it was thought that a phased truthful approach was best, with the aim of full disclosure perhaps by the mid-teens. This means a strategy in which each *piece* of information given is *in itself* truthful, so that there is no need for backtracking at a later date. For example, to introduce a notion such as "malformed ovaries" and then to have to modify this to "gonads" or "testicular tissue" if a teenager happens to find out later about her XY chromosomes was felt to be a recipe for disaster and likely to generate a great deal of mistrust and anger. Similarly, to hint vaguely to a 14 year old, who has already been told that she is infertile and has had her "ovaries" removed, that she "may need another (unspecified, but in fact a vaginoplasty) operation at some stage" just sets up more questions than it answers. It is also very important that there should not be long gaps where no information is given and in which doubts/questions and insecurities will arise.

Parents should not have to cope with all this on their own. The meeting discussing disclosure urged parents to push for professional psychological counselling so that the medical system is encouraged to put more emphasis on this element of the equation.

Adult issues

Meeting others

The best therapy (together with psychological counselling) is to be in touch with others who are similarly affected, and yet this has been the action that, in the past, many doctors have been least willing to facilitate. This vital step is unlikely to happen if the truth about the condition remains an "unspeakable monster" in the clinic and/or within the family.

Most support groups seem to be set up and run by women. We have failed to get the significant number of men with PAIS who have contacted us to get together and form any sort of concrete mutual support facility for men in the way that AISSG was set up by women. A man who co-founded (with a woman) an intersex advocacy organization told us that in his experience most support groups set up/run by men are not successful. A high percentage of doctors are men and have traditionally been reluctant to put patients/families in touch with others affected and/or have been scathing about the role of support groups. Is there something in the male psyche that does not appreciate the benefits of peer support?

Normalization and empowerment

By far the most frequent comments we receive from affected adults, on contacting the support group, are that they are "absolutely amazed that there are others with the same story" and (usually after attending their first group meeting) that they "no longer feel like a one-off freak". A 37 year old, who had suffered secrecy and denial in her family, described at a group meeting in 1996 how finding the support group in late 1994, and at last being able to meet others with AIS who were "making a go of their lives," had enabled her, for the first time in her life, to feel as if she was part of the real world – a member of the human race instead of an outcast.

Patients become highly suspicious when doctors go "over the top" in emphasizing their normality, or their femaleness, and yet seem determined to prevent them from discussing things with other patients. Meeting others will definitely normalize things for the isolated patient.

There is a perception amongst some people that support groups are full of people who are miserable losers, who only meet together to complain and depress each other. This is not the case, with our group at least. You could say that those who make the effort to seek us out and come to meetings are in fact the most brave and resourceful of the lot, because, after all, most of them have already had to ferret out the basic diagnostic information about themselves from sources like the Internet. Yes, we get people who are in a desperate state and who cry throughout their first meeting; yet after one or two meetings, we find they are coming along mainly for the social activities.

A 39 year old with CAIS in the USA wrote:

Meeting other women with AIS, finding them to be normal, makes it easier to view yourself this way, I think this is what caused me to make great strides in coming to terms with AIS. When I started going to meetings in the UK, I would literally look around the room and think to myself "This is a group of great women about whom I don't feel the least discomfort that they have XY chromosomes or once had testes." By being able to find this so utterly acceptable in them, I came to be much more accepting of myself. It's like the other group members are a mirror of ourselves and when we like what we see in the mirror it becomes easier to appreciate ourselves and to understand how others could find AIS acceptable in us.

A 44 year old with PAIS wrote:

Prior to meeting AIS women, I had this impression that there were aspects of my physical looks, or a vibe I might put out that would make people think I was not a woman. Baggage. I'm overly sensitive to it, and it remains an issue . . . . And I remember regularly probing my face in the mirror from age 14 to 20-something, to see what was different. Was there something in my face that gave me away, that was subtle to me, but more obvious to those who looked at me – especially women, since they'd be the first to know, I thought. Today I don't think so. It has been a big change since the day I first asked ___ [CAIS 39 year old], at the [AISSG USA] group meeting in NYC in Sept 96, "Can you tell by looking at me?" I had wanted to ask someone that question for three decades. I've been in solitary confinement for all that time. Yep, I got parolled last year. My only visitor was my mother. Kidding aside, in some ways I view my current life as 'restarting' [last year] in Sept 96. I was 14 when I was given 'the story' by the doctor. Maybe there is a part of me that is only 15 years old inside today.

Patients talk about gaining a sense of empowerment via the support group, about gaining a label for their condition, about understanding the medical jargon at last (one of the aims of *ALIAS* is to bridge the divide between lay and professional). It is partly a case, as already mentioned in connection with parents, of knowing what the outer limits are and of gaining the reassuring knowledge that all the cards are on the table and that no gremlins are lurking in corners.

Exorcising the past

Hearing how others have exorcised what happened to them in childhood or adolescence often inspires people to seek out historical information. This is often a vital prerequisite to moving forward. At a group meeting, a father who works in a caring profession explained the steps involved in grieving and in coming to terms with a personal loss or problem. He pointed out that unless the problem and the accompanying pain are first faced in their entirety, and acknowledged, there is no chance of moving on to the next stage, which is one of dealing with them and ultimately accepting them.

Intersexed women increasingly seek access to their medical records. They may also need to come to terms with nonessential surgery, carried out earlier in life without their informed consent. They may follow the example of the group member who, as an aid to coming to terms with her condition, compiled what she calls her "workshop manual" containing all her support group literature, copies of letters between her clinicians, and her own thoughts on her experience of AIS. Seeing what was discussed about you, and possibly seeing clinical photographs of yourself, can be very painful indeed but it can also be cathartic and empowering in piecing the jigsaw together and moving on.

Words or terminology are tools for *communication* – of ideas, concepts, etc. – and this can break down if those involved are not talking on the same wavelength. Some doctors take scientific/biological terms (e.g. "gonads") and stretch their established meaning (the meaning they would use when talking to their clinician colleagues) to mean something a bit different when talking to patients. This is in a well-intentioned but misguided attempt to conceal diagnostic information and/or to soften the blow for their patients. However, this can have adverse practical consequences apart from any considerations of emotional pain, for example raising false hopes.

Some affected adults contact the medical specialists who treated them as youngsters in order to "level the playing field" at last. This can be beneficial for both parties, patient and doctor. A 25 year old with CAIS emailed (Anon., 1999a):

. . . this week I got a phone call from the surgeon who did my gonadectomy 8 years ago. I had been trying to contact him for the past year, wanting to get copies of my charts . . . but he always avoided me and never returned my calls. I was going home for Easter and really wanted to confront him, his avoiding me has made me all the more annoyed at everything.

What I *was* most upset about was the fact that he had told me that he was removing my ovaries. For the following six and a half years, I was puzzled and then extremely angry that he hadn't preserved any of my eggs so that one day I might have my own surrogate child with my own genetic input. So it was with some relief in that respect when I found out about AIS and the fact that I never *had* ovaries, there *were* no eggs to harvest.

So I arranged to have a conflab with him, educate him somewhat on disclosure and throw some support group literature at him and tell him to educate himself, and I was looking forward to it, to being in control over that which he took so much control of before! I planned to walk in there looking brilliant, tall, proud and every bit like I'm coping with this "terrible news" that he felt like he had to keep from me all those years ago.

OK, the consultation.... No nerves at all; I walked in, shook his hand firmly and was pleasantly surprised to see that I was actually taller than him. One down to me!... I told him that I had been angry that he never thought to harvest any eggs from my 'ovaries', for future surrogacy. His reply? "I never told you that you had ovaries, I said gonads". So I was supposed to presume they weren't ovaries based on the non-information I was given?

To give him his dues, he was apologetic, never denied that I should have been told the truth . . . he rubbed his eyes a lot and told me he admired me. So I guess that's that, and that's another thing out of the way. I'm sending him the AISSG factsheet and the most recent *ALIAS*. He said that he's never encountered this before except as a med student in Canada years and years ago and I'm the only AIS patient he had. Everyone, you are all stars and I am so happy to be "one of you".

It seems that all this talking in euphemisms ("ovaries", "hysterectomy", "broken X chromosome" etc.) and the stretching/reinterpreting of an established meaning of words results in communication breakdown, dialogue failure and even elective mutism in medical consultations; it also deprives people of an honest and truthful baseline from which to sort out their options and make life decisions.

Informed consent

A 22-year-old woman with AIS emailed the support group (Anon., 1999b) saying:

The doctors I have spoken to are so vague, that it seems that they don't fully understand this disease or its effects on the patient. They have always been hiding something from me.

She explained how she had been told that during a vaginoplasty the surgeon would also be repairing her clitoromegaly. When she woke up she learned that the surgeon had decided she did not need the latter procedure. She said:

Now after reading more of this [AISSG] literature and speaking with him at the follow up appointment; [I see that] he was in some way trying to hold off the final surgery because he wasn't sure if there would be a loss of sensation to the clitoris. He actually tried to trick me, a 20-year-old woman at the time, instead of discussing all of my possible options. The more I read on this [AISSG web] site the more I know about my condition.

A 43 year old with the complete form of AIS wrote to the support group in mid 2000 (Anon., 2000a).

During the late 1970s when I was first investigated (aged 21) I was lied to and my testes were removed without my permission. I was simply told that they were going to remove some "lumps". If I had been a complete man the doctor would never have dared do such a thing. I do not understand why having a genetic defect somehow gives doctors the right to ignore my basic rights as a human being. When I found out what had been done to me (a few years later) I felt like I had been betrayed and mutilated.... If I sound angry it is just that they were difficult experiences...I have always lived in so much fear (it is a taboo subject even in my family) that I felt like I had committed some great crime.

After my testes were removed I experienced a range of psychological symptoms including: hot sweats, depression, mood swings and a distinct feeling of being generally unwell; even though I was taking oestrogens. My depression was not due to my discovery of having AIS because the doctors had lied to me and I did not know....I would go to the medics and beg them to give me my testosterone back and they refused again and again. I was convinced that it was the cause of my depression because I remembered how different I felt before and after the gonadectomy. Eventually I met Prof Jacobs and Dr Conway at the Middlesex [Hospital, London] and have not looked back. After 10 long years of depression I got the hormones, and straight away began to feel as happy and well as I had felt before the op.

I am still angry that it took me that long – angry that a doctor can tell me lies, remove all the testosterone that my body had naturally produced for 21 years, replace it with synthetic oestrogens and then refuse to give me my testosterone back! It doesn't take a genius to work out that this sudden and complete change in my hormones would have some effect, and no-one even bothered to check up on how I was coping.... Although I realise that the testosterone has no effect upon my tissues, there has been no research to see if it is active with regard to the brain and general mood. The team at the Middlesex have been great, they are the only medics I have met who genuinely want to help and ask me what it is I feel I need...

I could have understood if I had been a child, but I was 21 when I was operated on and what they did to me was not only unethical, but illegal. There is not much in this world that belongs to me but I feel strongly that once I become an adult my body is definitely mine...I am just so glad now that I never gave up fighting.

Confidence and communication

An adult with AIS at an early group meeting likened her family situation to "a trick done with mirrors" where "the parents project their unease and the child reflects it back (compounded by the probable unease of the treating physician) so that the whole issue gets passed around like a hot potato". It was also described as "a huge pink elephant in the middle of the sitting room but whose presence no one would ever acknowledge".

She later wrote to another AIS woman:

To save your parents from mental anguish and having to deal with things, you shouldered more of the burden yourself – inverse to the way 'family' is supposed to work. I remember repeatedly thinking as a teenager "How am I going to get myself out of this?" What I meant was not how would I make it all go away (I knew that was an impossibility). Rather I thought "How am I going to summon up the courage to get the help I need, how am I going to find the strength to talk about it?" (even though I didn't yet know the truth and know what 'it' was), "and how the hell am I ever going to build a normal relationship?" I couldn't even imagine telling anyone I was unable to have children and didn't have pubic hair – the two things I actually knew and understood at that age.

The image of being painted into a corner was vivid in my mind since the age of 12 or 13. It haunted me until age 36. I never saw any way out of the corner except by taking my life, until I came across the letter [from another woman with AIS, in a medical journal, giving the support group contact details]. The letter wasn't just a release from a corner, it was a release from the prison that was my mind, a place where everything was locked shut inside and could find no freedom of expression. And when I read the description, in *ALIAS* No. 1, of "... the process of hearing oneself actually saying out loud those words that you thought would forever remain as circling thoughts in your head", I convulsed with sobbing (the word convulsing is not an exaggeration; I had never cried from so deep a place, or as intensely as when I read that quote). Nothing I ever read so brilliantly depicted how I felt about my life experience and the ordeal of keeping it all locked inside my mind.

The quote referred to was actually as follows:

I have found, late in life, that there is in fact considerable power and healing ability in the actual process of articulating or verbalising one's fears about such things, almost irrespective of any response from the listener – it's the process of hearing oneself actually saying out loud those words that you thought would forever remain as circling thoughts in your head.

If the patient has never articulated the words describing her condition to "safe" people like parents, counsellors and other affected people, then she will not be able to play an active role in managing her treatment when face to face with a doctor in a threatening environment. This is especially true when she has just had her bodily deficiencies highlighted by a nurse, technician or receptionist asking about her last period (known within the support group as "the mother of all questions") or a cervical smear test, has had to wait in an infertility clinic area plastered with baby photographs from grateful parents, or has had to undergo scrutiny from doctors in training. She is more likely to behave as a defensive, monosyllabic child who wants to get out of the room as quickly as possible, rather than the intelligent communicative adult that she most likely is in other areas of her life.

A woman with CAIS wrote (Anon., 1997f):

I recently came to the realisation that because I'd never actually had the wherewithal to say the words "I have AIS" out loud in front of another human being, or to admit to having had testes, I'd never been able to claim 'ownership' of my condition. Well, I might perhaps have mumbled my diagnosis incoherently, fighting back the tears, when occasionally in adulthood a new doctor, surrounded by an army of students, would ask "Well what do we have here then, perhaps you'd like to tell us about your problem?" but I had never actually articulated the words spontaneously and clearly, and felt reasonably OK about it – until the third support group meeting in March 1996. This was a very momentous event in my life. I was in my late 40s.

Personal empowerment means that patients are more likely to communicate effectively with the doctor in the clinic, more likely to meet the clinician half-way and develop an equal partnership. This should make the doctor's job easier.

If the pink elephant is acknowledged in the clinic situation also, then at least there's a chance of an adult-to-adult exchange with the doctor. Talking with others enables it to be integrated into one's persona, so that it is no longer a huge externalized burden or monster, always held at arm's length and waiting to crush you at any moment. It lessens the fear of breaking down in front of the doctor at the mere mention of your condition because that's the only time the words are ever spoken out loud.

Some patients know a lot about their condition – from their private research, not necessarily from doctors – but are just not used to *articulating* any of this to other people, so that while they may be intellectually in control, they may be a disaster in the emotional arena. The patient may have spent many months steeling herself for an informed discussion during, say, an annual clinic visit but may retreat back into her shell if she finds that her efforts are not reciprocated or taken seriously.

A 37 year old with CAIS wrote:

I hate going to the doctor and getting blank stares when I tell them I have AIS, even when I spell it out – 'androgen insens...' And even when I revert to 'testicular feminization' they don't have the correct details for the correct syndrome. A senior resident I saw today (Stanford is a teaching hospital) thought I'd had a uterus and a dual set of gonads – ovaries *and* testes. When the head of the department (one of the top urogynecology experts) came in he didn't recognise 'androgen insensitivity' either but knew much more about the medical details when I said 'testicular feminization'. "Good lord, how long has the name been changed?" he said. I hate the feeling that a bunch of doctors are going home tonight to drag out the textbooks, and with young doctors I hate the slightly shocked look when they finally do understand that it's an intersex condition.

Sometimes I am proud of how much I have learned about AIS in the year since I discovered the truth and I am glad to show off my knowledge and my ability to talk about such an upsetting subject, but there are times when I really don't want to know more about this than my doctors. It didn't bother me to have to educate my family doctor, but *these* guys are supposed to be on top of things. They were nice guys, kind, respectful, considerate, but I was still quite upset.

The senior guy asked me why this information is kept from patients and I explained that the medical community has believed that we are incapable of handling the testes/karyotype information. The room was full of male doctors and he said "Well, we all have Y chromosomes and they work quite well for *us*." Well, I had a *large* laugh at *that*. I told them that Y chromosomes don't work so well when you have AIS, have been raised as a female, and quite want to stay that way.

I now find it useful to make sure that a new specialist knows ahead of time that I have AIS, before I come in. When I have to see a new one, I call ahead and ask to speak to the nurse when I make the appointment. I tell her I have AIS and say it used to be called testicular feminization but patients find that term very offensive. I make the nurse or receptionist take a very detailed message about my having AIS and ask if the doctor can call me back to confirm if he or she has ever had an AIS patient before. It prepares them (the nurse has no clue what I'm talking about but the message seems to get passed on clearly) and also warns the doctor in advance of my preference in terminology. I usually get a call back and it gets the awkward moment of recognition out of the way on the phone – where I can't see the slack-jawed, bug-eyed, dumb-ass look that comes over most of them, until they finally connect 'AIS' with the old term, and with testes, XY chromosomes, etc. Residents are especially good at this facial expression.

Women with AIS often come across doctors who cling to the out-dated terminology. The mother of an infant with CAIS visited her GP in 2001 and was annoyed to see the words "Testicular Feminization" in sky-high letters on the computer screen displaying her daughter's medical records. When she asked for it to be changed to "Androgen Insensitivity" the GP said "Oh, we don't use that term here in the UK, I'm afraid. It's a trendy Americanism". We told the mother to inform him that it was an *American* gynaecologist

(Morris) who assigned the *old term* to the condition before its true aetiology (target cell insensitivity) was discovered.

Autonomy/responsibility

Secrecy and poor communication deny patients their right to know about health risks associated with their condition and to seek monitoring/treatment. Another very common cry from new group members is "I didn't even know about the increased incidence of osteoporosis in AIS ... [or] ... about carrier status ... until I joined the support group". Some were not prescribed HRT following early orchidectomy, and now, osteoporotic in early middle-age, are considering legal action.

People gain information via the group that helps them take responsibility for their own health care. They are encouraged to persuade clinicians that they are at risk of osteoporosis and need bone density scans, even though they might be much younger than the usual, post-menopausal group considered most at risk. They learn how to obtain a certificate exempting them from UK prescription charges on the basis of having a condition requiring long-term (HRT) therapy. They hear of the amazing benefits of vaginal oestrogen cream in alleviating, even curing, cystitis, and in facilitating the use of vaginal dilators, even though many specialists will tell them that systemic oestrogen should suffice.

Contact with others can also influence more dramatic treatment choices. Individuals may feel a lot better about their own bodies when they find that the problems/issues are by no means unique, read intersex discourses and realize that some individuals actually take pride in identifying as intersexed, intergendered, etc. This means that some patients may then decide they do not want the genital surgery that seemed at one point (when the doctor was the only one doing the talking about her AIS) to be the only answer.

A 27-year-old woman with PAIS emailed to a group of AIS women:

I never had the clitoral recession surgery myself, although I certainly would be a candidate for one ... I don't know if I just had enlightened doctors who saw no need to 'normalize' me or what, but it was an un-subject and never discussed at all.

I was/am a pretty traumatized kid over the whole AIS thing, especially the enlarged clitoris, which I never spoke of to anyone. The last mention to another human being about it, before finding the [AIS email] circle and especially___ [another group member in similar situation], was my Mom telling me as a young kid not to worry about it, that I would grow into it. (Wrong, Mom, but it was a nice try.) The idea of someone seeing me naked, someone seeing that 'thing' mortified me to a degree I still haven't conquered. I shut off the entire idea of relationships and sex for this lifetime because

I didn't think I would ever find someone who could understand or accept it, not that I would have thought about giving anyone half a chance to come to any understanding or acceptance.

Now, as I climb toward that mystical age 30 mark, I feel like I'm finally getting my life into some kind of order and coming to believe in the fact that I can have a normal, happy life. Since finding the support group and the [AIS email discussion] circle, I'm a lot happier with my lot in life and realize that I'm glad I didn't risk the loss of sensitivity through the surgery. I realize now that it is not impossible to find someone who would understand and love me for me, and who would not worry, to the extent that I do, about the size of my clitoris. It bothers me a lot that I can't be totally sure whether B.C. (Before Contact) [with the group] I would have gotten the surgery, but with the realizations I've come to since then, I'm glad that I didn't do it. More than anything, I want to make sure that someone who does it has had the chance for those realizations that came to me relatively late in life.

Finding their voice

Finding their voice at last, via support/advocacy groups, has enabled XY women to inform clinicians of their real concerns. For a long time doctors have been talking *about* them without actually talking *with*, or listening *to* them. So what are the burning issues for AIS adults?

Overall, the main concerns of XY women seem to be (i) the major problem of secrecy, leading to isolation with lack of information and support; (ii) the devastating effects of being displayed as a freak in front of medical students and being subjected to medical photography; (iii) the immensely stigmatizing medical terminology used (supposedly behind their backs but which can be seen in the medical section of any academic bookshop, e.g. "genetic males" or "XY males" (with "males" used as a noun), "male pseudohermaphrodite", "undermasculinized males", "undervirilized males", "hairless pseudofemale", "sexually infantile" (referring to nipples), etc.); and (iv) lack of certain female bodily attributes. Generally these are the things that doctors and parents dismiss, gloss over or fail to acknowledge as being traumatizing. The issues that, in the longer term and with appropriate support, seem lesser concerns are the XY chromosomes and the testes (neither are discussed much at our meetings), infertility in many cases, and inherent gender identity (in CAIS at least). That is, all those things on which doctors and parents concentrate their thoughts/anxieties.

It seems that the medical profession has been worrying for years about what might be called a "deficient maleness" in conditions like AIS (and even talk about it in these terms in their research papers, even when describing girls/women with the complete form of AIS), whereas patients have been mainly concerned with their "lack of female attributes" and this is what they talk about at meetings: things like (i) lack of menstruation as a rite of passage, absence of pubic hair (in CAIS) and presence of pale underdeveloped nipples (all much more overt and everyday reminders of their "difference" than chromosomes or gonads – and a source of great anxiety for most AIS women); (ii) vaginal length, and size of clitoris and labia; (iii) sexual response and experience, testosterone and libido; (iv) HRT preparations; (v) comparison of body features (height, length of limbs, size of hands, feet, teeth); (vi) body odour (general lack of in CAIS?), etc.

One thing that everyone notices at our meetings is how one can dispense with all niceties and get down to the nitty gritty straight away, in stark contrast to how most affected women operate in their normal lives, even with women friends. I think most feel they missed out completely on adolescence, and on "girly" comparisons like this, because of feeling so stigmatized, marginalized and unusual. By meeting others you gain a sense of belonging to a peer group at last and can share commonalities but, importantly, it also shows you that there is as much variety between XY women as between women in general and that not everything about yourself that you are unhappy about is due to AIS, or Swyers, or whatever (the "AIS bucket" phenomenon).

Youngsters with CAIS may well be very confused and anxious about their physical/functional differences, compared with other girls, but underlying gender identity is not as fragile as many doctors/parents seem to think. The way to resolve the former is to allow discussion, counselling and meetings with others. Overemphasis by doctors/parents on essential "femaleness" in CAIS is unnecessary and is, in itself, likely to convey a sense of acute unease to the affected person.

There seems to have been a "mythologizing" of CAIS promoted via an overemphasis of these patients' femininity, both in the literature and in dialogues between doctors and parents/patients. There seems to have been an idea going around that AIS women are somehow more attractive, and behave in a more feminine way, than other women merely because of their complete insensitivity to male hormones (the old "air stewardesses, models and movie stars with AIS" notion). Whether true or not, these ideas are probably popular because they make the syndrome seem more remarkable and they reassure those people who are uncomfortable with the idea of an XY woman. But such notions are of little help to the affected women themselves and many members ask that we remove them from our literature.

We suggest infertility to be no more of an issue than in women who are infertile for other reasons, except that those with AIS have to shoulder this burden from an early age (maybe this makes it easier in adult life). Most support group contacts in long-term partnerships seem to have dealt with, or plan to deal with, this via adoption, surrogacy, etc. The burdens are probably "stacked", with unresolved vaginal hypoplasia possibly taking precedence over infertility in those who have this additional deficiency.

Sex talk

A common complaint by adult women to the group is that the doctors will *certainly* talk about infertility, will *probably* pluck unsubstantiated reassurances out of the air about gender identity, *may* talk about gonads and chromosomes, but the one thing they *never* discuss fully (beyond glib exhortations of "normality") is the patient's fitness for sex and relationships: topics that are at the forefront of the patient's mind. The group can provide help in the emotional, "you're-not-the-only-one" type of support but it cannot offer the much needed specialized psychosexual counselling, although psychosexual therapists occasionally attend our meetings.

A 39 year old with CAIS submitted her story for our website.

I've learned what little I know about AIS through dribs and drabs over the years, even though I was diagnosed with what I now know as CAIS at 16 or 17 . . .

I did not have intercourse until I was 34 and I believe the social retardation I suffered as a result of how my diagnosis was handled severely affected my personality, my ability to form intimate relationships and my self perception as a woman. I was given what everyone euphemistically referred to as a "hysterectomy". But I heard the words, "short vagina" said in passing, with no explanation and no elaboration. And it dramatically affected how I saw myself. I was so embarrassed by the very thought of it – how can you bring yourself to discuss *that* with a middle-aged white guy? Your mother? Anyone? I pretended it didn't matter and though my mother explained all the scientific stuff to me, I was only interested in the practical effect of it all: I couldn't have sex.

Well – I knew I could try but that it would be humiliating. So I didn't. For worse (or for better) I didn't *dare* "go all the way" with anyone – through college, through law school, and for years as a lawyer. And the longer I went a virgin, the more difficult it was to subject myself to the humiliation of someone rejecting my sex. All types of scenarios were played out in my head: "What??? No hair? What's wrong with you? I can't get it in!!! Oh my God! What's that scar? Testes?????", etc.

As I write this, I know it sounds so ridiculous. But I always felt I had so much more explaining to do than any other girl and I couldn't imagine how I could finesse the way I looked and how my body was made without diverting the romantic mood. My fears continued to

escalate. By 34, I felt I was a freak, or would be perceived as one. But I took a huge risk and planned to have sex just to get it over with . . . So inhibited was I that it took him over three hours of massaging me to achieve penetration . . . . As it was, it turned out to be a positive experience. One of the happiest memories I think I'll ever have is driving home on a sunny day, age 34, knowing that I had had sex. How pathetic it would seem to most people, but it was the first time I felt that I was normal. If only I had known it was possible decades earlier, my self concept might have evolved . . .

. . . there seems to be an effect on my psyche that remains from all those years of not being able to connect in that way. Am I imagining this? I try, but I think that now I'll always be too independent to form the kind of romantic, emotional, sexual attachment that most other people take for granted.

If anyone has been through this, please let me know. I'm sure there are psychological implications that haven't been explored. One of the first steps is having someone to identify with. That's what is so great about this [AISSG] website . . . . [I] hope that one day I can get over it. But it's hard and the rejection – if it ever happened – would reach such fearful magnitudes that I might never trust anyone ever again. Which explains my dilemma, but doesn't solve it.

Even younger women, born in more liberal times, have the same problems. A 23-year-old woman wrote from overseas.

I have the very same experiences as ___ [on the website]. I am quite good-looking, smart girl, successful and attractive. My only problem is that I have never had sex or a real relationship with men. All my merry friends would be shocked by this fact. I try to avoid lying to them, I just don't talk about sex with my friends . . . .

For much of this dilemma (knowing myself this is a bit stupid), I blame the doctors who made my diagnosis. I was thirteen, and there had been infertility – probably exactly AIS – in my mother's side of the family, so there were some doubts there might be something wrong in me too . . . . I was diagnosed to have "testicular feminization". The young male doctor displayed a figure of my chromosomes, told I had a genotype of a male but appearance of a female. "The patient has a short, blind vagina and there's some risk of a tumor if it's not operated", I heard during the process . . . . It came clear I cannot have children, but simply not a single word of sex. Nobody offered me any counseling, nobody explained to me what this peculiar condition might be.

It's been ten years now since the first diagnosis. I haven't been at gynecologist's even once. I haven't had sex or relationships or talked to anyone about it . . . It's only now I have found out that there actually *is* reasonable information about this and there are other names to it than this "testicular feminization", which I feel somehow inappropriate. And what's most important, I have found out there is a lot of other people with AIS too.

I know the doctors are not the big bad devil in this trauma, nor is my AIS. It is a complicated mix of many things . . . Still, I think that it would have been easier to grow up if the doctors would have treated me as a real living and feeling person, not as a medical freak, and if somebody would have talked to me seriously about me, genders and sex. Now they really made me feel like sexual outcast. They made me think that, for example, school lessons of sex issues were not meant to me: teachers speaked about sex of another species, the species of the normal. Anyway, the problem was not that I was told about my AIS. It is good to know that. I had always known there was something special in my body or my gender, and the diagnosis makes many things clear which was a true relief. The problem was the way it was told . . . . I just was hinted I was a monster to other people, and that's what I think is unforgivably cruel.

Vaginal hypoplasia

Decisions concerning vaginal hypoplasia involve questions of the timing of intervention and the method used. We have the impression that treatment in childhood is more often advocated in the USA than in the UK. But at a UK AISSG meeting, two paediatric endocrine nurses outlined an ethical problem involving a child (late childhood) in their care whose parents wanted to schedule a gonadectomy and a vaginoplasty at the same time. The parents were being secretive with their child and were not allowing the medical staff to give her any information that might allow her to give informed consent. The adults with AIS at the meeting felt that these parents were feeding their own anxieties about the whole issue, and that this would be patently obvious to the child, whose long-term interests would not be served by the proposed action. It seems more sensible to delay treatment until the patient is wanting to be prepared for sexual activity and can play a part in the choice of treatment.

There seems to have been an overemphasis on surgical vaginoplasty methods at the expense of less-invasive methods in which the patient has some control of and involvement in the process: methods such as the Frank manual pressure dilation technique (first described in 1938) or surgically assisted pressure dilatation methods like the Vecchietti procedure, a method that the AIS Support Group has been encouraging doctors and patients to look into for some years now (Anon., 1996e–g, 1998c–e, 1999c,d).

The founder of the US AISSG told us in 1998:

The McIndoe operation and Baldwin intestinal transposition are still very much the favored surgical alternatives to this day. Last week a mother of a teenager in S. California contacted me to tell me these were the two suggested methods presented by surgeons in a major metropolitan teaching hospital near L.A. I quickly sent the mom information about the "modified Vecchietti" method and suggested she inquire why this alternative had not been suggested. I'm really curious about what the surgeon's response will be when the mother presents this alternative.

I suspect that the Vecchietti isn't 'high tech' enough to appeal to most surgeons' interests – viz. they would not feel they had really accomplished anything by performing the procedure because they assess 'accomplishment' more in terms of the technical marvels of their operations and less in terms of the end results achieved by their patients. It strikes me that as both the MRKH support groups and our group promote the Vecchietti it will result in the failure to suggest this as an option being malpractice – even if the surgeon has legitimate reasons (can't imagine what they'd be) for favoring the Baldwin or McIndoe.

It could be argued that the use of surgical vaginoplasty is another example of doctors seeking to control everything themselves, to wave a magic (surgical) wand? Pressure dilatation can produce results that are as good, if not superior, to the most successful surgical outcome. The neovagina is created from stretching existing vaginal tissue without any cutting, so it retains its innervation, it lubricates naturally and involves no scarring. However, it does require a lot of psychological backup and support, because motivation to perform the rather tedious procedure twice a day is all important and is difficult to sustain. Very few gynaecology departments have this backup in place. As with general psychological support, the emotional needs of women coping with vaginal hypoplasia have been sadly neglected by the medical profession and this is where a multidisciplinary approach is so important.

A lot of genital surgery in children has been fuelled by anxiety over the performance aspects of males with a small penis. However, because medicine has not shown the same degree of concern about the capacity of female sexual "equipment" (and, therefore, no corresponding imperative to *masculinize* those in whom vaginal length falls short of the norm), there are some who, showing no outward signs of the panic-inducing deficient maleness, did not have their nonstandard genital morphology even properly recognized until relatively late and who have lived their life believing it precluded them from sexual relationships. A middle-aged woman with CAIS wrote (Anon., 1998f):

I discovered by self-examination in my early teens that my vagina was almost non-existent and told myself I could never have relationships. Every gynaecologist I saw following my eventual CAIS diagnosis, and clinical recognition of my anatomical problem, in my late teens, advised me against treatment unless I was about to get married or had a regular boyfriend (and I only saw one or two such clinicians; I felt far too much of a freak to go near them any more than necessary). But they didn't offer me any counseling to help me form such a relationship (and I felt far too traumatized and freakish to speak out in consultations, beyond answering 'yes' and 'no'). Everyone was so busy going on about how I was a normal female, in spite of my AIS, that I just didn't *dare* challenge this by asking how on earth I was going to have sex with a 1 cm vagina.

And no one mentioned the non-surgical pressure-dilation method until I had eventually undergone two plastic surgery operations (McIndoe skin graft and William's vulvo-vaginoplasty), which I now regret since they left me with scarring, and some disfigurement, without really helping matters. Being able to *talk* about the vaginal problem, and my whole AIS situation, would have been a lot more use to me.

She described her anguish at the reaction of a partner to her disclosure about her situation (Anon., 1997g). She also said:

At first (before the discussion turned angry) he did try to comfort me, and to be helpful, and said that in his experience, and in discussions with friends, he'd come to the conclusion that it wasn't what you *had* that mattered but what you *did* with what you had; and that maybe I should be adopting a different paradigm and thinking 'sensation' rather than thinking 'morphology'. At the time, I thought "what a stupid and unhelpful idea", but on reflection some months later I decided it was possibly one of the more sensible things he'd ever said (!) and I began to wish that I'd had a chance earlier in my life to discuss this possible mindset with a psycho-sexual counselor – since our high-tech medical system hadn't seemed able to provide me with a vagina at the time when one might have been of use to me in developing some view of myself as a sexual person, in the sense recognized by this society.

It is important that any young woman considering treatment for her vaginal hypoplasia should be given the opportunity to discuss the options not only with her specialist but also with *other women* who have undergone various types of treatment.

A woman in her mid thirties with AIS emailed:

I went through the McIndoe [skin graft vaginoplasty] surgery at 18.... The doctor didn't give me appropriate forms (dilators) for home use [after the surgery], so I had one thumb-sized form and one large wide one which I could never insert fully. Why he couldn't obtain appropriately-sized dilators prior to or shortly after the surgery, I don't know, but this was the major obstacle I never overcame. The pain of trying to use these forms at home, with no real help from the doctor, and a difficult examination in his office with the speculum, made me rule out sex entirely. I feel saddened that the surgery was carried out without adequate discussion and preparation beforehand. No mention was made of using pressure dilation before surgery, or the possibility, or necessity, of using sexual intercourse as a means of dilation/maintenance.

The negative experience with this surgery, and with the particular physician, resulted in me not seeking medical attention for over 18 years [she has never been prescribed HRT] and the complete avoidance of friendships with men. If the vaginal issue hadn't been the major problem, I think I would have lived a more normal social (sexual) life... but the fears of difficult or impossible vaginal intercourse, just made sexual contact out of the question for me. Besides this, I never understood how a girl with no pubic hair, and

two very prominent abdominal scars, and now two large skin-graft scars, could explain the situation to a man and not lie, freak out the man, totally turn him off, suffer rejection, etc.

The support group meetings have given me hope toward leading a more normal life. Just hearing everyone expressing their sexuality, in their myriad ways, has made me feel better. I find myself accepting myself more, and am not as uncomfortable talking to men.... In a way, it's a shame I didn't feel this way in my 20s.... It is difficult to imagine starting an emotional or physical relationship for the very first time in one's late 30s, but it is perhaps more of a psychological barrier than a physical one. The emotional and physical isolation can only be harmful. Now that the information about dilators and Vecchietti procedure is more widespread, the vaginal issues can perhaps be better addressed.

Hormone replacement therapy

It has been our observation that HRT is such an individual thing that this is the one area in which there is almost no point in women discussing "pros" and "cons" amongst themselves, other than perhaps issues relating to delivery method (e.g. tablets versus patches). A number of XY women are experimenting, under medical supervision, with testosterone-based HRT. There is also the (so far unanswered) question as to whether or not progesterone has benefits for patients without a uterus.

Rights of carriers

In AIS, denial and secrecy also cause problems for XX women in the family who might be carriers and who have a right to be made aware their potential carrier status so that they can make informed reproductive choices.

A 37-year-old woman with PAIS was at a UK support group meeting with her carrier sister. The sister related how she only learnt about AIS when she became pregnant in her thirties (even though her AIS sister had been diagnosed in her teens). She would very much have liked the chance to rehearse her feelings about all the implications/choices (prenatal tests, abortion, etc.) *before* becoming pregnant.

A 49 year old with CAIS emailed to the support group (Anon., 2001c):

Today my niece – the daughter of my non-AIS sister (my other sister and I have AIS) – announced she is "with child". She is 3.5 months pregnant. This should be great news to me yet my blood turned cold because my non-AIS sister *could* be a carrier.... I only found out about carriers last year when I got more info about AIS when I joined the group.

My non-AIS sister had a carrier test a year ago but still has had no result. We will chase tomorrow but lack of funding makes these delays happen. The big problem is... if she *is* a carrier, my niece could also be a carrier and the baby could be AIS. Is this right do you know? I am so worried. My niece had said she did not ever intend to have a baby. We had agreed not to tell her [about AIS] until we got the results of the carrier test but now it's too late.

Both my sisters have the denial factor – won't discuss AIS. My non-AIS sister has said I must not tell my niece now. She says – and she has a good point – that the stress involved could upset my niece and so damage the baby. She says that she may *not* be a carrier. Also that the baby could be a boy, or OK [XX noncarrier female] anyway.

Sorry . . . this is a tricky one to follow but I could really do with some advice here. It is an ethical dilemma. And a no-win situation. After the last group meeting I was all set to tell my niece about my condition too . . . What do you think I should do?

It sometimes works the other way round. At the same group meeting, a 35 year old with CAIS who had learnt her diagnosis late in life – not from a doctor or from her parents but in a letter from a cousin – tearfully explained how other people in her family (e.g. carriers) had been told more about her condition than she had. Being ostracized had been far more painful to her than the diagnostic knowledge itself.

In 2000, the website of the British Association of Paediatric Surgeons was displaying an article (MacKinnon, 1998) giving recommendations on truth disclosure in AIS, saying:

The diagnosis, if proved, may not lead to any immediate benefit to the patient or alteration in management. It could be argued for some families that investigations under such circumstances are not in the patient's interest.

When doctors advocate secrecy or half-truths like this, an obvious question is what about the rights of XX female relatives to know about their possible carrier status? Imagine the anger all round when a baby's AIS diagnosis is communicated to the parents and the mother's sister suddenly realises she herself must have AIS, and that no-one was brave enough to tell either her or her XX sister earlier in life so that they could each deal with the actuality and the possibility, respectively, in a useful way.

A father wrote to us in 2002.

First of all, thank you for the information that your organization has provided over the web, it has been invaluable. I am a father with an infant with CAIS. I found out by way of a hernia operation [on our baby]. My wife has a 25-year-old sister who also has CAIS but we have only just found out what it actually is. She was originally diagnosed with the older title, testicular feminisation, but was told at the time that it was a one off and a freakish event by her doctor. She was also very much misinformed on her condition and basically grew up thinking she was a freak, all because her doctor didn't look into it but merely assumed he knew all there was to know. So you could imagine the surprise we all had when we learnt what it actually was, through my little girl, ___ [baby's name].

How do doctors know what information may or may not be in the patient's interest? It is the sowing of these early seeds of secrecy and ignorance that may result, in 20, 30, 40, even 50 years time, in these "babies" being severely traumatized by reading words like "male pseudohermaphrodite" upside down in their medical notes. They may be too petrified to bring up the subject until later in life when they finally contact a support group saying: "Well, it seems the doctors never told my parents anything . . . so they never discussed it with me . . . so I've just lived in the belief I was a one-off freak, for all this time."

If doctors put their energy into helping us to publicize to society that these conditions/states actually *exist* in Nature, and that it is not so bad for people with access to a support group, then there would not be this perceived need to keep certain parts of the truth from certain parents/patients. It just seems like yet more paternalism and "doctoring" of information, with the medical profession once again setting themselves up as the gatekeepers of diagnostic information without, apparently, even considering involving clinical psychologists.

As AIS becomes less of a closet issue within families, there will be an increased demand for carrier testing services to enable XX female relatives to make reproductive choices. To date this has only been available on an ad hoc basis, as a favour on the back of genetic research into the androgen receptor gene, for which funding is now drying up.

Telling/educating others

The question of what to tell friends, partners and other family members is a major issue for XY women. Through discussions with women at support group meetings and by email it has become clear that *preparation* is all important. By the time the affected person comes to tell others, she should have reached some resolution of her feelings about her condition by having talked at length with other affected women, with counsellors, psychotherapists etc. and should have had a chance to rehearse, in these nonthreatening situations, what she might say when facing those with whom she is emotionally involved.

The worst situation is for the woman to be using the process of revelation as a primary means of resolving her own conflicts. If the teller is not used to talking about her condition, the exchange is likely to be fraught with additional complexities, with the listener having to cope with the woman's probable distress as well as having to deal with his or her own reaction, and with the teller then getting mixed signals reflected back from the confidant/e in a "hall of mirrors" scenario. If the woman herself is comfortable with her situation and can "spill the beans" in a confident, almost light-hearted manner, then the listener is far more likely to have a positive reaction, which in turn helps the "bean-spiller".

A middle-aged woman with CAIS wrote (Anon., 1997f):

It's almost unbelievable that in middle-age I should find myself agonizing over what, if anything, to tell my first ever real boyfriend about my condition. And that someone with whom I was emotionally involved had to be the very first human being to whom I'd ever articulated the words; and so late in life. In the emotional breakdown precipitated by my eventual disclosure of the truth to him – some two years after the early failure of the relationship [severe vaginal hypoplasia having made intercourse impossible] – I also found myself bringing up the subject of my medical condition with my parents for the first time, only to find that my father couldn't understand the medical basis of it at all and my mother wouldn't even try, still refusing to acknowledge my condition as being anything other than a fertility problem.

The same principle applies to parents who have the task of revealing the truth to their daughter. They really owe it to the listener to have sorted out their own feelings and conflicts as much as possible long before they embark on the telling.

The timing of telling others is very problematic for adult women. If it's a potential partner, do you tell them on the first date on the principle that if they can't cope with it upfront, then there's no future in the relationship? Do you tell when things get serious and sex is involved (particularly relevant in the case of vaginal hypoplasia or a larger than average clitoris)? Do you wait until the relationship seems likely to be long term and issues of fertility come into play? Telling a partner *early* risks jeopardizing the relationship. Telling a partner *late* risks accusations of lack of trust.

How *much* should one divulge: just the infertility, or the whole bag of tricks including the testes and XY chromosomes? How does the average androgen-sensitive man-in-the-street process the notion of an XY woman with testes? Whose needs are being served by a decision to tell? Does the other person have a right to know or is telling only advisable if it causes the affected woman herself pain to keep secrets from a loved one? It presents many dilemmas that women need to have explored beforehand.

Summary

Adult women with AIS and similar conditions have made enormous progress since the early–mid 1990s in coming out of the closet, gaining confidence, influencing medical practice and changing social attitudes. Intersex is now something of a hot topic in popular magazines and TV programmes. It is gratifying to see the number of psychological studies that are now underway and that a shift away from the medicalization of these conditions is taking place. The main problem area, in the eyes of the support group, is the continuing isolation amongst parents of infants and young children, and the huge ignorance of many GPs. Future decision making could also encompass issues of assisted conception brought about by advances in genetics.

REFERENCES

Anon. (1995a). Surgery – for whose benefit? *ALIAS* No. 3. Winter 1995.

(1995b). Can/should doctors counsel? *ALIAS* No. 1. Spring 1995.

(1995c). Multidisciplinary approach. *ALIAS* No. 1. Spring 1995.

(1996a). Malignancy risks. *ALIAS* No. 5. Summer 1996.

(1996b). Low bone density in AIS. *ALIAS* No. 6. Winter 1996.

(1996c). Letter to America. *ALIAS* No. 4. Spring 1996.

(1996d). A search for support. *ALIAS* No. 4. Spring 1996.

(1996e). Vaginal aplasia treatments. *ALIAS* No. 4. Spring 1996.

(1996f). Vecchietti video. *ALIAS* No. 5. Summer 1996.

(1996g). Vecchietti re-visited. *ALIAS* No. 6. Winter 1996.

(1997a). Puberty at six? *ALIAS* No. 9. Autumn 1997.

(1997b). Parent problems. *ALIAS* No. 10. Winter 1997.

(1997c). A mother's story. *ALIAS* No. 7. Spring 1997.

(1997d). Reading the words. *ALIAS* No. 9. Autumn 1997. [Also available on Debates/Discussions page of AISSG website http://www.medhelp.org/www/ais/43_debates.htm#textbooks.]

(1997e). Hearing the words. *ALIAS* No. 9. Autumn 1997. [Also available on Debates/Discussions page of AISSG website http://www.medhelp.org/www/ais/43_debates.htm#textbooks.]

(1997f). Saying the words. *ALIAS* No. 9. Autumn 1997. [Also available on Debates/Discussions page of AISSG website http://www.medhelp.org/www/ais/43_debates.htm#textbooks.]

(1997g). Plumbing problem perception. *ALIAS* No. 7. Spring 1997.

(1998a). Doing the right thing. *ALIAS* No. 11. Spring 1998.

(1998b). Truth disclosure discussion. *ALIAS* No. 12. Summer 1998.

(1998c). Vaginal hypoplasia. *ALIAS* No. 11. Spring 1998.

(1998d). 3rd US meeting. *ALIAS* No. 13. Autumn 1998.

(1998e). Vaginal hypoplasia discussion. *ALIAS* No. 13. Autumn 1998.

(1998f). Sensational paradigm? *ALIAS* No. 11. Spring 1998.

(1999a). Digging out your doc. *ALIAS* No. 15. Summer 1999.

(1999b). Webbed feat? *ALIAS* No. 15. Summer 1999.

(1999c). A vote for Vecchietti. *ALIAS* No. 14. Spring 1999.

(1999d). Vaginoplasty vs dilation. *ALIAS* No. 14. Spring 1999.

(2000a). ALIAS/website reactions. *ALIAS* No. 17. Summer 2000.

(2000b). A moan about mothers. *ALIAS* No. 16. Spring 2000.

(2001a). Old paradigm? *ALIAS* No. 18. Spring 2001.

(2001b). New Paradigm? *ALIAS* No. 18. Spring 2001.

(2001c). Carrier Status. *ALIAS* No. 19. Summer 2001.

Chase C (1995). Affronting reason. In *Looking Queer: Image and Identity in Lesbian, Bisexual, Gay and Transgendered Communities*, Atkins D, ed., pp. 205–220. Haworth, Binghamton, NY.

— (1999). Rethinking treatment for ambiguous genitalia. *Pediatr Nurs* 25, 451–455.

Dreger A D (1998). *Hermaphrodites and the Medical Invention of Sex*. Harvard University Press, Cambridge, MA.

Dreger A D (ed.) (1999). *Intersex in the Age of Ethics*. [Collection of articles from a special intersex issue of *J Clin Ethics* 9, No. 4, plus additional material.] University Publishing Group, Hagerstown, MD. http://www.upgbooks.com.

Fausto-Sterling A (1993). The five sexes: why male and female are not enough. *The Sciences*, March/April. [See also http://biomed.brown.edu/Faculty/F/Fausto-Sterling.html]

Foley S, Morley G W (1992). Care and counseling of the patient with vaginal agenesis. *Female Patient*, 17, 73–80. [Also available at http://www.isna.org/articles/foley-morley.html]

Holmes M (1994). Re-membering a queer body. *Undercurrents* May, 11–13 [Faculty of Environmental Studies, York University, Ontario, Canada; transcript available on AISSG website http://www.medhelp.org/www/ais/43_debates.htm#re-membering]

Kessler S (1990a). The medical construction of gender: case management of intersexed infants. *Signs* (*J Women Culture Soc*) Autumn. [Precis of the article is on AISSG website http://www.medhelp.org/www/ais/articles/kessler.htm]

— (1990b). *Lessons From the Intersexed*. Rutgers University Press, New Brunswick, NJ.

MacKinnon A E (1998). *Androgen Insensitivity Syndrome: How Much to Tell Families of Girls with Inguinal Hernia Regarding the Possible Diagnosis*. British Association of Paediatric Surgeons' website (2000). http://www.baps.org.uk.

Mantel H (1995). *A Change of Climate*. Penguin Books, London.

Money J (1987). Psychologic considerations in patients with ambisexual development. *Semin Reprod Endocrinol* 5, 307–313.

Morris J M (1953). The syndrome of testicular feminization in male pseudo-hermaphrodites. *Am J Obstet Gynecol* 65, 1192–1211.

Nahman M R (2000). Embodied stories, pragmatic lives: intersex body narratives on the net. MA Thesis, York University, Toronto.

Sandberg D (1995/6). Letter. In *Hermaphrodites with Attitude*. Autumn/Winter. [Newsletter of Intersex Society of North America http://www.isna.org]

Schober J M (1998). Long-term outcome of feminizing genitoplasty for intersex. In *Pediatric Surgery and Urology: Long-term Outcomes*. Saunders, London.

Slocum V (1995). Slaying the dragon [letter]. In *Hermaphrodites with Attitude*. Summer. [Newsletter of Intersex Society of North America http://www.isna.org]

Warne G L (1997). *Complete Androgen Insensitivity Syndrome*. [Patient/parent booklet] Department of Endocrinology and Diabetes, Royal Children's Hospital, Victoria, Australia. [Copies available from the AIS Support Group.]

Wilson B E, Reiner W G (1999). Management of intersex: a shifting paradigm. In *Intersex in the Age of Ethics*, Dreger A D, ed., [Collection of articles from a special intersex issue of *J Clin Ethics* 9, No. 4, plus additional material.] University Publishing Group, Hagerstown, MD. http://www.upgbooks.com.

RESOURCE SOURCES

Androgen Insensitivity Syndrome Support Group (AISSG) Newsletter *ALIAS*, website http://www.medhelp.org/www/ais.

Intersex Society of North America (ISNA) website http://www.isn.org.

Intersex Support Group International (ISGI) website http://www.isgi.org.

Part III

Management of specific disorders

18

Disorders of growth and puberty

Cristina Traggiai and Richard Stanhope

Department of Paediatric Endocrinology, Great Ormond Street Hospital for Children and The Middlesex Hospital, London, UK

Introduction

Puberty is defined as the acquisition of secondary sexual characteristics associated with a growth spurt and resulting in the attainment of reproductive function. The endocrine events of puberty commence many years before the onset of phenotypic puberty (see Ch. 4). The onset of puberty is characterized by nocturnal luteinizing hormone (LH) release. It is a result both of increased pituitary sensitivity to gonadotrophin-releasing hormone (GnRH) caused by prolonged unopposed oestrogen exposure of the gonadotrophic cells and of gonadal hormone secretion. In boys, spermatogenesis is initiated at stage 3, and menarche in girls occurs during late puberty. Initial menstrual cycles are usually anovulatory, which is associated with irregular and often painful periods. Precocious puberty is defined as the development of sexual characteristics before the age of eight years in girls and nine years in boys. Delayed puberty is defined when there is no sign of puberty at the age of 13.4 years in girls and 14 years in boys (2SD above the mean of chronological age for the onset of puberty).

It is important to recognize the harmony of normal events (consonance) of puberty; when it is absent, an endocrine disorder should be suspected. The loss of consonance has been described as one of the first signs of an endocrine disease (e.g. hypothyroidism, Cushing's syndrome, gonadal dysgenesis), in the absence of more obvious manifestations (Stanhope et al., 1986).

Disorders of pubertal development

The classification of disorders of pubertal development are described in Table 18.1.

Premature sexual maturation

Premature thelarche

Isolated premature thelarche

There are two forms of isolated premature thelarche, the classical and nonclassical forms. The onset of the classical form is usually under the age of two years (especially in the second half of the first year of life) and is continuous from the breast development that occurs under the influence of circulating maternal oestrogens in breast-feeding girls, with no other signs of puberty (absent pubic hair, normal growth velocity and bone age). It has an incidence of 21/100 000 persons/year (Van Winter et al., 1990). There is a temporary activation of the hypothalamic–pituitary–gonadal axis, and it is predominantly related to secretion of follicle-stimulating hormone (FSH) rather than LH. There are cycles at about six-weekly intervals, with waxing and waning of breast size, and the condition "burns itself out" after a few years (Stanhope et al., 1988). No treatment is required (Stanhope, 2000). The "atypical" or nonclassical isolated premature thelarche, which affects older girls, with occasional menstrual withdrawal bleeding tends to be associated with progression to central precocious puberty and may have longer-term sequelae although puberty and fertility are described as being normal (Pasquino et al., 1995).

Other forms of premature thelarche

A different condition is represented by slowly progressive precocious puberty (Fontoura et al., 1989), also known as thelarche variant (Stanhope and Brook, 1990) or exaggerated thelarche (Garibaldi et al., 1993). Such girls have breast changes as with premature thelarche but also have accelerated bone age and growth velocity and occasionally some

Paediatric and Adolescent Gynaecology, ed. Adam Balen et al. Published by Cambridge University Press.
© Cambridge University Press 2004.

Table 18.1. Classification of disorders of pubertal development

	Types
Premature sexual maturation	
Premature thelarche	Isolated premature thelarche (classical or nonclassical, atypical, forms)
	Slowly progressive precocious puberty (thelarche variant, exaggerated thelarche)
Isolated premature menarche	
Premature adrenarche	
Precocious puberty	Gonadotrophin-dependent form
	Gonadotrophin-independent form
Delayed puberty	
Pubertal delay	Constitutional growth and pubertal delay
	Secondary to chronic illness
Pubertal failure	Hypogonadotrophic hypogonadism
	Hypergonadotrophic hypogonadism

pubic hair development. We know little about the natural history of this condition, although final stature is unaffected. Treatment is not helpful and psychological difficulties are rare.

Isolated premature menarche

Isolated premature menarche comprises cyclical uterine withdrawal bleeding with no other signs of sexual maturation (Heller et al., 1979). The aetiology is unknown; there is an activation of the hypothalamic–pituitary – gonadal axis and it is related to FSH secretion, with increased sensitivity of the endometrium to oestrogens, which are at too low concentration to produce breast development (Heller et al., 1979). Some authors have reported the presence of ovarian follicular cysts (Blanco-Garcia et al., 1985). It is, however, important to exclude the presence of a local lesion of the genital tract, McCune–Albright syndrome (premature menarche may rapidly be followed by vulvovaginal and breast changes), exogenous administration of oestrogens and child abuse. There do not appear to be any long-term sequelae to either puberty or fertility (Murran et al., 1983).

Premature adrenarche

Premature adrenarche (or premature pubarche) is defined as precocious development of sexual hair (pubic hair,

axillary hair or both) before eight years of age in girls or nine years of age in boys, with no other signs of sexual maturation. There is an increased frequency between five and eight years of age. The aetiology is unknown, but there is a selective adrenal androgen activation and the condition is associated with the development of the zona reticularis of the adrenal cortex. Premature adrenarche is more common in girls than in boys and in black than in white racial groups (Silverman et al., 1952). Familial transmission is rare (Lee et al., 1987). The pubic hair, which is mostly limited to the labia majora in girls, is usually dark, straight or curly, and coarse (Ibanez et al., 1992). Other clinical symptoms may include skin changes, acne, adult-type perspiration and a deepening of the voice (Thamdrup, 1955). Such children may be taller than normal girls and their bone age may often be advanced (Silverman et al., 1952); however, some authors have noted a normal height and a normal bone age (Thamdrup, 1955). Plasma levels of dehydroepiandrosterone (DHEA-S) and Δ^4-androstendione and urinary 17-ketosteroids are elevated for age to the range normally seen in older pubertal children (Korth-Schtz et al., 1976). Long-term sequelae may be early puberty (Ibanez et al., 1992) peripubertal hirsutism and/or polycystic ovary syndrome (Ibanez et al., 1993). Premature adrenarche is an important condition to recognize but requires no treatment; the long-term potential sequelae (hyperinsulinism, hirsutism, obesity, menstrual disturbance) are beginning to be appreciated.

Precocious puberty

Precocious puberty is defined as the development of sexual characteristics before the age of eight years in girls and nine years in boys.

Gonadotrophin-dependent precocious puberty

Gonadotrophin-dependent precocious puberty (central precocious puberty (CPP)) is characterized by activation of the hypothalamic–pituitary–gonadal axis, with increased pulsatile release of LH, increased LH response to GnRH, and elevation of circulating gonadal sex steroid concentrations. Hypothalamic hamartoma, astrocytoma, optic glioma, pineal tumours, arachnoid cyst and CNS malformations have been reported as organic causes of CPP. The pathogenesis is unknown; it has been suggested that transforming growth factor α may be involved in the active stimulation of GnRH secretion in organic CPP (Junier et al., 1991). The idiopathic form of CPP occurs in 74% of the girls (Cisternino et al., 2000), and in 60% of the boys, who are more likely to have an occult intracranial tumour than girls

(De Sanctis et al., 2000). High risk factors for the presence of an intracranial tumour are a young age of onset (under the age of three years), high serum LH concentrations not associated with the development of an LH surge and high leptin concentrations, but it is impossible to exclude an intracranial lesion without performing a magnetic resonance scan (Chemaitilly et al., 2001). The treatment of hypothalamic hamartoma is generally pharmacological (see below), as surgical intervention is difficult and does not usually lead to resolution of the early puberty. The hamartoma usually remains the same size.

Early puberty in children who have been adopted from developing countries has been reported. The aetiology is unknown but different factors have been postulated as cause of this early sexual maturation: genetic potential, changes of environment (from an underprivileged to a privileged one) (Proos et al., 1991) insulin-like growth factor 1 (IGF-1), leptin (Virdis et al., 1998), exposure to dichlorodiphenyltrichloroethane (DDT) (Krstevska-Konstantinova et al., 2001) or a rapid increase in fat mass (causing a rapid increase of free sex steroid concentrations).

Therapy is with a GnRH agonist, which has the paradoxical action of inducing downregulation of pituitary GnRH receptors and desensitization of pituitary gonadotrophs, with suppression of spontaneous and stimulated pituitary gonadotrophin secretion. A recovery of the hypothalamic–pituitary–gonadal axis in a few weeks is seen at the end of treatment (Jay et al., 1992). The GnRH agonist may be given either by daily subcutaneous or intranasal administration or by a long-acting subcutaneous or intramuscular depot given every four weeks at a dosage of 3.75 mg or every 12 weeks at 11.25 mg. A withdrawal bleeding may occur within 1 month, but none should be seen thereafter. Cyproterone acetate (100 mg/m^2 daily in two doses for two to three weeks, to be started before the first GnRHa injection) may be useful to prevent the spotting. This treatment results in a fall of gonadal sex steroid levels into the prepubertal range, arrested or regression of secondary sexual development, a complete cessation of menses, slowed growth velocity and retarded skeletal maturation (Boepple et al., 1986). There are few side effects of GnRH agonist treatment in childhood; those that occur can include local reactions, headache, migraine, photophobia and reduced self-esteem. Growth hormone may be added to the treatment of some short girls, or those with a marked reduction of growth velocity (Tatò et al., 1995). Some questions need to be clarified for girls after stopping therapy: there are few data on the prevalence of polycystic ovaries, on bone mineral density (BMD) and obesity (Tatò et al., 2001). A reversible reduction of BMD

during treatment has been shown in some studies, but it has not been confirmed in others. An increased incidence of polycystic ovary morphology on ultrasound scan has been reported in CPP after stopping GnRH analogue therapy; it is not clear if this condition is caused by the disease itself, by the treatment or by a degree of adrenal hyperactivity (Tatò et al., 2001).

Gonadotrophin-independent precocious puberty
Gonadotrophin-independent precocious puberty (GIPP) is characterized by pubertal sex steroid concentrations in the presence of prepubertal or suppressed gonadotrophins. In patients with this condition, especially those without a family history, the possibility of disorders of the gonad or adrenal gland or an autonomous secretion of gonadotrophins by a tumour should be excluded. Prepubertal girls with pseudoprecocious puberty may have an isolated ovarian functional cyst caused by McCune–Albright syndrome (irregular areas of skin pigmentation, polyostotic fibrous dysplasia, and GIPP). In this syndrome, the mutation in the α-subunit of the G_s-protein leads to the constitutive activation of adenylyl cyclase in various tissues, including the ovary, with the characteristic ultrasound picture (large asymmetric ovaries) and autonomous ovarian activation. It may present with abdominal pain and loss of the normal consonance of puberty, with early uterine bleeding. Ovarian surgery should be avoided or should be very conservative in cases of ovarian torsion.

Functioning gonadal tumours (sex cord tumour and Sertoli cell tumour) presenting as GIPP have been described in Peutz–Jeghers syndrome (Zung et al., 1998). GIPP has been reported in two girls with hypomelanosis of Ito; it has been postulated that chromosomal polyploidy affects the gonad in the same way as it does the skin (Daubeney et al., 1993).

Testotoxicosis is GIPP in males. It is characterized by pubertal development of the tubules with proliferation of Leydig cells to the appearance of normal adult testes; it is autosomal recessive, and a mutation of the LH receptor has been found in some families (Kremer et al., 1993).

Exposure to oestrogens in food, drugs or cosmetics may cause iatrogenic GIPP. Activating mutations of the LH receptor in boys have been described as a possible cause of gonadotrophin-independent sexual precocity (with normal prepubertal or suppressed LH and FSH levels and variable testosterone levels). In contrast, the same mutations allow normal ovarian function in prepubertal and adult females (Latronico et al., 2000), probably because FSH is the dominant gonadotrophin for ovarian follicle maturation. Ovarian, adrenal or LH/chorionic

Table 18.2. Treatment of gonadotrophin-independent precocious puberty

Drug	Properties	Effects	Dosage	Side effects
Cyproterone acetate	Potent progestin (hydroxyprogesterone derivate) and antiandrogen	Suppression of gonadal and adrenal steroidogenesis: antigonadotrophic	$100\,mg/m^2$ daily in two or three divided doses	Drowsiness, fatigue and tiredness (caused by cortisol insufficiency); gynaecomastia; liver damage (large doses)
Ketoconazole	Fungicidal agent	Steroid biosynthesis inhibitor	200 mg three times a day	Rash; vomiting, diarrhoea
Spironolactone	Mineralocorticoid receptor antagonist	Antiandrogen and antimineralocorticoid	50–100 mg twice daily	Fatigue; hyperkalaemia; menstrual disturbance
Testolactone	Aromatase inhibitor	Inhibition of the conversion of testosterone to oestrogens	35 mg/kg daily in three divided doses	Abdominal pain; headache; diarrhoea; increased liver enzymes

gonadotrophin-secreting tumours (granulosa cell, sex cord, masculinizing, adrenal rest, hilus cell, lipid cell) have all been reported in GIPP.

Treatment is summarized in Table 18.2.

Delayed puberty

Delayed puberty is defined as when there is no sign of puberty at the age of 13.4 years in girls and 14 years in boys (2SD above the mean of chronological age for the onset of puberty).

Pubertal delay
Constitutional growth and pubertal delay
Constitutional delay in growth and puberty is the commonest condition presenting to a paediatric endocrinologist. It is characterized by a positive family history, short stature, delayed puberty, delayed epiphyseal maturation and a relatively short upper body segment (Albanese and Stanhope, 1995a). Height prognosis is in the appropriate range for the parental centiles. In severely delayed puberty, growth of the upper body segment is impaired and remains short even at final adult height and this probably explains the adult height deficit in constitutional delayed puberty (Albanese and Stanhope, 1995b).

Although constitutional delay of growth and puberty is usually a clinical diagnosis, if the normal consonance of puberty is lost or if there is extreme bone age delay, thyroid function tests should be performed. In girls, a karyotype is essential (to exclude Turner's syndrome or androgen insensitivity syndrome).

Treatment is usually offered for psychological reasons in order to help the adolescent with seriously delayed puberty and short stature. A short course of androgen, with depot

testosterone (25–50 mg intramuscularly every month for four to six months), to induce a growth spurt and onset of pubertal development, or a low-dose anabolic steroid (e.g. oxandrolone 1.25–2.5 mg daily for six months) in younger boys, may be offered.

The problem is less common in girls, and low-dose oestrogen (2–4 µg daily of ethinylestradiol or transcutaneous oestrogens for, at least, six months) may be offered. The onset of breast development associated with a growth spurt rapidly resolves the problem. Treatment usually needs to be continued until the stage of pubertal development is greater than could be explained by the administered dose of exogenous oestrogen, indicating that the girl is in spontaneous puberty.

Secondary to chronic illness
Practically all chronic illnesses result in pubertal delay if they are of sufficient intensity and duration, especially because improved treatment leads to prolonged life expectation. If the disease starts in the prepubertal period, a decrease of growth rate and pubertal delay has been reported; if the disease starts during puberty, pubertal development may arrest or regress. Leptin levels correlate with body mass index and it is hypothesized that leptin has a permissive role in pubertal development and may signal onset of puberty throughout the hypothalamic–pituitary axis and peripheral hormones (Kiess et al., 2000). Leptin seems necessary but not essential for normal pubertal maturation to proceed. In boys, rising serum leptin levels precede the onset of puberty and are highest in the early stages of puberty. In contrast, in girls, leptin levels generally increase steadily with pubertal development. In some diseases, treatment has been recognized as the cause of

pubertal delay (e.g. corticosteroid therapy can cause growth delay and delay epiphyseal and pubertal maturation in patients with severe asthma). The growth retardation in children with chronic renal failure is caused by elevated concentrations of IGF binding proteins (IGFBP), which inhibit the bioavailability of the IGFs. After renal transplantation, growth retardation is associated with low plasma growth hormone (GH) levels, with normal diurnal rhythm of GH, IGF-1, IGF-2, and IGFBP-1 secretion; prednisone therapy is associated with inhibition of cartilage and bone matrix formation and of IGFBP-3 secretion. High–normal plasma levels of biologically active LH and elevated plasma levels of immunoreactive LH in uraemic children have been reported; but changes of LH secretion are reversible after renal transplantation. In adolescents with chronic renal disease, delayed puberty has been reported in both sexes, with testicular atrophy, hypospermatogenesis, infertility and impotence in men and anovulation, infertility and menstrual disturbance in women (Hokken-Koelega et al., 2001).

In patients affected by β-thalassaemia major, short stature is caused by iron toxicity and bone dysplasia by desferrioxamine and endocrine disorders (GH deficiency, hypothyroidism, defect of IGF-1 synthesis, hypogonadism and neurosecretory dysfunction). Hypogonadism is caused by iron overload and by free radicals (secondary to siderosis) in the pituitary and gonadotroph cells, or more rarely in the gonads (Caruso-Nicoletti et al., 2001).

In hypo- and hyperthyroidism, thyroxine concentrations directly influence puberty through actions at hypothalamic and/or higher brain centres that control LH secretion. Diabetic females have a higher probability of delayed menarche if the onset of diabetes is before puberty, or a higher risk for development of menstrual disturbances if the onset is after puberty (Yeshaya et al., 1995).

Impairment of growth and delayed puberty in patients with inflammatory chronic bowel disease have been reported. Chronic undernutrition and inflammatory mediators (interleukin-6 and interleukin-1) secreted from the inflamed gut are associated with short stature. Inhibition of GnRH secretion and gonadal steroidogenesis may cause pubertal delay. Recent studies have shown that interleukin-6 and interleukin-1 can inhibit steroidogenesis in both the ovaries and testes (they can reach the gonads by way of the circulation or through the response to bacterial toxins); they can also inhibit the secretion of GnRH by activating hypothalamic neural circuits containing corticotrophin-releasing hormone and vasopressin (Griffiths, 1998).

Langerhans' cell histiocytosis often presents with diabetes insipidus. GH deficiency and gonadotrophin deficiency associated with diabetes insipidus can occur in severe cases of Langerhans' cell histiocytosis. Precocious puberty has also been reported in a patient with Langerhans' cell histiocytosis (Nanduri et al., 2000).

Amenorrhoea (primary and secondary), oligomenorrhoea, short luteal phases and anovulation can occur in the female athlete. The aetiology is not well understood, but it seems to be linked with low body fat stores and nutrition. There is a decrease in GnRH pulses from the hypothalamus, which in turn decreases the pulsatile secretion of LH and FSH and suppresses gonadal maturation. In runners, mild hyperandrogenism can cause delayed puberty; oestrogen replacement therapy is often prescribed in amenorrhoeic athletes, but loss of skeletal integrity may not be completely reversible (Warren and Shantha, 2000; see also Ch. 39).

In children treated for oncological diseases, growth and pubertal delay may result from damage to the hypothalamic–pituitary axis or the gonads. Patients who have received high doses (> 30 Gy) of cranial, craniospinal or total body irradiation are likely to develop GH deficiency within two to five years from cessation of treatment. Low doses of cranial irradiation (18–24 Gy) can cause precocious puberty, especially in girls, with a shorter growth spurt leading to a loss in final height. Delayed puberty has been reported after high doses (> 40 Gy) used to treat solid tumours adjacent to the hypothalamus (Rappaport et al., 1982).

There is a correlation between pubertal development and age (the immature hypothalamus may be more sensitive to irradiation), the dose of radiation given, different regimens and fractionation of irradiation (Hokken-Koelega et al., 1993; Locatelli et al., 1993). Irradiation of the gonads from spinal irradiation could potentially cause oligo/azoospermia with total doses of 6 Gy; Leydig cell damage is common after total doses > 20 Gy (Castillo et al., 1990). No long-term side effects on height, bone mineral density, body composition and bone maturation were found in patients with leukaemia treated with chemotherapy alone. Chemotherapy may cause growth retardation, but catch-up growth occurs after cessation of treatment (van der Sluis et al., 2000). Gonadal damage after cyclophosphamide (dose related and may be reversible) and busulphan (the association may cause permanent ovarian failure) is well documented in adults, but it seems that prepubertal and pubertal ovaries are more resistant than adult ovaries (Kumar et al., 1972). Ovaries are more resistant than testes, and Leydig cells are more resistant than seminiferous tubules and Sertoli cells (Hughes et al., 1980).

Early menopause has been reported as well. The possibility of using GnRH agonists to prevent ovarian damage has been proposed although of uncertain benefit.

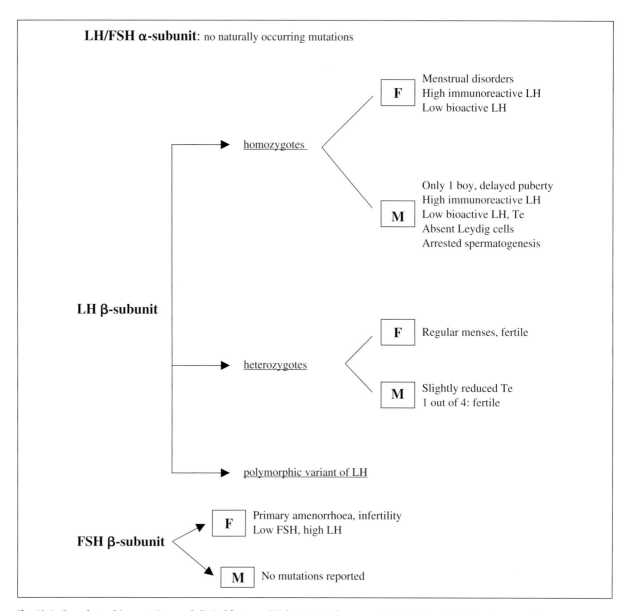

Fig. 18.1. Gonadotrophin mutations and clinical features. LH, luteinizing hormone; FSH, follicle-stimulating hormone; Te, testosterone; M, male, F, female.

Pubertal failure

Hypogonadotrophic hypogonadism

Hypogonadotrophic hypogonadism (HH) is characterized by low levels of sex steroids and gonadotrophin secretion. Idiopathic HH is the most common form. Abnormalities in GnRH secretion and action can result from lesions at different points on the pathways: impaired migration of GnRH-secreting neurons during development; defective GnRH synthesis, release and processing; or mutations affecting the receptor. Mutations have been identified in several genes, giving rise to mutant proteins (KAL; DAX1; related orphan nuclear receptor; steroidogenic factor-1;

leptin and prohormone convertase-1; the GnRH receptor; the pituitary transcription factors HESX-1, LHX3 and PROP-1; FSH; and LH) (Achermann and Jameson, 2001). The clinical features are vague and it is often difficult to distinguish between constitutional delay of growth and puberty and HH, especially in the early teenage years. A useful clinical sign is the growth deceleration after stopping a course of testosterone in children who fail to enter into puberty on their own. The endocrine distinction between HH, especially if partial, and constitutional delay is difficult to make. The best indication is provided by combining the results of a test for GnRH stimulation of LH release

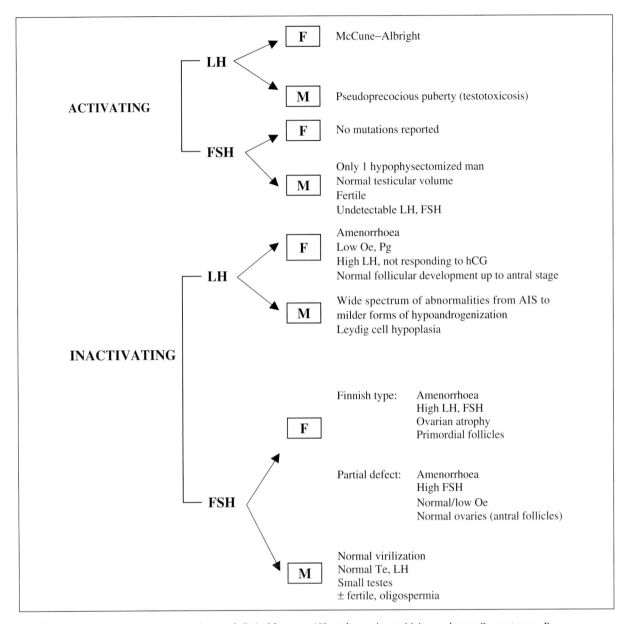

Fig. 18.2. Gonadotrophin receptor mutations and clinical features. AIS, androgen insensitivity syndrome; Oe, oestrogen; Pg, progesterone; Te, testosterone; hCG, human chorionic gonadotrophin; F, female; M, male.

(LHRH stimulation test: (100 μg or 2.5 μg/kg intravenous LHRH with blood taken at 20, 30 and 60 minutes) and a human chorionic gonadotrophin (hCG) test (1500 U intramuscular for 3 days and serum testosterone measured on day one and four). The interpretation of the LHRH test depends on the stage of puberty. The prepubertal child shows a small increment in LH and FSH up to 2–3 U/l. The response in early and mid-puberty is greater, particularly for LH. An absent response suggests gonadotrophin deficiency, but the test is unreliable in prepuberty and in

the child with simple delayed puberty. An exaggerated response, particularly with elevated basal levels, is obtained in precocious puberty and in gonadal failure. The normal testosterone response to the hCG test depends on the age of the patient. In infancy, a normal testosterone increment may vary from 2 to 10- or even 20-fold. In childhood, the increment is between 5- and 10-fold; during puberty, as the basal concentration is higher, the increment is less, 2- to 3-fold. If there is no response to a short hCG test (after three days), a prolonged test should be performed (after

Prepubertal

Short stature — *Dysmorphic features:*
Turner's syndrome
- Karyotype
Bone dysplasia
- Skeletal survey
Syndromes
- Genetics/chromosomes

No dysmorphic features:
Growth hormone deficiency
- Glucagon test
- Bone age
Hypothyroidism
- Thyroid function test
- Bone age
Cushing's syndrome
- Cortisol
Intracranial tumours
- Magnetic resonance scan
Chronic gonadotrophin β-subunit deficiency
- Follow-up
Chronic disease
- Improvement of disease and/or therapy
Ovarian failure
- Karyotype
- Pelvic ultrasound

Normal/tall stature — Androgen insensitivity syndrome
- Karyotype
Ovarian failure
- Karyotype

Arrested or regression of puberty

No consonance — Growth hormone deficiency
Hypothyroidism
Cushing's syndrome
Intracranial tumours

Consonance — Chronic disease
Chronic steroid therapy

Fig. 18.3. Flow chart for assessment of delayed puberty.

three weeks) (Dunkel et al., 1985). Some clinical features, such as anosmia, disturbance of colour vision and dyskinesis, may indicate a diagnosis of Kallmann's syndrome (X-linked). During fetal development, GnRH-releasing neurons and olfactory neurons originate in the olfactory placode and migrate through the cribriform plate to their final positions in the hypothalamus and olfactory bulb, respectively. The gene *KAL* encodes a protein that facilitates neuronal growth and migration. Cryptorchidism (three times greater than in idiopathic HH), unilateral renal agenesis, synkinesia (mirror-image movements), sensorineural deafness and icthyosis have been described in this syndrome (Quinton et al., 2001).

Prader–Willi syndrome is an autosomal dominant disease (defect on chromosome 15) characterized by decreased fetal activity, obesity, muscular hypotonia, men-

tal retardation, short stature, small hands and feet, micropenis, cryptorchidism and HH.

In recent years, gonadotrophin and gonadotrophin receptor mutations have been described (Achermann and Jameson, 2001). The phenotypic expression of these mutations is not well characterized and is variable (Figs. 18.1 and 18.2). LH and FSH have a common α-subunit (mapped on chromosome 6) and different β-subunits (LH-β on chromosome 19, and FSH-β on chromosome 11) (de Roux et al., 2001; Themmen et al., and Huhtaniemi, 2000; see also Ch. 3).

Hypergonadotrophic hypogonadism

Hypergonadotrophic hypogonadism is characterized by low levels of sex steroids and high circulating levels of gonadotrophin concentration. Gonadal dysgenesis is the most common cause. Turner's syndrome (45,X0 karyotype or Turner's mosaic 45,X0/46,XX), "pure" gonadal dysgenesis (XX karyotype), XY gonadal dysgenesis and multiple X chromosomes have been recognized as causes.

Turner's syndrome is a common sex chromosome abnormality and causes gonadal dysgenesis (Ch. 19). The major concerns in management of this syndrome are achievement of adequate final height (timing and duration of treatment with GH, oxandrolone, oestrogens), the timing of pubertal development, bone strength (as it seems that spontaneous puberty leads to a shorter final height, a course with agonist GnRH has been proposed) and fertility (the fetuses of women with Turner's syndrome who are fertile have a higher risk of developing congenital malformations; Guarnieri et al., 2001).

XX "pure" gonadal dysgenesis is characterized by gonadal failure alone but it may also be associated with sensorineural deafness (Perrault syndrome). XY gonadal dysgenesis is autosomal recessive (some may have an *SRY* mutation). Multiple X chromosome syndrome is extremely rare, with skeletal dysplasia, neurodevelopmental delay and gonadal failure. Patients with gonadal dysgenesis with a Y or Y fragment in their karyotype have a higher risk of developing gonadal cancer than patients without such abnormalities; surgical removal of the gonads must be performed.

Androgen insensitivity syndrome (AIS) is a defect of the androgen receptor caused by a gene defect in the X chromosome. There is a wide range of clinical manifestations in 46,XY individuals, from complete female external genitalia (complete AIS) to degrees of partial masculinization (partial AIS) (see Ch. 20 for greater details). The production and secretion of androgens are normal. Gonadectomy is required to eliminate the risk of gonadal malignancy. Although an adequate serum concentration of testosterone (basal or after hCG stimulation test) excludes a biosynthetic defect in testosterone production, a low testosterone (basal

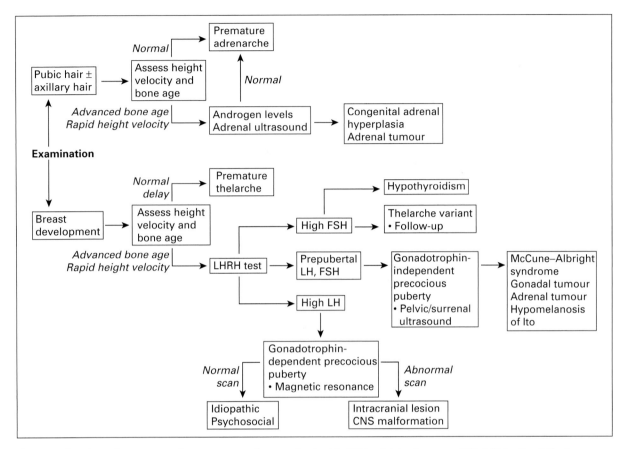

Fig. 18.4. Flow chart of assessment of premature sexual maturation in girls. LH, luteinizing hormone; FSH, follicle-stimulating hormone; LHRH, LH-releasing hormone.

or after hCG stimulation test) does not always exclude AIS. Basal LH and testosterone values are highly variable and might not be increased during early infancy (Ahmed et al., 1999). Patients with AIS are not strictly hypogonadal as they produce testosterone and this may be aromatized to oestrogen and induce satisfactory breast development, but of course they have no pubic hair in complete AIS because of the nonfunctioning androgen receptor.

Assessment of disorders of growth and puberty

Flow charts for assessment of delayed puberty and premature sexual maturation are summarized in Figs. 18.3 and 18.4, respectively.

REFERENCES

Achermann J C, Jameson J L (2001). Advances in the molecular genetics of hypogonadotropic hypogonadism. *J Pediatric Endocrinol Metab* 14, 3–15.

Ahmed S F, Cheng A, Hughes I A (1999). Assessment of the gonadotrophin–gonadal axis in androgen insensitivity syndrome. *Arch Dis Child* 80, 324–329.

Albanese A, Stanhope R (1995a). Investigation of delayed puberty. *Clin Endocrinol* 43, 105–110.

(1995b). Predictive factors in the determination of final height in boys with constitutional delay of growth and puberty. *J Pediatr* 126, 545–550.

Blanco-Garcia M, Evain-Brion D, Roger M, Job C L (1985). Isolated menses in prepubertal girls. *Pediatrics* 76, 43–47.

Boepple P A, Mansfield M J, Wierman M E et al. (1986). Use of a potent, long acting agonist of gonadotropin-releasing hormone in the treatment of precocious puberty. *Endocr Rev* 7, 24–33.

Caruso-Nicoletti M, De Sanctis V, Cavallo L et al. (2001). Management of puberty for optimal auxological results in β-thalassaemia major. *J Pediatr Endocrinol Metab* 14, 939–944.

Castillo L A, Craft A W, Kernahan J et al. (1990). Gonadal function after 12-Gy testicular irradiation in childhood acute lymphoblastic leukaemia. *Med Pediatr Oncol* 18, 185–189.

Chemaitilly W, Trivin C, Adan L et al. (2001). Central precocious puberty: clinical and laboratory features. *Clin Endocrinol* 54, 289–294.

Cisternino M, Arrigo T, Pasquino A M et al. (2000). Etiology and age incidence of precocious puberty in girls: a multicentric study. *J Pediatr Endocrinol Metab* 13, 695–701.

Daubeney P E F, Pal K, Stanhope R (1993). Hypomelanosis of Ito and precocious puberty. *Eur J Pediatr* 152, 715–716.

De Roux N, Milgrom E (2001). Inherited disorders of GnRH and gonadotropin receptors. *Mol Cell Endocrinol* 179, 83–87.

De Sanctis V, Corrias A, Rizzo V et al. (2000). Etiology of central precocious puberty in males: the results of the Italian Study Group for Physiopathology of Puberty. *J Pediatr Endocrinol Metab* 13, 687–693.

Dunaif A, Thomas A (2001). Current concepts in the polycystic ovary syndrome. *Annu Rev Med* 52, 401–419.

Dunkel L, Perheentupa J, Virtanen M, Maenpaa J (1985). Gonadotropin-releasing hormone test and human chorionic gonadotropin test in the diagnosis of gonadotropin deficiency in prepubertal boys. *J Pediatr* 107, 388–392.

Fontoura M, Brauner R, Prevot C, Rappaport R (1989). Precocious puberty in girls: early diagnosis of a slowly progressing variant. *Arch Dis Child* 64, 1170–1176.

Garibaldi L R, Aceto T Jr, Weber C (1993). The pattern of gonadotropin and estradiol secretion in exaggerated thelarche. *Acta Endocrinol* 128, 345–350.

Griffiths A M (1998). Inflammatory bowel disease. *Nutrition* 14, 788–791.

Guarneri M P, Abusrewwil S A S, Bernasconi S et al. (2001). Turner's syndrome. *J Pediatr Endocrinol Metab* 14, 959–965.

Heller M E, Dewhurst J, Grant D B (1979). Premature menarche without the evidence of precocious puberty. *Arch Dis Child* 54, 472–475.

Hokken-Koelega A C, van Doorn J W, Hahlen K et al. (1993). Long term effects of treatment for acute lymphoblastic leukaemia with or without cranial irradiation on growth and puberty: a comparative study. *Pediatr Res* 33, 577–582.

Hokken-Koelega A C S, Saenger P, Cappa M, Greggio N (2001). Unresolved problems concerning optimal therapy of puberty in children with chronic renal diseases. *J Pediatr Endocrinol Metab* 14, 945–952.

Hughes I A, Napier A, Thompson E N (1980). Pituitary–gonadal function in children treated for acute lymphoblastic leukaemia. *Acta Paediatr Scand* 69, 691–692.

Ibanez L, Virdis R, Potau N et al. (1992). Natural history of premature pubarche: an auxological study. *J Clin Endocrinol Metab* 74, 254–257.

Ibanez L, Potau N, Virdis R et al. (1993). Postpubertal outcome in girls diagnosed of premature pubarche during childhood: increased frequency of functional ovarian hyperandrogenism. *J Clin Endocrinol Metab* 76, 1599–1603.

Jay N, Mansfield M J, Blizzard R M et al. (1992). Ovulation and menstrual function of adolescent girls with central precocious puberty after therapy with gonadotrophin-releasing hormone agonists. *J Clin Endocrinol Metab* 75, 890–894.

Junier M P, Ma Y J, Costa M E et al. (1991). Transforming growth factor alpha contributes to the mechanism by which hypothalamic injury induces precocious puberty. *Proc Natl Acad Sci USA* 88, 9743–9747.

Kiess W, Muller G, Galler A et al. (2000). Body fat mass, leptin and puberty. *J Pediatr Endocrinol Metab* 13, 717–722.

Korth-Schutz S, Levine L S, New M I (1976). Evidence for the adrenal source of androgens in precocious adrenarche. *Acta Endocrinol* 82, 342–352.

Kremer H, Mariman E, Otten B J et al. (1993). Cosegregation of missense mutations of the luteinizing hormone receptor gene with familial male-limited precocious puberty. *Hum Mol Genet* 2, 1779–1783.

Krstevska-Konstantinova M, Charlier C, Craen M et al. (2001). Sexual precocity after immigration from developing countries to Belgium: evidence of previous exposure to organochlorine pesticides. *Hum Reprod* 16, 1020–1026.

Kumar R, Biggart J D, McEvoy J, McGeown M G (1972). Cyclophosphamide and reproductive function. *Lancet* i, 1212–1214.

Latronico A C, Lins T S, Brito V N et al. (2000). The effect of distinct activating mutations of the luteinizing hormone receptor gene on the pituitary–gonadal axis in both sexes. *Clin Endocrinol* 53, 609–613.

Lee P A, Migeon C J, Bias W B, Jones G S (1987). Familial hypersecretion of adrenal androgens transmitted as a dominant, non-HLA linked trait. *Obstet Gynecol* 69, 259–264.

Locatelli F, Giorgiani G, Pession A, Bozzola M (1993). Late effects in children after bone marrow transplantation: a review. *Haematology* 78, 319–328.

Murran D, Dewhurst J, Grant D B (1983). Premature menarche: a follow-up study. *Arch Dis Child* 58, 142–143.

Nanduri V R, Bareille P, Pritchard J, Stanhope R (2000). Growth and endocrine disorders in multisystem Langerhans' cell histiocytosis. *Clin Endocrinol* 53, 509–515.

Pasquino A M, Pucarelli I, Passeri F et al. (1995). Progression of premature thelarche to central precocious puberty. *J Pediatr* 126, 11–14.

Proos L A, Hofvander Y, Tuvemo T (1991). Menarcheal age and growth pattern of Indian girls adopted in Sweden. *Acta Paediatr Scand* 80, 852–858.

Quinton R, Duke V M, Robertson A et al. (2001). Idiopathic gonadotrophin deficiency: genetic questions addressed through phenotypic characterization. *Clin Endocrinol* 55, 163–174.

Rappaport R, Brauner R, Czernichow P et al. (1982). Effect of hypothalamic and pituitary irradiation on pubertal development in children with cranial tumors. *J Clin Endocrinol Metab* 54, 1164–1168.

Silverman S H, Migeon C, Rosemberg E, Wilkins L (1952). Precocius growth of sexual hair without other secondary sexual development; 'premature pubarche', a constitutional variation of adolescence. *Pediatrics* 10, 426–432.

Stanhope R (2000). Premature thelarche: clinical follow-up and indication for treatment. *J Pediatr Endocrinol Metab* 13, 827–830.

Stanhope R, Brook C G D (1986). Clinical diagnosis of disorders of puberty. *Br J Hosp Med* 35, 57–58.

(1990). Thelarche variant: a new syndrome of precocious sexual maturation? *Acta Endocrinol* 123, 481–486.

Stanhope R, Adams J, Brook C G D (1988). Fluctuation of breast size in isolated premature thelarche. *Acta Paediatr Scand* 74, 454–455.

Tatò L, Saggese G, Cavallo L et al. (1995). Use of combined Gn-RH agonist and hGH therapy for better attaining the goals in precocious puberty treatment. *Horm Res* 44, 49–54.

Tatò L, Savage M O, Antoniazzi F et al. (2001). Optimal therapy of pubertal disorders in precocious/early puberty. *J Pediatr Endocrinol Metab* 14, 985–995.

Thamdrup E (1955). Premature pubarche: a hypothalamic disorder? Report of 17 cases. *Acta Endocrinol* 18, 564–607.

Themmen A P N, Huhtaniemi I T (2000). Mutations of gonadotropins and gonadotropin receptors: elucidating the physiology and pathophysiology of pituitary–gonadal function. *Endocr Rev* 21, 551–583.

van der Sluis I, van der Heuvel-Eibrink M M, Hahlen K et al. (2000). Bone mineral density, body composition, and height in long term survivors of acute lymphoblastic leukemia in childhood. *Med Pediatr Oncol* 35, 415–420.

Van Winter J T, Noller K L, Zimmerman D, Melton L J (1990). Natural history of premature thelarche in Olmsted County, Minnesota, 1940 to 1984. *J Pediatr* 116, 278–280.

Virdis R, Street M E, Zampolli M et al. (1998). Precocious puberty in girls adopted from developing countries. *Arch Dis Child* 78, 152–154.

Warren M P, Shantha S (2000). The female athlete. *Baillières Best Prac Res Clin Endocrinol Metab* 14, 37–53.

Yeshaya A, Orvieto R, Dicker D et al. (1995). Menstrual characteristics of women suffering from insulin-dependent diabetes mellitus. *Int J Fertil Menopausal Stud* 40, 269–273.

Zung A, Shoham Z, Open M et al. (1998). Sertoli cell tumor causing precocious puberty in a girl with Peutz–Jeghers syndrome. *Gynecol Oncol* 70, 421–424.

19

Turner's syndrome

Per-Olof Janson[1], Marie-Louise Barrenäs[2], Berit Kriström[2], Charles Hanson[1], Anders Möller[3], Kerstin Wilhelmsen-Landin[4] and Kerstin Albertsson-Wikland[2]

[1] Department of Obstetrics and Gynaecology, Institute of the Health of the Woman and Child, University of Göteborg, Sweden
[2] Göteborg Pediatric Growth Research Centre, Institute of the Health of the Woman and Child, University of Göteborg, Sweden
[3] Department of Psychology, University of Göteborg, Sweden
[4] Endocrine division, Sahlgrenska University Hospital, Göteborg, Sweden

Introduction

Turner's syndrome (TS) is the most common sex chromosome disorder among women, affecting 1 out of 2000 liveborn girls (Gravholt et al., 1996). The main characteristics of TS include short stature and failure to enter puberty; this resuts from an accelerated rate of atresia of ovarian follicles, causing gonadal insufficiency and infertility. There is also a wide range of additional morbidities associated with the syndrome, as many other organ systems and tissues may be affected to a lesser or greater extent. Therefore, the variability of amount and degree of medical and psychosocial problems between individuals is great and the effects on health and quality of life vary from slight to profound. The need for hormone replacement therapy (HRT) to promote growth and puberty gives the paediatric endocrinologist the most central role when caring for and treating girls with TS. Among women of adult age with TS, counselling on fertility problems puts the focus on the specialists in reproductive medicine and clinical genetics, who are important members of a multidisciplinary network of different specialists in the counselling team.

Genetics

TS is a combination of clinical features caused by complete or partial loss of the second sex chromosome, with or without cell line mosaicism. It is believed that over 50% of the women with TS have a complete loss of one X chromosome (i.e. monosomy 45,X), while 20% have one normal X chromosome together with a structurally altered X chromosome. Such alterations may, for instance, be a loss of a part of the chromosome, a deletion, usually of the short arm, or a so-called isochromosome (i.e. a loss of the short arm and a duplication of the long arm (46,X,i(Xq)); Gravholt et al., 2000; Held et al., 1992). Approximately 30% of the individuals with TS have a mosaicism (i.e. a mixture of normal cells and cells with only one X chromosome (45,X/46,XX); alternatively cells may have 45,X in one cell line and a structurally altered X chromosome together with a normal X chromosome in the other (45,X/46,Xder(X)). Recent studies indicate that the number of girls and women with low-frequency mosaicism may be greater than previously believed (Hanson et al., 2001; Larsen et al., 1995; Leonova and Hanson, 1999). It was also suggested that all those with TS are mosaics, and that fetuses with true monosomy 45,X do not survive to term (Held et al., 1992) as more than 99% of all pregnancies with monosomy X abort (Hook and Warburton, 1983). The risk of monosomy X is not directly related to the maternal age as is the case with many other fetal chromosomal abberations. Cell lines with a male genotype as well as cells with structural alterations of the Y chromosome may be included in mosaicisms of individuals with TS. Such individuals have a potentially increased risk of developing a malignant tumour of the ovary (gonadoblastoma) and should, therefore, be considered for prophylactic gonadectomy (Gravholt et al., 2000; Manuel et al., 1976; Verp and Simpson, 1987).

Usually, the different Turner karyotypes (monosomy, mosaicism and structural deletion) are determined by analysing the frequencies of different cell lines using conventional karyotyping on lymphocytes. To exclude mosaicism involving less than 10% of all cells, at least

Paediatric and Adolescent Gynaecology, ed. Adam Balen et al. Published by Cambridge University Press.
© Cambridge University Press 2004.

30 cell metaphases must be evaluated. If the karyotype is still normal but the suspicion of TS remains, other cells than lymphocytes may be used, for instance fibroblasts. If marker chromosomes are observed, their origin can be determined, for example by using polymerase chain reaction (PCR). X/Y interphase fluorescence in situ hybridization (FISH) can be used in addition to routine karyotyping to identify Y chromosome material and to assess the level of mosaicism (100 nuclei analysed), which may be used to give a prognosis (Hanson et al., 2001).

Age at diagnosis

Early diagnosis is important if HRT is to be optimized. TS should be considered in any female patient with unexplained growth failure and/or pubertal delay. The diagnosis of TS requires the presence of characteristic physical findings in association with a complete or partial absence of the second X chromosome, with or without cell line mosaicism. One-third of the girls with TS are diagnosed at birth because of their typical physical features such as growth retardation, oedema of the hands and/or feet, nuchal folds (webbed neck), low hairline, low-set ears, small mandible, ptosis, micrognathia, left-sided cardiac anomalies, coarctation of the aorta, shield chest and feeding problems. Another third are diagnosed during childhood, and karyotyping is recommended in girls with an unexplained short stature, recurrent otitis media problems, cubitus valgus, short fourth metacarpal, high-arched palate, characteristic facies, ptosis and epicanthic folds. The remaining third are diagnosed during adolescence. TS should be suspected in teenage girls exhibiting an unexplained short stature, absence of puberty, pubertal arrest, or primary or secondary amenorrhoea with elevated levels of follicle-stimulating hormone (FSH) in addition to other TS stigmata. The diagnosis of TS can also be made in adult women; features suggestive of TS are short stature, oligomenorrhoea, infertility, habitual abortion, cardiac anomalies, hypertension, hypothyroidism, osteoporosis and early age-related hearing loss. TS may also be diagnosed prenatally by certain ultrasound findings such as growth retardation, increased nuchal translucency, cystic hygroma, coarctation of the aorta, left-sided cardiac defects, brachycephaly, renal anomalies, polyhydramnios and oligohydramnios. TS should also be suspected if maternal serum concentrations of α-fetoprotein, human chorionic gonadotrophin, inhibin A, and unconjugated oestriol are abnormal. A high probability of spontaneous miscarriage is seen in fetuses with a 45,X karyotype.

Paediatric aspects: short stature

The majority of girls with TS have short stature, resulting from a mild intrauterine growth retardation and/or growth failure during infancy, childhood and adolescence; during the last, such women frequently fail to undergo a normal pubertal growth spurt (Davenport et al., 1999; Karlberg et al., 1993). Without growth-promoting treatment, the average adult height of European women with TS is 20 cm (8 inches) below their healthy peers regardless of their ethnicity. Most girls with TS are not growth hormone (GH) deficient. However, the amount of the biologically most active GH isoform (22 kDa) has been shown to be reduced (Boguszewski et al., 1997).

In the neonatal period, hand and feet nuchal oedema and/or coarctation of the aorta raise the suspicion of TS. However, the clinical signs are often sparse; consequently, it is recommended that all girls with unexplained failure to thrive or short stature, irrespective of age, should have a karyotype performed. When the TS diagnosis is established, there are TS-specific growth curves from different countries for monitoring growth.

With modern growth-promoting therapy, combining GH sometimes with the nonaromatizable steroid oxandrolone and, at an appropriate height and age, with a very low initiating dose of oestrogen for pubertal induction, an adult height in the low normal range often can be achieved (Nilsson et al., 1996; Rosenfeld et al., 1998; Sas et al., 1999). As the optimal treatment is still unclear, therapy with GH, oxandrolone when needed and induction of puberty should be directed by a paediatric endocrinologist. The GH treatment is usually initiated as soon as the girl with TS has a reduced height velocity and a concomitant disease such as hypothyroidism or coeliac disease has been excluded or properly treated. The aim with the growth-promoting treatment is to reach a height in accordance with her peers at the age of puberty, and to be able to initiate puberty at a normal age. However, this is not always possible and in those cases a delicate choice between height and pubertal development has to be made in consultation with the girl.

The GH dosage recommended at present is 0.05 mg/kg daily in young girls. From the age of nine years, addition of low-dose oxandrolone (< 0.05 mg/kg daily) may be considered if height or growth velocity is low. However, there is considerable individual variation in growth response to GH treatment; therefore, the effect is monitored and adjusted when needed by the endocrinologist at regular intervals not exceeding three to six months. Prediction models for individualizing the GH dosage are available and may in the near future be used for guidance in GH treatment (Ranke et al., 2000).

Management of puberty

Most girls with TS will not experience a spontaneous pubertal development, as more than 90% are affected by ovarian insufficiency. Failure to enter puberty is a common reason for why TS is diagnosed. Only 10–15% have a spontaneous puberty and 2–5% will have spontaneous menses, but they will often experience a premature menopause. Usually, these patients are mosaics. If puberty starts spontaneously, oxandrolone treatment should be stopped.

Hormonal induction of feminization should mimic normal pubertal development as closely as possible. To assess gonadal function, serum gonadotrophin levels are determined at 9–11 years of age. High levels imply ovarian failure and a minimal possibility for spontaneous pubertal development. As oestrogen therapy causes the bone epiphyses to fuse within two years, which will limit the longitudinal bone growth, the priorities of the patient with TS must be established before therapy is started. If growth promotion is more important than early puberty, then oestrogen therapy should not be started until height has been maximized. Nevertheless, for psychological reasons, oestrogen therapy should start no later than 15 years of age. Oestrogen may be administered orally or transdermally. If oral oestrogen is given, hepatic function should be monitored. The initial dose should be low (one-sixth to one-quarter of the adult dose) and increased gradually (at intervals over three to six months). Doses should be individualized and adjusted to the response such as Tanner stage, bone age and uterine growth. When vaginal bleeding first occurs, or after 12–24 months of oestrogen therapy, a progestogen such as medroxyprogesterone can be added in order to establish menstrual cycles. In TS patients with spontaneous menses, the function of the ovaries should be analyzed (using serum levels of FSH and luteinizing hormone (LH)), because perimenstrual anovulation may lead to endometrial hyperplasia. Contraceptive advice should be provided, because women with TS may get pregnant without medical intervention. Routine counselling for prevention of sexually transmitted diseases is important and also genetic counselling.

Transitional phase

During infancy, childhood and adolescence, the paediatric endocrinologist is the key professional responsible for early diagnosis, treatment and care of the girl with TS. The goal is that these girls shall achieve a psychosocial development, a final height and puberty as close to normal as possible. The transition from paediatric to adult healthcare supervision occurs gradually and when growth and pubertal development are completed, usually by the age of 18 years. In late adolescence, questions arise about sexuality, fertility, contraception, sexually transmitted diseases and HRT. Accordingly, this time period is perceived by girls with TS as sensitive and delicate, leaving the safe and often familiar relationship with the paediatric endocrinologist to start a new contact with a gynaecologist. During the two to three years of transition, collaboration between the paediatric endocrinologist and a gynaecologist with special knowledge about fertility and TS is of great value to the patient. At the first visit to the gynaecologist, information is collected about the previous medical history including former and ongoing hormonal treatment. Later on, as the gynaecologist will be the physician taking the main responsibility for the woman throughout life, discussions take place concerning the lifelong need for oestrogen treatment, sexuality, fertility, family planning etc. Later, a pelvic ultrasound of the uterus, ovaries and follicles is recommended. The experience of having seen one's own uterus may increase the feeling of being normal, an important psychological aspect (Bryman et al., 1998). The gynaecologist is also responsible for the referral to other medical specialists according to standard recommendations for TS. Because of the great number of additional health problems associated with TS, a multidisciplinary Turner team of professionals is recommended (Fig. 19.1).

Gynaecology, fertility and reproductive technologies

In individuals with TS there is an accelerated loss of oocytes from the ovaries after the 18th week of fetal life and over the first postnatal months or years (Weiss, 1971). The mechanisms behind this phenomenon are not known. It appears that genes on the second X chromosome are responsible for ovarian maintenance rather than ovarian differentiation (Simpson and Rajkovic, 1999). Another explanation, suggested by Speed (1988), is that an unbalanced chromosome content in germ cells will result in meiotic arrest in metaphase I followed by atresia. Individuals with TS have normal vaginas, uteri and Fallopian tubes and in most 45,X adults with gonadal dysgenesis the normal gonad is replaced by a white fibrous streak 2 to 3 cm long and about 0.5 cm wide, located in the position ordinarily occupied by the ovary. On histological examination, there is a dense fibrous stroma indistinguishable from normal ovarian

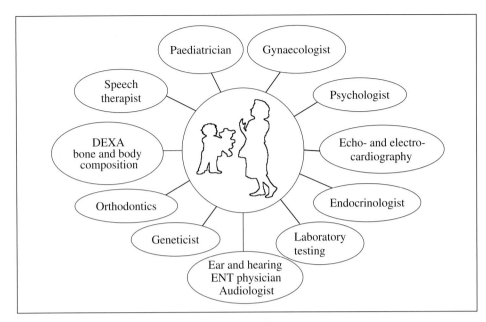

Fig. 19.1. The multidisciplinary team responsible for the care and management of women with Turner's syndrome in Sweden. ENT, ear, nose and throat; DEXA, dual-energy X-ray absorptiometry.

stroma. However, 5–10% of girls with TS still have follicles in their ovaries at the time of puberty and undergo pubertal development and begin spontaneous menstruation. Such girls can also get pregnant although it is an exceptional event estimated to occur in only 2% (Tarani et al., 1998). Healthy children have been reported from both those with monosomy X and those with mosaicism (Schwack and Schindler, 2000). However, spontaneous abortions, stillbirths and chromosomal defects have been reported to occur frequently in women with TS (King et al., 1978; Nielsen et al., 1979; Swapp et al., 1989), and TS can be transmitted from mother to daughter (Tarani et al., 1998). A conclusion that can be drawn from the sparse literature on this issue is that sexually active young women with TS need contraception (Hovatta, 1999) and that the conceptions occurring in women with TS may result in abortions or in high-risk pregnancies. Another factor affecting the fertility of spontaneously menstruating women with TS is premature ovarian failure early in adult life (Christin-Maitre et al., 1998).

The treatment options for the majority of women with TS and an infertility problem are adoption or ovum donation. There are generally no legal obstacles for couples who wish to adopt a child, since women with TS are mentally healthy and nowadays also stay physically fit with proper medical care. Ovum donation, which was introduced by a group in Melbourne in 1984 (Lutjen et al., 1984), is in some countries still prohibited by law. In other countries, subjects with TS

have been included in oocyte donation programmes with results comparable to those in other recipients (Khastgir et al., 1997). Although some authors have reported lower pregnancy rates in women with TS than other women with "spontaneous" premature ovarian failure, this has been attributed to decreased endometrial receptivity (Rogers et al., 1992; Yaron et al., 1996) or to a possible 21-hydroxylase deficiency (Cohen et al., 1999). Foudila et al., (1999) reported 20 pregnancies in 19 women with TS to whom oocytes had been donated by unpaid volunteers. The clinical pregnancy rate per transfer of fresh embryos was 46% and the implantation rate was 30%. The corresponding figures for frozen embryos were 28% and 19%, respectively. The total rate of spontaneous abortion was 40%. The delivered babies all survived and had a gestational age from 36 to 39 weeks and a mean birth weight among singletons of 2852 g. The authors point out that pregnancies in women with TS are not without risk and recommend special attention to cardiovascular disease (cardiac ultrasonography and magnetic resonance imaging of the heart and great vessels before treatment and during the first trimester of pregnancy). Indeed, maternal death has been reported from cardiac complications. The short stature of women with TS also increases the risk of fetopelvic disproportion, perhaps indicating that an elective caesarean section should be the safest mode of delivery. Multiple pregnancy must be avoided, and indeed the Finnish group (Foudila et al., 1999) recommend single embryo transfer. It is recommended that childbearing should be completed at an early age.

The attitudes of women with TS towards oocyte donation are probably very positive, as shown by Westlander et al. (1998) in a study preceding an anticipated change of restrictive law in Sweden, but further investigations on a more global level are necessary.

A future option for fertility preservation in individuals with TS might be freezing and thawing of subcortical ovarian biopsies containing immature oocytes (Hovatta et al., 1996; Newton et al., 1996). The cryopreserved ovarian biopsies could, after thawing, either be autotransplanted back to the woman at a later stage in her reproductive life or be subject to attempts at in vitro maturation of the oocytes, followed by in vitro fertilization and embryo transfer. Although there is experimental evidence in animals of successful retransplantation of cryopreserved ovarian tissue (Gosden et al., 1994), it has so far not been used clinically in patients with TS. Limitations to the application of ovarian autotransplantation in these patients are the difficulty in obtaining ovarian tissue with a sufficient number of oocytes, an inherent increased risk of spontaneous abortions and perhaps also an increased risk of transmission of genetic defects.

At present, in vitro maturation of cryopreserved immature human oocytes has not been successful, although this type of treatment might be a future possiblity, primarily not for those patients with TS for the same reasons as those given above (increased risk of spontaneous abortions and transmission of genetic defects), but rather for children and young adults who undergo gonadotoxic treatment for malignancy (Janson, 2000; see also Ch. 33).

It is recommended that young women with TS receive proper information about HRT, contraception, sexuality and sexually transmitted diseases as for women in general.

Women with TS enter sexual relationships at a later age, and less frequently than other women (Wide Boman et al., 2001). One reason might be feelings of being different. However, it has also been reported that women with TS are married as often as other women and are employed or study full time more often than women in general (Landin-Wilhelmsen et al., 1999).

Today, most women with TS are on oestrogen replacement therapy, which has a protective effect on osteoporosis and possibly also against cardiovascular disease (Landin-Wilhelmsen et al., 1999, 2000). The combination of cyclical oestrogen and progestogen is recommended. Usually, adult women with TS require at least 2 mg 17β-oestradiol daily. Side effects of weight gain and breast tenderness may occur, and the medication must be adjusted so that compliance is optimal. If HRT is complicated by irregular

bleeding, then an ultrasound and an endometrial biopsy should be considered. Recommendations for breast evaluation, self-examination and mammography are the same as for women in general.

Morbidity and the need for multidisciplinary management

TS has been associated with a number of diseases and congenital malformations, which may have a slight or profound effect on quality of life (Fig. 19.2 and Table 19.1). The interindividual variability within the syndrome is great, but some conditions have been linked to karyotype. Usually, congenital cardiac malformations and hearing loss occur more frequently among those with monosomy 45,X, while endocrine diseases, hypertension and arteriosclerosis are evenly distributed among those with 45,X and mosaicism. Approximately 50% of all deaths are caused by cardiovascular diseases occurring 6–13 years earlier than expected, TS women with 45,X living for fewer years than non-45,X (Naeraa et al., 1995).

Cardiac anomalies occur in approximately 75% of fetuses with TS and 30% of living patients with TS (Lacro et al., 1988), and more frequently in monosomy 45,X than in other karyotypes. Obstructive lesions of the left side of the heart dominate, the most common heart malformations being bicuspid aortic valves and coarctation of the aorta. Atrial and ventricular septal defects are less frequent. Aortic root dilatation is seen in approximately 5% of all these patients. Case reports on aortic dissection have been presented, and risk factors include pregnancy, delivery, hypertension and age. Hypertension is found more frequently in TS than the general population, even in the absence of cardiac or renal malformations.

Obesity (higher waist-to-hip ratio, more abdominal fat and less lean body mass) is also increased in TS compared with other women for the same body mass index (BMI) (Gravholt et al., 2000). As a result, women with TS have an altered body composition, reminiscent of the male body composition. Physical activity is reduced. These risk factors may partially explain the increased occurrence of diabetes mellitus, insulin resistance and glucose intolerance in TS. In women on HRT, blood lipids (cholesterol and triglycerides) do not differ from controls (Landin-Wilhelmsen et al., 2000).

Endocrine diseases, especially thyroiditis, are overrepresented in TS and 10–30% of these women develop hypothyroidism (Sylvén et al., 1991).

Coeliac disease, elevated hepatic enzyme levels in serum (alanine aminotransferase, gamma-glutamyltransferase,

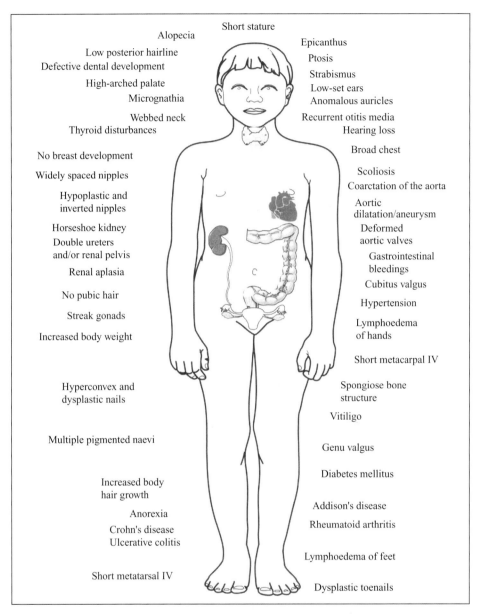

Short stature
Alopecia
Low posterior hairline
Defective dental development
High-arched palate
Micrognathia
Webbed neck
Thyroid disturbances

Epicanthus
Ptosis
Strabismus
Low-set ears
Anomalous auricles
Recurrent otitis media
Hearing loss

No breast development
Widely spaced nipples
Hypoplastic and inverted nipples
Horseshoe kidney
Double ureters and/or renal pelvis
Renal aplasia
No pubic hair
Streak gonads
Increased body weight

Broad chest
Scoliosis
Coarctation of the aorta
Aortic dilatation/aneurysm
Deformed aortic valves
Gastrointestinal bleedings
Cubitus valgus
Hypertension
Lymphoedema of hands
Short metacarpal IV

Hyperconvex and dysplastic nails
Multiple pigmented naevi
Increased body hair growth
Anorexia
Crohn's disease
Ulcerative colitis
Short metatarsal IV

Spongiose bone structure
Vitiligo
Genu valgus
Diabetes mellitus
Addison's disease
Rheumatoid arthritis
Lymphoedema of feet
Dysplastic toenails

Fig. 19.2. Schematic summary of disorders in Turner's syndrome. (With permission of Dr Lisskulla Sylvén.)

alkaline phosphatase) and cirrhosis of the liver are seen more frequently in TS than among controls (Gravholt et al., 1998; Ivarsson et al., 1999; Sylvén et al., 1991). Moreover, TS women are five times more likely to develop cancer of the colon and the rectum compared with non-TS women, possibly because TS has been associated with ulcerative colitis. No other cancers are reported with excess frequency.

The occurrence of skeletal anomalies, osteoporosis and fractures (both osteoporotic during adulthood and non-osteoporotic fractures during childhood) is increased in TS (Gargantini et al., 1988). Bone mineral content is decreased

in adults, but normal in girls with TS. Interestingly, TS women taking HRT seem to have better bone mineral density (BMD) than those who do not (Sylvén et al., 1991). BMD and the prevalence of osteoporosis and fractures did not differ between a female random population sample and a group of women with TS, who were younger than 45 years of age and taking HRT including growth-promoting and continuous oestrogen therapy. The karyotype was not different in those with or without osteoporosis and fractures (Landin-Wilhelmsen et al., 1999). Common skeletal malformations include short fourth metacarpal bone, cubitus

Table 19.1. The prevalence and relative risk of different clinical features in Turner's syndrome

Disorder/disease	Prevalence %	Relative risk
Short stature	95–100	≥ 1000
Amenorrhoea, infertility	95–98	≥ 1000
Physical abnormalities		
Congenital malformations of the heart	16–50	10–99
Coarctation of the aorta	5	100–999
Aortic root dilation	5	
Congenital malformations of the urinary system	37–60	5–9
Neck and thorax		
Short neck	80	5–9
Pterygium colli (webbed neck)	25	≥ 1000
Low posterior hairline	40	
Broad chest with widely spread nipples	30	1–4
Skeletal anomalies	35–75	10–99
Osteoporosis	80	10–99
Fractures	16–45	1–4
Skin, mouth and teeth		
Lymphoedema of hands/feet at birth or later	25	
Micrognathia (small mandibular bone)	60	10–99
High-arched palate	25–70	10–99
Multiple pigmented naevi	25	
Early teeth eruption and malformed teeth	Not reported	
Eyes, vision, ears, hearing, voice problems		
Strabismus, amblyopia and ptosis	20	
Requiring glasses	73	
Minor deformity or low-set external ears	23–70	1–4
Recurrent otitis media (girls)	48–85	10–99
Mild or moderate sensorineural hearing loss	48–84	10–99
Speech and voice problems	Not reported	
Endocrine disorders		
Thyroiditis	15	10–99
Hypothyroidism	10–30	5–9
Diabetes mellitus	5	1–4
Other diseases		
Hypertension requiring treatment	22	5–9
Elevated hepatic enzymes	33	10–99
Coeliac disease	5–15	10–99
Cancer of the colon and the rectum	5–15	5–9
Mental retardation	9	

Source: Compiled from Gotzsche et al., 1994; Gravholt et al., 1998; Landin-Wilhelmsen et al., 2001; Lippe, 1991; Sylvén et al., 1991.

valgus, micrognathia, genu valgum, a small mid-face and a high-arched palate. Also congenital hip dislocation, degenerative arthritis of the hips and scoliosis occur in TS.

Ear and hearing problems are often seen in TS. The external, middle and inner ear may be affected and problems occur more frequently in those with monosomy 45,X than with mosaicism (Barrenäs et al., 1999). In one-third of those with TS, a mild malformation of the outer ear or low-set ears is observed. Approximately two-thirds of TS girls suffer from recurrent otitis media problems, including temporary conductive hearing loss. Usually, the inner ear hearing function is normal in girls and young women. In adult women, a slowly progressive, age-dependent, mild or moderate sensorineural hearing loss is often found. A 27-year-old woman with monosomy 45,X or isochromosomy 46,X,i(Xq) is expected to have the same hearing as a 43-year-old woman with mosaicism, who, in turn, has a hearing loss equal to that in 60-year-old Swedish women (46,XX).

Strabismus, amblyopia and ptosis are common in TS, and two-thirds of TS patients use glasses. Early teeth eruption and malformed teeth are common. Other dental abnormalities may occur because of the small and retrognathic mandible and malocclusion. Speech and voice problems can occur. Skin problems such as numerous pigmented naevi and increased risk of keloid formation are common.

Recommendations

Cardiology

At the time of diagnosis, all individuals, regardless of age, should have a cardiac evaluation, including a complete physical examination and an echocardiogram and also a renal ultrasound. A cardiologist should follow patients with a cardiovascular malformation. Otherwise, a cardiovascular physical examination and echocardiogram, with particular attention paid to the aortic root, should be repeated approximately every five years throughout adult life. Patients and physicians should be aware that chest pain may be the initial symptom of aortic root dissection. Blood pressure should be monitored at each physical examination, and hypertension treated according to current treatment regimens. Diuretics having negative effects on insulin tolerance should be avoided. Both before and during spontaneous or assisted pregnancy, careful monitoring under the guidance of a cardiologist is advised. It is also recommended that childbearing in women with TS should be completed early.

Endocrinology

In adult women with TS, BMD (dual-energy X-ray absorptiometry of, at minimum, the femoral neck and the lumbar spine) should be measured at the initial visit and repeated every five years. An oral daily calcium intake of at least 1.0 g is recommended, as is weight-bearing exercise. If osteoporosis is present already at the initial examination, or if there is a significant deterioration in bone mass, oestrogen treatment should be considered. The level of thyrotrophin, total or free thyroxine, haemoglobin, fasting blood glucose, lipid profile, liver enzymes and renal function should be measured at the time of diagnosis and at intervals of one or two years thereafter. Physical activity should be increased, overweight reduced and dyslipidaemia treated with diet and specific lipid-lowering drugs.

Ears, nose and throat

As a result of recurrent otitis media, many girls with TS require close contact with an ear nose and throat (ENT) specialist. Otitis media in TS should be treated and followed up carefully, since recurrent otitis media may progress to mastoiditis and/or cholesteoma formation. Insertion of grommets should often be considered. Hearing aids are recommended for patients with hearing loss. An audiogram should be performed every five years. Short girls with recurrent otitis media should be referred to a paediatric endocrinologist if TS has not been diagnosed previously. Referral to a speech therapist is recommended for those with speech or voice problems.

Teeth and vision

Ophthalmologic evaluation should be part of the regular physical examination.
An orthodontic examination should occur at 8–10 years of age.

Psychosocial aspects

Girls and women with TS can nowadays, with the right treatment and support, live a good life. The possibilities of medical treatment today mean that TS is not associated with as many difficulties as earlier generations have experienced. However, the variation in the group is wide for psychological problems. When discussing problems related to TS, it is necessary to strive for a balance between, on the one side, pointing out special problems and, on the other side, the risk of stigmatization that exists.

Along the developmental process, there are some periods when there is an increased risk of TS-related complications. During infancy, it is rather common for girls with TS to have difficulties in eating (chewing, swallowing, vomiting, etc.) and they are often reported as crying a lot (Mathisen et al., 1992; Starke et al., 2002). At preschool age, there are risks for behavioural problems like hyperactivity and aggressiveness (McCauley et al., 1995). School children may have learning difficulties. TS is not associated with generally lower intelligence, except for the few girls with a small ring X chromosome. However, persons with TS more often have problems with spatial, perceptual and mathematical/numerical tasks (Rovet, 1993). Usually their verbal performance is normal. This may lead to an inconsistency with regard to their intellectual abilities that might induce problems in assessment and expectancies in school work. In these years, the social situation for the girls may include difficulties with friendship, either because of withdrawal or of aggressiveness (McCauley et al., 1995; Pavlidis et al., 1995; Wide Boman et al., 2000). In teenage years, girls with TS usually have a retarded physical development and do not enter puberty at the same time as other girls. Although clearly female in their gender identification, this can lead to insecurity about their own body and its functioning: thoughts about not being able to become a "normal" grown-up woman with intimacy and sexuality, a partner, children and so on. This, in its turn, can result in difficulties in peer relations (McCauley et al., 1995; Swillen et al., 1993; Wide Boman et al., 1998). There is then a risk of social isolation, downheartedness and problems in identity development.

Also parents can be worried about these aspects of the psychosocial development of their daughters, and the psychosocial problems may interfere with family life. The importance of the family climate in promoting the psychosocial development of the girls is emphasized in studies (Blin and Bühren, 1990; Chen et al., 1981; Molinari and Ragazzoni, 1996; Mullins et al., 1991; Nielsen, 1989).

The young woman will face challenges regarding independence, sexuality, partners and fertility, sometimes leading to social withdrawal and depression (Downey et al., 1989; Wide Boman et al., 2001). The older woman may face problems regarding her health and possible medical complications; existential questions related to ageing without children and family sometimes appear. Again there are risks for depression and social withdrawal.

Recommendations

As is evident from the text above, the problems described most frequently are not of a kind that easily present openly to the healthcare providers. Because of that, it is important to be aware of, and explicitly look for, the existence of possible problems for the single girl, family or woman.

The process of diagnosis includes several steps: the medical examination, waiting for answers, meeting with the physician and getting information. This is a stressful life situation for the parents (Starke et al., 2002), sometimes leading to crisis reactions. So they need to receive information and support, and sometimes crisis intervention, not only on one occasion but repeatedly. The parents need information on what is known about TS and its risks and complications; they also need to know about treatment possibilities and the uncertainty of prediction of the individual's development. It is very important that the parents have repeated opportunities to talk about their worries and to put subsequent questions and also that their observations are taken seriously and into consideration in the clinical practice. As a continuing process during childhood, the parents need to know about aspects of TS in order to be prepared to help their daughters. Direct measures for the girls include examination of learning capabilities and, if needed, special help in school work (often necessary in mathematics), investigation of emotional status and of self-perception and support in social situations. All girls need counselling and some need psychotherapy.

All measures, including (or especially) the medical ones, have a psychological meaning to the patient and her parents. This fact should be taken into consideration for every single measure taken with the patient. The transition of the teenage girl from the paediatric clinic to the women's clinic needs special consideration since it is a step from childhood to adulthood, from one culture to another. This is true for both counselling and practical arrangements. It is important not to lose contact with the girl/young woman when she moves from paediatric to adult care.

In late puberty and for the adult women, thoughts and concerns about relationships, partners and reproduction arise. The older woman might worry about medical complications, dysfunction such as hearing loss and the accelerated ageing process. All these concerns may need to be addressed by counselling.

In the multidisciplinary team caring for TS patients, psychological and social competencies are needed. It is of great value for the girl, her parents and the adult woman with TS to have the opportunity to sit down and discuss issues where life and TS meet, especially around those critical points in the development outlined above.

Case reports

There are several case reports in the literature regarding TS. Most of them describe pregnancies, gonadoblastomas and cardiac malformations as well as other rare diseases. There are interesting findings in relation to karyotype. Tarani et al. (1998) reviewed the pregnancy rate and found that out of 160 pregnancies in 74 TS women, 29% ended in

spontaneous abortion. Only 38% of all pregnancies resulted in healthy babies. The spontaneous pregnancy rate was 2% in TS and occurred mostly in those with mosaicism containing 46,XX. None of the pregnant TS women had a Y chromosome mosaicism.

Gravholt et al. (2000) described 14 patients among 114 TS women with Y chromosome material present in their karyotype. Ten went through ovariectomy. Only one of them had gonadoblastoma, hence the incidence of gonadoblastoma was 10% in TS with Y chromosome material in their study. This is lower than previously reported but the authors emphasized the need for prospective studies.

Lin et al. (1998) made a thorough review of the literature regarding aortic dilatation, dissection and rupture in TS. They found 68 published cases with these findings. Concomitant congenital cardiac malformation or hypertension was present in 90% of those patients. However, 10% had no predisposing factor. Two died suddenly from aortic dissection during an assisted pregnancy. Almost one-third of patients were below 21 years of age. Cardiac malformations are frequently found in TS and overrepresented in TS with 45,X karyotype (Landin-Wilhelmsen et al., 2001). The risk for acute aortic dissection must be considered in patients who participate in assisted pregnancy programmes.

In the Göteborg Turner Centre, two TS women have suffered acute aortic dissection. One had treated hypertension, and a known small aortic insufficiency detected by echocardiography, and died at the age of 28 with acute aortic dissection. The other TS woman experienced the aortic dissection during the seventh month of a pregnancy and both mother and baby survived. This woman had a Y chromosome mosaicism in both buccal cells and lymphocytes. She had an oophorectomy, but no gonadoblastoma was found.

REFERENCES

Barrenäs M-L, Nylén O, Hanson C (1999). The influence of karyotype on the auricle, otitis media and hearing in Turner syndrome. *Hear Res* 138, 163–170.

Blin J, Bühren A (1990). New aspects of counselling and care of patients afflicted with Ullrich–Turner syndrome. Results of a pilot project. *J Psychosom Obstet Gynaecol* 11, 91–100.

Boguszewski C, Jansson C, Boguszewski M et al. (1997). Increased proportion of circulating non-22-kilodalton growth hormone isoforms in short children: a possible mechanism for growth failure. *J Clin Endocrinol Metab* 82, 2944–2948.

Bryman I, Granberg S, Möller A, Wide-Boman U (1998). Valuable medical information and experience of patients from vaginal ultrasound in women with Turner syndrome. In *Proceedings of the 12th World Congress of Pediatric and Adolescent Gynecology*, Helsinki, Finland.

Chen H, Faigenbaum D, Weiss H (1981). Psychosocial aspects of patients with the *Ullrich–Turner* syndrome. *Am J Med Genet* 8, 191–203.

Christin-Maitre S, Vasseur C, Portnoi M F, Bouchard P (1998). Genes and premature ovarian failure. *Mol Cell Endocrinol* 145, 75–80.

Cohen M A, Suaer M V, Lindheim S R (1999). 21-Hydroxylase deficiency and Turner syndrome: a reason for administered endometrial receptivity. *Fertil Steril* 72, 937–939.

Davenport M L, Punyasavatsut N, Gunther D, Savendahl L, Stewart P W (1999). Turner syndrome: a pattern of early growth failure. *Acta Paediatr* 88, 118–121.

Downey J, Ehrhardt A A, Gruen R, Bell J J, Morishima A (1989). Psychopathology and social functioning in women with Turner syndrome. *J Nerv Mental Dis* 177, 191–201.

Foudila T, Söderström-Anttila V, Hovatta O (1999). Turner syndrome and pregnancies after oocyte donation. *Hum Reprod* 14, 532–535.

Gargantini L, Weber G, Braggion F, Cazzuffi M A (1988). Bone mineral content in Turner's syndrome. *Pediatr Res* 23, 127.

Gosden R G, Baird D T, Wade J C, Webb R (1994). Restoration of fertility to oophorectomized sheep by ovarian autografts stored at –196 degrees C. *Hum Reprod* 9, 597–603.

Gotzsche C O, Krag Olsen B, Nielsen J, Sorensen K E, Kristensen B O (1994). Prevalence of cardiovascular malformations and association with karyotypes in Turner's syndrome. *Arch Dis Child* 71, 433–436.

Gravholt C H, Juul S, Naeraa R W, Hansen J (1996). Prenatal and postnatal prevalence of Turner's syndrome: a register study. *Br Med J* 312, 16–21.

(1998). Morbidity in Turner syndrome. *J Clin Epidemiol* 51, 147–158.

Gravholt C H, Fedder J, Naeraa R W, Muller J (2000). Occurrence of gonadoblastoma in females with Turner syndrome and Y chromosome material: a population study. *J Clin Endocrinol Metab* 85, 3199–3202.

Hanson L, Bryman I, Albertsson-Wikland K, Barrenäs M-L, Janson P-O, Hanson C (2001). Mosaicism in Turner syndrome: an extended genetic analysis in women with Turner syndrome. *Hereditas* 134, 153–159.

Held K R, Kerber S, Kaminsky E et al. (1992). Mosaicism in 45,X Turner syndrome: does survival in early pregnancy depend on the presence of two sex chromosomes? *Hum Genet* 88, 288–294.

Hook E B, Warburton D (1983). The distribution of chromosomal genotypes associated with Turner's syndrome: livebirth prevalence rates and evidence for diminished fetal mortality and severity in genotypes associated with structural X abnormalities or mosaicism. *Hum Genet* 64, 24–27.

Houvatta O (1999). Pregnancies in women with Turner's Syndrome. The Finnish Medical Society Duodecim. *Ann Med* 31, 106–110.

Hovatta O, Silye R, Krausz T et al. (1996). Cryopreservation of human ovarian tissue using dimethylaminphoxide and propantheline–sucrose as cryoprotectant. *Hum Reprod* 11, 1268–1272.

Ivarsson S A, Carlsson A, Bredberg A et al. (1999). Prevalence of coeliac disease in Turner syndrome. *Acta Paediatr* 88, 933–936.

Janson P-O (2000). Possibilities of fertility preservation in children and young adults undergoing treatment for malignancy. *Acta Obstet Gynecol Scand* 79, 240–243.

Karlberg J, Albertsson-Wikland K, Naeraa R W, Rongen Westerlaken C, Wit J C (1993). Reference values for spontaneous growth in Turner girls and its use in estimating treatment effect. In *Basic and Clinical Approach to Turner Syndrome*, Hibi I, Takano K, eds., pp. 83–92. Elsevier Science, Amsterdam.

Khastgir G, Abdalla H, Thomas A, Korea L, Latarche L, Studd J (1997). Oocyte donation in Turner's syndrome: an analysis of the factors affecting the outcome. *Hum Reprod* 12, 279–285.

King C R, Mageyis E, Bennett S (1978). Pregnancy in Turner syndrome. *Gynecol Obstet* 52, 617–624.

Lacro R V, Jones K L, Benirschke K (1988). Coarctation of the aorta in Turner syndrome: a pathologic study of fetuses with nuchal cystic hygromas, hydrops fetalis, and female genitalia. *Pediatrics* 81, 445–451.

Landin-Wilhelmsen K, Bryman I, Windh M, Wilhelmsen L (1999). Osteoporosis and fractures in Turner syndrome: importance of growth promoting and oestrogen therapy. *Clin Endocrinol* 51, 497–502.

Landin-Wilhelmsen K, Sylvén L, Berntorp K et al. (2000). Swedish cardiac morbidity study in Turner syndrome. In *Optimizing Health Care for Turner Patients in the 21st Century*, Saenger P, Pasquino A M, eds., pp. 137–144. Elsevier Science, Amsterdam.

Landin-Wilhelmsen K, Bryman I, Wilhelmsen L (2001). Cardiac malformations and hypertension, but not metabolic risk factors, are common in Turner syndrome. *J Clin Endocrinol Metab* 86, 4166–4170.

Larsen T, Gravholt C H, Tillebeck A et al. (1995). Parental origin of the X chromosome, X chromosome mosaicism and screening for 'hidden' Y chromosome in 45,X Turner syndrome ascertained cytogenetically. *Clin Genet* 48, 6–11.

Leonova J, Hanson C (1999). A study of 45,X/46,XX mosaicism in Turner syndrome females: a novel primer pair for the (CAG)n repeat within the androgen receptor gene. *Hereditas* 131, 87–92.

Lin A E, Lippe B M, Geffner M E et al. (1986). Aortic dilatation, dissection and rupture in patients with Turner's syndrome. *J Pediatr* 109, 820–826.

Lippe B (1991). Turner syndrome. *Endocrinol Metab Clin North Am* 20, 121–152.

Lutjen P, Trounson A, Luton J, Findlay J, Wood C, Renon P (1984). The establishment and maintenance of pregnancy using in vitro fertilization and embryo donation in a patient with primary ovarian failure. *Nature*, 307, 174–175.

Manuel M, Katayama P K, Jones H W Jr (1976). The age of occurrence of gonadal tumours in intersex patients with a Y chromosome. *Am J Obstet Gynecol* 124, 293–300.

Mathisen B, Reilly S, Skuse D (1992). Oral motor dysfunction and feeding disorders of infants with Turner syndrome. *Dev Med Child Neurol* 34, 141–149.

McCauley E, Ross J L, Kushner H, Cutler G (1995). Self-esteem and behaviour in girls with Turner syndrome. *J Dev Behav Pediatr* 16, 82–88.

Molinari E, Ragazzoni P (1996). Diagnostic and therapeutic perspectives in Turner syndrome. *Acta Med Auxol* 28, 111–118.

Mullins L, Lynch J, Orten J, Youll L (1991). Developing a program to assist Turner syndrome patient and families. *Soc Work Health Care* 16, 69–79.

Naeraa R W, Gravholt C H, Hansen J, Nielsen J, Juul S (1995). Mortality in Turner Syndrome. In *Turner Syndrome in a Life Span Perspective: Research and Clinical Aspects*, Albertson-Wikland K, Ranke M B, eds., p. 323. Elsevier Science, Amsterdam.

Newton H, Anbard Y, Rutherford A et al. (1996). Low temperature storage and grafting of human ovarian tissue. *Hum Reprod* 11, 1487–1491.

Nielsen J (1989). What more can be done for girls and women with Turner syndrome and their parents? *Acta Paediatr Scand* 356, 93–100.

Nielsen S, Sillesen I, Hansen K B (1979). Fertility in Turner's syndrome. Case report and review of literature. *Br J Obstet Gynaecol* 86, 829–833.

Nilsson K O, Albertsson-Wikland K, Alm J et al. (1996). Improved final height in girls with Turner's syndrome treated with growth hormone and oxandrolone. *J Clin Endocrinol Metab* 81, 216–221.

Pavlidis K, McCauley E, Sybert V P (1995). Psychosocial and sexual functioning in women with Turner syndrome. *Clin Genet* 47, 85–89.

Ranke M B, Lindberg A, Chatelain P et al. (2000). Prediction of long-term response to recombinant human growth hormone (GH) in Turner syndrome: development and validation of mathematical models. *J Clin Endocrinol Metab* 85, 11, 4212–4218.

Rogers P A W, Murphy C R, Leeton J, Hoise M J, Beaton L (1992). Turner's syndrome patients lack tight junctions between uterine epithelial cells. *Hum Reprod* 7, 883–885.

Rosenfeld R G, Attie K M, Frane K et al. (1998). Growth hormone therapy of Turner's syndrome: beneficial effect on adult height. *J Pediatr* 132, 319–324.

Rovet J F (1993). The psychoeducational characteristics of children with Turner syndrome. *J Learn Disabil* 26, 333–341.

Sas T C, de Mulinck Keizer-Schrama S M, Stijnen T et al. (1999). Normalization of height in girls with Turner syndrome after long-term growth hormone treatment: results of a randomized dose-response trial. *J Clin Endocrinol Metab* 84, 4607–4612.

Schwack M, Schindler A E (2000). Turner syndrome (monosomy) and pregnancy. *Z Gynäkol* 122, 103–105.

Simpson J L, Rajkovic A (1999). Ovarian differentiation and gonadonal failure. *Am J Med Genet* (*Semin Med Genet*), 89, 186–200.

Speed R M (1988). The possible role of meiotic pairing anomalise in the atresia of human fetal oocytes. *Hum Genet* 78, 260–266.

Starke M, Albertsson-Wikland K, Möller A (2002). Parent's experiences of receiving the diagnosis of Turner's syndrome – an explorative and retrospective study. *Patient Educ Counselling* 47, 347–354.

(2003). Parent's descriptions of development and problems associated with having an infant with Turner syndrome – a retrospective study. *Patient Educ Counselling*, in press.

Swapp G H, Johnston A W, Watt J L Couzin D A, Stephens G S (1989). A fertile woman with non-mosaic Turner's syndrome: six cases and a review of the literature. *Br J Obstet Gynaecol* 96, 876–880.

Swillen A, Fryns J P, Kleczkowska A, Massa G, Vanderschueren-Lodeweyckx M, van den Berghe H (1993). Intelligence, behaviour and psychosocial development in Turner syndrome. *Genet Counselling* 4, 7–18.

Sylvén L, Hagenfeldt K, Bröndum-Nielsen K, von Schoultz B (1991). Middle-aged women with Turner's syndrome. Medical status, hormonal treatment and social life. *Acta Endocrinol* 125, 359–362.

Tarani L, Lampariello S, Raguso G et al. (1998). Pregnancy in patients with Turner's syndrome: six new cases and review of literature. *Gynecol Endocrinol* 12, 83–87.

Weiss L (1971). Additional evidence of gradual loss of germ cells in the pathogenesis of streak ovaries in Turner syndrome. *J Med Genet* 8, 540–544.

Verp M S, Simpson J L (1987). Abnormal sexual differentiation and neoplasia. *Cancer Genet Cytogenet* 25, 191–218.

Westlander G, Janson P-O, Tängfors U, Bergh C (1998). Attitudes of different groups of women in Sweden to oocyte donation and oocyte research. *Acta Obstet Gynecol Scand* 77, 317–321.

Wide Boman U, Möller A, Albertsson-Wikland K (1998). Psychological aspects of Turner syndrome. *J Psychosom Obstet Gynaecol* 19, 1–18.

(2000). Self-perception, behaviour and social functioning in Swedish girls with Turner syndrome: a population-based study. *Göteborg Psychol Rep* (Göteborg University) 30, 1–12.

Wide Boman U, Bryman I, Halling K, Möller A (2001). Women with Turner syndrome: psychological well-being, self-rated health and social life. *J Psychosom Obstet Gynaecol* 22, 113–122.

Yaron Y, Ochshorn Y, Amit A, Yovel I, Kogosowski A, Lessing J B (1996). Patients with Turner's syndrome may have an inherent abnormality affecting receptivity in oocyte donation. *Fertil Steril* 65, 1249–1252.

20

Androgen insensitivity syndromes

Jarmo Jääskeläinen and Ieuan A. Hughes

Department of Paediatrics, Addenbrooke's Hospital, Cambridge

Introduction

Androgen insensitivity syndromes (AIS) arise from target tissue resistance to androgen action. The clinical manifestations of androgen resistance vary from external genitalia that are completely female to degrees of partial masculinization. These syndromes are the most common identifiable cause of male undermasculinization.

Role of androgens in sex determination

After development of the testis (sex determination), which is not androgen dependent, the events of male sex differentiation involve two pathways, one inhibitory and one stimulatory. The principal function of the inhibitory pathway is to cause regression of the Müllerian ducts and thus to repress the development of female internal genitalia (Fallopian tubes, uterus, and upper third of the vagina). This process occurs between six and eight weeks' gestation, mediated by anti-Müllerian hormone (Josso and Clemente, 2003). The stimulatory events of male sex differentiation require high levels of androgens and a functional androgen receptor (AR). Testosterone is thought to be critical in stabilizing the Wolffian duct system to prevent its involution and to induce differentiation into the epididymides, vasa deferentia and seminal vesicles. Stabilization of the Wolffian ducts occurs between 9 and 13 weeks' gestation, when testosterone is secreted from the testes, mostly under the control of placental chorionic gonadotrophin. Dihydrotestosterone (DHT) cannot be involved in this process, as the 5α-reductase enzyme that converts testosterone into DHT is not yet expressed in these tissues (Wilson et al., 1993). On the contrary, 5α-reductase is expressed already at this stage of development in the prostate, prostatic urethra

and external genital primordia, and their development is DHT dependent (Imperato-McGinley et al., 1992).

Testicular descent is another critical event in male sex differentiation. This occurs in two morphologically distinct, hormonally regulated phases (Hutson et al. 1994). During the abdominal phase, the testes relocate from the original high abdominal position to the base of the abdomen. This transabdominal descent is mediated by contraction and outgrowth of the gubernaculum. The process is testis but not androgen dependent. Targeted deletion studies in mice have identified insulin-3 (Insl3), also known as Leydig insulin-like hormone, as a factor crucial for transabdominal descent (Nef and Parada, 1999).

The second phase of the process, the inguinoscrotal phase, corresponds to the migration of the testes and epididymis through the inguinal canal into the scrotum and this phase is regulated by a combination of hormonal and mechanical factors. Androgens induce gubernacular regression by inducing the disappearance of the extracellular matrix, leading to a condensation of fibrous material and an increase in cell density. It is hypothesized that the combination of regression of the gubernaculum and abdominal pressure caused by the growth of the viscera push the testes down through the inguinal canal (Frey et al., 1983). The gubernaculum contains high levels of AR and is considered the primary site of androgen action in testicular descent (Bentvelsen and George, 1993).

Androgen insensitivity syndrome: a hormone resistance state

Hormone resistance is diagnosed when circulating concentrations of serum hormones are high but there is little or

Paediatric and Adolescent Gynaecology, ed. Adam Balen et al. Published by Cambridge University Press.
© Cambridge University Press 2004.

no clinical effect. In addition to androgens, steroid hormone resistance states have been reported for glucocorticoids (Vingerhoeds et al., 1976), mineralocorticoids (Corvol and Funder, 1994), oestrogens (Smith et al., 1994) and progesterone (Keller et al., 1979). The vitamin D and thyroid hormone receptors belong to the same nuclear transcription factor family as the steroid receptors, and resistance to both of these hormones has also been described (Hughes et al., 1988; Refetoff et al., 1993).

Resistance to androgens, either testosterone or its 5α-reduced product DHT, leads to AIS. Classically, the disorder is caused by a mutation in the X-linked gene for AR, which is essential for androgen action (reviewed in Ahmed et al., 2000; Griffin, 1992).

AIS is the most common specific cause for male undermasculinization, but the estimates of its prevalence have varied widely, depending on the method of ascertainment. Jagiello and Atwell (1962) estimated the prevalence of complete AIS (CAIS) as 1:62 400 genetic males, based on the prevalence of inguinal hernia in phenotypic females in London and accepting the fact that one in five patients with this syndrome do not present with an inguinal or labial swelling. Later, a group in Denmark reported a higher prevalence for AIS, 1:20 400 genetic males, calculated from the number of primarily diagnosed cases with the disorder (Banksboll et al., 1992). In a recent Dutch study, which included only cases with a proven molecular diagnosis of AIS, the incidence was 1:99 000 genetic males (Boehmer et al., 2001a).

Historical aspects

There were numerous isolated case reports of individuals with probable AIS as early as the 1800s and early 1900s, but Dieffenbach (1912), an American geneticist, was the first to note the hereditary pattern of the syndrome. Pettersson and Bonnier (1937) concluded that the affected persons are genetic males. However, it was the comprehensive report of Morris in 1953 that clearly defined the syndrome (then known as testicular feminization syndrome). He recognized that this syndrome is a specific, inherited disorder and it is the most common cause of male pseudohermaphroditism. In his review of 82 cases of AIS, Morris specified the characteristic features of the syndrome: female habitus, breast development and other secondary sex characteristics, absent or scanty axillary and pubic hair, female external genitalia, absence of internal female genitalia, and bilateral undescended testes with the production of oestrogen and androgen (Morris, 1953). Lawson Wilkins noticed in 1950 that the pathophysiology of AIS was an insensitivity to androgens, as his affected 46,XY patient failed

to show signs of virilization in response to testosterone treatment (Wilkins, 1950). Later, he reported that the hair follicles in the axillary and pubic areas, although anatomically normal, were unresponsive to local or parenteral administration of androgens, and the beard, voice and clitoris were similarly unresponsive and so the basic defect in the hairless pseudofemale type is end-organ unresponsiveness to androgens (Wilkins, 1957). In the 1960s, Southern et al. showed normal testosterone levels in affected individuals (Southern, 1961) and in the 1970s the aetiology of AIS became feasible at the cellular level when androgen-binding assays in genital skin fibroblasts were established (Keenan et al., 1975). The breakthrough in the understanding of the molecular pathogenesis took place in 1988 when the human *AR* complementary DNA was cloned (Chang et al., 1988; Lubahn et al., 1988) and already in the same year the first *AR* mutation associated with CAIS was reported (Brown et al., 1988).

Clinical presentation

Complete androgen insensitivity syndrome

CAIS is the classical manifestation of AIS. By definition, there are no visible clinical signs of androgen action and the subjects with CAIS are born with normal female external genitalia, though the clitoris, labia minora and labia majora may be underdeveloped. If prenatal examinations are performed, CAIS can be suspected already prenatally, when the karyotype (46,XY) of the fetus does not match with the female phenotypic sex. Birth weight is reduced compared with healthy newborns with 46,XY karyotype (de Zegher et al., 1998). After birth, most subjects (up to 76%) are diagnosed early when inguinal hernias or inguinal or labial swellings in an apparently female infant are discovered to contain testes (Viner et al., 1997). All in all, inguinal hernias have been reported to be present in 90% of patients with CAIS, and in most cases hernias are bilateral (Viner et al., 1997). Estimates of the incidence of AIS in female infants with hernias have ranged from 1 to 12%, suggesting that any girl with an inguinal hernia should have a karyotype performed or CAIS otherwise excluded (Jagiello and Atwell, 1962; Pergament et al., 1973). However, many subjects with CAIS are not suspected of having the diagnosis until the onset of puberty, when breast development is normal but pubic and axillary hair development is not. Menarche, initially considered late, never occurs.

If not diagnosed by this time, CAIS can present after puberty as a gonadal tumour in an amenorrhoeic female (Manuel et al., 1976). Some affected individuals develop normal female (obviously androgen dependent) sexual hair

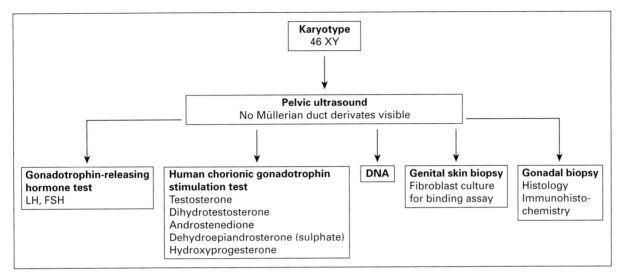

Fig. 20.1. Suggested investigations in a suspected case of androgen insensitivity syndrome. LH, luteinizing hormone; FSH, follicle-stimulating hormone.

at puberty and even more CAIS patients have some fine, silky pubic hair (Tanner 2) and scant axillary hair after puberty, developing under the influence of factors other than AR action (Boehmer et al., 2001a). The physical appearance is solely feminine and affected individuals have a feminine body image and sexual orientation (Wisniewski et al., 2000). Compared with normal females, mean adult height is increased (Varrela et al., 1984; Zachmann et al., 1986).

Partial androgen insensitivity syndrome

In 1947, Reifenstein reported an X-linked familial syndrome of hypospadias, infertility, and gynaecomastia in association with normal 17-ketosteroid excretion and high serum follicle-stimulating hormone (FSH) concentrations (Reifenstein, 1947). Thereafter, several patients with 46,XY karyotype with a variable degree of undermasculinization have been reported. Partial AIS (PAIS) includes a broad spectrum of male undermasculinization. In the most severe form of PAIS, the external genitalia are nearly normal female, except for clitoromegaly and/or posterior labial fusion. At the other extreme, the genitalia may be morphologically normal male, though small, or there may be simple coronal hypospadias or a prominent midline raphe of the scrotum.

Subjects with the mildest phenotypic form of AIS, also called minimal AIS (MAIS), are born with normal male external genitalia. At puberty, MAIS takes two phenotypic forms. In one, spermatogenesis and fertility are impaired; in the other, spermatogenesis is normal or sufficient to preserve fertility. In both, gynaecomastia, high-pitched voice,

sparse sex hair and impotence may be noted (Migeon et al., 1984; Pinsky et al., 1989).

Diagnosis

The diagnosis of AIS is based on clinical findings, endocrine evaluation and family history (Fig. 20.1). The diagnostic criteria for AIS include:
- male (46,XY) karyotype
- presence of testes with histology in accordance with testicular differentiation
- normal testosterone production and metabolism
- absence of Müllerian duct remnants
- undermasculinized external genitalia.
  Additional criteria for CAIS include:
- normal female external genitalia
- spontaneous feminization (but no menses) at puberty before gonadectomy with no virilization despite normal or high male levels of testosterone.

Strict criteria for AIS include also an identified mutation in the *AR* gene; this is relevant especially in the case of PAIS (Viner et al., 1997; Zachmann et al., 1986).

A complete diagnostic evaluation, therefore, includes karyotype analysis, pelvic ultrasonography, basal and human chorionic gonadotrophin (hCG)-stimulated serum testosterone, DHT and androstenedione as well as basal and gonadotrophin-releasing hormone (GnRH (or LHRH))-stimulated serum luteinizing hormone (LH) and FSH concentrations. Genital skin fibroblast culture is useful for AR functional studies, including androgen-binding assay, and it also serves as a source of DNA and mRNA for genetic analyses. Gonadal biopsy is valuable in the differential diagnosis; gonads of a patient with AIS usually show normal testicular differentiation, unlike the situation in gonadal dysgenesis.

As the syndrome is inherited in an X-linked recessive manner, the patients are expected to have 46,XY karyotype and, therefore, only one (defective) copy of the AR gene. However, CAIS has now been reported also in a 47,XXY female as a result of uniparental isodisomy (Uehara et al., 1999).

Generally, children and postpubertal (nongonadectomized) patients have normal or high basal and hCG-stimulated serum testosterone and DHT, as well as high LH concentrations (Ahmed et al., 1999). Furthermore, in patients with PAIS, the physiological postnatal surge of LH and testosterone during the first three postnatal months is either normal or exaggerated. However, in patients with CAIS, basal testosterone and both basal and GnRH-induced serum LH concentrations can be markedly low in infancy, and retained testosterone biosynthesis can only be detected by monitoring the testosterone response to hCG (Bouvattier et al., 2002).

Oestrogen production mainly by the testes and, to a lesser extent, by aromatization of androstenedione and testosterone in peripheral tissues is increased in individuals with AIS to about twice that of normal males as a result of increased LH stimulation of Leydig cells. Plasma or urinary levels of oestrogens are at the upper limit of normal or elevated compared with those in normal males (Quigley et al., 1995). Sex hormone binding globulin (SHBG) levels are comparable to those in normal females (Tremblay et al., 1972). Urinary steroid profiling is useful in differentiating AIS from defects in androgen biosynthesis.

Mutational analysis is a useful tool to confirm the diagnosis, but it is labour intensive and available only in research laboratories. AR mutations (currently more than 300 reported) are spread throughout the gene comprising eight exons. Therefore, the only way to find a mutation is to screen the protein-coding region of AR by analytical techniques such as single-strand conformational polymorphism (SSCP) and/or sequencing analysis (Gottlieb et al., 1999). Screening can reveal a mutation in more than 80% of those with CAIS when the diagnosis has been made on the basis of clinical findings, biochemical evaluation and family history. By comparison, in those with PAIS, even when optimally investigated, mutational analysis is positive in less than a third (Ahmed et al., 2000). The androgen-binding assay reveals an absence of binding in the majority of those with AIS. Cell lines are a useful source of RNA when analysing for the noncoding region AR mutations.

The binding assay can be useful in the investigation of PAIS where the full clinical and biochemical features may not be as specific (Ahmed et al., 2000).

Differential diagnosis

The differential diagnosis for AIS includes several conditions leading to impaired androgen production and metabolism. CAIS is a relatively clear entity and it only rarely leads to diagnostic problems if the initial diagnostic investigations are adequate. On the contrary, PAIS is a clinically heterogeneous disorder and presents a more complicated diagnostic problem.

Defects in steroid biosynthesis and metabolism can cause male undermasculinization. In 17β-hydroxysteroid dehydrogenase deficiency, the final step in testosterone biosynthesis (from androstenedione to testosterone) is impaired and 5α-reductase deficiency impairs the peripheral conversion of testosterone to DHT (Andersson et al., 1991; Saez et al., 1971). Androgen biosynthesis is also deficient in three rare conditions: 3β-hydroxysteroid dehydrogenase, P450c17 (17α-hydroxylase) and steroidogenic acute regulatory protein (StAR) deficiencies, which cause congenital adrenal hyperplasia and are thus associated with deficient cortisol biosynthesis (Lin et al., 1995; Rheaume et al., 1991; Yanase et al., 1991). Leydig cell hypoplasia resulting from mutations inactivating the LH receptor and congenital gonadotrophin deficiency are other rare specific causes for deficient testosterone production (Kremer et al., 1995). If gonadal histology is not available, disorders of gonadal differentiation, gonadal dysgenesis and extremely rare true hermaphroditism must also be included in the differential diagnosis (Berkovitz, 1992).

Studying androgen receptor function in vitro

Several assays to study different aspects of AR function have been reported. Two of these assays are commonly used: androgen-binding assay and AR $trans$-activation assay.

Studies of androgen binding in cultured genital skin fibroblasts have been utilized for the diagnosis of AIS for many years and elucidated the cause of AIS at the cellular level in many cases. A 2–3 mm genital skin biopsy intended for AR studies can be taken under local anaesthetic from the labia, which contains preferential expression of the AR. Alternatively, skin from the prepuce or labioscrotal folds can be obtained at the time of surgery. After culturing an adequate number of cells, which takes a minimum of six to eight weeks, the cells are incubated with a radiolabelled androgen (DHT, mibolerone, or metribolone are the most commonly used) in the presence or absence of an excess

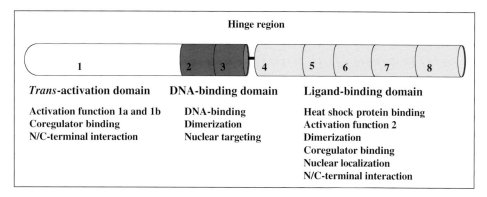

Fig. 20.2. The androgen receptor functional domains. Numbers 1–8 refer to the eight androgen receptor gene exons.

of the nonradiolabelled ligand. Several parameters (maximal ligand binding capacity, ligand dissociation constant, thermolability) can then be measured.

The effect of the identified mutation on AR-dependent *trans*-activation can also be studied. The AR-expressing plasmid (either normal or mutated) is transfected into a mammalian cell line (which itself does not express AR) together with a hormone response element (HRE) in construct with a suitable reporter vector. The transfected cells are then incubated with the ligand and thereafter the reporter activity is assayed. There are also a few reports where the *trans*-activation assay has been performed on patient fibroblasts, by transfecting the HRE–reporter (but not the AR), to study the patient's endogenous androgen signalling pathway. This kind of approach is useful as it may explain the molecular defect in AIS when no mutation can be found in *AR*, as in the case of a coactivator defect (Adachi et al., 2000; McPhaul et al., 1993).

Pathogenesis

The androgen receptor

The AR is an intracellular transcription factor that belongs to the steroid/nuclear receptor superfamily (Evans, 1988). Four of these receptors, AR, glucocorticoid receptor, mineralocorticoid receptor and progesterone receptor, are closely related and even have an ability to activate gene transcription via the same HRE. AR interacts directly with its target genes as a hormone–receptor complex and regulates their transcription.

Human *AR* has been localized to chromosome Xq11-12. It is approximately 90 kb long, but only about 2750 nucleotides code for the AR protein of 919 amino acid residues. The AR protein migrates during gel electrophoresis as 110 kDa and 112 kDa proteins, the latter representing

the phosphorylated form of AR (Brown et al., 1989; Chang et al., 1988; Jenster et al., 1994; Lubahn et al., 1988). The gene is divided into eight exons, and the first exon includes coding for two homopolymeric amino acid, polyglutamine and polyglycine repeats, which both are polymorphic in length (Andrew et al., 1997; Lumbroso et al., 1999) (Fig. 20.2).

Like all nuclear receptors, the AR protein consists of four major functional domains: the N-terminal transactivation domain (NTD, encoded by exon 1), the DNA-binding domain (DBD, encoded by exons 2 and 3), the hinge region or bipartite nuclear localization signal (encoded by exons 3 and 4) and the C-terminal ligand-binding domain (LBD, encoded by exons 4 to 8). In addition to their principal functions, these major domains embody subsidiary functions affecting receptor dimerization, nuclear localization and transcriptional regulation (Brinkmann, 2001). When activated by the ligand, the ligand–receptor complex translocates into the nucleus and binds to specific genomic DNA sequences in the regulatory regions of AR-regulated genes. Binding of the androgen–AR complex activates or represses the expression of androgen-regulated proteins (Fig. 20.3).

The AR, like other steroid hormone receptors, has two major *trans*-activation domains: activation function-1 (AF-1) in the N-terminal region and activation function-2 (AF-2) in the C-terminal region. These interact with the androgen target genes directly as well as indirectly by means of intermediary coactivators. AF-1 is autonomous and ligand independent, whereas AF-2 is ligand dependent (Thompson et al., 2001).

Also located in the AR N-terminal domain are motifs that form, in part, the interface for the interaction of NTD with the LBD. These motifs interact with different regions of the LBD to stabilize the hormone–receptor complex. The AF-2 of AR is transcriptionally weak but the cross-talk between the NTD and LBD regions is needed for optimal AR

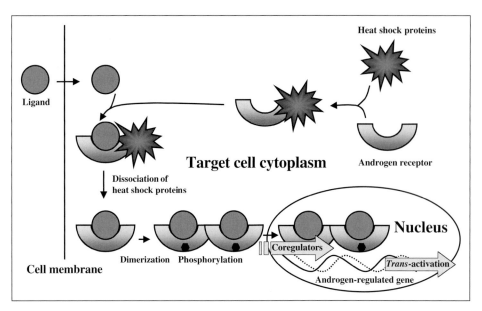

Fig. 20.3. The androgen receptor signalling pathway. The unliganded receptor is located in the cytoplasm. After a cascade of events, it is translocated into the nucleus where it activates androgen-responsive target genes.

function. It is not clear whether this interaction is direct or partially bridged via coregulators (He et al., 2000).

The crystal structures of the AR protein DBD and LBD have been reported. The LBD comprises 12 helices and a small β-sheet arranged in a so-called α-helical sandwich, a kind of fold that up to now has only been observed for the LBDs of nuclear receptors (Matias et al., 2000; Sack et al., 2001).

AR is expressed in various human tissues, and AR defects have been recognized also in conditions other than AIS, such as the X-linked motor neuron disorder known as Kennedy's disease and prostate cancer.

Androgen receptor gene mutations and polymorphisms
More mutations have been identified in *AR* than in the genes for any of the other steroid receptors: more than 270 different mutations in *AR* leading to AIS have been reported (Gottlieb et al., 1999) (Fig. 20.4; see also regularly updated *AR* mutation database at http://www.mcgill.ca/androgendb). Most of the mutations (almost two thirds) are single base pair mutations leading to an amino acid substitution in the LBD. About 20% of the mutations are located in the DBD, and although the NTD is the largest AR domain, it is affected by less than 15% of all the mutations. Intron splice-site mutations and large deletions spanning several exons account for less than 10% of the reported mutations. De novo mutations occur at a high rate (up to 30%), and there is evidence that every third de

novo mutation may have occurred at a postzygotic stage, leading to a somatic mutation (Hiort et al., 1998). Normal androgen binding does not exclude a mutation in AR or a disruption in androgen action. First, amino acid substitutions in the first three exons (including NTD and DBD) do not lead to abnormal binding of the ligand. Furthermore, a mutation in the LBD may lead to disruption of androgen action without affecting ligand binding by disturbing interactions between the C- and N-termini (Thompson et al., 2001). A mutation in the LBD may also affect the stability of AR homodimerization or interactions with coregulators.

The polymorphic trinucleotide repeat segment $(CAG)_n$ encoding a polyglutamine tract in the N-terminal domain of the AR has been shown to affect AR function in vitro: AR function is reduced by increasing length of $(CAG)_n$. Long repeat lengths are associated with reduced spermatogenesis (Tut et al., 1997). Furthermore, AR $(CAG)_n$ length seems to contribute to causal factors for genital abnormalities in mild cases of AIS, possibly with multifactorial aetiology. However, it does not seem to be able to lead to moderate or severe undermasculinization as the sole causative factor (Lim et al., 2001).

Androgen receptor coregulators
Nuclear receptor coregulators are coactivators or corepressors required by nuclear receptors for efficient transcriptional regulation (McKenna et al., 1999). Broadly defined,

coactivators are molecules that interact with nuclear receptors and enhance their *trans*-activation. Corepressors lower the transcription rate at target genes. By the end of year 2000, 45 different AR coregulators (more than 30 coactivators) had been reported (see androgen receptor mutations database at http://www.mcgill.ca/androgendb). Most of these coactivators interact also with other nuclear receptors and many interact with other coregulators, making a complex network. Theoretically, disrupted coactivator signalling could also lead to AIS in humans, but no such patient with an AR coregulator mutation has yet been reported. However, one female subject with CAIS has now been reported in whom the transmission of the activation signal from the AF-1 region of the AR was disrupted but no mutation was found in the *AR* gene, suggesting that a coactivator interacting with this region was lacking in this patient (Adachi et al., 2000).

Pathophysiology of AIS

Testicular development occurs normally in the androgen-insensitive fetus, and immature germ cells are present in the testes at birth and during childhood (Bale et al., 1992). However, there is a progressive decline of germ cell numbers with increasing age, and in adulthood, no germ cells are present in the testes of affected adults with CAIS (Rutgers and Scully, 1991).

Müllerian duct regression (being androgen independent) is generally normal and the patients lack a uterus, Fallopian tubes and a cervix. In some patients, however, rudimentary segments of the Müllerian ducts, such as diminutive Fallopian tubes, are found by ultrasonography or laparotomy (Gottlieb et al., 1999). In theory, patients with CAIS should also lack the upper, Müllerian duct-derived portion of the vagina, and hence have a shortened vagina. However, many patients with CAIS have satisfactory coitus without dyspareunia. Wolffian duct differentiation is thought to be testosterone dependent, and, therefore, these patients should lack vasa deferentia, epididymides, seminal vesicles and ejaculatory ducts. However, patients with CAIS may have structures that are macroscopically identified as Wolffian duct derivates and histologically resemble vestigial Wolffian ducts. These structures can be present without expressed AR protein (Boehmer et al., 2001a). However, there is also some recent evidence suggesting that well-developed and stabilized Wolffian ducts can be present in CAIS, if the mutation does not affect the N-terminal domain (Martin et al., 2000).

Testicular descent occurs to some extent in individuals with AIS, and the testes can be located anywhere along the pathway from the abdomen to the scrotum.

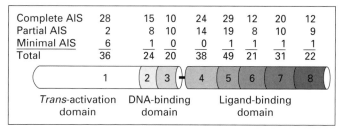

Fig. 20.4. The number of different androgen receptor gene mutations identified by 2002 associated with androgen insensitivity syndromes (AIS). Mutations are classified according to their location (exons 1–8) and to the predominant phenotype associated with the mutation. Large deletions (>1 exon), 5; splice mutations, 13; total mutations, 259.

Gonadal neoplasia

Testicular tumours of germ cell and nongerm cell (Sertoli cell and interstitial or Leydig cell) precursors occur with increased frequency in individuals with AIS; it is still unclear whether the incidence is any greater than that in simple cryptorchidism (Quigley et al., 1995). There is evidence that the occurrence of carcinoma in situ (CIS), also known as intratubular germ cell neoplasia, is increased already in children and adolescents with AIS (Cassio et al., 1990; Muller and Skakkebaek, 1984). In adults, this lesion has been well characterized. It is commonly seen adjacent to germ cell tumours; in half of the cases it progresses to invasive germ cell neoplasia within five years if orchidectomy is not performed (Ramani et al., 1993). Muller and Skakkebaek (1984) reported CIS in the testes in three of eight (38%) consecutive patients with CAIS aged two months, 13 years and 14 years. This finding led them to recommend gonadal biopsy as soon as the syndrome is diagnosed. Should the biopsy reveal CIS, they advocated immediate gonadectomy. Cassio et al. (1990) evaluated the histology of the removed gonads in 17 female subjects with AIS, aged 1–18 years. They found CIS in 8/17 (47%) of their patients and in 6/8 the lesion was bilateral. The youngest subject with this lesion was five years old. However, in two later studies, none of a total of 36 children or adolescents with AIS had carcinoma CIS (Bale et al., 1992; Ramani et al., 1993).

The overall risk for true neoplastic gonadal lesions (most often malignant germ cell tumours, seminomas) has been estimated to be 5–22% when all age groups are combined (Manuel et al., 1976; Morris and Mahesh, 1963; Rutgers and Scully, 1987; Scully, 1981). However, in subjects less than 25 years, the risk is much lower: less than 5%. In the literature, there are only nine subjects aged less than 20 years with gonadal neoplasia (and only one aged less than 10 years) (Chen et al., 1999, 2000; Handa et al., 1995; Horcher et al., 1983; Hurt et al., 1989; Manuel et al., 1976; Morris and

Mahesh, 1963; Perez-Palacios and Jaffe, 1972; Rutgers and Scully, 1987). After the age of 25 years, the risk is expected to rise rapidly and by the age of 50 years it is as high as 33% (Manuel et al., 1976).

Management

Management is complex and depends upon the degree of clinical manifestation, the molecular defect and decisions of early management (such as sex of rearing) (Box 20.1).

Box 20.1 Recommendations for practice

- Appropriate tests to confirm a diagnosis should be performed before gonadectomy.
- The risk for gonadal tumours is increased and gonadectomy is necessary in patients raised female; this should be done by early adulthood.
- Hormone replacement therapy with oestrogens is necessary in gonadectomized females, progestins should not be necessary.
- After the diagnosis is confirmed, counselling appropriate for an X-linked recessive disorder should be offered.

Decision of sex of rearing

In CAIS, the sex of rearing, as the phenotype, is uniformly female. In PAIS, the phenotype of the newborn can vary from an apparent female with a slightly enlarged clitoris to a male with a mild penile hypospadia and/or well-masculinized though small external genitalia. In the extreme cases, the decision on the sex of rearing is straightforward. However, between these extremes are all grades of frank external genital ambiguity that require delicate decision making in order to choose a sex of rearing that is compatible with surgical, anatomical constraints and with some predictive information concerning the probable balance between virilization and feminization at puberty (Ahmed et al., 2000; Gottlieb et al., 1999; Griffin, 1992). The sex chosen depends not only on anatomical but also on cultural considerations. The decision should be made on the basis of the clinical status, endoscopy, karyotype and steroid hormone assays. Although AR molecular binding and *trans*-activation analyses provide valuable information on the function of the mutant receptor, the information is not immediately available to help the decisions about sex of rearing. The results do

have the potential to predict responsiveness to androgens at the time of puberty in those raised male, and to provide guidance about dose and type of androgens that can be used therapeutically. There are also some grading schemes for clinical classification, which can be used in the decision making. Quigley et al. (1995) developed a phenotypic classification for AIS based on the Prader classification for congenital adrenal hyperplasia (Fig. 20.5). In this system, the genital phenotype of an individual with AIS is graded 1–7 in order of increasing severity of androgen resistance and thus increasingly more female phenotype. In this classification, grades 1–3 refer to male phenotype and grades 4–7 to female phenotype. Grade 4 refers to individuals with ambiguous phenotype, with severely limited masculinization evidenced by phallic structure that is intermediate between a clitoris and a penis, and labioscrotal folds with or without rugation and posterior fusion. It has been suggested that individuals with grade 1–3 AIS should be raised male, and those with grade 4–7 female (Diamond and Sigmundson, 1997).

Surgery

In CAIS, the external genitalia are unambiguously female and no early surgery is necessary. The vagina is short in this condition but surgical vaginal elongation is not indicated in most cases. Vaginal elongation can either be achieved digitally or by using dilators, and when this is done, most women are capable of normal intercourse (Boehmer et al., 2001a).

As the risk of gonadal neoplasia is clearly increased in AIS, it is generally agreed that the testes should be removed in the case of female sex of rearing. The main controversy centres on the timing of gonadectomy. In many centres, the accepted practice is to leave the testes in place until after puberty has been completed. Another option is to remove the testes as soon as the diagnosis is confirmed, preferably already at infancy, or later in childhood.

There are arguments supporting both early and late removal of the testes (see also Ch. 17). Evidence in favour of early gonadectomy include the high risk of CIS in the testes observed already in childhood (Cassio et al., 1990; Muller and Skakkebaek, 1984). If gonadectomy is performed early, the psychological stress from the potential for malignancy may be less. If the diagnosis is clear and gonads are located in inguinal hernias, gonadectomy can be performed together with herniorrhaphy. Testes located in the groin and manifest as lumps may also be upsetting for a girl and hence warrant early removal (Duckett, 1995). A satisfactory response to exogenous oestrogen replacement at puberty also favours early gonadectomy.

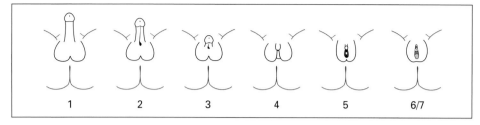

Fig. 20.5. The grading scheme for clinical classification of androgen insensitivity syndrome. Grades are numbered 1–7 in order of increasing severity of undermasculinization. Grade 1 represents normal prenatal masculinization. Grades 6/7 refer to normal female phenotype. In grade 7, no pubic hair is present in adulthood. (Classification adapted from Quigley et al., 1995.)

There are also arguments and evidence in favour of late gonadectomy. True gonadal neoplasia is rare until after puberty (Manuel et al., 1976) and if gonads are not removed, spontaneous development of female secondary characteristics at puberty occurs satisfactorily. Furthermore, prepubertal low serum concentrations of oestrogens may be important for higher central nervous system centres involved in the development of sexual identity and for bone mineralization (Collaer and Hines, 1995; Soule et al., 1995).

Hormone replacement

Female sex of rearing

In patients with female sex of rearing, oestrogen substitution is necessary after gonadectomy. If gonads are removed before the onset of puberty, the oestrogen replacement therapy should begin around 11 years of age or as indicated by patient preference. A number of replacement regimens are available, as discussed in Chapters 18 and 19. It is generally considered that progesterone substitution is not needed in the absence of the uterus, but this is not uniform practice (Warne and Hughes, 1995).

Male sex of rearing

If male sex of rearing is considered for a 46,XY infant with ambiguous genitalia, it is important to demonstrate that the genital tissues can respond to androgen and the penis will be capable of growing at puberty. The phallus should be measured and photographed and then 25 mg testosterone administered by intramuscular injection every four weeks for up to three injections. An adequate response is an increase in stretched penile length into the normal range (Burstein et al., 1979).

In many cases of PAIS, it is possible to overcome the functional defects of certain mutant ARs by pharmacotherapy with appropriate androgens or other steroids. It may also be possible to increase the concentration of deficient, but otherwise normal, AR by increasing the rate of synthesis or decreasing the rate of degradation. Some *AR* missense

mutations express androgen binding and/or *trans*-activation defects that are conditional on being exposed to a particular type of androgen (Kaufman et al., 1990; Pinsky et al., 1984). For example, a 46,XY patient with an *AR* missense mutation M807T has been reported (Ong et al., 1999). This patient was born with severely undermasculinized external genitalia. In vitro assays showed that AR *trans*-activation could be restored with DHT but not with testosterone. Accordingly, in vivo, no response in penile size was observed after treatment with testosterone, but local treatment with DHT gel led to a significant masculinization of the external genitalia. Thus, in vitro functional assays can help to identify the subset of patients with ambiguous genitalia who could respond well to androgen therapy, providing them an option to be reared in accordance with their chromosomal sex. It is anticipated that knowledge of the AR LBD crystal structure will result in the development of a new generation of androgen-like compounds that modulate AR function in a more specific manner.

Counselling and long-term outcome

It is a difficult and challenging task to explain AIS to a family (see Ch. 17). The essential message is that the girl with AIS is healthy but destined to be infertile, as she has no uterus. It is also important to state that the gonads (testes) are abnormal (in regard to the sex of rearing) and should be removed at some stage. It is also important to state the need for long-term oestrogen substitution treatment from the onset of puberty. The terms "testicular feminization" or "male pseudohermaphroditism" are confusing and should not be used when counselling the patient and/or her family.

Genetic counselling

AIS is a heritable disorder with significant consequences; consequently genetic counselling should be offered to the families of affected individuals. The AR is encoded by an

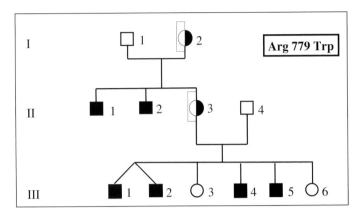

Fig. 20.6. A family tree of a patient with androgen insensitivity syndrome (AIS). Filled squares indicate AIS individuals; semi-filled circles indicate carrier females.

X-chromosomal gene and AIS follows an X-linked recessive pattern of inheritance. Therefore, for any carrier female, there is a 1:2 chance of a child with 46,XY karyotype being affected, and a 1:2 chance of a 46,XX child being a carrier. Though delayed puberty and/or reduced or asymmetric development of pubic and axillary hair occur in some AIS carriers, most 46,XX female carriers of AR mutations are healthy and fertile; therefore, carrier status detection is not possible based on clinical and laboratory data (Hiort et al., 1993). The polymorphic (in length) polyglutamine (CAG) and polyglycine (GGC) regions in the first exon have been used for genetic counselling of CAIS families when there is a clear family history (Davies et al., 1995) (Fig. 20.6). However, almost 30% of AR mutations are de novo mutations and a high proportion of these (about every third) arise postzygotically. Therefore, only direct analysis and identification of the mutation of the AR gene in the proband and family can provide a reliable basis for genetic counselling (Hiort et al., 1998). Furthermore, once a precise AR mutation is defined in an affected family, it is possible to perform prenatal diagnosis by analysing the appropriate region of the AR gene in DNA obtained by chorionic villus sampling.

Androgen receptor genotype does not always predict the phenotype

So far, AR is the only gene in which mutations associated with AIS have been identified. However, AIS is a heterogeneous syndrome both phenotypically and genotypically. In CAIS, phenotypic variation is very rare; only one family with coexistence of CAIS and PAIS has been so far described (Rodien et al., 1996). In contrast, phenotypic variability is common in PAIS. The AR mutations database includes 25 cases where an identical AR mutation is associated with significant phenotypic diversity (Gottlieb et al., 2001) and

significant phenotypic variation has been reported in up to one-third of families with PAIS (Boehmer et al., 2001a). Identical mutations have been associated with different PAIS phenotypes in the same kindred, even to such an extent that siblings with the same AR mutation have been assigned a different sex of rearing (Batch et al., 1993). Phenotypic variability may be a result of somatic mosaicism (Holterhus et al., 1997). Variable expression of other genes necessary for androgen biosynthesis and metabolism (such as 5α-reductase) may contribute to the phenotypic variation (Boehmer et al., 2001b).

Fertility

Clearly, in the absence of a uterus, a female patient with CAIS (or severe PAIS), is destined to be infertile.

In PAIS patients with male sex of rearing, testes show both qualitative and quantitative disturbances of spermatogenesis, and generally patients with PAIS, including those with even mild forms of PAIS, are considered infertile. However, several recent reports show that in nongonadectomized patients with PAIS and male sex of rearing, fertility is sometimes restored. As expected, mutations associated with restored fertility show only partial loss of function when examined in vitro (Chu et al., 2002; Giwercman et al., 2000; Knoke et al., 1999; Pinsky et al., 1989; Tsukada et al., 1997).

Psychosexual aspects

Females with CAIS overwhelmingly perceive themselves as highly feminine and not masculine throughout development. They also report their sexual attraction, fantasies and experiences are best described as female heterosexual (Wisniewski et al., 2000).

Most adult women are also satisfied with their sexual functioning, and libido and ability to experience orgasms are generally not a problem for women with CAIS (Wisniewski et al., 2000). Many women get married and become mothers through adoption. The incidence of homosexuality is low in women with AIS, which supports the hypothesis that the sex chromosomes per se do not directly contribute to the psychosexual orientation, whereas hormonal deandrogenization and morphological demasculinization may do so (Money et al., 1984).

Bone mineral density

The role of androgens in skeletal maturation and bone mineralization is not as clear as that of oestrogens. Men bearing mutations in the genes for the oestradiol receptor or aromatase fail to undergo accelerated growth during puberty and show profound deficits in adult bone mass (Bilezikian et al., 1998; Smith et al., 1994). However, the present data on bone mineralization in patients with AIS are not yet conclusive. All published reports show that adult CAIS patients have bone mineral densities lower than healthy female subjects (Bertelloni et al., 1998; Marcus et al., 2000; Munoz-Torres et al., 1995; Soule et al., 1995). Bone mineral densities are lower than in healthy female subjects already before gonadectomy; when adequate substitution of oestrogens is given, the patients show moderate deficits in bone mineralization, averaging close to $-1SD$ from normative means. The severe osteopenia (bone mineral density $< -2SD$) in some females may reflect a component of inadequate oestrogen replacement rather than androgen lack alone (Marcus et al., 2000). All in all, it seems that androgens have a role in bone mineralization independent from oestrogens. However, there are still many unresolved questions. It is not yet established whether gonadectomy in early childhood combined with oestrogen substitution to induce puberty is more or less deleterious for bone mineralization than late gonadectomy combined with oestrogen substitution started after gonadectomy.

Box 20.2 Key points

- Androgen insensitivity syndrome (AIS) is the most common recognized cause of undermasculinization in a 46,XY individual.
- As a rule, AIS is caused by a mutation in the androgen receptor gene, which is located on the X chromosome.
- Up to 30% of AIS results from a de novo mutation in the *AR* gene; therefore, family history can be negative.
- The phenotype may vary from female with normal external genitalia (complete AIS) to male with impaired spermatogenesis (minimal AIS).
- A female with complete AIS has normal external genitalia and lower vagina, but uterus and Fallopian tubes are not present.
- Generally, patients present with normal/high male serum concentrations of testosterone and dihydrotestosterone. However, serum baseline androgen concentrations may be low, especially in early infancy.

REFERENCES

* Indicates key references.

Adachi M, Takayanagi R, Tomura A et al. (2000). Androgen-insensitivity syndrome as a possible coactivator disease. *N Engl J Med* 343, 856–862.

Ahmed S F, Cheng A, Hughes I A (1999). Assessment of the gonadotropin-gonadal axis in androgen insensitivity syndrome. *Arch Dis Child* 80, 324–329.

*Ahmed S F, Cheng A, Dovey L et al. (2000). Phenotypic features, androgen receptor binding, and mutational analysis in 278 clinical cases reported as androgen insensitivity syndrome. *J Clin Endocrinol Metab* 85, 658–665.

Andersson S, Berman D M, Jenkins E P, Russell D W (1991). Deletion of steroid 5 alpha-reductase 2 gene in male pseudohermaphroditism. *Nature* 354, 159–161.

Andrew S E, Goldberg Y P, Hayden M R (1997). Rethinking genotype and phenotype correlations in polyglutamine expansion disorders. *Hum Mol Genet* 6, 2005–2010.

Bale P N, Howard N J, Wright J E (1992). Male pseudohermaphroditism in XY children with female phenotype. *Pediatr Pathol* 12, 29–49.

Banksboll S, Qvist I, Lebech P E, Lewinsky M (1992). Testicular feminization syndrome and associated gonadal tumors in Denmark. *Acta Obstet Gynecol Scand* 71, 63–66.

Batch J A, Davies H R, Evans B A, Hughes I A, Patterson M N (1993). Phenotypic variation and detection of carrier status in the partial androgen insensitivity syndrome. *Arch Dis Child* 68, 453–457.

Bentvelsen F M, George F W (1993). The fetal rat gubernaculum contains higher levels of androgen receptor than does the postnatal gubernaculum. *J Urol* 150, 1564–1566.

Berkovitz G D (1992). Abnormalities of gonadal determination and differentiation. *Semin Perinatol* 16, 289–298.

Bertelloni S, Baroncelli G I, Federico G, Cappa M, Lala R, Saggese G (1998). Altered bone mineral density in patients with complete androgen insensitivity syndrome. *Horm Res* 50, 309–314.

Bilezikian J P, Morishima A, Bell J, Grumbach M M (1998). Increased bone mass as a result of estrogen therapy in a man with aromatase deficiency. *N Engl J Med* 337, 599–603.

Boehmer A L, Brinkmann A O, Bruggenwirth H et al. (2001a). Genotype versus phenotype in families with androgen insensitivity syndrome. *J Clin Endocrinol Metab* 86, 4151–4160.

Boehmer A L, Brinkmann A O, Nijman R M (2001b). Phenotypic variation in a family with partial androgen insensitivity syndrome explained by differences in 5alpha dihydrotestosterone availability. *J Clin Endocrinol Metab* 86, 1240–1246.

Bouvattier C, Carel J C, Lecointre C et al. (2002). Postnatal changes of T, LH, and FSH in 46,XY infants with mutations in the *AR* gene. *J Clin Endocrinol Metab* 87, 29–32.

Brinkmann A O (2001). Molecular basis of androgen insensitivity. *Mol Cell Endocrinol* 179, 105–109.

Brown C J, Goss S J, Lubahn D B et al. (1989). Androgen receptor locus on human X chromosome: regional localization to Xq11-12 and description of a DNA polymorphism. *Am J Hum Genet* 44, 264–269.

Brown T R, Lubahn D B, Wilson E M, Joseph D R, French F S, Migeon C J (1988). Deletion of the steroid-binding domain of the human androgen receptor gene in one family with complete androgen insensitivity syndrome: evidence for further genetic heterogeneity of this syndrome. *Proc Natl Acad Sci USA* 85, 8151–8155.

Burstein S, Grumbach M M, Kaplan S (1979). Early determination of androgen responsiveness is important in the management of microphallus. *Lancet* ii, 983–986.

Cassio A, Cacciari E, D'Errico A (1990). Incidence of intratubular germ cell neoplasia in androgen insensitivity syndrome. *Acta Endocrinol* 123, 416–422.

Chang C S, Kokontis J, Liao S (1988). Molecular cloning of human and rat complementary DNA encoding androgen receptors. *Science* 240, 324–326.

Chen C P, Chern S R, Wang T Y, Wang W, Wang K L, Jeng C J (1999). Androgen receptor gene mutations in 46,XY females with germ cell tumors. *Hum Reprod* 14, 664–670.

Chen C P, Chern S R, Chen B F, Wang W, Hwu Y M (2000). Hamartoma in a pubertal patient with complete androgen insensitivity syndrome and R(831)X mutation of the androgen receptor gene. *Fertil Steril* 74, 182–183.

Chu J, Zhang R, Zhao Z et al. (2002). Male fertility is compatible with an Arg840Cys substitution in the AR in a large Chinese family affected with divergent phenotypes of AR insensitivity syndrome. *J Clin Endocrinol Metab* 87, 347–351.

Collaer M L, Hines M (1995). Human behavioral sex differences: a role for gonadal hormones during early development? *Psychol Bull* 118, 55–107.

Corvol D, Funder J (1994). The enigma of pseudohypoaldosteronism. *J Clin Endocrinol Metab* 79, 25–26.

Davies H R, Hughes I A, Patterson M N (1995). Genetic counselling in complete androgen insensitivity syndrome: trinucleotide repeat polymorphisms, single-strand conformation polymorphism and direct detection of two novel mutations in the androgen receptor gene. *Clin Endocrinol* 43, 69–77.

de Zegher F, Francois I, Boehmer A L et al. (1998). Androgens and fetal growth. *Horm Res* 50, 243–244.

Diamond M, Sigmundson H K (1997). Management of intersexuality. *Arch Pediatr Adolesc Med* 151, 1046–1050.

Dieffenbach H (1912). Familiaerer Hermaphroditismus. [Inaugural Dissertation.] Stuttgart, Germany.

Duckett J W (1995). Editorial: yolk sac tumor in a case of testicular feminization syndrome. *J Ped Surg* 30, 1367–1368.

Evans R M (1988). The steroid and thyroid hormone receptor superfamily. *Science* 240, 889–895.

Frey H L, Peng S, Rajfer J (1983). Synergy of abdominal pressure and androgens in testicular descent. *Biol Reprod* 29, 1233–1239.

Giwercman A, Kledal T, Schwartz M et al. (2000). Preserved male fertility despite decreased androgen sensitivity caused by a mutation in the ligand-binding domain of the androgen receptor. *J Clin Endocrinol Metab* 85, 2253–2259.

Gottlieb B, Pinsky L, Beitel L K, Trifiro M (1999). Androgen insensitivity. *Am J Med Genet* 89, 210–217.

Gottlieb B, Beitel L K, Trifiro M A (2001). Variable expressivity and mutation databases: The androgen receptor gene mutations database. *Hum Mutat* 17, 382–388.

Griffin J E (1992). Androgen resistance – the clinical and molecular spectrum. *N Engl J Med* 326, 611–618.

Handa N, Nagasaki A, Tsunoda M et al. (1995). Yolk sac tumor in a case of testicular feminization syndrome. *J Pediatr Surg* 30, 1366–1367.

He B, Kemppainen J A, Wilson E M (2000). FXXLF and WXXLF sequences mediate the NH_2-terminal interaction with the ligand binding domain of the androgen receptor. *J Biol Chem* 275, 22986–22994.

Hiort O, Huang Q, Sinnecker G H et al. (1993). Single strand conformation polymorphism analysis of androgen receptor gene mutations in patients with androgen insensitivity syndromes: application for diagnosis, genetic counselling, and therapy. *J Clin Endocrinol Metab* 77, 262–266.

Hiort O, Sinnecker G H, Holterhus P M, Nitsche E M, Kruse K (1998). Inherited and de novo androgen receptor gene mutations: investigation of single-case families. *J Pediatr* 132, 939–943.

Holterhus P M, Bruggenwirth H T, Hiort O et al. (1997). Mosaicism due to a somatic mutation of the androgen receptor gene determines phenotype in androgen insensitivity syndrome. *J Clin Endocrinol Metab* 82, 3584–3589.

Horcher E, Grunberger W, Parschalk O (1983). Classical seminoma in a case of testicular feminization syndrome. *Prog Pediatr Surg* 16, 139–141.

Hughes M R, Malloy P J, Kieback D G et al. (1988). Point mutations in the human vitamin D receptor gene associated with hypocalcemic rickets. *Science* 242, 1702–1705.

Hurt W G, Bodurtha J N, McCall J B, Ali M M (1989). Seminoma in pubertal patient with androgen insensitivity syndrome. *Am J Obstet Gynecol* 161, 530–531.

Hutson J M, Baker M, Terada M, Zhou B, Paxton G (1994). Hormonal control of testicular descent and the cause of cryptorchidism. *Reprod Fertil Dev* 6, 151–156.

Imperato-McGinley J, Sanchez R S, Spencer J R, Yee B, Vaughan E D (1992). Comparison of the effects of the 5 alpha-reductase inhibitor finasteride and the antiandrogen flutamide on prostate and genital differentiation: dose–response studies. *Endocrinology* 131, 1149–1156.

Jagiello G, Atwell J (1962). Prevalence of testicular feminization. *Lancet* i, 329.

Jenster G, de Ruiter P E, van der Korput H A, Kuiper G G, Trapman J, Brinkmann A O (1994). Changes in the abundance of androgen receptor isotypes: effects of ligand treatment, glutamine-stretch variation, and mutation of putative phosphorylation sites. *Biochemistry* 33, 14064–14072.

Josso N, Clemente N (2003). Transduction pathway of anti-Mullerian hormone, a sex-specific member of the TGF-beta family. *Trends Endocrinol Metab* 14, 91–97.

Kaufman M, Pinsky L, Gottlieb B et al. (1990). Androgen receptor defects in patients with minimal and partial androgen resistance classified according to a model of androgen–receptor complex energy states. *Horm Res* 33, 87–94.

Keenan B S, Meyer W J, Hadjian A J, Migeon C J (1975). Androgen receptor in human skin fibroblasts. Characterization of a specific 17beta-hydroxy-5alpha-androstan-3-one–protein complex in cell sonicates and nuclei. *Steroids* 25, 535–552.

Keller D W, Wiest W G, Askin F B, Johnson L W, Strickler R C (1979). Pseudocorpus luteum insufficiency: a local defect of progesterone action on endometrial stroma. *J Clin Endocrinol Metab* 48, 127–132.

Knoke I, Jakubiczka S, Lehnert H, Wieacker P (1999). A new point mutation of the androgen receptor gene in a patient with partial androgen resistance and severe oligozoospermia. *Andrologia* 31, 199–201.

Kremer H, Kraaij R, Toledo S P et al. (1995). Male pseudohermaphroditism due to a homozygous missense mutation of the luteinizing hormone receptor gene. *Nat Genet* 9, 160–164.

Lim H N, Nixon R M, Chen H, Hughes I A, Hawkins J R (2001). Evidence that longer androgen receptor polyglutamine repeats are a causal factor for genital abnormalities. *J Clin Endocrinol Metab* 86, 3207–3210.

Lin D, Sugawara T, Strauss J F III et al. (1995). Role of steroidogenic acute regulatory protein in adrenal and gonadal steroidogenesis. *Science* 267, 1828–1831.

*Lubahn D B, Joseph D R, Sullivan P M, Willard H F, French F S, Wilson E M (1988). Cloning of human androgen receptor complementary DNA and localization to the X-chromosome. *Science* 240, 327–330.

Lumbroso R, Beitel L K, Vasiliou D M, Trifiro M A, Pinsky L (1999). Codon-usage variants in the polymorphic $(GGN)_n$ trinucleotide repeat of the human androgen receptor gene. *Hum Genet* 101, 43–46.

Manuel M, Katayama K P, Jones H W Jr (1976). The age of occurrence of gonadal tumors in intersex patients with a Y chromosome. *Br Med J* 288, 1419–1420.

Marcus R, Leary D, Schneider D L, Shane E, Favus M, Quigley C A (2000). The contribution of testosterone to skeletal development and maintenance: lessons from the androgen insensitivity syndrome. *J Clin Endocrinol Metab* 85, 1032–1037.

Martin H, Hodapp J, Williams M, Ransley P G, Hughes I A (2000). Stabilisation of Wolffian ducts in androgen insensitivity: evidence in vivo for a constitutively active androgen receptor. *Pediatr Res* 49 (Suppl.), 52A.

Matias P M, Donner P, Coelho R et al. (2000). Structural evidence for the ligand specificity in the ligand binding domain of the human androgen receptor. *J Biol Chem* 275, 26164–26171.

McKenna N J, Lanz R B, O'Malley B W (1999). Nuclear receptor coregulators: cellular and molecular biology. *Endocr Rev* 20, 321–344.

McPhaul M J, Deslypere J P, Allman D R, Gerard R D (1993). The adenovirus-mediated delivery of a reporter gene permits the assessment of androgen receptor function in genital skin fibroblast cultures. Stimulation of Gs and inhibition of G(o). *J Biol Chem* 268, 26063–26066.

Migeon C J, Brown T R, Lanes R, Palacios A, Amrhein J A, Schoen E J (1984). A clinical syndrome of mild androgen insensitivity. *J Clin Endocrinol Metab* 59, 672–678.

Money J, Schwartz M, Lewis V G (1984). Adult erotosexual status and fetal hormonal masculinization and demasculinization: 46,XX congenital virilizing adrenal hyperplasia and 46,XY androgen-insensitivity syndrome compared. *Psychoneuroendocrinology* 9, 405–414.

Morris J M (1953). The syndrome of testicular feminization in male pseudohermaphrodites. *Am J Obstet Gynecol* 65, 1192–1211.

Morris J M, Mahesh V B (1963). Further observations on the syndrome, 'testicular feminization'. *Am J Obstet Gynecol* 87, 731–748.

Muller J, Skakkebaek J E (1984). Testicular carcinoma in situ in children with the androgen insensitivity (testicular feminisation) syndrome. *Br Med J* 288, 1419–1420.

Munoz-Torres M, Jodar E, Quesada M, Escobar-Jimenez F (1995). Bone mass in androgen-insensitivity syndrome: response to hormonal replacement therapy. *Calcif Tissue Int* 57, 94–96.

Nef S, Parada L F (1999). Cryptorchidism in mice mutant for Insl3. *Nat Genet* 22, 295–299.

Ong Y C, Wong H B, Adaikan G, Yong E L (1999). Directed pharmacological therapy of ambiguous genitalia due to an androgen receptor gene mutation. *Lancet* 354, 1444–1445.

Perez-Palacios G, Jaffe R B (1972). The syndrome of testicular feminization. *Pediatr Clin North Am* 19, 139–141.

Pergament E, Heimler A, Shah P (1973). Testicular feminisation and inguinal hernia. *Lancet* ii: 740–741.

Pettersson G, Bonnier G (1937). Inherited sex-mosaic in man. *Hereditas* 23, 49–69.

Pinsky L, Kaufman M, Killinger D W, Burko B, Shatz D, Volpe R (1984). Human minimal androgen insensitivity with normal dihydrotestosterone-binding capacity in cultured genital skin fibroblasts: evidence for an androgen-selective qualitative abnormality of the receptor. *Am J Hum Genet* 36, 965–978.

Pinsky L, Kaufman K, Killinger D W (1989). Impaired spermatogenesis is not an obligate expression of receptor-defective androgen resistance. *Am J Med Genet* 32, 100–104.

*Quigley C A, De Bellis A, Marschke K B, el-Awady M K, Wilson E M, French F S (1995). Androgen receptor defects: historical, clinical, and molecular perspectives. *Endocr Rev* 16, 271–321.

Ramani P, Yeung C K, Habeebu S S (1993). Testicular intratubular neoplasia in children and adolescents with intersex. *Am J Surg Pathol* 17, 1124–1133.

Refetoff S, Weiss R E, Usala S J (1993). The syndromes of resistance to thyroid hormone. *Endocr Rev* 14, 348–399.

Reifenstein E C (1947). Hereditary familial hypogonadism. *Proc Am Fed Clin Res* 3, 86.

Rheaume E, Lachance Y, Zhao H F et al. (1991). Structure and expression of a new complimentary DNA encoding the almost exclusive 3 beta-hydroxysteroid dehydrogenase/delta 5-delta 4-isomerase in human adrenal and gonads. *Mol Endocrinol* 5, 1147–1157.

Rodien P, Mebarki F, Mowszowicz I et al. (1996). Different phenotypes in a family with androgen insensitivity caused by the same M780I point mutation in the androgen receptor gene. *J Clin Endocrinol Metab* 81, 2994–2998.

Rutgers J L, Scully R E (1987). Pathology of the testis in intersex syndromes. *Semin Diagn Pathol* 4, 275–291.

(1991). The androgen insensitivity syndrome (testicular feminization): a clinicopathological study of 43 cases. *Int J Gynecol Pathol* 10, 126–144.

Sack J S, Kish K F, Wang C et al. (2001). Crystallographic structures of the ligand-binding domains of the androgen receptor and its T877A mutant complexed with the natural agonist dihydrotestosterone. *Proc Natl Acad Sci USA* 98, 4904–4909.

Saez J M, De Peretti E, Morera A M, David M, Bertrand J (1971). Familial male pseudohermaphroditism with gynaecomastia due to testicular 17-ketosteroid reductase defect. I. Studies in vivo. *J Clin Endocrinol Metab* 32, 604–610.

Scully R E (1981). Neoplasia associated with anomalous sexual development and abnormal sex chromosomes. *Pediatr Adolesc Endocrinol* 8, 203–217.

Smith E P, Boyd J, Frank G R et al. (1994). Estrogen resistance caused by a mutation in the estrogen-receptor gene in a man. *N Engl J Med* 33, 1056–1061.

Soule S G, Conway G, Prelevic G M, Prentice M, Ginsburg J, Jacobs H S (1995). Osteopenia as a feature of the androgen insensitivity syndrome. *Clin Endocrinol* 43, 671–675.

Southern A L (1961). The syndrome of testicular feminization: a report of three cases with chromatographic analysis of the urinary neutral 17-ketosteroids. *Ann Intern Med* 55, 925–931.

Thompson J, Saatcioglu F, Janne O A, Palvimo J J (2001). Disrupted amino- and carboxyl-terminal interactions of the androgen receptor are linked to androgen insensitivity. *Mol Endocrinol* 15, 923–35.

Tremblay R R, Foley T P Jr, Corvol P et al. (1972). Plasma concentration of testosterone, dihydrotestosterone, testosterone–oestradiol binding globulin, and pituitary gonadotrophins in the syndrome of male pseudo-hermaphroditism with testicular feminization. *Acta Endocrinol* 87, 331–341.

Tsukada T, Inoue M, Tachibana S, Nakai Y, Takebe H (1997). An androgen receptor mutation causing androgen resistance in undervirilized male syndrome. *J Clin Endocrinol Metab* 79, 1202–1207.

Tut T G, Chadessy F J, Trifiro M A, Pisnky L, Yong E L (1997). Long polyglutamine tracts in the androgen receptor are associated with reduced *trans*-activation, impaired sperm production, and male infertility. *J Clin Endocrinol Metab* 8, 3777–3782.

Uehara S, Tamure M, Nata M et al. (1999). Complete androgen insensitivity in a 47,XXY patient with uniparental disomy for the X chromosome. *Am J Med Genet* 86, 107–111.

Varrela J, Alvesalo L, Vinkka H (1984). Body size and shape in 46,XY females with complete testicular feminization. *Ann Hum Biol* 11, 291–301.

*Viner R M, Teoh Y, Williams D M, Patterson M N, Hughes I A (1997). Androgen insensitivity syndrome: a survey of diagnostic procedures and management in the UK. *Arch Dis Child* 77, 305–309.

Vingerhoeds A C, Thijssen J H, Schwarz F (1976). Spontaneous hypercortisolism without Cushing's syndrome. *J Clin Endocrinol Metab* 43, 1128–1133.

Warne G L, Hughes I A (1995). The clinical management of ambiguous genitalia. In *Clinical Paediatric Endocrinology*, Brook C G D ed., pp 53–68. Blackwell Science, Oxford, UK.

Wilkins L (1950). Heterosexual development. In *The Diagnosis and Treatment of Endocrine Disorders in Childhood and Adolescence*, Wilkins L ed., pp. 256–279. Charles C Thomas, Springfield, IL.

  (1957). Abnormal sex differentiation: hermaphroditism and gonadal dysgenesis. In *The Diagnosis and Treatment of Endocrine Disorders in Childhood and Adolescence*, Wilkins L ed., p. 258. Charles C Thomas, Springfield, IL.

Wilson J D, Griffin J E, Russell D W (1993). Steroid 5 alpha-reductase 2 deficiency. *Endocr Rev* 14, 577–593.

*Wisniewski A B, Migeon C J, Meyer-Bahlburg H F et al. (2000). Complete androgen insensitivity syndrome: long-term medical, surgical, and psychosexual outcome. *J Clin Endocrinol Metab* 85, 2664–2669.

Yanase T, Simpson E R, Waterman M R (1991). 17 alpha-hydroxylase/17,20-lyase deficiency: from clinical investigation to molecular definition. *Endocr Rev* 12, 91–108.

Zachmann M, Prader A, Sobel E H et al. (1986). Pubertal growth in patients with androgen insensitivity: indirect evidence for the importance of estrogens in pubertal growth of girls. *J Pediatr* 108, 694–697.

21

Rokitansky syndrome and other Müllerian anomalies

D. Keith Edmonds

Queen Charlotte's Hospital, London, UK

Introduction

This chapter relates to a wide range of Müllerian anomalies, which divide themselves into obstructive and nonobstructive disorders and aplasias. Müllerian aplasia is also known as the Mayer–Rokitansky–Küster–Hauser syndrome (MRKH or simply Rokitansky syndrome). This was first given its eponym by Hauser and Schreiner in 1961 (based on a review of the postmortem reports of Mayer (1829), Rokitansky (1838) and Küster (1910)).

Aetiology

The development of the normal female reproductive tract requires differentiation and development of the Müllerian ducts. These arise within the embryo only if there is an absence of the Y chromosome. During embryological development, both Müllerian and Wolffian ducts are present and remain so until the developing fetus is around 150–200 mm in length. In the presence of a gonad that has differentiated into a testis, the Sertoli cells produce anti-Müllerian hormone, which causes regression of the Müllerian ducts and persistence of the Wolffian ducts. The absence of a Y chromosome and, therefore, the failure of testicular development means that the Müllerian ducts persist; the failure to produce testosterone means that the Wolffian ducts regress. The genetic control of this development is poorly understood, but the association with other abnormalities and some familial developments suggest that there are genetic factors that determine abnormalities of this development and only rarely has it been suggested that these abnormalities are environmental. At a molecular level, the information is again poor, although certain developmental genes, e.g. *HOXA 13*, seem to be involved in some way.

In complete Müllerian aplasia (the Rokitansky–Küster–Hauser syndrome), the genetic and molecular basis of the problems that arise are still to be elucidated. It is almost certain that this has polygenic, multifactorial inheritance, as there has so far been no success in detecting individual genes in studies of affected individuals. The recurrence risk in first-degree relatives is suggested to be between 1 and 2%. It is possible that a dominant or recessive gene still could be discovered to explain this, but the majority of cases will only be explained by a polygenic inheritance.

Transverse vaginal septa result from failure of the urogenital sinus and the Müllerian duct derivatives to meet or canalize; this has been deduced from the fact that these septae are at predicted sites and that the superior surfaces of the septa are lined by cells derived from Müllerian epithelium and the inferior surfaces are lined by squamous epithelium, which has its origin in the urogenital sinus. It has been accepted since the early 1960s that this disorder involves an autosomal recessive gene (McKusick et al., 1964). This was demonstrated in the Amish, and other familial patterns have been suggested in other populations (Chitayat et al., 1987). However, the gene itself has yet to be cloned and, therefore, it is unclear whether all of these disorders in all populations are caused by the same gene, or whether there may be different genes involved. In the McKusick syndrome, the region of chromosome 20 p12 has been localized as the likely target area for this genetic aberration.

Longitudinal vaginal septae result from fusion defects of the paramesanephric ducts, which fail to fuse at their lower border and duplication of development thereafter

Paediatric and Adolescent Gynaecology, ed. Adam Balen et al. Published by Cambridge University Press.
© Cambridge University Press 2004.

occurs. The genetic basis of this remains equally confused; although family aggregates of this disorder are described, the prevalence of the disorder in sisters is only around 2% (Elias et al., 1984). These data, however, are very difficult to analyse, as many cases may be unrecognized as they do not necessarily cause a functional disorder. It is, therefore, likely that incomplete fusion is again a polygenic, multifactorial disorder.

Epidemiology

The prevalence of congenital malformations of the Müllerian system has been variously estimated between 0.1 and 3% (Golan et al., 1989; Sanfilippo, 1986). However, the incidence depends on the population that has been studied and the circumstances that lead to that investigation of the population. For example, if the population being investigated has a history of habitual abortion or infertility, the prevalence of uterine abnormalities can be as high as 12% (Zanetti, 1978). Population-based studies are lacking for uterine anomalies. There have been only two population-based studies on the incidence of Müllerian aplasia. One is reported by Evans et al., (1981), suggesting an incidence of around 1:10 000, but this study failed to define the specific syndromes that were being studied. The first population-based study on incidence by definition of the Rokitansky syndrome or total Müllerian aplasia reported the incidence at 1:5000 (Aittomaki et al., 2001) in Finland between 1960 and 1969. The incidence in Finland may not necessarily reflect the incidence in other populations and further studies are required to define this more clearly.

Pathophysiology

Uterine and vaginal abnormalities range from a minor defect that has almost no clinical importance to the complete absence of the vagina and uterus. In between, there can be any degree of impaired development of the uterus and vagina. The paramesonephric (Müllerian) system develops on the lateral surface of the urogenital ridges and they develop alongside the mesonephric ducts. Both the mesonephric and paramesonephric ducts are interdependent and the absence of one will prevent the development of the other. The paramesonephric ducts grow down caudally and then move medially to fuse with the opposite side in the midline on the posterior wall of the urogenital sinus. It is probable that the fusion occurs at the level of the uterine isthmus and then development proceeds caudally

and towards the cephalad at the same time. Midline absorption begins at the isthmus, subsequently unifying the cervix and vagina. The lower end of the paramesonephric duct then proliferates and the tissue moves caudally to invade the posterior wall of the urogenital sinus, forming the Müllerian tubercle. The most inferior part of this grows down towards the vagina and will eventually form the upper two-thirds of the vagina. Simultaneously, the urogenital sinus grows in a cephalad direction to meet the Müllerian tubercle, and these form themselves into the sinovaginal bulbs. The upgrowth will form the lower third of the vagina. The union of the two parts then results in a solid core, which undergoes canalization, giving rise to the patent vagina.

If the paramesonephric ducts fail to form, then there is failure of uterine development on that side, although the urogenital sinus will be present. If both paramesonephric ducts fail to form, then there is no functional uterus or vagina present. The association with mesonephric duct formation gives rise to the high incidence of renal anomalies in association with Müllerian anomalies. If the paramesonephric ducts are present, but fail to fuse, then duplication of the system results and hemi-uteri and hemi-vaginas may occur. Variations of anomaly may include uterus didelphus with a duplex vaginal system at one end of the spectrum or a single vagina, single cervix, single uterus with a small septum within it at the other end of the spectrum. Failure of the development of the urogenital sinus will result in vaginal atresia at its lower end, with a normal upper third of vagina, cervix and uterus above.

Clinical presentations

Müllerian agenesis

It is uncommon for Müllerian agenesis to be diagnosed prior to puberty, when secondary sexual characteristics develop without the onset of menses. Patients with these problems have normal ovarian function and, therefore, the development of the breast, pubic hair, axillary hair and the growth spurt are all normal. Failure to have any evidence of menses usually means that the girls present initially at around age 13 or 14 years. Too often they present to their general practitioners with this history and are told that it is likely that they will not require any treatment and that spontaneous menses will occur before the age of 16 and to return if this is not the case. This is an illogical management strategy and any girl who presents at any age with concern over her menses should be thoroughly examined to exclude congenital abnormalities and to allay effectively the fears and anxieties of both the parents and the child. Inspection of the vulva without digital examination will reveal the clinical picture of a vaginal dimple and no evidence of a vaginal passage.

Imperforate hymen

Girls with an imperforate hymen usually present with cyclical (monthly) abdominal pain caused by the retention of menstrual fluid within the vagina. Again, secondary sexual characteristics are normal and examination of the vulva reveals a bulging, blue membrane, which transilluminates the retained menstrual blood.

Transverse vaginal septae

In transverse vaginal septae, obstruction to the outflow tract again causes cyclical abdominal pain, but the reduced capacity of the vagina means that distension occurs quite quickly and the haematocolpos that results may well mean that a mass is palpable abdominally. Although a blood clot may occur within the uterus (a haematometra), this is generally small and the uterus itself does not become physically enlarged. Retrograde menstruation may occur and, as a result of this, endometriosis may arise, including the formation of endometriomata. Pelvic pain on a cyclical and chronic basis may result from this. Examination of the vulva in these circumstances may reveal a normal looking vulva, depending on the level of the transverse septal defect. The higher the septum, the more the lower part of the vagina has formed and, therefore, it may be difficult to see the obstructive element. When it is visible, it differs from an imperforate hymen in being pink, as the membrane is thick and does not allow transillumination (see Ch. 11).

Longitudinal vaginal septae

In longitudinal vaginal septae, one hemi-uterus and hemi-vagina function normally and there is an obstructed outflow of the other hemi-system. These girls present with normal menses and increasingly severe cyclical abdominal pain. Clinical examination often reveals an abdominopelvic mass, which represents the obstructed hemi-haematocolpos. Again, retrograde menstruation may result in endometriosis unilaterally and endometriomata may also form (see Ch. 10).

In all forms of obstructive outflow tract disorder, acute urinary retention may be a presenting clinical finding, caused by obstruction of the urethra by the haematocolpos.

Rudimentary horns

When a hemi-uterus has a noncommunicating horn, the obstruction to outflow gives the same cyclical abdominal pain picture, but without a pelvic mass, as there is no upper vagina into which the rudimentary horn can drain. Again, endometriosis may result from retrograde menstruation.

Imaging

In all cases of cyclical abdominal pain or primary amenorrhoea, a detailed image of the pelvis is essential in making the diagnosis. The most common way of imaging is with realtime ultrasound and in experienced hands the images required to diagnose the problem can easily be ascertained (see Ch. 10). Occasionally, imaging with ultrasound may be inconclusive and in these circumstances the use of magnetic resonance imaging should be considered. Here, detailed studies of the pelvis may be put together to identify an abnormality. There is no place for computed tomography scanning in the management of these disorders.

Associated conditions

As mentioned above renal and urinary tract abnormalities are commonly associated with Müllerian duct anomalies, as the development of both systems is intimately related. A number of syndromes associated with Müllerian aplasia have been described:
- Wolf–Hirschenhorn syndrome
- fascio-auricular vertebral syndrome
- Klippel–Feil syndrome
- MURCS syndrome
- urogenital dysplasia.

Incomplete Müllerian fusion, which spans everything from the bicornuate uterus through to uterus-didelphus and all degrees of incomplete fusion between these two, has also been associated with a number of syndromes:
- Apert syndrome
- Beckwith–Wiedemann syndrome
- cordal regression
- cloacal extrophy
- de Lange's syndrome
- Fryn's syndrome
- Meckel's syndrome
- prune belly syndrome
- Roberts' syndrome
- Rüdiger's syndrome

- triploidy
- trisomy 13
- trisomy 18
- urogenital dysplasia.

This wide range of associated conditions implies that the renal tract should be investigated in every patient presenting with a Müllerian anomaly. This investigation can probably be limited initially to a renal ultrasound, to establish that there are two functional kidneys. In some circumstances, intravenous urography could be carried out, but the importance of the findings in the presence of two functional kidneys demonstrated on ultrasound is limited. Duplication of ureters is probably of little importance, unless there is some functional abnormality with the kidney and, therefore, the use of intravenous urography in these circumstances is probably not justified. When one kidney is missing, more detailed urological examination should be carried out to establish whether or not there are horseshoe kidneys, pelvic kidneys, or other renal abnormalities, as these may be of much greater functional importance. In addition, the position of the kidney becomes paramount when deciding how to proceed with any surgical abdominal or pelvic procedure in the future.

Management

Medical management

These conditions do not lend themselves to medical management in terms of the resolution of their abnormality. However, in the acute situation, when girls present with acute or acute-on-chronic cyclical pelvic pain, the use of the continuous oral contraceptive pill, or gonadotrophin-releasing hormone (GnRH) analogues to prevent any further menstrual loss may be useful while the patient is prepared for the reconstructive surgery that they need. In many circumstances, this may totally obliterate the symptoms and the progress of any endometriosis and allow planned surgical reconstruction to be carried out at leisure.

Management of the Rokitansky syndrome

The approach to management in Rokitansky syndrome falls into two strategies: a nonsurgical approach using vaginal dilators and a surgical approach involving vaginoplasty.

Nonsurgical approach

In the author's opinion, the nonsurgical approach should be attempted in all patients with Rokitansky syndrome

prior to any attempt at a surgical reconstruction (Frank's procedure: Frank 1938; Rock 1997). The author's experience of nearly 220 patients with the Rokitansky syndrome has demonstrated that this nonsurgical approach results in 85% of patients achieving sexual intercourse and sexual satisfaction within relationships. The use of the vaginal dilator requires supervision by a clinical nurse specialist who is trained in this technique (see also Ch. 13). The technique involves the use of graduated glass, perspex or plastic vaginal dilators (see Fig. 13.1, p. 148) that are placed at the apex of the dimple of vaginal skin and pressure is exerted by the patient in order to stretch the vaginal skin into the space where the vagina should have been. This must be carried out under supervision initially and probably requires admission to hospital for suitable supervision and also suitable psychological support at the same time. The technique involves using the dilators on three occasions per day, each time for 15–20 minutes. Vaginal length may be achieved for satisfactory intercourse within six to eight weeks, although on occasions this may take longer, depending on the application of the patient. However, the resulting vagina is made of normal vaginal skin, is supple and is as close to the normal vagina as can be achieved. From a psychological point of view, this is a major achievement for these young women, as they are able then to have the confidence that their vagina is normal.

Surgical management (see also Ch. 11)
When patients fail to create a vagina with the use of dilators, a surgical approach may be required. There are numerous techniques that have been described, including partial- and full-thickness skin grafting, the use of amnion to line a vaginoplasty site, the use of oxidated cellulose, peritoneum (the Davidoff operation), skin flaps from the vulva, Vecchietti's procedure and the use of both large and small bowel.

Vaginoplasty
Vaginoplasty involves the creation of a neovaginal space between the urethra, bladder and rectum. The vaginal dimple is incised transversely and digital dissection on the lateral aspect allows the space between the two to be dissected free. It is important that the surgeon reaches the pelvic peritoneum in order to minimize the risk of subsequent vaginal shortening. Once the neovagina has been created, a number of different materials can be used to line this. A full-thickness or partial-thickness skin graft may be used (the McIndoe procedure; Ashworth et al., 1986) or amnion or other artificial materials may be used. These materials are placed over a mould that is made to fit the vagina and is usually made of soft foam rubber. The use of solid moulds should be discouraged because of the risk of damage to

the bladder neck and the risk of vesico-neovaginal fistula. The patient has a urethral catheter, which remains in place for five to seven days until the patient is returned to the operating theatre for inspection of the graft site. At this time, a further graft may be applied or, if the graft site is satisfactory, the patient may have the mould removed and begin the use of dilators. Failure to use the dilators adequately will mean that the neovagina will shorten and the end result is a shorter vagina than had been achieved surgically.

After three months, sexual intercourse may begin and on days when this does not occur the dilators should be used. At six months, the dilators can be ceased and only during prolonged periods of sexual inactivity should patients need to revert to the use of the dilators to avoid subsequent contracture.

The results of this surgical approach gives about a 80% success rate, but serious complications may occur. These include infection, haemorrhage, fistula formation and failure of the graft to become viable. Complications from this procedure occur in approximately 10% of patients (Alessandrescu et al., 1996). It is, therefore, essential that patients are counselled prior to surgery with regard to the complications that can occur and that consent is clearly laid down in terms of complications.

Bowel

In some circumstances, where the perineum is flat or the vaginal dimple is extremely short, there may be a place to consider the use of bowel to create a vaginal tube. This is a major procedure involving the isolation of a loop of bowel, which may be caecum, sigmoid colon or small bowel, and an anastomosis of the remaining bowel. The isolated segment is then swung on its pedicle to be attached at its lower end to the vulva and the upper end is closed. A number of reports of the use of bowel to create the vagina have been described and some surgeons have advocated this as the primary procedure. However, a recent report from Syed et al. (2001), indicating the incidence of diversion colitis in this procedure, counselled that this technique should be used only in extreme circumstances, because the complication rates are so high. Patients report chronic vaginal discharge from their bowel loop as a common problem. Adenocarcinoma has also been described in a loop of bowel used for this purpose (Andryzowicz, 1985; Hiroi et al., 2001). Numerous case reports and very small series have been reported, with similar success to other techniques of around 80%.

Skin flaps

At the present time, the Wei flap is probably the commonest skin-flap technique, but the use of this as a primary procedure ought to be questioned. This procedure involves the dissection of two elongated skin flaps on the lateral wall of the vulva and the mobilization of the graft, which is swung on its base from either side to line the neovaginal space. The defect created by the flap is then closed, to allow vulval healing. The advantage of this technique is that it does involve a full-thickness graft and, therefore, reduces the incidence of vaginal contracture during healing. It may well be very helpful to use these flap techniques when other surgical techniques have failed, but individual patients need to be assessed on their merits.

Vecchietti procedure

In the Vecchietti procedure (Vecchietti, 1979), an olive attached to a wire system is used gradually to dilate the neovaginal space. In Vecchietti's original procedure, a laparotomy was performed through a lower transverse abdominal incision. The olive was placed in the vaginal dimple and two polypropylene or wire sutures were placed through the olive and then brought out through the potential neovaginal space, through the pelvic cavity and out through the abdominal wall (see p. 148). Here they were attached to a ratchet mechanism that would allow increased pressure to be exerted in order to bring the olive further into the neovaginal space, thereby stretching the vaginal skin in a similar manner to that achieved with vaginal dilators. Fedele et al. (1996) have described this technique using a laparoscopic approach and report excellent results. The efficacy of this technique is difficult to establish, as these patients have not previously tried vaginal dilators without any surgical intervention. The results, therefore, are similar to those for vaginal dilators and there would seem to be little advantage in using this technique as a primary procedure for the creation of a neovagina. However, it is well merited in circumstances where the patient is not able to create a vagina and a reasonable dimple exists to allow this technique chance of success.

Complications of this technique seem to vary with the operator but are described as damage to the ureters and rupture of the olive through the upper pole of the vagina in some circumstances.

Long-term results in Rokitansky syndrome

The assessment of long-term results following both the nonsurgical and surgical approach are somewhat limited, although it would seem that about an 80% success rate can be expected from any one of the techniques. In using a selective approach to surgery, one is able to use a nonsurgical approach in a high percentage of patients and only around 15% of patients who use the nonsurgical approach will need to proceed to a surgical one. As the surgical techniques described above each have around about an 80% success rate, it is likely, therefore, that following a nonsurgical then surgical approach would achieve a successful result from therapy for 95–96% of patients, allowing them to have a satisfactory sex life. It is imperative, however, that it is understood that these results are achieved by surgeons who perform these techniques regularly, and such audit does not allow us to comment on procedures performed occasionally. The case for centres of excellence for this type of surgery has been made elsewhere.

The long-term sequelae following the nonsurgical approach includes the occasional report of vaginal prolapse (Matsui et al., 1999), although this is very uncommon and its incidence is unknown. In the Rokitansky syndrome, small rudimentary anlaga may be present. These represent remnants of the paramesonephric duct and occasionally they may develop leiomyomata. If there is active endometrial tissue within, cyclical pain may occur and surgical removal (often laparoscopically) is indicated.

Complications have also been reported for surgical neovaginal approaches, including squamous cell carcinomas and epithelial neoplasia. An instance of the human immunodeficiency virus transmission through a neovagina has also been reported (Kell et al., 1992).

Obstructive disorders

Complete duplication of the genital tract may lead to a midline vaginal septum. Patients may experience dyspareunia as a result of this and the septum may need to be excised. This procedure involves excision of the septum, both anteriorly and posteriorly, and care must be taken that the septum is excised in its entirety to the point where the two cervices join. If this is not removed completely, then resultant dyspareunia may ensue and further surgical revision may be necessary (see also Ch. 11).

Longitudinal vaginal septae
Longitudinal vaginal septae also require excision. Again, the septum should be removed in its entirety, in order to ensure, first, that there is long-term adequate drainage and, second, that there is no resultant dyspareunia in the long term. The failure to remove the septum in its entirety may mean that any ostium that is created reseals and having opened the hemi-uterus to the bacteria in the normal hemi-uterus, the risk of pyometra is very high and subsequent septicaemia may result. Again, this type of surgery must be performed correctly the first time. This should not be performed by occasional surgeons.

Transverse vaginal septae
Transverse vaginal septae may occur at three levels, as has previously been described, and the higher the septum, the more difficult it is to reconstruct a functional vagina. In the absence of the lower third of the vagina, the septum can be excised and a vaginal advancement made with ease; the resultant anastomosis should really not stenose. The use of vaginal dilators after surgery may be useful to avoid this happening. Mid and upper vaginal septae present a much more difficult surgical challenge and the anastomosis after excision of the septum may be very difficult. Occasionally, Z-plasties may be required in order to minimize the tension between the opposing ends of the vagina and the resultant surgery; it is very difficult to avoid stenosis subsequently. Again, the use of dilators may become important in the postoperative period to try to achieve a good result.

Rudimentary uteri
Rudimentary horns need to be surgically excised, as there is no place for attempting any unifying procedure. The procedure is usually straightforward and subsequent reconstruction of the uterus is achieved. The hemi-uterus that remains is normally functional.

Long-term outcome in obstructive disorders
The long-term outcome of patients with obstructive disorders has been poorly described. It would seem, however, that the surgical results in terms of sexual success would suggest that low vaginal septae and longitudinal vaginal septae have a very good prognosis, whereas those with high obstructive problems have much less satisfactory results. Reported series of long-term follow-up are small and, therefore, it is difficult to give a definitive figure of success (Alttaran et al., 1999; Rock et al., 1982).

Cervical agenesis

Cervical agenesis is a very rare condition where a functional uterus exists without a cervix, causing an outflow tract abnormality; there are only rare case reports and theories. Attempts to retain the uterus via surgical anastomosis over stents, to try and create a neocervix, have only been successfully performed since around 1980 and the success rate over this time for those centres that have reported their series is around 50%. The remaining patients have finally had a hysterectomy. Recent advice from the North American Society of Pediatric and Adolescent Gynecology advocates that attempts to try and salvage these uteri should not be made and that a hysterectomy should be advised as a primary procedure. The author feels very differently and that a 50% success rate is worth discussing with patients and allowing them to choose the strategy that they feel would best suit them (Edmonds, 1999). This is an extremely difficult decision and may be one that can be delayed by the use of the oral contraceptive pill or GnRH analogues to allow the patients time to consider their decision. Any attempt to perform this type of surgery should only be made by surgeons with experience in this technique.

Fertility

Patients with the Rokitansky syndrome have no functional uterine tissue and, therefore, conception is impossible. However, they are endocrinologically normal. The use of a surrogate mother to allow women with this condition the opportunity to reproduce has occurred since the early 1990s. Reports from the USA and the UK indicate a high success of around 45% in these womens' reproductive performance with surrogates. The follow-up of babies born through surrogacy in vitro fertilization shows that approximately 50% of babies were female and ultrasound examination of these female infants has revealed normal uteruses in all cases so far. A multifactorial inheritance in this condition, as mentioned under the genetics above, would suggest that the risk of recurrence in these circumstances is likely to be around 2% and, therefore, the small numbers of babies born so far (approximately 100 reported) means that it is still likely that this recurrence rate will indeed occur (Beski et al., 2000).

Uterine abnormalities

Most reports on Müllerian anomalies of the uterus have not documented any increase in infertility. Patients with a unicornuate uterus have a poor reproductive performance, however, in terms of spontaneous miscarriage and preterm delivery. In unicornuate uteruses, the spontaneous miscarriage rate is approximately 44%, with only a term birth rate of 40%. In patients with didelphic uteri, the miscarriage rate is increased and the preterm labour rate is also increased, but not to the same extent as with the unicornuate uterus and most of these losses are those associated with preterm birth. This high rate of preterm labour has prompted some practitioners to advocate performing an elective cervical cerclage, but there are no prospective studies looking at the efficacy of this and at the present time cervical cerclage should only be recommended if there is evidence of cervical incompetence.

Psychological and psychosexual aspects

The Rokitansky syndrome

The diagnosis of Müllerian aplasia is one that causes both parents and child enormous psychological trauma. The prospect of having no vagina and no reproductive ability often leads to acute depression, a feeling of worthlessness and doubts about gender (see also Ch. 14). Patients feel cheated of their chance of being able to reproduce, which they view, not unreasonably, as a fundamental human right and of course they are resentful of the fact that they are unable to perform the normal sexual act. These impact very significantly on the teenager, who is already struggling with the changes from childhood through puberty to adulthood. Not surprisingly, these changes may lead to considerable behavioural difficulties, and the involvement of a trained psychologist is extraordinarily important in the management of these patients. The planning of the management of these girls should be intimately linked to the opinion and preparation by the psychologist, and the success of treatment is influenced greatly by these aspects of care. The ability to persevere with the use of dilators or undergo a reconstructive surgical procedure requires considerable preparation and only when the adolescent is psychologically ready to undertake this arduous treatment should it be started.

The parents of these patients are also traumatized by this news and they also need strong and integrated psychological support. The use of parent self-help groups and patient self-help groups have proved to be invaluable in the management of these patients. With careful psychological care and an integrated approach between the clinicians, psychologists and nurse practitioners, the long-term results have proved to be highly satisfactory. Although the fertility issue and some of the sexual issues will remain for life, much of the quality-of-life issues that are associated with this condition can be overcome: a caring and compassionate approach will reap its rewards.

Obstructive disorders

As most of the surgical procedures that are performed for obstructive disorders result in resolution of the problem, it is unusual for those affected to have psychological or sexual difficulties in the long term. However, inappropriate surgery may result in complications that can be quite damaging psychologically to these women, and the focus on their abnormality may result in an abnormal attitude towards their genital tract. Here a sensitivity to the difficulties that these adolescents are facing, and again the involvement of a psychologist, may well be extremely helpful.

The long-term results ought to be satisfactory in the vast majority of cases.

Box 21.1 Key points

- Müllerian aplasia has a polygenic multifactorial inheritance.
- The prevalence of congenital malformations of the Müllerian system vary between 0.1 and 3%.
- The incidence of Müllerian aplasia is 1 in 5000.
- Müllerian agenesis presents as primary amenorrhoea in the presence of normal secondary sexual characteristics.
- Obstructive outflow tract disorders present with cyclical abdominal pain in the presence of secondary sexual characteristics.
- Realtime ultrasound is the most reliable way of assessing these congenital malformations.
- Müllerian aplasia is best treated by the nonsurgical use of vaginal dilators. Surgical approaches should be reserved for those patients who fail with the nonsurgical approach.
- Obstructive disorders need surgical treatment in which primary surgery has the highest chance of long-term success.
- Müllerian agenesis has a huge psychological impact on all patients. The involvement of a psychologist as part of a multidisciplinary team approach is essential.

REFERENCES

*Indicates key references.

Aittomaki K, Eroila H, Kajanoja P (2001). A population based study of the incidence of Müllerian aplasia in Finland. *Fertil Steril* 76, 624–625.

Alessandrescu D, Peltecu G C, Buhimschi C S, Buhimschi I A (1996). Neocolpopoiesis with split thickness skin graft as a surgical treatment for vaginal agenesis: retrospective review of 201 cases. *Am J Obstet Gynecol* 175, 131–138.

Andryjowicz E, Qizilbash M B (1985). Adenocarcinoma in a caecal neo-vagina. *Gynecol Oncol* 21, 235.

Ashworth M F, Morton K E, Dewhurst J, Lilford R J, Bates R G (1986). Vaginoplasty using amnion. *Obstet Gynecol* 65, 443–446.

*Attaran M, Falcone T, Gidwani G (1999). Obstructive Müllerian anomalies. In *Congenital Malformations of the Female Genital Tract*, Gidwani G, Falcone T, eds., pp. 155–158. Lippincott, Williams & Wilkins, Philadelphia, PA.

Beski S, Gorgy A, Venkat G, Craft I L, Edmonds K (2000). Gestational surrogacy, a feasible option for patients with Rokitansky syndrome. *Hum Reprod* 15, 2326–2328.

Chitayat D, Hahm S Y, Marion R W et al. (1987). Further delineation of the McKusick–Kaufman hydrometrocolpos–polydactyly syndrome. *Am Med J Dis Child* 141, 1133–1136.

Edmonds D K (1999). Diagnosis, clinical presentation and management of cervical agenesis. In *Congenital Malformations of the Female Genital Tract*, Gidwani G, Falcone T, eds., pp. 169–176. Lippincott, Williams & Wilkins, Philadelphia, PA.

Elias S, Simpson J L, Carson S A, Malinak L R, Buttram V C (1984). Genetic studies in incomplete Müllerian fusion. *Obstet Gynecol* 63, 276–279.

*Evans T, Poland M, Boving R (1981). Vaginal malformations. *Am J Obstet Gynecol* 141, 910–920.

Fedele L, Bianchi S, Tozzi L, Borruto F, Vignali M (1996). A new laparoscopic procedure for the creation of a neo-vagina in Mayer–Rokitansky–Küster–Hauser syndrome. *Fertil Steril* 66, 854–857.

Frank R T (1938). The formation of an artificial vagina without operation. *Am J Obstet Gynecol* 35, 1053–1055.

*Golan A, Langer R, Bukovsky I, Caspi E (1989). Congenital anomalies of the Müllerian system. *Fertil Steril* 51, 747–755.

Hauser G A, Schreiner W E (1961). Das Mayer–Rokitansky–Küster syndrome. *Schweiz Med Wochenschr* 91, 381–384.

Hiroi H, Yasugi T, Matsumoto K et al. (2001). Mucinous adenocarcinoma arising in a neo-vagina using the sigmoid colon thirty years after operation. *J Surg Oncol* 77, 61–64.

Kell P D, Barton S E, Edmonds D K, Boag F C (1992). HIV infection in a patient with the Mayer–Rokitansky–Küster–Hauser syndrome. *J Roy Soc Med* 85, 706–707.

Matsui H, Seki K, Sekiya S (1999). Prolapse of the neo-vagina in Mayer–Rokitansky–Küster–Hauser syndrome. *J Reprod Med* 44, 548–550.

McKusick V A, Bauer R L, Koop C E, Scott R B (1964). Hydrometrocolpos as a simply inherited malformation. *J Am Med Assoc* 189, 813–816.

*Rock J A (1997). Surgery for anomalies of the Müllerian ducts. In *Te Linde's Operative Gyneoclogy*, 8th edn, Rock J A, Thompson J D, eds., pp. 687–729. Lippincott-Raven, Philadelphia, PA.

*Rock J A, Zacur H A, Dlugi A M, Jones H W, Te Linde R W (1982). Pregnancy success following surgical correction of imperforate hymen complete vaginal septum. *Obstet Gynecol* 59, 448–451.

Sanfilippo J S, Wakim N G, Schikler K N, Yussman M A (1986). Endometriosis in association with uterine anomaly. *Am J Obstet Gynecol* 154, 39–43.

Song R, Wang X, Zhou G (1982). Reconstruction of the vagina with sensory function. *Clin Plast Surg* 9, 105–109.

Syed H A, Malone P S, Hitchcock R J (2001). Diversion colitis in children with colpovaginoplasty. *Br J Urol* 87, 857–860.

Vecchietti G (1979). Le neovagin dans le syndrome de Rokitansky–Küster–Hauser. *Rev Med Suisse Romande* 99, 593–601.

Zanetti E, Ferrari L R, Rossi G (1978). Classification and radiographic features of uterine malformations. Hysterosalpingogram study. *Br J Radiol* 51, 161–170.

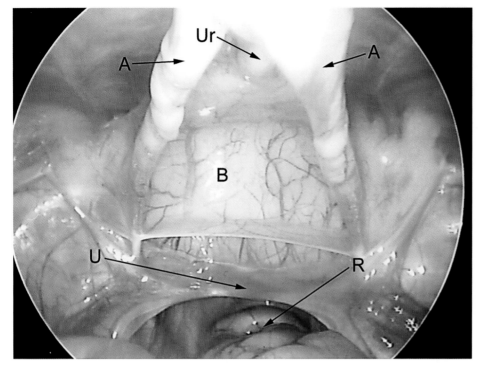

Fig. 7.2. Laparoscopic view of the bladder. This image was taken during a diagnostic laparoscopy of a 2-year-old girl, with the viewer looking towards the patient's toes. Underneath the peritoneal folds lie (anterior–posterior) the urachus (Ur), obliterated umbilical arteries (A), bladder (B), uterus (U) and rectum (R).

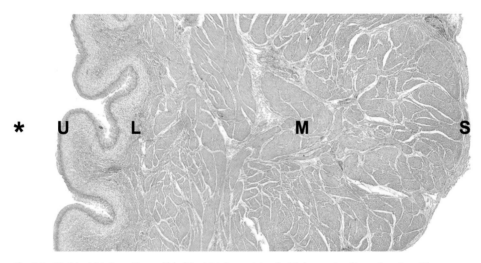

Fig. 7.3. Bladder histology. Normal bladder histology, stained with haematoxylin and eosin, with urothelium (U), lamina propria (L), detrusor muscle (M) and outer serosa (S); (⋆) denotes the lumen of the bladder.

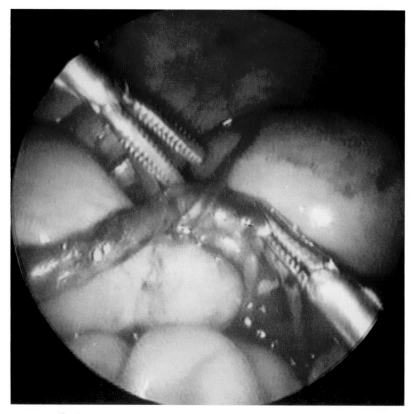

Fig. 12.5. Prenatally diagnosed torsion of an ovarian cyst. Laparoscopic view in a 1-week-old newborn.

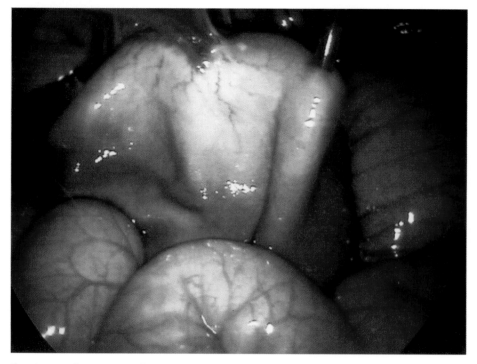

Fig. 12.7. Needle aspiration of large benign ovarian cyst in laparoscopic view. The needle is seen entering and draining the cyst at "one o'clock".

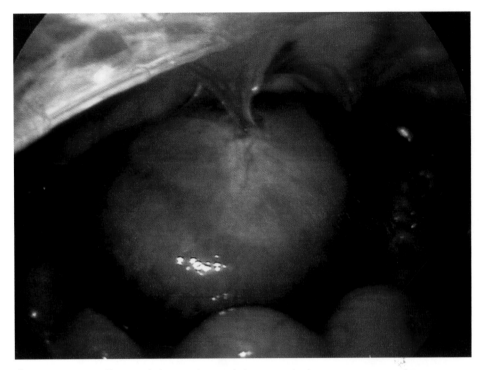

Fig. 12.8. Long-standing torted giant ovarian cyst in laparoscopic view.

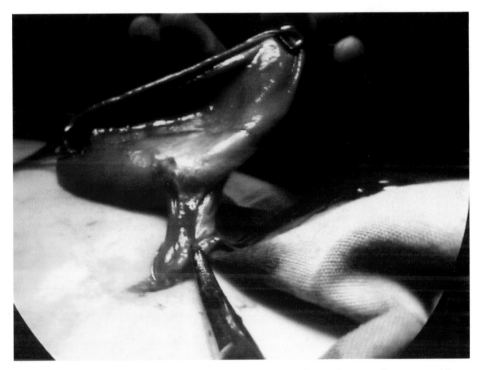

Fig. 12.9. A large ovarian cyst delivered outside the abdominal wall through a 1.5 cm long suprapubic incision after laparoscopic guided percutaneous needle aspiration.

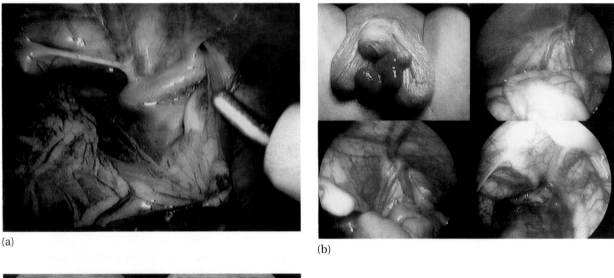

(a)

(b)

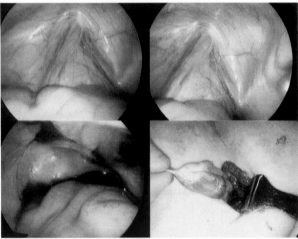

(c)

Fig. 12.10. Laparoscopy and intersex. (a) True hermophrodite. Laparoscopic view in a newborn showing ovo-testes and an inguinal hernia. (b) Partial androgen insensitivity. External and laparoscopic views showing relatively normal vas and vessels and no signs of Müllerian duct remnants. (c) Complete androgen insensitivity. Laparoscopic views showing relatively normal vas and vessels entering the left and right internal rings and no signs of Müllerian structures. External views showing a relatively normal looking testes within an inguinal hernia sac.

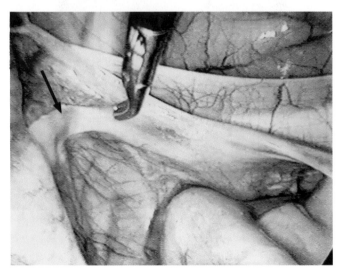

Fig. 12.11. An early gonadoblastoma in a 14-year-old girl with Turner's syndrome. Arrow indicates site of early changes.

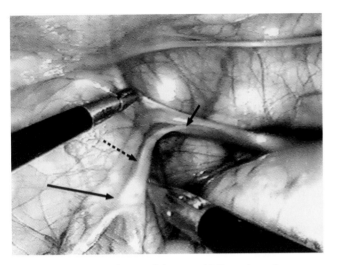

Fig. 12.12. Streak gonad in an adolescent with Turner's syndrome in laparoscopic view; note the ill-defined nature of the gonads. Small solid arrow indicates medial aspect of the left gonad extending almost onto the body of the uterus; broken arrow indicates narrow mesentery between the gonad and the Fallopian tube; long solid arrow indicates the lateral aspect of the gonad, which is almost inseparable from the fimbrial end of the tube.

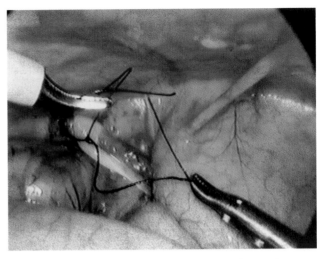

Fig. 12.13. A simple lateral trans-positioning of the left normal ovary above and lateral to the iliac vessels in laparoscopic view.

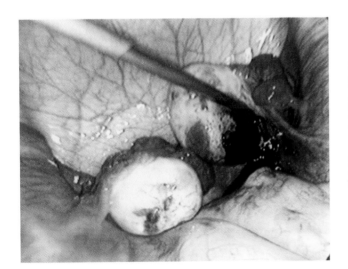

Fig. 12.14. Ovulation induced minor intraperitoneal haemorrhage, causing an acute abdomen in a 14-year-old girl.

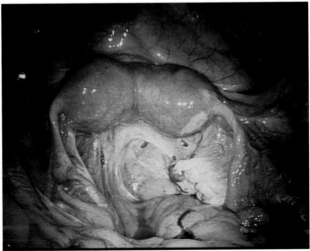

Fig. 12.15. A generalized view of the pelvis in a patient with a bicornuate uterus.

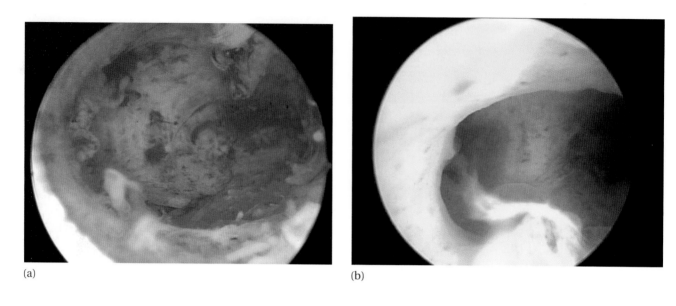

(a)

(b)

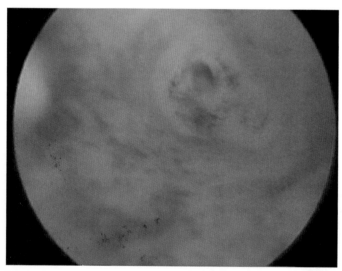

(c)

Fig. 12.16. A hysteroscopic view of a normal uterine cavity. (a) The normal cavity. (b) A bicornuate uterine cavity. (c) An uterine cavity with only one ostia (patient had a second noncommunicating accessory uterus).

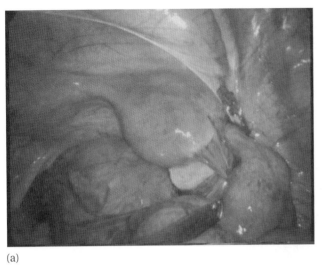

(a)

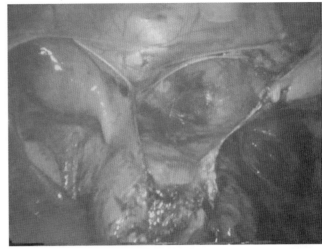

(b)

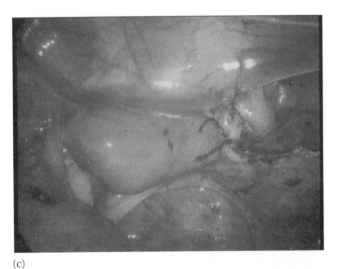

(c)

Fig. 12.17. Removal of an accessory uterine horn. (a) The normal uterus is on the left of the picture. The other uterus is the accessory horn to be excised. (b) The uterovesical fold has been reflected and the accessory uterus is partially dissected. (c) The accessory uterus has been excised.

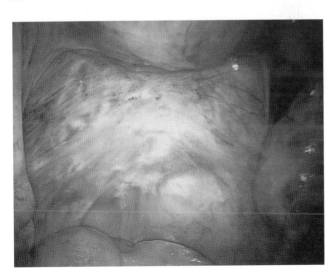

Fig. 12.18. A view of the pelvis in a patient with endometriosis and an obliterated pouch of Douglas.

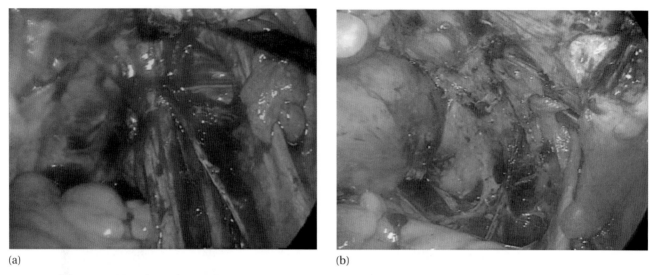

(a)

(b)

Fig. 12.19. Excision of an endometrial node. (a) A rectovaginal endometriotic nodule partly dissected free of surrounding structures prior to excision. (b) The view of the pelvis after the nodule has been excised.

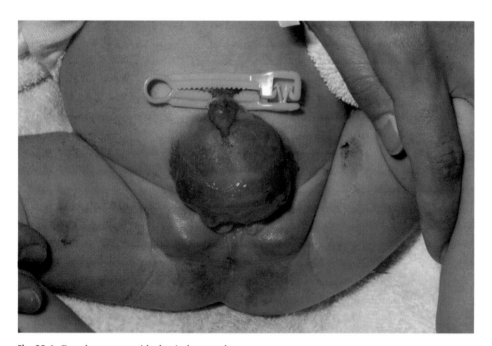

Fig. 23.1. Female neonate with classical exstrophy.

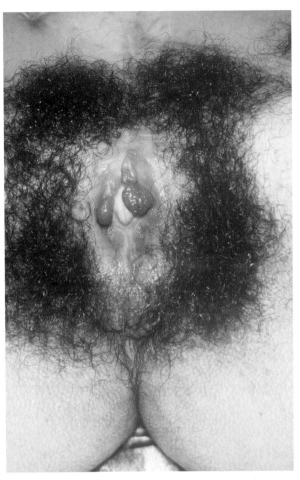

Fig. 23.3. Clinical photograph to show the labia in exstrophy.

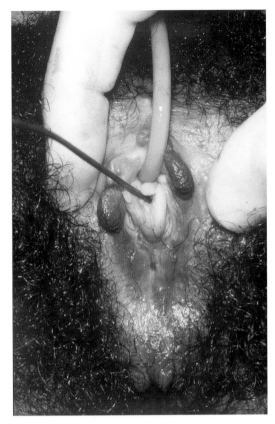

Fig. 23.4. Clinical photograph of the female perineum in exstrophy to show the bifid clitoris and labia. There is a probe in the introitus.

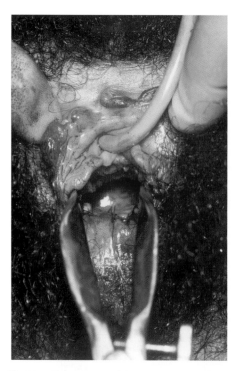

Fig. 23.6. Enlargement of the introitus by episiotomy.

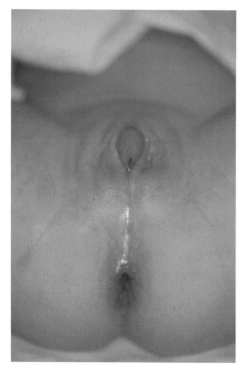

(a)

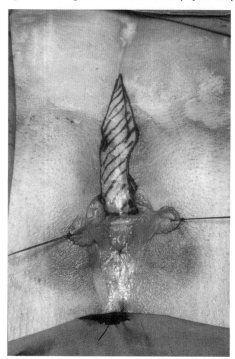

Fig. 23.7. Preoperative photograph to show the incision for the reconstruction of the supra pubic area and introitus in a female. The supra pubic scar is excised. The labia are united anteriorly. The hair-bearing flaps are rotated to cover the defect. An episiotomy is made and sutured open.

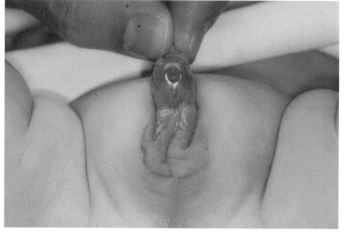

(b)

Fig. 24.4. Perineum in congenital adrenal hyperplasia. (a) Typical anatomy. (b) Perineum with a markedly enlarged penoclitoral organ, scrotalized labia major and an absent vaginal opening.

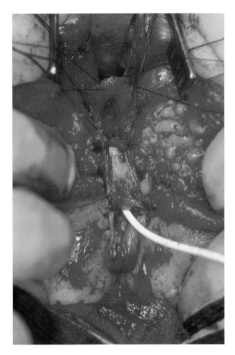

Fig. 24.9. Passerini's procedure.

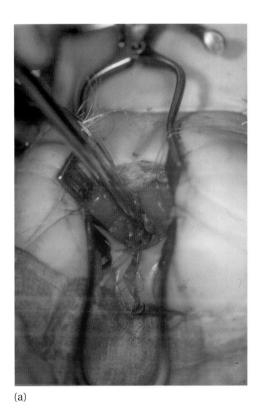

(a)

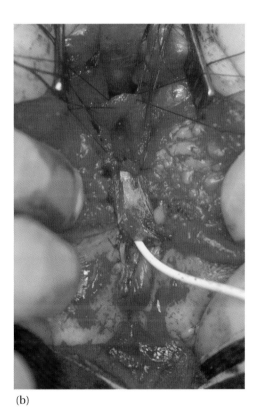

(b)

Fig. 24.11. Posterior sagittal approach to the urogenital sinus. (a) The bougie is in the vagina. The rectum is wide open.
(b) Reconstruction of the anterior wall of the vagina using the mucosa of the urogenital sinus.

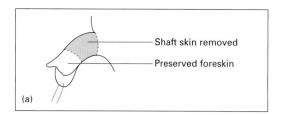

(a) Shaft skin removed / Preserved foreskin

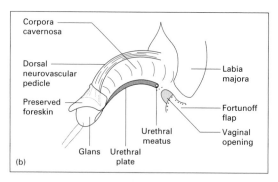

(b) Corpora cavernosa / Dorsal neurovascular pedicle / Preserved foreskin / Glans / Urethral plate / Urethral meatus / Labia majora / Fortunoff flap / Vaginal opening

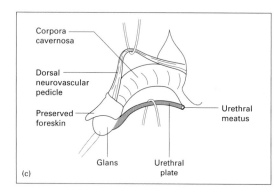

(c) Corpora cavernosa / Dorsal neurovascular pedicle / Preserved foreskin / Glans / Urethral plate / Urethral meatus

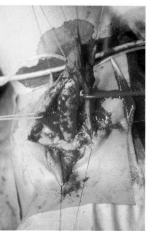

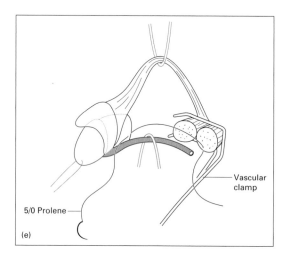

(e) 5/0 Prolene / Vascular clamp

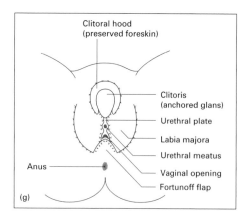

(g) Clitoral hood (preserved foreskin) / Clitoris (anchored glans) / Urethral plate / Labia majora / Urethral meatus / Vaginal opening / Fortunoff flap / Anus

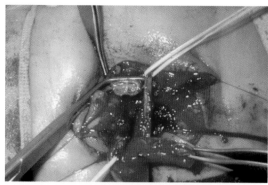

(d)

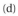

(f)

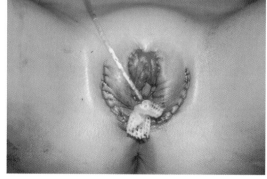

(h)

Fig. 24.13. (*opposite*) The penoclitoral organ. (a) Saddle incision line on the penoclitoral organ. (b) The penoclitoral organ with the glans (clitoris), the dorsal neurovascular pedicle, the two corpora cavernosa and the urethral plate. (c) Dissection of the penoclitoral organ. (d) Operative view of the dissected penoclitoral organ. Neurovascular pedicle (blue sling) and urethral plate (red sling). (e,f) Excision of the midpart of the corpora cavernosa to reduce the length of the penoclitoral organ. (g,h) final cosmetic appearance of the perineum after surgical correction.

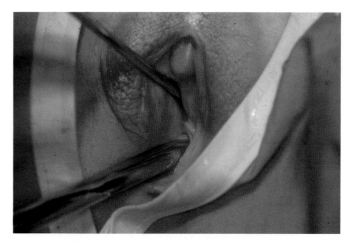

Fig. 24.14. Satisfactory long-term surgical outcome of surgery for a low urogenital sinus.

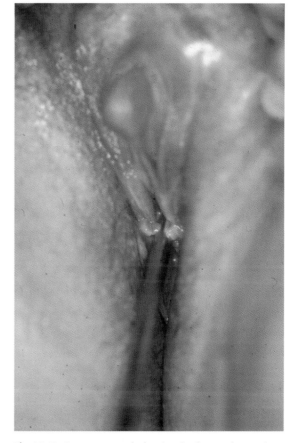

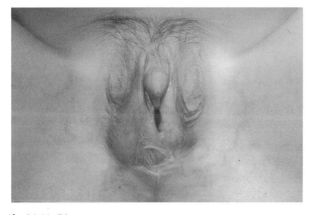

Fig. 24.16. Disaster.

Fig. 24.15. Long-term result showing the deep and posterior location of the vaginal introitus (bougie), the too long mucosal slide between the base of the clitoris and the urethral meatus. The clitoris is too big and sticks out.

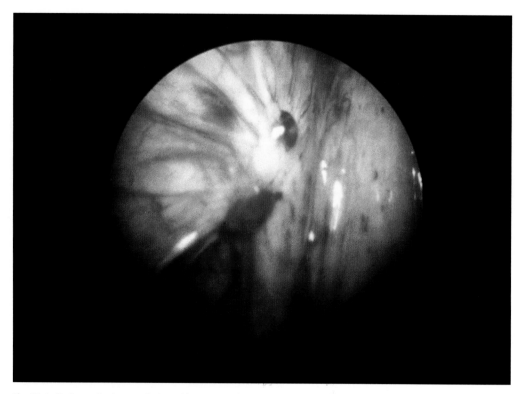

Fig. 29.1. Red papules in association with peritoneal puckering and scarring. (Courtesy of R. W. Shaw, Slide Atlas of Endometriosis, 1994.)

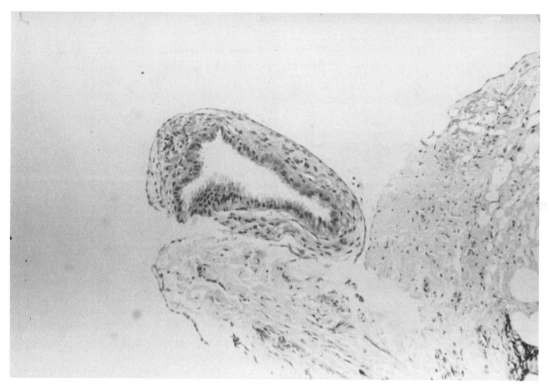

Fig. 29.2. High-power section of peritoneum with gland lined with endometrium-like epithelium and surrounded by stroma and haemorrhage. (Courtesy of R. W. Shaw, Slide Atlas of Endometriosis, 1994.)

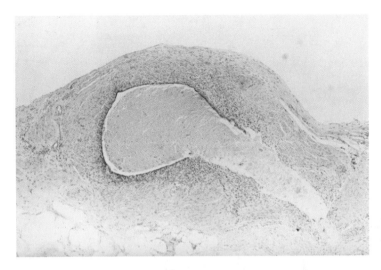

Fig. 29.3. Biopsy from peritoneal yellow-brown lesion showing fibrous tissue with a small blood-filled endometriotic gland. (Courtesy of R. W. Shaw, Slide Atlas of Endometriosis, 1994.)

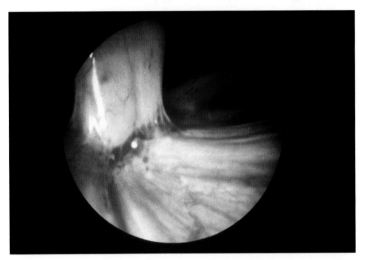

Fig. 29.4. White scarification with active red lesions involving the right round ligament. (Courtesy of R. W. Shaw, Slide Atlas of Endometriosis, 1994.)

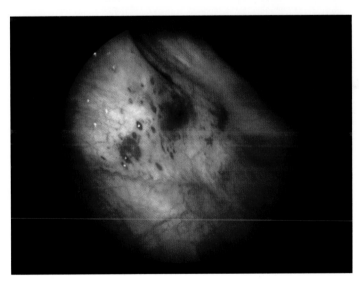

Fig. 29.5. Peritoneal fluid is a frequent finding in cases of mild or minimal endometriosis. Aspiration is advised to allow for a full inspection of the pouch of Douglas. (Courtesy of R. W. Shaw, Slide Atlas of Endometriosis, 1994.)

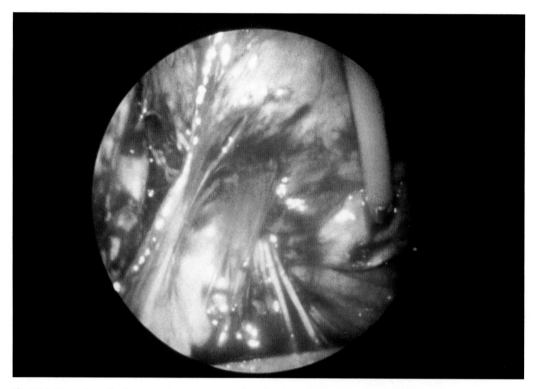

Fig. 29.6. Extensive adhesions seen in association with endometriosis. (Courtesy of R. W. Shaw, Slide Atlas of Endometriosis, 1994.)

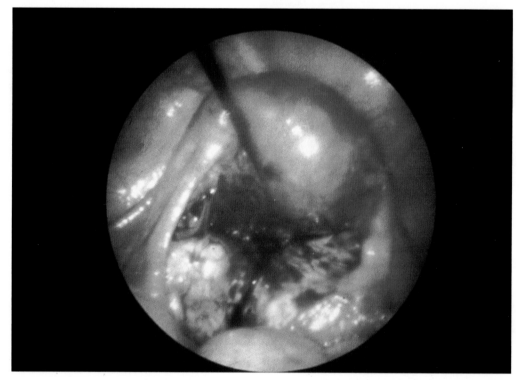

Fig. 29.7. Bilateral ovarian endometrioma adherent to each other and to the posterior uterine wall. (Courtesy of R. W. Shaw, Slide Atlas of Endometriosis, 1994.)

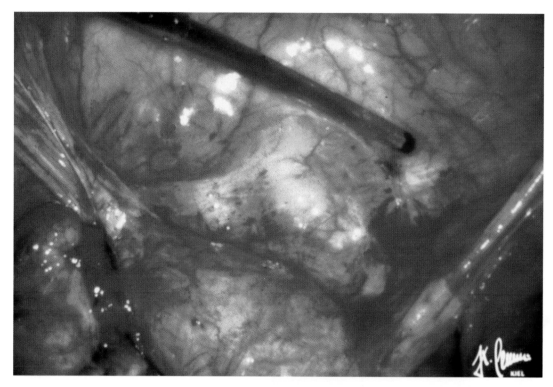

Fig. 29.8. Laproscopic local destructive treatment of endometriotic deposits.

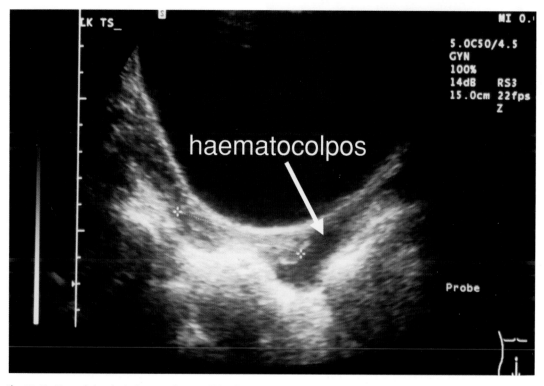

Fig. 29.10. Transabdominal ultrasound scan of blood in a haematocolpos in a 13 year old girl with an imperforate hymen.

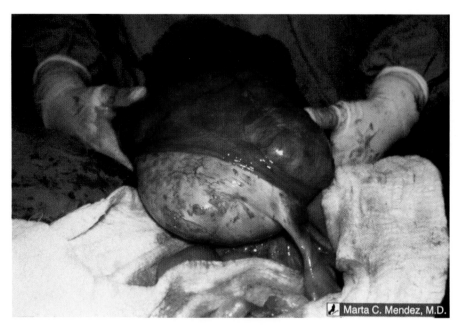

Fig. 29.11. Mesenteric cyst of the small bowel.

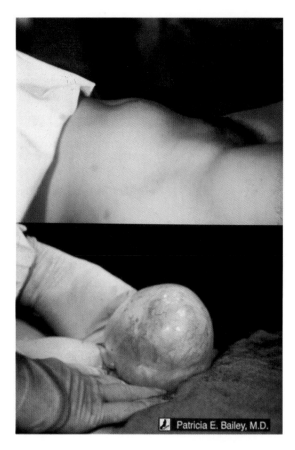

Fig. 29.12. Preoperative and intraoperative views of a 13-year-old girl with a large dermoid cyst. (Courtesy of the North American Society for Pediatric and Adolescent Gynecology, 1996.)

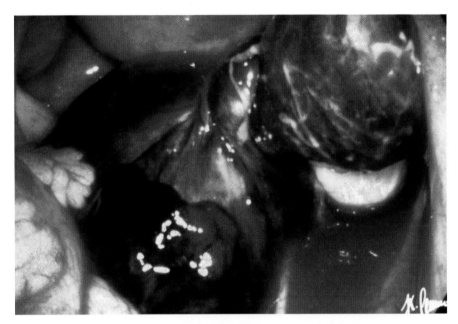

Fig. 29.13. Dysgerminoma of the ovary in an adolescent girl. (Courtesy of the North American Society for Pediatric and Adolescent Gynecology, 1996.)

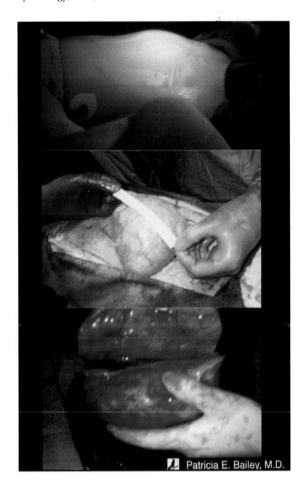

Fig. 29.14. Preoperative and intraoperative views of a 15-year-old girl with a dysgerminoma measuring 14 cm in diameter. (Courtesy of the North American Society for Pediatric and Adolescent Gynecology, 1996.)

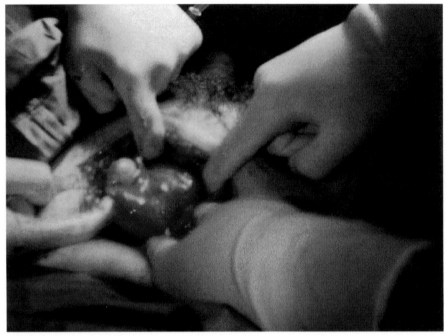

(a)

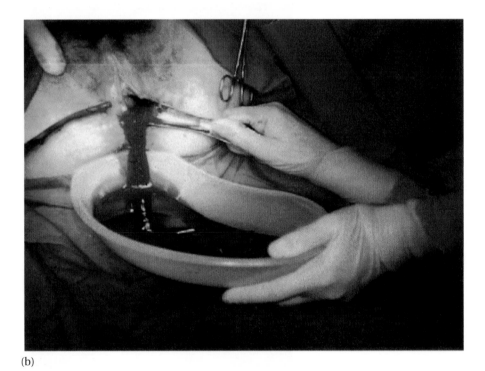

(b)

Fig. 29.15. A 13-year old postmenarchal girl presenting with pelvic pain and a pelvic mass caused by an obstructed hemivagina with a non-communicating septum and unrecognized uterine didelphys. (a) Small uteri lying above haematocolpos; (b) drainage of obstructed hemivagina on right; (c) longitudinal vaginal septum following drainage (note original vaginal orifice on left through which ongoing menstruation was evident); (d) view of pelvic organs following excision of longitudinal vaginal septum.

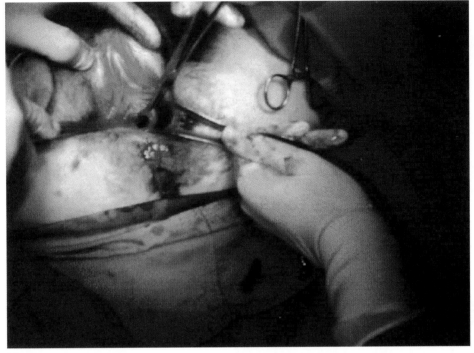

(c)

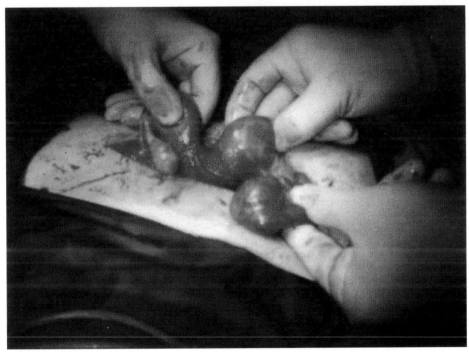

(d)

Fig. 29.15. (*Cont.*)

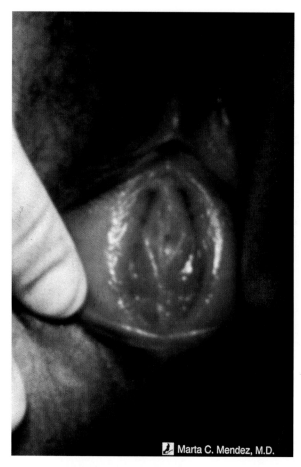

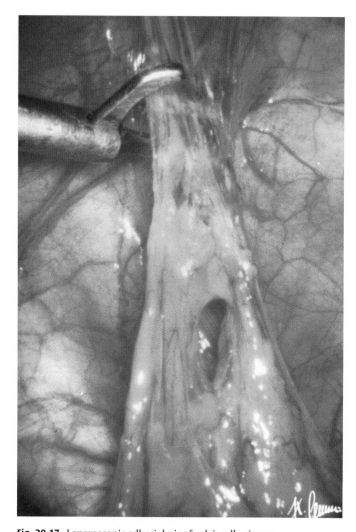

Fig. 29.16. Clinical appearance of a transverse vaginal septum behind the patient's normal hymen and completely distinct from this. (Courtesy of the North American Society for Pediatric and Adolescent Gynecology, 1996.)

Fig. 29.17. Laparoscopic adhesiolysis of pelvic adhesions as a consequence of pelvic inflammatory disease.

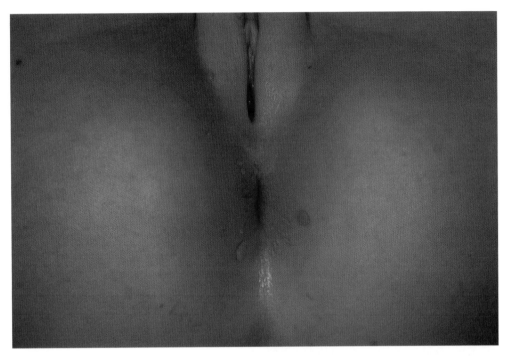

Fig. 35.1. Anogenital warts. Vulval and perianal warts in a 3-year-old child. (Copyright: Addenbrooke's Hospital, Cambridge.)

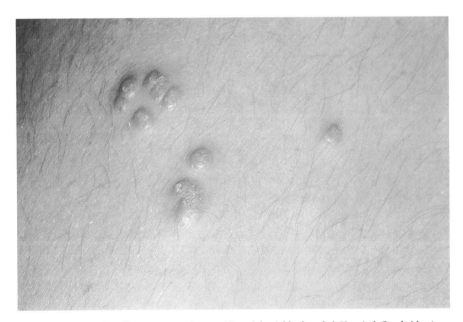

Fig. 35.2. Papules of molluscum contagiosum. (Copyright: Addenbrooke's Hospital, Cambridge.)

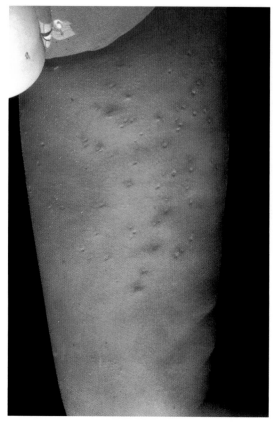

Fig. 35.3. Depressed scars following infection with molluscum contagiosum. (Copyright: Addenbrooke's Hospital, Cambridge.)

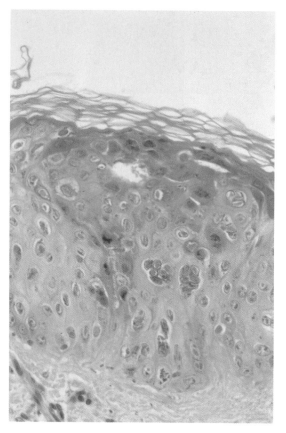

Fig. 35.4. Herpes simplex. Vulval biopsy showing epidermal cell necrosis and giant cell formation in herpes simplex infection.

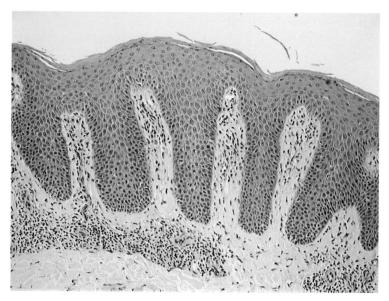

Fig. 35.5. Lichen simplex. Vulval biopsy showing epidermal thickening (acanthosis), mild hyperkeratosis and a chronic inflammatory cell infiltrate in the dermis. (Courtesy of Dr Ed Rytina, Histopathologist, Addenbrooke's Hospital, Cambridge.)

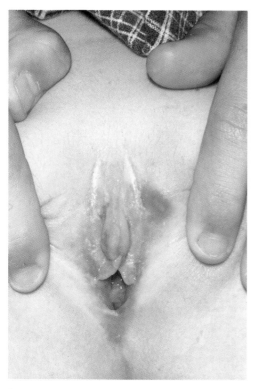

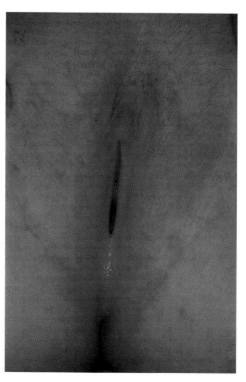

Fig. 35.6. Lichen sclerosus. Vulva of 6-year-old girl with whitish change, erythema and erosions. (Copyright: Addenbrooke's Hospital, Cambridge.)

Fig. 35.7. Lichen sclerosus. Vulva of 10-year-old girl after use of topical steroid. The lichen sclerosus is quiescent, but there is some smoothening of the vulval contours and erythema with some telangiecteses. (Copyright: Addenbrooke's Hospital, Cambridge.)

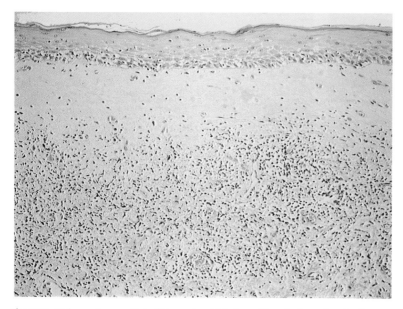

Fig. 35.8. Lichen sclerosus. Vulval biopsy in which the epidermis shows basal cells vacuolation. In the upper dermis, telangiectatic blood vessels are present in the homogeneous collagen and chronic inflammation persists in the lower dermis. (Courtesy of Dr Ed Rytina, Histopathologist, Addenbrooke's Hospital, Cambridge.)

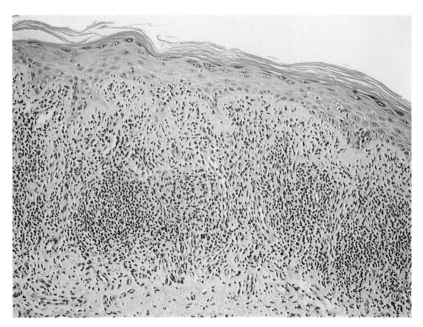

Fig. 35.9. Lichen planus. Vulval biopsy in which the epidermis has a 'saw-tooth' lower border and a band-like inflammatory cell infiltrate lies in the upper dermis. (Courtesy of Dr Ed Rytina, Histopathologist, Addenbrooke's Hospital, Cambridge.)

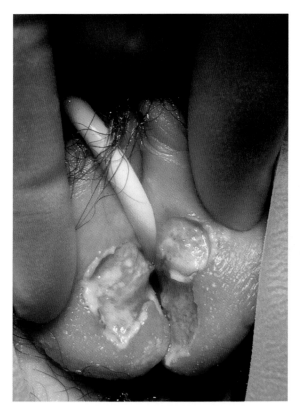

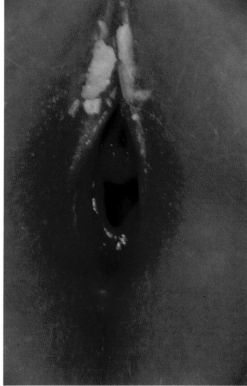

Fig. 35.10. Lipschütz ulcers in a 13-year-old child. (Copyright: Addenbrooke's Hospital, Cambridge.)

Fig. 36.1. Vulvitis in a prepubertal girl.

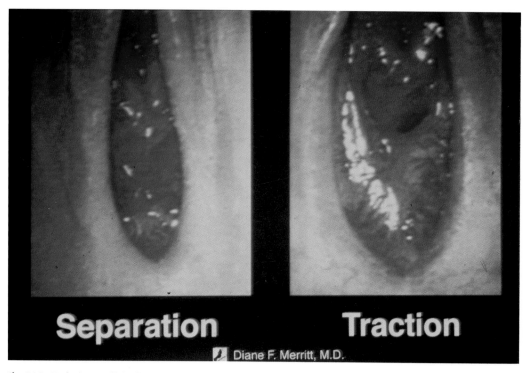

Fig. 36.3. Techniques of labial separation and lateral traction for viewing the hymen of a prepubertal girl.

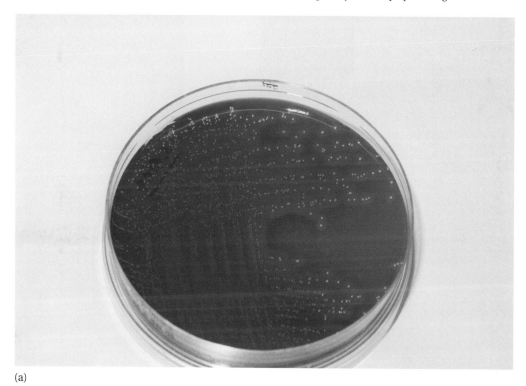

(a)

Fig. 36.6. Group A streptococci. (a) Beta-haemolysis on blood agar. (b) Gram film showing characteristic Gram-positive cocci in chains.

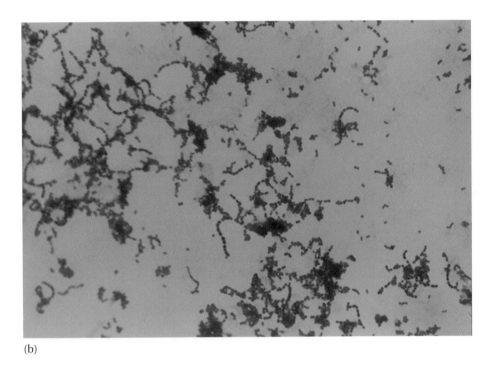

(b)

Fig. 36.6. (*Cont.*)

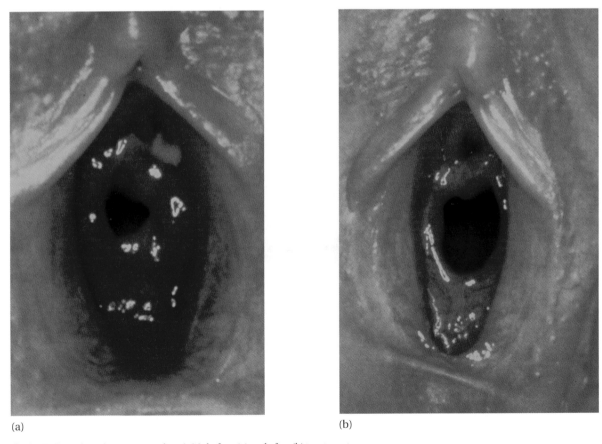

(a)

(b)

Fig. 36.7. Prepubertal streptococcal vaginitis before (a) and after (b) treatment.

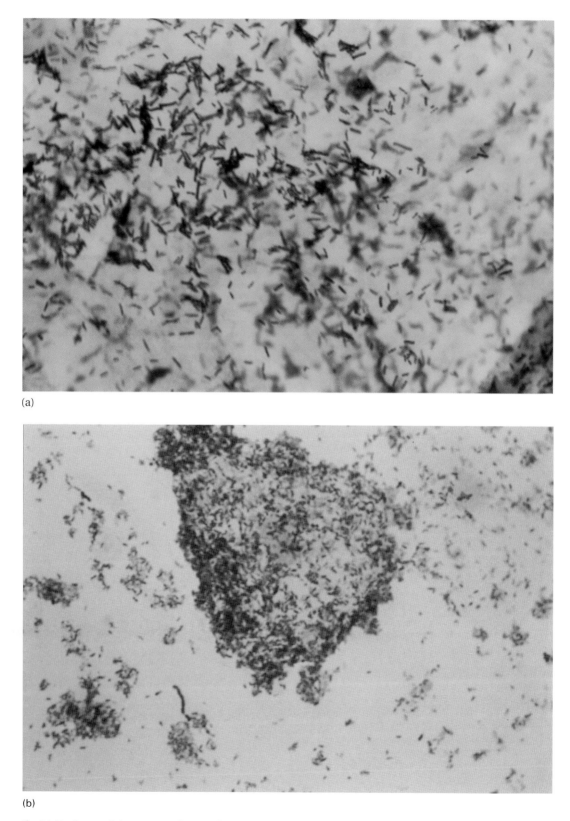

(a)

(b)

Fig. 36.10. Gram staining (a) Normal vagina flora (grade 1). (b) Clue cell (grade 3) in bacterial vaginosis.

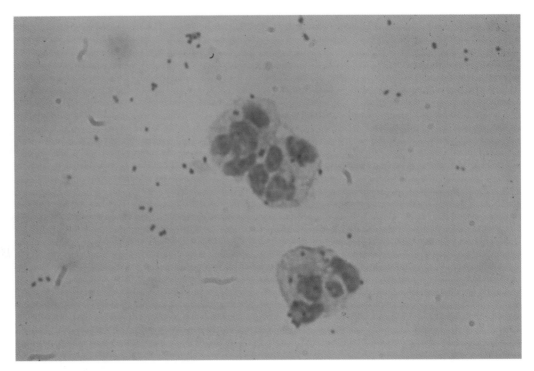

Fig. 36.12. Gram film of endocervical secretions showing Gram-negative intracellular diplococci in *Neisseria gonorrhoeae* infection.

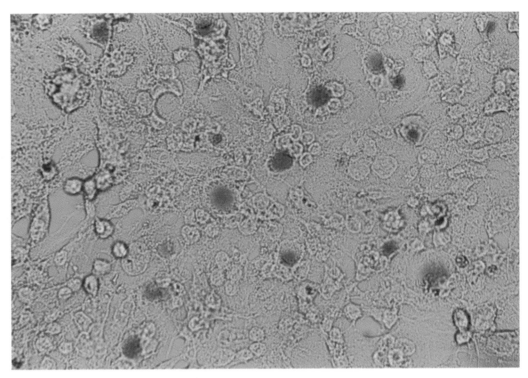

Fig. 36.14. McCoy cells showing typical intracytoplasmic inclusions of *Chlamydia trachomatis*, stained with iodine.

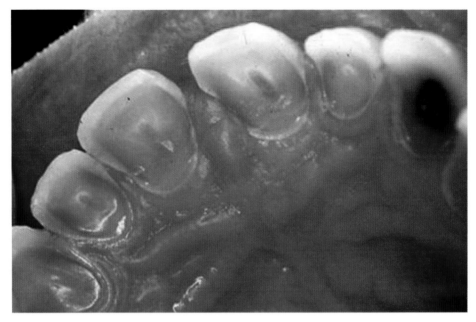

Fig. 38.2. Severe tooth erosion in bulimia nervosa. (Courtesy of Professor J. Treasure.)

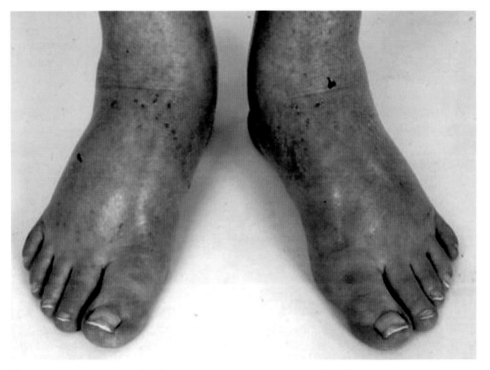

Fig. 38.3. Poor circulation and oedema in anorexia nervosa. (Courtesy of Professor J. Treasure.)

Acrocyanosis

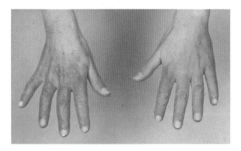

Fig. 38.4. Acrocyanosis in anorexia nervosa. (Courtesy of Professor J. Treasure.)

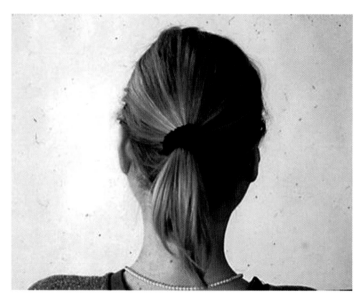

Fig. 38.5. Parotid gland enlargement caused by repeated vomiting. (Courtesy of Professor J. Treasure.)

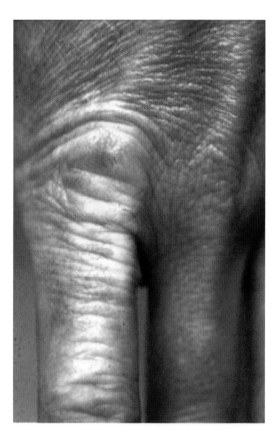

Fig. 38.6. Russell's sign caused by self-induced vomiting. (Courtesy of Professor J. Treasure.)

The XY female

Catherine L. Minto

The Elizabeth Garrett Anderson and Obstetric Hospital and University College London, UK

Introduction

In most pregnancies, fetal sexual development progresses smoothly down one of two paths leading to a male infant with an XY karyotype, scrotal testes and standard male genitalia or a female infant with an XX karyotype, ovaries and a uterus, and standard female external genitalia. However human fetal sexual determination and differentiation is complex and can be diverted from these dual standard pathways at a multitude of different points. When such a diversion occurs, the developing fetus can either switch over to the other pathway or blend the two, resulting in the birth of an intersex child.

Named androgynes by the Greeks, and later hermaphrodites by the Romans, no clear definition exists for the term "intersex", and correspondingly incidence figures vary greatly according to the conditions included (Blackless et al., 2000; Duckett et al., 1993; Quigley et al., 1995). In this chapter, the term intersex is used to mean a person with a mix or blend of the physically defining features (i.e. karyotype, gonadal structure, internal genitalia and external genitalia) usually associated with standard males and females. The term intersex, therefore, covers a diverse range of conditions encompassing individuals with standard male or female genitalia, who may have a variety of internal genital organs and karyotypes, and also those with ambiguous external genitalia. There are currently over 15 recognized intersex conditions, and in many of these there is an XY karyotype or some cells that are XY (Table 22.1). While there is currently debate over the optimal sex of rearing for some of these conditions (Blackless et al., 2000), in the past many of these children were raised as females. Those intersex conditions with XX chromosomes,

for example congenital adrenal hyperplasia caused by 21-hydroxylase deficiency (one of the commonest intersex conditions; see Ch. 24), are not discussed further in this chapter.

Various classifications of intersex conditions have been proposed, for example the terminology true hermaphroditism, female pseudohermaphroditism and male pseudohermaphroditism. As we have learnt more of the mechanisms of fetal sexual development, and of the aetiology behind many intersex conditions, these older categories are becoming less useful with the realisation that each intersex condition requires individual consideration. This chapter first provides an overview of aetiology and discusses the general area where each of these intersex conditions, incorporating XY chromosomal material, has diverted from the standard XY fetal development pathway. Then each condition is considered individually in more detail. Broad themes that relate to the management of many of these conditions are considered in more detail in other chapters and are only briefly mentioned here.

Aetiology

A brief glance at Fig. 22.1 will illustrate the variety of aetiologies that can lead to an XY female. The development of gonadal structures, followed by gonadal production of sex steroid hormones and anti-Müllerian hormone (AMH) along with the cellular response to these hormones, largely determines the features of each intersex condition, including external genital appearance, internal genital structures and fertility potential. The key to understanding the aetiology of XY female conditions lies in realising the early

Paediatric and Adolescent Gynaecology, ed. Adam Balen et al. Published by Cambridge University Press.
© Cambridge University Press 2004.

Table 22.1. Intersex conditions with an XY karyotype

Intersex condition	Internal genital organs	External genitalia appearance	Karyotype
5α-Reductase-2 deficiency	Testes	Variable from clitoral enlargement to ambiguous, to male with hypospadias and micropenis	46,XY
17β-Hydroxysteroid dehydrogenase deficiency	Testes	Variable from clitoral enlargement to ambiguous, to male with hypospadias and micropenis	46,XY
17-Hydroxylase deficiency	Testes	Female	46,XY
Complete androgen insensitivity syndrome	Testes	Female	46,XY
Congenital lipoid adrenal hypoplasia	Testes	Female	46,XY
Denys–Drash syndrome	Streak or dysgenetic testes	Female to ambiguous	46,XY
Frasier syndrome	Streak	Female to ambiguous	46,XY
Gonadal agenesis	Absent	Female	46,XY
Leydig cell hypoplasia	Testes with absent/diminished Leydig cells	Variable from normal female, to clitoral enlargement, to ambiguous, to male genitalia with micropenis	46,XY
Mixed gonadal dysgenesis	Bilateral dysgenetic testes, unilateral testis with contralateral streak, or dysgenetic testis.	Variable from clitoral enlargement, to ambiguous, to normal male appearance	45,X/46,XY
Mosaic Turner's syndrome	Bilateral streak gonads	Female	45,X/46,XY
Partial androgen insensitivity syndrome	Testes	Variable from normal female, to clitoral enlargement, to ambiguous, to normal male appearance	46,XY
Smith–Lemli–Opitz syndrome		Female to ambiguous	46,XY
Swyer's syndrome	Bilateral streak gonads	Female	46,XY
True hermaphroditism	Variable: consists of ovarian and testicular tissue, either separately or combined in ovotestes	Variable from normal female, to clitoral enlargement, to ambiguous, to normal male appearance	71% XX 20% XX/XY 7% XY

activity of testis development and subsequent production of testosterone and AMH, contrasted with the more passive role of later ovarian development and the lack of any ovarian activity required for female fetal external genital development.

Structural abnormalities in the gonad

Sex determination occurs at fertilization. At around 4 weeks, the undifferentiated gonad or genital ridge develops medial to the developing mesonephros. Already germ cells, originating in the yolk sac wall, have been migrating towards the genital ridge, and by week 4 these are found in the indifferent gonad. In an XY zygote, expression of the *SRY* gene on the Y chromosome, and other autosomal genes (e.g. *WT1*, *SOX9*, *SF1*; see Ch. 2), direct the indifferent gonad to become a testis (Berta et al., 1990). If *SRY* or one of these other autosomal testis-determining genes does not activate, the female pathway will continue and streak or

dysgenetic gonads will develop. The rest of the pathway of female development then proceeds smoothly, including the full development of the uterus and Fallopian tubes, as streak gonads do not produce AMH. If the abnormal gene only affects gonadal development, as in *SRY* mutations, then the resulting condition is Swyer's syndrome, also called complete XY gonadal dysgenesis (McElreavey et al., 1999). In this condition, it has been suggested that ovarian differentiation may commence but is not sustained because there is not a second X chromosome or perhaps because a requirement for certain ovarian-determining genes is not met (Russell et al., 1982). When testis-determining genes that also control the development of other structures are affected, then the complete sex reversal seen in Swyer's syndrome will occur in association with other abnormalities. In Denys–Drash syndrome (Jadresic et al., 1990) and Frasier syndrome (Barbaux et al., 1997), sex reversal is associated with renal abnormalities and alteration in the *WT1* (Wilms' tumour) gene. In campomelic dysplasia,

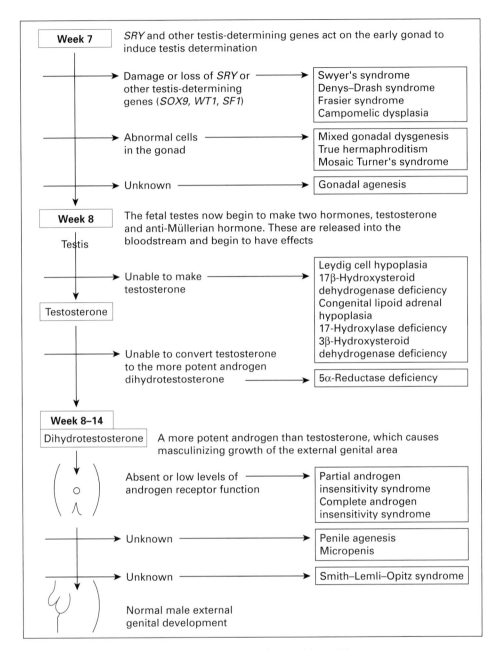

Fig. 22.1. Human sexual development and intersex conditions with an XY karyotype.

alterations in *SOX9* lead to skeletal anomalies and sex reversal (Schafer et al., 1995).

It is at this point during embryological development that other intersex conditions may also occur. It is probable that gonadal agenesis occurs at this early stage, leading to the same features as Swyer's syndrome although with the absence of any gonadal tissue (Mendonca et al., 1994). At this point also, atypical cell lines in the gonad, for example 45,X cell lines, may lead to abnormal testicular development in one or both gonads. In mosaic Turner's syndrome,

some XY cells in the streak gonad, composed predominantly of 45,X cells, can lead to an increased incidence of gonadal malignancy (Canto et al., 2000). Mixed gonadal dysgenesis has a mosaic 45,X/46,XY karyotype but is without the somatic features of Turner's syndrome. In this condition, the gonads can be a unilateral streak or dysgenetic testis with a structurally normal testis on the other side, or bilateral dysgenetic testes. The term "dysgenetic testis" means that the testis is abnormal in its structural components and has poor function, i.e. fails to produce adequate testosterone levels for normal sexual development. Subsequent development depends on testicular function, with those individuals that have poor testosterone production often having ambiguous genitalia with full or partial uterine development, depending on local AMH concentrations at the Müllerian duct (Berkovitz and Seeherunvong, 1998). In prenatally detected mosaic 45,X/46,XY fetuses, the majority (95%) are born with normal male genitalia, although with a high risk of gonadal dysgenesis (27%) (Chang et al., 1990). True hermaphroditism, the name given to a heterogeneous group of aetiologies that result in both testicular and ovarian determination in one individual, also has its origins at this stage in fetal development. In some cases, the karyotype is 46,XX/46,XY and the likelihood is that this is a chimera, an individual where two zygotes have fused to form one fetus with two distinct cell lines (Walker et al., 2000). Mosaicism and disruption in the genes controlling testicular and ovarian determination are also causes of true hermaphroditism (Slaney et al., 1998).

Errors in gonadal function

If normal testicular determination has been set in motion, Sertoli cells are the first to begin development and produce AMH, which promotes the local regression of Müllerian structures (uterus, Fallopian tubes and upper portion of the vagina). In the mixed gonadal structure conditions described above, the degree of Müllerian regression follows the quantity of AMH production from each gonad. In mixed gonadal dysgenesis with a unilateral testis, often a unicornuate uterus will have developed on the side of the dysgenetic gonad. Similarly, in true hermaphroditism, the extent and conformation of uterine and vaginal development is dependent on AMH production from both gonads.

Soon after Sertoli cell development, Leydig cells differentiate and start to secrete testosterone at 8 weeks, probably as a result of stimulation by placental chorionic gonadotrophin (hCG) (Rey and Picard, 1998). In the second and third trimesters, stimulation of Leydig cell testosterone production continues under the influence of fetally produced luteinizing hormone (LH). The circulating testosterone diffuses into cells of the Wolffian ducts and by binding to the androgen receptor causes development of the Wolffian structures (the vas deferens, seminal vesicles and epididymis); however, in other tissues testosterone has to undergo conversion in order to exert its androgenic effects. In the brain, testosterone is aromatized to to 17β-oestradiol and binds to oestradiol receptors to produce male-type CNS organisation, which is believed to lead to typical male behaviours after birth. At the external genitalia and prostate, intracellular conversion of testosterone

to dihydrotestosterone (DHT) by the enzyme 5α-reductase is necessary for male development (Imperato-McGinley, 1994). The intersex condition 5α-reductase deficiency results from reduced or absent function of this enzyme, leading to ambiguous genitalia at birth (Zhu et al., 1998).

A complete failure of the testes to produce testosterone will result in a switch to the female development pathway, although normal Sertoli cell function with AMH production will eliminate any Müllerian structures. Partial testosterone production will result in lower levels of testosterone available at the target tissues for conversion to DHT, and so the genital development will be ambiguous. In Leydig cell hypoplasia (also called Leydig cell agenesis), a failure of the Leydig cell response to hCG leads to either partial or complete absence of Leydig cell differentiation and correspondingly low or absent levels of testosterone production. The phenotypic spectrum of the condition is from normal female genitalia through to male genitalia with micropenis and primary hypogonadism. This condition has been shown in some affected families to result from mutations in the gene for the LH receptor (Stavrou et al., 1998), although in others the molecular cause remains elusive (Zenteno et al., 1999).

The pathway of steroid hormone biosynthesis in the Leydig cell, from cholesterol to testosterone, requires various proteins and enzymes to function correctly (Fig. 22.2) (Rumsby, 1997). The first step in this process, cholesterol movement to the inner mitochondrial membrane, requires the StAR (steroid acute regulatory) protein. Genetic mutations in the gene encoding StAR cause congenital lipoid adrenal hypoplasia, a condition with severe impairment of both adrenal and gonadal steroid hormone biosynthesis, and consequent female external genitalia in XY fetuses associated with mineralocorticoid and glucocorticoid deficiency (Bose et al., 1996). Mutations in the cholesterol side-chain cleavage enzyme (also called P450scc) have previously been thought to be lethal early in gestation, however, recently a mutation has been discovered in an XY female subject with adrenal insufficiency (Tajima et al., 2001). The next two enzymatic steps in the pathway, 17α-hydroxylase and 17,20-lyase, are both performed by the same enzyme (also called P450c17 or CYP17). These two steps are also required for adrenal cortisol synthesis, and so 17α-hydroxylase deficiency and 17,20-lyase deficiency (which usually occur together; Yanase, 1995) result in an intersex condition associated with adrenal hyperplasia and later hypertension (Geller et al., 1997). The other enzyme in this pathway required for both adrenal and gonadal steroid hormone biosynthesis is 3β-hydroxysteroid dehydrogenase type II. Deficiency of this enzyme leads to a severe type of congenital adrenal hyperplasia with salt wasting

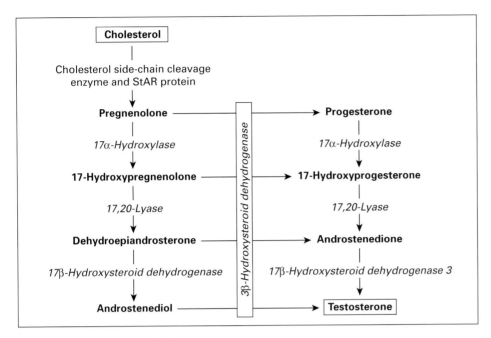

Fig. 22.2. Testosterone biosynthesis.

and variable ambiguity of the external genitalia in XY individuals (Pang, 2001). The last enzyme required to produce testosterone in the testis is 17β-hydroxysteroid dehydrogenase (17β-HSD, see below). This enzyme is not required for adrenal hormone biosynthesis, and so a deficiency results in variable genital ambiguity at birth with absent Müllerian structures (Boehmer et al., 1999; Zhu et al., 1998).

At this point in sexual development, if any genetic or environmental influence acts to destroy testicular structure or function completely, resulting in loss of both testes, then an intersex condition may occur. As the testes have already functioned, the condition is called embryonic testicular regression syndrome, and some degree of genital virilization and/or Müllerian duct regression would be expected depending on the timing of the loss of function (Josso and Briard, 1980; Marcantonio et al., 1994).

End-organ insensitivity to androgens

The final requirement for successful completion of male sexual differentiation is that the target cells are capable of fully responding to androgens, permitting growth of the genital tubercle, genital swellings and urethral fold to form the glans penis, scrotum, urethral tube and shaft of the penis, respectively. Complete loss of androgen receptor function, either through disruption of the androgen receptor structure (Ahmed et al., 2000) or its associated receptor elements (Adachi et al., 2000), results in complete androgen insensitivity syndrome (CAIS). If some receptor function

can occur, the genital appearance will vary from ambiguous to nearly male, and the designation is partial androgen insensitivity syndrome (PAIS) (Quigley et al., 1995).

Miscellaneous conditions

At these end stages of fetal sexual differentiation, other conditions may occur, for example micropenis (Ludwig, 1999) and penile agenesis (Oesch et al., 1987), for which we currently have little evidence of aetiology. Developmental disorders of the cloaca, such as cloacal exstrophy and bladder exstrophy, can also result in disruption to external genital development. There are also the rare cases of traumatic loss of the penis in neonatal or infant life (Bradley et al., 1998). In the past, children with these conditions were often reassigned to a female sex of rearing as penile reconstruction surgery was felt to be less successful than feminizing genital surgery (Duckett and Baskin, 1993). However this management is now being reevaluated and there are serious concerns over the long-term outcomes of infant sex reassignment in these conditions (Calikoglu, 1999; Reilly and Woodhouse, 1989).

Ethical considerations and general issues in the management of intersex conditions

Intersex states have both fascinated and disturbed humanity throughout history. While some cultures have revered their intersex members, many more have stigmatized or even, like the Romans, eliminated those displaying intersex features (Keller, 1940). Throughout the latter half of the twentieth century, medical practice has chosen hormonal drugs and surgery to try and relieve intersex features, in an attempt to normalize these conditions back into the standard category of male or female that society accepts (Donahoe, 1987; Duckett and Baskin, 1993; Rosenfield et al., 1980). The results of this management have remained largely unquantified (Creighton and Minto, 2001) and are now being contested (Chase, 1998) and reexamined at many levels (Creighton et al., 2001; Dreger, 1998; Schober, 1998). While the pathways of sexual differentiation and determination lead to an understanding of the basic aetiology behind many intersex conditions, what remains poorly understood is the variation in both physical and psychological development for many intersex conditions.

One problem remains the poor understanding of how an individual's adult sexual identity and gender develops (Zucker, 1999). Is biology an overriding factor with most aspects of future gender already imprinted at birth by the fetal hormone environment (Diamond et al., 1996)? Or is gender malleable and heavily influenced by postnatal events, for example the genital appearance or the sex-of-rearing assigned in infancy and reinforced by parental and societal attitudes (Money, 1985)? The truth probably lies somewhere between these two extremes; however, these fundamental questions over human development remain debated (Diamond and Sigmundson, 1997; Dreger, 1998), and correspondingly the management of intersex conditions remains imperfect.

Currently, for many intersex infants presenting with ambiguous genitalia, despite state-of-the-art genetic tests and innovative surgical techniques, clinicians remain unable to answer accurately such vital questions as what gender will this child choose to live as in the future or what is the potential growth of this phallus?

Academic debates also question whether intersex conditions are truly birth defects that need correction and dispute the practice of childhood surgery to normalize genitalia on both an ethical and evidence-based rationale (Diamond and Sigmundson, 1997). Other controversies have centred on the amount of information given to individuals about their intersex condition. Until relatively recently, it was accepted practice for clinicians to mislead both parents and patients about these conditions, based on the assumption that knowing the reality of these conditions would be psychologically disastrous (Edmonds, 1989). These policies of secrecy and deception over intersex diagnoses, reinforced by societies' ignorance of these conditions and general taboos over sexual issues, has led

to many adult patients being unaware of their true condition. The ethics and long-term effects of these policies of nondisclosure are discussed in more depth in other chapters, and most clinicians now agree that withholding the diagnosis is both ethically wrong and detrimental for patients, and practise full disclosure in a supported environment. However, this previous withholding of information on intersex conditions has inevitably hampered data collection on the various long-term outcomes of clinical interventions, and we are left with only biased cohort evaluation, case reports and clinical experience to guide current management. While we await more robust evidence, clinicians must remain open-minded and impartial, presenting all the management options to their patients in a nonpaternalistic manner.

Gonadectomy

For the majority of conditions discussed in this chapter, gonadectomy will be advised, often at an early age. While gonadectomy is indicated in conditions with dysgenetic gonads because of the high risk of gonadal malignancy, and in conditions such as PAIS where the patient will be raised female (where the aim is to avoid irreversible virilization around puberty), the indications for early gonadectomy in other conditions such as CAIS are not so clear. Once gonadectomy has been performed, hormone replacement therapy is advised because of the health risks involved in becoming deficient in sex steroids at a young age. As this hormone replacement therapy will need to be taken for several decades and will have both benefits and risks this information needs discussion. In the past, some patients have not been fully informed as to the reasons for their gonadectomy, or the true nature of their gonadal tissue. Without this type of information, true informed consent for gonadectomy is impossible. Just as in any other medical condition, patients have the right to decide their own management and it is important to provide accurate estimates on malignant risk, along with information on both the condition and the gonadal type, so that patients can make fully informed decisions. During gonadectomy in CAIS, 5α-reductase deficiency and 17β-hydroxysteroid dehydrogenase deficiency, essentially normal testicular tissue that may include germ cells, is being removed. In these cases consideration should be given to the future fertility options of these patients, and cryopreservation of gonadal tissue may be appropriate.

Multidisciplinary intersex clinics

Every intersex person, or family, should be referred to an expert multidisciplinary clinical team. Proper investigation

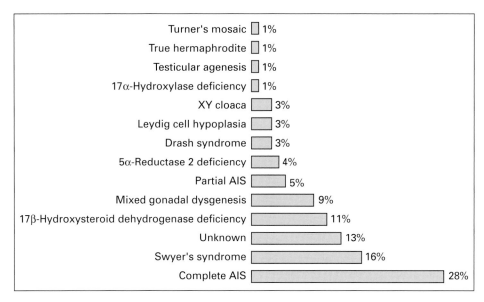

Fig. 22.3. An audit of the range of diagnoses in XY female intersex patients ($n = 47$) seen in a specialist adult intersex clinic. (NB: This may not accurately reflect the prevalence of each condition in the UK population due to referral bias.) AIS, androgen insensitivity syndrome. (Minto et al., 2003a.)

and accurate diagnosis are important and can be complex. In some cases, the aetiology of the intersex state will not be accurately determined because of limitations in our current knowledge; however, the misdiagnosis of conditions will be limited by referral to an expert centre. Full information on the intersex condition should be available, and information should be communicated in a supportive environment with the expertise of a clinical psychologist, who is an integral part of the expert intersex team. Clinical psychological support should also be available in an ongoing manner, as the psychological aspects of living with an intersex condition can impact in many areas of life, including personal relationships, sexual function and self-esteem. Literature on the available national support groups should be provided (The Androgen Insensitivity Support Group, http://www.medhelp.org/www/ais/) and contact with other affected individuals or families offered. Where an inherited condition is diagnosed, genetic counselling for the relevant family members should be available. Any surgery offered, including vaginoplasty, clitoral surgery and gonadectomy, should be presented with full information on both the potential benefits and the risks of the procedure.

The range of conditions and accurate diagnosis

With increased understanding of the control of gonadal differentiation and steroid hormone production, greater accuracy is now possible in determining the diagnoses of intersex conditions. Previously, the majority of XY females

presenting with primary amenorrhoea were assigned a diagnosis of CAIS. However, while this remains the commonest XY female condition (Fig. 22.3), inadequate investigation of these complex conditions can often lead to misdiagnosis and inappropriate management. Ongoing review of the diagnosis is important, especially for adolescents or adults where the diagnosis was made in childhood. In one recent nationwide study in the Netherlands where the diagnoses of 49 patients with an assigned diagnosis of AIS were reviewed, the diagnosis was changed in 35% (Boehmer et al., 2001).

Complete androgen insensitivity syndrome (see Ch. 20)

Morris originally called CAIS testicular feminization in 1953. He characterized the condition and postulated, wrongly, that the testes in these women produced a feminizing factor (Morris, 1953). The condition actually occurs because the body is unable to respond to androgens; consequently, for many years now "androgen insensitivity syndrome" has replaced "testicular feminization" as a more accurate term. In the complete form, the androgen receptor does not function, hence despite high testosterone production from the testes, no masculinizing effects will be seen. In the majority of cases the condition is caused by a mutation in the gene for the androgen receptor, located at Xq11-12, leading to the inability of androgen to bind to the androgen receptor; alternatively it can be caused

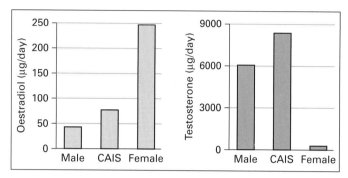

Fig. 22.4. Comparison of mean population sex steroid levels in males, females with complete androgen insensitivity syndrome (CAIS), and normal females in the luteal phase. (Adapted from Soule et al., 1995.)

by defective action of the receptor after androgen binding (Griffin, 1992). In two-thirds of those affected, the mutation is inherited from the mother, and the condition follows an X-linked recessive pattern. Carrier females are not expected to show any clinical effects, because the normal androgen receptor gene on their second X chromosome is functional; however, some carriers occasionally exhibit reduced amounts of pubic hair, presumably because of inactivation of their normal X chromosome in those cells (Griffin, 1992).

The incidence of CAIS varies according to the population studied, with estimates ranging from 1 in 40 800 (Bangsboll et al., 1992) to 1 in 120 000 (Quigley et al., 1995). Presentation is most often with primary amenorrhoea (around 45%) or an inguinal hernia (around 35%) in childhood (Rutgers and Scully, 1991). A minority is diagnosed through family screening or prenatal discordance between ultrasound determined sex and karyotype, or some may present with sexual problems, postcoital vaginal tears, a pelvic mass or infertility. Because of the complete insensitivity of the body to androgens, women with CAIS have a normal female appearance and normal female gender development; other features are:

- female external genitalia
- XY karyotype
- minimal or absent pubic and axillary hair
- absent uterus and Fallopian tubes
- bilateral intraabdominal or inguinal testes
- normal breast development
- high levels of endogenous testosterone production
- hypoplastic or absent Wolffian structures.

Many of those affected are said to be taller than average for a female. Clinical features developing at puberty, such as hirsutism, clitoromegaly and full axillary or pubic hair growth, rule out the diagnosis of CAIS. In rare families,

both PAIS and CAIS can result from the same androgen receptor gene mutation. Endocrine investigation will show high serum testosterone concentrations, and oestradiol concentrations lower than the female population range but usually higher than the male range (Fig. 22.4) (MacDonald et al., 1979). These oestradiol levels are produced both by the testes directly and by peripheral aromatization of testosterone, and they ensure adequate breast development at puberty. In many cases, breast development in CAIS is thought to be greater than average, probably because of a lack of testosterone inhibition on breast growth. Follicle-stimulating hormone (FSH) levels are usually normal or slightly raised. LH levels are elevated, reflecting the lack of recognition of testosterone feedback at the hypothalamus and pituitary, and the continued drive by LH to the testes to produce testosterone. In prepubertal children with CAIS, the testosterone and gonadotrophin levels are often within the normal range.

Both Müllerian and Wolffian structures are usually absent in CAIS but can sometimes remain as rudimentary structures. These can occasionally cause cystic paragonadal masses. In one study of 40 patients with CAIS, 35% had at least one Fallopian tube and 18% had a rudimentary midline uterus (Rutgers and Scully, 1991). No individuals with CAIS have been reported with a functional uterus. Vaginal development is also variable, with many of those with CAIS reported as having vaginal hypoplasia. The vagina is thought to be composed of a urogenital portion and a Müllerian portion. As the testes in a fetus with CAIS are thought to produce normal amounts of AMH, the Müllerian portion of the vagina should regress, leaving a shortened vagina without a cervix at the vault. The normal range of vaginal lengths in the general population have been reported as 11.1 ± 1.0 cm (Weber et al., 1995) and lengths in CAIS have been reported from 2 to 11 cm. The external genital appearance is normal, although sometimes the clitoris and labia are said to be small. Pubic hair can be variable but is markedly reduced in comparison with the general population, and usually Tanner grade 1 or 2 in quantity and distribution. The majority of hairs are fine vellus hairs rather than thickened sexual-type hairs.

The testes in CAIS are often intra-abdominal; however, up to 20% may be inguinal or occasionally found in the labia (Rutgers and Scully, 1991). Germ cells are thought to be progressively lost with age, falling from normal levels at aged 5 years to less than 30% of testes having scattered spermatogonia in adult life (Rutgers and Scully, 1991). Testicular pathology shows Leydig cell hyperplasia in the majority, with haematomatous nodules and Sertoli cell adenomas in some (Rutgers and Scully, 1991). The lifetime risk of malignant testicular tumours in CAIS has been reported as being 2–9% (Manuel et al., 1976; Rutgers and Scully, 1991). Malignant tumours are mainly seminomas (germ cell tumours) but more rarely Sertoli cell or Leydig cell tumours have been reported. The majority of gonadal malignancy occurs in those over the age of 50 years; however, a malignant tumour has been reported in a 14-year-old child (Hurt et al., 1989). The risk of gonadal malignancy is low prior to puberty, with cumulative risk estimated as <1% at 12 years, 2–5% from 20 to 30 years, rising to 30% at 50 years (Manuel et al., 1976; Rutgers and Scully, 1991; Verp and Simpson, 1987).

Clinical management

The psychological aspects of living with CAIS are covered in more detail in other chapters and are of paramount importance in clinical management. Psychological reactions to being diagnosed with CAIS have not been subjected to much research; however, recent work has shown that the initial reactions of anger, shock, grief and shame can be strong and persist for many years, in both parents and affected individuals. In one study of 10 adult women with CAIS, 90% still had feelings of shame an average of 26.5 years after learning of their diagnosis (Slijper et al., 2000). The XY karyotype may be difficult to come to terms with and may lead to a negative self-image. Other difficulties arise when passing through puberty, when some girls will feel isolated from peers because of their primary amenorrhoea, and unhappy with their lack of pubic hair. These reactions may affect social behaviour, formation of close relationships and sexual function. Long-term psychological support must, therefore, be available for affected children and their parents, for adolescents, and for adults.

Osteopenia (low bone mineral density) and osteoporosis are often seen in CAIS. It is well known that oestrogens are required for bone mineral density acquisition and maintenance; however, the role of androgens is less clearly understood. The confounding factor of oestrogen deficiency in some subjects with CAIS, owing to prepubertal gonadectomy associated with reduced amount of hormone replacement therapy, leads to problems in elucidating the role of androgens in acquiring bone mass (Soule et al., 1995). A recent study of 22 women with CAIS has shown that even with excellent compliance with oestrogen replacement therapy, lumbar spine bone mineral density is a mean 1 standard deviation from the population normal range (Marcus et al., 2000). Consequently, clinical management of CAIS should include appropriate screening of bone mineral density.

Timing of gonadectomy has been a controversial management issue in CAIS for many years. The indications for gonadectomy are the risk of malignant change in the testes and the possible discomfort from inguinal or labial testes. Location of the testes should be confirmed prior to surgery, by suitable imaging studies, and most intra-abdominal testes should be removed laparoscopically. In prepubertally diagnosed patients, some clinicians believe that gonadectomy should be performed as soon as the diagnosis is made (Batch et al., 1992), often at the time of an inguinal hernia repair. However, the risk of malignancy in childhood and adolescence is small, and the testes in CAIS are normally functioning endocrine organs producing adequate oestrogen levels for breast growth and other oestrogen-mediated pubertal events. Gonadectomy at this time prevents fully informed consent from the patient. It also necessitates hormone replacement treatment throughout adolescence, a possible time of poor compliance, and requires hospital attendances for monitoring of growth. Additionally, the acquisition of bone mass throughout puberty might be deficient in CAIS relative to other females, and it has been suggested that conventional oestrogen replacement regimens after prepubertal gonadectomy may be insufficient to maximize the gain in adolescent bone mass (Marcus et al., 2000). Other clinicians believe that the testes should be preserved through puberty to allow natural feminization, and then a gonadectomy performed postpubertally (Quint and Strickland, 2001). Critics of this management argue that it might be psychologically better for the gonadectomy to be performed in childhood rather than in adolescence, which might be a difficult time for a girl to come to terms with the information that she has internal testes (Batch et al., 1992). They also argue that delayed gonadectomy risks the development of a gonadal malignancy, with the youngest reported case in CAIS at 14 years (Hurt et al., 1989), and is unnecessary because of the availability of hormone replacement treatment.

If gonadectomy has been performed, hormone replacement therapy is required for general health and well-being, and for maintenance of bone density. This therapy is not thought to need a progestogen component because of the absence of a uterus, and it is generally given on a continuous basis. Most clinicians prescribe oestrogens because of sporadic reports of benefit from some CAIS individuals; a few women prefer to mimic their previous endogenous hormone environment prior to gonadectomy by taking parenteral high-dose testosterone replacement.

Another major consideration in the management of CAIS is vaginal hypoplasia, and the possible effect that this can have on sexual function. A recent study has shown a high prevalence of sexual dysfunction in CAIS (Minto et al., 2003a). Both psychological factors (e.g. negative self-perceptions of genital normality) and physical factors (e.g. vaginal hypoplasia) are thought to be predisposing factors.

In the same study, examination of a group of 20 women with CAIS detailed a mean vaginal length of 8.4 cm (range 6–11 cm) but all had previously undergone treatment for vaginal hypoplasia or were sexually active (Minto et al., 2003a). The range of vaginal length prior to intervention or sexual activity in CAIS remains unknown. Indications for treatment of vaginal hypoplasia are prevention of vaginal mucosa laceration, and associated haemorrhage, and improvement of sexual function. At present, there have been no prospective studies of the impact of vaginal hypoplasia interventions on sexual function in CAIS. Retrospective studies with unobjective assessments of sexual function in small samples have shown a benefit (Costa et al., 1997). Options for treatment of vaginal hypoplasia are self-dilatation therapy or surgical vaginoplasty. Concomitant psychological support is likely to improve outcomes. Prior to sexual activity, a thorough genital examination by an experienced gynaecologist, sometimes performed under anaesthetic, will provide an estimate of vaginal size and configuration. This allows vaginal hypoplasia interventions to be considered and is also an opportunity for reassurance on other aspects of genital appearance. The first-line treatment in most should be vaginal dilators, where an individual creates or lengthens the vagina with pressure (Ch. 13). Available studies claim anatomical success rates of dilatation therapy in the region of 80%, although they do not consider compliance or sexual function (Ingram, 1981). Dilators of various types have been used, and the most commonly used today are plastic dilators in a range of widths and lengths (see Fig. 13.1, p. 148). Treatment regimens vary but the schedule usually involves daily or tri-weekly sessions, of 15–30 minutes' duration, where the dilator is used to exert sustained pressure to the vaginal vault (see Ch. 13). The vaginal mucosa usually stretches, and the vaginal length is increased as new mucosal cells grow. Advantages of the method are the absence of surgical risk and fibrotic scar tissue, and the psychological advantage of the subject being in control and enlarging her own vagina. The disadvantages are the commitment and time taken to achieve a result, and the distaste that some patients feel towards dilatation.

Surgical vaginoplasty is usually reserved for those choosing not to use dilators or those unable to achieve adequate vaginal length with dilator treatment. There are many options of surgical vaginoplasty (Table 22.2), and the vast array of techniques attests to the lack of a single procedure with definably superior results. Outcome studies are scarce and most series in the literature are by a proponent of a certain technique reviewing the outcome of their series of cases, and concentrating mainly on surgical techniques and immediate postoperative outcome. There are very few adult sexual function outcome data, or information on

Table 22.2. Commoner vaginoplasty methods

Type	Description
Bowel	A pouch of ileum or colon with an intact vascular supply is brought down to a dissected space on the perineum
Skin graft	A split-thickness skin graft is laid into a dissected space in the perineum
Peritoneum	Peritoneum is brought down into a dissected space in the perineum
Vecchietti	Via a laparoscopic procedure, the vaginal vault is attached to a tension device on the lower abdominal wall and daily increases of tension lead to rapid stretching of the vagina from a small dimple to a larger vagina
Amnion	Amnion is laid as a graft material into a dissected space in the perineum
Williams	The labia majora are sutured to form an external pouch; no deep dissection is required

adjunctive therapies used with surgery such as oestrogen cream or vaginal dilators.

Apart from osteoporosis, there are currently no other long-term health concerns recognized in CAIS. There has been the suggestion of a theoretical increased risk of breast cancer in CAIS, as tumour formation is thought to be increased with increased oestrogenic and decreased androgenic stimulation (Ahmed et al., 2000). Currently, there have been no reports of breast cancer in CAIS, and so this risk remains unquantified. Both carrier detection and prenatal testing for CAIS may be available for some families, mainly where the androgen receptor mutation has been identified in the index case.

Partial androgen insensitivity syndrome

PAIS is less clearly defined than CAIS, and represents a more heterogeneous group, ranging from a predominantly female genital appearance to normal male genital appearance with associated lack of spermatogenesis (Table 22.3) (Quigley et al., 1995). Diagnosis can be complex and requires the exclusion of testosterone biosynthesis defects and 5α-reductase deficiency. The basic defect is thought to lie at the level of the androgen receptor, with partial function available. However, in contrast to CAIS, less than one-third of subjects with a clinical diagnosis of PAIS are currently found to have an androgen receptor mutation (Ahmed et al., 2000). Within families with PAIS that have an identified androgen receptor mutation, phenotype can vary widely, illustrating the current lack of ability to predict phenotype from genetic studies.

Table 22.3. Classifications of androgen insensitivity syndrome[a]

Authors	Types described									
Sinnecker et al. (1997)	Type 1		Type 2		Type 3	Type 4		Type 5		
	Normal male genitalia		Male-type genitalia		Ambiguous genitalia: phallus, genital folds, urogenital sinus or perineal hypospadias	Female-type genitalia		Normal female genitalia		
	Type 1a Defect in spermatogenesis	Type 1b 1a and/or defect in pubertal virilization	Type 2a Isolated hypospadias	Type 2b Micropenis, severe hypospadias and bifid scrotum		Type 4a Clitoromegaly, partial labial fusion, urogenital sinus	Type 4b Mild clitoromegaly, partial labial fusion, vaginal and urethral perineal openings	Type 5a Development of some sexual-type pubic hair at puberty	Type 5b No sexual-type pubic or axillary hair at puberty	
Quigley et al. (1995)	Type 1	Type 2	Type 3		Type 4	Type 5		Type 6	Type 7	
	Normal male genitalia	Mild abnormality in male genitalia (e.g. isolated hypospadias)	More severe abnormality in male genital appearance: micropenis, perineal hypospadias, bifid scrotum, undescended testes		phallus, genital folds, urogenital sinus	Severe abnormality in female genitalia: posterior labial fusion, urethral and vaginal perineal openings and clitoromegaly		Normal female genitalia, with variable amount of sexual-type pubic hair at puberty	Normal female genitalia with absence of sexual-type pubic hair at puberty	
Shkolney et al. (1999)	MAIS					PAIS		CAIS		
	Male external genitalia; may have gynaecomastia, high-pitched voice, reduced pubic hair and/or impaired spermatogenesis					Variable degree of ambiguity of external genitalia		Completely female external genitalia		

[a]The vertical alignment indicates the overlap between the divisions into subtypes by various authors.

Various classification systems have been devised for PAIS (Table 22.3), and presentation will usually vary according to the degree of androgen insensitivity. Those presenting with genital ambiguity (Quigley types 3 to 5) should be identified at birth as intersex and undergo appropriate investigations. Others with mild clitoromegaly or labial fusion may be missed at birth and will usually present with primary amenorrhoea and virilizing signs at puberty. Endocrine investigations will show similar findings to CAIS, with normal or raised male-range levels of testosterone and oestrogens and usually raised LH levels (Quigley et al., 1995). A variable degree of Wolffian duct development is seen.

Sex of rearing and surgical intervention in management of PAIS

Infant sex of rearing assignment is controversial in PAIS, with very few published outcomes of adult gender identity. One recent study has shown a problem with female gender development in 43% (three out of seven) of infants with PAIS reared as female (Sinnecker et al., 1997). Previous studies, promoting the importance of early genital surgery in stabilizing gender development, showed that of 32 XY intersex infants raised female, 9 of 23 (39%) requested reassignment

to male in adult life (Money et al., 1986). The difficulty with interpretation of these studies is the variety of factors possibly impacting on gender development, ascertainment bias (six subjects in the latter study were specifically referred with gender identity problems) and the lack of a definitive diagnosis available in most cases recorded as "PAIS". While more outcome data are eagerly awaited, in neonates diagnosed with PAIS the sex of rearing decision for parents and clinicians is extremely difficult. Because it is impossible to predict how a phallus will respond to pubertal testosterone treatment, and with the likely diagnosis of PAIS, many clinicians currently will advise a female sex of rearing for those with Quigley types 3 to 6 (Table 22.3).

If a decision to rear as female has been made, the next dilemma involves surgical intervention. Both gonadectomy and feminizing genitoplasty need to be considered; however, the indications for each are different. Gonadectomy is usually advised to prevent inappropriate production of gonadal androgens in a child that is being raised female. Androgenic effects in the body, for example deepening of the voice and male hair distribution, can be irreversible. Other indications for gonadectomy in PAIS are the possible discomfort of inguinal or labial testes, the abnormal cosmetic appearance of labial gonads in a female and the risk of testicular malignancy. The position of the testes will vary, but proportionately more testes would be expected to have descended to the inguinal ring or labia, with the increased androgen stimulation, compared with the situation in CAIS. As in CAIS, accurate localization of gonads by examination and appropriate imaging studies is essential to plan the surgical approach if gonadectomy is chosen. The risk of malignant change in the testes in PAIS is largely unknown, and as in CAIS may be related to the abnormal position of the gonads or to other differences in the testes. Studies of small samples of PAIS subjects have suggested a similar malignancy risk as CAIS with the incidence of tumours thought to be low prior to 20 years of age (approximately 3%) rising to 46% after the age of 40 years (Manuel et al., 1976). A more recent study has shown a high rate of intratubular germ cell neoplasia (a form of carcinoma in situ) in 73% (8 out of 11) of cases of PAIS studied, 62.5% of whom were prepubertal (Cassio et al., 1990). Studies of malignancy risk in intersex conditions from review of published cases are often open to ascertainment bias, and usually of small sample size; consequently, accurate figures for malignancy risks remain unknown.

Cosmetic surgery to make the genital area look more feminine was historically performed to stabilize gender and psychosexual development (Hampson, 1955); however, there is currently no evidence to show that either adult gender identity or psychosexual development have any association with childhood genital appearance. Studies that have looked at intersex adults who grew up without feminizing surgery, that is with genitalia that were either ambiguous in appearance or opposite to their sex of rearing, suggest that adult gender identity development is independent of genital appearance, and that the sex of rearing has more impact (Ellis, 1945; Money et al., 1955). Currently most clinicians consider that childhood genital surgery is indicated in those with a higher degree of genital ambiguity to avoid the assumed psychological distress of passing through childhood and adolescence with abnormal-looking genitalia. The evidence that feminizing surgery will improve psychological outcomes is lacking, with dismally few adult outcome studies in intersex conditions available (Creighton and Minto, 2001).

There are also risks and potential negative outcomes associated with surgery, and it is imperative that these are openly discussed with parents and patients, along with the potential benefits of surgery (Table 22.4). The most obvious risk of surgery is that both gonadectomy and feminizing genitoplasty are irreversible, and both will remove tissue that is potentially precious to the patient in the future, especially if a male gender identity develops. Other risks relate to cosmetic results, stenosis and scar tissue formation, and the possibility of damaged adult sexual function. Currently,

Table 22.4. Risks and benefits of feminizing surgery in intersex

Benefits	Risks
Stability in gender development	Damage to sexual function
Prevention of psychological distress from ambiguous genital appearance	Creation of psychological distress from undergoing childhood hospitalization, surgery and genital examination; possible lack of control over or consent for surgical interventions and stigmatization and isolation of the child
	Surgical complications: urinary tract dysfunction, malignancy in graft material, vaginal discharge from graft material
Good cosmetic outcomes	Poor cosmetic outcomes
Gender development in accordance with assigned sex of rearing	Gender development not concordant with sex of rearing, and irreversible surgery has been performed
Relief of parental anxiety	Damage to parent–child relationship
Stability in psychosexual development	Instability in psychosexual development
Vaginal introitus for adult penetrative sexual intercourse	Stenotic or fibrosed vaginal introitus causing dyspareunia
Vaginal passage for menstrual flow	Obstruction to menstrual flow from postsurgical scarring and fibrosis

there are few outcome data on any of these risks, although recent work has shown that adults who underwent clitoral surgery have a higher incidence of orgasmic dysfunction than those who did not (Minto et al., 2003b). Currently for adolescents and adults with clitoromegaly considering clitoral reduction surgery for dissatisfaction with cosmetic appearance, sexual dysfunction, or socially distressing erections, the surgical risk of damage to clitoral sensation and future orgasmic capacity is estimated at 25% (Minto et al., 2003b).

Many of those with PAIS will have no vaginal introitus, or a vagina of only a few centimetres depth. Generally, vaginoplasty is now avoided in childhood, because of the risks of surgery and the likely lack of relevance of a vaginal introitus in gender, psychosexual and general social development throughout childhood. A genital examination, often under anaesthetic, is usually performed at an appropriate time for the patient, usually after puberty, to determine vaginal, urethral and perineal structure and configuration. The options for enlarging or creating the vagina are essentially the same as in CAIS, although success with vaginal dilatation is usually difficult to achieve when the perineum is flat and without a vaginal dimple.

The psychological management of PAIS is as for other intersex conditions. Long-term health risks are largely unknown, although the osteopenia seen in CAIS seems to not be a feature of PAIS, presumably through partial androgen action on bone (Marcus et al., 2000). As for CAIS, there is a theoretically increased risk of breast cancer in PAIS, and two patients have been reported with breast cancer in PAIS associated with mutations in a specific region of the DNA-binding area of the androgen receptor gene (Ahmed et al., 2000).

Swyer's syndrome (complete or pure 46,XY gonadal dysgenesis)

In this condition, first described by Swyer in 1955, the gonad has undergone abnormal differentiation, culminating in bilateral dysgenetic streak gonads. The alternative titles of "complete" and "pure" 46,XY gonadal dysgenesis refer to the lack of any genital ambiguity or any features of Turner's syndrome, respectively. Histologically, the thin gonadal streaks are similar to those found in Turner's syndrome and are composed of ovarian-type stroma without any follicles. They do not produce AMH or steroid hormones during fetal or later life, and so the uterus and Fallopian tubes develop normally and the external genital appearance is female. Any signs of in utero androgen action on the genitalia, such as partial labial fusion or a urogenital sinus, exclude this diagnosis and suggest that the subject has partial gonadal dysgenesis or another intersex condition. At puberty, these streaks again fail to produce any sex steroid hormones, and the usual presentation is with primary amenorrhoea and lack of breast development, often with tall stature; other features include:
- female external genitalia
- XY karyotype
- normal Fallopian tubes and uterus (often described as small or infantile prior to oestrogenic hormone replacement therapy)
- bilateral intra-abdominal streak gonads
- delayed thelarche, or poor pubertal breast development
- normal pubic and axillary hair development at puberty
- low levels of oestrogen and high gonadotrophin levels
- absent Wolffian structures.

Pubic hair development is normal, and vaginal length is predicted to be within the normal range. Endocrine investigation will show low oestrogen and testosterone levels, with raised gonadotrophin levels.

Occasionally Swyer's syndrome has been reported occurring in families, either with other cases of Swyer's syndrome or with the partial form of gonadal dysgenesis, as an autosomal recessive trait; however, most cases are sporadic. Genetic analysis has shown that only approximately 20–30% of those affected have mutations or deletions of *SRY*, and it is assumed that the majority will have disruption of other genes important in controlling testis determination (Kwok et al., 1996). The streak gonads have a high risk of tumour formation, with the commonest being dysgerminomas and gonadoblastomas. The risk of malignancy has been estimated as 30–37.5%, and gonadoblastomas have been reported as early as 6 years of age (Dewhurst et al., 1971; Verp and Simpson, 1987). Malignant gonadal tumours are seen more frequently and at an earlier age in conditions with dysgenetic gonads compared with other intersex conditions, and gonadectomy is, therefore, recommended as soon as the diagnosis is made. Occasionally the clinical features of Swyer's syndrome can be distorted by the presence of an oestrogen-secreting tumour (e.g. gonadoblastoma) causing breast development.

Women with Swyer's syndrome have normal female gender identity development, and for the few cases diagnosed in infancy or childhood, there is no doubt over the appropriateness of a female sex of rearing. Clinical management includes starting hormone replacement therapy as soon as the diagnosis is confirmed. This therapy will need to have both oestrogen and progestogen components. The oestrogen should stimulate both uterine and breast growth, and the onset of menstruation. Fertility is possible with in vitro fertilization and donor oocytes. Often breast growth remains poor despite the oestrogen replacement and the option of breast augmentation surgery should be offered. The psychological aspects of living with Swyer's syndrome are similar in some respects to those of CAIS, although there is also the risk of poor body image because of the lack of breast development, which may additionally impact on both sexual function and quality of life. As in other intersex conditions, psychological support by an expert clinical psychologist is an integral part of treatment for many patients.

Other forms of XY gonadal dysgenesis

The term "dysgenetic" means that the gonad is both abnormal in its structural components and has poor function, and this definition encompasses both streak gonads and gonads that look more like testes but fail to function sufficiently to complete male sexual differentiation. All of these conditions have a similar gonadal malignancy risk to that seen in Swyer's syndrome, and either gonadectomy or surveillance of preserved gonadal tissue is essential. The majority will present with genital ambiguity in infancy, and decisions on the appropriate sex of rearing can be difficult and depend on various features in each individual. The issues surrounding cosmetic genital surgery are the same as those discussed above in PAIS. Pubertal change, in the absence of gonadectomy, is usually virilization, and breast development would raise the concern of an oestrogen-secreting tumour.

Partial gonadal dysgenesis

In partial gonadal dysgenesis, also called dysgenetic male pseudohermaphroditism, there is partial androgen secretion by dysgenetic testes or streak gonads. The karyotype is 46,XY, and genital appearance is usually ambiguous. The degree of internal Müllerian and Wolffian structure development depends on the quality of testicular function in intrauterine life. Aetiology in this condition remains largely unknown. A gonadoblastoma has been reported in an infant with partial gonadal dysgenesis at the age of 15 months (Berkovitz and Seeherunvong, 1998).

Mixed gonadal dysgenesis

In mixed gonadal dysgenesis, the karyotype is usually mosaic 45,X/46,XY. Gonadal structure is often a streak on one side with a contralateral testis. The development of internal and external genitalia reflects the gonadal function in utero and ranges from normal male external genitalia to ambiguous genital appearance.

Gonadal function depends on the structure of the gonads and, presumably, on the karyotype of cells within the gonad. Streak, dysgenetic or normal testicular tissue can develop. Some of the clinical features of Turner's syndrome, such as short stature, can be present. Malignant risk is increased, commonly gonadoblastoma.

True hermaphroditism

True hermaphroditism is defined as the presence, in one person, of both ovarian tissue with Graafian follicles and testicular tissue containing distinct tubules. The condition is not a discrete clinical entity, but rather a heterogeneous group of aetiologies that result in both testicular and ovarian determination in one individual. The gonads can be bilateral ovotestes, an ovotestis with a normal contralateral ovary or testis, or an ovary with a contralateral testis. Although rare in the UK, it forms a larger proportion of the

intersex cases in some African countries (Wiersma, 2001). The karyotype is variable; however, less than 30% of subjects with true hermaphroditism will have an XY karyotype or an XX/XY karyotype. It has been suggested that 46,XY true hermaphroditism and 46,XY partial gonadal dysgenesis may be different manifestations of the same condition, and that in the latter the gonads might be ovotestes in utero that cannot be sustained and degenerate into dysgenetic gonads or streaks. The risks of malignancy remain largely unknown, with estimates of between 5 and 10% (Verp and Simpson, 1987; Verp et al., 1992).

There is no consensus on the optimal sex of rearing in true hermaphroditism, and each case needs to be considered individually. There has been a report of a male true hermaphrodite fathering a child and several cases reported in the literature of women with true hermaphroditism achieving pregnancies (Krob et al., 1994).

Leydig cell hypoplasia

Leydig cell hypoplasia or agenesis is a rare condition with a wide clinical phenotype, ranging from normal female genitalia through to male genitalia with micropenis and primary hypogonadism. The main features of the condition are female or ambiguous genitalia in an XY individual. Investigation will show high LH levels associated with low testosterone levels that fail to rise with hCG stimulation. Gonadal histology will show absent or decreased numbers of Leydig cells. Müllerian structures will be absent, owing to normal fetal testicular AMH production, and Wolffian structures are usually present. The condition is thought to be caused by a defect in LH receptor function leading to a failure of Leydig cell differentiation and, therefore, a deficiency of fetal androgen production. Loss-of-function mutations within the LH receptor gene at 2p21 have now been found in some, but not all, with this condition, and the resulting phenotype is thought to be related to the completeness of loss of receptor function.

Where complete loss of receptor function has occurred, the clinical presentation is lack of breast development and primary amenorrhoea. As in CAIS, some degree of vaginal shortening is expected as a result of the action of AMH; in contrast to CAIS, pubic and axillary hair growth should be normal. The gonadal malignancy risk is unknown. For those with a complete type of receptor function loss it is predicted that adult gender identity will be female but there have been no formal studies to confirm this. In XX females with homozygous mutations in the LH receptor gene, genital appearance is normal, and breast development occurs at puberty; however, menstrual irregularity or amenorrhoea occur and are associated with infertility (Arnhold et al., 1999).

5α-Reductase deficiency

5α-Reductase deficiency is an autosomal recessive condition that has been extensively described in populations in the Dominican Republic (Imperato-McGinley et al., 1974) and Papua New Guinea (Herdt and Davidson, 1988) but is also seen in many other ethnic groups including African-American, Mexican, European, Middle Eastern and Turkish. The classic presentations are either at birth with ambiguous genitalia or later with an apparent change in appearance from female to male at puberty, with virilization, phallic growth and primary amenorrhoea. The condition is caused by a defect in the type 2 isoenzyme of 5α-reductase, and many defects in the gene at 2p23 have been found. Previously in the UK, management of cases diagnosed in infancy has been assignment to a female sex of rearing, with orchidectomy, feminizing genitoplasty and pubertal oestrogen therapy. However, practice varies worldwide and it may be that a male sex of rearing might be preferable in some cases.

The study of subjects with this condition has, like many other intersex conditions, been instrumental in increasing the understanding of sexual differentiation in humans. There are at least two isoenzymes of 5α-reductase, and it is the type 2 isoenzyme that is necessary for conversion of testosterone to DHT in the cells of the prostate and genital area during fetal development. Without the type 2 isoenzyme, the cells of the genital area and prostate fail to undergo male differentiation despite high circulating levels of testosterone, and the result is a predominantly female appearance at birth with rudimentary prostatic tissue. Intriguingly, Wolffian duct development seems only to require testosterone and so vas deferens, epididymis and seminal vesicles are normally developed in this condition. Other androgenic responses that do not require DHT will also occur in the fetus with 5α-reductase deficiency, such as aromatization of testosterone in brain cells to 17β-oestradiol, which may cause predetermination of male-type behaviour.

There is quite a range of phenotypic variation at birth in the condition, possibly reflecting different levels of enzyme function with specific mutations. At birth, the genital appearance is often clitoromegaly with labioscrotal folds and either a urogenital sinus or separate perineal vaginal and urethral openings: hence the old name of "pseudovaginal perineoscrotal hypospadias" (PPSH). However, some patients may have a more virilized genital appearance at birth,

with micropenis and penile hypospadias. The gonads are usually inguinal or labioscrotal, and descent occurs after puberty. Müllerian structures are absent and the vagina is predicted to be shortened as a result of the fetal testicular secretion of AMH. The diagnosis is made by examination of urinary steroid metabolites (low ratio of 5α to 5β reduced C19 steroids) and an increased plasma testosterone to DHT ratio. Plasma testosterone and gonadotrophin levels are normal or slightly raised.

At puberty – if gonadectomy has not been performed – body shape becomes more masculine, the voice deepens, spermatogenesis occurs and there is usually marked phallic growth to lengths of between 4 and 8 cm (Randall, 1994). It is not entirely clear why fetal virilization fails and yet pubertal virilization occurs in this condition. At puberty, there is increased genital expression of the weaker type 1 isoenzyme, which is not expressed in fetal life, and this may lead to DHT production. Alternatively, the high pubertal levels of testosterone may lead to sufficient androgen receptor activation in the genital cells. Other cells seem to remain dependent on metabolism of testosterone to DHT, and the prostate remains rudimentary, female pattern pubic hair occurs, and there are reduced amounts of body and facial hair. Adult gender and psychosexual outcomes are variable in the cases reported in the literature so far; many have developed male gender identities, and in those raised female there seems to be a greater chance of sex reassignment than in other intersex conditions (Imperato-McGinley, 1979; Canto et al., 1997). Several cases of paternity have now been reported in this condition (Katz et al., 1997); this, together with the available data on gender outcomes, seems to be growing evidence to consider male sex assignment for those diagnosed as neonates, irrespective of phallic size.

For female adolescents and adults with this condition, management is similar to PAIS and may include genital cosmetic procedures, interventions to enlarge the vagina and hormone replacement therapy. Expert clinical psychological management is especially important in 5α-reductase deficiency as the adult outcomes, in terms of adult gender identity, satisfaction with management, quality of life and sexual function, remain unknown. While a high incidence of gender identity problems might be expected, there have only been reports on small numbers of individuals with this condition in the literature, and it is important to take into account the potential publication bias of reporting the cases where a change of gender has occurred. Additionally, in the majority of cases reported where a male gender identity developed in adult life, the subjects had not undergone childhood gonadectomy and, therefore, were exposed to high levels of androgens at both the neonatal and pubertal gonadal androgen surges; this may alter gender outcomes.

17β-Hydroxysteroid dehydrogenase-3 deficiency

There are currently nine isolated human 17β-HSD enzymes (Adamski and Jakob, 2001) – also called 17-ketosteroid reductases. They regulate the bioavailability of sex steroid hormones in the body by catalysing the final step in the production of all androgens and oestrogens, the reduction of androstenedione to testosterone (Fig. 22.2). This step is vital for male sex determination in the fetus. A homozygous disruption of the gene for 17β-HSD-3, which is located on 9q22, leads to decreased or absent fetal testicular testosterone production. This autosomal recessive intersex condition has been described in detail in some inbred communities, such as an Arab community in Gaza where the incidence of 17β-HSD-3 deficiency approaches 1 in 200–300 births (Rosler et al., 1996).

Generally, the genital appearance at birth is female in appearance or mild clitoromegaly (Boehmer et al., 1999; Zhu et al., 1998). Occasionally, the appearance can be more typically male, with micropenis and labioscrotal folds. There seems to be wide phenotypic variation even within families with the same mutation, perhaps implying that there is wide variation in individual capacity for extragonadal testosterone formation. The karyotype is XY and there are normal but undescended testes. In the past, this condition was often misdiagnosed as CAIS in childhood; however, pubic hair growth should be normal and virilizing changes occur at puberty. As in 5α-reductase deficiency, it remains unclear how masculinizing effects occur at puberty when they have failed during fetal life. One theory is that other isoenzymes such as 17β-HSD-5 might lead to peripheral conversion to testosterone at puberty. Endocrine investigation will show a low testosterone to androstenedione ratio (< 0.8) that persists after hCG stimulation (Faisal et al., 2000). Such low ratios can also be seen in other causes of abnormal testicular function, but not in AIS. Müllerian structures are absent, although, surprisingly, Wolffian structures are normally formed, possibly because there is an alternative pathway for testosterone synthesis in the Wolffian ducts. Management is similar to that discussed for PAIS and 5α-reductase deficiency.

REFERENCES

Adachi M, Takayanagi R, Tomura A et al. (2000). Androgen-insensitivity syndrome as a possible coactivator disease. *N Engl J Med* 343, 856–862.

Adamski J, Jakob F J (2001). A guide to 17beta-hydroxysteroid dehydrogenases. *Mol Cell Endocrinol* 171, 1–4.

Ahmed S F, Cheng A, Dovey L et al. (2000). Phenotypic features, androgen receptor binding, and mutational analysis in 278 clinical cases reported as androgen insensitivity syndrome. *J Clin Endocrinol Metab* 85, 658–665.

Arnhold I J P, Latronico A C, Batista M C, Mendonca B B (1999). Menstrual disorders and infertility caused by inactivating mutations of the luteinising hormone receptor gene. *Fertil Steril* 71, 597–601.

Bangsboll S, Qvist I, Lebech P E, Lewinsky M (1992). Testicular feminization syndrome and associated gonadal tumours in Denmark. *Acta Obstet Gynecol Scand* 71, 63–66.

Barbaux S, Niaudet P, Gubler M C et al. (1997). Donor splice-site mutations in *WT1* are responsible for Frasier syndrome. *Nat Genet* 17(4), 467–470.

Batch J A, Patterson M N, Hughes I A (1992). Androgen insensitivity syndrome. *Reprod Med Rev* 1, 131–150.

Berkovitz G D, Seeherunvong T (1998). Abnormalities of gonadal differentiation. *Baillières Clin Endocrinol Metab* 12, 133–142.

Berta P, Hawkins J R, Sinclair A H et al. (1990). Genetic evidence equating SRY and the testis-determining factor. *Nature* 348, 448–450.

Blackless M, Charuvastra A, Derryck A, Fausto-Sterling A, Lauzanne K, Lee E (2000). How sexually dimorphic are we? Review and synthesis. *Am J Hum Biol* 12, 151–166.

Boehmer A L, Brinkmann A O, Sandkuijl L A et al. (1999). 17 Beta-hydroxysteroid dehydrogenase-3 deficiency: diagnosis, phenotypic variability, population genetics, and worldwide distribution of ancient and de novo mutations. *J Clin Endocrinol Metab* 84, 4713–4721.

Boehmer A L, Bruggenwirth H, van Assendelft C et al. (2001). Genotype versus phenotype in families with androgen insensitivity syndrome. *J Clin Endocrinol Metab* 86, 4151–4160.

Bose H S, Sugawara T, Strauss J F, III, Miller W L (1996). The pathophysiology and genetics of congenital lipoid adrenal hyperplasia. International Congenital Lipoid Adrenal Hyperplasia Consortium. *N Engl J Med* 335, 1870–1878.

Bradley S J, Oliver G D, Chernick A B, Zucker K J (1998). Experiment of nurture: ablatio penis at 2 months, sex reassignment at 7 months, and a psychosexual follow-up in young adulthood. *Pediatrics* 102, E9.

Calikoglu A S (1999). Should boys with micropenis be reared as girls? *J Pediatr* 134, 537–538.

Canto P, Vilchis F, Chavez B et al. (1997). Mutations of the 5 alpha-reductase type 2 gene in eight Mexican patients from six different pedigrees with 5 alpha-reductase-2 deficiency. *Clin Endocrinol* 46, 155–160.

Canto P, de la Chesnaye E, Lopez M et al. (2000). A mutation in the 5′ non-high mobility group box region of the SRY gene in patients with Turner syndrome and Y mosaicism. *J Clin Endocrinol Metab* 85, 1908–1911.

Cassio A, Cacciari E, D'Errico A et al. (1990). Incidence of intratubular germ cell neoplasia in androgen insensitivity syndrome. *Acta Endocrinol* 123, 416–422.

Chang H J, Clark R D, Bachman H (1990). The phenotype of 45,X/46,XY mosaicism: an analysis of 92 prenatally diagnosed cases. *Am J Hum Genet* 46, 156–167.

Chase C (1998). Surgical progress is not the answer to intersexuality. *J Clin Ethics* 9, 385–392.

Costa E M, Mendonca B B, Inacia M, Arnhold I J, Silva F A, Lodovici O (1997). Management of ambiguous genitalia in pseudohermaphrodites: new perspectives on vaginal dilation. *Fertil Steril* 67, 229–232.

Creighton S M, Minto C L (2001). Managing intersex. *Br Med J* 323, 1264–1265.

Creighton S M, Minto C L, Steele S J (2001). Objective cosmetic and anatomical outcomes at adolescence of feminising surgery for ambiguous genitalia done in childhood. *Lancet* 358, 124–125.

Dewhurst C J, Ferreira H P, Gillett P G (1971). Gonadal malignancy in XY females. *J Obstet Gynaecol Br Commonwealth* 78, 1077–1083.

Diamond M, Sigmundson H K (1997). Sex reassignment at birth. Long-term review and clinical implications. *Arch Pediatr Adolesc Med* 151, 298–304.

Diamond M, Binstock T, Kohl J V (1996). From fertilization to adult sexual behavior. *Horm Behav* 30, 333–353.

Donahoe P K (1987). The diagnosis and treatment of infants with intersex abnormalities. *Pediatr Clin North Am* 34, 1333–1348.

Dreger A D (1998). 'Ambiguous sex' – or ambivalent medicine? Ethical issues in the treatment of intersexuality. *Hastings Cent Rep* 28, 24–35.

Duckett J W, Baskin L S (1993). Genitoplasty for intersex anomalies. *Eur J Pediatr* 152(Suppl. 2), S80–S84.

Edmonds D K (1989). Intersexuality. In *Dewhurst's Practical Paediatric and Adolescent Gynaecology*, Edmonds D K, ed., pp. 6–26. Butterworths, London.

Ellis A (1945). The sexual psychology of human hermaphrodites. *Psychosom Med* 7, 108–125.

Faisal A S, Iqbal A, Hughes I A (2000). The testosterone: androstenedione ratio in male undermasculinization. *Clin Endocrinol* 53, 697–702.

Geller D H, Auchus R J, Mendonca B B, Miller W L (1997). The genetic and functional basis of isolated 17,20-lyase deficiency. *Nat Genet* 17, 201–205.

Griffin J E (1992). Androgen resistance: the clinical and molecular spectrum. *N Engl J Med* 326, 611–618.

Hampson J G (1955). Hermaphroditic genital appearance, rearing and eroticism in hyperadrenocorticism. *Bull Johns Hopkins Hosp* 96, 265–273.

Herdt G H, Davidson J (1988). The Sambia 'Turnim-Man': sociocultural and clinical aspects of gender formation in male pseudohermaphrodites with 5-alpha-reductase deficiency in Papua New Guinea. *Arch Sex Behav* 17, 33–56.

Hurt W G, Bodurtha J N, McCall J B, Ali M M (1989). Seminoma in pubertal patient with androgen insensitivity syndrome. *Am J Obstet Gynecol* 161, 530–531.

Imperato-McGinley J (1979). Androgens and the evolution of male gender identity among male PSH with 5 alpha reductase deficiency. *N Engl J Med* 300, 1233–1237.

(1994). 5-Alpha-reductase deficiency: human and animal models. *Eur Urol* 25(Suppl. 1), 20–23.

Imperato-McGinley J, Guerrero L, Gautier T, Petterson R E (1974). Steroid 5-alpha-reductase deficiency in man. An inherited form of male pseudohermaphroditism. *Science* 186, 1213–1215.

Ingram J M (1981). The bicycle seat stool in the treatment of vaginal agenesis and stenosis: a preliminary report. *Am J Obstet Gynecol* 140, 867–873.

Jadresic L, Leake J, Gordon I et al. (1990). Clinicopathologic review of twelve children with nephropathy, Wilms tumor, and genital abnormalities (Drash syndrome). *J Pediatr* 117, 717–725.

Josso N, Briard M L (1980). Embryonic testicular regression syndrome: variable phenotypic expression in siblings. *J Pediatr* 97, 200–204.

Katz M D, Kligman I, Cai L Q et al. (1997). Paternity by intrauterine insemination with sperm from a man with 5alpha-reductase-2 deficiency. *N Engl J Med* 336, 994–997.

Keller R (1940). Historical and cultural aspects of hermaphroditism. *Ciba Symp* 2, 466–470.

Krob G, Braun A, Kuhnle U (1994). True hermaphroditism: geographical distribution, clinical findings, chromosomes and gonadal histology. *Eur J Pediatr* 153, 2–10.

Kwok C, Tyler-Smith C, Mendonca B B et al. (1996). Mutation analysis of the 2 kb 5' to *SRY* in XY females and XY intersex subjects. *J Med Genet* 33, 465–468.

Ludwig G (1999). Micropenis and apparent micropenis – a diagnostic and therapeutic challenge. *Andrologia* 31, 27–30.

MacDonald P C, Madden J D, Brenner P F, Wilson J D, Siiteri P K (1979). Origin of estrogen in normal men and in women with testicular feminization. *J Clin Endocrinol Metab* 49, 905–916.

Manuel M, Katayama P K, Jones Jr H W (1976). The age of occurrence of gonadal tumours in intersex patients with a Y chromosome. *Am J Obstet Gynecol* 124, 293–300.

Marcantonio S M, Fechner P Y, Migeon C J, Perlman E J, Berkovitz G D (1994). Embryonic testicular regression sequence: a part of the clinical spectrum of 46,XY gonadal dysgenesis. *Am J Med Genet* 49, 1–5.

Marcus R, Leary D, Schneider D L, Shane E, Favus M, Quigley C A (2000). The contribution of testosterone to skeletal development and maintenance: lessons from the androgen insensitivity syndrome. *J Clin Endocrinol Metab* 85, 1032–1037.

McElreavey K, Fellous M (1999). Sex determination and the Y chromosome. *Am J Med Genet* 89, 176–185.

Mendonca B B, Barbosa A S, Arnhold I J, McElreavey K, Fellous M, Moreira-Filho C A (1994). Gonadal agenesis in XX and XY sisters: evidence for the involvement of an autosomal gene. *Am J Med Genet* 52, 39–43.

Minto C L, Liao L M, Conway G S, Creighton S M (2003a). Sexual function in adult women with complete androgen insensitivity syndrome. *Fertil Steril* 80, 157–164.

Minto C L, Liao L M, Woodhouse C R, Ransley P G, Creighton S M (2003b). The effect of clitoral surgery on sexual outcome in individuals who have intersex conditions with ambiguous genitalia: a cross-sectional study. *Lancet* 361, 1252–1257.

Money J (1985). Pediatric sexology and hermaphroditism. *J Sex Marital Ther* 11, 139–156.

Money J, Hampson J G, Hampson J L (1955). An examination of some basic sexual concepts: the evidence of human hermaphroditism. *Bull Johns Hopkins Hosp* 97, 301–319.

Money J, Devore H, Norman B F (1986). Gender identity and gender transposition: longitudinal outcome study of 32 male hermaphrodites assigned as girls. *J Sex Marital Ther* 12, 165–181.

Morris J M (1953). The syndrome of testicular feminization in male pseudohermaphrodites. *Am J Obstet Gynecol* 65, 1192–1211.

Oesch I L, Pinter A, Ransley P G (1987). Penile agenesis: a report of six cases. *J Pediatr Surg* 22, 172–174.

Pang S (2001). Congenital adrenal hyperplasia owing to 3 beta-hydroxysteroid dehydrogenase deficiency. *Endocrinol Metab Clin North Am* 30, 81–99.

Quigley C A, De Bellis A, Marschke K B, el Awady M K, Wilson E M, French F S (1995). Androgen receptor defects: historical, clinical, and molecular perspectives. *Endocr Rev* 16, 271–321.

Quint E H, Strickland J L (2001). Management quandary. Testicular feminization. *J Pediatr Adolesc Gynecol* 14, 99–100.

Randall V A (1994). Role of 5 alpha-reductase in health and disease. *Baillières Clin Endocrinol Metab* 8, 405–431.

Reilly J M, Woodhouse C R (1989). Small penis and the male sexual role. *J Urol* 142, 569–571.

Rey R, Picard J-Y (1998). Embryology and endocrinology of genital development. *Clin Endocrinol Metab* 12, 17–33.

Rosenfield R L, Lucky A W, Allen T D (1980). The diagnosis and management of intersex. *Curr Probl Pediatr* 10, 1–66.

Rosler A, Silverstein S, Abeliovich D (1996). A (R80Q) mutation in 17 beta-hydroxysteroid dehydrogenase type 3 gene among Arabs of Israel is associated with pseudohermaphroditism in males and normal asymptomatic females. *J Clin Endocrinol Metab* 81, 1827–1831.

Rumsby G (1997). Molecular biology of steroid biosynthesis. In *Molecular Endocrinology. Genetic Analysis of Hormones and their Receptors*, Rumsby G, Farrow S M, eds., pp. 179–202. BIOS Scientific, Oxford, UK.

Russell M H, Wachtel S S, Davis B W et al. (1982). Ovarian development in 46,XY gonadal dysgenesis. *Hum Genet* 60, 196–199.

Rutgers J L, Scully R E (1991). The androgen insensitivity syndrome (testicular feminisation): a clinicopathological study of 43 cases. *Int J Gynecol Pathol* 10, 126–144.

Schafer A J, Dominguez-Steglich M A, Guioli S et al. (1995). The role of SOX9 in autosomal sex reversal and campomelic dysplasia. *Philos Trans Roy Soc Lond B Biol Sci* 350, 271–277.

Schober J M (1998). Early feminizing genitoplasty or watchful waiting. *J Pediatr Adolesc Gynecol* 11, 154–156.

Sinnecker G H, Hiort O, Nitsche E M for the German Collaborative Intersex Study Group (1997). Functional assessment and clinical classification of androgen sensitivity in patients with mutations of the androgen receptor gene. *Eur J Pediatr* 156, 7–14.

Slaney S F, Chalmers I J, Affara N A, Chitty L S (1998). An autosomal or X linked mutation results in true hermaphrodites and 46,XX males in the same family. *J Med Genet* 35, 17–22.

Slijper F M, Frets P G, Boehmer A L, Drop S L, Niermeijer M F (2000). Androgen insensitivity syndrome (AIS): emotional reactions of parents and adult patients to the clinical diagnosis of AIS and its confirmation by androgen receptor gene mutation analysis. *Horm Res* 53, 9–15.

Soule S G, Conway G, Prelevic G M, Prentice M, Ginsburg J, Jacobs H S (1995). Osteopenia as a feature of the androgen insensitivity syndrome. *Clin Endocrinol* 43, 671–675.

Stavrou S S, Zhu Y S, Cai L Q et al. (1998). A novel mutation of the human luteinizing hormone receptor in 46,XY and 46,XX sisters. *J Clin Endocrinol Metab* 83, 2091–2098.

Swyer G (1955). Male pseudohermaphroditism: a hitherto undescribed form. *Br Med J* i, 709–710.

Tajima T, Fujieda K, Kouda N, Nakae J, Miller W L (2001). Heterozygous mutation in the cholesterol side chain cleavage enzyme (p450scc) gene in a patient with 46,XY sex reversal and adrenal insufficiency. *J Clin Endocrinol Metab* 86, 3820–3825.

Verp M S, Simpson J L (1987). Abnormal sexual differentiation and neoplasia. *Cancer Genet Cytogenet* 25, 191–218.

Verp M S, Harrison H H, Ober C et al. (1992). Chimerism as the etiology of a 46,XX/46,XY fertile true hermaphrodite. *Fertil Steril* 57, 346–349.

Walker A M, Walker J L, Adams S, Shi E, McGlynn M, Verge C F (2000). True hermaphroditism. *J Paediatr Child Health* 36, 69–73.

Weber A M, Walters M D, Schover L R, Mitchinson A (1995). Vaginal anatomy and sexual function. *Obstet Gynecol* 86, 946–949.

Wiersma R (2001). Management of the African child with true hermaphroditism. *J Pediatr Surg* 36, 397–399.

Yanase T. 17 Alpha-hydroxylase/17,20-lyase defects (1995). *J Steroid Biochem Mol Biol* 53, 153–157.

Zenteno J C, Canto P, Kofman-Alfaro S, Mendez J P (1999). Evidence for genetic heterogeneity in male pseudohermaphroditism due to Leydig cell hypoplasia. *J Clin Endocrinol Metab* 84, 3803–3806.

Zhu Y S, Katz M D, Imperato-McGinley J (1998). Natural potent androgens: lessons from human genetic models. *Baillières Clin Endocrinol Metab* 12, 83–113.

Zucker K J (1999). Intersexuality and gender identity differentiation. *Annu Rev Sex Res* 10, 1–69.

23

The gynaecology of the major genitourinary anomalies

Christopher R. J. Woodhouse

The Institute of Urology and the Hospital for Sick Children, Great Ormond St, London, UK

Introduction

There are three congenital genitourinary anomalies that have a serious impact on female sexual and reproductive function: exstrophy, spina bifida and the cloacal anomalies. It is true that spina bifida is primarily a neurological condition, but in practice it is the urological complications that dominate childhood and adolescence. The urologist usually manages the overall care.

Classical exstrophy has been recognized for about 2000 years and has been the subject of voluminous surgical literature since the middle of the last century. The results of exstrophy reconstruction, both functional and cosmetic, have improved considerably since the 1980s. The present adult women who were born with exstrophy would usually have had an early diversion and, if they wished, a continent reconstruction when such surgery became available. Few of them would have had a reconstruction that allowed them to void naturally and fewer still will have maintained that ability into their third decade (Woodhouse and Redgrave, 1996). Now, in specialist centres, primary reconstruction is undertaken in the first hours of life. Continence and spontaneous voiding are the norm; reconstruction with intestine and intermittent clean self-catheterization (ICSC) are sometimes needed.

With this general improvement has come the realization that exstrophic patients grow up and want to work, marry and have children. Exstrophy is an isolated anomaly in otherwise normal children. They grow up normally and, anecdotally, are intelligent and well-motivated adults. While the sexuality and erectile deformities of males have been well recognized, the female genitalia have been less well studied (in part because there are fewer affected girls).

Psychological reviews have indicated that patients are concerned about the appearance of their genitalia and it is now known that reconstruction can give a near normal appearance.

Spina bifida, at least in its more severe forms, is a complete contrast to exstrophy. The apparently isolated spinal anomaly produces a cascade of motor and sensory problems affecting every bodily function. Hydrocephalus is a common association leading to low IQ. There may be neurological problems above the spinal level giving, amongst other things, poor manual dexterity. There is a steady deterioration in almost all functions with growth, particularly through adolescence.

The adult population that is available for study was born in the 1950s and 1960s. Early surgery on all babies to close the spinal defect was just beginning. It would be hoped that long-term outcomes for babies born now would be better, if only because of more aggressive management of the neuropathic bladder. It is difficult, now, to appreciate the difference that the ileal conduit made to the management of the child with spina bifida when it was introduced by Bricker at the beginning of the 1950s. Until then, dribbling incontinence, chronic infection and renal failure had been the norm. Manual expression was used by the dedicated parent with variable success. Afterwards, children were "dry" and dilated kidneys returned to normal. The literature of the period is replete with papers eulogizing the Bricker operation.

Since the 1980s, almost all children with a neuropathic bladder will have had some active management aimed at preserving the kidneys, avoiding diversion and maintaining continence. McGuire has particularly drawn attention to the importance of the leak point pressure. This is the

Paediatric and Adolescent Gynaecology, ed. Adam Balen et al. Published by Cambridge University Press.
© Cambridge University Press 2004.

detrusor pressure at which incontinence occurs. If this pressure is below 40 cm H_2O, upper tract deterioration is unlikely (Raz et al., 1988). Treatment has been aimed at reduction of the storage pressure below this figure and maintenance of continence by ICSC, antimuscarinic drugs and, when necessary, bladder augmentation. A few patients will have had an artificial urinary sphincter implanted or a continent suprapubic diversion. The formation of an ileal conduit or the use of manual expression now are rare.

Exstrophy

In both males and females, the obvious anomaly of the open bladder (Fig. 23.1, colour plate) is associated with abnormalities of the pelvic bones and of the genitalia. There is a rare and more minor variation called epispadias in which the bladder defect consists solely of an absence of the bladder neck. The genitalia still have the same anomalies, though often to a lesser degree. A sagittal section of the pelvic organs is shown in Fig. 23.2. It will be seen that the vagina, introitus and anus are each displaced anteriorly. The vagina is shorter than normal, seldom measuring more than 5–6 cm, but of normal calibre. The uterus, which is in an almost normal anatomical position, enters superiorly so that the cervix is in the anterior vaginal wall. The ovaries and tubes are normal (Woodhouse and Hinsch, 1997).

Appearances in the adult

Uncorrected, the labia and introitus appear to be structures of the lower anterior abdominal wall (Fig. 23.3, colour

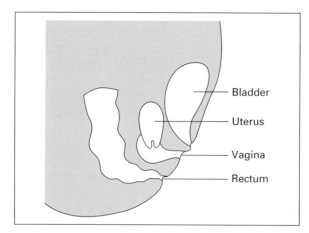

Fig. 23.2. Diagram to show a sagittal section of the female pelvis in exstrophy.

plate). The introitus is narrow (Fig. 23.4, colour plate). The narrowing is posterior and is a more substantial layer than the normal hymen, probably being a continuation of the posterior wall of the vagina. The anus is in the position of the normal vagina. The labia, particularly minora, are bifid and rudimentary. At present in adults with exstrophy, the pubic area is nearly always recessed from the uncorrected divarication of the pubic bones. The pubic hair lies on either side of the midline (Fig. 23.5).

The abnormality is variable; in some females, the labia are almost in the correct anatomical position. Those with a working bladder generally have a more normal appearance; otherwise, the original severity of the epispadias seems irrelevant.

Reconstruction

The object of the genital reconstruction is to unite the two halves of the clitoris and to fuse the anterior ends of the labia to make a fourchette. It is not possible to move the vagina posteriorly to its usual anatomical position, but labial and pubic reconstruction does disguise the abnormality reasonably well. The main data come from the 42 adult female patients with classical exstrophy reported from the author's adolescent urology clinic. The women were born between 1953 and 1980 and are now aged 21 to 48 (Woodhouse and Hinsch, 1997).

The method of surgical reconstruction has evolved over the last 15 years. Early in the series, there was less emphasis on the closure of the labia anteriorly, and a number of vaginoplasties were thought to be necessary.

Although the parts of the reconstruction are described separately, they are usually performed together. They are: the fusion of the labia anteriorly, opening of the introitus and reconstruction of the mons pubis.

Vaginoplasty. In spite of the very narrow introitus, the vagina above is of normal calibre. An episiotomy is made posteriorly from the introitus until a two to three finger opening has been created (Fig. 23.6, colour plate). It is usually possible to close the vaginal mucosa to the perineal skin directly but if not a flap of mucosa from the medial aspect of the labia can be rotated on each side to close the defect.

Vulvoplasty. The two halves of the clitoris (assuming that they can be identified) and the anterior ends of the labia are united to make a fourchette. No attempt is made to move the vagina posteriorly to its usual anatomical position. A diamond-shaped area of skin/mucosa is outlined anterior to the labia and extended down onto the anterior ends of each labus and hemi-clitoris (Fig. 23.7, colour

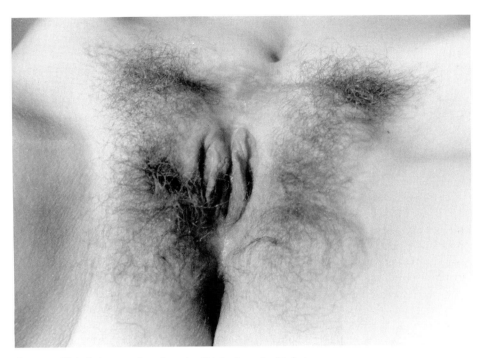

Fig. 23.5. Clinical photograph to show the distribution of pubic hair.

plate). This diamond and the underlying fatty tissue are excised. The defect is then closed longitudinally with fine absorbable sutures.

Monsplasty. It is most important, either in infancy or in adolescence, to rotate hair-bearing flaps of skin and fat to cover the midline defect. The flaps may be based laterally or inferiorly (Fid et al., 1993; Marconi et al., 1993; Ship and Pelzer, 1972). If there is too little skin available, larger flaps can be created by the use of skin expanders (Fid et al., 1993). The only problem with the use of tissue expanders (or using flaps under tension) is that the number of hair follicles is not increased. Therefore, although good skin cover is achieved, the pubic triangle can look a little "bald". The scarred and non-hairy skin from the midline is excised. This excision may be continuous with that from the anterior end of the labia. The flaps of hair-bearing skin, including all of the subcutaneous fat, are then mobilized and rotated to fill the defect (Fig. 23.8). An example of postoperative appearance is shown in Fig. 23.9. It is important to note that the position of the vagina is only disguised by the mons and the pubic hair: if the hair is parted, the labia can still be seen as structures of the lower abdominal wall.

Considering the fairly obvious abnormality of the vagina, both in position and appearance, it is surprising that more

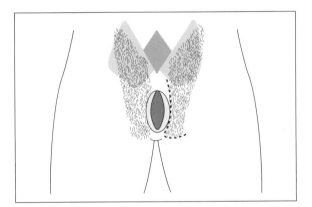

Fig. 23.8. Rotation of hair flaps to reconstruct the mons in exstrophy.

emotional problems are not seen. I am only aware of one patient in my series who has severe problems. Several females note that the rather broad perineum, which is a consequence of the outward rotation of the pelvis, makes the wearing of modern narrow crotched bathing costumes impractical.

As with males, there is now a tendency to reconstruct the genitalia in infancy or childhood. Hohenfelner's group suggest opening of the introitus and uniting the labia at three or four years of age (Stein et al., 1995). This

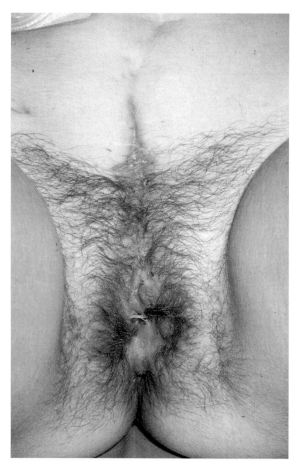

(a)

allows easy drainage of secretions and, later, menstrual flow. The more natural appearance in the school years is welcome.

Contemporary techniques of primary reconstruction recognize the distribution of hair-bearing skin and position it appropriately. Unfortunately, the benefit of such surgery may be lost if many revision operations cause unsightly midline scars later on. Excellent results from early reconstruction have been reported in 21 of 25 girls reviewed after puberty (Stein et al., 1995). However, most of these patients had been diverted and did not have the sequence of revision operations that is so common after primary reconstruction.

Intercourse

It is almost impossible for intercourse to take place unless the introitus has been opened. Thereafter, it should be normal. In my own patients, 34 have had sexual intercourse, including all of the 30 patients who have had introital reconstruction. Only 4 of 12 patients who have not been reconstructed claim to have had intercourse. Thirty two patients are married or have a regular partner.

The vagina runs directly posteriorly so that when the patient is standing the vagina is almost parallel with the floor. It is also rather shorter than usual. These arrangements normally do not interfere with intercourse. However, in a few patients the upward angle of the erect penis

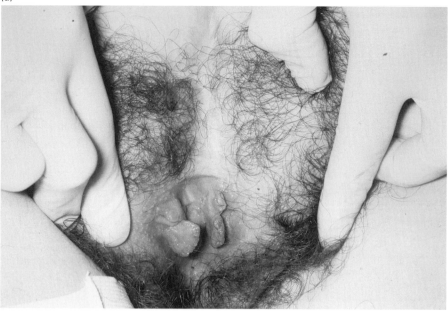

(b)

Fig. 23.9. Postoperative clinical photograph. (a) At rest. (b) The position of the labia is only disguised by their anterior union and the position of the pubic hair.

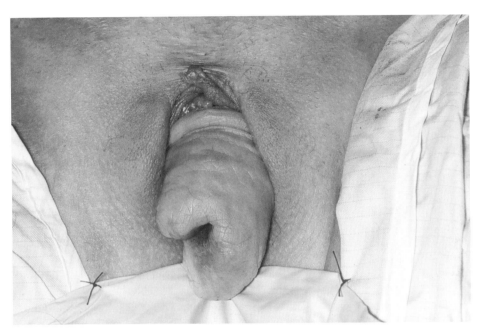

Fig. 23.10. Clinical photograph of an exstrophy patient with procedentia.

appears to impinge on the cervix and causes dyspareunia. Orgasm has been said to be normal in all patients. In the same series, all of the 19 patients over 18 years were said to have had intercourse but three considered it unpleasant. The source of unpleasantness was not given (Stein et al., 1996).

Fertility and pregnancy

The cervix enters the superior wall of the vagina and is close to the introitus: this must contribute to the ease with which the women appear to get pregnant. It is essential to explain to the patients at an early stage that fertility is normal.

Pregnancy has a poor reputation in females with exstrophy probably because of the literature review from 1722 to 1958 by Clemston (1958). There were only 49 live births from 64 pregnancies and two maternal deaths. Considering the level of obstetric care in the first 200 years of the review, these figures might indicate that pregnant exstrophy patients did quite well!

Contemporary results are better. In a combined series of 22 patients from my own series and the current literature there were 32 pregnancies. Two ended in spontaneous abortion and two in therapeutic abortion. There was only one obstetric catastrophe, which was the intrauterine death of twins. There were 27 livebirths. None of the offspring have had exstrophy or epispadias (Woodhouse, 1999).

Pregnancy and delivery can be normal. Elective caesarean section should be done in patients with a working bladder or with an artificial urinary sphincter (11 of the 27 deliveries mentioned above). The principle problem is subsequent uterine prolapse.

Inheritance

It has been reported from a postal survey of clinics throughout the world that 1 in 70 offspring have exstrophy or epispadias (Shapiro et al., 1984). This figure must represent the worst that can be expected. Screening pregnancies for fetuses with exstrophy is reasonably easy at 20–22 weeks. Advising the parents on whether or not to terminate an affected fetus at this late stage is almost impossible. Fetal ultrasound at 18 to 20 weeks may show that the bladder does not fill. This, combined with a low umbilicus and ambiguous genitalia if the fetus is male, should raise the possibility of exstrophy.

In view of the difficulties with ultrasound diagnosis, fetoscopy seems justified for suspected cases. In two pregnancies, classical exstrophy has been confirmed on fetoscopy (Dhillon, personal communication, 1997).

Uterine prolapse

The defective pelvic floor, open pelvic ring and poor uterine supports make prolapse common (Fig. 23.10). It is a considerable problem to correct (Blakeley and Mills, 1981; Dewhurst et al., 1980). Seven of my patients have had a total procedentia, one of whom had never had intercourse or a pregnancy. It may be found in up to 50% of patients after pregnancy. The uterus should not be removed as it is the only solid organ in the pelvis that has any hope of holding up the pelvic floor.

For the repair of procedentia, the most successful procedure is the gortex wrap. The sacral promontory is exposed. A strip of gortex is sutured to the periosteum. The end is passed around the cervix through the base of the broad ligament and brought back to the sacrum (Farkas et al., 1993). This procedure has been successful in all cases, with follow-up to a maximum of six years.

Hohenfelner advocates fixation of the uterus to the anterior abdominal wall in childhood. This is said to prevent prolapse but still allow normal pregnancy (Stein et al., 1995). Two women were able to have normal pregnancies without prolapse, while one of two women who did not have a fixation had slight prolapse after delivery. This "prophylactic surgery" may well be helpful. However, once prolapse has occurred, I have not found an anterior fixation to be an effective repair.

Spina bifida

Spina bifida is the common term given to a group of spinal cord anomalies properly called neural tube defects. It presents a complete contrast to exstrophy. Although the neurological abnormality appears to be isolated, just as the exstrophy defect is a bladder and genital abnormality, the effects of spina bifida involve almost every area of the body. Furthermore, there is a natural tendency for the secondary effects progressively to deteriorate. The gynaecological problems, therefore, have to be considered against a background of many other defects. Furthermore, about a half of the patients will have the visible problem of a permanent wheelchair existence, which often raises considerable prejudice in society – there are those who feel that sexual relationships are inappropriate for those in wheelchairs. At the worst end of the social spectrum, sexual abuse of disabled women is common.

Incidence

For women in general and spina bifida girls in particular, one of the great success stories of the last 20 years has been the discovery of the prophylactic role of folic acid. The incidence of all neural tube defects in babies in the Western world has diminished in this period. Even before the dis-

covery of the protective effects of folic acid, the overall incidence had been falling. In a recent study from the UK, it was shown that the incidence of neural tube defects started to fall about 18 years before the use of folic acid began to rise. The incidence fell from about 225/100 000 live births to about 48/100 000 livebirths between 1972 and 1990. The number of sales of folic acid was less than 100 000 per year until 1990, rising to 1.2 million per year by 1996 (Kadir et al., 1999).

However, the main protection against the conception of a baby with a neural tube defect is to give the mother folic acid supplements in the three months before conception and for the first trimester (Czeizel and Dudas, 1992; MRC Vitamin Study Research Group, 1991). The Department of Health in the UK now recommends that women who are at high risk of conceiving a baby with a neural tube defect should take 5 mg per day while 0.4 mg per day is sufficient for other women (Lloyd, 1992).

In spite of this prophylaxis, there remains a small risk of an affected pregnancy. At least one cause appears to be an inborn error of folic acid metabolism, which was found in 16 women who gave birth to two successive babies with myelomeningocele in spite of prophylaxis (Wild et al., 1994).

The use of selective termination of pregnancy in cases of neural tube defect is as much a social as a medical issue. In a series in South Australia between 1966 and 1991, the prevalence of affected pregnancies did not change but the number of affected livebirths fell by 84% from 2.29 to 0.35/1000 (Chan et al., 1993).

The number of adults with spina bifida is decreasing for two reasons. First, the use of folic acid and of selective termination have reduced the incidence of the condition. Second, babies born with spina bifida (at least on current data) have a reduced life expectancy, with 40% dying before adult life (Hunt, 2000). Nonetheless, there remains a substantial number of women with major disability from spina bifida who have particular gynaecological problems.

Sexuality

The sexual development of handicapped patients has received little attention. The most obvious public attention arises when there is a moral or ethical problem. For example, a difficult area of community policy is how to prevent unwanted pregnancies and sexual abuse in affected girls of low intelligence.

Those with severe congenital disabilities often fail to develop normal sexuality because of lack of privacy and dependence on others for normal daily living. They have low social and sexual confidence. Surprisingly, however, even those who can walk and whose spina bifida is "hidden" have major sexual problems. They will have uncertain bladder and bowel control, which leads to an unwillingness to mix with their peers on an equal basis. It is most important not to imagine that an apparently minor level of neurological disability means that sexuality is normal (Glass and Soni, 1999).

In general, the sexual function that depends on the brain is intact, while that which depends on the spinal cord will be damaged in line with the neurological level.

When children are brought up in the mainstream of education and integrated in school, the social results are excellent. In a study to compare 11 dimensions of self-image in adolescents with spina bifida with those of their peers, there was no difference in ten. Unfortunately, the eleventh was the dimension of sexuality, which was significantly below normal, especially in females (Cartwright et al., 1993).

Adolescents with spina bifida are often ignorant of even very straightforward aspects of sexuality that should be taught within the family. The ordinary facts of reproductive life often are not given. Up to 23% of girls do not know about the hygienic management of menstruation (Blum et al., 1991; Dorner, 1997). It is not surprising, therefore, that adolescents have very little sexual contact.

However, patients and their parents have a desire to learn about sexual development that is not fulfilled by doctors. In response to specific questions 95% of teenage patients and 59% of their parents felt that they had inadequate knowledge. Only a quarter of girls had had any sexual experience and, most disturbingly, 37% reported that they had been sexually abused.

Sexual function

In females, as in males, sexual function, as defined by sexual sensation and orgasm, is dependent on neurological level. Only a small number of girls have been investigated and it is difficult to define sexuality in terms that severely affected spina bifida girls can understand. Most with levels below L2 are thought to have normal sexual sensations, as are most with urinary continence. Only about 20% of those with higher levels or with urinary incontinence have normal sexual function (Cass et al., 1986).

I have noted that some women appear to have powerful contractions of the detrusor in response to sexual stimulation or orgasm. The contractions are painful if the bladder is empty and cause incontinence if any urine is present. They are not abolished by clam cystoplasty, but they are if the bladder is removed and a substitution cystoplasty performed (unpublished data).

Marriage and fertility

In spite of the rather gloomy findings in adolescents, many women with spina bifida establish long-term relationships and marriage. In a study from South Wales, 15 of 23 women had married and four were in a long-term relationship. Two of the married women divorced but one remarried. 11 women had had 11 children, several miscarriages and one still birth. Of the eight single women only four were felt to have no prospects of forming a stable relationship. It is interesting to note that these outcomes were unrelated to continence (Laurence and Beresford, 1975).

Fertility is thought to be normal. The main problem is, of course, the risk of a neural tube defect in the offspring (discussed above). Folic acid prophylaxis considerably reduces the risk. A secondary cause is the obesity commonly seen in adolescents with spina bifida. Unfortunately, the incidence of neural tube defect pregnancies is nearly double in women who are obese at the time of conception (body mass index $> 29\,kg/m^2$) (Shaw et al., 1996).

There have been several reports of favourable pregnancy outcomes in females with spina bifida, though one group summarized their experiences with difficult pregnancies in (medically) difficult patients from difficult (socially deprived) families (Richmond et al., 1987). Several specific problems have been identified. Urinary tract infections are almost inevitable; bladder function and mobility often deteriorate, though not permanently; the deformed and, often, small pelvis makes accommodation of the fetus difficult, leading to premature labour and an increased need for caesarean sections (Richmond et al., 1987; Rietberg and Lindhout, 1993).

In a series of 20 pregnancies, 35% were delivered before 37 weeks. Eight required a caesarean section, all for obstetric indications, most commonly disproportion (Rietberg and Lindhout, 1993). Four of five wheelchair-bound women required caesarean section compared with eight of 18 walkers (Arata et al., 2000).

Family planning

There are several special problems in family planning for women with spina bifida apart from the issues of folic acid and pregnancy difficulties. Although most patients, especially if supported by caring parents, are able to understand contraception, there are some who cannot give informed consent and who would be unable to use simple barrier techniques. This is a problem for society as well as for doctors and has been considered by the courts. It remains unethical for doctors to carry out treatment without the consent of a patient.

As screening for neural tube defects is offered to women, particularly those at risk, it would seem logical that those who themselves had spina bifida would take up the offer. There is little guidance in the literature. However, a survey reported in the correspondence section of a journal gave some interesting insight. A series of 114 women with spina bifida (48% in wheelchairs) were asked if they would have screening when pregnant. Only 39 said that they would accept screening and only nine would have a termination if they were found to have a fetus with a neural tube defect. The study was not peer reviewed and took place in Northern Ireland at a time when abortion was illegal. Even so, it does indicate that a desire for a termination is not universal and certainly cannot be presumed.

Doctors may have to consider the ability of a severely affected spina bifida patient to bring up a family. It is not part of the doctor's duty to censure. However, it is sometimes important to advise on practical issues of family upbringing, especially if the woman is single. At the very least, the appropriate social service agencies should be alerted in good time so that proper housing and social support can be arranged.

Although spina bifida is primarily a neurological condition, overall care in adults tends to lie with the urologist. Many will have had urinary reconstructions with intestine. The urine from such a reservoir gives a false-positive pregnancy test in 57% of women (and, curiously, in 71% of men). Pregnancy can only reliably be tested by measurement of blood human chorionic gonadotrophin levels.

All pregnant women with such reservoirs should have shared care by the urologist and by an obstetrician with appropriate experience. The urological complications of pregnancy are generally reversible after delivery. However, a special watch must be kept for ureteric obstruction. The pedicles of the intestine used for bladder reconstruction are likely to lie in front of the gravid uterus and are much at risk with caesarean section. Emergency sections should be avoided at all costs. If a caesarean is performed, a urologist should be on hand to guard the reconstruction.

The genitalia are not abnormal but the pelvic floor innervation obviously is. It is not surprising to find a high incidence of pelvic prolapse even in young nulliparous women. In a preliminary investigation, five of eight patients were found to have the cervix within 2 cm of the introitus and three had a rectocoele (Dutta et al., 2001).

Latex allergy

Paediatric urologists with a large practice in spina bifida are well aware of the problems of latex allergy. Sophisticated strategies have been established to identify patients at risk

and to avoid the serious problems of anaphylaxis especially under anaesthetic. Gynaecologists are much less aware of this potentially fatal problem.

Although there is a general recognition that children with spina bifida are particularly at risk, the reasons are unclear. It is tempting to think that the increased number of surgical procedures is to blame. It appears to be true that in a group with a 60% incidence of latex allergy, those that were allergic had had 50% more operations than those that were negative (Ellsworth et al., 1993). However, there are probably other factors to consider. The presence of latex-specific IgG was found in 25% of a group of European patients with spina bifida aged 2–40 years. Multivariate analysis showed that atopy, especially to pears and kiwi fruit, and a history of five or more operations were significantly and independently associated with latex allergy (Bernardini et al., 1998). When controlled for age and the number of operations, the incidence of latex allergy is five times greater in spina bifida than in other groups (Ziylan et al., 1996).

About a third of spina bifida patients will have a history of allergic reactions to latex products (Ellsworth et al., 1993). The level of awareness of the problem amongst these children and their families is low and so the symptoms should be specifically sought. In some cases, the association is obvious, but in others it may be obscure, such as itchy eyes while using washing-up gloves or genital reactions to condoms. In occasional patients there is acute anaphylaxis under anaesthetic.

During medical procedures, latex use should be reduced to a minimum. There are important warning signs that may alert the clinician to the problem in a previously unsuspected case. In a group of five children (from 17) who were undergoing transurethral bladder stimulation and urodynamics, all had coughing or sneezing for several minutes before bronchospasm and generalized allergic reactions developed (Schneck and Bellinger, 1993).

All who have a suggestive history or unexplained hypotensive episodes under anaesthetic should undergo skin testing and measurement of latex-specific IgE. A latex-free medical environment should be created for patients found to be at risk. In all of four patients on the author's service who presented with anaphylaxis under anaesthetic, further operations have been uneventful in a latex-free operating theatre (unpublished data).

As the incidence is so high in patients with spina bifida, a specific enquiry should be made for symptoms in all patients. Minor reactions can be treated with bronchodilators, antihistamines and, occasionally, steroids. It should be remembered that minor reactions may be the forerunners of major anaphylaxis. Obstetric units should have a protocol to create a latex-free environment.

Cloaca and urogenital sinus

The *cloaca maxima* was the main drain of ancient Rome. A great innovation at the time. The term cloaca is used to cover a wide spectrum of conditions in which the drainage of the urinary, genital and gastrointestinal tracts is through a single perineal orifice (true cloaca) or where the urinary and genital tracts are combined (urogenital sinus).

The most severe form of cloaca is rare. It is often associated with other major congenital anomalies especially of the cardiovascular system. With all three channels coalescing, there is almost never an anal sphincter and seldom a urethral one. In intermediate forms, the urethral sphincter is normal. Because there is no endocrine association, the internal genitalia are often normal. The urinary anomalies are potentially lethal and the reconstructive surgery in childhood is technically very difficult. There is, therefore, very little information on the long-term outcomes.

Surgery in infancy is aimed primarily at preserving life and only incidentally at separating the three channels. Diversion of both urinary and faecal tracts is usually essential. It will often be possible to create a continent bladder though emptying may require intermittent catheterization. A continent rectum is more difficult and many children remain clean only by a process of "controlled constipation" or continue with a colostomy (Hendren, 1986).

The reconstructive surgery has improved somewhat since the late 1970s. It is possible to achieve social urinary continence in about 80% of patients with or without the use of intermittent self-catheterization. Faecal continence remains a challenge and is achieved in about 60%. There is still little information about the genital outcome (Warne et al., 2002).

The condition must be distinguished from cloacal exstrophy, which is a severe variant of ectopia vesicae and has nothing in common with congenital adrenal hyperplasia (CAH). However, the commonest of this rare group of anomalies is associated with CAH (Ch. 24). 21-Hydroxylase deficiency is the cause for 90% of those affected and of these between a half and two-thirds will have salt loss owing to reduced aldosterone production. The anus and rectum are normal. The anatomy of the common path of the vagina and urethra, known as the urogenital sinus, ranges from a complete male type of urethra with a high union of the vagina to a confluence close to a perineal introitus. The urethral sphincters are likely to be normal.

Almost all those affected are identified at birth or, occasionally, in utero. Infants with CAH who have a 46,XX genotype will be raised female. Because of the block in adrenal synthesis of steroids, the level of fetal androgens is high. The external genitalia are ambiguous with an enlarged clitoris, which is not corrected with even the most meticulous endocrine control after birth. Surgery in infancy is aimed at the separation of the two tracts and is considered in Ch. 24. Recent controversy about the sexual outcome in intersex patients has cast doubt about the extent to which the genitalia should be altered in infancy.

It is becoming clear from animal work and from clinical observation that the brain is the most dominating organ in sexual orientation (Diamond, 1996; Glassberg, 1999). It is, therefore, not surprising that babies exposed to androgens in utero should exhibit some behaviour more often associated with boys.

In an early observational study, it was shown that CAH women grew up as "tom-boys" and had little interest in role rehearsal for marriage and motherhood (Ehrhardt et al., 1968). Even though some of these women had been treated late and with less completeness than would be the case now, the same group made similar, but less strong, findings more than 10 years later (Ehrhardt and Meyer-Bahlburg, 1981).

It is difficult to separate the effects of androgen exposure in utero from that of genital surgery, long-term medication and frequent hospital visits. Several control groups have been used and, although none is ideal, a consistent pattern has emerged. When women with CAH were compared with those with juvenile-onset diabetics the differences are very small, with similar sex role play and feelings of self-esteem. This suggests that some of the problem may lie in the chronic nature of the endocrine illness and the medical supervision that is required (Mosely et al., 1989). However, when compared with their sisters or female cousins, it becomes clear that women with CAH are less feminine and less secure in their female role. In growing up, CAH girls show less inclination to play as, or to form friendships with, other girls, sometimes to the extent of cross-dressing. As adults, although having similar marriage rates, they have fewer experiences of "true love", up to 20% at least fantasize about homosexual relationships and have intercourse less often. Up to 13% have gender identity disorder and occasional individuals change to a male gender role. The effects are most marked in those with the salt-losing form of CAH (Dittmann et al., 1992; Slijper et al., 1998; Zucker et al., 1996).

Sexuality

Scientific study of female sexuality is a comparatively new field at least as far as the surgeon is concerned. Well-known researchers such as Kinsey or Masters and Johnson recorded female sexual behaviour and normal sexual physiology. It is only in the 1990s that there has been detailed work on female sexual dysfunction (Berman et al., 1999).

Table 23.1. The number of women who have a patent vagina after primary surgery

Authors	Technical	No.	Patency after primary surgery	Patency after further surgery	Intercourse
Azziz et al., 1986	Total	42	5	33	33 (62%)
Bailez et al., 1992	Easy	25	6	13	11 (44%)
	Difficult	13	0	1	0
Alizai et al., 1999	Total		0	2	0
Krege et al., 2000	Easy	20	14	6	4 of 9^a
	Difficult	7	4	2	2 of 6^a

^{a}Intercourse only considered in patients over 15 years of age who completed a questionnaire.

Some follow-up on vaginoplasty has been limited to assessments of patency, penetration and fertility without considering the quality of the sexual experience. Papers refer to the vagina being "satisfactory" without saying to whom it was satisfactory or by what means satisfaction was measured. Such limited assessment may not be totally invalid. The strictly surgical results could be thought of purely in terms of the ability to create a "vagina" where none previously existed.

The timing of vaginal reconstruction appears to have been a matter of contention for at least 25 years. It would seem that only a minority of children are reconstructed in a single operation in infancy or early childhood (Azziz et al., 1986). In looking at the long-term follow-up of 16 women (of an original 32 children) Lattimer's group concluded in 1976 that the results of vaginoplasty were so poor that operation should not be done before puberty (Sotiropoulos et al., 1976).

However, feminizing genitoplasty in infancy remains a standard procedure, though surgery to reduce the size of the clitoris has become less radical with time. The results of single-stage feminizing genitoplasty in infants have been widely reported (Rink and Adams, 1998). They are better in those with a low confluence of the vagina and urethra.

Table 23.1 shows the number of women who have a patent vagina after primary surgery and the additional number patent after revision surgery. In two of the papers it is possible to divide the patients into those with a low confluence (easy) and a high confluence (difficult). In the study by Alizai et al. (1999), the mean age of the patients was 13.1 years; although all were postpubertal all were thought to be too young for intercourse to be considered. In the

study by Krege et al. (2000), intercourse was only considered in 15 patients over 15 years who completed a questionnaire (Alizai et al., 1999; Azziz et al., 1986; Bailez et al., 1992; Krege et al., 2000). It can be difficult to work out exactly what surgery was done, when and to whom! It would seem that of 85 evaluable patients, 50 were having sexual intercourse (59%). When feminizing genitoplasty is done in infancy, additional surgery around puberty is often required – in all of the patients in the series of Alizai et al. (1999). With or without additional surgery after puberty, non-salt losers are nearly twice as likely to achieve satisfactory intercourse (87% versus 46%) (Azziz et al., 1986). It will be seen later that the pregnancy rate appears to be higher than the intercourse rate. This anomalous statistic is because the pregnancy rate is given as a percentage of those women who are having intercourse.

The quality of intercourse and its frequency seem to be less good in women with CAH than in controls. Even in the "surgical" papers, it is said that intercourse may be infrequent. All the evidence shows the great importance of the clitoris in achieving orgasm. After vaginal reconstruction, about 50% of women will be able to achieve orgasm, but almost always with clitoral stimulation (Krege et al., 2000). With a natural vagina treated by regular dilatation all women can achieve orgasm, but if the clitoris has been amputated only 71% can do so (Costa et al., 1997). This emphasizes the need to preserve the clitoris.

There is some evidence that surgery even to reduce the size of the clitoris in adults impairs sexual sensation. A very small group of four women who had experienced normal sexual intercourse before clitoral surgery has been reported. After standard surgery for clitoral reduction, one maintained normal sexual function, two had difficulty in achieving an orgasm and one was anorgasmic (Schober, 1999a).

If such damage can occur when operating on the comparatively large adult clitoris, it is likely that the same, or worse, damage may occur when such surgery is done in infants. In patients from my hospital, we have identified 18 women born with ambiguous genitalia who had undergone clitoral reduction in infancy and nine similar women who had had no clitoral surgery. Not all of them had CAH. Mean global function scores (as assessed by GRISS modified sexual function inventory) were worse in those who had had clitoral surgery. Twenty eight percent of the clitoral surgery patients were anorgasmic (C. L. Minto, unpublished data).

When considering clitoral reduction in adults, it is most important to establish that which the woman wishes to achieve. The probable damage to sexual sensation must be clearly pointed out.

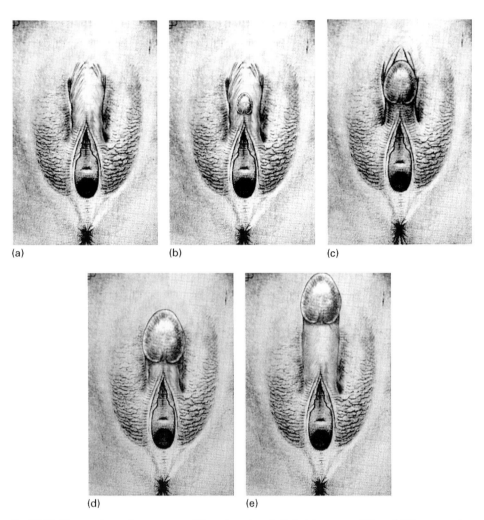

Fig. 23.11. The spectrum of appearance of the external genitalia in intersex conditions. (a) Near normal; (b) minor clitoral hypertrophy; (c) hypertrophy of the glans of the clitoris and early masculinization of the labial folds; (d) hypertrophy of the clitoral shaft; (e) development of a distinct shaft of the glans. (Courtesy of Dr J. M. Schober.)

Inadequate vagina

The external genitalia show varying degrees of masculinization. In female neonates they appear to be completely male but with no gonads in the scrotum. In adults, the spectrum is illustrated in Fig. 23.11. If the vagina has failed adequately to develop or is absent, a variety of techniques for reconstruction may be used (see also Ch. 22). None has been shown to produce an ideal substitute for the natural organ. In a review of the literature on vaginoplasty, Schober (1999a) found that follow-up assessment was usually confined to the observation that penetrative intercourse was possible with no attempt to measure its quality. It seems unlikely that any substitute would have the same sexual sensation as the natural vagina.

If the vagina is present but narrow, every effort should be made to enlarge it by progressive self-dilatation. In adults with enthusiasm, it is possible to enlarge a vagina from 5 mm to 10 cm with sufficient diameter for intercourse, over several months, with graded acrylic moulds. The advantage of this technique is that the vagina has normal physiological function, including lubrication during intercourse (Costa et al., 1997).

There is some conflict about the wisdom of routine dilatation of the vagina after genitoplasty in infancy. Krege et al. (2000) suggested that it should not be a routine if only because of the psychological problems that it may cause (though they offer no evidence for this fear). Gearhart and, even more strongly, Hendren recommend dilatation

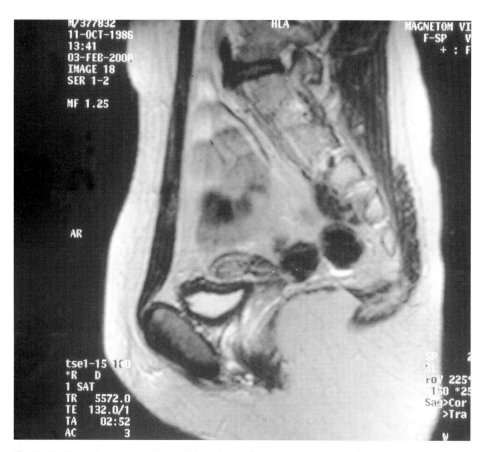

Fig. 23.12. Magnetic resonance image of the pelvis to show a normal uterus and a rudimentary vagina.

to prevent postoperative stenosis (Bailez et al., 1992). In spite of this, all of Hendren's patients required further minor surgery at puberty to allow intercourse.

Unfortunately, the perineal tissues may be so scarred that dilatation is not possible. Occasionally, it may be possible to dilate the vagina under anaesthetic sufficiently that the woman can maintain its calibre with regular dilatation or intercourse. When dilatation is possible, the outcome for sexual intercourse appears satisfactory in the small number of cases that have been reported: in one series, all of three women with CAH were able to have satisfactory intercourse and two became pregnant. In contrast, 50% patients (none of whom had CAH) who had various forms of reconstruction complained of bleeding with intercourse (Costa et al., 1997).

If reconstructive surgery is required, careful definition of the extent of the problem is required. The external genitalia and vagina are best defined by examination under anaesthetic by all of the surgeons likely to be involved in the reconstruction: gynaecologist, plastic surgeon and urologist. The cystoscope can be used to inspect the vagina

above a narrow introitus, often finding that the upper part of the vagina is normal. The internal genitalia are best defined by magnetic resonance imaging (Fig. 23.12). In the small number of girls with normal internal genitalia and no vagina, the timing of surgery is critical and must be performed before the menarche. If the window of opportunity is missed, menstruation can be suppressed temporarily with gonadotrophin-releasing hormone agonists.

A narrow vagina may be augmented with bowel or skin. A bowel augmentation will normally be done by a urologist used to using bowel for bladder reconstruction. A piece of ileum equal in length to the existing vagina and with a long enough pedicle to reach the introitus is selected. It is opened on its antimesenteric border. The vagina is opened longitudinally either anteriorly or posteriorly and sutured "face to face" with the ileum.

Intestinal vaginoplasty is seldom needed for patients with CAH. The results quoted for other diagnoses are said to be good, but follow-up has been confined to establishing that intercourse takes place without undue difficulty. Up to 70% of women who had an intestinal vagina formed in infancy report the ability to have intercourse, with a 10% incidence of dyspareunia (Hensle and Dean, 1992).

A skin augmentation is seldom indicated in CAH. It is usually done by a plastic surgeon using skin from the medial aspect of the thigh. The technique was originally described by Sir Archibald McIndoe in 1938. There have been several modifications, but the principle remains the same: a cavity is created in the position of the vagina and lined with meshed split skin on a mould. The initial complication rate is high as the the skin fails to take in about 65% of patients. Most will require at least one revision procedure and final surgery is best left until after puberty. About 75% of patients are able to have intercourse (and some of the remainder may be unwilling rather than unable). Self-dilatation with a mould is usually needed in periods of sexual inactivity (Hojsgaard and Villadsen, 1995).

A variety of other tissues have been used as free grafts to line a vagina that has been split open longitudinally. Many of the series are small and the results unpredictable (Schober, 1999b).

Schober (1999a), in an extensive review of the literature, questioned not only the validity of the follow-up in terms of critical evaluation of female sexuality but even whether such surgery should be performed in childhood. Although it is correct to evaluate the quality of intercourse as well as possible to decide which technique is the best, it must be remembered that such surgery is only done to enable penetrative intercourse to take place: it might be said that poor intercourse may be better than none at all.

The timing of reconstruction is very important. All of the techniques seem to require some dilatation during childhood. Intestinal vaginas require douching to wash out the mucus. Surgery to enlarge the vagina may be needed at puberty. All of this is done to maintain an organ that, it may be hoped, will not be used for 14 years or more. Perhaps the most compelling argument against surgery in infancy is the risk of neoplasia. In her review, Schober (1999a) identified five patients with squamous cell carcinoma of skin vaginas and four patients with adenocarcinoma of intestinal vaginas between 1927 and 1994. The women were between 25 and 30 years of age and the carcinomas were detected between 8 and 25 years after reconstruction. This makes them very rare cancers and none of the relatively large series of vaginal reconstruction reported any cases. Nonetheless, the risk remains and a good case can be made for deferring elective surgery until a woman can give her own consent.

Fertility

The wide spectrum of adrenal enzyme deficiencies is covered in Chapter 24. Women with 21-hydroxylase deficiency,

Table 23.2. Pregnancies in those with congenital adrenal hyperplasia (CAH) reported in the English literature from 1956 to 1997

	Simple virilizing	Salt wasting	Unspecified	Totals
Women	34	10	18	62
Pregnancies	48	15	28	91
Therapeutic abortion	1	4	6	11
Spontaneous abortion	7	1	5	13
Ectopic pregnancy	1			1
Vaginal delivery of normal child	10	4	2	16
Caesarean delivery of normal child	19	6	14	39
Unspecified delivery of normal child	9			9
Vaginal delivery of CAH child	1			1
Still pregnant at publication			1	1

Source: Adapted from the review by Lo et al. (1999) updated to 1999 (Klingensmith et al., 1977; Lo et al., 1999; Zacharin, 1999).

11β-hydroxylase deficiency and 3β-hydroxylase deficiency are potentially fertile. However, infrequent ovulation compounded by poor compliance with steroid replacement therapy reduces the likelihood of pregnancy. The ovulation rate per cycle is only about 40%, with a good correlation between plasma testosterone and 17-hydroxyprogesterone levels (Premawardhana et al., 1997).

Until the 1980s, although the fertility rate was known to be about 60%, reports of successful pregnancy in salt losers were uncommon (Klingensmith et al., 1977). In a relatively large and unselected series of 80 women (half being salt losers), 40 were having heterosexual intercourse. Fifteen of twenty five with simple virilization had 25 pregnancies producing 20 normal children. In contrast, only 1 of 15 with salt-wasting CAH became pregnant and she had an elective termination (Mulaikal et al., 1987).

It would seem that better steroid management has improved prospects for those with salt-wasting CAH. In a more recent series three of five with salt-wasting CAH and two of three with simple virilizing CAH who were sexually active had eight successful pregnancies (Premawardhana et al., 1997). The outcome of pregnancies in a review of the literature from 1956 to 1997 is shown in Table 23.2 (Lo et al., 1999).

Although fertility is associated with early and optimal management of the endocrine defects, delayed therapy in mild cases can still have a good outcome. In the series of Klingensmith et al. (1977) none of the four patients first treated after 20 years of age were able to conceive. However, mild CAH may be found in women with menstrual dysfunction and clinical evidence of excess androgen. The diagnosis should be considered in short, hirsute women with infrequent or absent menstruation. Initiation of treatment in adult life not only establishes normal menstruation but may allow conception in up to 64% of women (Birnbaum and Rose, 1984; Bissada et al., 1987).

Circulating androgen levels in pregnant women with CAH increase. In some cases, it may be necessary to increase steroid medication (for example to 15 mg per day of prednisolone). Placental aromatase activity has been shown to be normal. As maternal androgens undergo aromatization to oestrogen in the placenta, a female fetus will be protected and her genitalia will be normal (Lo et al., 1999).

Screening

It is possible to screen pregnant women for a fetus with CAH. As the condition occurs in 1 in 14 000 livebirths, it would be difficult to justify universal screening. However, it is caused by a genetic defect (deletion or conversion of CYP21) that may occur in families. Therefore, in pregnancies in high-risk mothers, the defect can be sought for in amniotic fluid. The index case will usually be a CAH child born to the mother. As the inheritance follows an autosomal recessive pattern, the risk of a further CAH baby is 25%.

Techniques for fetal diagnosis are improving with time but are already highly specific. The problem is that treatment of the mother must begin before a confirmed diagnosis is available. In a suspect pregnancy, treatment with oral dexamethasone should be started when pregnancy is confirmed at about the fourth or fifth week of gestation ($20\,\mu g/kg$ pre pregnancy maternal weight in two or three divided doses daily).

Chorionic villus sampling (CVS) can be done at about six weeks. In a series of 31 pregnancies, a correct result was obtained in 30 and one was equivocal (Karaviti et al., 1992). Fetal karyotype should be available at about eight weeks and treatment stopped if the fetus is male. DNA analysis should be available by about 10 weeks when treatment is stopped for unaffected fetuses.

Amniocentesis may be done at about 15 weeks. Karyotype, DNA analysis of amniotic cells and (in women who are not already on dexamethasone) 17α-hydroxprogesterone can be determined by week 20. A correct prenatal diagnosis was made in all of 55 fetuses in 54 pregnancies (including the one that was indeterminate on CVS) in the series of Karaviti et al. (1992).

CVS is considered to be the ideal method as the result is available earlier. However, it is not possible in all obstetric units and in some cases the mother may present too late in pregnancy.

Follow-up has shown that the genitalia of affected and unaffected fetuses, and the growth milestones in childhood are normal. Even treatment started as late as 13 weeks of gestation is effective. This indicates that dexamethasone treatment of the mother allows correct genital development of affected female fetuses and does not damage the genitalia of others when given unnecessarily early in pregnancy while awaiting a diagnosis (Karaviti et al., 1992).

The future

Merely because the outcomes from the psychosexual point of view have been unsatisfactory does not mean that past management of CAH was wrong. The metabolic and structural effects of the single enzyme defect are devastating and, in the case of the salt-losing form, potentially lethal. The damage that is inflicted in utero cannot, in the present state of our knowledge, be undone.

There is no "right answer" to the question of gender assignment at birth. At present, Western society is not sophisticated enough to accept a child of indeterminate gender. Parents, relatives, schools, registrars and government officials demand a declaration. Once made, the declaration is, in all ways, very hard to change. It would be quite difficult to ignore the fact that infants with CAH who are 46,XX are fertile as females but not as males.

It could be said, therefore, that, in this impossibly difficult situation, to make such an individual as "female" as possible is the best form of damage limitation. It is possible that a failure to establish a firm gender identity in infancy would worsen the psychosexual morbidity, even beyond that which is currently found.

The current controversy about gender assignment has raised some most important issues, not least the question that the previously held views on gender assignment cannot be accepted without evidence. It seems correct, on the basis of a doctor's obligation to do no harm, to limit the surgery on the genitalia to that which is necessary for physical health. Where surgery is required on the lower urinary tract, it would be difficult to avoid exteriorizing the vagina even if later enlargement is needed. With even the limited outcome results available today, it is difficult to justify clitoral reduction or radical vaginoplasty in infants.

Box 23.1 Key points

Exstrophy
- The perineal orifices are displaced anteriorly so that the introitus is almost a structure of the lower abdominal wall.
- The labia are not fused anteriorly and the clitoris is bifid.
- The introitus is narrowed and requires, at least, an episiotomy before intercourse can take place.
- The external genitalia should be reconstructed.
- Fertility is normal.
- The incidence of prolapse, amounting to procedentia, is about 50% by adult life and may occur even in the nulliparous woman.
- Prolapse is almost impossible to repair if a hysterectomy has been performed so this should not occur.

Spina bifida
- The incidence of spina bifida is decreasing.
- Patients are poorly informed about sexuality and intercourse.
- Intercourse and orgasm are probably normal if the spinal level is at L2 or below.
- Long-term partnerships are common in spite of continuing incontinence.
- Fertility is probably normal but prophylactic folic acid must be prescribed to limit the risk of the fetus having a neural tube defect.
- Pregnancy and delivery are difficult because of the pelvic deformity.
- The incidence of latex allergy is high.

Urogenital sinus
- The commonest cause is congenital adrenal hyperplasia.
- The development of that which is conventionally thought to be normal female gender behaviour is impaired even with good endocrine control.
- There is controversy at present about the need for, and timing of, feminizing genitoplasty. Surgery in infancy should probably be kept to a minimum. Definitive vaginoplasty should probably be delayed until adolescence.
- There is increasing evidence that clitoral reduction impairs the sexual response: the clitoris should not be removed from infants.
- About 60–80% of women with simple virilizing and 50% of salt-losing women are fertile.

REFERENCES

*Indicates key references.

Alizai N, Thomas D F M, Lilford R J, Batchelor A G G, Johnson N (1999). Feminizing genitoplasty for congenital adrenal hyperplasia: what happens at puberty? *J Urol* 161, 1588–1591.

Arata M, Grover S, Dunne K, Bryan D (2000). Pregnancy outcome and complications in women with spina bifida. *J Reprod Med* 45, 743–748.

Azziz R, Mulaikal R M, Migeon C G, Jones H W, Rock J A (1986). Congenital adrenal hyperplasia: long term results following vaginal reconstruction. *Fertil Steril* 46, 1011–1014.

Bailez M M, Gearhart J P, Migeon C G, Rock J A (1992). Vaginal reconstruction after initial construction of the external genitalia in girls with salt wasting adrenal hyperplasia. *J Urol* 148, 680–684.

Berman J R, Berman L, Goldstein I (1999). Female sexual dysfunction: incidence, pathophysiology, evaluation and treatment options. *Urology* 54, 385–391.

Bernardini R, Novembre E, Lombardi E et al. (1998). Prevalence of and risk factors for latex sensitisation in patients with spina bifida. *J Urol* 160, 1775–1778.

Birnbaum M D, Rose L I (1984). Late onset adrenocortical hydroxylase deficiencies associated with menstrual dysfunction. *Gynecol Obstet* 63, 445–451.

Bissada N K, Sakati N, Woodhouse N J Y, Morcos R R (1987). One stage complete reconstruction of patients with congenital adrenal hyperplasia. *J Urol* 137, 703–705.

Blakeley C R, Mills W G (1981). The obstetric and gynaecological complications of bladder exstrophy and epispadias. *Br J Gynaecol Obstet* 88, 167–173.

Blum R W, Resnick M D, Nelson R, St Germaine A (1991). Family and peer issues among adolescents with spina bifida and cerebral palsy. *Pediatrics* 88, 280–285.

Cartwright D B, Joseph A S, Grenier C E (1993). A self image profile analysis of spina bifida adolescents in Louisiana. *J Louisiana State Med Soc* 145, 394–402.

*Cass A S, Bloom D A, Luxenberg M (1986). Sexual function in adults with myelomeningocele. *J Urol* 136, 425–426.

Chan A, Robertson E F, Haan E A (1993). Prevalence of neural tube defects in South Australia, 1966–91, effectiveness and impact of prenatal diagnosis. *Br Med J* 307, 703–706.

Clemston C A B (1958). Ectopia vesicae and the split pelvis. *J Gynecol Obstet* 65, 973–981.

Costa E M, Mendonca B B, Inacio M, Arnhold I J, Silva F A, Lodovici O (1997). Management of ambiguous genitalia in pseudohermaphrodites: new perspectives on vaginal dilatation. *Fertil Steril* 67, 229–232.

Czeizel A E, Dudas I (1992). Prevention of the first occurrence of neural tube defects by periconceptional vitamin supplementation. *N Engl J Med* 327, 1832–1835.

Dewhurst J, Topliss P H, Shepherd J H (1980). Ivalon sponge hysteropexy for genital prolapse in patients with bladder exstrophy. *Br J Gynaecol Obstet* 87, 67–69.

Diamond M (1996). Sex assignment considerations. *J Sex Res* 22, 161–174.

Dittmann R W, Kappes M E, Kappes M H (1992). Sexual behaviour in adolescent and adult females with congenital adrenal hyperplasia. *Psychoneuroendocrinology* 17, 153–170.

Dorner S (1997). Sexual interest and activity in adolescents with spina bifida. *J Child Psychol Psychiatry* 18, 229–237.

Dutta S C, Franke J J, Fleischer A C, Trusier L, Brock J W (2001). *Pelvic Prolapse in Young Adult Females with Spina Bifida*, pp. 36–37. AUA, New Orleans, MI.

Ehrhardt A A, Meyer-Bahlburg H F L (1981). Effects of prenatal sex hormones on gender related behaviour. *Science* 211, 1312–1318.

Ehrhardt A A, Evers K, Money J (1968). Inflence of androgens and some aspects of sexually dimorphic behaviour in women with the late treated adrenogenital syndrome. *Johns Hopkins Med J* 123, 115–122.

Ellsworth P I, Merguerian P A, Klein R B, Rozycki A A (1993). Evaluation and risk factors of latex allergy in spina bifida patients: is it preventable?. *J Urol* 150, 691–693.

Farkas A G, Shepherd J E, Woodhouse C R J (1993). Hysterosacropexy for uterine prolapse with associated urinary tract abnormalities. *J Gynecol Obstet* 13, 358–360.

Fid J F, Rosenberg P, Rothaus K (1993). The use of tissue expanders in the final reconstruction of the infra pubic midline scar, mons pubis and vulva after bladder exstrophy repair. *Urology* 41, 426–430.

Glass C, Soni B (1999). Sexual problems of disabled patients. *Br Med J* 318, 518–521.

Glassberg K I (1999). Editorial: gender assignment and the paediatric urologist. *J Urol* 161, 1308–1310.

Hendren W H (1986). Repair of cloacal anomalies: current techniques. *J Pediatr Surg* 21, 1159–1176.

Hensle T W, Dean G E (1992). Vaginal replacement in children. *J Urol* 148, 677–679.

Hojsgaard A, Villadsen I (1995). McIndoe procedure for congenital vaginal agenesis: complications and results. *Br J Plastic Surg* 48, 97–102.

Hunt G M (2000). Open spina bifida: outcome for a complete cohort treated unselectively and followed into adulthood. *Dev Med Child Neurol* 32, 108–118.

Kadir R A, Sabin C, Whitlow B, Brockbank E, Economides D (1999). Neural tube defects and periconceptional folic acid in England and Wales: retrospective study. *Br Med J* 319, 92–93.

Karaviti L P, Mercado A B, Mercado M B et al. (1992). Prenatal diagnosis/treatment in families at risk for infants with steroid 21-hydroxylase deficiency (congenital adrenal hyperplasia). *J Steroid Biochem Mol Biol* 41, 445–451.

Klingensmith G J, Garcia S C, Jones H W, Migeon C G, Blizzard R M (1977). Glucocorticoid treatment of girls with congenital adrenal hyperplasia: effects on height, sexual maturation and fertility. *J Pediatr* 90, 996–1004.

Krege S, Walz K H, Hauffa B P, Körner I, Rübben H (2000). Long term follow up of female patients with congenital adrenal hyperplasia from 21-hydroxylase deficiency, with special emphasis on the results of vaginoplasty. *Br J Urol Int* 86, 253–259.

Laurence K M, Beresford A (1975). Continence, friends, marriage and children in 51 adults with spina bifida. *Dev Med Child Neurol* 17(Suppl. 35), 123–128.

Lloyd J (1992). *Folic Acid and the Prevention of Neural Tube Defects*. Department of Health, London.

Lo J C, Schwitzgebel V M, Tyrrell J B et al. (1999). Normal female infants born of mothers with classic congenital adrenal hyperplasia due to 21-hydroxylase deficiency. *J Clin Endocrinol Metab* 84, 930–936.

Marconi F, Messina P, Pavanello P (1993). Cosmetic reconstruction of the mons veneris and lower abdominal wall by skin expansion as the last stage of surgical treatment of bladder exstrophy. *Plastic Reconstruct Surg* 91, 551–555.

Mosely M, Bidder R, Hughes I A (1989). Sex role behaviour and self image in young patients with congenital adrenal hyperplasia. *Br J Sex Med* 16, 72–75.

*MRC Vitamin Study Research Group (1991). Prevention of neural tube defects: results of the MRC vitamin study. *Lancet* 338, 131–135.

*Mulaikal R M, Migeon C G, Rock J A (1987). Fertility rates in female patients with congenital adrenal hyperplasia due to 21-hydroxylase deficiency. *N Engl J Med* 316, 178–182.

Premawardhana L D, Hughes I A, Read G F, Scanlon M F (1997). Longer term outcome in females with congenital adrenal hyperplasia (CAH): the Cardiff experience. *Clin Endocrinol* 20, 690–694.

Raz S, McGuire E J, Erlich R M et al. (1988). Fascial sling to correct male neurogenic sphincter incompetence: the McGuire–Raz approach. *J Urol* 139, 528–531.

Richmond D, Zaharievski I, Bond A (1987). Management of pregnancy in mothers with spina bifida. *Eur J Obstet Reprod Biol* 25, 341–345.

Rietberg C C, Lindhout D (1993). Adult patients with spina bifida cystica: genetic counselling, pregnancy and delivery. *Eur J Obstet Reprod Biol* 52, 63–70.

Rink R R, Adams M (1998). Feminizing genitoplasty: the state of the art. *World J Urol* 16, 212–218.

Sawyer S M, Roberts K V (1999). Sexual and reproductive health in young people with spina bifida. *Dev Med Neurol* 41, 671–675.

Schneck F X, Bellinger M (1993). The innocent cough or sneeze: the harbinger of serious latex allergy in children during bladder stimulation and urodynamics. *J Urol* 150, 687–690.

Schober J M (1999a). Feminising genitoplasty for intersex. In *Paediatric Surgery and Urology: Long Term Outcomes*, Stringer M D, Oldham K T, Mouriquand P D E, Howard E R, eds., pp. 549–558. Saunders, London.

Schober J M (1999b). Quality of life studies in patients with ambiguous genitalia. *World J Urol* 17, 249–252.

Shapiro E, Lepor H, Jeffs R D (1984). The inheritance of the exstrophy/epispadias complex. *J Urol* 132, 308–310.

Shaw G M, Velie E M, Schaffer D (1996). Risk of neural tube defect-affected pregnancies among obese women. *J Am Med Assoc* 275, 1093–1096.

Ship A G, Pelzer R H (1972). Reconstruction of the female escucheon in exstrophy of the bladder. *Plastic Reconstruct Surg* 49, 643–646.

Slijper F M E, Drop S L S, Molenaar J C, de Muinck Keizer-Schrama M P F (1998). Long term psychological evaluation of intersex children. *Arch Sex Behav* 27, 125–144.

Sotiropoulos A, Morishima A, Homsy Y, Lattimer J K (1976). Long term assessment of genital reconstruction in female pseudo-hermaphrodites. *J Urol* 115, 599–601.

Stein R, Fisch M, Bauer H, Hohenfelner R (1995). Operative reconstruction of the external and internal genitalia in female patients with bladder exstrophy or incontinent epispadias. *J Urol* 154, 1002–1007.

Stein R, Hohenfellner K, Fisch M et al. (1996). Social integration, sexual behaviour and fertility in patients with bladder exstrophy – a long term follow up. *Eur J Pediatr* 155, 678–683.

Warne S, Wilcox D T, Ransley P G (2002). Nephro-urological outcome for cloaca patients. *Br J Urol Int* 89(Suppl. 2), 55.

Wild J, Seller M J, Schorah C J, Smithells R W (1994). Investigation of folate intake and metabolism in women who have had two pregnancies complicated by neural tube defects. *Br J Gynaecol Obstet* 101, 197–202.

Woodhouse C R J (1999). Sexual function in congenital anomalies. In *Textbook of Erectile Dysfunction*, Carson C C, Kirby R S, Goldstein I, eds., pp. 613–625. Isis Medical Media, Oxford.

*Woodhouse C R J, Hinsch R (1997). The anatomy and reconstrction of the adult female genitalia in classical exstrophy. Br *J Urol* 79, 618–622.

Woodhouse C R J, Redgrave N G (1996). Late failure of the reconstructed exstrophy bladder. *Br J Urol* 77, 590–592.

Zacharin M (1999). Fertility and its complications in a patient with salt losing congenital adrenal hyperplasia. *J Pediatr Endocrinol Metab* 12, 89–94.

Ziylan H O, Ander A H, Alp T et al. (1996). Latex allergy in patients with spinal dysraphism: the role of multiple surgery. *Br J Urol* 78, 777–779.

*Zucker K J, Bradley S J, Oliver G, Blake J, Fleming S, Hood J (1996). Psychosexual behaviour of women with congenital adrenal hyperplasia. *Horm Behav* 30, 300–318.

24

Congenital adrenal hyperplasia

Gerard S. Conway[1] and Pierre D. E. Mouriquand[2]

[1] Department of Endocrinology, Middlesex Hospital, London
[2] Claude-Bernard University–Lyon I and Hospital Debrousse, Lyon, France

Characteristics of congenital adrenal hyperplasia and medical treatment

GERARD S. CONWAY

Overview of the adrenal gland

The adrenal glands are triangular in shape, measuring $3\,cm \times 5\,cm \times 1\,cm$, and are sited above each kidney. The central adrenal medulla is responsible for production of adrenaline and noradrenaline. This portion of the adrenal may be dysplastic early in the natural history of congenital adrenal hyperplasia (CAH) and in time the hyperplastic cortex takes over and the medulla becomes atrophic (Merke et al., 2000a). Absence of the adrenal medulla is thought to be of no consequence because catecholamines are also produced throughout the nervous system.

The adrenal cortex is responsible for the production of three types of steroid; glucocorticoids (cortisol), mineralocorticoids (aldosterone) and androgens. CAH refers to defects in one of the enzyme steps in the adrenal steroidogenesis pathways, which mediate the alterations to the basic four carbon rings in the substrate cholesterol.

Cholesterol is the substrate for all steroid hormones (Miller, 1991). It is taken up by adrenal cells via receptors for low and high density lipoprotein (LDL and HDL, respectively), the abundance of which is increased by the action of adrenocorticotrophic hormone (ACTH). The scheme of adrenal steroid production is presented in Fig. 24.1. The conversion of cholesterol to cortisol occurs in five stages.

1. Cholesterol side-chain cleavage (cholesterol desmolase; gene designation: *CYP11A1*) is the rate-limiting step in the cortisol pathway. Cholesterol is delivered by StAR protein (steroidogenic acute regulatory protein) to the mitochondria where the side-chain cleavage enzyme is located. The electron transfer process, which results in removal of the side chain at C20, produces the cortisol precursor pregnenolone.

2. 3β-Hydroxysteroid dehydrogenase (3βHSD) converts pregnenolone to progesterone, 17-hydroxyprogesterone to 17-hydroxypregnenolone and dehydroepian-drosterone (DHEA) to androstenedione in the smooth endoplasmic reticulum of the cell.

3. 17-Hydroxylase (gene *CYP17*) catalyses the hydroxylation of pregnenolone and progesterone to their 17-hydroxy counterparts. For products destined for the androgen pathway, *CYP17* is also responsible for 17,20-lyase activity, producing the C19 group of compounds: 17-hydroxypregnenolone to DHEA.

4. 21-Hydroxylase (gene *CYP21*) is responsible for the conversion of 17α-hydroxyprogesterone to 11-deoxycortisol in the cortisol pathway and progesterone to deoxycorticosterone in the mineralocorticoid pathway. Defects in this enzyme are responsible for 90% of cases of CAH.

5. 11β-Hydroxylase makes the final conversion of 11-deoxycortisol to cortisol (gene *CYP11B1*).

All forms of CAH are inherited as autosomal recessive conditions. This chapter will focus on 21-hydroxylase deficiency. The features of the rare forms of CAH are listed in Table 24.1 for reference.

21-Hydroxylase deficiency

Genetics

CAH caused by 21-hydroxylase deficiency is one of the most common inherited diseases, with an incidence of

Paediatric and Adolescent Gynaecology, ed. Adam Balen et al. Published by Cambridge University Press.
© Cambridge University Press 2004.

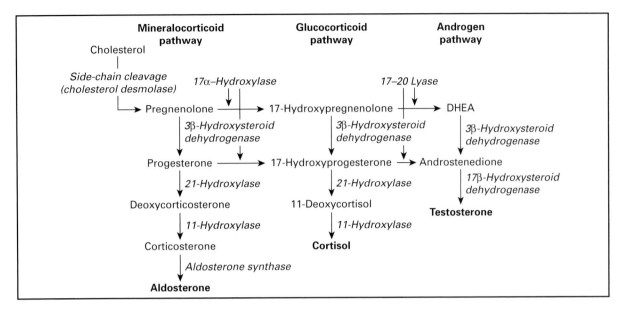

Fig. 24.1. Pathways of adrenal steroid biosynthesis. DHEA, dehydroepiandrosterone.

approximately 1:14 000 births, extrapolating to 4000 individuals in the UK (Rumsby et al., 1992). Carrier status is found in about 1:80 individuals. In some populations, such as Alaskan Eskimos, the incidence of classical CAH is raised threefold, and in others, such as Jews of Eastern European decent, there is a higher incidence of mild gene mutations leading to nonclassical CAH.

The reason why CAH is so common is related to the unusual gene structure (White and Speiser, 2000). The gene for 21-hydroxylase (*CYp21*) is located on chromosome 6 in the middle of the histocompatibility (HLA) complex (Fig. 24.2). There are two adjacent copies of the gene – an active copy and an inactive copy – a "pseudo-gene". Most of the mutations causing 21-hydroxylase deficiency are the result of malalignment of these two similar genes during recombination at meiosis. This malalignment can either cause genetic material to be deleted from the active 21-hydroxylase gene or it can cause the insertion of pseudo-gene material into the active gene sequence (gene conversion). Depending on the genetic background of the local population, as many as 20% of individuals with CAH may appear to have no detectable mutation at routine screening.

Pathophysiology

The diminished function of the 21-hydroxylase enzyme results in cortisol deficiency, which, in turn, causes an increase in ACTH secretion through lack of negative feedback by cortisol to the pituitary and hypothalamus (Auchus, 2001). The raised circulating ACTH concentration upregu-lates LDL and HDL receptors in the adrenal gland, as well as transcription of the side-chain cleavage enzyme, which is normally the rate-limiting step in cortisol production. The cortisol precursors proximal to the 21-hydroxylase block are substrates for the androgen pathway and their accumulation increases the drive to androgen production. The goal of treatment, therefore, is to replace glucocorticoid, suppressing ACTH and removing the excess drive to androgen production.

When the loss of 21-hydroxylase enzyme activity is severe, aldosterone is also lacking, causing a chain of events: salt wasting, volume depletion, hypotension, reduced renal blood flow and raised plasma renin activity. Aldosterone is replaced with fludrocortisone, which allows normal sodium retention; the effectiveness of this therapy can be measured by the suppression of plasma renin activity to the normal range.

Diagnosis of congenital adrenal hyperplasia

Plasma 17-hydroxyprogesterone concentration
17-Hydroxyprogesterone is the cortisol precursor immediately proximal to the 21-hydroxylase block. It is unambiguously raised in severe forms of CAH and can be measured on heel prick samples taken for population screening for phenylketonuria and hypothyroidism (Clague and Thomas, 2002); this analysis is not routine in the UK. In milder forms of CAH, measurements of circulating concentrations of 17-hydroxyprogesterone might overlap with the normal range and greater discrimination can be

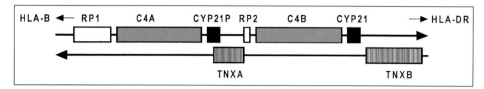

Fig. 24.2. The region on chromosome 6p21.3 to show duplication of genes. CYP21, 21-hydroxylase gene; CYP21P, 21-hydroxylase pseudo gene; RP1 and RP2, genes encoding a nuclear protein and a truncated counterpart, respectively; TNXB and TNXA, tenascin-X gene and a truncated counterpart, respectively.

Table 24.1. Synopsis of the rare forms of congenital adrenal hyperplasia

Enzyme deficiency (Gene)	Clinical picture
11β-Hydroxylase deficiency (*CYP11B1*)	Virilization is similar to 21-hydroxylase deficiency but salt wasting does not occur. 11-Deoxycortisol, which has mineralocorticoid activity, accumulates, causing hypertension as early as 2 years of age
Aldosterone synthase deficiency (*CYP11B2*)	Only the production of aldosterone is affected; individuals present with salt wasting
17α-Hydroxylase deficiency (*CYP17*)	This enzyme block caused deficiency of cortisol, androgens and oestrogen. Increased adrenocorticotrophic hormone drives the mineralocorticoid pathway. Deoxycorticosterone causes hypertension and hypokalaemic alkalosis; corticosterone prevents symptomatic cortisol deficiency. 46,XX females fail to enter puberty with raised gonadotrophins. Affected 46,XY individuals are feminized without a uterus
3β-Hydroxysteroid dehydrogenase deficiency (*HSD3B2*)	This proximal block in the steroid pathway leads to lack of cortisol, aldosterone, potent androgens and oestrogen, resulting in salt-wasting, mild female virilization and undervirilized males. Late-onset forms also occur
StAR protein deficiency (lipoid hyperplasia) (*STAR*)	Severe deficiency of all steroid groups. Both 46,XX and 46,XY have a female external appearance: genetic males have no uterus

offered with measurements during a synacthen test, using 250 μg synthetic ACTH. A cut-off of 30 pmol/l has been defined, above which the diagnosis of late-onset CAH can be made.

Urinary steroid profile with gas chromatography and mass spectrometry

The abundance of various steroid precursors and metabolites can be shown in the urine with gas chromatography and mass spectroscopy. In 21-hydroxylase deficiency, there is a characteristic change in the chromatography profile, with peaks representing the build-up of steroid precursors analogous to 17-hydroxyprogesterone and pregnenolone.

Genetic screening

While mutation screening of *CYP21* is available, because of a significant false-negative rate in mutation detection (approximately 10–20%), genetic definition of CAH cannot be taken as definitive (Krone et al., 1998). Therefore, the diagnosis is based on the above biochemical measurements and there is no requirement for routine genetic confirmation.

Prenatal genetic diagnosis and treatment is relevant mainly to mothers who have already had one child with CAH and not to women *with* CAH, whose children are at a very low risk of inheriting this recessive condition (New et al., 2001). Dexamethasone is started as early as possible in the at-risk pregnancy while the results of genetic analysis of a chorionic villus sampling is awaited. Dexamethasone is then stopped if male fetuses or females negative for mutation screening are detected. Dexamethasone is chosen because it crosses the placenta and is aimed at suppressing the fetal adrenal. While this strategy is effective in reducing the severity of ambiguous genitalia there is some concern over the long-term safety for children exposed to dexamethasone in utero (Seckl and Miller, 1997; Miller, 1999a).

Clinical spectrum of 21-hydroxylase deficiency throughout life

The typical picture of CAH is variable from the severest classical form, presenting with neonatal salt wasting, to mild androgen excess in women who may present any time from adolescence to the fifth decade with nonclassical or late-onset CAH (White and Speiser, 2000). Intermediate forms of CAH present with virilization mediated by androgen excess in childhood. This spectrum of phenotype is broadly, but not precisely, paralleled by the severity of the mutation in *CYP21*, and the magnitude of deficiency of enzyme activity (Hughes, 1998).

Presentation in early childhood

In simple virilizing CAH, an individual escapes the effect of aldosterone and cortisol deficiency and presents with androgen excess as a child (Bridges et al., 1994). Androgen excess causes accelerated growth but also mediates early closure of the epiphyses, leading to compromised final height. Girls present with enlargement of the clitoris and early appearance of pubic hair. Boys present with early penile enlargement, but with no accompanying testicular development because the source of androgens is adrenal – hence "pseudo" precocious puberty as opposed to true precocious puberty, which arises from testicular androgen production. Because of tall stature and muscular development, boys appear older than their years, causing problems with peer relationships.

Classical congenital adrenal hyperplasia in adolescence

Adolescence is a difficult time for any individual with a chronic disease (Speiser, 2001). Children take particular notice of an unusual appearance, especially if it affects aspects of gender or maturity. Psychological support and support group contact are especially important over this time. In this age group, a girl with CAH may experience hirsutism and obesity. Boys, although generally having an easier time of it, have to adjust to being the tallest in their peer group before puberty, to becoming the shortest as their epiphyses close. Psychological disturbance may often manifest itself in poor compliance.

Various metabolic quirks make the control of CAH through adolescence especially difficult. It has long been recognized that the therapeutic window between suppression of excess androgens and the Cushingoid effect of excess glucocorticoids is very narrow in adolescence. Hence teenage girls may be both hirsute *and* obese. One reason for this is that adolescents metabolize cortisol more quickly than younger children or adults, so that dosing of glucocorticoids may have to be more precise and more frequent (Charmandari et al., 2001).

Once a final height has been attained, boys with CAH tolerate adrenal androgen excess well. As a consequence, compliance is often poor and long-term follow-up neglected in males. Indeed, in our adult CAH clinic at the Middlesex Hospital, the ratio of female to male is approximately 4:1.

Late onset or non-classical congenital adrenal hyperplasia

The mildest form of CAH is almost completely restricted to female presentation with hyperandrogenism (Moran et al., 2000). The late-onset form is fairly distinct from classical CAH in terms of mutation analysis of *CYP21* (Deneux et al., 2001; Rumsby et al., 1998) where the mutation giving rise to V281L predominates (Speiser et al., 2000). Women with late-onset CAH present with hirsutism and oligomenorrhoea and form a subgroup (approximately 1%) of women with polycystic ovary syndrome (PCOS). In fact, a polycystic ovary morphology is present on ultrasound in nearly all individuals with CAH to the eyes of an experienced ultrasonographer. Presumably, the polycystic ovarian morphology develops in response to ovarian androgen excess, or perhaps the result of ACTH-responsive tissue within the ovary analogous to adrenal rests found in the testis (see below). In the 1980s, definition of this subgroup of women with PCOS was thought to be important because treatment with glucocorticoids might be appropriate. In fact, women with late-onset CAH probably do better with conventional ovarian suppression (i.e. the combined oral contraceptive pill) and antiandrogen therapy, so the clinical need for screening for this condition has diminished.

Clinical features

Salt-wasting crisis

In severe mutations, aldosterone synthesis is compromised. The usual presentation is with the salt-wasting crisis, comprising hypotension, hyponatraemia and hyperkalaemia in the first few weeks of life. Aldosterone deficiency is reflected in increased plasma renin activity, resulting from volume depletion.

Ambiguous genitalia

Female fetuses exposed to excess androgens in utero present with enlargement of the clitoris and fusion of the labia, which take on the rugose appearance of the scrotum. Occasionally, masculinization of a female fetus is so complete that assignment of male gender is not questioned and some individuals have survived as 46,XX males only to be diagnosed later in life (Woelfle et al., 2002).

Genital surgery

The spectrum of female genital anatomy varies from minimal clitoral enlargement to a near normal male appearance with a urogenital sinus (UGS). In childhood, clitoral reduction or vaginoplasty might be required. In adolescence there is often need for revision of vaginoplasty. A repeat clitoral reduction should only be required if androgen excess is not controlled. In adults, revision of earlier surgery is occasionally required and dilators are the mainstay of management. There are few little long-term follow-up data on which to base the decision of the timing of genital surgery in CAH (Creighton et al., 2001; Krege et al., 2000; see below).

Gender issues

Issues of gender orientation often cause great concern but are not always addressed in routine clinic appointments. It is commonly documented that girls with CAH demonstrate more "rough and tumble" play and have more male friends than average (Berenbaum et al., 2000; Iijima et al., 2001). It is difficult to assess how these observations translate to adult sexuality (Meyer-Bahlburg, 2001). There are some women with CAH who are more comfortable with bisexual and homosexual relationships but this may, in some cases, have more to do with their concerns about the appearance of their genitalia, with feelings of vulnerability and apprehension of a sexual relationship with men.

In all women, testosterone levels can affect libido, although this effect is very unpredictable (Ehrhardt et al., 1968). Some women with CAH find that when testosterone levels are high, sex drive is increased. Reducing testosterone with a higher dose of cortisol treatment can reduce excessive sex drive. A low libido is a more difficult problem as it is rarely improved by changing the dose of treatment: counselling might be an answer here. (see also Chs. 14 and 37).

Fertility

Most women with CAH have polycystic ovaries on ultrasonography compared with the 25% of women without CAH who would be expected to have polycystic morphology (McKenna and Cunningham, 1995). It may be that high levels of testosterone in childhood cause the development of polycystic ovaries in some women but this is far from certain. Clearly adrenal testosterone can induce menstrual irregularity and anovulation, which can improve with higher doses of glucocorticoid but the balance of treatment in this instance can be very difficult.

Menstrual irregularity occurs in about 30% of women with non-salt-losing CAH and 50% of women with salt-losing CAH compared with 10% of women without CAH (Gordon, 1999). There is surprisingly little information about fertility in women with CAH and most of our knowledge on this subject comes from a time before modern fertility treatments. These "historical" data state that two-thirds of women with non-salt-losing CAH are fertile without the need for treatment whereas only 10% of women with salt-losing CAH are fertile (Krone et al., 2001; Meyer-Bahlburg, 1999; Mulaikal et al., 1987). Most specialists feel that the current prospects for fertility are better than these

figures would indicate (Miller, 1999b). If a woman with CAH has very irregular periods, then it is likely that specialist fertility treatment will be required. On the whole, fertility treatments will be the same as for women without CAH, with clomiphene citrate being the first choice and gonadotrophins or in vitro fertilization for resistant cases.

One point of detail that is often missed is the effect of moderately raised serum progesterone concentrations. In poorly controlled CAH, progesterone will accumulate in the same way as its 17-hydroxy counterpart. This has the effect of acting like a progesterone-only oral contraceptive, causing failure of implantation even if ovulation is induced (Holmes-Walker et al., 1995). Suppression of progesterone may require higher doses of glucocorticoid than average and in some instances can be very difficult to achieve.

For women with late-onset CAH, fertility problems are usually less marked. In the mildest forms, steroid treatment might be necessary in order to conceive but it may be possible to stop this treatment in pregnancy.

Pregnancy

Once pregnant, both the mother with CAH and her child should expect to be healthy in every way. Both glucocorticoid and mineralocorticoid doses may need to be increased in pregnancy, and labour must be covered with parenteral hydrocortisone. Placental aromatase converts testosterone to oestradiol, protecting the fetus from androgen excess, and destroys any excess hydrocortisone in the circulation. In a recent review of children born to mothers with CAH, all babies were healthy and normal (Lo et al., 1999). Two-thirds of babies were delivered by caesarean section and only one-third by vaginal delivery. One of the many reasons for caesarean sections may be related to concerns over earlier genital surgery. It is useful to evaluate genital scar tissue before pregnancy to inform women of the chances of a vaginal delivery (see below).

Congenital adrenal hyperplasia in men

The problems of weight gain and the side effects of treatment can affect men as much as women but are usually less, so the suppression of adrenal androgen excess is less critical in men. Short stature, which can result from difficulties in treatment of CAH in childhood, can be a particular psychological burden for men. High levels of testosterone in CAH can cause problems with aggression and excessive sex drive in men.

There are two important long-term consequences of CAH that only affect men, both of which are the result of too little treatment with cortisol. These are infertility and testicular enlargement. If adrenal suppression is inadequate, then high adrenal testosterone production will cause suppression of secretion of luteinizing hormone (LH) and follicle-stimulating hormone (FSH). The testes are then shut down, with suppression of spermatogenesis. Sperm production usually picks up if the glucocorticoid doses are increased. It can take several months for the sperm count to rise and occasionally oligospermia is not reversible (Murphy et al., 2001).

Testicular enlargement results from inadequate glucocorticoid treatment and it takes many years to occur (Cabrera et al., 2001; Stikkelbroeck et al., 2001). Normal testes contain a few adrenal cells with ACTH receptors. These cells can undergo hypertrophy under relentless ACTH drive. This enlargement is usually reversible if the dose of glucocorticoid is increased. Occasionally, urologists advise a biopsy of the enlarged testis because the condition mimics malignancy. Even though there is no documented increased risk of testicular cancer in CAH, it is reassuring to make this check.

Long-term outcomes

Life expectancy after the age of four appears to be normal (Swerdlow et al., 1998) and quality of life is well preserved (Jääskeläinen and Voutilainen, 2000). Some have recorded diminished bone mineral density resulting from excessive glucocorticoid treatment (Gussinye et al., 1997; Paganini et al., 2000) although adjustment for height has not always been conducted in these studies. Risk markers for coronary heart disease are not greatly disturbed (Botero et al., 2000).

Perhaps the most worrying long-term event in CAH is the appearance of adrenal tumours (Merke et al., 1999). Many anecdotal reports have raised this issue, but the prevalence of adrenal tumours is not yet clear in screening studies.

Treatment

Glucocorticoids

Three glucocorticoids are in general use. Dexamethasone, the most potent, is most likely to cause iatrogenic Cushing's syndrome (Table 24.2). Hydrocortisone, the shortest acting, often requires three divided doses, which in adolescents might increase the likelihood for poor compliance. Prednisolone, intermediate in both potency and half-life, may be optimal for many teenagers. Cortisone acetate is less readily available in the UK but is used widely in Europe; its potency is similar to that of hydrocortisone.

In childhood, dosage is titrated to growth velocity and body surface area (Merke and Kabbani, 2001). In adults, monitoring against blood levels of adrenal and reproductive hormones is required.

Table 24.2. Relative strengths of glucocorticoids

	Potency relative to hydrocortisone	Average daily dose (mg)
Hydrocortisone	1	20–30
Cortisone acetate	0.8	25–37.5
Prednisolone	5	5–10
Dexamethasone	40	0.5–0.75

In females, the androgens androstenedione and testosterone are probably the best parameters to follow. Androstenedione has the advantage of not being bound to sex hormone-binding globulin (SHBG), which can confound measurements of testosterone particularly in obese subjects where SHBG is low. 17-Hydroxyprogesterone, though commonly measured, is variable by the hour, which limits its value as random measurements of 17-hydroxyprogesterone can only be interpreted with precise knowledge of the timing of the previous dose of glucocorticoid.

In males, where testicular androgen production is proportionately greater, testosterone measurements are less useful although testosterone may be frankly raised. A more sensitive marker is suppression of LH and FSH by testosterone. Monitoring with gonadotrophins in men is also logical, as it is relevant to one of the late effects of CAH in males: spermatogenesis.

Fludrocortisone

The main issue for fludrocortisone replacement in the adolescent is that the requirement for this hormone diminishes quite sharply through teenage years. This phenomenon is a reflection of a general escape from salt requirement found in adults. For example, individuals with aldosterone resistance commonly escape the need for salt supplements in adult life. Indeed, with the increasing risk of hypertension in adults, it is generally safer to aim for slight underdosage with fludrocortisone than the converse. Excessive doses of fludrocortisone are reflected by suppression of plasma renin activity, hypokalaemia and hypertension. For this reason, it is our goal in management to aim for a plasma renin activity measurement in the upper end of the normal range.

Oral contraceptives

For a proportion of women with classical CAH, a regular menstrual cycle cannot be achieved without inducing Cushing's syndrome. In this situation, combined ovarian and adrenal suppression might be required, using the combined oral contraceptive. However, there is no evidence that the amenorrhoea associated with CAH might be sinister, in that endometrial hyperplasia is prevented by the raised concentration of progesterone in CAH. Indeed, progesterone hypersecretion can be very difficult to suppress in rare individuals and its endometrial effect analogous to the progesterone-only oral contraceptive can be insurmountable. At this centre, a nonsuppressible progesterone hypersecretion is an indication for adrenalectomy in those women seeking fertility.

Antiandrogens

Because of the difficulty in suppressing androgen excess without inducing Cushing's syndrome, there is logic in using antiandrogen blockade, allowing higher levels of circulating testosterone and lower doses of glucocorticoids (Merke et al., 2000b). Cyproterone acetate has been used for this indication but has a tendency to compound weight gain. Flutamide, although with a greater hepatotoxicity, is the antiandrogen of choice, being the most potent. In the experience of this centre, spironolactone and finasteride are not sufficiently potent for this indication.

Adrenalectomy

There is no consistent agreement as to the indication for adrenalectomy, which has occasionally been reported in CAH (Gmyrek et al., 2002). The difficulty comes with the fact that poor compliance is often a part of the failure of medical treatment. Poor compliance with glucocorticoids after adrenalectomy, however, may be life threatening, and there are anecdotal reports of death following adrenalectomy. However, adrenalectomy will convert an individual with CAH to one with Addison's disease, which is generally much easier to manage, particularly in a woman with intractable amenorrhoea and hyperandrogenism.

An adult congenital adrenal hyperplasia clinic

A clinic dedicated to CAH benefits from a multidisciplinary structure. Endocrinology, psychology, gynaecology and sex therapy all have a place and it is efficient to provide these in a one-stop service if possible. In addition, clinical nurse specialists are often best at providing support for the use of dilators and support groups can add pastoral care and advise on the structure of service provision.

In order to illustrate the management of adults with CAH we present here a profile of a single centre clinic. The Middlesex Hospital Adult CAH Clinic comprises 113 individuals aged between 17 and 73 (mean age 32). The distribution of the various subtypes of CAH is representative of their relative frequencies in most quoted series (Table 24.3).

Table 24.3. The types of congenital adrenal hyperplasia seen at the Middlesex Clinic

CAH subtype	No.
21-Hydroxylase deficiency	102
Classical salt wasting	59
Non-salt wasting	21
Late onset	22
11-Hydroxylase deficiency	4
17-Hydroxylase/17–20, lyase deficiency	3
3β-Hydroxysteroid dehydrogenase deficiency	2
StAR protein deficiency	2

Interestingly, only 27 (24%) of attendees are male, suggesting that many men become lost to follow-up in adult life.

One of the main outcomes of paediatric care is final height (Eugster et al., 2001; New, 2001). The mean (SD) height was reduced in women to 1.55 m (0.06) and men 1.67 m (0.07). There was no increase in final height in those of younger age to suggest that there had been any change in treatment outcome in recent years. There was no difference in final height between the three subtypes of 21-hydroxylase deficiency. Women tended to be more obese than men (mean body mass indices 27.1 and 25.7 kg/m^2, respectively).

The type of glucocorticoid use was hydrocortisone 42%, prednisolone 33% and dexamethasone 23%. The median daily dosage of glucocorticoids in hydrocortisone equivalents (Table 24.2) was 35 mg (range, 15–150) on arrival in clinic and fell to 25 mg (range, 15–40) over 1 year. The mean serum 17-hydroxyprogesterone at first visit was 65 pmol/l (range, 1–337; normal $<$ 20 pmol/l) and in women serum testosterone values were 3.4 nmol/l (range, 0.2–19.9; normal range, 0.7–3.7 nmol/l). There was no correlation between the recorded dose of glucocorticoid and the endocrine parameters, suggesting that compliance was a major determinant. A reduction in the dosage of glucocorticoid in women was achieved with the introduction of antiandrogens in 35% of women and in four who underwent bilateral adrenalectomy.

The median daily dosage of fludrocortisone in the salt-wasting subgroup was 200 µg (range, 25–300) falling to 150 µg (range, 25–200) after 1 year. The mean ambulant plasma renin activity was 8.2 pmol/l per h (range, 1.0–17.3) at first visit (normal range 0.8–4.3 pmol/l per h).

Control of symptoms in women can be measured in terms of menstrual cycle and hyperandrogenism. Too few had challenged fertility to provide a meaningful figure for this end point. With regard to menstrual cycle, 34% were amenorrhoeic, 26% oligomenorrhoeic and 39% achieved a normal menstrual cycle. With regard to hirsutism, 69% had minimal excess hair and 31% described hirsutism as an ongoing problem.

Surgical management of congenital adrenal hyperplasia

PIERRE D. E. MOURIQUAND

CAH is the most frequent cause of genital ambiguity in female children. The 21-hydroxylase deficiency (see above) is the most common enzyme defect described in this group of patients and represents 1 case for 12 500 births (Pang, 1997).

Beside the metabolic and endocrine disorders of CAH that require specific paediatric care from birth onwards, patients with CAH should be assessed and managed by the paediatric urologist from early childhood to improve the cosmetic appearance of the genital area and to provide a potentially normal sexual function during adulthood. The management of these patients requires a close collaboration between paediatric endocrinologists and surgeons.

There is no consensus about the surgical approach to CAH as some surgeons prefer to delay vaginoplasty until later in life while others favour a complete genital reconstruction during the first few months of life.

We exclude from this chapter 46,XX patients with CAH raised as male and 46,XY patients with CAH; neither will we describe surgery of adrenal glands, which has been discussed in some specific situations (Gunther et al., 1997; van Wyk et al., 1996).

Anatomy of congenital adrenal hyperplasia

The urogenital sinus

CAH is characterized by an abnormal confluence of the vagina and urethra (Figs. 24.3 and 24.4a (colour plate)). The vaginal cavity joins the posterior wall of the urethra at any level between the bladder neck (high UGS) and the very distal urethra (low UGS). Usually the higher the sinus, the smaller the vaginal cavity. UGS should be distinguished from female hypospadias, which is a rare malformation where the female urethra joins the anterior wall of the vagina at any level between the upper and lower part of the vagina. In severe female hypospadias, the urethra is often atretic as well as the bladder neck (Knight et al., 1995).

The penoclitoral organ

The clitoris is almost always enlarged and sometimes as big as a male child's penis (Fig. 24.4b, colour plate). The more

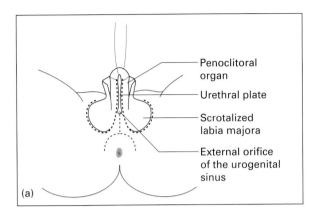

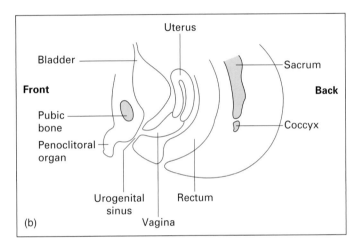

Fig. 24.3. Anatomy of congenital adrenal hyperplasia. (a) Perineum and incision lines (dotted line). (b) Sagittal anatomy of the pelvis.

virilized the child is, the longer is the urethral canal. Four elements need to be carefully identified: (i) the glans (i.e. the clitoris itself), (ii) the dorsal neurovascular bundle, (iii) the two corpora cavernosa, and (iv) the urethral plate. The glans will be preserved with its dorsal neurovascular bundle but the two corpora cavernosa will be removed. The urethral plate is abnormally long, extending from the orifice of the UGS up to the glans base. This excess of urethral tissue can be most useful to connect the anterior wall of the vagina to the perineum in those with high UGS (see below Passerini's technique).

The labia majora

The two labia majora are "scrotalized" (i.e. they look like scrotums separated in the midline by the urethral plate). There can be quite a lot of redundant, pigmented and crumpled tissue at this site.

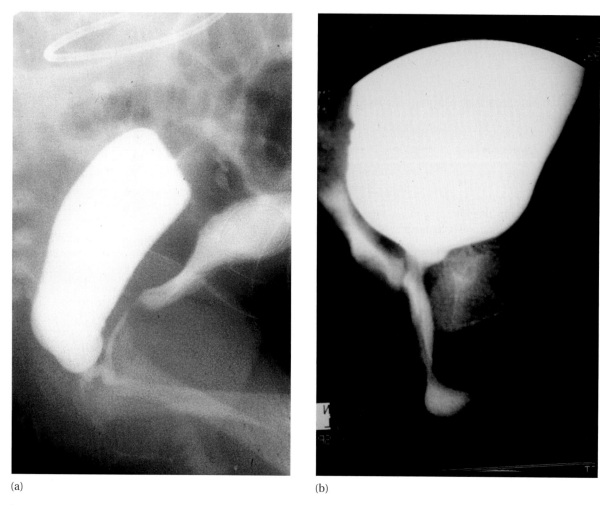

(a)   (b)

Fig. 24.5. Radiography in urogenital sinus. (a) Low urethrovaginal confluence; (b) high urethrovaginal confluence.

Principles of genital surgery

Although both medical monitoring and surgical techniques have improved substantially since the 1980s, genitoplasty for CAH is a difficult procedure that requires extensive experience and a highly specialized paediatric service. This explains why patients with CAH, along with all intersex patients, should be referred to specialized institutions. Surgery includes three main steps:

- opening of the vaginal cavity to the pelvic floor (vaginoplasty), which is definitely the most difficult part of the whole procedure as the vaginal "cul de sac" can be quite high (high UGS)
- reduction of the clitoral size, which is combined with anchoring of the preserved glans (i.e. clitoris) to the underlying deeper structures
- lowering of the two labia majora and the perineoplasty, which is important for the cosmetic appearance.

Patient age for surgery

Surgical repair is commonly programmed between 2 and 6 months of age, mainly for psychological reasons both for the parents and for the child. It is quite traumatic for the mother to see her daughter's abnormal genitalia at each nappy change. It is also believed that a nearly normal appearance of the external genitalia is important for the child to complete her "sexual identity"; the multifactorial determination of sexual identity, however, remains poorly understood. (See also Chs. 17 and 23 for further discussion of this controversy.) As detailed below, some surgeons prefer to defer vaginoplasty until puberty and restrict the procedure to a perineoplasty during the first few months of life.

Steroid supplementation

Adrenal function and steroid supplementation need to be carefully monitored before, during and after surgery as the procedure itself is an additional stress factor for the child (see the earlier part of this chapter).

Bowel preparation

Bowel preparation may be indicated if a vaginal substitution is planned.

Preoperative endoscopic and radiological assessment

The question to answer before starting the procedure is: How high is the UGS? To answer it, the child needs to be anaesthetized and examined both with a urethrocystoscope and a X-ray contrast study of the UGS (Fig. 24.5). In some cases, a Fogarty balloon catheter can be placed into the vaginal cavity, which will help its identification during the dissection.

Vaginoplasty with low urogenital sinus

Classical perineal approach

The classical perineal approach is illustrated in Figs. 24.3 and 24.6 (Hughes and Mouriquand, 1995; Mollard et al., 1990): the child is placed in a dorsal lithotomy position. A balloon bladder catheter is placed into the bladder. An inverted U-shaped incision line is outlined on the perineum (Fortunoff et al., 1964). The apex of the "U" is where the vaginal introitus should be. A midline incision is made

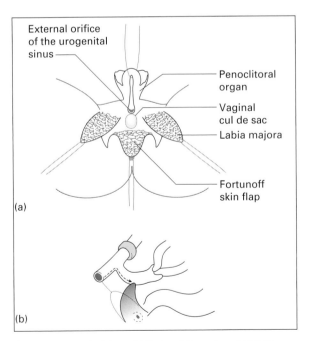

Fig. 24.6. Urogenital sinus. (a) Perineal dissection. (b) Midline sagittal opening and reconstruction of the posterior sagittal wall using the Fortunoff flap.

between the orifice of the UGS and the apex of the "U". Laterally the incision line follows the edges of the labia majora. The border between the labial tissue and the adjacent skin is very well defined (pigmented and crumpled labial surface). Anteriorly to the orifice of the UGS, the incision line follows the edges of the urethral plate. The incision line on the penoclitoral organ will be detailed below. An electric current section (diathermy) is used for all the skin incisions on the perineum because it is much neater and bloodless. The inverted U-shaped skin flap is freed with a substantial amount of underlying fat and held downward with a stay suture. The vertical midline incision opens the UGS and very often, in those with low UGS, allows the identification of the vaginal "cul de sac". The vagina is opened widely. Its posterior edge is sutured to the apex of the U-shaped skin flap, creating the posterior connection of the vagina to the pelvic floor. The mucosal anterior wall of the vagina remains in continuity with the distal mucosal posterior edge of the urethral meatus. On each side, the labia majora are extensively freed with their fatty tissue, being kept connected anteriorly only by two bridges of skin. They are both moved downwards and their apex is sutured to the low extremity of each vertical branch of the "U". The lateral walls of the vagina can then be sutured to the medial edges of each labia majora. A Jelonet mesh is left within the vagina for a couple of days.

Total urogenital sinus mobilization

Total urogenital sinus mobilization (Fig 24.7) was originally described by Peña in 1997 and aims at mobilizing the entire common urethrovaginal conduit (i.e. the UGS) until the junction between the urethra and vagina is exteriorized. The UGS is then excised and the urethral and vaginal edges sutured to the perineum. The operation originally described for cloacal malformations was subsequently used for UGS surgery (Jenak et al., 2001; Ludwikowski et al., 1999;

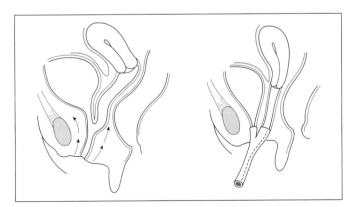

Fig. 24.7. Total urogenital sinus mobilization.

Rink and Yerkes, 2001). For this procedure, it is necessary that there is a short UGS (≤ 3 cm) and that the proximal urethra is adequate (Ludwikowski et al., 1999). Rink (2000) advised that it is useful to keep the mobilized UGS mucosal tissue instead of excising it as it can be opened on the ventral side and used to create a mucosa-lined vestibule. This operation can also be combined with a vaginal pull through procedure (see Passerini's procedure, below). Reserves were expressed by Hendren (2000) about this technique in case the vagina enters at either an intermediate or a high level, as he feared that mobilizing the vagina and UGS together, while amputating the distal UGS, might create a short urethral segment between the new vaginal opening and the bladder neck. This could increase the frequency of coitus-induced cystitis, which is known to be severe and more frequent in this group of patients. One should also be aware that urinary incontinence might be an issue later in some of these patients if the mobilization is too extensive.

Vaginoplasty with high urogenital sinus
Since the traditional perineal approach of high UGS described by Hendren and Crawford in 1969, several other techniques have been described to facilitate vaginal exposure and mobilization.

The Passerini procedure
The Passerini procedure is described in Figs. 24.8 and 24.9 (colour plate; Passerini-Glazel, 1989, 1998, 1999). After inserting a Fogarty balloon catheter into the vaginal cavity and placing a Foley catheter into the bladder, the incision is performed as above and the UGS is approached. The posterior wall of the urethra is dissected upwards making a large window through the fibers of the elevator ani. This wide space is important to avoid later vaginal stenosis by outer constriction. The confluence is then approached knowing that there is often no clear cleavage plane between the vagina and the urethra. It is, therefore, often

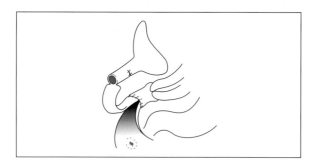

Fig. 24.8. Passerini's procedure.

necessary to open longitudinally the vaginal "cul de sac" where the Fogarty balloon can be felt. The junction between the urethra and the vagina is identified and the vagina can then be safely separated from the urethra. The posterior longitudinal incision should be generously extended to maximize the vaginal opening and reduce the risk of subsequent intrinsic vaginal stenosis. The next step is the clitoral reduction (see below) preserving intact the UGS tissues whose dorsal aspect is incised longitudinally down to the apex of the inverted "U" at the level of the future site of the urethral meatus. The V-shaped mucosal flap obtained is sutured to the base of the reduced clitoris while the remaining portion of the split UGS hangs down. The dorsal phallic skin is incised longitudinally down to its base, producing two rectangular flaps. These are rotated down and their medial edges are sutured to the lateral edges of the opened UGS. A wide rectangle is created with its central portion represented by the mucosal aspect of the split UGS. The combined phallic and UGS flaps are then progressively sutured to the vagina starting from the 12 o'clock position. A Fortunoff-type flap previously created from the perineal skin is then sutured at 6 o'clock to the vagina, completing the posterior wall of the distal vagina. In very severe cases when the vaginal cavity cannot be detached from the urethral wall, a transtrigonal detachment of the vagina can be performed and the reconstruction of the anterior vaginal wall can be performed as above using the transtrigonal exposure.

Variants of this technique using two lateral skin flaps have been described when the child has already had a previous clitoral reduction with no penile skin available (Parrott and Woodard, 1991).

The posterior sagittal approach
Following Peña's (1989) experience of cloacal anomalies, a high UGS can be approached through a posterior sagittal midline approach starting from the tip of the coccyx (which can be removed in severe cloacal anomalies) down to the orifice of the UGS through the rectum (Peña et al., 1992) with or without colostomy (Figs. 24.10 and 24.11 (colour plate)). Rink et al. in 1997 described a similar technique without division of the rectal wall. The penoclitoral surgery is performed first (see below) preserving the urethral plate and the penile skin for potential use as the anterior flap to the separated vagina (see Passerini's procedure). Rink and coworkers (Adams and Rink, 1998; Rink et al., 1997) then advocated the prone position with the legs spread and pelvis elevated on rolls. The U-shaped incision described above is the same, as is the midline dissection between the rectum and the UGS. As dissection proceeds, the rectum

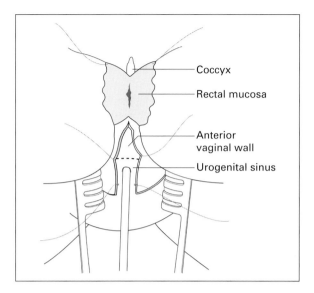

Fig. 24.10. Posterior sagittal approach to the urogenital sinus.

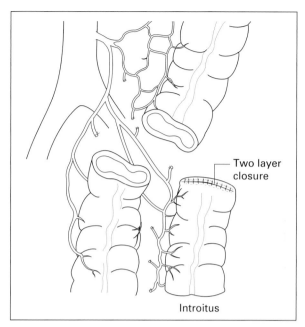

Fig. 24.12. Colovaginoplasty using the sigmoid colon.

is retracted with a Deavor retractor and does not require incision or division. The UGS is opened posteriorly in the midline from the meatus to the vaginal confluence. The distal atretic vagina is opened on its posterior aspect into the more normal proximal vagina. The anterior wall of the vagina is dissected away from the proximal urethra and bladder. This position also provides excellent vision for tubularization of the urethra, which is done in several layers with fine resorbable sutures over a Foley catheter. Healthy fatty tissue can be brought from either side together in the midline to separate the urethra and the vagina. The posterior perineal flap is sutured to the opened posterior vagina. When a preputial flap is available, it is sutured to the opened anterior vagina. If not available, a labial flap is constructed to reach the anterior vagina. This flap may be developed on either side.

Bowel vaginal replacement

In rare cases, the residual vaginal cavity is too small to be connected to the pelvic floor and a vaginal substitution appears necessary to bridge the gap. Paediatric urologists much favour intestinal substitution (Fig. 24.12) to replace the vagina rather than using local perineal skin flaps or other techniques, as they believe that regular vaginal dilatations (needed with the latter technique) are particularly badly accepted by children. The technique consists in isolating a short segment (10–20 cm) of either ileum or sigmoid colon. The mesentery of this bowel segment is extensively dissected upwards in order to connect this neovagina with minimal tension. Ileum is favoured by some for

infants whereas sigmoid colon is preferred for vaginal reconstruction in adolescents (Hensle et al., 1998; Hitchcock and Malone, 1994; Tillem et al., 1998; Wesley and Coran, 1992).

Other surgeons (Patil and Mathews, 1995) have suggested a composite vaginoplasty using bowel for the proximal vagina and expanded skin with tissue expanders.

Other types of vaginal substitution

1. *Vaginal tract without skin graft.* Creating a vaginal tract by dissecting a perineal pouch or space between bladder and rectum was originally described by Dupuytren in 1817 (Schober, 1999). This procedure regained popularity in 1994 when Jackson and Rosenblatt (see Schober, 1999) reported four patients in which Intercede, an absorbable adhesion barrier, was placed over a mould to create the cavity. Good results were reported in all four. However, all patients had to use the mould continuously for three to six months after surgery and for 15 minutes, three times a day thereafter.

2. *Split-thickness grafts.* These were developed by Counsellor and by McIndoe (cited in Schober, 1999). This technique requires a transperineal incision to provide space between the bladder and the rectum. A mould covered with a split-thickness skin graft is then placed. Regular dilatations are needed to keep the vaginal cavity patent. These vaginoplasties require lubrication. The satisfaction rate

has been reported as high as 90% in the sexually active population (cited in Schober, 1999).

3. *Skin flap vaginoplasty*. This technique moves skin flaps on a pedicle or base to the operative site. The full-thickness skin flaps can be obtained from the pudendal thigh, fasciocutaneous flap, a rectus abdominus flap, a labial flap or buttock flaps. Although there are very few series published, stenosis, small vaginal size and poor lubrication seem to be a major drawback of these reconstructions, which can only be attempted after puberty.

4. *Vaginoplasties using amnion, peritoneum and bladder mucosa*. These approaches have also been reported (cited in Schober, 1999).

Clitoral reduction

Clitoral reduction is the second step in the classical approach to CAH (Fig. 24.13, colour plate). Continuing the incision previously described for the vaginoplasty, the incision line follows the edges of the urethral plate up to the glans cap. The foreskin and the shaft skin can be both used for the reconstruction of the anterior vaginal wall, as described above in Passerini's technique, but in most cases, we advocate the saddle skin incision on the dorsum of the penis (Mollard et al., 1981). This incision consists of removing the mid-portion of the shaft skin to expose the two corpora cavernosa. The foreskin is carefully preserved to reconstruct the clitoral hood and the labia minora. As described above in the anatomy, the dorsal neurovascular bundle innervating and irrigating the glans (i.e. the clitoris) is carefully dissected off the dorsal aspect of the corpora cavernosa. Fine sharp scissors allow the dissection of this dorsal pedicle starting from the lateral aspect of each corpora. This pedicle is quite broad and represents a large strip of tissue running along the dorsum of the penis. This strip needs to be fully dissected from the glans down to the base of the penis. On the ventral side of the penis, the urethral plate is also lifted off from the ventral aspect of the corpora cavernosa from the glans cap down to the perineum. Once this dissection is completed, a vascular clamp is placed at the base of both corpora cavernosa along their pubic bone attachments. The penile portion of the corpora is excised keeping their distal ends attached to the glans. The remaining distal segments of corpora are then anastomosed to the crura and the clamp is removed. The glans is then deeply anchored to the inner surface of the symphysis and the adjacent perineal tissues. The dorsal aspect of the foreskin is sutured to the pubic skin reconstituting the clitoral hood. The lateral aspects of the foreskin are sutured to each side of the urethral plate mimicking the labia minora.

Other authors (Glassberg and Laungani, 1981) have advocated the use of corporeal plication to reduce the size of the penoclitoral organ. The long-term results of these procedures are unsatisfactory, with insufficient clitoral reduction and pain at erection.

Labial plasty

Once the vagina is connected to the pelvic floor and the penoclitoral organ reduced in size, both labia majora are lowered giving a more normal female appearance to the whole perineum (Fig. 24.13h colour plate).

Postoperative care

The Foley catheter is kept in place for 7 to 10 days. The vaginal mesh is removed on the second postoperative day. Antibiotic cover is advised during the procedure and continued for a few days.

Spraying local antiseptics (aqueous chlorhexidine) on the perineal wound is recommended at each nappy change in order to keep the area perfectly clean. The clitoral hood often becomes dusky or black and oedematous a few hours after surgery, but a few days later its appearance comes back to normal. Postoperative vaginal dilatations are no longer recommended as they are very poorly accepted by both parents and the child.

Outcome of surgery

There are few data concerning the long-term outcomes of the procedures used for female genitoplasty.

The cosmetic appearance of the perineum

In our experience, clitoral reduction, lowering of the labia majora and perineoplasty gives average to good long-term cosmetic results (Fig. 24.14, colour plate). However, the clitoris is often too big and sticks out because it is not sufficiently anchored ventrally when erect. Complementary procedures are sometimes needed to reduce the size of the clitoris by excision of a ventral section of spongiform tissue. The strip of urethral mucosa sitting between the base of the clitoris and the urethral opening is often too long, creating a mucosal slide (Fig. 24.15, colour plate). It could be improved by reducing the length of the urethral plate or by plicating it. Complete disasters occur and may result from inappropriate techniques or inexperienced surgeons (Fig. 24.16, colour plate).

The vagina, subsequent sex life and related psychological problems

The vagina, the subsequent sexual life and related psychological problems are the real issues to be considered when assessing the results of this surgery. Most patients will require a vaginal revision at puberty because of a narrow introitus and/or for more extensive reconstruction because of vaginal stricture or vaginal insufficiency. In some cases, the urethral and the vaginal openings look very deeply located and too close. This probably explains the higher incidence of urinary tract infections in this group of patients when they start sexual activity. In patients with vaginal substitution, mucous discharge is a recognized problem but it is generally not thought to be a serious complication. However, diversion colitis has been recently reported in 3 of 18 children who underwent colovaginoplasty (Syed et al., 2001). Local irrigations using a solution of short-chain fatty acids or steroid enemas and mesalazine may help to reduce these unpleasant symptoms. Substitutive vaginoplasties that are too long can lead to chronic inflammation, with severe discharge and bleeding, and may well require subsequent surgical reduction.

Alizai et al. (1999) in Leeds reported disappointing late results in 14 girls who underwent genital reconstruction early in childhood. They highlighted the importance of close follow-up and challenged the prevailing assumption that total correction can be achieved with a single operation in infancy. Although simple exteriorization of a low vagina can reasonably be combined with cosmetic correction of virilized external genitalia in infancy, they believed that in some cases it may be best to defer definitive reconstruction of the intermediate or high vagina until after puberty.

Krege et al. (2000) reported intravaginal stenosis in 9 of 25 patients (36%) and suggested that vaginoplasty should not be performed in infants but only at adolescence.

Creighton (2001) also reported poor results of this surgery with increasing evidence of patient dissatisfaction. She suggested that clinicians working in this field should step back and review their practice. Surgery may not be necessary. We need much more information to allow clinicians and parents to make informed decisions, and for this purpose multicentre research on long-term outcomes is essential (see also Ch. 25). Other authors (Vates et al., 1999) judged the functional, social and psychosexual outcomes of vaginal reconstruction more positively. Mulaikal et al. (1987) reported that out of 80 patients with CAH, 40 had a satisfactory introitus and regular heterosexual intercourse. However 87% of those with salt-losing CAH and 50% of those with non-salt-losing CAH are single. Among those with CAH who were sexually active, 60% were reported as fertile. There is no increase of homosexuality reported among the CAH group (Kuhnle, 1995).

Summary

Feminizing genitoplasty procedures have changed quite dramatically since the 1980s but little is known about the long-term outcomes. If techniques have much improved, we have made little progress in terms of surgical indications. The major problem we all meet in genital surgery for intersexuality is our poor knowledge of the parameters determining "sexual identity". For many years, surgeons and endocrinologists thought that the external body appearance was crucial to establish sexual behaviour. We know nowadays that the establishment of "sexual identity" is far more complex and probably starts in utero. Endocrine factors such as the testosterone peak registered in male babies after birth are probably as important as the genetic factors, the environmental, cultural and educational factors, to establish the sexual profile. It is mandatory to develop multicentre and multidisciplinary studies in this field even knowing that they are extremely difficult to set up, mainly for psychological reasons. Taking the medical history and examining an adult patient who underwent genital surgery in early childhood to establish her sexual behaviour is a very delicate enterprise that can be very traumatic for the patient and may cause irreversible psychological damage if not conducted with great care, tact and expertise. One needs to say very few words to destroy someone else. The approach to intersexuality is changing, as reflected by the outstanding work of Tina Schober (1998, 1999) and William Reiner (2001) but there is still no consensus.

REFERENCES

Adams M C, Rink R C (1998). Posterior prone sagittal approach to the high vagina. *Dialog Pediatr Urol* 21, 3–4.

Alizai N K, Thomas D F M, Lilford R J, Batchelor A G G, Johnson N (1999). Feminizing genitoplasty for congenital adrenal hyperplasia: What happens at puberty? *J Urol* 161, 1588–1591.

Auchus, R J (2001). The genetics, pathophysiology, and management of human deficiencies of P450C17. *Endocrinol Metab Clin North Am* 30, 101–119, vii.

Berenbaum S A, Duck S C, Bryk K (2000). Behavioral effects of prenatal versus postnatal androgen excess in children with 21-hydroxylase-deficient congenital adrenal hyperplasia. *J Clin Endocrinol Metab* 85, 727–733.

Botero D, Arango A, Danon M, Lifshitz F (2000). Lipid profile in congenital adrenal hyperplasia. *Metabolism* 49, 790–793.

Bridges N A, Christopher J A, Hindmarsh P C, Brook C G (1994). Sexual precocity: sex incidence and aetiology. *Arch Dis Child* 70, 116–118.

Cabrera M S, Vogiatzi M G, New M I (2001). Long term outcome in adult males with classic congenital adrenal hyperplasia. *J Clin Endocrinol Metab* 86, 3070–3078.

Charmandari E, Hindmarsh P C, Johnston A, Brook C G (2001). Congenital adrenal hyperplasia due to 21-hydroxylase deficiency: alterations in cortisol pharmacokinetics at puberty. *J Clin Endocrinol Metab* 86, 2701–2708.

Clague A, Thomas A (2002). Neonatal biochemical screening for disease. *Clin Chim Acta* 315, 99–110.

Creighton S (2001). Surgery for intersex. *J Roy Soc Med* 94, 218–220.

Creighton S M, Minto C L, Steele S J (2001). Objective cosmetic and anatomical outcomes at adolescence of feminising surgery for ambiguous genitalia done in childhood. *Lancet* 358, 124–125.

Deneux C, Tardy V, Dib A et al. (2001). Phenotype-genotype correlation in 56 women with nonclassical congenital adrenal hyperplasia due to 21-hydroxylase deficiency. *J Clin Endocrinol Metab* 86, 207–213.

Ehrhardt A A, Evers K, Money J (1968). Influence of androgen and some aspects of sexually dimorphic behavior in women with the late-treated adrenogenital syndrome. *Johns Hopkins Med J* 123, 115–122.

Eugster E A, Dimeglio L A, Wright J C, Freidenberg G R, Seshadri R, Pescovitz O H (2001). Height outcome in congenital adrenal hyperplasia caused by 21-hydroxylase deficiency: a meta-analysis. *J Pediatr* 138, 26–32.

Fortunoff S T, Lattimer J K, Edson M (1964). Vaginoplasty technique for female pseudohermaphrodites. *Surg Gynecol Obstet* 118, 545–548.

Glassberg K I, Laungani G (1981). Reduction clitoroplasty. *Urology* 27, 604–605.

Gmyrek G A, New M I, Sosa R E, Poppas D P (2002). Bilateral laparoscopic adrenalectomy as a treatment for classic congenital adrenal hyperplasia attributable to 21-hydroxylase deficiency. *Pediatrics* 109, E28.

Gordon C M (1999). Menstrual disorders in adolescents: excess androgens and the polycystic ovary syndrome. *Pediatr Clin North Am* 46, 519–543.

Gunther D F, Bukowski T P, Ritzen E M, Wedell A, Van Wyk J J (1997). Prophylactic adrenalectomy of a three-year-old girl with congenital adrenal hyperplasia: Pre- and postoperative studies. *J Clin Endocr Metab* 82, 3324–3327.

Gussinye M, Carrascosa A, Potau N et al. (1997). Bone mineral density in prepubertal and in adolescent and young adult patients with the salt-wasting form of congenital adrenal hyperplasia. *Pediatrics* 100, 671–674.

Hendren W H (2000). A dissenting viewpoint concerning total urogenital mobilization. *Dialog Pediatr Urol* 23, 4–5.

Hendren W H, Crawford J D (1969). Adrenogenital syndrome: the anatomy of the anomaly and its repair. Some new concepts. *J Pediatr Surg* 4, 49–58.

Hensle T W, Reiley E A (1998). Vaginal replacement in children and young adults. *J Urol* 159, 1035–1038.

Hitchcock R J I, Malone P S (1994). Colovaginoplasty in infants and children. *Br J Urol* 73, 196–199.

Holmes-Walker D J, Conway G S, Honour J W, Rumsby G, Jacobs H S (1995). Menstrual disturbance and hypersecretion of progesterone in women with congenital adrenal hyperplasia due to 21-hydroxylase deficiency. *Clin Endocrinol* 43, 291–296.

Hughes I A (1998). Congenital adrenal hyperplasia – a continuum of disorders. *Lancet* 352, 752–754.

Hughes I A, Mouriquand P D E (1995). Ambiguous genitalia in the newborn. *Surgery* 13, 265–271.

Iijima M, Arisaka O, Minamoto F, Arai Y (2001). Sex differences in children's free drawings: a study on girls with congenital adrenal hyperplasia. *Horm Behav* 40, 99–104.

Jääskeläinen J, Voutilainen R (2000). Long-term outcome of classical 21-hydroxylase deficiency: diagnosis, complications and quality of life. *Acta Paediatr* 89, 183–187.

Jenak R, Ludwikowski B, Gonzales R (2001). Total urogenital sinus mobilization: a modified perineal approach for feminizing genitoplasty and urogenital sinus repair. *J Urol* 165, 2347–2349.

Knight H M L, Phillips N J, Mouriquand P D E (1995). Female hypospadias: a case report. *J Pediatr Surg* 30, 1738–1740.

Krege S, Walz K H, Hauffa B P, Körner I, Rübben H (2000). Long-term follow-up of female patients with congenital adrenal hyperplasia from 21-hydroxylase deficiency, with special emphasis on the results of vaginoplasty. *Br J Urol Int* 86, 253–259.

Krone N, Roscher A A, Schwarz H P, Braun A (1998). Comprehensive analytical strategy for mutation screening in 21-hydroxylase deficiency. *Clin Chem* 44, 2075–2082.

Krone N, Wachter I, Stefanidou M, Roscher A A, Schwarz H P (2001). Mothers with congenital adrenal hyperplasia and their children: outcome of pregnancy, birth and childhood. *Clin Endocrinol* 55, 523–529.

Kuhnle U (1995). The quality of life in adult female patients with congenital adrenal hyperplasia: a comprehensive study of the impact of genital malformations and chronic disease on female patients life. *Eur J Pediatr* 154, 708–716.

Lo J C, Schwitzgebel V M, Tyrrell J B et al. (1999). Normal female infants born of mothers with classic congenital adrenal hyperplasia due to 21-hydroxylase deficiency. *J Clin Endocrinol Metab* 84, 930–936.

Ludwikowski B, Oesch Hayward I, Gonzales R (1999). Total urogenital sinus mobilization: expanded applications. *Br J Urol Int* 83, 820–822.

McKenna T J, Cunningham S K (1995). Adrenal androgen production in polycystic ovary syndrome. *Eur J Endocrinol* 133, 383–389.

Merke D P, Kabbani M (2001). Congenital adrenal hyperplasia: epidemiology, management and practical drug treatment. *Paediatr Drug* 3, 599–611.

Merke D P, Bornstein S R, Braddock D, Chrousos G P (1999). Adrenal lymphocytic infiltration and adrenocortical tumors in a patient with 21-hydroxylase deficiency. *N Engl J Med* 340, 1121–1122.

Merke D P, Chrousos G P, Eisenhofer G et al. (2000a). Adreno-medullary dysplasia and hypofunction in patients with classic 21-hydroxylase deficiency. *N Engl J Med* 343, 1362–1368.

Merke D P, Keil M F, Jones J V, Fields J, Hill S, Cutler G B Jr (2000b). Flutamide, testolactone, and reduced hydrocortisone dose maintain normal growth velocity and bone maturation despite elevated androgen levels in children with congenital adrenal hyperplasia. *J Clin Endocrinol Metab* 85, 1114–1120.

Meyer-Bahlburg H F (1999). What causes low rates of child-bearing in congenital adrenal hyperplasia? *J Clin Endocrinol Metab* 84, 1844–1847.

(2001). Gender and sexuality in classic congenital adrenal hyperplasia. *Endocrinol Metab Clin North Am* 30, 155–171, viii.

Miller W L (1991). Congenital adrenal hyperplasias. *Endocrinol Metab Clin North Am* 20, 721–749.

(1999a). Congenital adrenal hyperplasia in the adult patient. *Adv Intern Med* 44, 155–173.

(1999b). Dexamethasone treatment of congenital adrenal hyperplasia in utero: an experimental therapy of unproven safety. *J Urol* 162, 537–540.

Mollard P, Juskiewenski S, Sarkissian J (1981). Clitoridoplasty in intersex: a new technique. *Br J Urol* 53, 371–373.

Mollard P, Mouriquand P D E, Viguier J L (1990). Chirurgie des ambiguités sexuelles. Techniques, indications, résultats. *Pédiatrie* 45, 87–93.

Moran C, Azziz R, Carmina E et al. (2000). 21-Hydroxylase-deficient nonclassic adrenal hyperplasia is a progressive disorder: a multicenter study. *Am J Obstet Gynecol* 183, 1468–1474.

Mulaikal R M, Migeon C J, Rock J A (1987). Fertility rates in female patients with congenital adrenal hyperplasia due to 21-hydroxylase deficiency. *N Engl J Med* 316, 178–182.

Murphy H, George C, de Kretser D, Judd S (2001). Successful treatment with ICSI of infertility caused by azoospermia associated with adrenal rests in the testes: case report. *Hum Reprod* 16, 263–267.

New M I (2001). Factors determining final height in congenital adrenal hyperplasia. *J Pediatr Endocrinol Metab* 14(Suppl. 2), 933–937.

New M I, Carlson A, Obeid J et al. (2001). Prenatal diagnosis for congenital adrenal hyperplasia in 532 pregnancies. *J Clin Endocrinol Metab* 86, 5651–5657.

Paganini C, Radetti G, Livieri C, Braga V, Migliavacca D, Adami S (2000). Height, bone mineral density and bone markers in congenital adrenal hyperplasia. *Horm Res* 54, 164–168.

Pang S (1997). Congenital adrenal hyperplasia. *Endocrinol Metab Clin North Am* 26, 853–891.

Parrott T S, Woodard J R (1991). Abdominoperineal approach of the high, short vagina in the adrenogenital syndrome. *J Urol* 146, 647–648.

Passerini-Glazel G (1989). A new 1-stage procedure for clitoridovaginoplasty in severely masculinized female pseudohermaphrodites. *J Urol* 142, 565–568.

(1998). Vaginoplasty in severely virilized CAH females. *Dialog Pediatr Urol* 21, 2–3.

(1999). Feminizing genitoplasty. *J Urol* 161, 1592–1593.

Patil U, Mathews R (1995). Use of tissue expanders in vaginoplasty. *Dialog Pediatr Urol* 18, 6–8.

Peña A (1989). Surgical management of persistent cloaca: results in 54 patients with a posterior sagittal approach. *J Pediatr Surg* 24, 590–598.

(1997). Total urogenital mobilisation – an easier way to repair cloacas. *J Pediatr Surg* 32, 263–268.

Peña A, Filmer B, Binilla E, Mendez M, Stolar C (1992). Transanorectal approach for the treatment of urogenital sinus: preliminary report. *J Pediatr Surg* 27, 681–685.

Reiner W G (2001). Psychological and psychiatric aspects of genitourinary conditions. In *Pediatric Urology*, Gearhart J P, Rink R C, Mouriquand P D E, eds., pp. 696–704. Saunders Philadelphia, PA.

Rink R C (2000). Total urogenital mobilization (TUM). *Dialog Pediatr Urol* 23, 2–3.

Rink R C, Yerkes E B (2001). Surgical management of female genital anomalies, intersex (urogenital sinus), and cloacal anomalies. In *Pediatric Urology*, Gearhart J P, Rink R C, Mouriquand P D E, eds., pp. 659–685. Saunders, Philadelphia, PA.

Rink R C, Pope J C, Kropp B P, Smith E R, Keating M A, Adams M C (1997). Reconstruction of the high urogenital sinus: early perineal prone approach without division of the rectum. *J Urol* 158, 1293–1297.

Rumsby G, Skinner C, Honour J W (1992). Genetic analysis of the steroid 21-hydroxylase gene following in vitro amplification of genomic DNA. *J Steroid Biochem Mol Biol* 41, 827–829.

Rumsby G, Avey C J, Conway G S, Honour J W (1998). Genotype–phenotype analysis in late onset 21-hydroxylase deficiency in comparison to the classical forms. *Clin Endocrinol* 48, 707–711.

Schober J M (1998). Feminizing genitoplasty for intersex. In *Pediatric Surgery and Urology: Long Term Outcomes*, Stringer M D, Mouriquand P D E, Oldham K T, Howard E R, eds., pp. 549–558. Saunders, Philadelphia, PA.

(1999). Long-term outcomes and changing attitudes to intersexuality. *Br J Urol Int* 83(Suppl. 3), 39–50.

Seckl J R, Miller W L (1997). How safe is long-term prenatal glucocorticoid treatment? *J Am Med Assoc* 277, 1077–1079.

Speiser P W (2001). Congenital adrenal hyperplasia: transition from childhood to adulthood. *J Endocrinol Invest* 24, 681–691.

Speiser P W, Knochenhauer E S, Dewailly D, Fruzzetti F, Marcondes J A, Azziz R (2000). A multicenter study of women with nonclassical congenital adrenal hyperplasia: relationship between genotype and phenotype. *Mol Genet Metab* 71, 527–534.

Stikkelbroeck N M, Otten B J, Pasic A et al. (2001). High prevalence of testicular adrenal rest tumors, impaired spermatogenesis, and Leydig cell failure in adolescent and adult males with congenital adrenal hyperplasia. *J Clin Endocrinol Metab* 86, 5721–5728.

Swerdlow A J, Higgins C D, Brook C G et al. (1998). Mortality in patients with congenital adrenal hyperplasia: a cohort study. *J Pediatr* 133, 516–520.

Syed H A, Malone P S J, Hitchcock R J (2001). Diversion colitis in children with colovaginoplasty. *Br J Urol Int* 87, 857–860.

Tillem S M, Stock J A, Hanna M K (1998). Vaginal construction in children. *J Urol* 160, 186–190.

van Wyk J J, Gunther D F, Ritzen E M et al. (1996). The use of adrenalectomy as a treatment for congenital adrenal hyperplasia. *J Clin Endocr Metab* 81, 3180–3189.

Vates T S, Fleming P, Leleszi J P, Barthold J S, Gonzales R, Perlmutter A D (1999). Functional, social and psychosexual adjustment after vaginal reconstruction. *J Urol* 162, 182–187.

Wesley J R, Coran A G (1992). Intestinal vaginoplasty for congenital absence of vagina. *J Pediatr Surg* 27, 885–889.

White P C, Speiser P W (2000). Congenital adrenal hyperplasia due to 21-hydroxylase deficiency. *Endocr Rev* 21, 245–291.

Woelfle J, Hoepffner W, Sippell W G et al. (2002). Complete virilization in congenital adrenal hyperplasia: clinical course, medical management and disease-related complications. *Clin Endocrinol* 56, 231–238.

25

Long-term sequelae of genital surgery

Sarah Creighton

Elizabeth Garrett Anderson and Obstetric Hospital,
University College London Hospitals, London, UK

Introduction

The role of genital surgery in the treatment of intersex conditions is under intense scrutiny at present. The need for genital surgery must be urgently evaluated. The advent of well-organized support groups for intersex conditions has given patients the confidence to express their concerns and a platform from which to do so. There is increasing evidence from the patient support groups of dissatisfaction with surgery (AISSG, 2001; *The Times*, 2001). Adult patients feel damaged by their genital surgery, which in many cases was done before they were old enough to consent or to understand the long-term implications. In addition, some more thoughtful surgeons are recommending greater caution with the surgical approach to the treatment of intersex conditions (Schober, 1998). Patient dissatisfaction has led to a call in some quarters for a moratorium on genital surgery (ISNA, 2001).

Crucial to the debate on the role of genital surgery are data on the long-term outcome of surgery. Unfortunately, there are very few studies of adult patients with intersex conditions that look at psychosexual function and outcome. Although surgeons operate with the intention of improving the psychosocial and psychosexual outcome, there is little long-term follow-up of these children into adult life to confirm that this approach is the correct one. There is no evidence base on which to plan treatment and counsel patients. This may be because surgery is performed by paediatric surgeons who would not then follow their patients into adulthood. However, the adult outcome of other paediatric operations has been followed without obvious difficulty. It is more likely that long-term follow-up

studies on intersex patients have been hampered by the widespread policy of nondisclosure, which makes honest and open assessment impossible. Gynaecologists who take over the care and later surgery of these women also have a duty to provide good follow-up data; however, again few gynaecologists have provided any results.

If clinical practice is to improve, it requires careful evaluation of accurate long-term data. The areas of surgery currently under review are:
- surgery for ambiguous genitalia
- treatment for the absent or shortened vagina.

Surgery for ambiguous genitalia

Aims of surgery

Since the work of John Money in the 1950s (Money et al., 1955, 1957), the aim of genital surgery has been to normalize the cosmetic appearance of the genitals. Surgery has focused on cosmetic appearance rather than future sexual function. This is in the belief that a good psychosexual and psychosocial outcome is facilitated by genitals appropriate to the chosen sex of rearing. Since John Money's work, it has become routine to recommend feminizing genital surgery to all infants with ambiguous genitalia raised female. The operation most commonly done is a feminizing genitoplasty to reduce clitoral size and create a vagina. The operation is performed at the age of 12 to 18 months and there are several techniques described (Ch. 24).

Although generally accepted by clinicians and parents as a logical approach, there is no evidence to support the fact that this is an effective treatment.

Paediatric and Adolescent Gynaecology, ed. Adam Balen et al. Published by Cambridge University Press.
© Cambridge University Press 2004.

Clitoral surgery

The clitoris is an erotically important sensory organ. However, sexual response is multifactorial and the exact contribution of the clitoris to orgasm is not yet understood. Our understanding of the clitoris has increased recently. It has been demonstrated that the corpora and crura are much larger than previously thought, surrounding two-thirds of the urethra and extending into the vaginal vestibule. Further work on the neuroanatomy of the human fetal clitoris has demonstrated an extensive network of nerves completely around the tunica, with multiple perforating branches entering the dorsal aspect of the corporeal body and glans (Baskin et al., 1999). It is clear that any incision on the clitoris risks damage to the innervation of the clitoris and potentially to future sexual function. The exact nature of this damage has not yet been evaluated.

There are three main types of clitoral operations:
- clitorectomy or clitoral amputation
- clitoral recession
- clitoral reduction.

Clitorectomy removes all that can be seen of the clitoris. The skin from the prepuce and clitoral hood may be used elsewhere if a vaginoplasty is performed at the same time. The glans and corpora are removed and there is no attempt to preserve the nerve supply. Although commonly used in the past, this procedure has become less popular. However, there are reports in the literature suggesting its use relatively recently, even in the UK.

Clitoral recession does not remove any of the clitoral tissue but folds it back up under the symphysis pubis. Although the nerve connections in theory remain intact, many patients complained of painful erections and this procedure has also fallen into disuse.

Clitoral reduction is described in Chapter 24. The aim is to preserve the neurovascular bundle and interfere as little as possible with sensation. This is the procedure most commonly performed today.

Unfortunately for the purposes of literature review, most papers do not make it clear which operation has been performed.

Sexual function after childhood clitoral surgery

There are over 70 papers on clitoral surgery in the literature. However, even where follow-up data are given and comments made on psychosexual well-being, no details are given of methodology. Long-term results may be reported on very young patients who have not had an opportunity to be sexually active. Conclusions are very general such as "clitoral sensation normal in all" (Allen et al., 1982) or "in all 10 the clitoris has normal sensation to touch" (Oesterling

et al., 1987). Some surgeons seem at the least overoptimistic in describing genital surgery as achieving "near normal cosmetic and functional results" (Rink and Adams, 1998).

Attempts have been made to determine whether preserving the neurovascular bundle preserves sensation. Gearhart et al. (1985) reported six patients with normal pudendal nerve latencies before and after clitoral reduction. These patients were all children and so will not have had a psychosexual evaluation. In response Chase (1986) reported several adult women with impaired sexual function and yet normal pudendal nerve latencies after clitoral surgery. This may be because sensation to the clitoris is carried in unmyelinated and small myelinated fibres and not in large myelinated fibres assessed by this technique.

Three studies have looked in more detail at psychosexual function in intersex women after genital surgery. The first by Dittman et al. (1992) compared 34 women with congenital adrenal hyperplasia (CAH) to their non-CAH sisters. The CAH group were less likely to be sexually active and less likely to experience orgasm. May et al. (1996) looked at 19 women with CAH and compared them with a control group of women with diabetes. Again, those with CAH had significantly less sexual experience and had worse satisfaction scores. They were more likely to report problems with penetration and less likely to experience orgasm. They attributed their difficulties to their surgery.

Most recently, Minto et al. (2003) studied 37 adult women with a history of ambiguous genitalia. Of the group, 24 had undergone feminizing genital surgery and 13 had avoided surgery. Overall sexual function scores were poor in both groups when compared with a standard UK population of women. However, there were significant differences between the two groups. Those who had clitoral surgery were significantly less likely to achieve orgasm (26% were anorgasmic) compared with those who had not had surgery (0% anorgasmic). There was no difference in outcome with the type of clitoral procedure performed, although numbers of different procedures were small.

These three studies suggest that surgery to the clitoris not only does not improve sexual function but may, in fact, be detrimental to it. It is important that this information is available to clinicians and parents making decisions about surgery. Surgery is irreversible and at present decisions are made purely on the cosmetic appearance of the genitalia. However, although a clitoris looks large on a small baby, the appearance relative to the rest of the genitals will change as the child grows older. Consideration must be given to deferring clitoral surgery, particularly in mild to moderate clitoromegaly. An adolescent or adult patient may request surgery because of discomfort or dissatisfaction with the appearance and can than be able to make their own decision with full knowledge of the implications of surgery.

Vaginal surgery for ambiguous genitalia

Feminizing genital surgery traditionally includes a vaginoplasty. This may be done using skin flaps made from tissue left over from the clitoral reduction or other surgeons use a "pull-through" technique (Ch. 24). Surgery is usually performed at the age of 12 to 18 months and the aim of the surgery is to normalize the appearance of the genitalia. The long-term aim of surgery would be to allow passage for menstruation and tampon use and later sexual activity.

The literature is lacking in detailed follow-up for vaginoplasty and most work has been done on women with CAH. Older studies reported a reasonable outcome, with Azziz et al. (1986) reporting satisfactory intercourse – defined as the ability to have comfortable intercourse – in 62% of patients. This study did not look at sexual satisfaction or the ability to orgasm. The same unit subsequently reported an inadequate vaginal introitus in 35% of patients and cite this as a reason for less-frequent heterosexual activity and subsequent fertility (Mulaikal et al., 1987). Subsequent studies have warned of a worse outcome than previously thought. Alizai et al. (1999) studied 14 girls with CAH after puberty and found that all but one would need further surgery for comfortable intercourse. Creighton et al. (2001) looked at 44 adolescents with prior surgery for ambiguous genitalia and again found 98% would need further treatment to the vagina for tampon use or intercourse. They also comment on the number of repeat procedures during childhood, with children having two or three vaginal or clitoral operations prior to adolescence.

The vagina is not necessary for a young girl prior to menstruation or sexual intercourse. It has been suggested that the absence of a vagina would be noticed by the child, her carers and her peers and would be detrimental to her. This is not confirmed by those women with Mayer–Rokitansky–Küster–Hauser syndrome or androgen insensitivity syndrome who present with primary amenorrhoea. These women may have complete absence of the vagina, which has not been identified and has not caused psychological or developmental problems. It would seem logical, therefore, to defer surgery until later in life in the majority of cases. This may need to be prior to menstruation in some women (e.g. CAH) or prior to sexual activity in those women who will not menstruate. This should limit the total number of operations an individual will undergo and allow the patient to consent and be involved in the decision for surgery.

Vaginal dilators after vaginoplasty

Dilatation in infants and prepubertal girls
Some units advocate routine use of vaginal dilators after vaginoplasty even in infants. Unfortunately, there is no evidence that regular dilator use improves the long-term outcome. Concerns have been raised about the effects on a child and her family if the parents are advised to dilate their daughter's vagina regularly. It is possible that this may cause psychological difficulties. In addition, there are anecdotal reports of families under investigation by social services after the child has described her vaginal dilatation to nonfamily members. The amount of distress this can cause must not be underestimated. In view of the fact that there is no long-term evidence of benefit, the routine use of dilators in prepubertal girls is not recommended. This also adds weight to the argument to defer vaginoplasty to the older age group, where dilatation – if recommended – is more appropriate and acceptable (see also Ch. 13).

Dilatation in adolescent and adult women after vaginoplasty
The situation is different in an adolescent or adult patient who has undergone vaginoplasty prior to embarking on a sexual relationship. Some types of vaginoplasty such as skin-graft vaginoplasties are particularly prone to contracture. It is likely that this risk is reduced by dilators at least until a regular sexual relationship is established.

Treatment for the absent or short vagina

An absent or short vagina most commonly occurs in Mayer–Rokitansky–Küster–Hauser syndrome and androgen insensitivity syndrome. The aim of treatment is to create a vagina suitable for penetrative sexual intercourse. Intercourse should not be painful and should be enjoyable and satisfying.

Vaginal dilators

The first line of treatment should be vaginal dilators, as described in Ch. 13. Most units accept that they are the treatment of first choice. There are, however, few good long-term studies. Available studies claim success rates in the region of 80%, although they do not consider compliance or sexual function (Costa et al., 1997; Ingram, 1981). However, despite lack of data on sexual function, the low incidence of side effects would make this treatment a logical first choice, with surgery reserved for those women unable to achieve adequate vaginal length via dilators.

Surgical options

There are numerous surgical procedures for vaginoplasty (see also Ch. 21). Most techniques have their proponents and most series in the literature concentrate on surgical techniques and immediate postoperative outcome. There are few adult sexual function outcome data. There is no information on adjunctive therapies used with surgery, such as oestrogen cream or vaginal dilators. The following procedures are still used.

Williams' vulvovaginoplasty

The surgery is simple and relatively noninvasive and may be indicated if perineal dissection is impossible. Short-term satisfactory results are reported (Williams, 1976) but there are no long-term follow-up data available. Anecdotally, patients complain that the vagina is too short and there is no feeling of penetration. Dilators are difficult to use because of the angle of the external vagina.

Lining of a neovagina

The McIndoe–Reed procedure, which comprises creation of a vaginal space and lining with a split skin graft, is probably the most widely used procedure (Ch. 21). There are follow-up reports of this technique although none contain objective assessment of sexual function. However "normal sexual function" has been reported in 80–90% of women after this technique (Rock et al., 1983). Complications include vaginal soreness and dryness. Contracture is common and difficult to treat. Cali and Pratt (1968) reported on 113 women one to seven years following vaginoplasty with skin grafting: 90% were satisfied with their sexual function although 42% had some degree of contracture.

Other tissues have been used to line the neovagina, such as amnion. Short-term reports are good but there are no long-term data containing assessment of sexual function (Ashworth et al., 1986).

Vaginal intestinal replacement

Intestine has been used in vaginal replacement for nearly 100 years (Baldwin, 1904). Initial complications were major and included death and the technique fell out of favour for 60 years or so. More recently, the technique has become widely used for vaginal replacement in intersex conditions and also following pelvic exenteration for cancer. There are small studies reporting good success rates. Martinez-Mora et al. (1992) reported on 19 patients undergoing sigmoidovaginostomy with follow-up ranging from 1 to 15 years. A good result was reported for 18 patients, with one developing a stricture of the vaginal perineal introitus. Coitus and orgasm were reported as "normal" in all women, but no details given of how this was assessed.

Vecchietti technique

The Vecchietti technique is not as yet available in the UK although it is widely used in Europe. It combines elements of dilatation and vaginal surgery. Pressure is applied on the vaginal dimple by an acrylic olive. Threads from the olive are passed through the potential neovaginal space and the abdominal wall and connected to a traction device. The device is tightened over 8 to 10 days. Reported success rates are high (Veronikis et al., 1997) although there are few long-term data and no assessment of sexual function after the procedure.

Malignancy risk

More recent concern has focused on malignancy risk following vaginoplasty. So far, there have been at least 19 published case reports of malignancy in women following vaginoplasty for absent vagina (Table 25.1). Vaginal cancer is reported with the McIndoe–Reed vaginoplasty, when the malignancy is a squamous cell carcinoma, and also with intestinal vaginoplasty, when the malignancy is more commonly an adenocarcinoma. Primary vaginal cancer in the general female population is very rare and usually presents in the seventh decade of life. Vaginal cancer in women with a neovagina presents at a much earlier age, with most occurring in women in their thirties and forties (Lawrence, 2001). The interval from vaginoplasty to development of cancer is approximately 20 years.

It is difficult to know how best to screen women with a neovagina for malignancy. It would seem sensible to examine this group vaginally on a yearly basis. However, some intestinal vaginas can be very capacious and thorough assessment may not be possible in the outpatient setting. These patients may require vaginoscopy under general anaesthetic. Cytological screening can also be difficult to interpret. Most cancer cases reported in the literature presented with symptoms of discharge and bleeding. It is very important that such symptoms are taken seriously in this group of women and vaginoscopy and biopsy performed readily.

There have been no reports of vaginal cancer in women using dilators alone.

Summary

Many factors affect the psychosocial and psychosexual well-being of those with intersex disorders and related conditions. In the past, surgery was regarded as the cornerstone of treatment. Parents and clinicians viewed surgery to some

Table 25.1. Reported cases of malignancy following creation of a neovagina

Source	Age at vaginoplasty	Age at diagnosis of cancer	Type of vaginoplasty	Type of cancer
Ritchie, 1929	13	26	Small bowel	Adenocarcinoma
Lavand and Homme, 1938	18	33	Colon	Adenocarcinoma
Jackson, 1959	17	25	Skin graft	Squamous cell carcinoma
Krieg and Goltner, 1966	27	71	Colon	Adenocarcinoma
Cali and Pratt, 1968	18	26	Skin graft	Squamous cell carcinoma
Duckler, 1972	17	36	Skin graft	Squamous cell carcinoma
Rotmensch et al., 1983	28	33	Skin graft	Squamous cell carcinoma
Jaeger and Engle, 1984	28	52	Colon	Adenocarcinoma
Rummel et al., 1985	17	29	Skin graft	Squamous cell carcinoma
Imrie et al., 1986	17	29	Skin graft	Squamous cell carcinoma
Hopkins and Morley, 1987	18	42	Skin graft	Squamous cell carcinoma
Balzer and Zander, 1989	28	43	Skin graft	Squamous cell carcinoma
Auber et al., 1989	20	59	Small bowel	Adenocarcinoma
Balik et al., 1992	19	38	Peritoneum	Squamous cell carcinoma
Munkarah et al., 1994	21	42	Skin graft	Mucinous adenocarcinoma
Bobin et al., 1999	22	43	Ingrowth/cleavage	Squamous cell carcinoma
Schult et al., 2000			Skin graft	Squamous cell carcinoma
Hiroi et al., 2001	23	53	Sigmoid	Adenocarcinoma
Lowe et al., 2001			Skin graft	Squamous cell carcinoma

extent as a "cure". Unfortunately, this can lead to neglect of other areas, especially the psychological issues. There are few long-term data on surgical outcome, and follow-up of patients has been hampered by the policy of nondisclosure of diagnosis. Patient satisfaction with surgery will be affected by other factors, discussed elsewhere in this textbook, such as nondisclosure and secrecy, repeated genital examinations, being exhibited as a curiosity for medical students and medical photography (Creighton et al., 2002). These may all lead to a poor body image, a lack of self-confidence and general unhappiness.

Despite the difficulty with accurate assessment, it is becoming clearer that surgery does not seem to improve sexual satisfaction. There are emerging data that it may damage sexual function. If this is indeed true, and in the absence of any evidence that feminizing surgery benefits psychosocial outcome, then the option of deferring cosmetic genital surgery must be discussed with the family (Box 25.1). Truthful information must be given to the patient and their family from the outset. Adequate and informed psychological support should be available to all families whether or not they elect to have surgery.

We have failed dismally in the past to provide adequate information to allow parents and patients to make fully informed decisions. Reparation can only come with well-organized multicentre follow-up studies involving adult patients who have and have not had surgery, to assess gynaecological, sexual and psychological well-being. At least then we can begin to understand the full implications of caring for patients with intersex conditions and adjust our clinical services accordingly to provide the best possible care (Box 25.2).

Box 25.1 Recommendations for practice

- Vaginal dilators are the treatment of choice for the absent or short vagina in adolescent and adult patients.
- Vaginoplasty can be deferred until adolescence in the majority of patients.
- Parents of infants with ambiguous genitalia considering genital surgery must be aware of the potential implications for future sexual function. The option of no surgery should be discussed.
- Vaginal discharge and bleeding in a patient with an intestinal or skin graft vaginoplasty must be investigated as these symptoms may indicate malignancy.
- Reconstructive genital surgery is complex and should only be performed in specialist centres.

Box 25.2 Key points

- Objective data on the long-term outcomes of genital surgery in intersex conditions is lacking.
- There are no data demonstrating that feminizing surgery improves psychosocial outcome.
- There is increasing evidence that clitoral surgery damages sexual function and may alter the ability to reach orgasm.
- The majority of children undergoing reconstructive genital surgery will need further treatment in adolescence or adult life.
- Vaginal cancer may occur after vaginoplasty with skin graft and intestine.

REFERENCES

*Indicates key references

AISSG (Androgen Insensitivity Syndrome Support Group) (2001). www.medhelp.org/www/ais.

*Alizai N K, Thomas D F M, Lilford R J, Batchelor G G, Johnson F (1999). Feminizing genitoplasty for adrenal hyperplasia: what happens at puberty. *J Urol* 161, 1588–1591.

Allen L E, Hardy B E, Churchill B M (1982). The surgical management of the enlarged clitoris. *J Urol* 128, 351–354.

Ashworth M F, Morton K E, Dewhurst J, Lilford R J, Bates R G (1986). Vaginoplasty using amnion. *Gynecol Obstet* 67, 443–446.

Auber G, Carbonara T, Di Boito L, Patriarca S (1989). Carcinoma of the neovagina following a Baldwin–Mori operation for congenital absence of the vagina. *J Obstet Gynaecol* 10, 68.

Azziz R, Mulaikal R M, Migeon C J, Jones H W, Rock J A (1986). Congenital adrenal hyperplasia: long term results following vaginal reconstruction. *Fertil Steril* 46, 1011–1014.

Baldwin J F (1904). The formation of an artificial vagina by intestinal transposition. *Ann Surg* 40, 398.

Balik E, Maral I, Sozen U, Bezirciogli I, Tugsel Z, Velibes D (1992). Karzinom in einer Davydov Neovagina. *Geburt Frauenheilk* 52, 68.

Baltzer J, Zander J (1989). Primary squamous cell carcinoma of the neovagina. *Gynecol Oncol* 35, 99–103.

*Baskin L S, Erol A, WuLi Y, Kurzrock E, Cunha G R (1999). Anatomical studies of the human clitoris. *J Urol* 162, 1015–1020.

Bobin J, Zinzindohoue C, Naba T, Isac S, Mage G (1999). Primary squamous carcinoma in a patient with vaginal agenesis. *Gynecol Oncol* 74, 293–297.

*Cali R W, Pratt J H (1968). Congenital absence of the vagina: long term results of vaginal reconstruction in 175 cases. *Am J Obstet Gynecol* 100, 752–763.

Chase C (1996). Letter of response. *J Urol* 156, 1139.

Costa E M, Mendonca B B, Inacia M, Arnhold I J, Silva F A, Lodovici O (1997). Management of ambiguous genitalia in pseudo-hermaphrodites: new perspectives on vaginal dilation. *Fertil Steril* 67, 229–232.

*Creighton S, Minto C L, Steele S J (2001). Feminizing childhood surgery for ambiguous genitalia: objective cosmetic and anatomical outcomes in adolescence. *Lancet* 358, 124–125.

*Creighton S, Alderson J, Brown S, Minto C L (2002). Medical photography: ethics, consent and the intersex patient. *Br J Urol Int* 89, 67–72.

Dittman R W, Kappes M E, Kappes M H (1992). Sexual behaviour in adolescent and adult females with congenital adrenal hyperplasia. *Psychoneuroendocrinology* 17, 153–170.

Duckler L (1972). Squamous cell carcinoma developing in an artificial vagina. *Obstet Gynecol* 40, 35–38.

Gearhart J P, Burnett A, Owens J H (1995). Measurement of pudendal evoked potentials during feminising genitoplasty: technique and applications. *J Urol* 153, 486–487.

Hiroi H, Yasugi T, Matsumoto K et al. (2001). Mucinous carcinoma arising in a neovagina using the sigmoid colon thirty years after the operation: a case report. *J Surg Oncol* 77, 61–64.

Hopkins M, Morley G (1987). Squamous cell carcinoma of the neovagina. *Obstet Gynecol* 69, 525–527.

Imrie J, Kennedy J, Holmes J, MacGrouther D (1986). Intraepithelial neoplasia arising in an artificial vagina. *Obstet Gynecol* 93, 886–888.

Ingram J M (1981). The bicycle seat stool in the treatment of vaginal agenesis and stenosis: a preliminary report. *Am J Obstet Gynecol* 140, 867–873.

ISNA (Intersex Society of North America) (2001). www.isna.org.

Jackson G (1959). Primary carcinoma of an artificial vagina. *Obstet Gynecol* 14, 534–536.

Jaeger K, Engle C (1984). Karzinom in Kunstlicher Scheide bei kongenitaler Vaginalalpaise. *Krankenhausartz* 57, 491–493.

Krieg H, Goltner E (1966). Primares Karzinom in einer kunstlic Scheid. *Z Gynakol* 88, 1575–1578.

Lavane Homme P (1939). Complication tardive apparue au niveau d'vagin artificial. *Brixelles Med* 19, 14015.

Lawrence A (2001). Vaginal neoplasia in a male-to-female transsexual: case review of the literature and recommendations for cytologic screening. *Int J Transgend* 5, 1.

Lowe M P, Ault K A, Sood A K (2001). Recurrent carcinoma in situ of a neovagina. *Gynecol Oncol* 80, 403–404.

Martinez-Mora M, Isnard R, Castellevi A, Lopez-Orte P (1992). Neovagina in vaginal agenesis: surgical methods and long term results. *J Pediatr Surg* 27, 10–14.

*May B, Boyle M, Grant D (1996). A comparative study of sexual experiences. *J Health Psychol* 1, 479–492.

Minto C, Creighton S, Woodhouse C (2001). Long-term sexual function in intersex conditions with ambiguous genitalia. British Association of Urological Surgeons Annual Meeting Dublin.

Minto C, Liao K L M, Woodhouse C R J, Ransley P G, Creighton S (2003). Sexual outcomes in intersex conditions with ambiguous genitalia: the effect of clitoral surgery. *Lancet* 361, 1367–1369.

Money J, Hampson J G, Hampson J L (1955). Hermaphroditism: recommendations concerning assignment of sex, change of sex and psychologic management. *Bull Johns Hosp* 97, 284–300.

(1957). Imprinting and establishment of the gender role. *Arch Neuro Psychiatry* 77, 333–336.

Mulaikal R M, Migeon C J, Rock J A (1987). Fertility rates in female patients with congenital adrenal hyperplasia due to 21-hydroxylase deficiency. *N Engl J Med* 316, 178–182.

Munkarah A, Malone J, Budev H, Evans T (1994). Mucinous adenocarcinoma arising from a neovagina. *Gynecol Oncol* 52, 275.

Oesterling J E, Gearhart J P, Jeffs R D (1987). A unified approach to early reconstructive surgery of the child with ambiguous genitalia. *J Urol* 138, 1079–1082.

Rink R, Adams M A (1998). Feminizing genitoplasty: state of the art. *World J Urol* 16, 212–218.

Ritchie R (1929). Primary carcinoma of the vagina following a Baldwin reconstruction operation for congenital absence of the vagina. *Am J Obstet Gynecol* 18, 794–799.

Rock J A, Reeves L A, Retto H et al. (1983). Success following vaginal creation for Mullerian agenesis. *Fertil Steril* 39, 809–813.

Rotmensch J, Rosensheim N, Dillon M, Murphy A, Woodruff S, (1983). Carcinoma arising in the neovagina: case report and review of the literature. *Obstet Gynecol* 61, 534–536.

Rummel H, Kuhn W, Heberling D (1985). Karzinomentstehun der Neovagina nach Vaginalplastik *Geburt Frauenheilk* 2, 124–125.

Schober J (1998). Early feminizing genitoplasty or watchful waiting. *J Ped Adolesc Gynecol* 11, 154–156.

Schult M, Hecker A, Lelle RJ, Senninger N, Winder G (2000). Recurrent rectoneovaginal fistula caused by an incidental squamous cell carcinoma of the neovagina in Mayer–Rokitanski–Küster–Hauser syndrome. *Gynecol Oncol* 77, 210–212.

The Times (2001). *Ethics and Gender.* June 26th Health Supplement.

Veronikis D K, McClure B G, Nichols D H (1997). The Vecchietti operation for constructing a neovagina: indications, instrumentations and techniques. *Obstet Gynecol* 90, 301–304.

Williams E A (1976). Uterovaginal agenesis. *Ann Roy Coll Surg Engl* 58, 226.

26

Amenorrhoea

Adam H. Balen

Department of Reproductive Medicine, The General Infirmary, Leeds, UK

Introduction

Amenorrhoea is the absence of menstruation, either temporarily or permanently. It may occur as a normal physiological condition, such as before puberty, during pregnancy, lactation or the menopause, or as a feature of a systemic or gynaecological disorder.

Primary amenorrhoea

The failure to menstruate by the age of 16 years in the presence of normal secondary sexual development, or 14 years in the absence of secondary sexual characteristics, warrants investigation. This distinction helps to differentiate reproductive tract anomalies from gonadal quiescence and gonadal failure (see earlier chapters). Primary amenorrhoea may be a result of congenital abnormalities in the development of ovaries, genital tract or external genitalia (see Chs. 20–24) or a disturbance of the normal endocrinological events of puberty (Ch. 18). Most of the causes of secondary amenorrhoea can also cause primary amenorrhoea if they occur before the menarche. Delayed puberty is often constitutional, but it is important to exclude primary ovarian failure or hypothalamic/pituitary dysfunction. Overall, it is estimated that endocrine disorders account for approximately 40% of primary amenorrhoea, the remaining 60% being the result of developmental abnormalities (Table 26.1).

Chapters 19 and 20–24 describe the causes of primary amenorrhoea other than those described below under secondary amenorrhoea. Many of these conditions will have presented either at birth or during childhood. Management should be in a specialized clinic that can provide a multidisciplinary approach to care.

Secondary amenorrhoea

Cessation of menstruation for six consecutive months in a woman who has previously had regular periods is the usual criterion for investigation. Women with secondary amenorrhoea must have a patent lower genital tract, an endometrium that is responsive to ovarian hormone stimulation and ovaries that have responded to pituitary gonadotrophins.

Examination and investigation of amenorrhoea

A thorough history and a careful examination of stature and body form, secondary sexual development and external genitalia should always be carried out before further investigations (Table 26.2) are instigated. A history of secondary amenorrhoea may be misleading, as the "periods" may have been the result of exogenous hormone administration. In most cases, however, a history of secondary amenorrhoea excludes congenital abnormalities. A family history of fertility problems, autoimmune disorders or premature menopause may also give clues to the aetiology.

A bimanual examination is inappropriate in a young woman who has never been sexually active, and examination of the external genitalia of an adolescent should be undertaken in the presence of the patient's mother. Furthermore, it may be more appropriate to defer any such examination from the first consultation in order to gain an

Paediatric and Adolescent Gynaecology, ed. Adam Balen et al. Published by Cambridge University Press.
© Cambridge University Press 2004.

Table 26.1. Classification of primary amenorrhoea

Causes	Conditions
Uterine	Müllerian agenesis (e.g. Rokitansky syndrome; Ch. 21)
Ovarian	Polycystic ovary syndrome (Ch. 27)
	Premature ovarian failure (usually genetic, e.g. Turner's syndrome; Chs. 19 and 30)
Hypothalamus *(hypogonadotrophic hypogonadism)*	Weight loss (Ch. 39)
	Intense exercise (e.g. ballerinas; Ch. 18)
	Idiopathic (Ch. 18)
Delayed puberty	Constitutional delay or secondary amenorrhoea (see text and Ch. 18)
Pituitary	Hyperprolactinaemia
	Hypopituitarism
Hypothalamic/ pituitary damage *(hypogonadism)*	Tumours (craniopharyngiomas, gliomas, germinomas, dermoid cysts)
	Cranial irradiation, head injuries (rare in young girls)
Systemic disorders	Chronic debilitating illness
	Weight loss
	Endocrine disorders (thyroid disease, Cushing's syndrome, etc.)

Table 26.2. Investigations for amenorrhoea

Type	Components
Physical examination	Note body mass index, pubertal development,
	Stigmata of polycystic ovary syndrome (PCOS) and other endocrine disease
Endocrine assessment	Pregnancy test if suspected
	Follicle-stimulating hormone, luteinizing hormone
	Prolactin
	Thyroid function tests
	Testosterone (if stigmata of PCOS)
	Further endocrinology only if above do not provide diagnosis
Pelvic imaging	Ultrasound: morphology of ovaries and endometrial thickness (for oestrogenization)
	Magnetic resonance imaging (MRI) if suggestion of complex developmental problem
Pituitary/hypothalamic imaging	MRI if indicated
Bone mineral densitometry	If at risk of osteoporosis
Karyotype	If premature ovarian failure

adolescent woman's confidence for future management. A transabdominal ultrasound examination of the pelvis is an excellent noninvasive method of obtaining valuable information in these patients. However, examination under anaesthetic is sometimes indicated, particularly in cases of intersex.

On establishing that the internal and external genitalia are normally developed, it is important to exclude pregnancy in women of any age. Measurement of height and weight should be done in order to calculate a patient's body mass index (BMI). The normal range is $20-25 \, \text{kg/m}^2$, and a value above or below this range may suggest a diagnosis of weight-related amenorrhoea (which is a term usually applied to *underweight* women).

A baseline assessment in all patients should include measurement of serum prolactin and gonadotrophin concentrations and an assessment of thyroid function. Prolactins levels may be elevated in response to a number of conditions, including stress, a recent breast examination or even having a blood test. However, the elevation is usually moderate and transient. A more permanent, but still moderate elevation (greater than 700 mU/l) is associated with hypothyroidism and is also a finding in some women with polycystic ovary syndrome (PCOS), where prolactin levels up to 2000 mU/l have been reported. PCOS may also result in amenorrhoea, which can create diagnostic difficulties, and hence of appropriate management, for those women with hyperprolactinaemia and polycystic ovaries. Amenorrhoea in women with PCOS is secondary to acyclical ovarian activity and continuous oestrogen production. A positive response to a progestogen challenge test, which induces a withdrawal bleed, will distinguish patients with PCOS-related hyperprolactinaemia from those with polycystic ovaries and unrelated hyperprolactinaemia, because the latter causes oestrogen deficiency and, therefore, failure to respond to the progestogen challenge (a pelvic ultrasound assessment of ovarian morphology and endometrial thickness will also provide the answer).

A serum prolactin concentration of greater than 1000 mU/l on two occasions warrants further investigation. Computed tomography (CT) or magnetic resonance imaging (MRI) of the pituitary fossa may be used to exclude a hypothalamic tumour, a nonfunctioning pituitary tumour compressing the hypothalamus (e.g. craniopharyngioma) or a prolactinoma (Fig. 26.1). Serum prolactin concentrations greater than 5000 mU/l are usually associated with a macroprolactinoma, which by definition is greater than 1 cm in diameter.

Serum measurements of oestradiol are unhelpful as its levels vary considerably, even in a patient with amenorrhoea. If the patient has sufficient oestrogen, the endometrium will be shed on withdrawal of an exogenous progestogen preparation (see above).

Serum gonadotrophin measurements help to distinguish between hypothalamic or pituitary failure and gonadal failure. Elevated gonadotrophin concentrations indicate a failure of negative feedback as a result of primary ovarian failure. A serum follicle-stimulating hormone (FSH) concentration of greater than 15 mU/l that is not associated with a preovulatory surge suggests impending ovarian failure. FSH levels of greater than 40 mU/l are suggestive of irreversible ovarian failure. The exact values vary according to individual assays, and so local reference levels should be checked.

An elevated luteinizing hormone (LH) concentration, when associated with a raised FSH concentration, is indicative of ovarian failure. However if LH is elevated alone (and is not attributable to the preovulatory LH surge), this suggests PCOS, which may be confirmed by a pelvic ultrasound scan (Ch. 27). Rarely, elevated LH in a phenotypic female may be caused by the androgen insensitivity syndrome (AIS; Ch. 20).

Failure at the level of the hypothalamus or pituitary is reflected by abnormally low levels of serum gonadotrophin concentrations and gives rise to hypogonadotrophic hypogonadism. Kallman's syndrome is the clinical finding of hyposmia and/or colour blindness associated with hypogonadotrophic hypogonadism. It is difficult to distinguish between hypothalamic and pituitary aetiology as both respond to stimulation with gonadotrophin-releasing hormone (GnRH). A skull X-ray is rarely performed nowadays as much more information is provided by CT or MRI.

Karyotyping of women with primary amenorrhoea or those under 30 years with gonadotrophin levels compatible with premature ovarian failure, should be performed, as some chromosomal abnormalities (e.g. Turner's syndrome) may be associated with premature ovarian failure. An autoantibody screen should also be undertaken in women with a premature menopause (under the age of 40 years) (Ch. 30).

A history of a recent endometrial curettage or endometriotis in a patient with normal genitalia and normal

endocrinology, but with absent or only a small withdrawal bleed following a progestogen challenge, is suggestive of Asherman's syndrome. A hysteroscopy will confirm the diagnosis.

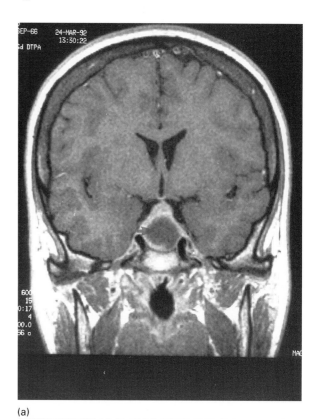

(a)

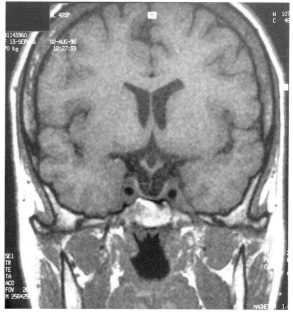

(b)

Fig. 26.1. Magnetic resonance image of a pituitary macroadenoma, T_1-weighted image after gadolinium enhancement. (a) The macroadenoma has a cystic central component (arrow) and there is suprasellar extension causing compression of the optic chiasm. (b) After 6 months of therapy with bromocriptine, the tumour has almost completely resolved. (Reproduced with permission from Balen A H, Jacobs H S (2003) *Infertility in Practice*, 2nd edn. Churchill Livingstone, London.)

Measurement of bone mineral density (BMD) is indicated in amenorrhoeic women who are oestrogen deficient. Measurements of density are made in the lumbar spine and femoral neck. The vertebral bone is more sensitive to oestrogen deficiency, and vertebral fractures tend to occur in a younger age group (50–60 years) than fractures at the femoral neck (70+ years). However, it should be noted that crush fractures can spuriously increase the measured BMD. A radiograph of the dorsolumbar spine is, therefore, often complimentary, particularly in patients who have lost height.

Amenorrhoea may also have long-term metabolic and physical consequences. In women with PCOS and prolonged amenorrhoea, there is a risk of endometrial hyperplasia and adenocarcinoma. If, on resumption of menstruation, there is a history of persistent intermenstrual bleeding or on ultrasound there is a postmenstrual endometrial thickness of greater than 10 mm, then an endometrial biopsy is indicated (Ch. 27).

Secondary amenorrhoea

The principal causes of secondary amenorrhoea are outlined in Table 26.3. The frequency with which these conditions present is given in Table 23.4.

Genital tract abnormalities

Asherman's syndrome is a condition in which intrauterine adhesions prevent normal growth of the endometrium (Asherman, 1950). This may be the result of a too vigorous endometrial curettage or may follow endometriotis. Typically amenorrhoea is not absolute, and it may be possible to induce a withdrawal bleed. Diagnosis and treatment by adhesiolysis is done hysteroscopically. Following surgery, a three month course of cyclical progesterone/oestrogen should be given. Some clinicians insert a Foley catheter into the uterine cavity for seven to ten days postoperatively, or an intrauterine contraceptive device for two to three months, in order to prevent recurrence of adhesions.

Cervical stenosis is an occasional cause of secondary amenorrhoea. It was relatively common following a traditional cone biopsy for the treatment of cervical intraepithelial neoplasia. However, modern procedures, such as laser or loop diathermy, have less postoperative cervical complications. Treatment for cervical stenosis consists of careful cervical dilatation: the concurrent use of laparoscopy and ultrasound may help to prevent the inadvertent creation of a false passage.

Table 26.3. Classification of secondary amenorrhoea

Cause	Conditions
Uterine	Asherman's syndrome
	Cervical stenosis
Ovarian causes	Polycystic ovary syndrome
	Premature ovarian failure (genetic, autoimmune, infective, radio/chemotherapy)
Hypothalamus *(hypogonadotrophic hypogonadism)*	Weight loss
	Exercise
	Chronic illness
	Psychological distress
	Idiopathic
Pituitary	Hyperprolactinaemia
	Hypopituitarism
	Sheehan's syndrome
Hypothalamic/ pituitary damage *(hypogonadism)*	Tumours (craniopharyngiomas, gliomas, germinomas, dermoid cysts)
	Cranial irradiation
	Head injuries
	Sarcoidosis
	Tuberculosis
Systemic disorders	Chronic debilitating illness
	Weight loss
	Endocrine disorders (thyroid disease, Cushing's syndrome, etc.)

Table 26.4. The aetiology of secondary amenorrhoea in 570 patients attending an endocrine clinic

Course	Percentage
Polycystic ovary syndrome	36.9
Premature ovarian failure	23.6
Hyperprolactinaemia	16.9
Weight-related amenorrhoea	9.8
Hypogonadotrophic hypogonadism	5.9
Hypopituitarism	4.4
Exercise-related amenorrhoea	2.5

Systemic disorders causing secondary amenorrhoea

Chronic disease may result in menstrual disorders as a consequence of the general disease state, weight loss or by the effect of the disease process on the hypothalamic–pituitary axis. Furthermore, a chronic disease that leads to immobility, such as chronic obstructive airways disease, may increase the risk of amenorrhoea-associated osteoporosis.

In addition, certain diseases affect gonadal function directly. Women with chronic renal failure have a discordantly elevated LH, possibly as a consequence of impaired clearance. Prolactin is also elevated in these women because of failure of the normal dopamine inhibition. Diabetes mellitus may result in functional hypothalamic–pituitary amenorrhoea and be associated with an increased risk of PCOS. Liver disease affects the level of circulating sex hormone-binding globulin, and thus circulating free hormone levels, thereby disrupting the normal feedback mechanisms. Metabolism of various hormones, including testosterone, are also liver dependent; both menstruation and fertility return after liver transplantation. Endocrine disorders such as thyrotoxicosis and Cushing's syndrome are commonly associated with gonadal dysfunction. Autoimmune endocrinopathies may be associated with premature ovarian failure, because of ovarian antibodies (Ch. 30).

Management of these patients should concentrate on the underlying systemic problem and on preventing complications of oestrogen deficiency. If fertility is required, it is desirable to achieve maximal health and where possible to discontinue teratogenic drugs.

Weight-related amenorrhoea

Weight can have profound effects on gonadotrophin regulation and release (see also more detailed accounts in Ch. 6). Weight disorders are also common. In one study, up to 35% of women attending an endocrine clinic had secondary amenorrhoea associated with weight loss. A regular menstrual cycle is unlikely to occur if the BMI is less than $19\,kg/m^2$. Fat appears to be critical to a normally functioning hypothalamic–pituitary–gonadal axis. It is estimated that at least 22% of body weight should be fat in order to maintain ovulatory cycles (Frisch, 1976). This level enables the extraovarian aromatization of androgens to oestrogens and maintains appropriate feedback control of the hypothalamic–pituitary–ovarian axis. Therefore, girls who are significantly underweight prior to puberty may have primary amenorrhoea, while those who are significantly underweight after puberty will have secondary amenorrhoea. The clinical presentation depends upon the severity of the nutritional insult and its age of onset. To cause amenorrhoea, the loss must be 10–15% of the woman's normal weight for height. Weight loss may result from a number of causes including self-induced abstinence, starvation, illness and exercise. However, whatever the precipitating cause, the net result is impairment of gonadotrophin secretion. Weight-related gonadotrophin deficiency is more pronounced with LH than FSH. This and the reduction in pulsatility of gonadotrophin secretion may result in a "multicystic" pattern in the ovary. This appearance is typical of normal puberty and is seen when there are several cysts (approximately 5–10 mm in diameter together with a stroma of normal density) (see Fig. 27.4, p. 346).

Anorexia nervosa is at the extreme end of a spectrum of eating disorders and is invariably accompanied by menstrual disturbance, and indeed it may account for between 15 and 35% of patients with amenorrhoea. Women with anorexia nervosa should be managed in collaboration with a psychiatrist, and it is essential to encourage weight gain as the main therapy (see also more detailed accounts in Chs. 38 and 39).

An artificial cycle may be induced with the combined oral contraceptive. However, this may corroborate in the denial of weight loss as the underlying problem. Similarly, while it is possible to induce ovulation with GnRH, or exogenous gonadotrophins, treatment of infertility in the significantly underweight patient is associated with a significant increase in intrauterine growth retardation and neonatal problems (van der Spuy, 1988). Furthermore, since three-quarters of the cell divisions that occur during pregnancy do so during the first trimester, it is essential that nutritional status is optimized before conception. Low birth weight is also now being related to an increased risk of cardiovascular disease, obstructive lung disease and schizophrenia in adult life.

Weight-related amenorrhoea may also have profound long-term effects on BMD. Oestrogen deficiency, reduced calcium and protein intake, reduced levels of vitamin D and elevated cortisol levels can all contribute to osteoporosis. The age of onset of anorexia nervosa is also important, as prolonged amenorrhoea before the normal age at which peak bone mass is obtained (approximately 25 years) increases the likelihood of severe osteoporosis.

Worldwide, involuntary starvation is the commonest cause of reduced reproductive ability, resulting in delayed pubertal growth and menarche in adolescents and infertility in adults. Acute malnutrition, as seen in famine conditions and during and after World War II, has profound effects on fertility and fecundity. Ovulatory function usually returns quickly on restoration of adequate nutrition. The chronic malnutrition common in developing countries has less profound effects on fertility but is associated with small and premature babies.

Psychological stress

Studies have failed to demonstrate a link between stressful life events and amenorrhoea of greater than two months. However, stress may lead to physical debility such as weight loss, which may then cause menstrual disturbance (see also more detailed accounts in Chs. 38 and 39).

Exercise-related amenorrhoea

Menstrual disturbance is common in athletes undergoing intensive training. Between 10 and 20% have oligomenorrhoea or amenorrhoea, compared with 5% in the general population. Amenorrhoea is more common in athletes under 30 years and is particularly common in women involved in the endurance events (such as long distance running). Up to 50% of competitive runners training 80 miles per week may be amenorrhoeic (Cumming and Rebar, 1983).

The main aetiological factors are weight and percentage body fat content, but other factors have also been postulated. Physiological changes are consistent with those associated with starvation and chronic illness. In order to conserve energy, there may be a fall in thyroid-stimulating hormone, a reduction in triiodothyronine and an elevation of the inactive reverse-triiodothyronine. Exercise also leads to a fall in circulating insulin and insulin-like growth factor 1 and, therefore, decreases their stimulation of the pituitary and ovary. Prolactin and circulating androgen levels show no consistent changes with exercise.

Ballet dancers provide an interesting, and much studied subgroup of sportswomen, because their training begins at an early age. They have been found to have a significant delay in menarche (15.4 compared with 12.5 years) and a retardation in pubertal development, which parallels the intensity of their training. Menstrual irregularities are common and up to 44% have secondary amenorrhoea (Warren et al., 1986). In a survey of 75 dancers, 61% were found to have stress fractures and 24% had scoliosis; the risk of these pathological features was increased if menarche was delayed or if there were prolonged periods of amenorrhoea.

These findings may be explained by delayed pubertal maturation resulting in attainment of a greater than expected height and a predisposition to scoliosis, as oestrogen is required for epiphyseal closure.

Exercise-induced amenorrhoea has the potential to cause severe long-term morbidity, particularly with regard to osteoporosis. Studies on young ballet dancers have shown that the amount of exercise undertaken by these dancers does not compensate for these osteoporotic changes (Warren et al., 1986). Oestrogen is also important in the formation of collagen, and soft tissue injuries are also common in dancers (Bowling, 1989).

Whereas moderate exercise has been found to reduce the incidence of postmenopausal osteoporosis, young athletes may be placing themselves at risk at an age when the attainment of peak bone mass is important for long-term skeletal strength. Appropriate advice should be given, particularly regarding diet, and the use of a cyclical oestrogen/progestogen preparation should be considered. It is important to enlist the support of both parents and trainers when trying to encourage a young athlete to modify her exercise programme and diet in order to reinstate a normal menstrual cycle with the aim of preventing long-term morbidity.

Hypothalamic causes of secondary amenorrhoea

Hypothalamic causes of amenorrhoea may be either primary or secondary. Primary hypothalamic lesions include craniopharyngiomas, germinomas, gliomas and dermoid cysts. These hypothalamic lesions either disrupt the normal pathway of prolactin inhibitory factor (dopamine), thus causing hyperprolactinaemia, or compress and/or destroy hypothalamic and pituitary tissue. Treatment is usually surgical, with additional radiotherapy if required. Hormone replacement therapy is required to mimic ovarian function; if the pituitary gland is damaged either by the lesion or by the treatment, replacement thyroid and adrenal hormones are required.

Secondary hypogonadotrophic hypogonadism may result from systemic conditions including sarcoidosis and tuberculosis, as well as following head injury or cranial irradiation. Sheehan's syndrome, the result of profound and prolonged hypotension on the sensitive pituitary gland, enlarged by pregnancy, may also be a cause of hypogonadotrophic hypogonadism in someone with a history of a major obstetric haemorrhage (Sheehan, 1939). It is essential to assess the pituitary function fully in all these patients and then instigate the appropriate replacement therapy. Ovulation may be induced with pulsatile subcutaneous GnRH (if the pituitary is intact) or human menopausal gonadotrophins (hMG). The administration of pulsatile GnRH provides the most "physiological" correction of infertility caused by hypogonadotrophic hypogonadism and will result in unifollicular ovulation, while hMG therapy requires close monitoring to prevent multiple pregnancy. Purified or recombinant FSH preparations are not suitable for women with hypogonadotrophic hypogonadism (or pituitary hypogonadism) as these patients have absent endogenous production of LH and so, while follicular growth may occur, oestrogen biosynthesis is impaired (Shoham et al., 1991). Therefore, hMG, which contains FSH and LH activity, is necessary for these patients.

Pituitary causes of secondary amenorrhoea

Hyperprolactinaemia is the commonest pituitary cause of amenorrhoea. There are many causes of mildly elevated serum prolactin concentrations, including stress, and a recent physical or breast examination. If the prolactin concentration is greater than 1000 mU/l then the test should be repeated; if prolactin is still elevated, it is necesary to image the pituitary fossa (CT or MRI scan). Hyperprolactinaemia may result from a prolactin-secreting pituitary adenoma or from a nonfunctioning "disconnection" tumour in the region of the hypothalamus or pituitary, which disrupts the inhibitory influence of dopamine on prolactin secretion. Large nonfunctioning tumours are usually associated with serum prolactin concentrations of less than 3000 mU/l, while prolactin-secreting macroadenomas usually result in concentrations of 8000 mU/l or more. Other causes include hypothyroidism, polycystic ovary syndrome (up to 2500 mU/l) and several drugs (e.g. the dopaminergic antagonist phenothiazines, domperidone and metoclopramide).

In women with amenorrhoea associated with hyperprolactinaemia, the main symptoms are usually those of oestrogen deficiency. In contrast, when hyperprolactinaemia is associated with PCOS, the syndrome is characterized by adequate oestrogenization, polycystic ovaries on ultrasound scan and a withdrawal bleed in response to a progestogen challenge test. Galactorrhoea may be found in up to a third of hyperprolactinaemic patients, although its appearance is neither correlated with prolactin levels nor with the presence of a tumour. Approximately 5% of patients present with visual field defects.

A prolactin-secreting pituitary microadenoma is usually associated with a moderately elevated prolactin (1500–4000 mU/l) and is unlikely to result in abnormalities on a lateral skull radiograph. By comparison, a macroadenoma, associated with a prolactin greater than 5000–8000 mU/l and by definition greater than 1 cm diameter, may cause typical radiological changes: an asymmetrically enlarged pituitary fossa, with a double contour to its floor and erosion of the clinoid processes. CT and MRI scans now allow detailed examination of the extent of the tumour and, in particular, identification of suprasellar extension and compression of the opitic chiasma or invasion of the cavernous sinuses. Prolactin is an excellent tumour marker and so the higher the serum concentration the larger the size of the tumour expected on the MRI scan. In contrast, a large tumour on the scan with only a moderately elevated serum prolactin concentration (2000–3000 mU/l) suggests a nonfunctioning tumour with "disconnection" from the hypothalamus.

The management of hyperprolactinaemia centres around the use of dopamine agonists, of which bromocriptine is the most widely used. Of course, if the hyperprolactinaemia is drug induced, stopping the relevant preparation should be recommended. This may not, however, be appropriate if the cause is a psychotropic medication, for example a phenothiazine being used to treat schizophrenia. In these cases, it is reasonable to continue the drug and prescribe a low-dose combined oral contraceptive preparation in order to counteract the symptoms of oestrogen deficiency. Serum prolactin concentrations must then be carefully monitored to ensure that they do not rise further.

Most patients show a fall in prolactin levels within a few days of commencing bromocriptine therapy and a reduction of tumour volume within six weeks. Longer-acting preparations (e.g. quinagolide, twice weekly cabergoline) may be prescribed to those patients who develop unacceptable side effects. Surgery, in the form of a transsphenoidal adenectomy, is reserved for drug resistance and failure to shrink a macroadenoma or if there are intolerable side effects of the drugs (the most common indication). Nonfunctioning tumours should be removed surgically and are usually detected by a combination of imaging and a serum prolactin concentration of less than 3000 mU/l. When the prolactin level is between 3000 and 8000 mU/l, a trial of bromocriptine is warranted. If the prolactin level falls, it can be assumed that the tumour is a prolactin-secreting macroadenoma. Operative treatment is also required if there is suprasellar extension of the tumour that has not regressed during treatment with bromocriptine and a pregnancy is desired. With the present day skills of neurosurgeons in transsphenoidal surgery, it is seldom necessary to resort to pituitary irradiation, which offers no advantages and necessitates long-term surveillance to detect consequent hypopituitarism (which is immediately apparent if it occurs after surgery) (Soule and Jacobs, 1995). If the serum prolactin is found to be elevated and the patient has a regular menstrual cycle, no treatment is necessary unless the cycle is anovulatory and fertility is desired. Amenorrhoea is the "bioassay" of prolactin excess and should be corrected for its sequelae, rather than for the serum level of prolactin (Soule and Jacobs, 1995).

Ovarian causes of amenorrhoea

Polycystic ovary syndrome is discussed in Ch. 27 and premature ovarian failure in Chs. 19 and 30.

Iatrogenic causes of amenorrhoea

There are many iatrogenic causes of amenorrhoea, which may be either temporary or permanent. These include malignant conditions that require either radiation to the abdomen/pelvis or chemotherapy. Both these treatments may result in permanent gonadal damage, the amount of damage being directly related to the age of the patient, the cumulative dose and the patient's prior menstrual status (Chs. 31 and 32).

Gynaecological procedures such as oophorectomy, hysterectomy and endometrial resection inevitably result in amenorrhoea. Hormone replacement should be prescribed for these patients where appropriate.

Hormone therapy itself can be deliberately used to disrupt the menstrual cycle. However, iatrogenic causes

Box 26.1 Key points

- Secondary amenorrhoea is usually considered to be amenorrhoea of six or more months' duration during reproductive years.
- Aetiology and treatment can be conveniently catagorized into hypothalamic, pituitary, ovarian or, uterine causes, or systemic illness, which in essence causes secondary hypothalamic amenorrhoea.
- Correct diagnosis is readily made if a logical protocol is applied.
- The polycystic ovary syndrome is the commonest cause of secondary amenorrhoea and is the only major cause of amenorrhoea that is *not* associated with oestrogen deficiency.
- The amenorrhoea of polycystic ovary syndrome should be treated in order either to enhance fertility or to prevent endometrial hyperplasia/adenocarcinoma (see Ch. 27).
- Oestrogen deficiency results in the long-term sequelae of osteoporosis and cardiovascular disease; consequently, the cause of amenorrhoea should be corrected early and hormone replacement therapy administered if necessary.
- Fertility can be achieved either after ovulation induction or, in premature ovarian failure, with oocyte donation/in vitro fertilization.

of ovarian quiescence have the same consequences of oestrogen deficiency as in any other aetiology. For example, the use of GnRH analogues in the treatment of oestrogen-dependent conditions (e.g. precocious puberty, endometriosis, uterine fibroids) results in a significant decrease in BMD in as little as six months, although the demineralization is reversible with the cessation of therapy, especially for the treatment of benign conditions in young women who are in the process of achieving their peak bone mass. The concurrent use of an androgenic progestogen, or low-dose oestrogen, may protect against bone loss.

Summary

In this chapter we have provided an overview of the causes of amenorrhoea and a description of the management of those conditions which are not covered elsewhere in this book. It is essential to provide the young woman with a diagnosis as quickly as possible so that a management plan can be formulated (Box 26.1).

REFERENCES

Asherman J G (1950). Traumatic intrauterine adhesions. *J Obstet Gynaecol Br Emp*, 57, 892–896.

Balen A H, Jacobs H S (2003). *Infertility in Practice*, 2nd edn. Churchill Livingstone, London.

Bowling A (1989). Injuries to dancers: prevalence, treatment and perception of causes. *Br Med J* 298, 731–734.

Cumming D C, Rebar R W (1983). Exercise and reproductive function in women. *Am J Indust Med* 4, 113–125.

Frisch R E (1976). Fatness of girls from menarche to age 18 years, with a nomogram. *Hum Biol* 48, 353–359.

Sheehan H L (1939). Simmond's disease due to post-partum necrosis of the anterior pituitary. *Q J Med* 8, 277.

Shoham Z, Balen A H, Patel A, Jacobs H S (1991). Results of ovulation induction using human menopausal gonadotropin or purified follicle-stimulating hormone in hypogonadotropic hypogonadism patients. *Fertil Steril* 56, 1048–1053.

Soule S G, Jacobs H S (1995). Prolactinomas: present day management. *Br J Obstet Gynaecol* 102, 178–181.

van der Spuy Z M, Steer P J, McCusker M, Steele S J, Jacobs H S (1988). Outcome of pregnancy in underweight women after spontaneous and induced ovulation. *Br Med J* 296, 962–965.

Warren M P, Brooks-Gunn J, Hamilton L H, Warren L F, Hamilton W G (1986). Scoliosis and fractures in young ballet dancers. *N Engl J Med* 314, 1348–1353.

27

The polycystic ovary syndrome and adolescent women

Adam H. Balen[1] and David Dunger[2]

[1]Department of Reproductive Medicine, The General Infirmary, Leeds, UK
[2] Department of Paediatrics, Addenbrooke's Hospital, Cambridge, UK

Introduction

The polycystic ovary syndrome (PCOS) is the commonest endocrine disturbance affecting women, yet it is only in the 1990s that we have begun to piece together a clearer idea of its pathogenesis (Balen, 1999). It has long been recognized that the presence of enlarged ovaries with multiple small cysts (2–9 mm) and a hypervascularized, androgen-secreting stroma are associated with signs of androgen excess (hirsutism, alopecia, acne), obesity and menstrual cycle disturbance (oligomenorrhoea or amenorrhoea). There is considerable heterogeneity of symptoms and signs amongst women with PCOS (Table 27.1) and for an individual these may change over time (Balen et al., 1995). The PCOS is familial (Franks et al., 1997) and various aspects of the syndrome may be differentially inherited. Furthermore, polycystic ovaries can exist without clinical signs of the syndrome, which may then become expressed over time. While ultrasound provides an excellent technique for the detection of polycystic ovaries, controversy still exists over the precise definition of PCOS and whether or not the diagnosis should require confirmation of polycystic ovarian morphology (Figs. 27.1–27.4).

Some argue that the definition of PCOS should be based on biochemical evidence of ovarian hyperandrogenism rather than the ultrasound appearance, as hyperandrogenism may exist in women who have normal ovarian morphology as detected by ultrasound. This view has been adopted in the USA and the 1990 National Institute of Health Conference on PCOS recommended that diagnostic criteria should include evidence of hyperandrogenism and ovulatory dysfunction in the absence of nonclassical adrenal hyperplasia and that evidence of polycystic

ovarian morphology is not essential. The definition of PCOS in the UK and Europe relies more heavily on the detection of polycystic ovarian changes on ultrasound and recognizes the spectrum from those with polycystic ovaries and no avert symptomatology right through to those with the most severe clinical and biochemical disorders. The diagnosis of PCOS is usually reserved for those women who exhibit an ultrasound picture of polycystic ovaries and who display one or more of the clinical symptoms (menstrual cycle disturbance, hirsutism, obesity, hyperandrogenism) and/or one or more of the recognized biochemical disturbances (elevated luteinizing hormone (LH), testosterone, androstenedione). This definition of PCOS requires exclusion of specific underlying diseases of the adrenal or pituitary glands (acromegaly, prolactinoma, congenital adrenal hyperplasia (CAH)) as these could predispose to similar ultrasound and biochemical features.

An international consensus meeting in 2003 held jointly by the European Society for Human Reproduction and Embryology (ESHRE) and the American Society for Reproductive Medicine (ASRM) agreed that two out of the following three criteria would define the PCOS:
- oligo-ovulation or anovulation (i.e. oligomenorrhoea or amenorrhoea)
- hyperandrogenism (clinical or biochemical)
- polycystic ovaries on ultrasound scan.

There are a number of interlinking factors that affect expression of PCOS. A gain in weight is associated with a worsening of symptoms, while weight loss will ameliorate the endocrine and metabolic profile and symptomatology (Clarke et al., 1995). Normal ovarian function relies upon the selection of a follicle, which responds to an appropriate signal (follicle-stimulating hormone (FSH)) in order to

Paediatric and Adolescent Gynaecology, ed. Adam Balen et al. Published by Cambridge University Press.
© Cambridge University Press 2004.

Table 27.1. The spectrum of clinical manifestations of polycystic ovary syndrome

Symptoms	Serum endocrinology	Possible late sequelae
Obesity	↑ Androgens (testosterone and androstenedione)	Diabetes mellitus
Menstrual disturbance	↑ Luteinizing hormone	Dyslipidaemia
Infertility	↑ Fasting insulin	Hypertension
Hyperandrogenism	↑ Prolactin	Cardiovascular disease
Asymptomatic	↓ Sex hormone-binding globulin	Endometrial carcinoma
	↑ Oestradiol, oestrone	Breast cancer

grow, become "dominant" and ovulate. This mechanism is disturbed in women with PCOS, resulting in multiple small cysts, most of which contain potentially viable oocytes but within dysfunctional follicles.

Elevations in serum concentrations of insulin are common in both lean and obese women with PCOS, even when allowance is made for differences in weight or body composition (Conway et al., 1992). Indeed, it is hyperinsulinaemia that many feel is the key to the pathogenesis of the syndrome (Dunaif 1997) as insulin stimulates androgen secretion by the ovarian stroma and appears to affect the normal development of ovarian follicles, both by the adverse effects of androgens on follicular growth and possibly also by suppressing apoptosis and permitting the survival of follicles otherwise destined to disappear. Insulin stimulates androgen secretion by the ovarian stroma, thus restricting follicular growth, and leads to suppression of liver production of sex hormone-binding globulin (SHBG), an important determinant of the free androgen index. The prevalence of diabetes in obese women with PCOS is approximately 11% (Conway 1990) and so a measurement of impaired glucose tolerance is important and long-term screening advisable. An underlying insulin resistance, promoting compensatory hyperinsulinaemia, could explain links with type 2 diabetes and risk of gestational diabetes.

Pathogenesis of polycystic ovary syndrome and puberty

High-resolution ultrasound scanning has made an accurate estimate of the prevalence of polycystic ovaries possible. Several studies have estimated the prevalence of polycystic ovaries in "normal adult" women and have found rates of 22–33% (Clayton et al., 1992; Farquhar et al., 1994;

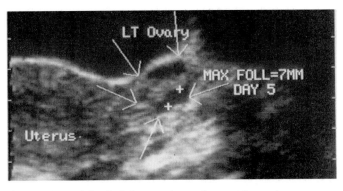

Fig. 27.1. Transabdominal ultrasound scan of a normal ovary in the early follicular phase of the menstrual cycle. (Reproduced with permission from Balen A H, Jacobs H S (2003). *Infertility in Practice*, 2nd edn. Churchill Livingstone, London.)

Michelmore et al., 1999; Polson et al., 1988) but it is not known at what age they first appear. Many of those women with polycystic ovaries detected by ultrasound do not have overt symptoms of PCOS. For example, in a study of 224 women randomly recruited from general practice surgeries and local universities, Michelmore et al. (1999) noted a prevalence of polycystic ovaries of around 33% but only 26% of the women fulfilled the European criteria for PCOS and only 4% the US criteria. Polycystic ovaries were associated with irregular menstrual cycles and significantly higher serum testosterone concentrations when compared with normal ovaries. Yet, only a small proportion of the women with polycystic ovaries (15%) had serum testosterone levels outside the normal range. Therefore, polycystic ovaries detected by routine screening in young women appears to be a rather benign condition with only marginal elevation of testosterone and few significant differences with respect to features of hyperandrogenism and menstrual cycle disturbance.

PCOS appears to have its origins during adolescence and is thought to be associated with increased weight gain during puberty (Balen and Dunger, 1995). However, the gene(s) involved has not yet been identified and the effect of environmental influences such as weight changes and circulating hormone concentrations, and the age at which these occur, are still being unravelled. Detecting polycystic ovaries in girls relies upon transabdominal scanning, which in adults failed to detect 30% of polycystic ovaries compared with 100% detection rate with a transvaginal scan (Fox et al., 1991). Bridges et al. (1993) performed 428 ovarian scans in girls aged between 3 and 18 years and found polycystic ovaries in 101 girls (24% of the total). The rate of detection of polycystic ovaries was 6% in six-year-old girls rising to 18% in those aged 10 years and 26% in those aged 15 years.

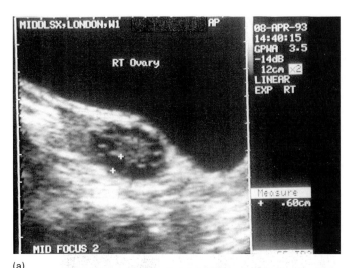

(a)

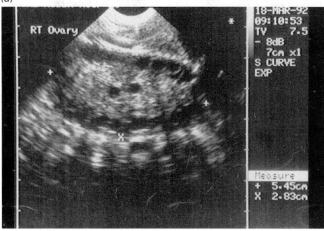

(b)

Fig. 27.2. Ultrasound scans of a polycystic ovary.
(a) Transabdominal; (b) transvaginal. (Reproduced with permission from Balen A H, Jacobs H S (2003). *Infertility in Practice*, 2nd edn. Churchill Livingstone, London.)

The implication of this study is that polycystic ovaries are present before puberty and are more easy to detect in older girls as the ovaries increase in size.

Prior to puberty, there appears to be two periods of increased ovarian growth. The first is at adrenarche in response to increased concentrations of circulating androgens and the second is just before and during puberty owing to rising gonadotrophin levels and the actions of growth hormone and insulin-like growth factor-1 (IGF-1) and insulin on the ovary. Sampaolo et al. (1994) reported a study of 49 obese girls at different stages of puberty, comparing their pelvic ultrasound features and endocrine profiles with 35 controls matched for age and pubertal stage. They found that obesity was associated with a significant increase in

uterine and ovarian volume. They also found obese postmenarchal girls with polycystic ovaries had larger uterine and ovarian volumes than obese postmenarchal girls with normal ovaries. Sampaolo et al. (1994) concluded that obesity leads to hyperinsulinism; this causes both hyperandrogenaemia and raised IGF-1 levels, which augments the ovarian response to gonadotrophins. This implies that obesity may be important in the pathogenesis of polycystic ovaries, but further study is required to evaluate this. It is known that obesity is not a prerequisite for PCOS. Indeed, in a series of 1741 women with polycystic ovaries in a study by Balen et al. (1995), only 38.4% of patients were overweight (body mass index (BMI) > 25 kg/m^2).

As well as an association between tall stature and obesity with PCOS, a high prevalence has also been noted in a number of conditions associated with hyperinsulinaemia. PCOS is common in subjects with genetic defects of the insulin receptor and congenital lypodystrophy. It has also been observed in children with glycogen storage disease treated with high doses of oral glucose and in adolescents with type 1 diabetes, where there are inappropriately high levels of circulating insulin. Consequently, during childhood as in adult life, high circulating levels of insulin from whatever cause may be a trigger for the subsequent development of polycystic ovaries.

Adrenarche

In the study reported by Bridges et al. (1993), adrenarche was associated with an increased prevalence of PCOS on ultrasound. Adrenarche has always been considered to be a benign condition but recent work from several groups has suggested that, along with premature pubarche, it may in some populations be associated with insulin resistance. In a series of elegant studies, Ibanez et al. (2000) have shown that girls presenting with premature adrenarche and pubarche may be more insulin resistant than controls and are at high risk of developing ovarian hyperandrogenism after menarche. This association was particularly strong in girls who were born small for gestational age. However, this sequence of low birth weight, premature pubarche, insulin resistance and ovarian hyperandrogenism is not necessarily associated with ovarian morphological features of polycystic ovaries; rather, small ovaries have been reported.

The association between PCOS and insulin resistance, together with links with type 2 diabetes and gestational diabetes, have led to the suggestion that PCOS could be related to a "thrifty ovary"; this would enhance fertility during periods of poor nutrition and only lead to infertility and associated problems with improved nutrition. Similarly, insulin

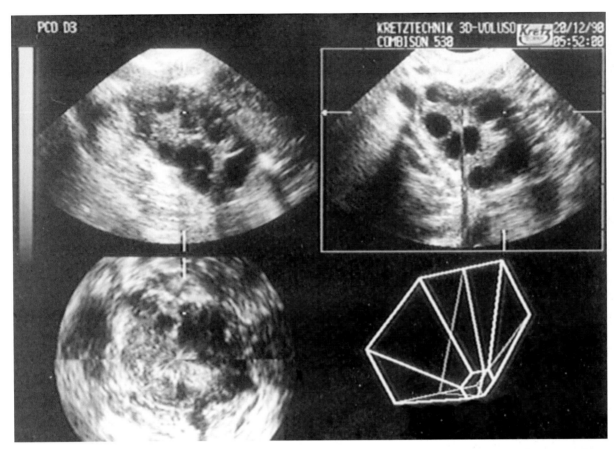

Fig. 27.3. Three-dimensional transvaginal ultrasound scan of a polycystic ovary. (Reproduced with permission from Balen A H, Jacobs H S (2003). *Infertility in Practice*, 2nd edn. Churchill Livingstone, London.)

resistance per se may be a survival mechanism whereby growth is maintained during poor nutrition, and risks for gestational diabetes and type 2 diabetes only become apparent with increased weight gain. The *INS* VNTR (variable number of tandem repeats) class III/III genotype, as well as links with PCOS, gestational diabetes and type 2 diabetes, may also represent a putative "thrifty genotype" by conferring larger size at birth and thus potentially increased perinatal survival in the face of maternal/fetal nutritional deprivation.

Larger birth weight has been associated with adult risk of polycystic ovaries in historical (Cresswell et al., 1997) and more contemporary cohorts (Michelmore et al., 2001). These data indicate that the risk for PCOS may originate in early prenatal development and could be influenced by both uterine environment and/or fetal genotype. The larger size at birth associated with *INS* VNTR III/III genotype may reflect intrinsic insulin resistance in the fetus. In other infants, larger size at birth could reflect fetal hyperinsulinaemia secondary to increased pla-

cental transfer of glucose, as observed in infants of diabetic mothers. Exposure to high levels of insulin, by either mechanism, could predispose to the development of polycystic ovaries.

Paradoxically, insulin resistance, ovarian hyperandrogenism and ovarian dysfunction have also been associated with *low birth weight*. These links with low birth weight and postnatal catch-up growth are seen not only in girls presenting with premature pubarche but also in nonselected low birth weight infants (Ibanez et al., 2000) and correspond to well-replicated low birth weight associations with type 2 diabetes risk (Hales et al., 1991). Our recent data indicate that this phenotype in girls with premature pubarche is independently associated with both low birth weight and the *INS* VNTR genotype class I allele, which, although associated with lower birth weight, confers increased postnatal insulin secretion and greater weight gain. However, this sequence of low birth weight, postnatal catch-up growth, hyperinsulinaemia and ovarian hyperandrogenism is not associated with polycystic ovarian changes,

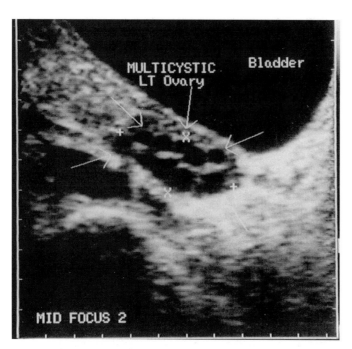

Fig. 27.4. Transabdominal ultrasound scan of a multicystic ovary. (Reproduced with permission from Balen A H, Jacobs H S (2003). *Infertility in Practice*, 2nd edn. Churchill Livingstone, London.)

but rather with small ovaries and reduced volume percentage of primordial follicles.

These apparently paradoxical pathways to the classical PCOS symptomatology of anovulation and ovarian hyperandrogenism (the one being associated with *higher birth weight*, class III *INS* VNTR genotype and polycystic ovaries on ultrasound, and the other with a *lower birth weight*, class I *INS* VNTR genotype and no polycystic ovarian changes) may accurately reflect the dichotomy in the definitions of PCOS.

There may well be important genetic and ethnic differences between populations that determine the severity and characteristics of the PCOS phenotype. Insulin resistance is thought to be particularly severe in Hispanic women with PCOS compared with nonHispanic women matched for age, weight and body composition. Within the UK, the Indian and Pakistani population appear to have a high background risk for insulin resistance and a high prevalence of PCOS (see review Balen and Michelmore, 2002).

Puberty

The prevalence of polycystic ovaries increases dramatically at puberty. Normal pubertal development is associated with an increase in insulin resistance, which is most marked in peripheral glucose uptake rather than hepatic glucose production. There is compensatory hyperinsulinaemia, which has an active rather than a passive role in pubertal growth and development. The high insulin levels lead to a gradual fall in SHBG and IGF-1 binding protein production by the liver. The exposure of the ovary to high levels of insulin may be important in ovarian development, directly or indirectly through falls in this binding protein and a rise in IGF-1. Insulin resistance at puberty is thought to be driven by increases in growth hormone secretion and both growth hormone and IGF-1 may be important for ovarian development.

Nobels and Dewailly (1992) suggested that PCOS resulted from the effects of the progressively rising levels of insulin and IGF-1 on the ovary during puberty. They speculated that polycystic ovarian changes may persist in some girls owing to an abnormal continuance of hyperinsulinaemia after puberty. However, this is only likely to be the case in those programmed or genetically predisposed to insulin resistance.

Excessive weight gain during puberty will lead to an exacerbation of any underlying insulin resistance and to compensatory hyperinsulinaemia. The trends towards an ever increasing prevalence of obesity during childhood and adolescence could increase the rate of expression of PCOS during puberty. The recent rise in the prevalence of type 2 diabetes presenting earlier during childhood in several ethnic minority groups in the USA and other parts of the world may also be accompanied by an increasing prevalence of PCOS.

Diagnosis in children and adolescents

There is an increasing awareness of the increased prevalence of PCOS in children with genetic forms of insulin resistance and in those with conditions such as glycogen storage disease and type 1 diabetes, where hyperinsulinaemia may be the result of therapy. However, the increasing background prevalence of obesity in Western society should also increase our awareness of the possibility of PCOS developing in genetically susceptible individuals in the UK. PCOS is likely to parallel the increasing prevalence of insulin resistance and type 2 diabetes that is currently being observed in the Asian population. Other ethnic groups known to be at increased risk of insulin resistance may also be at risk of PCOS. The sequence of low birth weight, premature pubarche and ovarian hyperandrogenism has, so far, only been described in a few populations, but more active investigation and follow-up of patients presenting with adrenarche or pubarche is indicated. Presentation of PCOS during adolescence is likely to be similar to that seen in adults with either menstrual disturbance or evidence of hyperandrogenism, acne and hirsutism. Acanthosis nigricans may be an important marker of insulin resistance. Cryptogenic CAH needs to be carefully excluded and evidence of polycystic ovaries ought to be sought on transabdominal ultrasound.

Although obesity and PCOS are clearly linked, the mechanism underlying the relationship is uncertain. Obesity is associated with hyperinsulinaemia and this could, by driving down levels of SHBG, lead to higher free androgen levels and an increase in symptomology. The association between obesity and raised free androgen levels is, however, even stronger in women with increased central obesity, a phenotype known to be associated with insulin resistance.

Leptin is a 167 amino acid residue peptide that is secreted by fat cells in response to insulin and glucocorticoids (see Ch. 6). Leptin is transported by a protein that appears to be the extracellular domain of the leptin receptor itself (Tartaglia et al., 1995). Leptin receptors are found in the choroid plexus, on the hypothalamus and ovary and at many other sites. Leptin decreases the intake of food and stimulates thermogenesis. Leptin also appears to inhibit the hypothalamic peptide neuropeptide Y, which is an inhibitor of gonadotrophin-releasing hormone (GnRH) pulsatility. Leptin appears to serve as the signal from the body fat to the brain about the adequacy of fat stores for reproduction. Therefore, menstruation will only occur if fat stores are adequate. Obesity, by comparison, is associated with high circulating concentrations of leptin and this, in turn, might be a mechanism for hypersecretion of LH in women with PCOS. To date, most studies have been in the leptin-deficient and consequently obese *Ob/Ob* mouse. Starvation of the *Ob/Ob* mouse leads to weight loss, yet fertility is only restored after the administration of leptin. Leptin administration to overweight, infertile women may not be as straightforward as it might initially seem because of the complex nature of leptin transport into the brain. Nonetheless, the role of leptin in human reproduction is an exciting area of ongoing research. Recently, there has been interest in whether abnormalities of leptin secretion could predispose to weight gain in women with PCOS. Evidence for "leptin resistance" (i.e. leptin levels that are greater than might be predicted by BMI) have been noted in PCOS and in a general population of women who were overweight. "Leptin resistance" is common in other insulin-resistant states and its role, if any, in the pathophysiology of PCOS is yet to be determined.

Family studies and genetics

Several studies have demonstrated an increased prevalence of PCOS in family members of affected individuals (see Franks et al., 2001). However, the heterogeneity of the syndrome, the lack of a universally accepted definition and the problem of identifying a possible male phenotype for the condition has complicated the interpretation of family and genetic studies. With the recent developments in molecular biology, the search for the genetic basis for the predisposition of PCOS has begun.

Initial genetic studies concentrated on excess androgen synthesis by the ovary as a primary cause for the abnormal biochemical profiles in PCOS. Abnormalities of the gene *CYP17* encoding 17β-hydroxylase/17,20-lyase gene, which regulate androgen synthesis in the ovary, has been proposed as a cause for the hyperandrogenism in PCOS. However, several studies have failed to confirm linkage within families.

Hyperinsulinaemia and insulin resistance are well-documented features of PCOS and have been shown to be more common in family members of women with PCOS. A recent study of the insulin gene minisatellite or the *INS* VNTR on chromosome 11p15.5, which regulates insulin gene expression, has demonstrated association with an anovulatory PCOS and hyperinsulinaemia. In particular it is the class III alleles inherited from the father that are most strongly linked to PCOS and to type 2 diabetes.

Genetic study of PCOS has identified links with insulin secretion and insulin action. Association has been reported with common allelic variation at the VNTR in the promoter region of *INS* (Waterworth et al., 1997). This locus has been variably associated with the risk of obesity, insulin resistance and type 2 diabetes. The identified association has been with the class III/III genotype, particularly in women who have anovulatory cycles and are hyperinsulinaemic (Waterworth et al., 1997). These associations are particularly evident where the III allele has been inherited from the father. A systematic screen of 37 candidate genes for PCOS have demonstrated linkage with follistatin, an activin-binding neutralizing protein (Urbanek et al., 1999). Amongst the actions of activin are promotion of follicular development, increased FSH production and pancreatic β-cell secretion of insulin. Subsequent research has not confirmed this association.

The study of Michelmore et al. (1999, 2001) reflected the rather benign characteristics of polycystic ovaries detected by routine screening in young women with only marginal elevation of testosterone and few significant differences with respect to features of hyperandrogenism and menstrual cycle disturbance. There were no differences in *INS* VNTR genotype between those with and without polycystic ovaries but the association between polycystic ovaries and larger size at birth was highly significant (p 0.004). The study did, however, confirm the profound heterogeneity of association between polycystic ovaries, birth weight and insulin sensitivity.

Heterogeneity of polycystic ovary syndrome

A few years ago we reported what remains in the literature as the largest series of women with polycystic ovaries detected by ultrasound scan (1800) who were attending a reproductive endocrinology clinic (Balen et al., 1995). All patients had at least one symptom of the PCOS and 38% were overweight (BMI $>$ 25 kg/m^2). Obesity was significantly associated with an increased risk of hirsutism, menstrual cycle disturbance and an elevated serum testosterone concentration. Obesity was also associated with an increased rate of infertility and menstrual cycle disturbance. Twenty six per cent of patients with primary infertility and 14% of patients with secondary infertility had a BMI of $>$ 30 kg/m^2.

Approximately 30% of the patients had a regular menstrual cycle, 50% had oligomenorrhoea and 20% had amenorrhoea. A rising serum concentration of testosterone was associated with an increased risk of hirsutism, infertility and cycle disturbance. The rates of infertility and menstrual cycle disturbance also increased with increasing serum LH concentrations greater than 10 IU/l. The serum LH concentration of those with primary infertility was significantly higher than that of women with secondary infertility and both were higher than that of those with proven fertility. Ovarian morphology appears to be the most sensitive marker of the PCOS, compared with the classical endocrine features of raised serum LH and testosterone, which were found in only 39.8% and 28.9% of patients, respectively, in this series (Balen et al., 1995).

Hypersecretion of LH occurs in approximately 40% of women who have polycystic ovaries. The risk of infertility and miscarriage is raised in these patients. Several hypotheses have been suggested to explain this oversecretion of LH. These include increased pulse frequency of GnRH, increased pituitary sensitivity to GnRH, hyperinsulinaemic stimulation of the pituitary gland and disturbance of the ovarian steroid–pituitary feedback mechanism. However, none of these fully explain hypersecretion of LH and it may be that leptin also has a role to play here.

Management of the polycystic ovary syndrome

Obesity

The clinical management of a women with PCOS should be focused on her individual problems. Obesity worsens both symptomatology and the endocrine profile and so obese women (BMI $>$ 30 kg/m^2) should be encouraged to lose weight. Weight loss improves the endocrine profile (Kiddy et al., 1989), the likelihood of ovulation and a healthy pregnancy. A study by Clark et al. (1995) looked at the effect of a weight-loss programme on women with at least a two year history of anovulatory infertility, clomiphene resistance and a BMI $>$ 30 kg/m^2. Weight loss had a significant effect on endocrine function, ovulation and subsequent pregnancy: 12 of the 13 subjects resumed ovulation, 11 becoming pregnant (five spontaneously). Fasting insulin and serum testosterone concentrations also fell. The advice for the adolescent girl with PCOS is to avoid weight gain because of the long-term impact of obesity on reproductive function and general health. It is thought that weight gain associated with the combination oral contraceptive (COC) may result in a greater rate of symptoms when discontinuing therapy – although there are no prospective data looking at young women with PCOS who are prescribed COC for symptom control compared with untreated young women with PCOS. There is, therefore, a feeling that the prescription of the COC should be limited and either general advice or the use of insulin-sensitizing agents (such as metformin) is favoured.

Eating disorders are common during adolescence and have been shown to be more prevalent in young women with PCOS (see Ch. 38).

Menstrual irregularity

The easiest way to control the menstrual cycle is the use of a low-dose COC preparation. This will result in an artificial cycle and regular shedding of the endometrium. An alternative is a progestogen (such as medroxyprogesterone acetate (Provera) or dydrogesterone (Duphaston)) for 12 days every one to three months to induce a withdrawal bleed. It is also important once again to encourage weight loss. As women with PCOS are thought to be at increased risk of cardiovascular disease a "lipid friendly" COC should be used. At present, the ideal COC has not been found, although there is hope for the new preparation Yasmin (Schering), which contains the antiandrogenic progestogen drosperinone and appears not only to suppress androgens but also to reduce blood pressure, in the context of a normal lipid profile.

In women with anovulatory cycles, the action of oestradiol on the endometrium is unopposed because of the lack of cyclical progesterone secretion. This may result in episodes of irregular uterine bleeding and, in the long term, endometrial hyperplasia and even endometrial cancer. An ultrasound assessment of endometrial thickness provides a bioassay for oestradiol production by the ovaries and conversion of androgens in the peripheral fat. If the endometrium is thicker than 15 mm, a withdrawal bleed should be induced; if the endometrium fails to shed then endometrial sampling is required to exclude endometrial hyperplasia or malignancy. The only young women to get endometrial carcinoma (< 35 years), which otherwise has a mean age of occurrence of 61 years in the UK, are those with anovulation secondary to PCOS or oestrogen-secreting tumours. Consequently, the adolescent with oligo/amenorrhoea should be provided with therapy to induce a menstrual bleed at least every three months.

Infertility

Infertility is unlikely to be an issue for the adolescent girl, although often questions are asked about future fertility, usually by anxious parents. The familial nature of the condition may also mean that other family members may have presented with infertility (e.g. mother or sisters). Health advice can be usefully given to the young woman, in particular to watch her weight, in order to minimize adverse consequences to reproductive health.

Ovulation can be induced with antioestrogens, such as clomiphene citrate (50–100 mg) on days 2–6 of a natural or artificially induced bleed (Fig. 27.5). While clomiphene is successful in inducing ovulation in over 80% of women, pregnancy only occurs in about 40%. Clomiphene citrate should only be prescribed in a setting where ultrasound monitoring is available (and performed) in order to minimize the 10% risk of multiple pregnancy (Fig. 27.6) and to ensure that ovulation is taking place (RCOG Guidelines, 1998). Once an ovulatory dose has been reached, the cumulative conception rate continues to increase for up to 10 to 12 cycles (Kousta et al., 1997).

The therapeutic options for patients with anovulatory infertility who are resistant to antioestrogens are either parenteral gonadotrophin therapy or laparoscopic ovarian diathermy. Because the polycystic ovary is very sensitive to stimulation by exogenous hormones, it is very important to start with very low doses of gonadotrophins and follicular development must be carefully monitored by ultrasound scans. The advent of transvaginal ultrasonography, with its higher resolution and clearer view of the developing follicles, has enabled the multiple pregnancy rate to be reduced

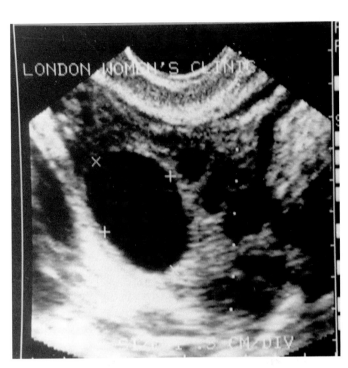

Fig. 27.5. Transvaginal ultrasound scan of unifollicular development in a polycystic ovary after ovarian stimulation. (Reproduced with permission from Balen A H, Jacobs H S (2003). *Infertility in Practice*, 2nd edn. Churchill Livingstone, London.)

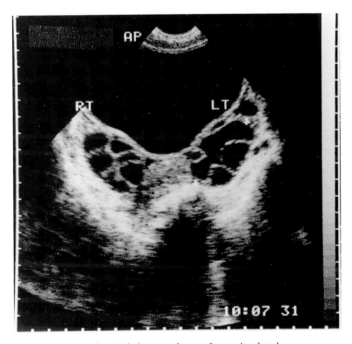

Fig. 27.6. Transabdominal ultrasound scan of overstimulated polycystic ovaries. (Reproduced with permission from Balen A H, Jacobs H S (2003). *Infertility in Practice*, 2nd edn. Churchill Livingstone, London.)

to approximately 7%. Cumulative conception and livebirth rates after six months have been reported as 62% and 54%, respectively, and after 12 months 73% and 62%, respectively (Balen et al., 1994). Close monitoring should enable treatment to be suspended if three or more mature follicles develop, as the risk of multiple pregnancy obviously increases.

Ovarian diathermy is free of the risks of multiple pregnancy and ovarian hyperstimulation and does not require intensive ultrasound monitoring. Laparoscopic ovarian diathermy has taken the place of wedge resection of the ovaries (which resulted in extensive periovarian and tubal adhesions), and it appears to be as effective as routine gonadotrophin therapy in the treatment of clomiphine-insensitive PCOS (Farquhar et al., 2002).

A number of pharmacological agents have been used to amplify the physiological effect of weight loss, notably metformin. This biguanide inhibits the production of hepatic glucose and enhances the sensitivity of peripheral tissue to insulin, thereby decreasing insulin secretion. It has been shown that metformin ameliorates hyperandrogenism and abnormalities of gonadotrophin secretion in women with PCOS (Nestler et al., 1996) and can restore menstrual cyclicity and fertility (Velazquez et al., 1997). Not all authors agree with these findings, particularly if there is no concurrent weight loss (Ehrmann et al., 1997). The insulin-sensitizing agent troglitazone also appears to improve significantly the metabolic and reproductive abnormalities in PCOS although this product has been withdrawn recently because of reports of deaths from hepatotoxicity. Newer insulin-sensitizing agents are currently being evaluated as is the phosphoglycan containing drug D-chiro-inositol.

Metformin is the most promising and safe sensitizer to insulin available in the UK at the present time and may have benefits for short- and long-term health, by improving obesity, hyperandrogenism, fertility, insulin sensitivity and lipid profile. There has been much publicity about its use and a recent Cochrane meta-analysis has indicated significant benefit on rates of ovulation both alone and when combined with clomiphene citrate (Lord et al., 2003). Insulin-sensitizing agents, such as metformin, might also play a role in the longer-term management of some of the other features and long-term health risks of PCOS.

Hyperandrogenism and hirsutism

The bioavailability of testosterone is affected by the serum concentration of SHBG. High levels of insulin lower the production of SHBG and so increase the free fraction of androgen. Elevated serum androgen concentrations stimulate peripheral androgen receptors, resulting in an

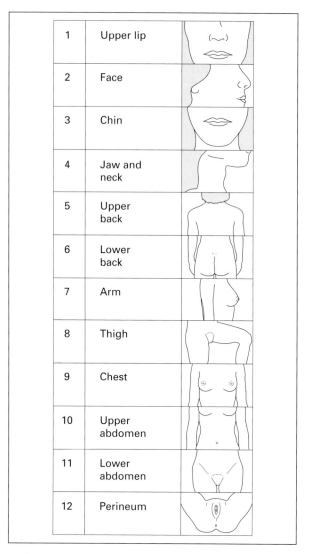

Fig. 27.7. Ferriman Gallwey score. Each area is given a score from 1 to 4 (1, mild; 2, moderate; 3, complete light coverage; 4, heavy coverage).

increase in 5α-reductase activity, which directly increases the conversion of testosterone to the more potent metabolite dihydrotestosterone. Symptoms of hyperandrogenism include hirsutism, which can be a distressing condition. Hirsutism is characterized by terminal hair growth in a male pattern of distribution, including chin, upper lip, chest, upper and lower back, upper and lower abdomen, upper arm, thigh and buttocks. A standardized scoring system, such as the modified Ferriman and Gallwey score, should be used to evaluate the degree of hirsutism before and during treatments (Fig. 27.7).

Treatment options include cosmetic and medical therapies. Medical regimens stop further progression of hirsutism and decrease the rate of hair growth. However, drug therapies may take six to nine months or longer before any benefit is perceived and so physical treatments, including electrolysis, waxing and bleaching, may be helpful while waiting for medical treatments to work. Symptoms of hyperandrogenism can be treated by a combination of an oestrogen (such as ethinylestradiol, or a COC) and the antiandrogen cyproterone acetate (50–100 mg). Oestrogens lower circulating androgens by a combination of a slight inhibition of gonadotrophin secretion and gonadotrophin-sensitive ovarian steroid production and an increase in hepatic production of SHBG, resulting in lower free testosterone. The cyproterone is taken for the first 10 days of a cycle (the "reversed sequential" method) and the oestrogen for the first 21 days. After a gap of exactly seven days, during which menstruation usually occurs, the regimen is repeated. As an alternative, the preparation Dianette (Schering) contains ethinylestradiol in combination with cyproterone, although at a lower dose (2 mg). Cyproterone acetate acts as a competitive inhibitor at the androgen receptor. Serum levels of LH, FSH, oestradiol, androstenedione, total and free testosterone are lowered while SHBG increases. However, there is an increase in triglycerides and apolipoproteins A1, A2, and B. Cyproterone acetate can cause liver damage, and liver function should be checked regularly. The newer preparation Yasmin (Schering; see above) appears to have a more favourable lipid and metabolic profile but is yet to be used extensively for the management of PCOS. Other antiandrogens such as spironolactone, ketoconazole and flutamide have been tried but are not widely used in the UK.

Long-term consequences of the polycystic ovary syndrome

The long-term risk of endometrial hyperplasia and endometrial carcinoma as a result of chronic anovulation and unopposed oestrogen has long been recognized. With increasing awareness of the metabolic abnormalities associated with the syndrome, there is concern regarding cardiovascular risk, type 2 diabetes and other long-term health implications in these women.

Obesity and metabolic abnormalities are recognized risk factors for the development of ischaemic heart disease in the general population, and these are also recognized features of PCOS. The idea that women with PCOS are at greater risk for cardiovascular disease is based on:
- higher insulin resistance than weight-matched controls
- the occurence of metabolic disturbances associated with insulin resistance, which are known to increase cardiovascular risk in other populations.

There is evidence that insulin resistance, central obesity and hyperandrogenaemia are features of PCOS and have an adverse effect on lipid metabolism. Women with PCOS have been shown to have dyslipidaemia, with reduced high density lipoprotein cholesterol and elevated serum triglyceride concentrations, along with elevated serum plasminogen activator inhibitor I concentrations. Consequently, evidence is mounting that women with PCOS may have an increased risk of developing cardiovascular disease and diabetes later in life, which has important implications in their management (see review by Rajkowa et al., 2000). These issues are of relevance when counselling the young woman with PCOS, together with her parents and, possibly also, sisters.

Summary

PCOS is one of the most common endocrine disorders, although its aetiology remains unknown (Box 27.1). This heterogeneous disorder may present, at one end of the spectrum, with the single finding of polycystic ovarian morphology as detected by pelvic ultrasound. At the other end of the spectrum symptoms such as obesity, hyperandrogenism, menstrual cycle disturbance and infertility may occur either singly or in combination. Metabolic disturbances (elevated serum concentrations of LH, testosterone, insulin and prolactin) are common and may have profound implications on the long-term health of women with PCOS.

PCOS is a familial condition and appears to have its origins during adolescence, when it is thought to be associated with increased weight gain during puberty. In the management of young women with menstrual disturbances or mild signs of hyperandrogenism, there is an increasing awareness amongst physicians about the possibility of PCOS. This awareness should be enhanced if there is a family history.

Women with PCOS are characterized by the presence of insulin resistance, central obesity, and dyslipidaemia, which appears to place them at a higher risk of developing diabetes as well as cardiovascular disease. Therapeutic interventions in the form of metformin and other insulin-sensitizing drugs appear to be potentially effective tools in ameliorating insulin resistance, with improvement in clinical and hormonal parameters, and possible reduction in cardiovascular risk. However, further evaluation is needed in adolescents. Encouraging weight loss remains the most effective first-line therapeutic intervention in these women – albeit hard to achieve. Further longitudinal studies need to be performed to investigate the natural history of PCOS and its sequelae for the health of women.

Box 27.1 Key points

- PCOS is the commonest endocrine disorder in women (approximate prevalence 10–15%).
- PCOS is a heterogeneous condition. Diagnosis is made by the ultrasound detection of polycystic ovaries and one or more of a combination of symptoms and signs: hyperandrogenism (acne, hirsutism, alopecia), obesity, menstrual cycle disturbance (oligo/amenorrhoea) and biochemical abnormalities (hypersecretion of testosterone, LH and insulin).
- Diagnosis made by two out of the following:
  - oligo- or amenorrhoea
  - hyperandrogenism (clinical or biochemical)
  - polycystic ovaries on ultrasound scan.
- Management is symptom orientated.
- If obese, weight loss improves symptoms and endocrinology and should be encouraged. A glucose tolerance test should be performed if the BMI is $> 30 \, kg/m^2$.
- Menstrual cycle control is achieved by cyclical oral contraceptives or progestogens.
- Ovulation induction may be difficult and require progression through various treatments, which should be monitored carefully to prevent multiple pregnancy. It may be achieved with clomiphene citrate, gonadotrophin therapy or laparoscopic ovarian diathermy.
- Hyperandrogenism is usually managed with ethinylestradiol in combination with cyproterone acetate (Dianette, Schering Healthcare). Alternatives include spironolactone, flutamide and finasteride, all of which have potential adverse effects.
- Insulin-sensitizing agents (e.g. metformin) are showing early promise but require further long-term evaluation and should only be prescribed by endocrinologists/reproductive endocrinologists.

REFERENCES

Balen A H (1999). The pathogenesis of polycystic ovary syndrome: the enigma unravels. *Lancet* 354, 966–977.

Balen A H, Dunger D (1995). Pubertal maturation of the internal genitalia. [Commentary.] *Ultrasound Obstet Gynecol* 6, 164–165.

Balen A H, Jacobs H S (2003). *Infertility in Practice*, 2nd edn. Churchill Livingstone, London.

Balen A H, Michelmore K (2002). Polycystic ovary syndrome: are national views important? *Hum Reprod* 17, 2219–2227.

Balen A H, Braat D D M, West C, Patel A, Jacobs H S (1994). Cumulative conception and live birth rates after the treatment of anovulatory infertility. An analysis of the safety and efficacy of ovulation induction in 200 patients. *Hum Reprod* 9, 1563–1570.

Balen A H, Conway G S, Kaltsas G et al. (1995). Polycystic ovary syndrome: the spectrum of the disorder in 1741 patients. *Hum Reprod* 10, 2705–2712.

Bridges N A, Cooke A, Healy M J R, Hindmarsh P C, Brook C G D (1993). Standards for ovarian volume in childhood and puberty. *Fertil Steril* 60, 456–460.

Clark A M, Ledger W, Galletly C et al. (1995). Weight loss results in significant improvement in pregnancy and ovulation rates in anovulatory obese women. *Hum Reprod* 10, 2705–2712.

Clayton R N, Ogden V, Hodgekinson J et al. (1992). How common are polycystic ovaries in normal women and what is their significance for the fertility of the population? *Clin Endocrinol* 37, 127–134.

Conway G S (1990). Insulin resistance and the polycystic ovary syndrome. *Contemp Rev Obstet Gynaecol* 2, 34–39.

Conway G S, Agrawal R, Betterridge D J et al. (1992). Risk factors for coronary artery disease in lean and obese women with polycystic ovary syndrome. *Clin Endocrinol* 37, 119–125.

Cresswell J L, Barker D J, Osmond C, Egger P, Phillips D I, Fraser R B (1997). Fetal growth, length of gestation, and polycystic ovaries in adult life. *Lancet* 350, 1131–1135.

Dunaif A (1997). Insulin resistance and the polycystic ovary syndrome: mechanisms and implication for pathogenesis. *Endocr Rev* 18, 774–800.

Ehrmann D A, Cavaghan M K, Imperial J, Sturis J, Rosenfield R L, Polonsky K S (1997). Effects of metformin on insulin secretion, insulin action and ovarian steroidogenesis in women with polycystic ovary syndrome. *J Clin Endocrinol Metab* 82, 1241–1247.

Farquhar C M, Birdsall M, Manning P, Mitchell J M (1994). Transabdominal versus transvaginal ultrasound in the diagnosis of polycystic ovaries on ultrasound scanning in a population of randomly selected women. *Ultrasound Obstet Gynaecol* 4, 54–59.

Farquhar C M, Vandekerckhove P, Lilford R (2002). Laparoscopic "drilling" by diathermy or laser for ovulation induction in anovulatory polycystic ovary syndrome (Cochrane Review). *Cochrane Library*, issue 4, Oxford.

Fox R, Corrigan E, Thomas P A, Hull M G R (1991). The diagnosis of polycystic ovaries in women with oligo-amenorrhoea: predictive power of endocrine tests. *Clin Endocrinol* 34, 127–131.

Franks S, Gharani N, Waterworth D et al. (1997). The genetic basis of polycystic ovary syndrome. *Hum Reprod* 12, 2641–2648.

Franks S, Gharani N, McCarthy M (2001). Candidate genes in polycystic ovary syndrome. *Hum Reprod Update* 7, 405–410.

Hales C N, Barker D J, Clark P M et al. (1991). Fetal and infant growth and impaired glucose tolerance at age 64. *Br Med J* 303, 1019–1022.

Ibanez L, Potau N, Enriquez G, de Zegher F (2000). Reduced uterine and ovarian size in adolescent girls born small for gestational age. *Pediatr Res* 47, 575–577.

Kiddy D S, Hamilton Fairley D, Bush A et al. (1989). Characteristics of obese amenorrheic hyperandrogenic women before and after weight loss. *J Clin Endocrinol Metab* 68, 173–179.

Kousta E, White D M, Franks S (1997). Modern use of clomiphene citrate in induction of ovulation. *Hum Reprod Update* 3, 359–365.

Lord J M, Flight I H K, Norman R J (2003). Metformin in polycystic ovary syndrome: systematic review and meta-analysis. *Br Med J* 327, 951–955.

Michelmore K F, Balen A H, Dunger D B, Vessey M P (1999). Polycystic ovaries and associated clinical and biochemical features in young women. *Clin Endcrinol* 51, 779–786.

Michelmore K, Ong K, Mason S et al. (2001). Clinical features in women with polycystic ovaries: relationships to insulin sensitivity, insulin gene *VNTR* and birth weight. *Clin Endocrinol* 55, 439–446.

Nestler J E, Jakubowicz D J (1996). Decreases in ovarian cytochrome P450c17alpha activity and serum free testosterone after reduction of insulin secretion in polycystic ovary syndrome. *N Engl J Med* 335, 617–623.

Nobles F and Dewailly D (1992). Puberty and polycystic ovary syndrome: the insulin/insulin-like growth factor 1 hypothesis. *Fert Steril* 58, 655–666.

Polson D W, Adams J, Wadsworth J, Franks S (1988). Polycystic ovaries – a common finding in normal women. *Lancet* i, 870–872.

Rajkowha M, Glass M R, Rutherford A J, Michelmore K, Balen A H (2000). Polycystic ovary syndrome: a risk factor for cardiovascular disease? *Br J Obstet Gynaecol* 107, 11–18.

RCOG (Royal College of Gynaecologists) (1998). *Guidelines on the Initial Investigation and Management of Infertility.* RCOG Press, London.

Sampaolo P, Livien C, Montanari L, Paganelli A, Salesi A, Lorini R (1994). Precocious signs of polycystic ovaries in obese girls. *Ultrasound Obstet Gynecol* 4, 1–6.

Tartaglia L A, Dembski M, Weng X et al. (1995). Identification and expression cloning of a leptin receptor (OBR). *Cell* 83, 1263–1271.

Urbanek M, Legro R S, Driscoli D A et al. (1999). Thirty-seven candidate genes for polycystic ovary syndrome: strongest evidence is linkage with follistatin. *Proc Natl Acad Sci USA* 96, 8573–8578.

Velazquez E M, Acosta A, Mendoza S G (1997). Menstrual cyclicity after metformin therapy in PCOS. *Obstet Gynecol* 90, 392–395.

Waterworth D M, Bennett S T, Gharani N (1997). Linkage and association of insulin gene VNTR regulatory polymorphism with polycystic ovary syndrome. *Lancet* 349, 986–990.

28

Menstrual disorders in adolescent girls

Eleonora Porcu and Stefano Venturoli

Institute of Obstetrics and Gynaecology, University of Bologna, Italy

Introduction

In adolescence, anovulatory or oligo-ovulatory cycles are a common occurrence during the reproductive development process, and physiological hyperandrogenaemia is characteristic of this period of reproductive life. Oligo-anovulatory cycles may result in regular menstrual function when adulthood is reached or may be the first sign of an ongoing reproductive derangement. Anovulatory cycles in adolescence have a hyperandrogenic profile that correlates with increased mean luteinizing hormone (LH) levels, pulse amplitude and pulse frequency; there is also increased ovarian volume with a multicystic appearance. Although these endocrine findings probably represent a physiological condition in the first years after menarche, they may continue to the development of persistent reproductive disturbances. Individuals who ovulate and have regular cycles beginning at menarche, as well as those oligo-anovulatory adolescents who quickly normalize their cycles, have a more favourable reproductive prognosis.

The clinical implications of these common endocrine variations were examined in a longitudinal study of 34 girls from puberty to postmenarche and of 73 girls for one to seven years after menarche (Venturoli et al., 1986a,b, 1995).

Hormonal profiles of adolescents with irregular cycles

Of adolescents who have irregular cycles beginning at menarche but do not demonstrate other pathological features of androgen excess (such as obesity, acne,

hirsutism, or major emotional/psychiatric disorders), 30% will demonstrate levels of androstenedione and testosterone above the upper limit of normal (Venturoli et al., 1986a) (Fig. 28.1). Subjects with increased androgen levels are generally anovulatory, although the occasional ovulatory girl may demonstrate hyperandrogenaemia. Hence, the clinical significance of this finding during this period of life remains unclear. Besides increased androgen levels, anovulation may be associated with either increased LH levels (with approximately 30% of subjects having levels greater than those found in adults) or with normal circulating LH values. This would suggest that there are two different pathological mechanisms that may result in the development of adolescent oligo-anovulation.

Anovulatory girls with high LH levels also have increased LH pulse amplitude and pulse frequency, while anovulatory subjects with normal LH values have normal LH pulse frequency and amplitude, similar to that found in adolescents with regular ovulatory cycles (Venturoli et al., 1987). Neuroendocrine differences between anovulatory girls with high LH levels, and those with normal LH values are even more pronounced if one takes into account the circadian profiles of this gonadotrophin. Adolescents with high LH levels tend to demonstrate higher levels of this hormone in the afternoon, while increased nocturnal levels of LH are found in anovulatory girls with normal LH levels (Porcu et al., 1987) (Fig. 28.2). Both of these profiles differ from that found in ovulatory girls, who do not demonstrate any clear circadian variation in their LH levels. The presence of accentuated circadian variations in LH secretion is probably a marker of reproductive immaturity. These data, taken together, seem to suggest that increased LH secretion in adolescents results in an ovarian function that

Paediatric and Adolescent Gynaecology, ed. Adam Balen et al. Published by Cambridge University Press.
© Cambridge University Press 2004.

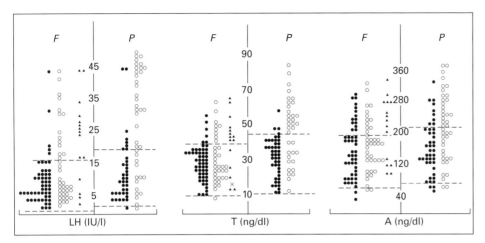

Fig. 28.1. Distribution of luteinizing hormone (LH), testosterone (T) and androstenedione (A) found in amenorrhoeic subjects (▲) on a random day and in subjects with irregular cycles (ovulatory (●) or anovulatory (○) during the follicular (F) and the premenstrual phases (P) with reference to the normal adult range (---). The percentages of subjects exceeding the adult range follow. Follicular phase: LH 20%, T 17%, A 29%, premenstrual phase: LH 35.8%, T 26%, A 33.7%; amenorrheic subjects: LH 73%, T 67%, A 67%. (From Venturoli et al., 1986a.)

is similar to that found in adults with the polycystic ovary syndrome (PCOS; see Ch. 27). In keeping with this assumption, when androgen levels are compared in adolescent subjects with high and normal LH values, it appears that higher testosterone and androstenedione levels are associated with increased LH secretion and increased LH pulsatility, supporting a mainly ovarian origin for adolescent hyperandrogenism.

The ovary in adolescence

Histological studies stress the similarity between pubertal or postpubertal ovaries and those found in women with PCOS (Merril, 1963). Besides the increased volume and multicystic appearance, these similarities include theca hyperplasia and luteinization, cystic and atretic follicles and cortical fibrosis. The value of ultrasound in the evaluation of the adolescent ovary is unclear. In our opinion, the ultrasound appearance of the ovary in adolescence cannot be rigidly classified. However, our experience suggests that some basic sonographic features can be identified: (i) homogeneous ovaries of normal or low volume, with few small cystic areas; (ii) multifollicular ovaries of normal of increased volume containing several cystic areas diffusely distributed throughout the ovary, 5–10 mm in diameter; (iii) polycystic ovaries with increased ovarian volume and many follicles, primarily distributed to the cortex, and an increased amount of

ovarian stroma; (iv) multifollicular and polycystic (as in (ii) and (iii)) but with an additional dominant follicle or a few lead follicles, which generally exceed 13 mm in diameter.

These four basic sonographic pictures can be observed in adolescence, although it should be noted that a wide spectrum and variation from these descriptions can be found.

During puberty and adolescence, a high follicular turnover does exist in the ovary, with waves of maturation and atresia. With increasing pubertal stage and chronological age, ovarian volume and the number of developing follicles increases. This process continues until the hypothalamic–pituitary–ovarian (HPO) development is completed. Ovarian volume increases and its internal structure changes, with a gradual increase in the number and size of the follicles and a progressive increase in the amount of stroma, derived from continued follicular atresia. The greater the duration of the maturational process, the more accentuated these ovarian features will be. The above-described ultrasound appearances are often the result of a transitional process from one type to another, which may be of variable duration. These transitions are probably the result of an improvement or worsening of the endocrine and metabolic milieu, resulting in either greater or lesser resemblance to the normal adult or PCOS ovary, respectively. The ovarian volume of adolescents with regular cycles does not appear to be any different from the ovarian volume of normal adults, while over 40% of girls

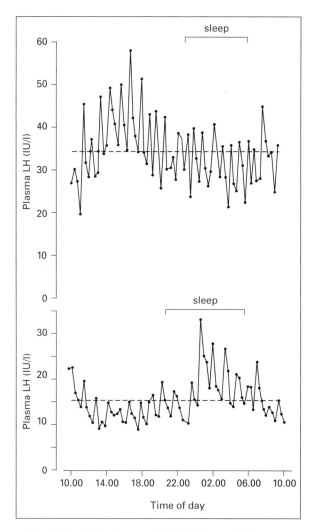

Fig. 28.2. Luteinizing hormone (LH) circadian profile in anovulatory adolescents with increased (upper panel) or normal (lower panel) LH levels. (From Porcu et al., 1987.)

with oligo-anovulation have mean ovarian volumes that are above the normal limit (Venturoli et al., 1984) (Fig. 28.3). Anovulatory adolescents with high LH levels have ovarian volumes that are significantly higher than oligo-ovulatory girls with normal LH values; in addition, 57% of adolescents with oligo-anovulation also have unhomogeneous ovaries because of the presence of multiple hypoechoic areas that exceed 3 mm in diameter. A clear-cut division between the central stromal area and the peripheral location of the follicles can be made in only 30% of those girls having unhomogeneous ovaries. We believe that multifollicularity of the ovary, increased ovarian volume, high LH and androgen levels, and oligo-anovulation are frequent findings and strongly interlinked in adolescents with oligo-anovulation (Venturoli et al., 1986b). Overall, anovulation

affected 30% of adolescents in our study, enlarged ovaries were present in 45%, unhomogeneous ovaries were present in 57%, high LH levels in 30%, and high androgen levels in 30%.

Long-term follow-up of ovulatory function in adolescents

The long-term outcome of ovulatory disorders in adolescents was examined in a longitudinal study of 73 adolescents with irregular cycles (Venturoli et al., 1995). Follow-up ranged from one to seven years postmenarche. Mean postmenarcheal age of the adolescents was 2.7 years at the first visit, and 5.5 years at their last follow-up visit. During follow-up, the prevalence of girls with regular ovulation increased from 11 to 36% among oligo-ovulatory adolescents who had high LH levels when first examined. Mean LH levels decreased during follow-up and 44% of girls had levels within the normal adult range at their last visit. Only a few girls who initially had elevated LH levels became ovulatory and normalized their LH values, thereby achieving a complete maturation of their HPO axis. This suggests that high LH-related anovulation is not always an irreversible condition in adolescence but can demonstrate spontaneous improvement. However, oligo-anovulatory girls with persistently high LH levels probably have a much less favourable reproductive prognosis. They generally do not demonstrate a change in ovarian function and their clinical condition evolves into the stereotypical PCOS of adulthood. During their last visit, many of those subjects with persistent elevations in LH levels were hyperandrogenic, with

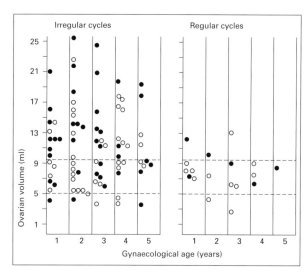

Fig. 28.3. Distribution of ovarian volume in girls with regular or irregular menstrual cycles (From Venturoli et al., 1984.)

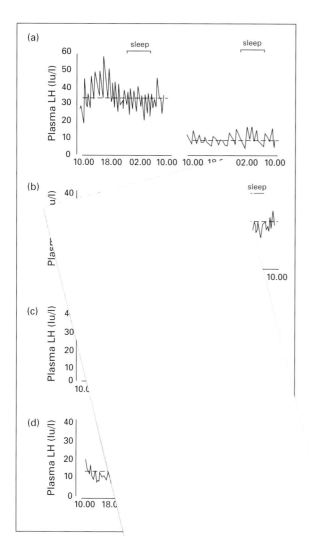

Fig. 28.4. Circadian lutein[...] adolescent. (a) At the gynae[...] subject was anovulatory wit[...] ovulatory at the last evaluati[...] when episodic LH secretion s[...] amplitude and frequency, and [...] variation with the highest level[...] An adolescent at the gynaecolog[...] years *(right)*. The anovulatory co[...] at the first examination persisted [...] LH patterns did not change except[...] adolescent at the gynaecological ag[...] *(right)*. At first examination, the sub[...] normal LH levels but she was ovulate[...] the accentuated circadian variation w[...] morning disappeared. (d) An adolesce[...] of 3 years *(left)* and 6 years *(right)*. The a[...] normal LH levels seen at the first examin[...] mean LH levels decreased and the circad[...] pronounced even though a nocturnal don[...] present. (Porcu et al., 1997.)

T and A values exceeding those of the normal adult range. Further maturation did not necessarily normalize their androgen levels, with hyperandrogenaemia becoming a permanent feature even among regularly ovulatory subjects.

The long-term follow-up of seven anovulatory girls with high LH levels showed that after a number of years three became regularly ovulatory with a reduction in their mean LH values, pulse frequency, pulse and amplitude (Venturoli et al., 1992). The increased levels of LH apparent during the daytime disappeared changing to normal adult LH circadian rhythm (Porcu et al., 1997) (Fig. 28.4).

A different reproductive outcome can be expected if there is little change in the function of the HPO axis. Ovarian volume and structure undergoes significant changes during adolescence, in concordance with neuroendocrine maturation. However, in our experience, these changes take place very slowly and are frequently incomplete in adolescence, with persistently irregular cycles. In particular, ovarian volume and the prevalence of dishomogeneity within the ovary does not seem to change significantly with increasing age, with these values remaining above the adult normal range in oligo-anovulatory girls. Only 22% of girls who had enlarged ovaries at their initial visit demonstrated a normalization of ovarian volume during follow-up, while the polycystic structure was substantially confirmed.

A very long follow-up assessment was undertaken for 13 females (Porcu et al., 2000). After 20 years, all but three women still had irregular cycles. Three became overweight and four developed hirsutism. LH levels normalized in 10 women while androgens remained above normal range in 2 subjects. Ovaries were further enlarged and polycystic [...] nine subjects. Four women were not willing to have a [...]gnancy. Two women had spontaneous pregnancy with [...]mal term delivery. Two women conceived but had early [...]ated miscarriages. Five women, after about three years [...]ertility, underwent assisted reproductive treatments.

[...]ry

[...]ent functional outcomes of adolescent ovulatory [...]n can be identified. The first is the result of a [...] increase in ovulatory frequency and regularity, [...]nates the adolescent oligo-ovulatory features [...]hes an adult endocrine and morphological [...] econd has persistence of oligo-anovulation, [...]ith the establishment of the endocrine and [...]orphological features of HPO axis immaturity, which constitutes the functional basis for the development of subsequent hyperandrogenic symptoms. In an adolescent with persistently irregular ovulatory cycles, the development of ovulatory abnormalities is linked to a progressive increase in ovarian volume until the ovary has a polycystic appearance ultrasonographically; this is accompanied by increasing androgen levels. While hyperandrogenaemia may have a role in the development of ovulatory cycles during this period of time, this benign physiological impact is of limited duration. The persistence of hyperandrogenaemia into adulthood appears to compromise the quality of reproductive function, even in the presence of regular ovulation, and may be the functional basis for the development of androgenic pathology and infertility.

REFERENCES

Merril J A (1963). The morphology of the prepubertal ovary: relationship to the polycystic ovary syndrome. *South Med J* 56, 225–231.

Porcu E, Venturoli S, Magrini O et al. (1987). Circadian variations of luteinizing hormone can have two different profiles in adolescent anovulation. *J Clin Endocrinol Metab* 65, 488–493.

Porcu E, Venturoli S, Longhi M, Fabbri R, Paradisi R, Flamigni C (1997). Chronobiologic evolution of luteinizing hormone secretion in adolescent developmental patterns and speculations on the onset of the polycystic ovary syndrome. *Fertil Steril* 67, 842–848.

Porcu E, Venturoli S, Giunchi S, Fratto R, Alfieri S, Caracciolo D (2000). Twenty year follow-up of adolescents with irregular cycles. *Fertil Steril* 74(Suppl 1), 89–90.

Venturoli S, Porcu E, Fabbri R, Paradisi R, Orsini L F, Flamigni C (1984). Ovaries and menstrual cycles in adolescence. *Gynecol Obstet Invest* 17, 219–222.

Venturoli S, Porcu E, Fabbri R et al. (1986a). Menstrual irregularities in adolescents: hormonal pattern and ovarian morphology. *Horm Res* 24, 269–279.

    (1986b). Ovarian multifollicularity high LH and androgen plasma levels and anovulation are frequent and strongly linked in adolescent irregular cycles. *Acta Endocrinol* 11, 368–372.

Venturoli S, Porcu E, Gammi L et al. (1987). Different gonadotropin pulsatile fashions in anovulatory cycles of young girls indicate different maturational pathways in adolescence. *J Clin Endocrinol Metab* 65, 785–791.

Venturoli S, Porcu E, Fabbri R et al. (1992). Longitudinal evaluation of the different gonadotropin pulsatile patterns in anovulatory cycles of young girls. *J Clin Endocrinol Metab* 76, 836–841.

    (1995). Longitudinal change of sonographic ovarian aspects and endocrine parameters in irregular cycles of adolescence. *Pediatr Res* 38, 974–980.

29

Pelvic pain, ovarian cysts and endometriosis in adolescent girls

Paul L. Wood

Kettering General Hospital, Kettering, UK

Introduction

The legacy of pelvic pathology and pelvic pain in adolescence is not inconsiderable in later life, with ramifications from both the actual pathological processes and their management. The main negative outcomes include subfertility, adhesion formation and chronic pelvic pain. Although these are in general well-recognized causative implications, the general awareness of their origins in the adolescent period is less well acknowledged. As a result, diagnosis may be delayed or treatment may be inappropriate, with consequent negative long-term outcomes for the individual. The lack of a consensus in the definition of chronic pelvic pain greatly hinders epidemiological studies. However, and despite limited data, the prevalence of chronic pelvic pain in the population appears to be high, with an annual prevalence in primary care in the UK of 38/1000 in women, a rate comparable to asthma (37/1000) and back pain (41/1000) (Zondervan & Barlow, 2000). The significance of two defined causes of pelvic pain in adolescence, endometriosis and ovarian cysts, will be explored first prior to an overall review of pelvic pain in this age group. The subject matter will nevertheless overlap throughout this chapter, given the inevitable close interrelationships that exist between pelvic pain, endometriosis and ovarian cysts. For instance, deep endometriosis, pelvic adhesions and ovarian cystic endometriosis are all independent predictors of pelvic pain (Porpora et al., 1999). Alternatively, obstructive anomalies of the female genital tract that preclude the outflow of menstruation and result in the collection of blood in the vagina and uterus also increase the likelihood of retrograde flow. These conditions will occur in young women soon after the menarche and

tend to result in the development of pelvic masses, endometriosis and/or abdominal pain. In addition, the long-term sequelae of endometriosis may influence fertility. A high index of suspicion is required in order to diagnose these congenital malformations early in young adolescents (Breech & Laufer, 1999) and ensure early surgical release of the obstruction.

Endometriosis

Pathophysiology

Endometriosis is a progressive disease affecting approximately 10% of women; it can result in dyspareunia, dysmenorrhoea, low back pain and subfertility (Wellbery, 1999). A genetic or familial tendency for the development of endometriosis has been reported, with a 6.9% rate of endometriosis in first-degree relatives of women with the disease compared with 1% in the control population (Simpson et al., 1981). Endometriosis is the commonest cause of chronic pelvic pain in adolescents, affecting up to 70% of girls with chronic pelvic pain unresponsive to medical management. This should, therefore, be strongly suspected in adolescent girls with chronic pelvic pain who are unresponsive to medication in the form of combined oral contraceptives and nonsteroidal anti-inflammatory agents. Approximately 10% of women affected by primary dysmenorrhoea will not respond to these simple measures and it is in this group that it is important to consider secondary causes of dysmenorrhoea (Coco, 1999). Although endometriosis is the commonest finding in teenagers not responding to these measures, Müllerian

Paediatric and Adolescent Gynaecology, ed. Adam Balen et al. Published by Cambridge University Press.
© Cambridge University Press 2004.

abnormalities and musculoskeletal causes must also be considered (Schroeder & Sanfilippo, 1999).

The characteristics of endometriosis in adolescence have been analysed based upon a series of 40 adolescents aged between 11 and 19 years (Audbert, 2000).

Two identifiable entities were noted.

1. Endometriosis associated with an obstructive genital anomaly. This is sometimes found in young patients for whom the severity of the endometriosis depends upon the delay in establishing the diagnosis. Retrograde menstrual flow has been listed as one of the pathophysiological processes in the development of endometriosis. These lesions may regress spontaneously, sometimes completely, when the anomaly has been surgically treated.

2. Endometriosis of adolescents aged 17 years and over and who present mainly with chronic pelvic pain or severe dysmenorrhoea.

Endometriosis of the Fallopian tube has been diagnosed in a child as young as 13 years within one month of the menarche (Yamamoto et al., 1997). An adenomyotic cyst within the myometrium of a 16-year-old girl has also been described (Tamura et al., 1996). The average interval between menarche and diagnosis of endometriosis in adolescents has been calculated as being of the order of 5.2 years (Liang et al., 1995). The endometriotic deposits are usually mild and are frequently atypical in appearance. The commonest lesions, however, are red and superficial (Reese et al., 1996). These lesions are potentially recurrent, and the possible consequences on subsequent fertility need to be studied further. Data suggest that it is not the actual size of ovarian cyst endometriosis that causes pelvic pain but rather the association with adhesions (Porpora et al., 1999). In addition, it appears that the pain of endometriosis has little relationship to the location or colour of the lesions and, importantly, the site of pain can extend beyond any visible lesions and onto what appears to be normal peritoneum (Demco, 1998).

In an effort to determine any increase in prevalence of endometriosis in patients with all Müllerian abnormalities, Ugur et al. (1995) reviewed patients attending a reproductive endocrinology clinic and compared these with a control group. These patients were then studied depending on whether the anomalies were obstructive or nonobstructive. Obstructive anomalies were confirmed as being associated more with endometriosis than were nonobstructive anomalies ($p < 0.001$). Those with nonobstructive anomalies did not have a higher prevalence of endometriosis compared with the control group ($p > 0.05$). Although endometriosis was not seen more frequently in patients with Müllerian abnormalities as a whole, outflow obstruction

was nevertheless shown to be an important contributory factor to the development of endometriosis. The evaluation of these patients contributes evidence in favour of the theories of retrograde menstruation and coelomic metaplasia in the origins of endometriosis but militates against a possible relation with a developmental defect of differentiation or migration of the Müllerian duct system during embryogenesis.

In a separate study, endometriosis was observed in 7/45 (16%) patients with uterine didelphys with no obstructive lesions. The author, however, considered that in the long term a didelphyic uterus per se was not associated with an increased frequency of endometriosis (Heinonen, 2000), a conclusion consistent with that reached by Ugur and his coworkers (1995).

Symptomatology

Endometriosis in adolescence commonly presents atypically. Clinical symptoms are often uncharacteristic and there is often no direct relationship between the extent of the disease and the severity of the symptoms. The leading symptoms of dysmenorrhoea and chronic pelvic pain do not have to occur synchronously with the menstrual cycle and may, therefore, be noncyclical (Stummvoll and Kapshammer, 1999). Alternatively the symptoms seen in teenagers may not differ from those such as dyspareunia seen in older women (Liang et al., 1995). Affected individuals may, in addition, present with gastrointestinal symptoms (Gidwani, 1989).

Diagnosis

Clinical history and examination

An actual clinical diagnosis of endometriosis tends to be difficult to make on meeting with the patient in clinic, although the history is often generally helpful. Pelvic examination in an adolescent can be difficult but a rectal examination may reveal pelvic tenderness, nodularity, fixity of the pelvic organs or an ovarian mass.

Ultrasound and other imaging techniques

Imaging techniques are often unable to provide the correct diagnosis but the assessment of the pelvis in young females includes the option of other imaging techniques apart from ultrasound (Barnewolt, 1998). Ultrasonographic criteria for the diagnosis of endometriomata include the identification of cystic structures with low, homogeneous echogenicity and the presence of a thick cystic wall with regular margins (Volpi et al., 1995). Cystic teratomata may, however, have similar appearances and result in false-positive results. The sensitivity of diagnosing endometriomata at transvaginal scanning has been estimated at 82.4%, with a specificity of 97.7%. The positive and negative predictive values were 94% and 92.8%, respectively, and the diagnostic accuracy was 93% (Volpi et al., 1995). Colour Doppler imaging has been used to try to differentiate between endometriomas and other adnexal masses to better effect than B-mode ultrasonography alone (Guerriero et al., 1998).

Biochemical screening

The sensitivity and specificity of serum carbohydrate antigen 125 (CA-125) for the diagnosis of endometriosis have been quoted as 61.1% and 87.5%, respectively (Chen et al., 1998) with elevated levels mainly in those with advanced endometriosis. CA-125 estimations may, therefore, be more useful in the follow-up of recurrence in patients with advanced endometriosis and in those who initially present with elevated CA-125 levels. As a test, however, CA-125 is not considered to be an effective screening tool for patients with dysmenorrhoea or for monitoring therapy.

Laparoscopy

Early diagnosis and therapy using laparoscopic techniques is recommended sooner rather than later, with investigation of symptoms even in adolescent girls (Stummvoll & Kapshammer, 1999). A retrospective analysis of the records of 129 adolescents and young women treated surgically revealed 22 (17%) with endometriosis. The main indications for surgical intervention were dysmenorrhoea, cyclical abdominal pain and cysts, which were later identified as being endometriotic in origin. The authors concluded that persistent abdominal pain in young women that does not respond to conventional therapy should be followed up by diagnostic laparoscopy or laparotomy as necessary (Zrubek et al., 1999).

The definitive diagnosis of endometriosis can still only be made at laparoscopy in the vast majority of women (Wellbery, 1999) and laparoscopy remains the gold standard. Newer techniques allow for microlaparoscopy with conscious sedation and have been presented as a safe and effective alternative to the established approach of conventional laparoscopy under general anaesthesia (Almeida et al., 1997). In general, adult laparoscopic equipment is used in adolescents rather than requiring the specialized equipment needed when performing laparoscopy in paediatric patients.

A retrospective analysis of girls aged 11–19 years admitted requiring ongoing investigations for pelvic pain following medical treatment found that 73% had endometriosis and that minimal disease was most commonly encountered (Reese et al., 1996). In another study, 35.2% (37) of

adolescents (aged 11–19 years) presenting with chronic or acute pelvic pain and right-sided lower abdominal pain were found to have endometriosis. The majority had early stage disease and the lesions tended to involve just one site or pelvic organ. Approximately one-third, however, had lesions at multiple sites, including the Pouch of Douglas, uterosacral ligaments and ovarian fossa (Emmert et al., 1998).

A study evaluating endometriosis specifically in an adolescent population (26 women aged 16–20 years) at laparoscopy and staged according to the American Society of Reproductive Medicine staging criteria showed that 61.6% were classified as having first-stage disease, 30.8% second stage and 3.8% third stage (Hassan et al., 1999).

Given that adolescents with chronic pelvic pain not responding to treatment with the oral contraceptive or non-steroidal anti-inflammatory agents are more likely to have endometriosis (Zydowicz-Mucha et al., 1999), and in view of the high rate of endometriosis, this group should be referred to a gynaecologist experienced with the subtle laparoscopic findings of atypical endometriosis. In this way, the correct diagnosis can be facilitated and the aetiology of the pelvic pain established so that appropriate therapy can be initiated (Laufer et al., 1997). Meticulous inspection of the pelvic peritoneal surfaces will often reveal superficial or atypical lesions in these patients (Figs. 29.1–29.7, colour plates). There may be a natural progression of endometriosis from atypical lesions in adolescence to classic lesions in adults (Propst & Laufer, 1999). Clear vesicles of atypical endometriosis have been seen in adolescents using laparoscopic visualization along with irrigation fluid. The fluid is used to identify and appreciate the three-dimensional configuration of these otherwise clear lesions. The use of irrigation fluid within the pelvis also allows light reflection to be excluded as a confounding variable in the diagnosis of these lesions (Laufer, 1997).

Management

Medical treatment designed to interfere with ovulation and induce amenorrhoea generally provides effective pain relief and is very much along the lines offered to adults with endometriosis, with the options of continuous high-dose oral progestogens or danazol. The recurrence rate following cessation of treatment, however, is high, and this type of treatment will not resolve those cases where infertility is an issue (Wellbery, 1999). On the whole, therefore, treatment in the teenage group does not really differ from that in older women.

The initial management of endometriosis at laparoscopy could also involve surgical resection or destruction at the time of diagnosis (Fig. 29.8, colour plate), followed by medical treatment. Up to 91.9% of endometriotic lesions identified in adolescents have been amenable to endocoagulation at the time of laparoscopy (Emmert et al., 1998).

Gonadotrophin-releasing hormone (GnRH) agonists should be considered for adolescents over the age of 16 who have completed pubertal maturation (Propst & Laufer, 1999). Add-back therapy in adolescents with endometriosis not responding to conventional therapy and requiring GnRH agonist treatment can be considered but this combination has not been specifically studied in the adolescent population. The ideal dose of add-back sex steroids in this group is yet to be delineated (Lubianca et al., 1998).

As a general rule, it would appear that treatment with a GnRH agonist following conservative surgery for mild to severe symptomatic endometriosis significantly prolongs the pain-free interval following surgery and does not adversely affect the reproductive prognosis (Hornstein, 1997; Vercellini et al., 1999).

Ovarian cysts

All types of ovarian tumours seen in the adult population can also be seen in children and adolescents, but the relative incidence of each entity varies considerably with age. Functional nonneoplastic cysts and masses are much more frequent in the adolescent and are generally follicular or corpus luteal in origin. The widespread availability and use of ultrasound has resulted in an increase in the detection rate of ovarian cysts in teenagers. Ovarian cysts in the teenage years may be asymptomatic but can be seen in association with menstrual irregularities, pain, urinary frequency, constipation or pelvic discomfort.

Kanizsai et al. (1998) found that ovarian cysts in children and adolescents were mostly unilateral, unilocular and simple, with the size varying between 3 and 5 cm in diameter with approximately one-third measuring more than 5 cm. A number will be found incidentally on ultrasound while scanning for other reasons, usually irregular bleeding. These cysts tend to resolve spontaneously in four or five weeks on average, and only a minority will require surgical treatment. Indications for surgery included the detection of complex cysts indicative of dermoid-type cysts or suspected malignancy, the actual size of the cysts, severe pelvic pain or a failure of the cyst to resolve or decrease in size spontaneously or in response to treatment, as measured using ultrasound (Kanizsai et al., 1998).

In the adolescent age group, neoplasms are more likely to be germ cell rather than epithelial in origin. Fortunately in children and adolescents, just 10% of ovarian tumours are

malignant. A complete history and clinical examination are vitally important. A solid component on ultrasound is the most statistically significant predictor of a malignant ovarian mass (Brown et al., 1998). Whenever an ovarian mass, be it physiological or neoplastic, benign or malignant, is diagnosed in an adolescent female, every effort must be made to preserve the reproductive function in that female in order to ensure future childbearing (Kozlowski, 1999).

Differential diagnosis

Other than for functional cysts relating to normal ovarian function, ovarian cysts can develop as a consequence of other external influences that might first become manifest as ovarian cysts. The McCune–Albright syndrome consists of a triad of polyostotic fibrous dysplasia, café-au-lait spots and endocrinopathies along with the development and regression of oestrogen-producing ovarian cysts, which lead to peripheral precocious puberty with breast development and vaginal bleeding. Those affected can display signs of juvenile hyperthyroidism, hyperparathyroidism and Cushing's syndrome.

Hypothyroidism per se can be associated with enlarged multicystic ovaries in adolescence, presenting with pelvic pain and a pelvic mass (Hansen et al., 1997) (Fig. 29.9).

The occurrence of multiple cysts of both ovaries has been described for the first time in childhood or adolescence in a patient with a gonadotroph adenoma with elevated levels of follicle-stimulating hormone (Tashiro et al., 1999). Massive thin-walled ovarian cysts after puberty, which have given rise to significant morbidity, have been described in patients previously treated for cloacal exstrophy (Geiger & Coran, 1998).

Although an adolescent may present with a cystic pelvic mass that on clinical examination and on ultrasonic investigation is consistent with an ovarian cyst, the presenting picture might prove to be particularly misleading. The differential diagnosis includes

- appendix abscess
- tuboovarian abscess
- hydrocolpos/haematocolpos (Fig. 29.10)
- distended bladder
- Wilms' tumour
- enlarged spleen
- mesenteric cyst (Fig. 29.11, colour plate)
- central precocious puberty
- McCune–Albright syndrome
- primary hypothyroidism.

An obstructed hemi-vagina in a case of unrecognized uterine didelphys may, for instance, result in a large collection of blood behind the obstructed hemi-vagina, which can

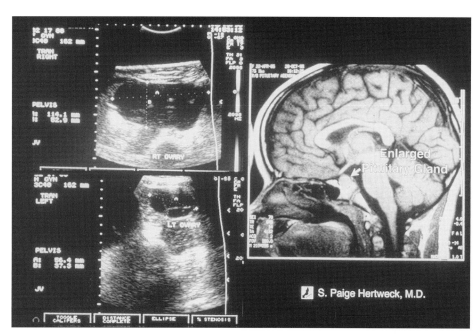

Fig. 29.9. Hypothyroidism and ovarian cysts: diffuse enlargement of the pituitary gland (magnetic resonance imaging) and bilaterally enlarged multicystic ovaries (ultrasound). (Courtesy of the North American Society for Pediatric and Adolescent Gynecology, 1996.)

present as a pelvic mass. This is obviously a more diffi-cult diagnostic problem than an imperforate hymen with haematocolpos and haematometra since the patient is still visibly menstruating from the revealed uterus and vagina. The diagnosis may then only be made at the time of an open laparotomy for a presumed ovarian cyst, at which time it is vital that the condition be recognized and the longitudinal vaginal septum excised. Another unusual presentation de-scribed in the literature relates to a painful groin swelling in a 14-year-old girl, which in reality was found to represent an incarcerated haemorrhagic ovarian cyst (Poenaru et al., 1999).

The commoner pathological ovarian cysts in adolescents

The more common pathological ovarian cysts seen in ado-lescents are:
1. germ cell tumours
2. epithelial tumours
3. sex cord stroma tumours.

Germ cell tumours

The commonest ovarian tumour in childhood is the benign cystic teratoma (dermoid cyst; Fig. 29.12, colour plate). Ul-trasound examination may provide clues as to the under-lying diagnosis but the diagnosis can be missed despite

imaging. Benign cystic ovarian teratomata may often be identified by a preoperative radiograph, which can reveal the presence of teeth within the pelvic mass (Ahmed, 1999). A diagnosis made in this way will, however, depend on the extent of enlargement of the cyst(s) and their degree of maturation. Treatment consists of excision of the cyst with ovarian reconstruction, thereby preserving reproduc-tive function as much as possible.

While dermoid cysts are mature teratomata, immature germ cell tumours (immature teratomata) can also occur. Immature teratomata are the third commonest of all germ cell tumours and account for 15% of these and 1% of all teratomas. These tumours contain elements from all three germ cell layers and are almost always unilateral. The me-dian age of presentation is 19 years and they usually present as stage 1 disease. The size of these tumours and the de-gree of differentiation are factors influencing survival. Uni-lateral salpingo-oophorectomy is an adequate treatment for stage 1A tumours. There are usually no useful tumour markers available and adjuvant chemotherapy is indicated. Whereas other germ cell tumours are bilateral in just 1% of cases, 10–15% of dysgerminomas are bilateral (Fig. 29.13, colour plate). These are malignant and treatment consists of salpingo-oophorectomy of the affected side and full ovarian malignancy staging (Fig. 29.14, colour plate). The place of adjuvant therapy after conservative surgery has been controversial, since irradiation can lead to infertility.

Adjuvant combination chemotherapy can, however, be as effective as adjuvant radiotherapy.

Endodermal sinus tumours account for 5% of all ovarian malignancies and are the second commonest germ cell tumour. These are usually exclusively unilateral with a median age of presentation of 19 years. Virtually all those affected have a raised serum α-fetoprotein and can present with abdominal pain, a raised temperature, vaginal bleeding and/or an abdominopelvic mass. Management is unilateral salpingo-oophorectomy: stage 1 tumours are the most common finding. These tumours are radioresistant and treatment consists of adjuvant combination chemotherapy.

Mixed germ cell tumours usually have more than one malignant germ component present at an early stage. The mean age of presentation is 16 years. Most are unilateral and are dealt with by unilateral salpingo-oophorectomy. Staging, cytoreduction and adjuvant chemotherapy are recommended.

A review of all ovarian germ cell tumours over a 16-year period in a tertiary referral centre revealed a complete response in 93% of patients. A majority, 80%, of those who subsequently relapsed were successfully salvaged. Advancing stage of the disease was the only significant adverse prognostic factor. None of the children subsequently delivered to these affected females were reported to have any congenital abnormalities. The review, therefore, indicates a high cure rate with combined surgery and chemotherapy and that conservative surgery and preservation of fertility are feasible (Ezzat et al., 1999).

Epithelial tumours

Mucinous or cystic cystadenomata are usually benign and account for no more than 10–20% of ovarian cysts in adolescence, most being diagnosed after the menarche. Conservative surgery is required, with particular care taken to ensure that there is no spillage of the mucinous contents since such spillage can result in long-term catastrophic complications of pseudomyxoma peritonei.

Sex cord stromal tumours

Juvenile granulosa cell tumours account for 3–5% of all ovarian tumours in children, with over 80% occurring under the age of 20 years. The size of the tumours can vary from 3 to 30 cm in diameter, and no correlation has been found between size and evidence of invasion (Aboud, 1997). Menstrual irregularity may be the only sign, although patients may present with an acute abdomen or a pelvic mass. The vast majority are unilateral and are usually stage 1A (Calaminus et al., 1997) since they tend to present early in view of their oestrogen production. They have a more favourable prognosis than the typical adult tumour,

although inevitably more advanced stages have a poor clinical outcome. Treatment consists of unilateral salpingo-oophorectomy as a staging exercise and those staged as 1A require surgery only. There is no effective modality of therapy determined for more advanced stages, with aggressive debulking plus carboplatin and etoposide chemotherapy showing encouraging results. The best treatment for aggressive and recurrent disease has yet to be determined (Powell & Otis, 1997) but multidrug chemotherapy including cisplatin-based regimens may be used to enhance treatment results (Savage et al., 1998). During chemotherapy, half the patients became amenorrhoeic but 96% resumed normal menstruation on completion of treatment (Perrin et al., 1999). Thecomas are regarded as benign tumours but granulosa cell tumours are characterized by a long natural history with a significant capacity to recur after an apparent clinical cure; consequently adequate follow-up is important (Aboud, 1997). Tumour recurrence can be dealt with by aggressive surgical removal followed by salvage chemotherapy such as bleomycin and taxol, with encouraging results (Powell et al., 2001).

If the adolescent presents with evidence of hirsutism or virilization, then a Sertoli–Leydig tumour should be considered. These tumours are usually unilateral and if well differentiated are treated by unilateral salpingo-oophorectomy.

Management

In the absence of symptoms and the presence of benign ultrasonic and biochemical parameters, ongoing observation with repeated ultrasound examination is a reasonable option for adolescent girls with such cysts (Grazyna et al., 1998). Tumour markers such as α-fetoprotein, human chorionic gonadotrophin and CA-125 are usually not elevated but should be checked upon diagnosis of a complex ovarian cyst and can be followed up accordingly if elevated prior to treatment.

In cases of solid or complex ovarian neoplasms, surgery is the rule even for benign disease. Ovarian cystectomy or unilateral salpingo-oophorectomy with great care to establish the absence of the disease in the remaining ovary is the usual procedure. Additional treatment for malignant ovarian tumours will depend on the type of malignancy and the stage of the disease.

Emergency surgery will be required in those with acute complications to ovarian cysts. Patients with simple ovarian cysts, mature cystic teratomas and normal ovaries are more likely to undergo torsion than those with other benign or malignant tumours (Templeman et al., 2000). Salpingo-oophorectomy has been the procedure of choice in torsion of an ovarian cyst. However, new data suggest that correction of the torsion alone (detorsion) may result in subsequent follicular function despite the predetorsion size of the ovary or colour of the adnexa, even if this is seen to be black. This is illustrated by a report of ovarian torsion seen in a young child (Eckler et al., 2000), which demonstrates the nature of this condition and highlights the ability of detorsion and stabilization to preserve what appeared to be a necrotic ovary at the time of initial presentation.

Laparoscopic removal of benign cystic teratomata (dermoid cyst) has been shown to be safe and beneficial in selected patients when performed by an experienced laparoscopic surgeon. The incidence of chemical peritonitis following such surgery is in the order of just 0.2% (Nezhat et al., 1999). Removal can be effected using enucleation and removal via a trochar sleeve, enucleation and removal within an impermeable sac, or enucleation and removal via a posterior colpotomy.

The size of benign ovarian cysts continues to be a limiting factor for laparoscopic surgery, with most surgeons opting for laparotomy for larger cysts. Eltabbakh and Kaiser (2000) described how they successfully dealt with a 22 cm benign ovarian cyst extending above the umbilicus in a 15-year-old girl using a laparoscopic approach. A prelaparoscopy cyst drainage was carried out using a suprapubic catheter with a coiled end (Bonanno catheter) in order to minimize leakage around the aspiration site, and this was followed by a laparoscopic cystectomy. It appears, therefore, that, with proper patient selection, laparoscopic surgery can be safely applied in a select group of patients with large, benign ovarian cysts.

For many young patients with nonmalignant ovarian lesions such as endometriomata, benign cysts and fibromas, these cysts can be treated laparoscopically, thereby avoiding a laparotomy (Mettler et al., 1997).

Pelvic pain

Pelvic pain is a common symptom in the adolescent female and can be acute or chronic. This differentiation is less helpful in adolescent patients than in older women.

The following discussion will concentrate primarily on the non-acute situation, although it is pertinent to point out that acute pain may represent a life-threatening situation and torsion, pelvic inflammatory disease and ectopic pregnancy must be considered. Consideration needs to be given to nongynaecological causes of acute abdominal pain, particularly gastrointestinal (e.g. acute appendicitis, mesenteric adenitis) and urinary (acute pyelonephritis, ureteric calculus) causes. Isolated or recurrent isolated torsion of the Fallopian tube presenting as an acute abdomen in adolescence has been described (Fig. 29.10). Such an occurrence should be considered in the differential

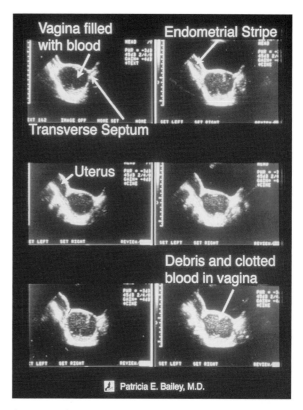

Fig. 29.10. Ultrasonography in a 14 year old girl demonstrating haematocolpos and haematometra (Courtesy of the North American Society for Pediatric and Adolescent Gynecology, 1996).

diagnosis of lower abdominal or pelvic pain since prompt surgical intervention may allow for preservation of the tube (Lineberry & Rodriguez, 2000; Raziel et al., 1999).

Primary dysmenorrhoea is a common finding in adolescence, with a frequency of 80–85% (Balbi et al., 2000; Hillen et al., 1999). Over half reported that their dysmenorrhoea limited their activities. Early menarche is associated with increased prevalence and severity of dysmenorrhoea, and a long and heavy menstrual flow is also associated with an increase in the severity of the pain. The management of menstrual disorders in adolescence is explored elsewhere. What is clear is that chronic pain has a negative psychological impact and the clinical interaction is often unsatisfactory for patients and doctors alike. One major difficulty is that each of the words "chronic pelvic pain" is open to a number of different definitions, thereby making any studies of the condition potentially disparate. The lack of consensus on definition is recognized as a major problem. Adolescents are, however, recognized as a subgroup who are known to suffer from recurrent chronic abdominal pain. A retrospective analysis of chronic pelvic pain in primary care identified a mean duration of symptoms in the those aged 13–20 years of 13.7 months (Zondervan et al., 1999).

The impact of pelvic pain on lifestyle and whether this affects schooling, sleep, exercise or family life needs to be considered. Equally, the presence of mood disturbances such as depression and anxiety need to be explored. Patients thus affected have a highly significant elevation in their hostility score when compared with normative data (Selfe et al., 1998). It might well be pertinent to enquire about psychological or social antecedents, although caution should be exerted before enquiring directly about childhood sexual abuse without a specific prompt from the patient. Women with a history of physical or sexual abuse, and particularly those with severe abuse, have been found to be much more likely to report somatic symptoms including pelvic pain. These women not only had more somatic symptoms but also increased functional disability (Leserman et al., 1998).

Those with the chronic pelvic pain syndrome have been found to have a significantly higher incidence of sexual abuse and severe psychological disturbances compared with women with the chronic vulvar pain syndrome or a healthy control group. Although women with vulvodynia were found to be psychologically similar to controls, those with chronic pelvic pain have been found to be younger and less well educated and were more likely to have a history of physical or sexual abuse, to report recent depression and to screen positive for current depression, to have more work absences and to have more somatic complaints (Reed et al., 2000). Others have also found sexual abuse to be a significant predictor of the chronic pelvic pain syndrome (Bodden-Heidrich et al., 1999). Other studies have also demonstrated that women with chronic pelvic pain have a higher incidence of past sexual abuse compared with women in a comparison pain group and with women with no pain (Collett et al., 1998). The prevalence of childhood sexual abuse has been reported to be as high as 26% (Jamieson & Steege, 1997) and 22% in women with chronic pelvic pain and a history of sexual victimization before the age of 15 years (Lampe et al., 2000). The latter also looked at the significance of physical and emotional trauma but found that there was no such association with chronic pelvic pain. Savidge & Slade (1997) have warned, however, that evidence that women with chronic pelvic pain without discernible pathology differ in personality, psychological state or life experiences from women with an identifiable cause for their pain, or those without chronic pelvic pain, is inconclusive.

A relationship between posttraumatic stress disorder and chronic pelvic pain has been mooted, both of which have been associated with specific alterations of the hypothalamic–pituitary–adrenal axis. Alterations to this axis seen in women with the chronic pelvic pain syndrome

Table 29.1. Causes of chronic pelvic pain in adolescent girls

	Causes
Endometrium	Endometriosis
Infection	Ovarian/parovarian cysts
	Pelvic inflammatory disease
	Pelvic adhesions
	Tuboovarian abscess
Congenital abnormalities	Müllerian tract/congenital obstructive anomalies
Pelvic congestion syndrome	–
Musculoskeletal dysfunction	Partial detachment of round ligament
	Postural problems/lower spine dysfunction
	Nerve entrapment
Gastrointestinal tract	Irritable bowel syndrome
	Appendicular inflammation
	Lactose intolerance
	Chronic constipation
	Inflammatory bowel disease
Urinary tract	Urethral syndrome/diverticulum
Psychosomatic problems	

partly parallel and partly contrast the neuroendocrine correlates of posttraumatic stress disorder but show marked similarity to findings in patients with other stress-related bodily disorders. The findings are suggestive that a lack of the protective properties of cortisol may be of relevance for the development of bodily disorders in individuals who are chronically stressed or traumatized (Heim et al., 1998).

Differential diagnosis

Although a common symptom, chronic pelvic pain is a particularly difficult condition to manage during adolescence. Laparoscopy failed to identify any abnormality in as many as 60% of adolescents undergoing investigation for chronic pelvic pain (Kontoravdis et al., 1999). Endometriosis was found in 25%, ovarian cysts in 7%, parovarian cysts in 3%, pelvic inflammatory disease in 3% and adhesions in 2%. The authors concluded that, although laparoscopy was a valuable and effective procedure in the diagnosis and management of chronic pelvic pain in a selected group of patients, not all adolescents referred to their clinic with a label of chronic pelvic pain underwent laparoscopy.

Causes of pelvic pain are given in Table 29.1. Causes other than for endometriosis and ovarian cysts are listed below.

Congenital abnormalities

Pelvic pain in a teenager with primary amenorrhoea can indicate Müllerian tract obstructive anomalies, such as an imperforate hymen or transverse vaginal septum (Figs. 29.15 and 29.16, colour plates). The latter is rarer, occurring in every 30 000 to 84 000 women, and is frequently associated with genitourinary, musculoskeletal and cardiac malformations plus congenital unilateral or bilateral tubal atresia (Polasek et al., 1995).

More rarely, congenital cervicovaginal aplasia (either isolated cervical or combined with partial or complete vaginal atresia) with a functioning endometrium can give rise to uncontrolled pelvic pain in adolescence (Badawy et al., 1997). Surgical canalization in selected patients with congenital cervical atresia can be successfully performed to provide patients with an opportunity for conservative management, resulting in normal menstrual bleeding, resolution of pelvic pain and some limited potential for fertility (Fujimoto et al., 1997).

A study of 49 women with uterine didelphys revealed an obstructive hemi-vagina in 18% (Heinonen, 2000). A unicornuate uterus with a functioning rudimentary horn can also result in severe pain (Dadhwal et al., 2000). Menstrual blood from the enclosed endometrial cavity within the residual horn can fill progressively, leading to a large haematosalpinx (Jaszczynski et al., 1995). Such obstructions result in pelvic pain that is difficult to diagnose given that the adolescent is seen to be menstruating in any event. It is only recourse to examination and imaging techniques that will allow for the correct diagnosis to be made, the obstruction released and the pain to be resolved. The value of ultrasound would, however, tend to be limited to diagnosing these malformations in the early stages of their manifestation; thereafter, the specific diagnosis is much more difficult to make using noninvasive methods.

Gastrointestinal tract

Symptoms suggestive of the irritable bowel syndrome include episodes of pain occurring more than once a month, an altered bowel habit, relief of pain with defaecation and abdominal distension associated with acute exacerbations and not just confined to the premenstrual phase. Deep dyspareunia has also been associated with the irritable bowel syndrome and it has been suggested that this is a more likely diagnosis if the onset of pain is several hours after intercourse. Symptoms from lactose intolerance can also masquerade or be misinterpreted as being gynaecological in origin (Blumenthal et al., 1981). Individuals thus affected tend to have gastrointestinal symptoms along with abdominal pain and improve when lactose is withdrawn from the diet. Chronic constipation needs to be considered in

the differential diagnosis although an altered bowel habit may in itself be a manifestation of gynaecological pathology such as endometriosis; consequently, a diagnosis of constipation per se does not exclude the presence of other pathology causing pain (Gidwani, 1989). Crohn's disease can present at a young age, with evidence that the mean age of onset of symptoms can be as young as 11.6 years (Castile et al., 1980). Although again there tends to be associated gastrointestinal symptoms, up to 7% of those affected may present with isolated abdominal pain. Appendicular problems need to be considered in the differential diagnosis of right-sided pelvic pain, both acute and chronic; appendicectomy at the time of exploratory surgery has been recommended in young patients with episodic, well-localized symptoms associated with systemic malaise (Chao et al., 1997).

Pelvic congestion

Pelvic congestion is a common finding in women with chronic pelvic pain (Papathanasiou et al., 1999) and tends to be associated with deep dyspareunia and postcoital aching. The pain is of a variable nature and location and can radiate through to the back or down the legs. This can be exacerbated while standing and relieved when lying down.

Infection

A high index of suspicion for pelvic infection and tuboovarian abscess is needed in sexually active adolescents, especially given the need for early diagnosis and treatment. Not all such cases will present with pelvic pain, a pelvic mass, a raised temperature and an increased white cell count; some may present with relatively mild abdominal pain (Huang et al., 1997). Although sexually transmissible infections are the commonest underlying problem, rarer infections such as tuberculosis (Klein et al., 1976), actinomycosis and coccidiomycosis (Saw et al., 1975) have been described in the literature as causing pelvic pain of obscure origin.

Urinary tract

The urethral syndrome has also been associated with pelvic pain. Chronic lower abdominal pain is one manifestation of the urethral syndrome, which improves when treatment is directed towards this syndrome. A urethral diverticulum can also present with pelvic pain (Romanzi et al., 2000).

Musculoskeletal causes

Patients with chronic pelvic pain have been found to have a common pattern of faulty posture associated with lifestyle factors, a majority of whom were shown to have improved in response to physical therapy treatment. Dysfunction of the lower spine can be a cause of pelvic pain in adolescents (Schaffer, 1995). Nerve entrapment, often involving the ilioinguinal or iliohypogastric nerves, can be associated with the specific localization of abdominal tenderness.

A case of partial detachment of the round ligament at its cornual insertion has been described in a 13-year-old female complaining of pelvic pain localized to the right lower abdominal quadrant (Baraldi & Ghirardini, 1998).

Examination

Abdominal examination may reveal specific sites of tenderness. One finger "trigger point" tenderness suggests nerve entrapment and can be confirmed by infiltration of local anaesthetic into the tender area. "Ovarian point tenderness" (lower abdominal lateral tenderness) may be seen in the pelvic congestion syndrome, but patients with the irritable bowel syndrome have similar abdominal tenderness. Nodularity, especially in the Pouch of Douglas, will indicate endometriosis. Alternatively, actual endometriotic deposits may be visible in the posterior fornix and the clinical diagnosis can be confirmed using an outpatient vaginal biopsy.

Dysfunction of the locomotor system needs to be considered when there is no organic cause for the pain, with specific examination looking for dysfunction of the sacroiliac joints, lumbar joints, pelvis and hips.

Investigations

Microbiology

Chronic pelvic infection is unlikely in this age group but cervical and vaginal swabs should be taken in adolescents who are sexually active. For a number of biological and psychosocial reasons, sexually active adolescents have the highest rate of sexually transmissible diseases of any sexually active age group (Braverman, 2000) and a higher rate of diagnosis of acute pelvic inflammatory disease than any other age group (Blythe, 1998). A significant number of teenagers exhibit only mild or vague symptoms, so a high index of suspicion is required by the physician to initiate treatment. Adolescents, in particular, require aggressive treatment of pelvic inflammatory disease to prevent the long-term sequelae (Rome, 1998). Laparoscopy may be required where significant pain persists despite aggressive treatment for pelvic inflammation confirmed by positive bacterial cultures or in those adolescents with a working diagnosis of recurrent pelvic inflammation without any other objective evidence. There should be sufficient objective evidence available before labelling an individual as suffering from chronic pelvic inflammatory disease.

Ultrasound

Ultrasound is frequently the initial, and sometimes only, imaging examination indicated. Ultrasound scanning is a simple technique but is often of limited value in these cases, notwithstanding that the subjects tend to be good candidates for ultrasonography, often with thin and unscarred abdominal walls and generally good tolerance to larger bladder volumes. The transabdominal approach is the obvious choice for any adolescent who is not sexually active, but the transvaginal approach is an option for those who are sexually active and emotionally mature. A negative examination might help to provide reassurance as to the absence of gross pelvic pathology and might result in the identification of dilated pelvic veins. In an attempt to understand the clinical outcome in patients with pelvic pain and normal pelvic ultrasound findings, Harris et al. (2000) found that pelvic pain improved or resolved in 66/86 patients (77%) although, unsurprisingly, improvement was less common in the group with chronic pain for an excess of six months (7/14). There are more limited indications for plain radiography, genitography, computed tomography and magnetic resonance imaging.

Laparoscopy

Unfortunately neither early endometriosis nor pelvic adhesions can be reliably detected by noninvasive techniques.

Ozaksit et al. (1995) attempted to evaluate the correlation of preoperative pelvic pain examination and ultrasonography with the laparoscopic finding in a group of adolescents with chronic pelvic pain. The predictive values of normal and abnormal findings at pelvic examination were 42.8% and 93.5%, respectively. Ultrasonography correlated with laparoscopy in 39/45 cases. The predictive value of normal findings at ultrasound was 60% and that of abnormal findings 92.4%. However, there were abnormal laparoscopic findings in half those cases where both pelvic examination and ultrasound scan were normal. Laparoscopy did reveal an abnormality in all patients who were identified as having an abnormal pelvic examination and abnormal ultrasound scan findings. The authors concluded that the clinical evaluation of chronic pelvic pain is highly predictive when combined with ultrasound, but that confirmation is best provided by laparoscopy.

The indications for laparoscopy have been explored earlier in this chapter and as a technique can provide reassurance if not an actual diagnosis of the cause of the pain.

Management

The analysis of risk factors for chronic pelvic pain is highly complicated owing to its multifactorial aetiology. For the young patient who presents with chronic pelvic pain, a multidisciplinary approach is essential to facilitate diagnosis and management. Where possible, organic disease such as endometriosis, adhesions and obstructive malformations should be identified and treated as indicated (Fig. 29.17, colour plate). The development of a treatment team, recognizing psychosocial and environmental factors and encouraging long-term relationships, is a critical component of the care of these patients and in the prevention of recurrent symptom formation and future disability. There is a recognized need to focus on psychopathology and relationship dysfunction and also on coping techniques and rehabilitation. The efficacy of a multidisciplinary approach for the treatment of chronic pelvic pain has been well documented. The gynaecologist will tend to focus on the coordination of care in difficult patients, the patient's awareness of improvements in pain reports and their function at school or work. Finally, it is helpful to reinforce consistent compliance with medication, on the basis that small improvements beget larger improvements in daily functioning (Economy & Laufer, 1999; Rickert & Kozlowski, 2000). The role of the psychiatrist will include an assessment of any psychosocial issues in the aetiology of the pain and to treat comorbid depression, anxiety, posttraumatic stress disorder, somatization, maladaptive coping and sexual dysfunction. Early and adequate attention to these factors is likely to reduce unnecessary invasive procedures, decrease disability and assist in cost-effective early rehabilitation. Reassurance may be given in the absence of a positive diagnosis or specific pathology. Although endometriosis and pelvic inflammatory disease are the commonest physical changes seen at laparoscopy in those with chronic pelvic pain, a note of caution needs to be struck in that a finding of mild endometriosis or adhesions might be coincidental and not causative. Under these circumstances, treatment directed to this end may fail to provide the necessary relief and thereby cause additional distress.

Calls have been made for more empirical use of medical treatment with a GnRH analogue given concerns that laparoscopy may be unnecessary, fruitless and even hazardous, besides being expensive (Lindheim, 1999). Endometriosis is the most frequent source of chronic pelvic pain and responds well to medical treatment. Use of GnRH agonists for six months can reduce the American Fertility Society endometriosis scores by half, with cure rates at five years of 75% of respondents who had minimal disease and 33% of responders with severe disease. This approach to empirical treatment remains controversial given the lack of exact knowledge of the underlying pathology and the side effects and costs of the medical treatments proposed.

However, there is also evidence that diagnostic la-

paroscopy can have beneficial effects in women with chronic pelvic pain and that these effects appear to be the result of psychological mechanisms. Patients undergoing laparoscopy for chronic right iliac fossa pain considered the procedure to have been worthwhile (32/41) even though in some cases it did not relieve their chronic pain (Chao et al., 1997). Pain reduction has been observed from before to after a diagnostic laparoscopy and regression analyses have confirmed that psychological factors would predict improvements in pain levels. Improvements in pain after laparoscopy were predicted by beliefs about pain and the change in each woman's evaluation of the seriousness of her condition. Further understanding of these mechanisms could help in the understanding and treatment of women with chronic pelvic pain (Elcombe et al., 1997).

Chiropractic treatment has been reported as helpful in a majority of those with dysfunction of the locomotor system (Hawk et al., 1997). Schaffer (1995) carried out a prospective single-group interventional study for women with chronic pelvic pain and found positive short-term effects. Acupuncture has been postulated as beneficial in young patients with severe chronic pain including that of endometriosis, but additional studies are needed to quantify the costs and effectiveness of this approach (Kemper et al., 2000).

Summary

Pelvic pain can have multiple sources and can be difficult to diagnose and treat. Boxes 29.1 and 29.2 summarize the recommendations for best practice and the key points, respectively, for this common condition.

Box 29.1 Recommendations for best practice

- Adolescents with persistent abdominal pain not responding to conventional therapy should be followed up by diagnostic laparoscopy.
- Hemi-obstructive congenital abnormalities should be excluded when faced with a cystic pelvic mass of apparent ovarian origin.
- In the absence of symptoms and in the presence of ultrasonic and biochemical evidence of benign disease, ongoing observation with repeated ultrasound examination is a reasonable option in adolescence. Surgery is the rule for solid or complex ovarian tumours.
- A multidisciplinary approach is essential for adolescents presenting with chronic pelvic pain to facilitate diagnosis and management.

Box 29.2 Key points

- Endometriosis is the commonest cause of chronic pelvic pain in adolescents, commonly presents atypically and the symptoms may be noncyclical.
- Laparoscopy remains the gold standard for diagnosis of endometriosis.
- Clear vesicles of atypical endometriosis have been identified in adolescents.
- A high index of suspicion is required to diagnose hemi-obstructive malformations in young adolescents.
- Ovarian cysts in children and adolescents tend to be unilateral, unilocular and simple.
- In adolescents, neoplasms are more likely to be germ cell than epithelial in origin, with 10% of ovarian tumours being malignant.
- Individuals with a history of physical or sexual abuse are more likely to report chronic pelvic pain.

REFERENCES

*Indicates key references.

Aboud E (1997). A review of granulosa cell tumours and thecomas of the ovary. *Arch Gynecol Obstet* 2594, 161–165.

Ahmed S (1999). Enlargement and maturation in benign cystic ovarian teratomata. *Pediatr Surg Int* 15, 435–436.

Almeida O D Jr, Val-Gallas J M, Browning J L (1997). A protocol for conscious sedation in microlaparoscopy. *J Am Assoc Gynecol Laparosc* 4, 591–594.

*Audbert A (2000). Characteristics of adolescent endometriosis. *Gynecol Obstet Fertil* 28, 450–454.

Badawy S Z, Prasad M, Powers C, Wojtowycz A R (1997). Congenital cervicovaginal aplasia with septate uterus and functioning endometrium. *J Pediatr Adolesc Gynecol* 10, 213–217.

Balbi C, Musone R, Menditto A et al. (2000). Influence of menstrual factors and dietary habits on menstrual pain in adolescence. *Int J Obstet Gynecol Reprod Biol* 91, 143–148.

Baraldi R, Ghirardini G (1998). Partial detachment of round ligament found at laparoscopy for chronic pain in a female adolescent. *J Pediatr Adolesc Gynecol* 11, 189–190.

Barnewolt C E (1998). Imaging techniques to assess the pelvis in young females. *Sem Pediatr Surg* 7, 73–81.

Blumenthal I, Kelleher J, Littlewood J (1981). Recurrent abdominal pain and lactose intolerance in childhood and adolescence. *Br Med J* 282, 2013–2014.

Blythe M J (1998). Pelvic inflammatory disease in the adolescent population. *Sem Pediatr Surg* 7, 43–51.

Bodden-Heidrich R, Busch M, Kuppers V, Beckmann M W, Rechenberger I, Bender H G (1999). Chronic pelvic pain syndrome (CPPS), and chronic vulvar pain syndrome (CVPS), evaluation of psychosomatic aspects. *J Psychosom Obstet Gynecol* 20, 145–151.

Braverman P K (2000). Sexually transmitted diseases in adolescents. *Med Clinics N Am* 84, 869–889.

*Breech L L, Laufer M R (1999). Obstructive anomalies of the female genital tract. *J Reprod Med* 44, 233–240.

Brown D L, Doubilet P M, Miller F H et al. (1998). Benign and malignant ovarian masses: selection of the most discriminating gray-scale and Doppler sonographic features. *Radiology* 208, 103–110.

Calaminus G, Wessalowski R, Harms D, Gobel U (1997). Juvenile granulosa cell tumours of the ovary in children and adolescents: results from 33 patients registered in a prospective co-operative study. *Gynecol Oncol* 65, 447–452.

Castile R, Telander R L, Cooney D R et al. (1980). Crohn's disease in children: assessment of the progression of disease, growth and prognosis. *J Paediatr Surg* 15, 462–469.

Chao K, Farrell S, Kerdemelidis P, Tulloh B (1997). Diagnostic laparoscopy for chronic right iliac fossa pain: a pilot study. *Aus N Z J Surg* 67, 789–791.

Chen F P, Soong Y K, Lee N, Lo S K (1998). The use of serum CA-125 as a marker for endometriosis in patients with dysmenorrhoea for monitoring therapy and for recurrence of endometriosis. *Acta Obstet Gynecol Scand* 77, 665–670.

Coco A S (1999). Primary dysmenorrhoea. *Am Fam Physician* 60, 489–496.

Collett B J, Cordle C J, Stewart C R, Jagger C (1998). A comparative study of women with chronic pelvic pain, chronic non-pelvic pain and those with no history of pain attending general practitioners. *Br J Obstet Gynaecol* 105, 87–92.

Dadhwal V, Mittal S, Kumar S, Barua A (2000). Hematometra in postmenarchal adolescent girls: a report of two cases. *Gynecol Obstet Invest* 50, 67–69.

Demco L (1998). Mapping the source and character of pain due to endometriosis by patient-assisted-laparoscopy. *J Am Assoc Gynecol Laparosc* 5, 241–245.

Eckler K, Laufer M R, Perlman S E (2000). Conservative management of bilateral asynchronous adnexal torsion with necrosis in a prepubescent girl. *J Pediatr Surg* 35, 1248–1251.

Economy K E, Laufer M R (1999). Pelvic pain. *Adolesc Med* 10, 291–304.

Elcombe S, Gath D, Day A (1997). The psychological effects of laparoscopy on women with chronic pelvic pain. *Psychol Med* 27, 1041–1050.

Eltabbakh G H, Kaiser J R (2000). Laparoscopic management of a large ovarian cyst in an adolescent. A case report. *J Reprod Med* 45, 231–234.

Emmert C, Romann D, Riedel H H (1998). Endometriosis diagnosed by laparoscopy in adolescent girls. *Arch Gynecol Obstet* 261, 89–93.

Ezzat A, Raja M, Babri Y et al. (1999). Malignant ovarian germ cell tumours – a survival and prognostic analysis. *Acta Oncol* 38, 455–460.

Fujimoto V Y, Miller J H, Klein N A, Soules M R (1997). Congenital cervical atresia: report of seven cases and review of the literature. *Am J Obstet Gynecol* 177, 1419–1425.

Geiger J D, Coran A G (1998). The association of large ovarian cysts with cloacal exstrophy. *J Pediatr Surg* 33, 719–721.

Gidwani G (1989). Endometriosis: more common than you think. *Contemp Pediatr* 6, 99–110.

Grazyna M B, Malgorzata J, Rzej M, Marek M, Marian S (1998). Ovarian cysts in adolescent girls: report of 196 cases. *Ginekol Pol* 69, 1218–1222.

Guerriero S, Ajossa S, Mais V, Risalvato A, Lai M P, Melis G B (1998). The diagnosis of endometriomas using colour Doppler energy imaging. *Hum Reprod* 13, 1691–1695.

Hansen K A, Tho S P, Hanly M, Moretuzzo R W, McDonough P G (1997). Massive ovarian enlargement in primary hypothyroidism. *Fertil Steril* 67, 169–171.

Harris R D, Holtzman S R, Poppe A M (2000). Clinical outcome in female patients with pelvic pain and normal pelvic US findings. *Radiology* 216, 440–443.

Hassan E, Kontoravdis A, Hassiakos D, Kalogirou D, Kontoravdis N, Creatsas G (1999). Evaluation of combined endoscopic and pharmaceutical management of endometriosis during adolescence. *Clin Exp Obstet Gynecol* 26, 85–87.

Hawk C, Long C, Azad A (1997). Chiropractic care for women with chronic pelvic pain: a prospective single-group intervention study. *J Manip Physiol Ther* 20, 73–79.

Heim C, Ehlert U, Hanker J P, Helhammer D H (1998). Abuse-related posttraumatic stress disorder and alterations of the hypothalamic–pituitary–adrenal axis in women with chronic pelvic pain. *Psychosom Med* 60, 309–318.

Heinonen P K (2000). Clinical implications of the didelphyic uterus: long-term follow-up of 49 cases. *Int J Obstet Gynecol Reprod Biol* 91, 183–190.

Hillen T I, Grbavac S L, Johnston P J, Straton J A, Keogh J M (1999). Primary dysmenorrhoea in young Western Australian women: prevalence, impact and knowledge of treatment. *J Adolesc Health* 25, 40–45.

Hornstein M D, Hemmings R, Yupze A A, Heinrichs W L (1997). Use of nafarelin versus placebo after reductive laparoscopic surgery for endometriosis. *Fertil Steril* 68, 860–864.

Huang A, Jay M S, Uhler M (1997). Tuboovarian abscess in the adolescent. *J Pediatr Adolesc Gynecol* 10, 73–77.

Jamieson D J, Steege J F (1997). The association of sexual abuse with pelvic pain complaints in a primary care population. *Am J Obstet Gynecol* 177, 1408–1412.

Jaszczynski P, Adamek K, Jawornik M (1995). An enormous oviduct haematoma coexisting with a residual uterus horn in an adolescent. *Gonekol Pol* 66, 249–252.

*Kanizsai B, Orley J, Szigetvari I, Doszpod J (1998). Ovarian cysts in children and adolescents: their occurrence, behavior, and management. *J Pediatr Adolesc Gynecol* 11, 85–88.

Kemper K J, Sarah R, Silver-Highfield E, Xiarhos E, Barnes L, Berde C (2000). On pins and needles? Pediatric pain patients' experience with acupuncture. *Pediatrics* 105, 941–947.

Klein T A, Richmond J A, Mishell D R Jr (1976). Pelvic tuberculosis. *Obstet Gynecol* 48, 99–104.

Kontoravdis A, Hassan E, Hassiakos D, Botsis D, Kontoravdis N, Creatsas G (1999). Laparoscopic evaluation and management of chronic pelvic pain during adolescence. *Clin Exp Obstet Gynecol* 26, 76–77.

Kozlowski K J (1999). Ovarian masses. *Adolesc Med* 10, 337–350.

Lampe A, Solder E, Ennemoser A, Schubert C, Rumpold G, Sollner W (2000). Chronic pelvic pain and previous sexual abuse. *Obstet Gynecol* 96, 929–933.

Laufer M R (1997). Identification of clear vesicular lesions of atypical endometriosis: a new technique. *Fertil Steril* 68, 739–740.

Laufer M R, Goitein L, Bush M, Cramer D W, Emans S J (1997). Prevalence of endometriosis in adolescent girls with chronic pelvic pain not responding to conventional therapy. *J Pediatr Adolesc Gynecol* 10, 199–202.

Liang C C, Soong Y K, Ho Y S (1995). Endometriosis in adolescent women. *Chang Xue Zhi* 18, 315–321.

Leserman J, Li Z, Drossman D A, Hu Y J (1998). Selected symptoms associated with sexual and physical abuse history among female patients with gastrointestinal disorders: the impact on subsequent health care visits. *Psychol Med* 28, 417–425.

Lindheim S R (1999). Chronic pelvic pain: presumptive diagnosis and therapy using GnRH agonists. *Int J Fertil Womens Med* 44, 131–138.

Lineberry T D, Rodriguez H (2000). Isolated torsion of the fallopian tube in an adolescent: a case report. *J Pediatr Adolesc Gynecol* 13, 135–137.

Lubianca J N, Gordon C M, Laufer M R (1998). 'Add-back' therapy for endometriosis in adolescents. *J Reprod Med* 43, 164–172.

Mettler L, Semm K, Shive K (1997). Endoscopic management of adnexal masses. *J Soc Lap Surg* 1, 103–112.

Nezhat C R, Kalyoncu Nezhat C H, Johnson E, Berlanda N, Nezhat F (1999). Laparoscopic management of ovarian dermoid cysts: ten years' experience. *Soc Lap Surg* 3, 179–184.

Ozaksit G, Caglar T, Zorlu C G et al. (1995). Chronic pelvic pain in adolescent women. Diagnostic laparoscopy and ultrasonography. *J Reprod Med* 40, 500–502.

Papathanasiou K, Papageorgiou C, Panidis D, Mantalenakis S (1999). Our experience in laparoscopic diagnosis and management in women with chronic pelvic pain. *Clin Exp Obstet Gynecol* 26, 190–192.

Perrin L C, Low J, Nicklin J L, Ward B G, Crandon A J (1999). Fertility and ovarian function after conservative surgery for germ cell tumours of the ovary. *Aus N Z J Obstet Gynaecol* 39, 243–245.

Poenaru D, Jacobs D A, Kamal I (1999). Unusual findings in the inguinal canal: a report of four cases. *Pediatr Surg Int* 15, 515–516.

Polasek P M, Erickson L D, Stanhope C R (1995). Transverse vaginal septum associated with tubal atresia. *Mayo Clinic Proc* 70, 965–968.

Porpora M G, Koninckx P R, Piazze J, Natili M, Colagrande S, Cosmi E V (1999). Correlation between endometriosis and pelvic pain. *J Am Assoc Gynecol Laparosc* 6, 429–434.

Powell J L, Otis C N (1997). Management of advanced juvenile granulosa cell tumour of the ovary. *Gynecol Oncol* 64, 282–284.

Powell J L, Connor G P, Henderson G S (2001). Management of recurrent juvenile granulosa cell tumour of the ovary. *Gynecol Oncol* 81, 113–116.

Propst A M, Laufer M R (1999). Endometriosis in adolescents. Incidence, diagnosis and treatment. *J Reprod Med* 44, 751–758.

Raziel A, Mordechai E, Friedler S, Schachter M, Pansky M, Ron-El R (1999). Isolated recurrent torsion of the Fallopian tube: case report. *Hum Reprod* 14, 3000–3001.

*Reed B D, Haefner H K, Punch M R, Roth R S, Gorenflow D W, Gillespie B W (2000). Psychosocial and sexual functioning in women with vulvodynia and chronic pelvic pain. A comparative evaluation. *J Reprod Med* 45, 624–632.

Reese K A, Reddy S, Rock J A (1996). Endometriosis in an adolescent population: the Emory experience. *J Pediatr Adolesc Gynecol* 9, 125–128.

Rickert V I, Kozlowski K J (2000). Pelvic pain. A SAFE approach. *Obstet Gynecol Clinics North Am* 27, 181–193.

Romanzi L J, Groutz A, Blaivas J G (2000). Urethral diverticulum in women: diverse presentations resulting in diagnostic delay and mismanagement. *J Urol* 164, 428–433.

Rome E S (1998). Pelvic inflammatory disease: the importance of aggressive treatment in adolescents. *Cleveland Clinic J Med* 65, 369–376.

Savage P, Constenla D, Fisher C et al. (1998). Granulosa cell tumours of the ovary: demographics, survival and the management of advanced disease. *Clin Oncol* 10, 242–245.

Savidge C J, Slade P (1997). Psychological aspects of chronic pelvic pain. *J Psychosom Res* 42, 433–444.

Saw E C, Smale L E, Einstein H, Huntington R W Jr (1975). Female genital coccidioidomycosis. *Obstet Gynecol* 45, 199–202.

Schaffer M (1995). Pelvic pain in girls and adolescents. In *Proceedings of the XI World Congress of Paediatric and Adolescent Gynaecology*, p. 130.

Schroeder B, Sanfilippo J S (1999). Dysmenorrhoea and pelvic pain in adolescents. *Pediatr Clinics N Am* 46, 555–571.

Selfe S A, Matthews Z, Stones R W (1998). *J Womens Health* 7, 1041–1048.

Simpson J L, Elias S, Malinak L R, Buttram V C Jr (1981). Hereditable aspects of endometriosis. 1. Genetic studies. *Am J Obstet Gynecol* 137, 327–331.

Shaw R W (1994). *A Slide Atlas of Endometriosis*. Parthenon, London.

Stummvoll W, Kapshammer E (1999). Clinical aspects of endometriosis. *Wein Med Wochenschr* 149, 358–360.

Tamura M, Fukaya T, Takaya R, Ip C W, Yajima A (1996). Juvenile adenomyotic cyst of the corpus uteri with dysmenorrhoea. *Tohoku J Exp Med* 178, 339–344.

Tashiro H, Katabuchi H, Ohtake H, Kaku T, Ushio Y, Okamura H (1999). A follicle-stimulating hormone-secreting gonadotroph adenoma with ovarian enlargement in a 10-year old girl. *Fertil Steril* 72, 158–160.

Templeman C, Fallat M E, Blinchevsky A, Hertwick S P (2000). Non-inflammatory ovarian masses in girls and young women. *Obstet Gynecol* 96, 229–233.

*Ugur M, Turan C, Mungan T et al. (1995). Endometriosis in association with Mullerian abnormalities. *Gynecol Obstet Invest* 40, 261–264.

Vercellini P, Crosignani P G, Fadini R, Radici E, Belloni C, Sismondi P (1999). A gonadotrophin-releasing hormone agonist compared with expectant management after conservative surgery for symptomatic endometriosis. *Br J Obstet Gynaecol* 106, 672–677.

Volpi E, de Grandis T, Zucccaro G, La Vista A, Sismondi P (1995). Role of transvaginal ultrasound in the detection of endometriomata. *J Clin Ultrasound* 23, 163–167.

Wellbery C (1999). Diagnosis and treatment of endometriosis. *Am Fam Physician* 60, 1752–62.

Yamamoto K, Mitsuhashi Y, Takaike T, Takase K, Hoshiai H, Noda K (1997). Tubal endometriosis diagnosed within one month after menarche: case report. *Tohoku J Exp Med* 181, 385–387.

Zondervan K, Barlow D H (2000). Epidemiology of chronic pelvic pain. *Best Practice Res Clin Obstet Gynaecol* 14, 403–414.

Zondervan K, Yudkin P L, Vessey M P, Dawes M G, Barlow D H, Kennedy S H (1999). Patterns of diagnosis and referral in women consulting for chronic pelvic pain in UK primary care. *Br J Obstet Gynecol* 106, 1156–1161.

Zrubek H, Sikorski M, Nasser M, Stachowicz, Chil A (1999). Endometriosis in adolescents and young women. Can we afford to delay the diagnosis? *Ginekol Pol* 70, 264–269.

Zydowicz-Mucha E, Palatynski A, Mikaszewska-Pietraszun J, Zawalski W (1999). Laparoscopic evaluation of adolescent girls suffering from algomenorrhoea and acyclic pelvic pain. *Ginekol Pol* 70, 260–263.

30

Premature ovarian failure and ovarian ageing

Colin J. Davis[1] and Gerard S. Conway[2]

[1]St Bartholomews and the Royal London Hospitals, London, UK
[2]University College Hospital and The Middlesex Hospital, London, UK

Introduction

The ovary is a particularly unusual organ in that it is programmed to expire long before the average age of death. As such, it provides a unique model of the ageing process. An ovary that fails prematurely might do so through some defect in its development or through accelerated ageing. Because it is difficult to distinguish between these possibilities, it is convenient to consider processes of dysgenesis and demise together. Various labels have been applied to the phenomenon of early failure of the ovary: *ovarian dysgenesis* is usually applied to those women who present with primary amenorrhoea; *premature ovarian failure* (POF) applies to those with secondary hypergonadotrophic amenorrhoea before the age of 40; and *early ovarian failure* applies to those who enter the menopause between the ages of 40 and 45. *Resistant ovary syndrome* and *occult ovarian failure* are hypergonadotrophic states without amenorrhoea but are usually considered to be part of this spectrum of disorders. POF has a prevalence of 1% and is defined as amenorrhoea of greater than six months' duration in the presence of raised gonadotrophins, follicle-stimulating hormone (FSH) greater than 40 IU/l, on at least two occasions and occurring before the age of 40 (Coulam et al., 1986). This contrasts with the mean age of menopause at 51 years (McKinlay et al., 1972).

Aetiology

The cause of POF in most instances is unclear; however two broad mechanisms can be considered, acquired or genetic aetiologies. Environmental damage can produce a clinical picture of ovarian failure through viral or autoimmune oophoritis, environmental toxins and iatrogenic causes such as pelvic surgery, radiation or chemotherapy. Mutations of genes encoding proteins vital for ovarian development may produce a spectrum of phenotype from ovarian dysgenesis to early menopause.

Ovarian development and function

There are a number of events necessary for normal gonadal development, with three of critical importance. First, migration of primordial sex cells by amoeboid movement from the yolk sac along the dorsal mesentery of the hindgut to the gonadal ridges occurs at 6 weeks of gestation. Second, differentiation of the gonadal ridge begins when primordial sex cells interact with resident somatic blastema in the gonad. Third, gamete maturation occurs after meiosis is resumed. The oocyte is held in prophase of the first meiotic division until ovulation, which might occur up to 40 years later. This prolonged state of suspended development might render the oocyte vulnerable to damage by various processes.

Meiosis converts oogonia into nondividing primary oocytes. The net effect is a germ cell peak of 6 million by 20 weeks of gestation (Baker, 1963). Subsequently, there is germ cell atresia and the remaining germ cells are invested by pregranulosa cells to form primordial follicles. The pregranulosa cells are initially spindle shaped but change to cuboidal cells and secrete mucopolysaccharides to form a translucent covering around the oocyte known as the zona pellucida (Chiquoine, 1960). These follicles are known as primary follicles and their subsequent growth is dependent on gonadotrophin stimulation. As they increase in size and

Paediatric and Adolescent Gynaecology, ed. Adam Balen et al. Published by Cambridge University Press.
© Cambridge University Press 2004.

373

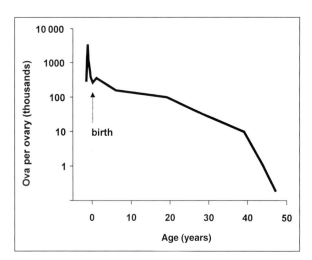

Fig. 30.1. Number of germ cells in one ovary over life. A peak of 3.5 million is reached in utero, falling to about 2 million at birth and 10 000 at the menopause transition.

become secondary follicles the pregranulosa cells become granulosa cells and develop FSH, oestrogen and androgen receptors (Huhtaniemi et al., 1987). At the same time, the theca interna cells develop luteinizing hormone (LH) cell surface receptors (May et al., 1980). The secondary follicles continue their growth, becoming late antral follicles during the postnatal prepubertal period. They develop a central antrum filled with sex steroids and granulosa-derived proteins. The process of primordial to late antral follicle development takes approximately 70 days.

At birth, each ovary contains 2 million germ cells but subsequently this figure falls to 400 000 by puberty (Jirasek, 1976) and less than 10 000 at the start of the perimenopausal period (Richardson et al., 1987) (Fig. 30.1). Menopause ensues as a direct result of exhaustion of the ovarian germ cell reserve (Gosden and Faddy, 1998). These two forms of atresia are categorized under the umbrella of apoptosis.

Apoptosis

The term apoptosis is derived from the Greek words *apo* and *ptosis* meaning to fall away from. It is used to describe a series of events resulting in developmental and homeostatic cell deaths controlled by the body and is distinguished from accidental cell death initiated by a noxious insult (Kerr et al., 1972). In cellular terms, it is characterized by separation of the cell from its neighbouring cells, loss of cell volume, chromatin condensation and margination along the nuclear envelope (nuclear pyknosis) and budding and fragmentation of the cell into plasma membrane-bound vesicles called apoptotic bodies (Frisch and Francis, 1994). The final outcome of the apoptotic body is phagocytosis by resident macrophages or neighbouring epithelial cells

(Bursch et al., 1990). This prevents secondary necrosis and inflammation from occurring, key components of pathological tissue injury (Majno and Joris, 1995).

The process of apoptosis is regulated by a number of genes and recent studies have characterized the sequence of stages involved (Cryns and Yuan, 1998; Goldstein, 1997; Li et al., 1997; Yang and Korsmeyer, 1996; Patel et al., 1996; Zou et al., 1997).

Aetiology of ovarian failure

The mechanisms of ovarian failure can be considered in terms of the processes of ovarian development, a pathogenetic classification (Table 30.1), or the frequency of clinical presentation (Table 30.2).

Potential mechanisms of gonadal dysfunction

The main errors that can occur in gonadal development and function are:
- presence of genetically active Y chromosome material and absence of two intact and genetically active X chromosomes in the germline

Table 30.1. Pathogenetic classification of primary ovarian failure

	Causes
Gonadal dysgenesis	Turner's syndrome: 45X and variants
	X chromosome translocation or deletion
Ovarian failure	Perrault's syndrome
	46,XX gonadal dysgenesis
Genetic associations	X chromosome defects: Turner's syndrome and variants
	Galactosaemia
	Fragile X syndrome premutations
	Blepharophimosis–ptosis–epicanthus inversus syndrome (BPES)
	Follicle-stimulating hormone receptor gene mutations
	Inhibin alpha gene defects
Autoimmune	Autoimmune polyendocrinopathy syndrome 1 (APECED)
	Autoimmune polyendocrinopathy syndrome 2
	Association with various autoimmune diseases
	Isolated autoimmune ovarian failure
Infection	Viral oophoritis
Iatrogenic	Chemotherapy
	Radiotherapy
	Pelvic surgery
Idiopathic	? Environmental toxins; smoking

Table 30.2. Causes of primary ovarian failure in 347 women attending the clinic at University College Hospital, London

Diagnosis	No.	Percentage
Environmental	190	55
Idiopathic sporadic	149	42.9
Autoimmune polyendocrinopathy types 1 and 2	27	7.8
Iatrogenic: chemotherapy, radiation, surgery	14	4.0
Genetic	157	45
Turner's syndrome	98	28.3
Idiopathic familial	30	8.6
Galactosaemia	17	4.9
Fragile X premutation	7	2.0
BPES (Blepharophimosis–ptosis–epicanthus inversus syndrome)	3	0.9
X chromosome breakpoints	1	0.3
Perrault's syndrome	1	0.3

- complete lack of migration of sex cells to the urogenital ridge
- migration of fewer than average sex cells
- incomplete mitosis of germ cells
- in utero damage to germ cells
- failure of development of normal granulosa cell layer
- failure of oogonia transformation into primary follicles, with arrested meiotic prophase
- lack of primary follicular response to fetal FSH.

Genetic causes of ovarian failure

Human genetic models of ovarian failure

A genetic basis for ovarian failure is suggested by the occurrence of families with two or more women affected with POF (Aittomaki, 1994; Coulam et al., 1983; Mattisson et al., 1984; van Kasteren et al., 1999a; Vegetti et al., 1998). With careful analysis of the family history, the prevalence of familial POF has been reported to be 19% (Davis et al., 2000). The mode of inheritance of idiopathic familial POF is usually impossible to define because of necessarily small pedigrees; autosomal dominant, X-linked dominant (van Kasteren et al., 1999a) and autosomal recessive (Aittomaki, 1994; Meyers et al., 1996) are each possible. We identified 30 cytogenetically normal families with idiopathic POF (Fig. 30.2). Five consanguineous pedigrees and one pedigree with transmission of susceptibility through fathers were identified and the inheritance pattern of these was assumed to be autosomal recessive and autosomal dominant,

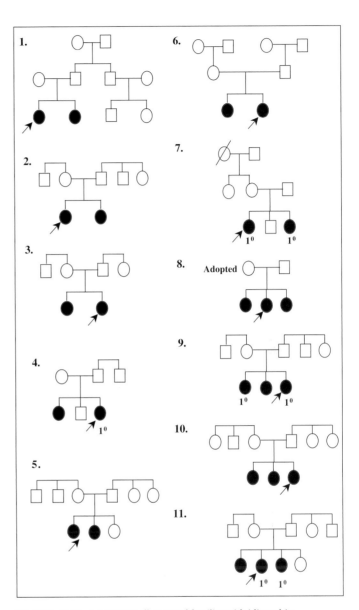

Fig. 30.2. Thirty cytogenetically normal families with idiopathic premature ovarian failure (POF). $\square$, male; $\bullet$, female with POF; =, consanguineous; 1^0, primary amenorrhoea; $\nearrow$, proband.

respectively. The remaining 24 pedigrees were grouped into "sibling only" pedigrees and "multiple generation" pedigrees (Fig. 30.2). When all 30 idiopathic families were considered together, there was a preponderance of female siblings of women with POF (ratio 2.6:1, corrected for ascertainment bias to 1.7:1, $p = 0.036$). Affected females of "sibling only" pedigrees were more likely to present with primary amenorrhoea and had a trend to earlier onset of secondary amenorrhoea compared with other inheritance patterns. Interestingly, a similar reduction in male siblings of affected females was found in a paper examining the

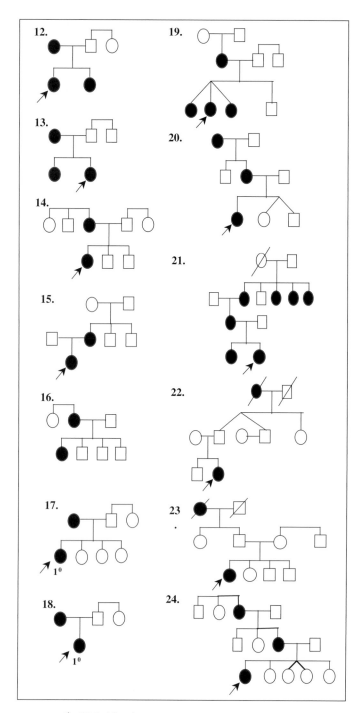

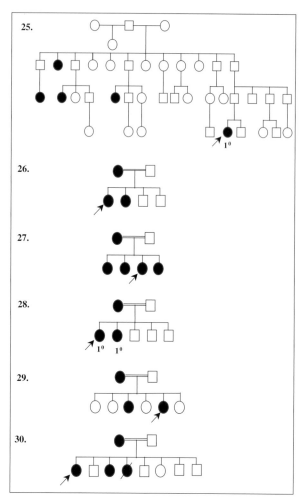

Fig. 30.2. (*Cont.*)

Fig. 30.2. (*Cont.*)

families of women with early (as opposed to premature) menopause (Cramer et al., 1995). In a second strategy, we have compared sex ratios across different causes of familial POF and demonstrated that the combined idiopathic series and the X chromosome defects group share a female preponderance, suggesting that a common mechanism is in play.

One biological explanation for an excess of females is through occult defects of the X chromosome. It has been postulated that ovary-determining genes on the X chromosome must escape X inactivation (Davis et al., 1998; Davison et al., 1998) and do not have homologues on the Y chromosome (Page et al., 1987). Therefore, males would be haplo-insufficient for these genes, some of which might have a vital extraovarian function. Males inheriting mutations of genes on the X chromosome would have to be nonviable. No male subject with a terminal deletion of the long arm of the X chromosome has been described. It has been postulated that essential genes necessary for life, such as glucose 6-phosphate dehydrogenase, are located on the long arm of the X chromosome and, therefore, haplo-insufficient males would be nonviable (Fitch et al., 1982). A detailed, precise family history of POF is essential for defining a subgroup of familial POF, which may allow the identification of inherited gene mutations resulting in the phenotype of ovarian failure.

Turner's syndrome

In the male, various genes have been identified as vital for spermatogenesis, with most lying on the Y chromosome (Sinclair et al., 1990). By analogy, it might be expected that many genes on the X chromosome are vital for normal ovarian development. Complete absence of one X chromosome results almost invariably in ovarian dysgenesis and primary or, more occasionally, secondary amenorrhoea (Pasquino et al., 1997). The fact that absence of an X chromosome is so deleterious to ovarian function, compared with a largely inactivated X chromosome in normal females, suggests that two intact alleles of ovarian-determining gene(s) on the X chromosome are required for normal function. Therefore, candidate loci causing POF should escape X inactivation (Chu and Connor, 1995). In general, it appears that abnormalities of the long arm of the X chromosome result in ovarian failure while those of the short arm affect stature as well (Sarto et al., 1973; Therman et al., 1990).

In Turner's syndrome, the initial germ cell multiplication in the first four to six weeks of ovarian development occurs normally but the subsequent round of germ cell apoptosis is accelerated (Singh and Carr, 1966). One major X chromosome locus for POF is on the short arm, Xp11.2-22.1 (Zinn et al., 1998). At least 15% of 45,X/46,XX individuals and 3–5% of 45,XO individuals menstruate (Simpson, 1975) but overall the prospect of fertility is relatively poor.

Critical regions of the X chromosome

The "critical region" hypothesis, proposed by Sarto et al. in 1973, identified the region Xq13-26 as vital for normal ovarian function. Two further reports confirmed this region as important for ovarian function, based on cytogenetic and clinical studies of patients with X/autosome translocations (Phelan et al., 1977; Summitt et al., 1978). Since then, the region has been refined to two ovarian determining loci, POF 1 at Xq26-27 (Krauss et al., 1987) and POF 2 at Xq13-21 (Powell et al., 1994). Yet further detail has been reported with the identification of 11 balanced X/autosome translocations associated with POF mapped to a yeast artificial chromosome (YAC) contiguent spanning most of Xq21 and corresponding to a 15 Mb region (Sala et al., 1997). A region of this size has been estimated to contain at least eight different genes in Xq21 involved in ovarian development, and interruption of such genes could cause POF. Deletions and translocations of the X chromosome are associated with

varying degrees of diminished reproductive capacity especially ovarian dysgenesis and/or POF (Fitch et al., 1982; Powell et al., 1994; Tharapel et al., 1993; Veneman et al., 1991). Spontaneous menstruation occurs in approximately 40% of 46,Xdel(X)(p11) individuals (Simpson, 1987). Krauss et al. (1987) reported a family of four women with an Xq deletion (q21.3-27); three of the women had POF and one had irregular menses at 31 years. Further evidence has been provided by Davison et al. (1998), who presented a family transmitting a stable deletion at Xq26.1. The early diagnosis of familial X chromosome deletions causing POF allowed for prediction of impending menopause and the opportunity of assisted conception.

Diaphanous X chromosome breakpoint gene

Bione et al. (1997, 1998) demonstrated a balanced X;12 translocation, t(X;12)q21;p1.3), in a POF family with a breakpoint in the last intron of the *diaphanous* (*DIA*) gene, a human homologue of the drosophila gene *diaphanous* (*dia*), mapped to Xq22 (Banfi et al., 1997; Bione et al., 1998). *dia* is ubiquitously expressed and conserved across species from yeast upwards. It encodes the FH1/FH2 protein family involved in cytokinesis and other actin-mediated morphogenetic processes, which are needed in the early stages of development. Interestingly, *dia* is inactivated and, therefore, contradicts the premise that POF genes escape X inactivation (Zinn et al., 1993). Mutant alleles of *dia* affect spermatogenesis and oogenesis and lead to sterility, with alteration in follicular cell proliferation in the female. Mutations in human *DIA* may interfere with mechanisms leading to cell follicle proliferation. Prueitt et al. (2000) have mapped nine Xq translocation breakpoints and identified *XPNPEP2* as a premature ovarian failure candidate gene. Further studies are needed to dissect the different genes located on the long arm of chromosome X involved in POF.

Single gene associations with POF

Abnormalities in the follicle-stimulating hormone receptor in primary ovarian failure

The inactivating point mutations of the FSH receptor are responsible for POF inherited as an autosomal recessive trait, as was first recognized in Finland (Aittomaki et al., 1995). The result is a mutation with a valine to alanine change and occurs on the short arm of chromosome 2. To date it has only been reported as a cause of POF with primary amenorrhoea in Finnish pedigrees (Aittomaki et al., 1995). The histological appearance of the ovaries of women with this mutation showed hypoplasia with scant primordial follicles but none had complete ovarian dysgenesis with streak ovaries (Aittomaki et al., 1996). The presence of follicles up to the preantral stage confirms the exclusive role of FSH in the terminal maturation of follicular growth.

The term "gonadotrophin resistance" has now been characterized in molecular terms by mutations blocking the gonadotrophin receptors (Conway et al., 1996). The prevalence of FSH receptor mutations in the UK is low and is a very rare cause of POF (Conway et al., 1997). This specific loss-of-function mutation has not been identified in other groups of women with ovarian failure (Conway et al., 1999; da Fonte Kolek et al., 1998; Layman et al., 1998). Men homozygous for this mutation have variable and sometimes satisfactory fertility. This contrasts with women, who have completely unresponsive hypoplastic ovaries (Tapanainen et al., 1997). Recently, a woman presenting with secondary amenorrhoea has been reported to have a heterozygous FSH receptor mutation. The mutation resulted in a partial loss of function of the receptor with secondary amenorrhoea and very high plasma gonadotrophin concentrations, contrasting with normal sized ovaries and antral follicles up to 5 mm at ultrasonography. Histological and immunohistochemical examination of the ovaries showed normal follicular development up to the small antral stage and a disruption at further stages. The patient was found to carry compound heterozygotic mutations of FSH receptor gene, resulting in Ile160Thr and Arg573Cys substitutions located, respectively, in the extracellular domain and in the third intracellular loop of the receptor. This observation suggests that a limited FSH effect is sufficient to promote follicular growth up to the small antral stage. Further development necessitates strong FSH stimulation. The contrast between very high FSH levels and normal sized ovaries with antral follicles may, therefore, be characteristic of such patients (Beau et al., 1998).

Galactosaemia

Galactosaemia is a clinically heterogeneous autosomal recessive inborn error of metabolism caused by total, or near-total, deficiency of galactose 1-phosphate uridyltransferase (GALT), resulting in extremely elevated levels of galactose 1-phosphate (Gal-1-P) (Sardhawalla and Wraith, 1987). Most commonly, the initial presentation is vomiting, jaundice and failure to thrive in the first week of life. The incidence of galactosaemia varies enormously in different populations throughout the world. It ranges from 1:30 000–40 000 livebirths in European countries where neonatal screening is undertaken (Murphy et al., 1999) to as few as 1:1 000 000 in Japan (Hirokawa et al., 1997).

Immediate treatment consists of ensuring a strict lactose-free diet. The problems arise from tissue accumu-

lation of Gal-1-P, which is the main toxic metabolite, and galactitol, which is toxic to the lens of the eye. Cardinal features are hepatomegaly, cataracts and mental retardation, growth delay and ovarian failure (Waggoner et al., 1990). The exact mechanism causing ovarian failure is not fully understood since some individuals will have only minimal ovarian dysfunction despite poor dietary restriction of lactose and galactose (Fraser et al., 1986). Gal-1-P accumulates in the ovary both pre- and postnatally in galactosaemic females and inhibits biochemical pathways involved in carbohydrate metabolism (Gitzelmann and Steinman, 1984). Evidence for a direct toxic effect of galactose to the ovary comes from a study showing a significant reduction in the number of medium or large ovarian follicles in the offspring of pregnant and nursing rats fed a 50% galactose diet (Chen et al., 1981). Interestingly, the rat testes were resistant to galactose and its metabolites.

The status of heterozygous females remains unclear, with conflicting evidence as to the risk of developing POF. Original work hypothesized that POF was associated with disorders of galactose metabolism (Cramer et al., 1989) and heterozygotes might experience POF (Sayle et al., 1996). Another study found no association between carrier status for galactosaemia and POF (Kaufman et al., 1993). A stage of resistant ovary syndrome is one pathway in the progression to irreversible POF in some with galactosaemia (Twigg et al., 1996). Studies examining ovarian biopsies in galactosaemic females confirm a reduction in the number of primary follicles but found no correlation with ovarian dysfunction (Robinson et al., 1984). The use of histological analysis is, therefore, not routinely indicated.

The gene *GALT* has been localized to position 13 on the short arm of chromosome 9 and spans 4.3 kb of DNA arranged into 11 exons (Shih et al., 1984). The most frequently cited mutations give rise to Gln188Arg, Lys285Asn, Ser135Leu and Asn314Asp. Gln188Arg is the most commonly occurring change in European populations, with a prevalence of approximately 64% (Elsas et al., 1993). It arises as a result of a mutation in codon 188, at a highly conserved position in exon 6 of the short arm of chromosome 9 (Reichardt and Woo, 1991). It is most prevalent in Ireland especially amongst the travelling population (Murphy et al., 1999), followed by Great Britain (Tyfield et al., 1999) and is associated with a severe biochemical phenotype and substantial if not complete loss in GALT activity (Fridovich-Keil and Jinks-Robertson, 1993).

Fragile X premutation

Fragile X syndrome is the most commonly inherited form of moderate learning difficulties in males and results from an expansion of the trinucleotide repeat sequence in the first exon of the gene *FMR1* (Xq27.3) (Bates and Howard, 1990). The full fragile X mutation occurs when the number of trinucleotide repeats is in excess of 200, gene transcription fails and the FMR1 protein is not expressed (Jacobs, 1991). In normal individuals, there are less than 60 trinucleotide repeats at this fragile site. The fragile X premutation occurs when between 60 and 200 trinucleotide repeat sequences are present and *FMR1* is transcribed (Devys et al., 1993). It has been hypothesized that expansion of the trinucleotide sequence at the premutation level interferes in some way with *FMR1* gene transcription in the fetal ovary, resulting in premutation carriers having a reduced number of oocytes at birth (Conway et al., 1995).

Women with POF are 10 times more likely than average to carry a fragile X premutation and it has been demonstrated that 3% of women with sporadic POF carry the fragile X premutation (Conway et al., 1998). The fragile X premutation is a genetic marker for familial POF in 13% of pedigrees and as such provides an important tool for the prediction of POF in as yet unaffected females. While the mechanism of ovarian failure remains obscure in women with the fragile X premutation, this association provides an example of X dominant inheritance (Allingham-Hawkins et al., 1999).

Blepharophimosis–ptosis–epicanthus inversus syndrome

Blepharophimosis–ptosis–epicanthus inversus syndrome (BPES) is rare condition first described by Vignes in 1889 and is characterized by typical facial features. These include a reduction on the horizontal length of the palpebral fissures (blepharophimosis), drooping of the eyelids (ptosis) and a skin fold running across the inner canthus (epicanthus inversus). It is transmitted in an autosomal dominant manner and is caused by disruption of chromosome 3 locus 3q23 either by deletion or translocation (Amati et al., 1995).

Ovarian failure occurs in approximately 50% of affected females. Two distinct types have been identified: type 1 in which penetrance is 100%, transmission is through males and all women are infertile; and type 2 where penetrance is 96.5%, transmission is through both sexes and females are fertile (Zolotogora et al., 1983). A variant of BPES is accompanied by POF in affected females and is likely to represent a contiguous gene syndrome (Oley and Baraitser, 1988). Women with BPES frequently enter a state of intermittent ovarian failure or "resistant ovary syndrome" (Fraser et al., 1988). Normal ovarian volume and large follicles persist long after the serum FSH concentration rises (Toomes and Dixon, 1998).

The region responsible for BPES has been mapped to a translocation breakpoint at 3q23 between primers D3S1316 and D3S1615 (Lawson et al., 1995). More recently, it has been refined to a 280 kb interval using a YAC (Toomes and Dixon, 1998). Both types of BPES have been mapped to the same locus (3q22-23), suggesting that ovarian failure is part of a spectrum of phenotype rather than a distinct entity (Amati et al., 1996). Recently, mutations of the forkhead transcription factor FOXL2 have been identified (Crisponi et al., 2001). These mutations produce a truncated protein. The target genes of FOXL2 are as yet unknown. FOXL2 could interact with members of the transforming growth factor β (TGF-β) family and, therefore, might be involved in follicle apoptosis.

Inhibin

Inhibin exerts its physiological effect by the negative feedback control of FSH, thereby affecting recruitment and development of ovarian follicles during folliculogenesis. Inhibin is a glycoprotein and is structurally related to the TGF-β superfamily (Vale et al., 1988). A variant of the gene for the inhibin α-subunit was found in three (7%) women from a group of 43 patients with POF, which contrasted with only 1 (0.7%) woman from a group of 150 controls. This variant results from an alanine to threonine substitution and is highly conserved across species, with the potential to affect FSH receptor binding and hence fulfils the criteria for a candidate gene mutation for POF (Shelling et al., 2000).

Perrault's syndrome

Perrault's syndrome is the combination of congenital deafness, gonadal dysgenesis and short stature and is inherited in an autosomal recessive manner. The genetic defect in Perrault's syndrome is yet to be defined.

Murine knockout models

An alternative strategy in identifying genetic causes of POF is the study of gene knockout animal models. Various genes in the reproductive system have been interrupted to produce knockout mice. Few of these have a phenotype that mimic human POF.

Connexin 37

Connexin 37 provides another example of the use of transgenic technology to identify candidate genes for POF. Connexins are proteins that form intercellular channels involved in gap junctions. Half of an intercellular channel is known as a connexon. Each connexon is a hexamer of subunit proteins called connexins. Connexin 37 is present exclusively in the ovary and makes up part of the gap junction between the ovum and the granulosa cells. Absence of this protein causes infertility of homozygous knockout mice but the role in humans is yet to be characterized (Simon et al., 1997).

Cyclin D_2

Cyclin D_2 is a D-type cyclin and is critical during the G_1 phase of the mammalian cell cycle. It is specifically induced by FSH via a cyclic AMP-dependent pathway. Knockout female mice deficient in cyclin D_2 are sterile owing to the inability of ovarian granulosa cells to proliferate normally in response to FSH. This contrasts with mutant males, who have hypoplastic testes but retain fertility (Sicinski et al., 1996).

Growth differentiation factor 9

Growth differentiation factor 9 (GDF-9) is a member of the TGF-β superfamily that originally was thought to be expressed only in the ovary (McGrath et al., 1995). Expression of GDF-9 mRNA has been recently found in nonovarian tissues in mice, rats and humans (Fitzpatrick et al., 1998). It is secreted from the oocyte and required for ovarian folliculogenesis. Female mice deficient in GDF-9 are infertile, and analysis of their ovaries reveals formation of primordial and primary one-layer follicles but a block in follicular development beyond the primary one-layer follicle stage (Dong et al., 1996). Recently, no mutations of the two exons of GDF-9 were identified in 15 Japanese women with POF (Takebayashi et al., 2000).

Zinc finger gene on the X chromosome

The zinc finger (ZFX) gene (locus Xp22.3-21.2) is the X chromosome homologue of the zinc finger Y chromosome (ZFY) gene. ZFX knockout mice exhibit infertility in both sexes and the female phenotype appears to be analogous to POF in humans (Luoh et al., 1997).

Human deleted in azoospermia-like 1 gene (DAZL1)

The human deleted in azoospermia (DAZ) gene family contains a cluster of DAZ genes on the Y chromosome and a single autosomal homologue, DAZL1 (DAZ-Like), that maps to chromosome 3p24. The DAZ gene located on the Y chromosome is the commonest molecularly defined cause of infertility in men. In mice, loss of function of the

homologue of DAZL1 results in the loss of male and female germ cells. Dazl1 protein is localized to prenatal and postnatal follicles. Human Dazl1 protein is expressed embryonically in germ cells of girls and in mature oocytes (Dorfman et al., 1999).

Acquired causes of primary ovarian failure

The acquired causes of POF are listed in Table 30.1 while Table 30.2 refers to this category under the umbrella of environmental causes and specifically relates to 347 women attending the ovarian failure clinic at the Middlesex Hospital London.

Environmental toxins

Ovarian dysfunction can result from environmental toxins through interruption of gonadotrophin-releasing hormone pulsatile release from the hypothalamus (Vermulen, 1993) as well as through alteration in oocyte number. A variety of toxins have been identified including alcohol, food, stress and viral infection. A previous infection such as varicella has been noted in up to 3.5% of patients with POF (Rebar and Connolly, 1996). Mumps is the best documented cause of POF (Grasso, 1976). Cytomegalovirus however, causes oophoritis in patients with immunocompromise such as acquired immunodeficiency syndrome (AIDS) (Familiari et al., 1991). The major environmental influence determining the age of menopause is smoking (Jick et al., 1977). Smoking advances the age of menopause by about 1.5 years (Brambilla and McKinlay, 1989).

Radiotherapy

Radiation-induced ovarian failure is dependent on the age of the patient as well as the dose received. The most significant effect occurs in the early phases of follicular development, thereby destroying oocytes and sparing mature follicles (Ogilvy-Stuart and Shalet, 1993). A radiation dose of 600 rad or more produces ovarian failure in greater than 90% of patients over the age of 40 years (Taylor et al., 1993). The ovaries of prepubertal girls are particularly resistant to irradiation (Shalet et al., 1976). For pregnancies following chemotherapy and/or radiotherapy, there is a slightly higher rate of miscarriage but no increased risk of congenital abnormalities (Averette et al., 1990).

Chemotherapy

Chemotherapeutic agents destroy rapidly dividing cells and in the ovary affect proliferating granulosa and theca cells of mature follicles (Gradishar and Schilsky, 1989). Ovarian failure is dependent on the dose and type of treatment and the age of the patient. Women less than 40 years of age are far less likely to develop ovarian failure than older individuals (Koyama et al., 1977). The prepubertal ovary is relatively resistant to the effects of alkylating agents (Chapman and Sutcliffe, 1981). Hormonal suppression of ovarian function has not, however, led to an improvement in ovarian preservation following chemotherapy (Ataya et al., 1995).

Alkylating agents have the greatest effect, causing permanent damage by altering cellular DNA of resting oocytes and proliferating cells (Epstein, 1990). Reversible ovarian failure has been reported in some instances following the use of cyclophosphamide and other alkylating agents for some childhood leukaemias (Siris et al., 1976). As with radiotherapy, the ovaries of older women are more sensitive to cytotoxic drug-induced damage (Bryne et al., 1987) and histopathological changes include cortical stromal fibrosis with loss or arrest of follicles (Nicosia et al., 1985).

The *Bax* gene has been implicated in potentiating the detrimental effects of chemotherapy through the apoptosis process. Knockout mice deficient for *Bax* have been shown to be resistant to the effects of chemotherapy and exhibit preserved primordial follicle numbers following chemotherapy (McCurrah et al., 1997). The potential for manipulation of this gene in humans is currently being investigated in relation to treatment of epithelial ovarian carcinoma (Strobel et al., 1998). The clinical implications of these findings are widespread and may offer future benefits in the human ovary (Perez et al., 1999).

Sphingomyelinase

Ceramide is directly involved in signalling somatic cell death as part of the apoptotic process. It is a sphingolid derived from sphingomyelinase-catalysed hydrolysis and is metabolized by ceramidase to sphingosine, which is then phosphorylated to sphingosine 1-phosphate (S1P). In a defining paper, Morita et al. (2000) tested the functional relevance of the sphingomyelin pathway in ovarian germ cell dynamics with the goal of developing in vivo approaches to control signalling pathways responsible for oocyte death in both normal and pathological conditions. Mice deficient for sphingomyelin phosphodiesterase 1 (SMPD1) had an increased ovarian reserve, as evidenced by hyperplasia of preantral, primary and primordial follicles, compared with wild-type mice. These findings indicate there is an ovarian-intrinsic cell death defect in the SMPD1-null mouse, and that enhanced survival of the developing germ cell line during organogenesis is the mechanism underlying the

substantially enlarged oocyte pool at birth. Deficiency of SMPD1 can be reproduced in oocytes by addition of a ceramide antagonist, S1P. Administration of S1P 2 hours prior to ionizing radiation resulted in a significant and dose-dependent preservation of ovaries, with complete protection of the quiescent (primordial) and growing (primary, preantral) follicles. Small-lipid pretreatment therapy (S1P), offers promise for clinical development to preserve normal ovarian function and fertility in young girls and reproductive-age women treated for cancer.

Surgical procedures

Clearly, bilateral oophorectomy will result in ovarian failure. Hysterectomy with conservation of ovaries has been shown to result in an earlier onset of menopause, probably because of disruption to the ovarian blood supply. It is not evident, however, whether ovarian surgery hastens the onset of ovarian failure.

Autoimmunity

The first cases of autoimmune disease and POF were described in 1954 (Guinet and Pommatau, 1954). In this initial series, POF occurred in conjunction with hypothyroidism and preceded Addison's disease by a number of years. Autoimmune Addison's disease is associated with POF in the polyendocrinopathies type I and II (APS type 1 and type 2). In one series of patients with APS type 1, 58% of women had POF (Ahonen et al., 1988). This contrasts with APS type 2, where the prevalence of POF is 5–10% (Neufeld et al., 1981). In a study examining the causes of POF and autoimmunity, APS types 1 and 2 were found in 3% of patients with POF (Betterle et al., 1993). Hypothyroidism has subsequently been shown to be the most commonly associated autoimmune disease (Alper and Garner, 1985). Other associated endocrine disorders include myaesthenia gravis, Crohn's disease, systemic lupus erythematosus, vitiligo and pernicious anaemia (Blizzard and Gibbs, 1968; Collen et al., 1979; de Moraes-Ruehsen et al., 1972; Lundberg and Persson, 1969). A study reporting on 215 ovarian biopsies in women with POF concluded that patients with adrenal disease were more likely to develop ovarian failure as a result of lymphocytic oophoritis (Hoek et al., 1997).

The presence of autoantibodies in patients with POF has been studied in a number of series (Chen et al., 1996; Wheatcroft et al., 1994). Their exact role in the pathogenesis of POF remains unclear but good evidence exists that ovarian antibodies can arise secondary to any form of ovarian insult (Wheatcroft and Weetman, 1997). Hypothyroidism and diabetes mellitus have been detected by biochemical screening in patients with karyotypically normal spontaneous POF (Anasti et al., 1998). A study characterizing 135 patients with idiopathic POF found evidence of positive autoimmunity in 31%, with the majority of the autoimmune group (90%) having antibodies against the thyroid gland. This was considered the best marker for antibody status (Conway et al., 1996). Uncontrolled studies and anecdotal cases of the return of ovarian function following the use of high-dose steroid immunosuppression have been reported (Coulam et al., 1981) but presently have no proven benefit and carry a significant risk of complications, such as osteoporosis.

A recent discovery has been the gene for the autoimmune regulator (AIRE), which has been isolated on the long arm of chromosome 21q22 (Nagamine et al., 1997). It is linked to APS type 1; however, the role of the AIRE protein is not known.

Clinical evaluation of primary ovarian failure

The theoretical and molecular aspects of ovarian failure discussed above must be born in mind when an individual first presents. The relative frequency of the various causes of hypergonadotrophic hypogonadism will vary depending on the local referral patterns and the intensity of investigation. Table 30.2 illustrates the pattern of causes in patients presenting to a specialist clinic in London.

History and examination

Early onset of ovarian failure will present with primary amenorrhoea and failure to progress through puberty. In some girls, the ovaries will be dysgenetic and appear as streaks while in others some ovarian tissue will be visible on ultrasound. Secondary amenorrhoea presenting before the age of 40 may be of sudden onset or have a prodromal menstrual irregularity. The symptoms of oestrogen deficiency, amenorrhoea, flushing, vaginal dryness and dyspareunia are variable and are usually less obvious in those with primary amenorrhoea. Depression and low self-esteem may be the result of both oestrogen deficiency and the label of premature menopause (Liao et al., 2000). Primary amenorrhoea can be defined as absent menarche after the age of 14.5 years, which is the 95th centile for the onset of menstruation. Secondary amenorrhoea is classically defined as amenorrhoea of at least six months' duration. Some women, however, appear to become stable with lesser degrees of ovarian failure, either with intermittent periods and a raised serum FSH concentration or with occult raised FSH with regular periods (Healy, 1994). The spectrum of ovarian failure spans the diagnostic labels of ovarian dysgenesis

through POF to resistant ovary syndrome, which are probably stages of the same process.

The only features of the history that are helpful in determining aetiology of ovarian failure are a positive family history, a concurrent autoimmune disorder or stigmata of one of the inherited conditions.

In many instances, a formal pedigree enquiry is required to determine other female family members who may be affected, particularly if the inheritance is passed through an unaffected male. Given the disappointing treatment options for established ovarian failure, it is important to identify females who are at risk of infertility so that they will be able to review their family planning. Of families transmitting POF, 13% are at risk of transmitting fragile X syndrome. Identifying this groups allows prevention of this disruptive form of mental retardation in males by genetic counselling or antenatal diagnosis (Conway et al., 1998; Murray, 2000).

Ten to thirty percent of women with POF already have a concurrent autoimmune disorder, the most common of which is hypothyroidism. In the sequence of the most common autoimmune associations found is APS type 2, where ovarian failure can occur at any stage. Consequently, a history should include symptoms of Addison's disease, hypothyroidism and diabetes in particular, with the less-common associations of autoimmune arthritides and inflammatory bowel disease being kept in mind. Further, women with established POF should be monitored for the later appearance of these conditions.

Examination may reveal a clue to an autoimmune background, perhaps through vitiligo or premature greying of scalp hair. Alternatively, signs of rheumatoid arthritis or systemic lupus erythematosus may be evident. The congenital associations of blepharophimosis and ptosis with BPES or deafness and short stature with Perrault syndrome should be considered. Occasionally, even Turner's syndrome can go undiagnosed in an individual who is mosaic with secondary amenorrhoea and rather few stigmata of the classical diagnosis.

Investigations

Some women appear to go through self-limiting, brief bouts of ovarian failure and for this reason two measurements of FSH some weeks apart should be taken before the diagnosis of POF is made. An FSH level higher than 50 mU/l has been used as a general definition of POF. However, this level can probably be lowered to 20 U/l as pregnancy is very rare at this level. Cytogenetic analysis is essential in women presenting with primary amenorrhoea, when chromosomal defects, usually a Turner variant or the presence of a Y chromosome, can be found in 40% (Sarto, 1974). It is rare for women with secondary amenorrhoea to have a chromosomal defect detectable by cytogenetic analysis, although when it does occur the prospects for predicting ovarian failure in as yet unaffected family members can be vital. Cytogenetic abnormalities, usually small deletions of the X chromosome, have been found in women presenting with amenorrhoea as late as 35 years of age (Davison et al., 1998).

The value of antibody screening is debatable as the sensitivity of the current tests for autoantibodies directed against the ovary is low. Only a small percentage of women show positive immunofluorescence against the ovary by standard methods while 20–30% are positive for thyroid autoimmunity (Conway et al., 1998). While the definition of an autoimmune aetiology may not alter management, it is very helpful for the patient to be able to define the process of ovarian destruction. Most importantly, though, is the need for long-term follow-up of women with positive autoimmunity in case they acquire another component of a polyendocrinopathy. At the very least, annual urinalysis, electrolyte and thyroid-stimulating hormone measurements are required in this group in order to screen for diabetes, Addison's disease and hypothyroidism.

Oestrogen deficiency is a major risk factor for osteoporosis and women with POF usually opt for long-term oestrogen replacement therapy. A measurement of bone mineral density is extremely useful in assessing the balance of the risks and benefits of an individual's oestrogen regimen. In some women with low bone density, follow-up bone density measurements will be required at intervals.

The place of ovarian biopsy and pelvic ultrasound is restricted to research. Neither investigation has been accepted as influencing management. While some investigators have found that the histological appearance of the ovary can predict fertility prospects (Zara et al., 1987), it remains the case that women with no ova visible on biopsy have spontaneously conceived, making the application of this procedure largely obsolete (Khastgir et al., 1994). Similarly, while pregnancy after the diagnosis of POF is more likely if the ovaries are still identifiable on ultrasonography, the event is so rare that the discrimination offered by this test is not routinely useful.

Treatment of primary ovarian failure

The diagnosis of POF in a young woman is a devastating event, even though the news is often received passively. At the very least, an early follow-up appointment is required in order to clarify the future prospects once the initial acute reaction has subsided. One of the most neglected aspects

of POF is the long-term psychological scar left by the diagnosis. This is especially true of younger women, who experience low self-esteem and depression that cannot be accounted for solely by oestrogen deficiency. Input from a clinical psychologist is a vital part of the early management process particularly because anger is often directed to the diagnosing physician, who is then unable to provide effective emotional support. The trauma of the diagnosis often returns as friends become pregnant, and follow-up counselling may be necessary long after the acute event. Low self-esteem, infertility and difficulties with oestrogen replacement commonly inflict stress upon partnerships.

Hormone replacement therapy

Women who experience an early menopause are at a reduced risk of breast cancer and thrombosis but increased risk of osteoporosis and cardiovascular disease. Much of this risk profile can be attributed to oestrogen deficiency. Young women with POF are often acutely symptomatic, with hot flushes, night sweats and vaginal dryness, and should be on hormone replacement therapy (HRT). Some of younger onset may require HRT for nearly 40 years. The degree to which this long-term administration of oestrogen prevents cardiovascular disease or increases risk of breast cancer is unknown in this female population, although the usual assumption is that these risks are returned to normal with HRT used up until the average age of the menopause.

The choice of oestrogen in the HRT formulation must be made on individual basis. Adolescents with primary amenorrhoea should be treated with low-dose unopposed oestrogens in gradually increasing dosage for some two years in order to mimic physiological onset of puberty. The optimal preparation for this manoeuvre is not established. In the UK, it has been traditional to use ethinylestradiol as this is the only preparation available in a sufficiently low dose. A more accurate mimic of physiology may be obtained, however, by cutting the matrix transdermal patches and starting with one sixth of a patch to initiate puberty. As the dose of oestrogen is increased, cyclical progesterone is introduced to induce menstruation.

Once cyclical therapy has been established, the choice of maintenance treatment lies between an oral contraceptive and HRT preparation. Remembering that occasional sporadic pregnancy can occur, some women might choose a combined oral contraceptive (COC) preparation. These, however, provide oestrogen only for three weeks out of four and many women are symptomatic of oestrogen deficiency in the pill-free week. Also, COCs supply supraphysiological oestrogen, which may increase the risk of thromboembolic events to a greater degree than HRT formulations, especially in women who smoke. Few direct comparisons of COC and HRT exist in the literature. For those women who are troubled by side effects from oral oestrogen, a transdermal preparation may be the answer, particularly for those with concurrent hypertension or with additional risk factors for thrombosis. Those women with particularly prominent vaginal symptoms may benefit from additional topical oestrogen in the form of a pessary, vaginal tablet or cream.

Progesterone is required for all women with an intact uterus in order to avoid endometrial hyperplasia induced by unopposed oestrogen. While some women might find the continuous combined form of oestrogen and progesterone replacement attractive as a way of avoiding menstruation, it must be remembered that the use of these preparations in young women has not been studied over the long term.

Options for fertility

Spontaneous return of ovarian function can occur in women with a firm diagnosis of POF and no particular feature predicts this rare event with great accuracy. Pregnancy has been recorded in 3–5% of women (Polansky and de Papp, 1976). Pregnancies have even been reported in women who have used the oral contraceptive as a form of oestrogen replacement and in some women who have no ova found on ovarian biopsy. A history of chemotherapy, evidence of autoimmunity or visible ovaries on ultrasonography all make the return of ovarian function slightly more likely.

There are some reports in the literature of induced pregnancies in women with POF. However, it is now clear that no medical treatment makes this rare event more likely. Conventional ovulation-induction treatments with, or without, suppression of gonadotrophins do not raise the fertility rate above background levels in women with POF (Check et al., 1990). HRT has a neutral effect on fertility in this group of women: in fact, most women who conceive do so while taking HRT (van Kasteren and Schoemaker, 1999). Uncontrolled studies have suggested that treatment with glucocorticoids might promote fertility, particularly in women who have an autoimmune aetiology for ovarian failure. However, a controlled European study has demonstrated the lack of effect of corticoids in treating infertility (van Kasteren et al., 1999b).

The advent of ovum donation has been a major breakthrough for women with ovarian failure over the past 10 years (Devroey et al., 1988). As the number of assisted reproduction centres offering ovum donation increases, more women will be able to take up this option. The success

rate of ovum donation is somewhat higher than that for standard in vitro fertilization, giving each couple a 30% chance of a pregnancy for each cycle of treatment (Ch. 34). Embryo donation offers an alternative strategy for achieving a normal pregnancy if there is subfertility in the male partner, while some couples require surrogacy or choose adoption.

There is increasing expectation that advanced assisted reproduction techniques might make it possible to utilize the very few eggs remaining in the ovary at the time of diagnosis of ovarian failure. So far, there have been no consistent successes with ovarian material (Aubard et al., 2001). Frozen sections of ovary might be used for later autotransplantation with a view to in vivo ovulation; alternatively, dispersed ova might be matured in vitro in preparation for fertilization. Until the methodology of these techniques are proven, cryopreservation should be reserved for use in limited circumstances such as chemotherapy (Ch. 33). It seems premature to offer cryopreservation to women presenting with non-iatrogenic ovarian failure in whom very little ovarian tissue remains at the time of diagnosis. Instead, women with established ovarian failure will have to wait for the establishment of in vitro maturation of oocytes.

REFERENCES

Ahonen P, Koskimies S, Lokki M L et al. (1988). The expression of autoimmune polyglandular disease type 1 appears associated with several HLA-A antigens but not with HLA-DR. *J Clin Endocrinol Metab* 66, 1151–1157.

Aittomaki K (1994). The genetics of XX gonadal dysgenesis. *Am J Hum Genet* 54, 844–851.

Aittomaki K, Lucerna J L D, Pakarinen P et al. (1995). Mutation in the follicle-stimulating hormone receptor gene causes hereditary hypergonadotrophic ovarian failure. *Cell* 82, 959–968.

Aittomaki K, Herva U-H, Juntunen K et al. (1996). Clinical features of primary ovarian failure caused by a point mutation in the follicle-stimulating hormone receptor gene. *J Clin Endocrinol Metab* 81, 3722–3726.

Allingham-Hawkins D J, Babul-Hirji R et al. (1999). Fragile X premutation is a significant risk factor for premature ovarian failure: the International Collaborative POF in Fragile X study-preliminary data. *Am J Med Genet* 83, 322–325.

Alper M M, Garner P R (1985). Premature ovarian failure: its relationship to autoimmune disease. *Obstet Gynaecol* 66, 27–30.

Amati P, Chomel J C, Nivelon-Chevalier A et al. (1995). A gene for blepharophimosis–ptosis–epicanthus inversus maps to chromosome 3q23. *Hum Genet* 96, 213–215.

Amati P, Gasparini P, Zlotogora J et al. (1996). A gene for premature ovarian failure associated with eyelid malformation maps to chromosome 3q22-q23. *Am J Hum Genet* 58, 1089–1092.

Anasti J N, Kalantaridou S N, Kimzey L M et al. (1998). Bone loss in young women with karyotypically normal spontaneous premature ovarian failure. *Obstet Gynaecol* 91, 12–16.

Ataya K, Rao L V, Lawrence E et al. (1995). Luteinising hormone-releasing agonist inhibits cyclophosphamide-induced ovarian follicular depletion in Rhesus monkeys. *Biol Reprod* 52, 365–372.

Aubard Y, Piver P, Pech J C, Galinat S, Teissier M (2001). Ovarian tissue cryopreservation and gynecologic oncology: a review. *Int J Obstet Gynecol Reprod Biol* 97, 5–14.

Averette H E, Boike G M, Jarrell M A (1990). Effects of cancer chemotherapy on gonadal function and reproductive capacity. *Can J Clin* 40, 199–209.

Baker T G (1963). A quantitative and cytological study of germ cells in the human ovary. *Proc Roy Soc Lond* 158, 417–433.

Banfi S, Borsani G, Bulfone A et al. (1997). Drosophila-related expressed sequences. *Hum Mol Genet* 6, 1745–1753.

Bates A, Howard P J (1990). Distal long arm deletions of the X chromosome and ovarian failure. *J Med Genet* 27, 722–723.

Beau I, Touraine P, Meduri G et al. (1998). A novel phenotype related to partial loss of function mutations of the follicle stimulating hormone receptor. *Clin Invest* 102, 1352–1359.

Betterle C, Rossi A, Dalla Pria S et al. (1993). Premature ovarian failure: autoimmunity and natural history. *Clin Endocrinol* 39, 35–43.

Bione S, Sala C, Manzini C et al. (1998). A human homologue of the *Drosophila melanogaster diaphanous* gene is disrupted in a patient with premature ovarian failure: evidence for conserved function in oogenesis and implications for human sterility. *Am J Hum Genet* 62, 533–541.

Blizzard R M, Gibbs J H (1968). Candidiasis: studies pertaining to its association with endocrinopathies and pernicious anaemia. *Paediatr* 42, 231–236.

Brambilla D J, Mckinlay S M (1989). A prospective study of factors affecting age at menopause. *J Clin Epidemiol* 42, 1031–1039.

Bryne J, Mulvihill J J, Myers M H et al. (1987). Effects of treatment on fertility in long-term survivors of childhood cancer. *N Engl J Med* 317, 1315–1321.

Bursch W, Kleine L, Tenniswood M (1990). The biochemistry of cell death via apoptosis. *Biochem Cell Biol* 68, 1071–1074.

Chapman R M, Sutcliffe S B (1981). Protection of ovarian function by oral contraceptive use in women receiving chemotherapy for Hodgkin's disease. *Blood* 58, 849–851.

Check J H, Nazari A, Nowroozi K, Shapse D, Chase J S, Vaze M (1990). Ovulation induction and pregnancies in 100 consecutive women with hypergonadotropic amenorrhea. *Fertil Steril* 53, 90.

Chen S, Sawicka J, Betterle C et al. (1996). Autoantibodies to steroidogenic enzymes in autoimmune polyglandular syndrome, Addison's disease and premature ovarian failure. *J Clin Endocrinol Metab* 81, 1871–1876.

Chen Y T, Mattison D R, Schulman J D (1981). Hypogonadism and galactosaemia. *N Engl J Med* 305, 464.

Chiquoine A D (1960). The development of the zona pellucida in mammalian ovum. *Am J Anat* 106, 149–169.

Chu C E, Connor J M (1995). Molecular biology of Turner's Syndrome. *Arch Dis Child* 72, 285–286.

Collen R J, Lippe B M, Kaplan S A (1979). Primary ovarian failure, juvenile rheumatoid arthritis and vitiligo. *Am J Dis Child* 133, 598–600.

Conway E, Hoppner W, Gromoll J et al. (1997). Mutations of the receptor gene are rare in familial and sporadic premature ovarian failure [Abstract]. *J Endocrinol* 152(suppl), 257.

Conway G S, Hettiarachchi S, Murray A et al. (1995). Fragile X premutations in familial premature ovarian failure. *Lancet* 346, 309–310.

Conway G S, Kaltsas G, Patel A, Davies M C, Jacobs H S (1996). Characterization of idiopathic premature ovarian failure. *Fertil Steril* 65, 337–341.

Conway G S, Payne N N, Webb J, Murray A, Jacobs P A (1998). Fragile X premutation screening in women with premature ovarian failure. *Hum Reprod* 13, 1184–1187.

Conway G S, Conway E, Walker C et al. (1999). Mutation screening and isoform prevalence of the follicle stimulating hormone receptor gene mutation in women with premature ovarian failure, resistant ovary syndrome and polycystic ovarian syndrome. *Clin Endocrinol (Oxf)* 51, 97–99.

Coulam C B, Kempers R D, Randall R V (1981). Premature ovarian failure. *Fertil Steril* 36, 238–240.

Coulam C B, Adamson S C, Annegers J F (1986). Incidence of premature ovarian failure. *Obstet Gynecol* 67, 604–606.

Coulam C B, Stringfellow S, Hoefnagel D (1983). Evidence for a genetic factor in the aetiology of premature ovarian failure. *Fertil Steril* 40, 693–695.

Cramer D W, Harlow B L, Barbieri R L et al. (1989). Galactose-1-phosphate uridyl transferase activity associated with age at menopause and reproductive history. *Fertil Steril* 51, 609–615.

Cramer D W, Huijuan X, Harlow B L (1995). Family history as a predictor of early menopause. *Fertil Steril* 64, 740–745.

Crisponi L, Deiana M, Loi A et al. (2001). The putative forkhead transcription factor FOXL2 is mutated in blepharophimosis/ptosis/epicanthus inversus syndrome. *Nat Genet* 27, 159–166.

Cryns V L, Yuan J (1998). The cutting edge: caspases in apoptosis and disease. In *When Cells Die. A Comprehensive Evaluation of Apoptosis and Programmed Cell Death*, Lockshin R A, Zakeri Z, Tilly J L, eds., pp. 177–210. Wiley-Liss, New York.

da Fonte Kolek M B, Batista M C, Russell A J et al. (1998). No evidence of the inactivating mutation (C566T) in the follicle stimulating hormone receptor gene in Brazilian women with premature ovarian failure. *Fertil Steril* 70, 565–567.

Davis C J, Davison R M, Conway G S (1998). Familial premature ovarian failure: clinical and genetic features. *Cont Rev Obstet Gynecol* 10, 289–294.

Davis C J, Davison R M, Payne N N et al. (2000). Female sex preponderance for idiopathic familial premature ovarian failure suggests an X chromosome defect. *Hum Reprod* 15, 2418–2422.

Davison R M, Quilter C R, Webb J et al. (1998). A familial case of X chromosome deletion ascertained by cytogenetic screening of women with premature ovarian failure. *Hum Reprod* 13, 3039–3041.

de Moraes-Ruehsen M, Blizzard R M, Garcia-Bunuel R et al. (1972). Autoimmunity and ovarian failure. *Am J Obstet Gynecol* 112, 693–703.

Devroey P, Wisanto A, Camus M et al. (1988). Oocyte donation in patients without ovarian function. *Hum Reprod* 3, 699–704.

Devys D, Lutz Y, Rouyer N (1993). The FMR-1 protein is cytoplasmic, most abundant in neurons and appears in carriers of a fragile X premutation. *Nat Genet* 4, 335–340.

Dong J, Albertini D F, Nishimori K et al. (1996). Growth differentiation factor-9 is required during early ovarian folliculogenesis. *Nature* 383, 485–486.

Dorfman D M, Genest D R, Reijo Pera R A (1999). Human *DAZL1* encodes a candidate fertility factor in women that localises to prenatal and postnatal germ cells. *Hum Reprod* 14, 2531–2536.

Elsas L J, Fridovich-Keil J L, Leslie N (1993). Galactosaemia: a molecular approach to the enigma. *Int Paediatr* 8, 101–109.

Epstein R J (1990). Drug induced DNA damage and tumour chemosensitivity. *J Clin Oncol* 8, 2062–2084.

Familiari U, Larocca L M, Tamburrini E et al. (1991). Premenopausal cytomegalovirus oophoritis in a patient with AIDS. *AIDS* 4, 458–459.

Fitch N, de saint Victor J, Richer C L et al. (1982). Premature menopause due to a small deletion in the long arm of the X chromosome: a report of three cases and a review. *Am J Obstet Gynaecol* 142, 968–972.

Fitzpatrick S L, Sindoni D M, Shughrue P J et al. (1998). Expression of growth differentiation factor-9 messenger ribonucleic acid in ovarian and non-ovarian rodent and human tissues. *Endocrinol* 139, 2571–2578.

Fraser I S, Greco S, Robertson D M (1986). Resistant ovary syndrome and premature ovarian failure in young women with galactosaemia. *Clin Reprod Fertil* 4, 133–138.

Fraser I S, Shearman R P, Smith A et al. (1988). An association between blepharophimosis, resistant ovary syndrome and true menopause. *Fertil Steril* 50, 747–751.

Fridovich-Keil J L, Jinks-Robertson S (1993). A yeast expression system for human galactose-1–phosphate uridylyltransferase. *Proc Natl Acad Sci USA* 90, 398–402.

Frisch S M, Francis H (1994). Disruption of epithelial cell-matrix interactions induces apoptosis. *J Cell Biol* 124, 619–626.

Gitzelmann R, Steinman B (1984). Galactosaemia: how does long-term treatment change the outcome? *Enzyme* 32, 37–46.

Goldstein P (1997). Controlling cell death. *Science* 275, 1081–1082.

Gosden R G, Faddy M J (1998). Biological basis of premature ovarian failure. *Reprod Fertil Dev* 10, 73–78.

Gradishar W J, Schilsky R L (1989). Ovarian function following radiation and chemotherapy for cancer. *Semin Oncol* 16, 425–436.

Grasso E (1976). Parotiti epodemiche pluricomplicate. *G Mal Infett Parasit* 26, 184–187.

Guinet P, Pommatau E (1954). Le pseudo-panhypopituitarisme par insuffisiences associees ovarienne, thyroidienne, et semenale. *Ann Endocrinol* 15, 327–332.

Healy D L (1994). Occult ovarian failure. *Curr Ther Endocrinol Metab* 5, 198–199.

Hirokawa H, Okano Y, Asada M et al. (1999). Molecular basis for phenotypic heterogeneity in galactosaemia: prediction of clinical phenotype from genotype in Japanese patients. *Eur J Hum Genet* 7, 757–764.

Hoek A, Schoemaker J, Drexhage H A (1997). Premature ovarian failure and ovarian autoimmunity. *Endocr Rev* 18, 107–134.

Huhtaniemi I, Yamamoto M, Ranta T et al. (1987). Follicle stimulating hormone receptors appear earlier in the primate testis than in the ovary. *J Clin Endocrinol Metab* 65, 1210–1214.

Jacobs P A (1991). Fragile X syndrome. *J Med Genet* 28, 809–810.

Jick H, Porter J, Morrison A S (1997). Relation between smoking and age of natural menopause. *Lancet* i, 1354–1355.

Jirasek J E (1976). Principles of reproductive embryology. In *Disorders of Sexual Differentiation. Aetiology and Clinical Delineation*, Simpson J L, ed., pp. 51–110. Academic Press, New York.

Kaufman F R, Devgan S, Donnell G N (1993). Results of a survey of carrier women for the galactosaemia gene. *Fertil Steril* 60, 727–728.

Kerr J F R, Wyllie A H, Currie A R (1972). Apoptosis: a basic biological phenomenon with wide-ranging implications in tissue kinetics. *Br J Cancer* 26, 239–257.

Khastgir G, Abdalla H, Studd J W (1994). The case against ovarian biopsy for the diagnosis of premature menopause. *Br J Obstet Gynaecol* 101, 96–98.

Koyama H, Wada T, Nishizaway et al. (1977). Cyclophosphamide-induced ovarian failure and its therapeutic significance in patients with breast cancer. *Cancer* 39, 1403–1409.

Krauss C, Turksoy R N, Atkins L et al. (1987). Familial premature ovarian failure due to an interstitial deletion of the long arm of the X chromosome. *N Engl J Med* 317, 125–131.

Lawson C T, Toomes C, Fryer A et al. (1995). Definition of the blepharophimosis, ptosis, epicanthus inversus syndrome critical region at chromosome 3q23 based on the analysis of chromosomal anomalies. *Hum Mol Genet* 4, 963–967.

Layman L C, Amde S, Cohen D P et al. (1998). The Finnish follicle stimulating hormone receptor gene mutation is rare in North American women with 46,XX ovarian failure. *Fertil Steril* 69, 300–302.

Li P, Nijhawan D, Budihardjo I et al. (1997). Cytochrome *c* and dATP-dependent formation of Apaf-1/caspase-9 complex initiates an apoptotic protease complex. *Cell* 91, 479–489.

Liao K L, Wood N, Conway G S (2000). Premature menopause and psychological well-being. *J Psychosom Obstet Gynaecol* 21, 167–74.

Lundberg P O, Persson V H (1969). Disappearance of amenorrhoea after thymectomy. A case report. *Acta Soc Med Uppsala* 74, 206–208.

Luoh S W, Bain P A, Polakiewicz R D et al. (1997). ZFX mutation results in small animal size and reduced germ cell number in male and female mice. *Development* 124, 2275–2284.

Majno G, Joris I (1995). Apoptosis, oncosis, and necrosis. An overview of cell death. *Am J Pathol* 146, 3–15.

Mattison D R, Evans M I, Schwimmer W B et al. (1984). Familial premature ovarian failure. *Am J Hum Genet* 36, 1341–1348.

May J M, McCarty K, Reichert L E et al. (1980). Follicle stimulating-hormone-mediated induction of functional luteinising/human chorionic gonadotrophin receptors during monolayer of porcine granulosa cells. *Endocrinol* 107, 1041–1049.

McCurrah M E, Connor T M, Knudson C M et al. (1997). Bax-deficiency promotes drug resistance and oncogenic transformation by attenuating p53-dependent apoptosis. *Proc Natl Acad Sci USA* 94, 2345–2349.

McGrath S A, Esquela A F, Lee S J (1995). Oocyte-specific expression of growth/differentiation factor-9. *Mol Endocrinol* 9, 131–136.

McKinlay S, Jeffreys M, Thompson B (1972). An investigation of age of menopause. *J Biosoc Sci* 4, 161–173.

Meyers C M, Boughman J A, Rivas M et al. (1996). Gonadal (ovarian) dysgenesis in 46,XX individuals: frequency of the autosomal recessive form. *Am J Med Genet* 63, 518–524.

Morita Y, Perez G I, Paris F et al. (2000). Oocyte apoptosis is suppressed by disruption of the *acid sphingomyelinase* gene or by sphingosine-1-phosphate therapy. *Nat Med* 6, 1109–1114.

Murphy M, McHugh B, Tighe O et al. (1999). Genetic basis of transferase-deficient galactosaemia in Ireland and the population history of the Irish Travellers. *Eur J Hum Genet* 7, 549–554.

Murray A (2000). Premature ovarian failure and the FMR1 gene. *Semin Reprod Med* 18, 59–66.

Nagamine K, Peterson P, Scott H S et al. (1997). Positional cloning of the APECED gene. *Nat Genet* 17, 393–397.

Neufeld M, Maclaren N K, Blizzard R M (1981). Two types of autoimmune Addison's disease associates with different polyglandular autoimmune (PGA) syndromes. *Medicine* 60, 355–362.

Nicosia S V, Matus-Ridley M, Meadows A T (1985). Gonadal effects of cancer therapy in girls. *Cancer* 55, 2364–2372.

Ogilvy-Stuart A L, Shalet S M (1993). Effect of radiation on the human reproductive system. *Environ Health Perspect* 101, 109–116.

Oley C, Baraitser M (1988). Blepharophimosis, ptosis epicanthus inversus syndrome (BPES). *J Med Genet* 25, 47–51.

Page D C, Mosher R, Simpson E M et al. (1987). The sex determining region of the Y chromosome encodes a finger protein. *Cell* 51, 1091–1104.

Pasquino A, Passeri F, Pucarelli I et al. (1997). Spontaneous pubertal development in Turner's syndrome. *J Clin Endocrinol Metab* 82, 1810–1813.

Patel T, Gores G J, Kaufmann S H (1996). The role of proteases during apoptosis. *FASSEB J* 10, 587–597.

Perez G I, Robles R, Knudson C M et al. (1999). Prolongation of ovarian lifespan into advanced chronological age by Bax-deficiency. *Nat Genet* 21, 200–203.

Phelan J P, Upton R T, Summitt R L (1977). Balanced reciprocal X-4 translocation in a female patient with early secondary amenorrhoea. *Am J Obstet Gynecol* 129, 607–613.

Polansky S, de Papp E W (1976). Pregnancy associated with hypergonadotropic hypogonadism. *Obstet Gynecol* 47, 47S–51S.

Powell C M, Taggart R T, Drumheller T C et al. (1994). Molecular and cytogenetic studies of an X: autosome translocation in a patient with premature ovarian failure and a review of the literature. *Am J Med Genet* 52, 19–26.

Prueitt R L, Ross J L, Zinn A R (2000). Physical mapping of nine Xq translocation breakpoints and identification of XPNPEP2 as a premature ovarian failure candidate gene. *Cytogenet Cell Genet* 89, 44–50.

Rebar R W, Connolly H V (1996). Clinical features of young women with hypergonadotrophic amenorrhoea. *Fertil Steril* 53, 804–810.

Reichardt J K, Woo S L (1991). Molecular basis of galactosemia: mutations and polymorphisms in the gene encoding human galactose-1–phosphate uridylyltransferase. *Proc Natl Acad Sci USA* 88, 2633–2637.

Richardson S J, Senikas V, Nelson J F (1987). Follicular depletion during the menopausal transition: evidence for accelerated loss and ultimate exhaustion. *J Clin Endocrinol Metab* 65, 1231–1236.

Robinson A C, Dockeray C J, Cullen M J et al. (1984). Hypergonadotrophic hypogonadism in classical galactosaemia: evidence of defective oogenesis. Case report. *Br J Obstet Gynaecol* 91, 199–200.

Sala C, Arrigo G, Torri G et al. (1997). Eleven X chromosome breakpoints associated with premature ovarian failure map to a 15-Mb YAC contig spanning Xq21. *Genomics* 40, 123–131.

Sardharwalla I B, Wraith J E (1987). Galactosaemia. *Nutr Health* 5, 175–188.

Sarto G E (1974). Cytogenetics of fifty patients with primary amenorrhoea. *Am J Obstet Gynecol* 119, 14–23.

Sarto G E, Therman E, Patau K (1973). X inactivation in man: a woman with t(Xq;12q+). *Am J Hum Genet* 25, 262–270.

Sayle A E, Cooper G S, Savitz D A (1996). Menstrual and reproductive history of mothers of galactosaemic children. *Fertil Steril* 65, 534–538.

Shalet S M, Beardwell C G, Morris-Jones P H et al. (1976). Ovarian failure following abdominal irradiation in childhood. *Br J Cancer* 33, 655–658.

Shelling A N, Burton K A, Chand A L et al. (2000). Inhibin: a candidate gene for premature ovarian failure. *Hum Reprod* 15, 2644–2649.

Shih L Y, Suslak L, Rosin I et al. (1984). Gene dosage studies supporting localisation of the structural gene for galactose-1-phosphate uridyl transferase (GALT) to band p13 of chromosome 9. *Am J Med Genet* 19, 539–543.

Sicinski P, Donaher J L, Geng Y et al. (1996). Cyclin D2 is an FSH-responsive gene involved in gonadal cell proliferation and oncogenesis. *Nature* 384, 470–474.

Simon A, Goodenough D, Li E et al. (1996). Female infertility in mice lacking connexin 37. *Nature* 385, 525–529.

Simpson J L (1975). Gonadal dysgenesis and abnormalities of the human sex chromosomes: current status of phenotypic karyotypic correlations. *Birth Defects* 11, 23–59.

(1987). Genetic control of sexual development. In *Advances in Fertility and Sterility* Vol. 3: *Releasing Hoemones and Genetics and Immunology in Human Reproduction*, Ratnam S S, Teoh

E S eds., pp. 165–173. [*Proceedings of the 12th World Congress on Fertility and Sterility*, 1986] Parthenon Press, Lancaster, UK.

Sinclair A H, Berta P, Palmer M S et al. (1990). A gene from the human sex-determining region encodes a protein with homology to a conserved DNA binding motif. *Nature* 346, 240–244.

Singh R P, Carr D H (1966). The anatomy and histology of XO human embryos and fetuses. *Anat Rec* 155, 369–383.

Siris E S, Leventhal B G, Vaitukaitis J L (1976). Effects of childhood leukaemia and chemotherapy on puberty and reproductive function in girls. *N Engl J Med* 294, 1143–1146.

Strobel T, Tai Y T, Korsmeyer S et al. (1998). BAD partly reverses paclitaxel resistance in human ovarian cancer cells. *Oncogene* 17, 2419–2427.

Summitt R L, Tipton R E, Wilroy R S et al. (1978). X-autosome translocations: A review. In *Sex Differentiation and Chromosomal Abnormalities*, Summitt R L, Bergsma D, eds., pp. 219–247. Alan R. Liss, for the National Foundation-March of Dimes 1978 BD:OAS XIV 6C.

Takebayashi K, Takakura K, Wang H Q et al. (2000). Mutation analysis of the growth differentiation factor-9 and-9B genes in patients with premature ovarian failure and polycystic ovary syndrome. *Fertil Steril* 74, 976–979.

Tapanainen J S, Aittomaki K, Min J et al. (1997). Men homozygous for an inactivating mutation of the follicle stimulating hormone (FSH) receptor gene present variable suppression of spermatogenesis and fertility. *Nat Genet* 15, 205–206.

Taylor A E, Schneyer A L, Sluss P M et al. (1993). Ovarian failure, resistance and activation. In *The Ovary*, Adashi E Y, Leung C K, eds., pp. 629–635. Raven, New York.

Tharapel A T, Erson K P, Simpson J L et al. (1993). Deletion (X) (q26.1-q28) in a proband and her mother: molecular characterisation and phenotypic–karyotypic deductions. *Am J Hum Genet* 52, 463–471.

Therman E, Susman B (1990). The similarity of phenotypic effects caused by Xp and Xq deletions in the human female: a hypothesis. *Hum Genet* 85, 175–183.

Therman E, Laxova R, Susman B (1990). The critical region on the human Xq: effects caused by Xp and Xq deletions in the human female: a hypothesis. *Hum Genet* 85, 455–461.

Toomes C, Dixon M J (1998). Refinement of a translocation breakpoint associated with blepharophimosis-ptosis-epicanthus inversus syndrome to a 280-kb interval at chromosome 3q23. *Genomics* 53, 308–314.

Twigg S, Wallman L, McElduff A (1996). The resistant ovary syndrome in a patient with galactosaemia: a clue to the natural history of ovarian failure. *J Clin Endocrinol Metab* 81, 1329–1331.

Tyfield L, Reichardt J, Fridovich-Keil J et al. (1999). Classical galactosaemia and mutations at the galactose-1-phosphate uridyl transferase (GALT) gene. *Hum Genet* 13, 417–430.

Vale W, Rivier C, Hsueh A et al. (1988). Chemical and biological characterisation of the inhibin family of proteins. *Rec Prog Horm Res* 44, 1–21.

van Kasteren Y M, Schoemaker J (1999). Premature ovarian failure: a systematic review on therapeutic interventions to restore ovarian function and achieve pregnancy. *Hum Reprod Update* 5, 483–492.

van Kasteren Y M, Hundscheid R D L, Smits F P M et al. (1999a). Familial idiopathic premature ovarian failure: an overrated and underestimated genetic disease? *Hum Reprod* 14, 2455–2459.

van Kasteren Y M, Braat D D et al. (1999b). Corticosteroids do not influence ovarian responsiveness to gonadotropins in patients with premature ovarian failure: a randomized, placebo-controlled trial. *Fertil Steril* 71, 90–95.

Vegetti W, Tibiletti M, Testa G et al. (1998). Inheritance in idiopathic premature ovarian failure: analysis of 71 cases. *Hum Reprod* 13, 1796–1800.

Veneman T F, Beverstock G C, Exalto N et al. (1991). Premature menopause of an inherited deletion in the long arm of the X chromosome. *Fertil Steril* 55, 631–634.

Vermulen A (1993). Environment, human reproduction, menopause and andropause. *Environ Health Perspect* 101, 91–100.

Waggoner D D, Buist N R, Donnell G N (1990). Long-term prognosis in galactosaemia: results of a survey of 350 cases. *J Inherit Metab Dis* 13, 802–818.

Wheatcroft N J, Weetman A P (1997). Is premature ovarian failure an autoimmune disease? *Autoimmunity* 25, 157–165.

Wheatcroft N J, Toogood A A, Li T C et al. (1994). Detection of antibodies to ovarian antigens in women with premature ovarian failure. *Clin Exp Immunol* 96, 122–128.

Yang E, Korsmeyer S J (1996). Molecular thanatopsis: a discourse on the BCL-2 family and cell death. *Blood* 88, 386–401.

Zara C, Bulgarelli C, Montanari L (1987). Laparoscopic ovarian biopsy in hypergonadotropic amenorrhea. *Acta-Eur-Fertil* 18, 49–53.

Zou H, Henzel W J, Liu X et al. (1997). Apaf-1, a human protein homologous to *C. elegans* CED-4, participates in cytochrome *c*-dependent activation of caspase-3. *Cell* 90, 405–413.

Zinn A R, Page D C, Fisher E M (1993). Turner's syndrome: the case of the missing sex chromosome. *Trends in Genet* 9, 90–93.

Zinn A R, Tonk V S, Chen Z et al. (1998). Evidence for a Turner syndrome locus or loci at Xp11.2-p22.1. *Am J Hum Genet* 63, 1757–1766.

Zolotogora J, Sagi M, Cohen T (1983). The blepharophimosis, ptosis, and epicanthus inversus syndrome: delineation of two types. *Am J Hum Genet* 35, 1020–1027.

31

Gynaecological cancers in childhood

Tito Lopes

Queen Elizabeth Hospital, Gateshead, UK

Introduction

Childhood cancers are rare, with approximately 1300 new cases a year in the UK (up to age 15) while in the USA the incidence is estimated at $15.1/10^5$ (less than age 20), accounting for approximately 2% of all cancers.

Because of their rarity, childhood cancers should be managed in tertiary referral centres, using a multidisciplinary approach with participation in national and international trials. Only in this way can management of these children improve along with advancing our knowledge and study of childhood cancers.

Various national and international organizations have been established in the last 40 years to advance the care of children with cancer. In the USA, the Children's Cancer Group (CCG) founded in 1955, the Pediatric Oncology Group (POG) created in 1980, the National Wilm's Tumour Study Group and the Intergroup Rhabdomyosarcoma Study Group (IRSG) have recently merged to form the Children's Oncology Group. In Europe the Société International d'Oncologie Pédiatrique (SIOP) was created in 1969.

In the UK, the Children's Cancer Study Group (UKCCSG) was created in 1977 and currently has 22 paediatric treatment centres within the UK. The proportion of children treated at UKCCSG centres has increased over recent years, as a result of tertiary referral, to approximately 80% of all children with cancer. A high proportion of these children are entered into clinical trials and as a result there has been an improvement in their survival, compared with those treated elsewhere.

Gynaecological malignancies in childhood and adolescence are extremely rare and only account for a small number of cases each year in the UK. As a result of centralization and rationalization since the 1970s, the management of gynaecological malignancies in childhood and adolescence has moved away from the care of the gynaecologist to the paediatric oncologist. The only cases likely to present to the gynaecologist today are those with ovarian tumours presenting in their late teens.

The commonest site for childhood gynaecological malignancies is the ovary, with the commonest histology being germ cell tumours. The vagina is the second most common site, invariably embryonal rhabdomyosarcomas. The incidence of clear cell adenocarcinomas of the vagina (and cervix) in childhood rose in the 1970s and 1980s as a result of maternal diethylstilbestrol (DES) ingestion in the 1950s and 1960s but has continued to decline in recent years. Other gynaecological tumours in childhood such as vulval and uterine tumours are extremely rare.

Ovarian malignancies

The incidence of ovarian cancers in children under the age of 15 years is approximately $1.7/10^6$. Less than 10% of these occur at age less than five years, approximately 20% in five to nine year olds and greater than 70% in girls aged 10–14 years (La Vecchia et al., 1983). Girls aged 15 to 19 years have a higher incidence of ovarian cancer, with a rate of $21/10^6$ (Ries et al., 2001). The vast majority (> 80%) of ovarian cancers are germ cell tumours followed by epithelial ovarian tumours, especially in the teens, followed by sex-cord stromal tumours.

Paediatric and Adolescent Gynaecology, ed. Adam Balen et al. Published by Cambridge University Press.
© Cambridge University Press 2004.

Table 31.1. The International Federation of Gynecologic Oncologists (FIGO) staging system for epithelial ovarian tumours

Stage	Characteristics
I	Tumour limited to the ovaries
A	One ovary, no ascites, intact capsule
B	Both ovaries, no ascites, intact capsule
C	Ruptured capsule, capsular involvement, positive peritoneal washings, or malignant ascites
II	Ovarian tumour with pelvic extension
A	Pelvic extension to uterus or tubes
B	Pelvic extension to other pelvic organs
C	Pelvic extension, plus findings indicated for stage IC
III	Tumour outside the pelvis, or positive nodes
A	Microscopic seeding outside the true pelvis
B	Gross deposits less than 2 cm
C	Gross deposits greater than 2 cm or positive nodes
IV	Distant organ involvement, including liver parenchyma or pleural space

Staging

Epithelial ovarian tumours are staged using the International Federation of Gynecologic Oncologists (FIGO) staging system. This is a surgico-pathological staging based on an accurate assessment at the time of primary surgery combined with the pathological findings. There are four stages and these are summarized in Table 31.1.

However with paediatric extragonadal germ cell tumours, because of similarities in the histogenesis, metastatic pattern and response to treatment, regardless of primary site other staging systems are used such as the TNM (primary tumour, regional nodes, metastases) and Brodeur staging systems (Brodeur et al., 1981) that are not specific to the ovary.

Presentation

The commonest presenting symptoms for ovarian cancers are abdominal pain and distension. Although the commonest symptom is pain, the incidence of malignancy in girls presenting with acute abdominal pain can be as low as 3%. This is much lower than in girls found to have an ovarian mass alone, where the incidence of malignant disease may be as high as 26% (Cass et al., 2001).

Ovarian cancers are most common in the second decade of life. As a result, in a group of girls aged less than 18 years presenting with an ovarian mass, the incidence of malignant disease was 2.9% in those presenting under the age of eight, compared with 33% in those presenting after eight years of age (Brown et al., 1993).

Some granulosa cell tumours secrete oestradiol and may present in prepubertal girls with precocious puberty. Several of the other nonepithelial tumours also produce specific enzymes or hormones, and these can be used as tumour markers to assist diagnosis and follow-up. Of the germ cell tumours dysgerminomas can produce lactic dehydrogenase, endodermal sinus tumours produce α-fetoprotein, while choriocarcinomas produce human chorionic gonadotrophin. Sex cord stromal tumours can produce oestrogen, testosterone and inhibin. CA125 may also be elevated in nonepithelial as well as epithelial ovarian malignancies.

In girls with persistent abdominal symptoms, a general and, where appropriate, a pelvic examination should be performed, along with an ultrasound scan to exclude ovarian masses. When an ovarian mass is identified, a computed tomographic or magnetic resonance scan, chest radiograph and a search for tumour markers should be performed prior to considering surgery.

Management

The primary treatment for ovarian cancers in childhood is conservative surgery followed by chemotherapy if required. The surgery should involve a staging laparotomy with careful assessment of the peritoneal cavity and retroperitoneal lymph nodes. The malignant ovary and any other disease present should be removed while preserving the uterus and remaining ovary. In cases where removal of all the disease is not possible or may comprise fertility, a diagnostic biopsy should be performed.

In early-stage tumours the need for, and type of, chemotherapy is dependent on the histology of the tumour. However for nonepithelial tumours, chemotherapy is increasingly withheld in the adjuvant setting, being reserved for patients with progressive disease or in those where the tumour markers fail to normalize following surgery. This approach is obviously dependent upon careful clinical, radiological and serological review but has the advantage that many patients avoid chemotherapy (or radiotherapy), and their potential complications such as secondary leukaemia and infertility.

Germ cell tumours

More than 60% of ovarian tumours in childhood and adolescence are of germ cell origin and one-third of them are malignant. They occur primarily in adolescents and young adults although they can occur in girls younger than 15 years of age. They are frequently unilateral and are curable if found and treated early. The use of combination chemotherapy after initial surgery has dramatically improved the prognosis for this tumour.

Pathology

Ovarian germ cell tumours show greater variety than do their counterparts arising in the testes. They include benign mature teratomas, immature teratomas and malignant germ cell tumours.

A simplified classification for germ cell tumours is:
- dysgerminoma
- endodermal sinus tumour
- embryonal carcinoma
- polyembryoma
- choriocarcinoma
- teratoma:
  —immature
  —mature: monodermal and highly specialized
  —mixed forms of the above.

The commonest paediatric malignant germ cell tumour is the dysgerminoma. This is uncommon in girls under 15 years of age, with most cases diagnosed in adolescence and young adulthood.

Prior to the advent of chemotherapy, the prognosis for germ cell tumours was generally poor. Endodermal sinus tumours of the ovary are particularly aggressive and prior to the widespread use of combination chemotherapy only 27% of patients with stage I endodermal sinus tumour were alive at 2 years (Gallion et al., 1979) and over 50% died within a year of diagnosis.

The management of ovarian immature teratomas has traditionally involved the use of adjuvant chemotherapy especially for high-grade tumours. However, the need for postoperative chemotherapy in children and adolescents with extracranial immature teratomas, including ovarian tumours, has been questioned. For this reason, the POG and CCG undertook a trial to try to answer this question. Between 1990 and 1995, 44 patients with ovarian immature teratomas were managed by surgery alone. Thirty-one patients had pure ovarian immature teratoma and 13 patients had ovarian immature teratoma with foci of yolk sac tumour. Follow-up included examination, measurement of the tumour markers alpha-fetoprotein and human chorionic gonadotrophin, and imaging. The four-year event-free and overall survival for the ovarian immature teratoma group and for the ovarian immature teratoma plus yolk sac tumour group was 97.7% and 100%, respectively (Cushing et al., 1999). The findings of this study would suggest that in most children with ovarian immature teratoma, chemotherapy should be reserved for those with relapse.

Similarly for girls with stage I dysgerminoma, a unilateral salpingo-oophorectomy conserving the uterus and other ovary should be performed with chemotherapy reserved for those 15–25% that recur. In those with advanced stage dysgerminoma, standard practice has been to remove as much disease as possible followed by chemotherapy. However, studies in adult women with dysgerminomas have shown that a unilateral salpingo-oophorectomy followed by chemotherapy results in high cure rates while maintaining fertility.

For patients with ovarian malignant germ cell tumours other than dysgerminoma or immature teratoma, treatment has generally involved surgical resection with postoperative chemotherapy. As with dysgerminomas, studies in adult women have demonstrated that surgery can be conservative with unilateral salpingo-oophorectomy followed by chemotherapy.

Chemotherapy combinations containing cisplatin, etoposide and bleomycin (PEB) have been the preferred treatment for germ cell tumours because of a low relapse rate and a short treatment time. However, a recent study by the UKCCSG has shown that substituting carboplatin for cisplatin, the JEB regimen, resulted in a 93.2% five-year survival for malignant extracranial germ cell tumours. The conclusion was that this regimen was more effective and less toxic than previous regimens including BEP (Mann et al., 2000).

Prognosis

The prognosis for germ cell tumours of the ovary is excellent, with five-year survivals of greater than 85% (Baranzelli et al., 2000) for all stages, rising to greater than 97% for early-stage immature teratomas (Cushing et al., 1999). From their studies, POG and CCG found that the primary site and stage of disease are the most significant factors related to prognosis. As a result, they have developed a new classification system for patients stratifying them into three risk groups.

Low risk. Patients with stage I malignant gonadal and extragonadal germ cell tumours, including stage I immature teratomas.

Intermediate risk. Patients with stage II–IV gonadal and stage II extragonadal germ cell tumours.

High risk. Patients with stage III and IV extragonadal germ cell tumours.

Patients with ovarian germ cell tumours will fall into either the low or intermediate risk depending on nodal or metastatic disease.

The SIOP studies on germ cell tumours found that, along with site and stage of the tumour, an α-fetoprotein level of greater than 10 000 ng/ml was also a significant poor prognostic factor for germ cell tumours (Baranzelli et al., 1999).

Sex-cord stromal tumours

The sex-cord stromal tumours are very rare in childhood. They are composed of granulosa cells, theca cells, fibroblasts and stromal cells, either singly or in combination, with the commonest being the granulosa cell tumour. The majority of these tumours present under the age of 10 years; because of the secretion of oestrogen by some tumours, 40–70% may present with precocious pseudopuberty. Other presenting symptoms include abdominal pain, distension and ascites (Calaminus et al., 1997; Cronje et al., 1998) Some of the tumours can be large and present with acute pain. The majority of sex-cord stromal tumours present with early disease and the prognosis tends to be good, particularly in those with precocious puberty. As with the germ cell tumours, primary treatment usually consists of conservative surgery with oophorectomy. Chemotherapy, usually platinum based, is reserved for advanced stage disease.

Nonovarian malignancies

The annual incidence of nonovarian malignancies in girls under the age of 15 years in the UK has been estimated at approximately $0.5/10^6$ female children (La Vecchia et al., 1984). In this series, which covered 16 years from 1962 to 1978, there were 55 cases identified. The majority presented under the age of five years, with 15 (27.3%) diagnosed under the age of one, and 25 (45.5%) between 1 and 4 years of age. The remaining 15 (27.3%) developed disease between the ages of 5 and 14 years. The distribution of the primary sites are given in Table 31.2. In 45 (81.8%), the tumour was a

Table 31.2. The distribution of primary sites of nonovarian malignancies in 55 girls under the age of 15 years in the UK

Site	No.
Vulva	9 (16.4%)
Vagina	28 (50.9%)
Cervix	3 (5.5%)
Corpus luteum	12 (21.8%)
Unspecified	3 (5.5%)

Source: From La Vecchia et al. (1984).

sarcoma, mostly of the botryoid subtype (26). There were seven (11.7%) carcinomas of which four were clear cell, and three (5.5%) were germ cell tumours.

Genital rhabdomyosarcoma

Incidence

Rhabdomyosarcoma, a malignant tumour of skeletal muscle origin, accounts for approximately 3.5% of the cases of cancer among children from birth to 14 years and 2% of those in adolescents and young adults 15 to 19 years of age. In the UK, this involves approximately 60 children each year. The most common primary sites for rhabdomyosarcoma are the head and neck, the genitourinary tract and the extremities.

Rhabdomyosarcoma of the female genital tract is exceedingly rare, as suggested above, with an incidence of less than $0.5/10^6$ female children. The vagina is the commonest site followed by the vulva and uterus.

The majority of these tumours present under the age of five years though cervical tumours typically present in the second decade.

Predisposing factors

The vast majority of cases occur sporadically with no recognized predisposing factor, although a small proportion are associated with genetic conditions that include the Li-Fraumeni cancer susceptibility syndrome (with germline *p53* mutations), neurofibromatosis type I and Beckwith–Wiedemann syndrome.

Pathology

Rhabdomyosarcomas are divided into several histological subsets: embryonal, embryonal botryoid and spindle cell subtypes, alveolar, anaplastic and undifferentiated (Qualman et al., 1998). The embryonal subtype is the most frequently observed histological subtype in children, accounting for approximately 60–70% of rhabdomyosarcomas of childhood. Tumours with embryonal histology typically arise in the head and neck region or in the genitourinary tract. Botryoid tumours represent about 10% of all rhabdomyosarcoma cases and are embryonal tumours that arise under the mucosal surface of body orifices such as the vagina, bladder, nares and biliary tract. As such, the majority of tumours of the female genital tract are of the botryoid subtype of embryonal rhabdomyosarcoma.

Table 31.3. The US Intergroup Rhabdomyosarcoma Study postsurgical grouping system

Group	Characteristics
I	Localized disease that is completely resected with no regional nodal involvement
II	
A	Grossly resected tumour with microscopic residual disease, but no regional nodal involvement
B	Regional disease with involved nodes, with complete resection and no residual disease
C	Regional disease with involved nodes, grossly resected, but with evidence of microscopic residual and/or histological involvement of the most distal regional node (from the primary site)
III	Incomplete resection (or biopsy only) of the primary site and, therefore, has gross residual disease
IV	Distant metastatic disease present at the time of diagnosis.

Approximately 20% of children with rhabdomyosarcoma have the alveolar subtype, with an increased frequency of this subtype noted in adolescents and in patients with primary sites involving the extremities, trunk and perineum/perirectal region. Undifferentiated sarcomas of soft tissue also occur in childhood and are treated similarly to alveolar rhabdomyosarcoma.

Staging

Different staging systems for rhabdomyosarcomas have been developed in the USA and Europe. In the USA, the Intergroup Rhabdomyosarcoma Group (IRSG) have traditionally assigned patients into different prognostic groups based on known risk factors. Trials have then been designed based on assignment of patients to these different prognostic groups.

The first three IRSG studies (IRS I–III) prescribed treatment based on a postsurgical grouping system with groups defined by the extent of disease and the extent of initial surgical resection (Table 31.3). SIOP in Europe, however, assessed the stage of disease using either a pretreatment or postsurgical TNM staging system (Table 31.4).

These two staging systems are based on different criteria but their reliability was found to be similar (Kappa index 0.78 for the SIOP; TNM and 0.82 for the IRSG grouping system (Rodary et al., 1989)). However, the IRSG system is based on surgery as the primary treatment and is also dependent on the extent of surgery performed. Although surgery remains the primary treatment option for the ma-

Table 31.4. The Société International d'Oncologie Pédiatrique (SIOP) staging of rhabdomyosarcoma based on either pretreatment or postsurgical TNM staging system

Stage	Subtype	Characteristics
Pretreatment staging		
I	T1	Tumour localized to organ or tissue of origin
	N0	No evidence of regional lymph node involvement
	M0	No evidence of metastases
II	T2	Tumour involving one or more contiguous organs or tissues or with adjacent malignant effusion
	N0	No evidence of regional lymph node involvement
	M0	No evidence of metastases
III	Any T	
	N1	Evidence of regional lymph node involvement
	M0	No evidence of metastases
IV	Any T	
	Any N	
	M1	Evidence of distant metastases
Postsurgical staging		
pT1		Tumour limited to organ or tissue of origin; complete excision with free margins
pT1		Tumour invasion beyond organ or tissue of origin; complete excision with free margins
pT3		Tumour incompletely resected
pT3a		Evidence of microscopic residual disease
pT3b		Evidence of macroscopic residual disease or diagnostic biopsy only

Note: T_1 primary tumor; N_1 lymph node involvement; M_1 metastasis.

jority of these tumours, this is not the case for tumours of the orbit or genitourinary system and as such is not ideal for gynaecological tumours.

In an attempt to use a pretreatment staging system, the IRSG developed a TNM-based pretreatment staging system based on retrospective data from IRSG II. Classification of patients by tumour size, clinical status of regional lymph nodes, presence or absence of metastatic disease and location of the primary tumour (at a favourable or unfavourable anatomic site) created four prognostically distinct staging categories that were relatively equal in size (Lawrence et al., 1997). Brief definitions for each stage are as follows.

Stage 1. Favourable localized disease involving the orbit or head and neck (excluding parameningeal sites), or nonbladder/nonprostate genitourinary region, or biliary tract. This stage includes nonmetastatic gynaecological rhabdomyosarcomas.

Stage 2. Localized disease of any unfavourable primary site not included in the stage I category. Primary tumours must be less than or equal to 5 cm in diameter, and there must be no regional nodal involvement.

Stage 3. Localized disease of any unfavourable primary site not included in the stage I category. These patients differ from stage II patients by having primary tumours greater than 5 cm and/or regional nodal involvement.

Stage 4. Metastatic disease at diagnosis. This stage includes metastatic gynaecological rhabdomyosarcomas.

The IRSG have used their modified TNM pretreatment staging combined with the clinical groups to develop prognostic groups for their current studies. Patients are classified for protocol purposes as low, intermediate or high risk. General definitions of each of these categories are as follows.

Low risk. Patients with localized embryonal rhabdomyosarcoma occurring at favourable sites (i.e. Stage 1) and patients with embryonal rhabdomyosarcoma occurring at unfavourable sites with either completely resected disease (i.e. clinical group I) or microscopic residual disease (i.e. clinical group II).

Intermediate risk. Patients with embryonal rhabdomyosarcoma occurring at unfavourable sites with gross residual disease (i.e. clinical group III), patients with metastatic embryonal rhabdomyosarcoma who are younger than 10 years and patients with nonmetastatic alveolar rhabdomyosarcoma or undifferentiated sarcoma at any site.

High risk. Patients with metastatic rhabdomyosarcoma or undifferentiated sarcoma at presentation excepting embryonal cases in children younger than 10 years.

The majority of gynaecological rhabdomyosarcomas fall into the low- and intermediate-risk groups.

Presentation

Most genital rhabdomyosarcomas present before the age of five years. Vaginal bleeding and discharge are the commonest presenting symptoms. The bleeding may be minimal or a sudden bright loss with clots, while the discharge is offensive and blood stained. A polypoid mass often resembling a bunch of grapes may fill the vagina and present at the introitus. At other times, it can present as a simple polyp or a haemorrhagic mass. Examination under sedation or general anaesthesia should be performed and a diagnostic

biopsy taken. Cystoscopy and rectal examination allow assessment of the extent of the disease.

Management

In the mid 1970s, the standard treatment for rhabdomyosarcomas of the female genital tract was radical surgery, usually in the form of exenterative surgery (Barber and Graber, 1973; Dewhurst, 1977). However, as a result of trials undertaken since then, the rate of hysterectomy has dropped to less than 25%.

For girls with primary tumours of the genital tract, the initial surgical procedure is now usually a diagnostic biopsy only followed by multiple agent chemotherapy, which invariably removes the need for primary radical surgery. For vulval or vaginal rhabdomyosarcomas, primary chemotherapy and adjunctive radiation when needed results in excellent disease-free survival and recent studies suggest that primary chemotherapy may reduce the need for definitive surgery in uterine tumours as well (Corpron et al., 1995; Martelli et al., 1999).

The IRSG recently reviewed 151 cases of rhabdomyosarcoma of the female genital tract treated in their IRSG protocols I–IV. Chemotherapy was predominantly vincristine, actinomycin D and cyclophosphamide (VAC) based. The rate of hysterectomy decreased from 48% in IRS-I/II to 22% in IRS-III/IV with an increase in the use of radiation therapy from 23% in IRS-II to 45% in IRS-IV. Many patients with primary vaginal tumours had radiation therapy delayed or omitted in later studies with excellent outcome. The conclusion was that localized female genital rhabdomyosarcoma is usually curable with combination chemotherapy, a conservative surgical approach and the use of radiotherapy for selected patients (Arndt et al., 2001).

Of patients treated in SIOP protocols MMT 84 and MMT 89 between 1984 and 1994, 38 girls with nonmetastatic rhabdomyosarcoma of the female genital tract were identified. The majority of the girls received primary chemotherapy with ifosfamide, vincristine and actinomycin D. Further treatment with surgery or radiotherapy was used only when there was incomplete remission or at the time of relapse. Thirteen patients (34%) were treated with chemotherapy alone and 17 patients (45%) required further local treatment. In patients with a complete response to primary chemotherapy, surgery or local radiotherapy was thought to be unnecessary (Martelli et al., 1999).

There are currently two phase III trials being undertaken by the IRSG. The first is a randomized study of VAC versus VAC alternating with vincristine, topotecan and cyclophosphamide in patients with intermediate risk disease. The second is a study on dactinomycin and vincristine with or without cyclophosphamide and/or radiotherapy in patients with low-risk rhabdomyosarcoma of embryonal or botyroid subtype.

Prognosis

In the recent IRSG article on 151 cases of rhabdomyosarcomas of the female genital tract (Arndt et al., 2001), the overall five-year survival was 82% (87% for locoregional disease). Analysis of prognostic factors revealed that an age of one to nine years at the time of diagnosis, noninvasive tumours, and the use of IRS-II or IRS-IV treatments was associated with significantly better outcome. Patients who were aged one to nine years did best, with a five-year survival of 98%. Patients outside of this age range benefited from more intensified therapy (five-year survival of 67% on IRS I/II compared with 90% on IRS III/IV) (Arndt et al., 2001).

In the series of 38 girls with nonmetastatic rhabdomyosarcoma of the female genital tract treated by SIOP, the overall five-year survival was 91%, which is comparable to the 87% reported above (Martelli et al., 1999).

Clear cell adenocarcinomas of the vagina and cervix

From 1940 through the 1960s, DES, a synthetic oestrogen, was given to pregnant women to try to prevent pregnancy complications and miscarriage. As a result, it is estimated that as many as three million women in the USA may have been exposed to DES in utero. In 1970, Herbst and Scully reported six cases of clear cell carcinoma of the vagina in adolescents and subsequently made the link with maternal exposure to DES (Herbst and Scully, 1970; Herbst et al., 1971). Fortunately, the cancer only develops in 0.1% of exposed females, with a peak incidence being in the late teens and early twenties, with a mean age at diagnosis of 20 years.

Although most young women with clear cell adenocarcinoma of the vagina had prenatal exposure to DES, some develop it without DES exposure. In a review of 318 cases of vaginal clear cell adenocarcinomas, 20% of the women had no evidence of DES exposure. Survival differed significantly between these women and those with DES exposure. Survival at five and ten years for DES-exposed women was 84 and 78%, respectively, compared with 69 and 60%, respectively, for non-DES cases (five years, $p = 0.007$; ten years, $p = 0.008$). The sites of disease recurrence also differed, with those not exposed to DES more likely to present with (or to develop later) distant metastases to the lungs (24% versus 9%) or to supraclavicular lymph nodes (8% versus 1.6%) (Waggoner et al., 1994).

Approximately one-third of the cases affect the cervix and the main symptom is abnormal vaginal bleeding. The tumour is similar to adult tumours, with the characteristic clear cells from the presence of glycogen in the cytoplasm. Most of the tumours are exophytic though some are submucosal and present with nodularity in the vagina only.

As DES has not been used in pregnancy since the early 1970s, this tumour is now exceedingly uncommon in adolescence.

Long-term sequelae

The most obvious potential long-term sequelae in girls treated for gynaecological tumours is the loss of fertility or ovarian function. Although the need for performing hysterectomy has fallen as a result of combination chemotherapy, this has been countered in some situations by an increased use of radiotherapy. In children requiring external beam radiotherapy to the pelvis, the option of ovarian transposition should be considered, placing the ovaries outside the radiation field. Uterine musculature and blood flow are irreversibly affected by high-dose irradiation in childhood, resulting in an increased incidence of nulliparity, fetal loss and intrauterine growth retardation (Critchley et al., 1992; see Ch. 32).

Careful monitoring of ovarian function in susceptible children should be performed and if there is evidence of ovarian failure, hormone replacement therapy is needed from expected puberty to menopause. This is essential for the development of secondary sex characteristics as well as long-term bone mineralization and cardiovascular protection.

Approximately 4% of survivors of childhood cancers will develop a second primary tumour within 25 years of the initial tumour. This is six times the expected number of cancers and is attributable to the carcinogenic effects of radiotherapy and certain cytotoxic drugs such as alkylating agents and anthracyclines.

Data on the educational, psychosocial and quality of life aspects of children surviving cancer is retrospective, limited and conflicting. Prospective evaluation of the consequences of new treatments is essential and strategies for long-term follow-up of survivors of childhood cancers are being developed (Wallace et al., 2001).

REFERENCES

Arndt C A, Donaldson S S, Anderson J R et al. (2001). What constitutes optimal therapy for patients with rhabdomyosarcoma of the female genital tract? *Cancer* 91, 2454–2468.

Baranzelli M C, Kramar A, Bouffet E et al. (1999). Prognostic factors in children with localized malignant nonseminomatous germ cell tumors. *J Clin Oncol* 17, 1212.

Baranzelli M C, Bouffet E, Quintana E, Portas M, Thyss A, Patte C (2000). Non-seminomatous ovarian germ cell tumours in children. *Eur J Cancer* 36, 376–383.

Barber H R, Graber E A (1973). Gynecological tumors in childhood and adolescence. *Obstet Gynecol Surv* 28(Suppl.), 357–381.

Brodeur G M, Howarth C B, Pratt C B, Caces J, Hustu H O (1981). Malignant germ cell tumors in 57 children and adolescents. *Cancer* 48, 1890–1898.

Brown M F, Hebra A, McGeehin K, Ross A J, III (1993). Ovarian masses in children: a review of 91 cases of malignant and benign masses. *J Pediatr Surg* 28, 930–931.

Calaminus G, Wessalowski R, Harms D, Gobel U (1997). Juvenile granulosa cell tumors of the ovary in children and adolescents: results from 33 patients registered in a prospective cooperative study. *Gynecol Oncol* 65, 447–452.

Cass D L, Hawkins E, Brandt M L et al. (2001). Surgery for ovarian masses in infants, children, and adolescents: 102 consecutive patients treated in a 15-year period. *J Pediatr Surg* 36, 693–699.

Corpron C A, Andrassy R J, Hays D M et al. (1995). Conservative management of uterine pediatric rhabdomyosarcoma: a report from the Intergroup Rhabdomyosarcoma Study III and IV pilot. *J Pediatr Surg* 30, 942–944.

Critchley H O, Wallace W H, Shalet S M, Mamtora H, Higginson J, Anderson D C (1992). Abdominal irradiation in childhood; the potential for pregnancy. *Br J Obstet Gynaecol* 99, 392–394.

Cronje H S, Niemand I, Bam R H, Woodruff J D (1998). Abdominal irradiation in childhood; the potential for pregnancy. *Obstet Gynecol Surv* 53, 240–247.

Cushing B, Giller R, Ablin A et al. (1999). Surgical resection alone is effective treatment for ovarian immature teratoma in children and adolescents: a report of the pediatric oncology group and the children's cancer group. *Am J Obstet Gynecol* 181, 353–358.

Dewhurst C J (1977). Tumors of the genital tract in childhood and adolescence. *Clin Obstet Gynecol* 20, 595–606.

Gallion H, van Nagell J R, Jr, Powell D F, Donaldson E S, Hanson M (1979). Therapy of endodermal sinus tumor of the ovary. *Am J Obstet Gynecol* 135, 447–451.

Herbst A L, Scully R E (1970). Adenocarcinoma of the vagina in adolescence. A report of 7 cases including 6 clear-cell carcinomas (so-called mesonephromas). *Cancer* 25, 745–757.

Herbst A L, Ulfelder H, Poskanzer D C (1971). Adenocarcinoma of the vagina. Association of maternal stilbestrol therapy with tumor appearance in young women. *N Engl J Med* 284, 878–881.

La Vecchia C, Morris H B, Draper G J (1983). Malignant ovarian tumours in childhood in Britain, 1962–78. *Br J Cancer* 48, 363–374.

La Vecchia C, Draper G J, Franceschi S (1984). Childhood non-ovarian female genital tract cancers in Britain, 1962–1978. Descriptive epidemiology and long-term survival. *Cancer* 54, 188–192.

Lawrence W, Jr, Anderson J R, Gehan E A, Maurer H (1997).). Pretreatment TNM staging of childhood rhabdomyosarcoma: a report of the Intergroup Rhabdomyosarcoma Study Group, Children's Cancer Study Group and Pediatric Oncology Group. *Cancer* 80, 1165–1170.

Mann J R, Raafat F, Robinson K et al. (2000). The United Kingdom Children's Cancer Study Group's second germ cell tumor study: carboplatin, etoposide, and bleomycin are effective treatment for children with malignant extracranial germ cell tumors, with acceptable toxicity. *J Clin Oncol* 18, 3809–3818.

Martelli H, Oberlin O, Rey A et al. (1999). Conservative treatment for girls with nonmetastatic rhabdomyosarcoma of the genital tract: a report from the Study Committee of the International Society of Pediatric Oncology. *J Clin Oncol* 17, 2117–2122.

Qualman S J, Coffin C M, Newton W A et al. (1998). Intergroup Rhabdomyosarcoma Study: update for pathologists. *Pediatr Dev Pathol* 1, 550–561.

Ries L A G, Eisner M P, Kosary C L et al. (2001). SEER cancer statistics review 1973–1998. National Cancer Institute, Bethesda, MD http://seer.cancer.gov/.

Rodary C, Flamant F, Donaldson S S (1989). An attempt to use a common staging system in rhabdomyosarcoma: a report of an international workshop initiated by the International Society of Pediatric Oncology (SIOP). *Med Pediatr Oncol* 17, 210–215.

Waggoner S E, Mittendorf R, Biney N, Anderson D, Herbst A L (1994). Influence of in utero diethylstilbestrol exposure on the prognosis and biologic behavior of vaginal clear-cell adenocarcinoma. *Gynecol Oncol* 55, 238–244.

Wallace W H, Blacklay A, Eiser C et al. (2001). Developing strategies for long term follow up of survivors of childhood cancer. *BMJ* 323, 271–274.

32

Late reproductive sequelae of treatment for childhood cancer

Angela B. Thomson[1], Hilary O.D. Critchley[2], Christopher J. H. Kelnar[2] and W. Hamish B. Wallace[1]

[1]Department of Haematology/Oncology, Royal Hospital for Sick Children, Edinburgh, UK
[2]Department of Developmental and Reproductive Sciences, University of Edinburgh, Edinburgh, UK

Introduction

Tremendous therapeutic advances in the management of childhood malignancies mean that the majority of children can realistically hope for long-term survival. Cancer in childhood is rare, with about 1400 new cases per year in the UK and a cumulative risk of 1 in 650 by the age of 15 years (Stiller, 1997; Wallace, 1997). With survival rates in excess of 70%, it is estimated that by the year 2010, 1 in 250 of the young adult population will be a long-term survivor of childhood cancer (Fig. 32.1) (Bleyer, 1990). However, the successful treatment of cancer in childhood with chemotherapy and or radiotherapy is associated with a number of unwanted side effects in later life (Wallace et al., 2001). Therefore, the major challenge faced by paediatric oncologists today is to sustain the excellent survival rates while striving to improve the quality of life of the survivors.

One of the most important issues for the survivors of childhood cancer is the impact of their disease and its treatment on reproductive function and the implications for the health of their offspring. In the female, chemotherapy and radiotherapy may damage the ovary and hasten oocyte depletion, resulting in loss of hormone production, truncated fecundity and a premature menopause (Meirow, 2000; Thomson et al., 2002). Infertility is one of the most commonly encountered and psychologically traumatic late complications of treatment for childhood cancer, and consequently, strategies to preserve fertile potential are being pursued. While semen cryopreservation is a successful and routine technique for preservation of male fertility, at least in sexually mature males, similar measures to retain fertile potential in females remain experimental (Meirow, 2000; Sanger et al., 1992; Thomson et al., 2002). Options for preservation of female fertility are limited and are dependent upon the sexual maturity of the patient. These involve invasive and expensive procedures at a time when a patient has active disease, is adjusting to a new diagnosis of cancer and is restricted by time constraints enforced by the need to start treatment.

Gametes may be cryopreserved as oocytes or embryos (Atkinson et al., 1994; Porcu et al., 1997). Oocytes, on the one hand, survive cryopreservation and thawing poorly and are associated with very low pregnancy rates (Porcu et al., 1997). On the other hand, embryo cryopreservation and pregnancy with assisted reproduction is more successful but requires a stable partner (Atkinson et al., 1994). Both options require ovarian stimulation and oocyte collection, which will delay the start of treatment and may compromise their outlook. For the young, sexually immature patients, for whom ovarian stimulation and oocyte retrieval is both technically challenging and ethically unacceptable, alternative strategies must be developed. Advances in assisted reproduction techniques have focused attention on preserving gonadal tissue for future use (Carroll and Gosden, 1993; Gosden, 1990; Gosden et al., 1994a; Nugent et al., 1997; Oktay et al., 1997, 2000a). Cryopreservation of immature ovarian tissue is the most promising option, with restoration of natural fertility and preservation of hormone production following autotransplantation, or maturation of oocytes in vitro in combination with assisted reproduction (Oktay et al., 1997, 2000a; see also Ch. 33). Harvesting and the potential future use of gonadal tissue is an exciting area of gamete biology that opens up new and unchartered territory for paediatric oncologists. Many scientific, ethical and legal issues remain to be addressed before techniques to preserve fertility are available (Wallace and Walker, 2001).

Paediatric and Adolescent Gynaecology, ed. Adam Balen et al. Published by Cambridge University Press.
© Cambridge University Press 2004.

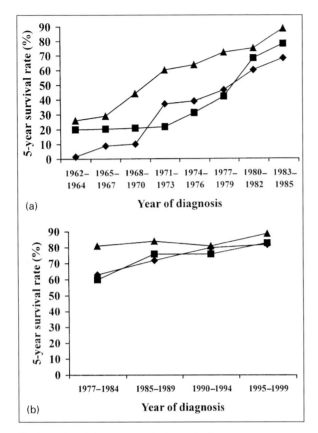

(a)

(b)

Fig. 32.1. Trends in 5-year survival rates for three common cancers: acute lymphoblastic leukaemia (♦), nonHodgkin lymphoma (■) and Wilms' tumour (▲). (a) From 1962 to 1985, there was a dramatic increase in 5-year survival. (b) From 1977 to 1999, there was a sustained improvement in 5-year survival.

In this chapter, we consider the impact of radiotherapy and chemotherapy treatment for childhood cancer on female reproductive function, strategies for preservation of fertile potential and implications for the health of the offspring.

Childhood cancer

Childhood cancers exhibit greater diversity in terms of anatomical site and histological type (Fig. 32.2) than adult cancers, where carcinomas of the breast, lung and gut predominate. Approximately one-third of all cancers in childhood are leukaemias, of which 80% are acute lymphoblastic leukaemia (ALL), followed by brain and spinal tumours, which account for about 25% of cases. Embryonal tumours (neuroblastoma, retinoblastoma, Wilms' tumour and hepatoblastoma) make up 15% of cases, and lymphomas 11% (both Hodgkin's and nonHodgkin's lymphomas). The remainder comprises bone (osteosarcoma

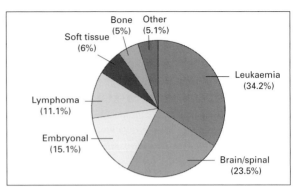

Fig. 32.2. Distribution of the major childhood cancers. (From Stiller, 1997.)

and Ewing's sarcoma) and soft tissue tumours (rhabdomyosarcoma), and a variety of more rare tumours. Leukaemia and embryonal tumours are more common in children under five years of age, in contrast to Hodgkin's disease and osteosarcomas, which peak in puberty and early adulthood (Stiller, 1997). Management of children with cancer is centralized in specialized paediatric oncology centres and treatment generally involves multiagent chemotherapy, either alone or in combination with surgery and or radiotherapy. The reproductive potential of the children depends not on the underlying diagnosis but upon the nature of the treatment they have received. Our awareness of the burden of obstetric and gynaecological problems experienced by cancer survivors is largely a result of retrospective studies evaluating the impact of treatment protocols. Although most of the past treatment protocols have been superseded, it is the children treated with these protocols that are now presenting with fertility issues, and some late effects may be progressive over time. Management of children with cancer requires an understanding of the gonadotoxic effects of therapy; counselling and, where possible, taking appropriate steps to preserve fertility; and long-term follow-up of the survivors and their offspring to determine whether they are at increased risk of adverse pregnancy outcome, genetic diseases and cancer. Acknowledgement of the need for prospective evaluation of continually evolving therapeutic regimens is necessary to further our understanding of the impact of treatment on long-term reproductive health.

Ovary

The human ovary is endowed with a fixed pool of primordial follicles, maximal at about five months of gestational age and with approximately two million oocytes present at birth. Follicle depletion, as a result of atresia and recruitment towards ovulation, leads to premature exhaustion of the follicle pool and menopause at a median age of 51 years. The fertile "window" in females is characterized by roughly 400 monthly ovulations of a mature oocyte (Block, 1952; Faddy et al., 1992). Ovarian failure and a premature menopause will arise from any cytotoxic insult, which either depletes the oocyte pool or hastens its decline (Byrne et al., 1992). Although the exact mechanisms of cytotoxic damage are uncertain, both chemotherapy and radiotherapy may inflict such an insult. The outcome following the insult will depend upon the extent of the injury and the age of the child at the time of treatment. Complete destruction of the oocyte pool in the prepubertal child will result in failure to undergo spontaneous pubertal development; destruction during puberty will be associated with arrest of pubertal development and, subsequently, primary amenorrhoea. Where the injury is sufficient to cause destruction of the oocyte pool in the postpubertal female, there will be premature ovarian failure. While normal progression through puberty, the onset of menarche and continuation of regular menstrual cycles are reassuring it is not predictive of a normal reproductive lifespan. Quantifying the magnitude of the insult and predicting the onset of ovarian failure has become a realistic possibility following radiotherapy but remains difficult to assess following chemotherapy. In a small number of cases, recovery of menstruation is seen, suggesting that additional mechanisms to cytotoxic follicle death may be involved. These women may still progress to a premature menopause and all patients will require long-term follow-up.

Extensive investigations are underway to establish the mechanisms underlying radiation- and chemotherapy-induced ovarian damage. From histological and immunohistochemical studies, it is apparent that the end result following cytotoxic insult is depleted follicle stores and ovarian atrophy (Chapman et al., 1979; Familiari et al., 1993; Marcello et al., 1990). In vitro studies have explored the direct effect of cytotoxic chemotherapy-induced damage on primordial follicles by exploring cortical ovarian slices removed from healthy women and exposed to cisplatinum (Meirow et al., 1998). Histology and immunohistochemistry staining demonstrated that cisplatinum induced pregranulosa cell swelling and changes consistent with apoptosis. Perez et al. (1997) have shown in mice that doxorubicin induces primordial follicle destruction by inducing apoptosis of the pregranulosa cells. The need for methods to prevent apoptotic germ cell destruction has initiated a search to map the apoptotic signalling pathway in an attempt to identify key inhibitory genes and proteins to block the pathway. Perez et al. (2000) demon-

Table 32.1. Radiotherapy-induced damage to the reproductive tract

Site	Effect
Cranial/total body irradiation	Hypogonadotrophic hypogonadism
Total body/abdomen/ pelvic	Ovarian failure ($LD_{50} < 2$ Gy): older women > 6 Gy; younger women > 20 Gy
	Uterine damage: decreased volume, decreased elasticity

strated in mice studies that members of the caspase gene family were required for oocyte death although the protein p53 was not required for drug-induced oocyte destruction. Further studies have demonstrated that intracellular potassium regulation may play a critical role in oocyte death. Potassium efflux during ovarian death appears early in oocytes and granulosa cells and may regulate a number of apoptotic events including caspase activity and internucleosomal DNA cleavage (Ataya and Ramahi-Ataya, 1993). Clearly more research is required to further our understanding of cytotoxic-mediated ovarian dysfunction in the hope that preventative strategies can be developed.

Radiotherapy-induced ovarian damage

Although used sparingly because of damage to growing tissues, radiotherapy is administered to obtain local disease control and to consolidate remission. Total body, craniospinal, abdominal or pelvic irradiation may cause ovarian and uterine dysfunction (Table 32.1). The degree of impairment is related to the radiation dose, fractionation schedule and age at time of treatment (Bath et al., 1999; Chiarelli et al., 1999; Lushbaugh and Casarett, 1976; Matsumoto et al., 1999; Sanders, 1991; Sanders et al., 1996; Thibaud et al., 1998; Wallace et al., 1989a,b, 1993). The number of primordial follicles present at the time of treatment and the dose of radiotherapy will determine the fertile "window" and dictate the age at menopause. A number of mathematical models have been proposed to explain the complex process of natural follicle decline based on a series of data describing the number of follicles present at different ages in humans (Block, 1953; Faddy et al., 1992; Richardson et al., 1987). For any given age, the size of the follicle pool can be estimated based upon this complex mathematical model of decline. In order to predict the age of menopause in patients following radiotherapy, the extent of the radiation-induced damage to the follicle pool can be determined. We have previously estimated the dose of radiation required to destroy 50% of the oocytes (LD_{50}) to be less than 4 Gy, based upon an exponential model of oocyte decay

(Wallace et al., 1989b). The mathematical model used to calculate this value is now believed to be an oversimplification, and current thinking is that follicle decay represents an instantaneous rate of temporal change based upon the remaining population pool, expressed mathematically as a differential equation (Faddy et al., 1983, 1992; Faddy and Gosden, 1996). Furthermore, we determined the LD_{50} to be 4 Gy from our original cohort of women, who were treated with 30 Gy at a median age of 4 years (range, 1.3–13.1) and in whom ovarian failure was detected at 12.7 years (range, 9.7–15.9). Given the high doses of irradiation administered, it is likely that ovarian failure would have occurred earlier but was undetectable clinically. This would have lead to an overestimate of the calculated LD_{50}. In a second study ovarian function was assessed in eight patients who had received total body irradiation (TBI) (14.4 Gy) at age 11.5 years (range, 4.9–15.1). Ovarian failure was defined as failure to undergo or complete pubertal development or the onset of secondary amenorrhoea in conjunction with persistently elevated gonadotrophin (follicle-stimulating hormone (FSH) and luteinizing hormone (LH) > 32 IU/l) and low oestradiol levels (< 40 pmol/l). Six of the eight subjects at age 13.15 years (range, 12.5–16) had ovarian failure (Bath et al., 1999). Based on these new data, where diagnosis of ovarian failure was more likely to reflect the true age of onset of ovarian failure, and a revised mathematical model of natural oocyte decline, we were able to determine the surviving fraction of oocytes following irradiation and estimate the LD_{50} of the human oocyte to be less than 2 Gy (Wallace et al., 2003). This explains sterilization with total depletion of primordial follicle reserve following high doses of radiotherapy and premature ovarian failure following lower doses that cause only partial depletion of the primordial follicle pool. Using this model, it is possible to predict the likely age of premature ovarian failure following a given dose of radiation at any age. This will enable us to counsel patients more appropriately with regard to reproductive function and, where possible, take measures to preserve fertility.

Total body irradiation

TBI, either alone or in combination with chemotherapy, is used as conditioning for bone marrow transplantation and may cause infertility (Bath et al., 1999; Matsumoto et al., 1999; Sanders et al., 1996; Thibaud et al., 1998). In a long-term follow-up of 708 females, median age 3 years (range, 1–17), after bone marrow transplantation (BMT), 532 had received TBI (10–15.75 Gy, single exposure or fractionated) and cyclophosphamide (200 mg/kg) and 176 were treated with cyclophosphamide (200 mg/kg) alone or with busulphan (16 mg/kg) as conditioning therapy. Ovarian

failure was observed in 90% of patients following TBI and 68% following chemotherapy only. Among an additional 82 patients treated prepubertally with the same regimens, ovarian failure was reported in 72% (Sanders et al., 1996).

Bath et al. (1999) studied the impact of TBI on ovarian function in childhood and adolescence. Ovarian function was assessed in eight patients who had received TBI (14.4 Gy) at age 11.5 years (range, 4.9–15.1). Six of the eight girls, at age 13.15 years (range, 12.5–16), had ovarian failure. Biochemical evidence of incipient ovarian failure was observed in two girls treated prepubertally, with clinically apparent preservation of ovarian function.

Matsumoto et al. (1999) studied ovarian function in 18 girls who had undergone bone marrow transplantation at 8.5 years (range, 4.5–15.3), before the onset of menarche, for a variety of haematological malignant ($n = 14$) and nonmalignant conditions ($n = 4$). Conditioning therapy involved a variety of chemotherapy agents and fractionated TBI, 8–12 Gy and 6–8 Gy for malignant and nonmalignant diseases, respectively. Twelve patients achieved menarche at a median age of 12.8 years (range, 10.8–14). Age at transplant was significantly younger in girls who achieved menarche than in those who developed primary amenorrhoea (mean (SD), 7.2 (0.5) versus 11.1 (1.7) years). The younger patient has a larger oocyte pool at the time of treatment and may have a shortened window of opportunity for fertility before developing a premature menopause. Furthermore, in five of the remaining six patients, gonadotrophin levels were elevated despite the onset of menses. This may reflect impending premature ovarian failure and truncated fecundity.

Abdominal or pelvic irradiation

Abdominal and pelvic irradiation may be used in the treatment of a variety of malignancies including Wilms' tumour, pelvic rhabdomyosarcoma and Ewing's sarcoma of the pelvis or spine, with the dose and volume dependent upon the diagnosis and tumour size. Ovarian function was reviewed sequentially in 53 females treated between 1942 and 1985 with surgery and external abdominal radiotherapy for an intraabdominal tumour. Ovarian failure was observed in 97% (37 of 38) of females following whole abdominal irradiation in childhood (20–30 Gy). Of the 37 women, primary amenorrhoea was reported in 71% and a premature menopause (median age 23.5 years) in the remainder (Wallace et al., 1989a). Of the 15 patients who received flank irradiation (20–30 Gy), median age at assessment 15.2 years, ovarian function was normal in all but one, in whom pubertal failure had occurred. In one patient who required sex steroid replacement therapy to achieve normal secondary sexual characteristics for pubertal failure following abdominal radiotherapy, there was evidence of recovery of ovarian function, with conception reported at age 22.7 years. In total, there were four documented conceptions: all patients had received whole abdominal irradiation (20–26.5 Gy), but all had mid-trimester miscarriages and subsequently underwent a premature menopause. Poor uterine function may have contributed to the failure to sustain pregnancy. It is well recognized that the prevalence of ovarian failure following whole abdominal radiotherapy has been unacceptably high, with the majority of patients failing to complete pubertal development without hormone replacement therapy. The introduction of flank irradiation from 1972 has resulted in significantly less pubertal failure but the onset of a premature menopause may occur with time.

A permanent menopause may be induced in women over 40 years following gonadal radiotherapy treatment with 6 Gy, while significantly higher doses are required to completely destroy the oocyte pool and induce ovarian failure in younger women and children (Lushbaugh and Casarett, 1976). This reflects the smaller follicle reserve in older patients and hence increased susceptibility to smaller doses of irradiation.

In a retrospective study of medical records of 830 long-term female survivors of childhood cancer, Chiarelli et al. (1999) evaluated the risk of premature menopause and infertility following abdominal/pelvic radiation and/or alkylating agent-based chemotherapy compared with those patients treated with nonsterilizing surgery alone. The results demonstrated that the risk of premature ovarian failure increased significantly with increasing dose of abdominal irradiation. The relative risk with doses < 20 Gy was 1.02, increasing to 1.37 with irradiation of 20–35 Gy and to 3.27 with doses > 35 Gy. The percentage of women with premature ovarian failure was 22% and 32% following radiation doses of 20–35 Gy and > 35 Gy, respectively.

Cranial and craniospinal irradiation

Cranial or craniospinal radiotherapy may be used in the treatment of some brain tumours and ALL with central nervous system (CNS) involvement. Scatter irradiation from craniospinal radiotherapy may directly affect ovarian function. Cranial irradiation may indirectly impair ovarian function by causing hypogonadotrophic hypogonadism. Gonadotrophins were elevated in 7 of 11 (64%) females who had received cranial irradiation (mean dose 32 Gy) for brain tumours (Livesey and Brook, 1988). Hypothalamic–pituitary function shows progressive compromise following high-dose cranial irradiation (> 30 Gy) and the risk of gonadotrophin deficiency is 60% by four years out from treatment (Littley et al., 1989). Low-dose CNS-directed ra-

diotherapy in the treatment of ALL has been associated with subtle perturbations in growth hormone secretion but there are a few reports assessing the impact on the secretion of other pituitary hormones in adulthood (Birkebaek et al., 1998; Brennan et al., 1998; Crowne et al., 1992). In a study on reproductive function following treatment for childhood ALL, women who had received prophylactic CNS radiation had a significantly lower first birth rate than those without irradiation, indicating that doses of 18–24 Gy to the brain may be a possible risk factor (Nygaard et al., 1991). The late effects of hypothalamic–pituitary–ovarian dysfunction are often subtle and may be progressive with time. Bath et al. (2001) reported decreased LH production, reduced LH surge and short luteal phases in a group of women treated with low-dose cranial irradiation (18–24 Gy) as CNS-directed therapy for ALL. For women exposed to low-dose cranial irradiation, regular menses does not ensure normal hypothalamic–pituitary function and early referral and detailed endocrine assessment is necessary if these women present with infertility.

Chemotherapy-induced ovarian damage

The ovary is generally less susceptible to the deleterious effects of cytotoxic chemotherapy than the testis; nevertheless, ovarian function may be significantly impaired following chemotherapy treatment for childhood cancer. Chemotherapy-induced ovarian dysfunction has been recognized for many years and was first described in humans following busulfan treatment of chronic myeloid leukaemia in 1956 (Louis et al., 1956). Since then a number of agents have been described as causing ovarian damage, including cis-platinum, procarbazine and the alkylating agents, such as chlorambucil and cyclophosphamide (Table 32.2).

Table 32.2. Gonadotoxic chemotherapy agents

Type	Drugs
Alkylating agents	Cyclophosphamide
	Ifosfamide
	Nitrosoureas, e.g. BCNU, CCNU
	Chlorambucil
	Melphalan
	Busulphan
Vinca-alkaloids	Vinblastine
Antimetabolites	Cytarabine
Platinum agents	Cis-platinum
Others	Procarbazine

Note: BCNU, 1,3-bis-(2-chloroethyl)-1-nitrosourea; CCNU, N-(2-chloroethyl)-N'-cyclohexyl-N-nitrosourea.

The extent of the damage to the reproductive organs is dependent upon the agent administered and dose received (Boumpas et al., 1993; Chapman et al., 1981; Clark et al., 1995; Mackie et al., 1996; Mok et al., 1998; Pasqualini et al., 1987; Siris et al., 1976; Teinturier et al., 1998; Wallace et al., 1989c; Waxman et al., 1982; Whitehead et al., 1983). However, as most treatments are delivered as multiagent regimens, often with synergistic toxicity, it can be difficult to determine the specific contribution of each individual agent. The impact of chemotherapy on ovarian function has been widely investigated and most clinical studies have focused on combination chemotherapy regimens used in the treatment of haematological malignancies, particularly Hodgkin's disease (Chapman et al., 1981; Clark et al., 1995; Mackie et al., 1996; Waxman et al., 1982; Whitehead et al., 1983). Occasionally, chemotherapeutic agents are administered as monotherapy, enabling the direct gonadotoxic effects of the agent to be studied, such as cyclophosphamide treatment of autoimmune diseases (Boumpas et al., 1993; Mok et al., 1998).

Although the mechanism of cytotoxic chemotherapy-induced damage to the ovary is uncertain, destruction of the fixed, nonrenewable oocyte pool is likely. Clinical studies have shown that age is an important factor in determining the outcome of ovarian function following chemotherapy. Older women have a much higher incidence of complete ovarian failure and permanent infertility compared with their younger counterparts (Fisher and Cheung, 1984; Moore, 2000). The impact of therapy on age was evaluated in 44 females treated with the combination chemotherapy regimen MVPP (nitrogen mustard (mechlorethamine), vinblastine, procarbazine, prednisolone) for Hodgkin's disease at a median age of 23 years. Regular menses were maintained in 39% (17 of 44; median age 22 years), oligomenorrhoea developed in 23% (10 of 44; median age 23 years) and amenorrhoea occurred in 39% (17 of 44; median age 30 years) during chemotherapy (Whitehead et al., 1983). The apparent resistance of the young ovary is likely to reflect the larger reserve of primordial follicles, but this must be regarded with caution, as the potential for the onset of a premature menopause remains.

Alkylating agents form an integral part of many treatment protocols and have long been recognized to impair gonadal function. One of the most widely studied of such agents is cyclophosphamide, which is frequently used in the treatment of many childhood malignancies. High-dose cyclophosphamide may be used as conditioning therapy before BMT either alone, where recovery is more likely, or in combination with other chemotherapeutic agents or TBI. Ovarian function, as defined by spontaneous menstruation and normal hormone profile without hormone sup-

plement, was assessed in 176 females following high-dose cyclophosphamide with or without high-dose busulphan and BMT (aged 13–58 years at transplant) (Sanders et al., 1996). Of the 103 women receiving cyclophosphamide alone (200 mg/kg), ovarian function was preserved in 56 (54%). The addition of busulphan (16 mg/kg) was associated with a higher prevalence of patients with ovarian dysfunction, with recovery observed in only 1 of 73 females. In the same study, Sanders et al. (1996) reported recovery of ovarian function in 28% (23 of 82) girls treated prepubertally with similar regimens.

Hodgkin's disease is one of the commoner malignancies presenting in adolescence and young adulthood and is curable in the majority of cases. A number of therapeutic regimens have been used successfully but are frequently associated with infertility. Treatment of Hodgkin's disease with established combination chemotherapy regimens – MVPP, MOPP (mechlorethamine, vincristine, procarbazine and prednisolone) or ChlVPP (chlorambucil, vinblastine, procarbazine and prednisolone) – results in ovarian failure in 19–63% (Chapman et al., 1981; Clark et al., 1995; Mackie et al., 1996; Waxman et al., 1982; Whitehead et al., 1983). Amenorrhoea is much more commonly encountered in women over 30 years (50–89%) than in younger women, in whom ovarian function appears to be preserved in 48–100%. In a large retrospective study following treatment with MOPP for Hodgkin's disease during childhood (< 16 years), normal menstrual function was reported in 87% (75 of 86) of girls. There was no effect on the age at menarche and ovarian function was preserved in all patients who had received only three courses of MOPP (Sy Ortin et al., 1990). In another study, ovarian function was assessed in 32 female survivors of childhood Hodgkin's disease. All subjects had received treatment with ChlVPP chemotherapy alone with no radiotherapy below the diaphragm, at a median age of 13.0 years (range, 9–15.2). Seventeen (53%) of the girls had raised gonadotrophin levels, 10 of whom had symptomatic ovarian failure and six received hormone replacement therapy. Nine women had 11 successful pregnancies, two of whom had previously had symptoms of ovarian failure with one requiring hormone replacement therapy (Mackie et al., 1996).

Alternative regimens may be used to treat Hodgkin's disease successfully that are less gonadotoxic. The ABVD combination (doxorubicin, bleomycin, vinblastine and dacarbazine), which contains neither an alkylating agent nor procarbazine, has been shown to be significantly less gonadotoxic. Brusamolino et al. (2000) observed that fertility was preserved in young women after four courses of ABVD chemotherapy followed by radiotherapy. Transient amenorrhoea was reported by 12 of 33 patients less than 45 years of age, and none of the 17 patients with permanent amenorrhoea was less than 25 years. The beneficial effects of reduced gonadotoxicity with the ABVD regimen are offset by the increased risk of cardiotoxicity associated with anthracyclines. Consequently, "hybrid" chemotherapy protocols have been introduced in an attempt to reduce the cumulative dose of any individual agent and hopefully reduce late sequelae. Treatment of 36 adolescents (median age at diagnosis 14 years) with the hybrid regimen COP/ABVD (five courses of COP (cyclophosphamide, vincristine and procarbazine) alternating with four courses of ABVD) and low-dose regional radiotherapy (20 Gy) was associated with preservation of ovarian function in the majority of patients. Ovarian failure occurred in 17% (6 of 36) patients and 10 patients have had a total of 17 pregnancies (Hudson et al., 1993).

Treatment for childhood ALL, the commonest childhood malignancy, is associated with an overall five-year survival rate of more than 75%. The successful treatment of ALL with combination chemotherapy appears to be associated with preservation of ovarian function in the majority (Green et al., 1989; Pasqualini et al., 1987; Siris et al., 1976). In a UK study of 40 girls treated for childhood ALL, all achieved adult pubertal development (median age at menarche 12.4 years) and 37 had regular menses (Wallace et al., 1993). Four patients had biochemical evidence of ovarian damage with raised gonadotrophins, three of whom had received craniospinal irradiation and one additional cyclophosphamide (4.48 g). None of the girls required hormone replacement therapy. There were 14 livebirths in nine long-term survivors, with no perinatal complications or serious congenital abnormalities and no reported cases of malignant disease in their offspring. A recent study has shown decreased LH excretion and short luteal phase in young women treated for ALL in childhood. This subtle ovulation disorder is probably related to low-dose cranial irradiation (Bath et al., 2001). Current treatment for standard risk ALL is unlikely to be sterilizing, but for patients who relapse treatment involves intensive chemotherapy, frequently with TBI and BMT and is likely to result in impaired fertility.

Ovarian failure following high-dose chemotherapy treatment as conditioning for BMT appears to be temporary. In a study of 43 women with aplastic anaemia, cyclophosphamide conditioning (200 mg/kg) resulted in amenorrhoea in all women, with 36 showing recovery of normal ovarian function 3–42 months after transplantation (Sanders, 1991). Ovarian function was normal in 95% of females treated prepubertally with cyclophosphamide (200 mg/kg) as conditioning therapy for BMT. However, doses in excess of 200 mg/kg may result in premature ovarian failure (Sanders, 1991). Studies are currently under-

way to evaluate the impact of ifosfamide, an analogue of cyclophosphamide, on ovarian function. Combination chemotherapy and continually evolving protocols require vigilant long-term follow-up of these patients to monitor the risk of late effects.

In a study to assess the impact of busulfan therapy, pubertal status and ovarian function was studied in 21 girls aged 11–21 years who had been treated with high-dose chemotherapy and autologous BMT without TBI for malignant tumours. Ten girls received busulfan ($600\,mg/m^2$) and melphalan ($140\,mg/m^2$) with or without cyclophosphamide ($3.6\,g/m^2$). The remaining 11 did not receive busulfan treatment. In 12 of the 21 girls (57%), there was clinical and biochemical evidence of ovarian failure; of these 12, 10 had received busulfan treatment, indicating the gonadotoxic nature of high-dose busulfan treatment (Teinturier et al., 1998).

Recovery of ovarian function

Despite regular menses, the "fertile window" may be reduced and the possibility of a premature menopause in childhood cancer survivors is of great concern. Several studies have demonstrated that a significant proportion of young patients with continued menstruation following cessation of chemotherapy were at risk of subsequently undergoing a premature menopause many years later (Byrne et al., 1992; Wallace et al., 1993). Chiarelli et al. (1999) evaluated the risk of premature menopause and infertility in 719 female cancer survivors who had regular menses at the end of treatment. Treatment with alkylating agents in addition to abdominal radiotherapy was associated with an increased risk of premature menopause (relative risk 2.58), with the risk increasing with increasing dose of both treatment modalities. The risk of early menopause was assessed in a retrospective study of 1067 long-term survivors of childhood and adolescent malignancy (< 20 years at diagnosis) who were menstruating at 21 years of age. Long-term cancer survivors, aged 13–19 years at diagnosis, demonstrated a risk of menopause four times greater than that of controls aged 21–25 years. The risk was dependent upon the modality of therapy. Following radiotherapy alone, the relative risk of developing a premature menopause during the early twenties was 3.7; after treatment with alkylating agents alone this was 9.2, with a 27-fold increased risk when both modalities of therapy were received. By 31 years of age, 42% of the group had reached menopause, in contrast to only 5% of the control group. Long-term follow-up will be necessary as a number of these young women may subsequently progress to a premature menopause (Byrne et al., 1992).

Table 32.3. Assessment of ovarian function

Ovarian dysfunction	Clinical outcome	Endocrine profile
Ovarian failure prepubertally	Delayed puberty	Undetectable prepubertally
	Primary amenorrhoea	From pubertal age: elevated FSH, reduced oestradiol
Ovarian failure during or after puberty	Arrested puberty Secondary amenorrhoea Menopausal symptoms	Elevated FSH; reduced oestradiol

Note: FSH, follicle-stimulating hormone.

Recovery of ovarian function is reported in a number of patients following cytotoxic chemotherapy- and radiotherapy-related amenorrhoea. Ovarian function may recover in two or three years in younger women, but recovery rarely occurs in older women with treatment-induced amenorrhoea (Bines et al., 1996; Chapman et al., 1979; Chatterjee et al., 1996). Younger age at BMT may predict return of ovarian function: Schimmer et al. (1998) reported a return of function in 29% (5 of 17) of patients 6–48 months after an initial period of amenorrhoea immediately following alkylating agent-based chemotherapy or TBI conditioning therapy and BMT. Histological studies of human ovarian tissue after chemotherapy have demonstrated ovarian atrophy and marked loss of primordial follicles (Familiari et al., 1993; Marcello et al., 1990). From a practical point of view, although recovery occurs in only a very small minority, young patients with treatment-induced amenorrhoea should be advised to continue with contraception.

Investigation of ovarian function

Clinical manifestations of ovarian damage depend upon the age of the child at the time of treatment (Table 32.3). Cytotoxic damage sustained prepubertally may result in failure to develop secondary sexual characteristics. If the child is peripubertal at the time of treatment, there may be arrest of pubertal development, with subsequent primary amenorrhoea. In postpubertal females, ovarian failure will manifest as secondary amenorrhoea, often with symptoms of oestrogen deficiency. Biochemically, ovarian failure is detected as elevated gonadotrophins and undetectable oestradiol. It must be remembered that FSH levels often fluctuate and FSH testing may need repeating.

Prediction of a premature menopause is difficult, although early follicular phase assay of FSH, oestradiol and inhibin B and ovarian ultrasound are potential tools to assess ovarian reserve. Elevated early follicular phase FSH with preservation of oestradiol production is characteristic of the perimenopause, the length of which may vary (Ahmed Eddiary et al., 1994; Sherman et al., 1976). Ovarian failure will require oestrogen replacement for pubertal induction and cyclical hormone replacement to relieve the symptoms of oestrogen deficiency (vaginal dryness, hot flushes and irritability), provide cardiovascular protection and optimize bone density. The loss of ovarian function following chemotherapy administration in postmenarcheal patients is associated with significant changes in libido and sexual function (Chapman et al., 1979). For those women with confirmed hypogonadotrophic hypogonadism after radiotherapy, ovulation induction may be achieved with pulsed gonadotrophin therapy. Women exposed to low-dose cranial irradiation should have early referral to gynaecologists and detailed endocrine assessment if they present with infertility.

Uterus

Radiotherapy-induced uterine damage

Recent data demonstrate that uterine function may be compromised following radiotherapy that involves the pelvis, regardless of the age at time of treatment. Reduced uterine volume and decreased elasticity of uterine musculature, possibly as a consequence of impaired vascularization, are found in girls receiving pelvic, abdominal and total body irradiation prepubertally (Bath et al., 1999; Critchley et al., 1992). Disruption of uterine characteristics may compromise implantation and continuation of pregnancy. Although successful pregnancies following radiotherapy are reported, the incidence of spontaneous miscarriage, premature delivery and intrauterine growth retardation is significantly increased (Bines et al., 1996; Larsen et al., 2000; Li et al., 1987; Wallace et al., 1989b). Sanders et al. (1996) reported an increased risk of spontaneous abortion in patients who had received TBI, with pregnancies ending in miscarriage in 38%. Of eight livebirths, five (63%) had preterm delivery and labour, four of whom were low birth weight and one very low birth weight. There was no increased incidence of congenital abnormalities (Sanders et al., 1996). For patients with oocyte depletion following TBI, oocyte donation is an option but outcome will invariably depend upon uterine characteristics and a small uterus is associated with poor outcome. Although data are limited, one study reported three cases of oocyte donation in women who had ovarian failure following treatment for haematological malignancies with BMT and TBI (Larsen et al., 2000). One woman with a uterus of normal or almost normal size delivered a healthy child in the 37th week of gestation. A second woman with severely diminished uterine volume had a second trimester miscarriage. The third woman had yet to conceive.

Following whole abdominal irradiation (20–30 Gy) in childhood, all pregnancies occurring in women with preserved ovarian function resulted in mid-trimester miscarriage (Wallace et al., 1989a). In a large study of 2083 survivors of childhood cancer, pregnancy outcome was compared in those patients treated for Wilms' tumour with or without abdominal irradiation (Hawkins and Smith, 1989). The spontaneous abortion rate was 22% in those exposed to radiotherapy compared with 6% in the unexposed group. Birth weight was also significantly reduced (mean of 500 g less) in the exposed compared with the unexposed group. In studies exploring the role of exogenous sex steroids, women with premature ovarian failure following TBI for childhood leukaemia and treated with physiological sex steroid replacement therapy have shown an increase in uterine volume and endometrial thickness (Bath et al., 1999; Critchley et al., 1990). This is encouraging for future fertility prospects and may be a useful way of assessing uterine function when considering these women for assisted reproductive techniques.

Chemotherapy and the uterus

Chemotherapy does not appear to have any significant lasting adverse effect on uterine function. Successful pregnancy, with no increased risk of miscarriage, and healthy offspring are reported following treatment with combination chemotherapy regimens (Nicholson and Byrne, 1993; Salooja et al., 2001).

Investigation of uterine function

Normal uterine shape, length and volume for pre-, peri- and postpuberty are well documented (Holm et al., 1995). Ultrasound scanning is a reliable noninvasive technique for assessing uterine size and shape, blood supply and endometrial thickness. Uterine artery blood flow may be assessed by Doppler scanning and resistance to flow expressed as the pulsatility index. Endometrial biopsy enables assessment of endometrial function using histological and immunocytochemistry techniques (Critchley et al., 1998; Snijders et al., 1992).

Maternal health during pregnancy

As the population of young adults of reproductive age who have received treatment for cancer increases, the side effects of chemotherapy and radiotherapy are of increasing concern. A number of therapeutic regimens are widely recognized to be associated with an increased risk of cardiac disease, renal impairment, musculoskeletal problems and endocrine and metabolic disturbances. Although there are no data to support an increase in maternal deaths during pregnancy, there is potentially an increased risk of illness burden owing to the side effects of cancer therapy, which must be addressed by the obstetrician when caring for the mother during her pregnancy (Robertson et al., 1994). Exposure to anthracyclines as part of successful treatment for childhood cancer requires regular echocardiography assessments during pregnancy.

Progeny

Overall there are reassuring reports that there is no increased incidence of either congenital abnormalities or childhood malignancy in children born to long-term survivors of childhood cancer (Hawkins et al., 1989; Li et al., 1979). However, these successful pregnancies mostly resulted from normally achieved conception. We do not know the consequences of circumventing the natural selection processes of normal sexual reproduction using assisted reproduction techniques, nor the effects of these techniques on the complex cascade of precisely timed molecular interactions of early embryonic development. Continued surveillance of the progeny of survivors of childhood cancer remains essential (Grundy et al., 2001a).

As with males, there is the theoretical risk that exposure to chemotherapeutic agents or irradiation may cause mutations and DNA changes to the oocyte. Animal studies have demonstrated high abortion and malformation rates related to different stages of oocyte maturation at the time of exposure to chemotherapy (Hawkins 1994; Salooja et al., 2001; Sanders et al., 1996). This has raised concerns regarding the use of assisted reproduction techniques and embryo cryopreservation in patients previously exposed to cancer therapy. Reassuringly, studies of pregnancy outcome in cancer survivors have not substantiated these concerns. There is no increased incidence of chromosomal or congenital abnormalities in offspring born to women exposed to cancer therapy (Hawkins 1994; Salooja et al., 2001; Sanders et al., 1996).

Table 32.4. Clinical and experimental strategies for preservation of reproductive function in girls undergoing treatment for childhood cancer

Clinical practice	Experimental strategies
Oophoropexy	Cryopreservation of oocytes
Embryo cryopreservation	Gonadotrophin suppression
	Inhibition of follicle apoptosis
	Cryopreservation of ovarian tissue

Fertility preservation

A number of strategies to protect the ovaries and preserve fertility during cancer therapy have been attempted with limited success (Table 32.4; see also Ch. 33). Limitation of radiation dose to the ovary is sometimes practised in adult women but in children is technically difficult. In young sexually mature females with partners, collection of mature oocytes for storage or fertilization and subsequent embryo cryopreservation is possible. For prepubertal girls, and the majority of young women, preservation of fertility remains experimental and harvesting and storage of gonadal tissue before commencing cancer therapy is the most promising option.

Advances in assisted reproduction and increasing interest in gamete extraction and maturation have focused attention on preserving gonadal tissue from children before sterilizing chemotherapy or radiotherapy, with the realistic expectation that future technologies will be able to utilize their immature gametes (Carroll and Gosden 1993; Gosden 1990; Gosden et al., 1994a; Guanasena et al., 1997; Oktay et al., 1997, 2000a). The impetus for preserving gonadal tissue follows on the heels of pioneering experiments in ewes together with media interest in the report of a successful autologous ovarian graft in a previously oophorectomized female (Gosden et al., 1994a). Such issues have inevitably raised questions from parents and oncologists about their possible application in children undergoing cancer therapies (Grundy et al., 2001b; Wallace and Walker 2001).

Established practices

Surgical translocation

Reducing the radiation dose to the ovary by shielding or removing the ovaries from the field of radiation (oophoropexy) may preserve ovarian function (Leporrier et al., 1987; Thomas et al., 1976). Repositioning the ovaries outside the field of radiotherapy is more applicable to the adult female of reproductive age with malignancies such as cervical cancer or occasionally for pelvic lymph node irradiation; its value in the prepubertal child is less clear.

Oophoropexy involves laparoscopic transposition of the ovaries (with blood supply intact) to a position behind the uterus, which acts as a shield, or to the paracolic gutters, away from the field of radiation, to minimize exposure. Experimentally, heterotopic ovarian autotransplantation has involved grafting the ovary to a distant site in the body and anastamosing blood vessels (Atkinson et al., 1994). The ovarian dose received during pelvic nodal irradiation for Hodgkin's disease can be limited from 44 Gy to 0.22–0.55 Gy by midline oophoropexy, and in women who are less than 25 years at the time of treatment, ovarian failure is infrequent (Sy Ortin et al., 1990). However, even where ovarian function is preserved, oocyte retrieval with assisted reproduction and surrogacy may be required to achieve a pregnancy as the uterus may also have been damaged by the radiation therapy. This will compromise the ability of the women to carry a pregnancy to term.

Storage of embryos or mature oocytes

The only established successful strategy currently available for preservation of female fertility is cryopreservation of embryos. Embryo cryopreservation and in vitro fertilization may be offered to women before treatment for cancer. Embryo banking has the advantage that it allows a number of embryos to be stored without a need for further in vitro fertilization cycles; however, this requires the patient to have a partner or to use donor sperm. On average, 10 oocytes are collected per cycle, limiting the number of embryos available for cryopreservation. The overall livebirth rate from a single cycle of treatment is 11% (Porcu et al., 1997). Cryopreservation of oocytes is an alternative possibility for women without a partner but is much less successful, with fewer than one baby born per 100 oocytes stored and as such remains experimental (Atkinson et al., 1994). The main disadvantage of embryo or oocyte storage is the requirement for superovulation with gonadotrophins, which will inevitably delay the commencement of cancer therapy.

Experimental strategies

Gonadotrophin suppression

One approach to preserving fertile potential was based on the original idea that the prepubertal ovary is quiescent and, therefore, protected from the cytotoxic effects of chemotherapy and radiotherapy, which destroy rapidly dividing cells. It was hypothesized that suppression of hypothalamic–pituitary–gonadal axis by administration of the gonadotrophin-releasing hormone (GnRH) analogues would render the ovary less susceptible. A number of studies have demonstrated that GnRH analogues inhibit chemotherapy-induced ovarian follicular depletion in rodents (Ataya and Ramahi-Ataya, 1993). Progesterone or GnRH agonists were shown to maintain fertility and fecundity rates comparable to those of untreated control animals (Montz et al., 1991). While it has since become clear that the prepubertal ovary is vulnerable to the deleterious effects of cytotoxic therapy, the mechanisms by which such hormonal manipulation may offer protection of ovarian function are unclear. It is likely that the relative "resistance" of the prepubertal ovary to cytotoxic therapy reflects the larger number of follicles present at the time of treatment rather than the avoidance of damage. In rodents, GnRH analogues prevent follicular growth and mitosis by blocking gonadotrophin induction. Although the exact mechanism is uncertain it may involve direct suppression of GnRH receptors in the ovary, with subsequent inhibition of recruitment of small follicles into the proliferating pool as well as atresia of the already developed follicles. However, there remains uncertainty about applicability in the human, particularly as the human ovary has significantly fewer numbers of GnRH receptors. Using a primate model, Ataya et al. (1995a,b) demonstrated that GnRH analogue cotreatment protected the Rhesus monkey from cyclophosphamide-induced ovarian damage by significantly reducing follicular decline compared with that in animals treated with cyclophosphamide alone (from 65% to 29%). These findings are supported by clinical studies that demonstrated that cotreatment of GnRH analogue with chemotherapy reduced primary ovarian failure to 1 in 44 (2.3%) compared with 26 out of 45 (58%) in the group treated with chemotherapy (with or without mantle field irradiation) only (Blumenfeld et al., 1996; Blumenfeld, 2000). In another study, Blumenfeld and coworkers (2000) were able to study the protective effects of GnRH agonists in patients undergoing cytotoxic alkylating agent-based treatment for systemic lupus erythematosus. Ovarian function was preserved in all eight women receiving GnRH agonists in conjunction with chlorambucil or cyclophosphamide, in contrast to five of the nine (56%) patients treated with chemotherapy only. Adjuvant treatment with a GnRH analogue to limit the gonadal toxic effects of otherwise successful treatment regimens is potentially attractive. However, this must be viewed with some caution as although GnRH analogues provided some protection against cyclophosphamide, no advantage was conferred against irradiation or high-dose chemotherapy as conditioning therapy for BMT, where ovarian failure was unpreventable irrespective of hormone suppression (Meirow, 1999). In the case of radiation, this may be in part explained by the different mechanism of gonadal damage induced by radiotherapy, namely the destruction of primordial follicles, which are not under the influence of gonadotrophins (Gosden et al., 1997a).

The judicious use of GnRH analogues may play a role in the appropriate patient group, such as young women and children subjected to alkylating agent-based chemotherapy for Hodgkin's disease.

Prevention of follicle atresia

Oocyte loss induced by anticancer therapy has been shown to occur by apoptosis; consequently, inhibition of the apoptotic pathway has been explored as a mechanism for preventing ovarian failure. Although the exact pathway remains to be elucidated, accumulating data support the role of ceramide in signalling somatic cell death. Ceramide is a sphingolipid second messenger derived from sphingomyelinase-catalysed hydrolysis, in addition to de novo synthesis. In turn, ceramide is metabolized and phosphorylated to give sphingosine 1-phosphate, which is believed to inhibit apoptosis in somatic cells. The role of the sphingomyelin pathway has also been studied in germ cells. Disruption of the gene encoding acid sphingomyelinase or treatment with sphingosine 1-phosphate attenuates apoptosis of primordial fetal oocytes, with increased oocyte numbers present at birth. Treatment of mice ooctyes with sphingosine 1-phosphate prevents chemotherapy-induced apoptosis in vitro. In vivo administration of sphingosine 1-phosphate confers resistance to radiation-induced apoptosis in mice, with pregnancy rates of 100% (Morita et al., 2000). While this may herald a new approach to preservation of ovarian function, further studies are necessary to explore the detrimental effects of such treatment on normal neurological function, as deletion of sphingomyelinase during normal fetal life leads to the development of symptoms similar to those of Neimann–Pick disease after birth.

Harvesting and future use of ovarian tissue

The only option potentially available for prepubertal children and the majority of young women is cryopreservation of ovarian tissue (see also Ch. 33). Human ovaries are too large and too fibrous to store in their entirety, because of poor penetration of the cryoprotectants. Hence, harvesting ovarian tissue may take the form of cryopreservation of slices of ovarian cortex, which are rich in primordial follicles, or cryopreservation of immature oocytes. Harvesting and cryopreservation of ovarian tissue is advantageous compared with embryo and oocyte storage for a number of reasons. Good survival rates and viability after thawing are similar whether primordial follicles are stored as slices or in isolation, in contrast to immature oocytes where survival is poor and increased rates of chromosomal abnormalities and spindle malformation are reported (Ludwig et al., 1999;

Oktay et al., 1997). Furthermore, hundreds of immature oocytes can be stored without the necessity of hormone stimulation and delay in commencing treatment.

Cryopreservation of ovarian tissue in rodents was first explored during the 1950s but was largely abandoned until the 1990s because of poor cryoprotectants and lack of automated cryopreservation machines (Green et al., 1956; Parkes and Smith, 1952; Parrot, 1960). With the advent of newer cryoprotectants such as dimethylsulphoxide, propanediol and ethylene glycol, interest in cryopreservation has been regenerated and the results encouraging. Transplantation of fresh and cryopreserved fetal ovarian tissue into adult syngeneic mice successfully restored fertility in up to 86% of the animals, comparable to that of controls (Cox et al., 1996). In other studies, similar successes have been reported with orthotopic transplantation of frozen–thawed ovarian tissue in the mouse (Candy et al., 2000; Shaw et al., 2000; Sztein et al., 1998). In 1994 pioneering experiments by Gosden and coworkers demonstrated equally encouraging results in sheep, which is more applicable to humans than the rodents as sheep and human ovaries share similar characteristics. Fresh and frozen–thawed cortical strips were autotransplanted onto the ovarian pedicle of oopherectomized sheep. Return of ovulation was evident within four months of transplantation and two successful pregnancies resulted, one from each of the fresh and frozen grafts, with healthy offspring (Gosden et al., 1994a). These studies also reported that reimplanted frozen or thawed cortical strips could restore normal oestrous cycles for at least 22 months (Baird et al., 1999). Further studies of frozen–thawed tissue autotransplants have shown that there is a drastic reduction in follicle reserve during the freezing and thawing and during the revascularization period: 7% and 65%, respectively, suggesting that the ovarian grafts will have a limited lifespan (Baird et al., 1999).

One potential strategy for the future use of the stored material would be to replant the ovarian tissue with the hope of restoring natural fertility and also maintaining sex steroid production. Autologous transplantation of fresh and frozen–thawed primordial follicles to the ovaries of sterile recipients has restored fertility, resulting in live healthy offspring in mice and sheep (Carroll and Gosden, 1993; Gosden et al., 1994a; Gosden, 1990; Guanasena et al., 1997). Human primordial follicles survive cryopreservation and return of ovarian hormonal activity has been achieved with reimplantation. However, no pregnancies have yet been reported and this procedure must be considered experimental (Oktay et al., 2000b; Radford et al., 2001). It is likely that ovarian grafts will have a limited lifespan, in which case transplantation should be delayed until fertility is desired.

Of major concern surrounding the autotransplantation of ovarian cortical strips is the potential for the ovarian tissue to harbour malignant cells capable of inducing a relapse of the disease upon reimplantation. This is particularly pertinent to haematological malignancies where blood-borne transport of malignant cells may seed the ovaries. Fresh and frozen–thawed ovarian tissue from diseased mice transmitted lymphoma when transplanted into healthy recipients (Shaw et al., 1996). In another study, human frozen–thawed ovarian cortical strips were collected from patients with Hodgkin's and nonHodgkin's lymphoma, ALL and acute myelocytic leukaemia and xenografted to severely immunodeficient mice. There was no evidence of disease recurrence in the tissue from patients with nonHodgkin's lymphoma but one xenograft of tissue from a patient with Hodgkin's disease (one of five) resulted in tumour recurrence. The results from ALL and acute myelocytic leukaemia xenografts were inconclusive (Kim et al., 1999). This highlights the risk of potential transmission of cancer cells and emphasizes the need to ensure adequate procedures are developed to enable storage of tumour-free tissue, and the careful selection of the appropriate patients from whom tissue should be harvested. It is clear that transmission of cancer cells will depend upon the type of cancer; cancers with a very low risk of metastasizing to the ovaries will constitute the group of patients in whom these strategies should be considered.

In view of the potential risk of transplanting tumour cells, a number of alternative strategies are being investigated. The risk of transplanting tumour cells can be eliminated by maturing the ovarian follicles in vitro followed by assisted reproduction (Gosden et al., 1997b; Oktay et al., 2000b). In vitro culture of secondary preantral follicles to antral stages using FSH stimulation has been successful in a number of species, including mouse, hamster, pig and humans (Abir et al., 1997; Eppig and Schroeder, 1989; Hovatta et al., 1996; Roy and Greenwald, 1989; Roy and Treasy, 1993; Spears et al., 1994). Maturation of secondary mouse follicles in vitro with fertilization of the oocytes has produced healthy offspring (Spears et al., 1994). Despite this, secondary follicles are few in number in human ovaries and development into early antral stages is associated with a very high rate of oocyte loss (Abir et al., 1997). Consequently, successful and realistic in vitro maturation of human tissues dictates the development of techniques to mature the much more abundant, primordial follicle (Abir et al., 1998; Hovatta et al., 1996). At present, this is limited by our current lack of knowledge of the signals involved in inducing primordial follicle growth into secondary follicles, although it is presumably mediated by interaction with surrounding stromal cells (Abir et al., 1997). Culture of primordial follicles may be approached by culture of ovarian cortical slices, which would maintain the structural integrity and enable interaction between follicles and surrounding stromal cells. Alternatively, primordial follicles could be isolated and cultured, which would have the advantage of allowing direct monitoring of follicular development. Culture of primary and primordial follicles to preovulatory and preantral stages, respectively, has been achieved in mice, with subsequent isolation and maturation of the secondary follicles. A live offspring was produced following in vitro fertilization in one mouse (Eppig and O'Brien, 1996). Cultures from enzymatically isolated primary and primordial follicles from mice, rats and pigs have yielded similar degrees of development (Cain et al., 1995; Eppig and O'Brien, 1996; Greenwald and Moor, 1989; Torrance et al., 1989). Isolated fresh and frozen–thawed human primordial follicles have been successfully maintained in culture for up to 5 days but no evidence of growth was observed (Oktay et al., 1997).

Heterotopic xenogeneic transplantation is an alternative strategy to eliminate the risk of reimplanting tissue that might harbour malignant cells. Studies have shown that the renal capsule of immunodeficient mice can successfully serve as a site for transplantation of ovarian slices from various species, including humans (Gosden et al., 1994b; Nugent et al., 1997; Weissman et al., 1999). Ovarian cortical slices from sheep, cats and marmosets have been transplanted to immunodeficient mice and developed to late antral stages, providing a model and a host for follicular development (Bosma et al., 1983; Candy et al., 1995). Oktay and colleagues (1998) have shown cryopreservation and xenografting of human ovarian tissue to be a viable proposition when they reported follicle survival rates of 50–80% for ovarian cortex donated by healthy patients, frozen for up to two months and then grafted under the kidney capsule of mice with severe combined immuno-deficiency (SCID) (Oktay et al., 1998). Similar studies transplanting human ovarian slices to SCID mice have produced similar results following administration of FSH (Gosden et al., 1994b; Oktay et al., 2001; Weissman et al., 1999). Weissmen and coworkers (1999) reported antral follicle development and oocyte retrieval after intramuscular xenografting of human ovarian tissue to nude mice. The advantage of using SCID mice is that they carry a mutation that renders them immunodeficient in both B and T cells; therefore, they are unable to reject grafts from foreign species (Bosma et al., 1983).

The above studies provided the impetus for ovarian transplantation trials in humans. These trials have explored both orthotopic and heterotopic transplantation (Oktay and Karlikaya 2000; Oktay 2001; Wells et al., 1976). In orthotopic transplantation, the tissue is grafted near to the infundibulopelvic ligament, which would enable natural pregnancy if the Fallopian tubes are intact. Heterotopic transplantation involves grafting of the tissue to the subcutaneous space above the brachioradialis fascia in the forearm, a technique that has been used successfully for parathyroid tissue for many years (Wells et al., 1976). Subcutaneous ovarian transplantation was successfully reported in two women before pelvic irradiation or following oophorectomy with preservation of endocrine function. Menopause was confirmed immediately following transplantation in both patients. In the first subject, follicle development was evident on ultrasound by 10 weeks and a dominant follicle developed each month during the 18 month follow-up. Percutaneous aspirations yielded a mature oocyte. In the second subject, follicle development resumed by 6 months and was associated with regular monthly menses during the 10 month follow-up (Oktay et al., 2001). Oktay and Karlikaya (2000) reported the reimplantation of cryopreserved ovarian tissue into a 29-year-old woman who had previously undergone bilateral oophorectomy for a nonmalignant condition. The ovarian tissue was divided into 80 pieces and sewn onto cellulose membranes in a pocket positioned beneath the pelvic peritoneum. Following gonadotrophin administration, follicular development was observed and ovulation was induced by administration of human chorionic gonadotrophin. Similar results were obtained following heterogenic transplantation of ovarian tissue beneath the skin of the forearm. In another study, Radford and co-workers (2001) studied orthotopic reimplantation of cryopreserved ovarian cortical strips after high-dose chemotherapy in a 36-year-old woman for a third recurrence of Hodgkin's lymphoma (Radford et al., 2001). Immediately after chemotherapy the woman was clinically and biochemically postmenopausal, but by seven months the hot flushes had abated and her hormone profile demonstrated an oestradiol surge one month later with subsequent menstruation. By nine months, her hormone profile returned to that of ovarian failure. Histological assessment of the ovarian cortical strips demonstrated only a few primordial follicles. The ovaries in this subject had previously been exposed to substantial amounts of cytotoxic chemotherapy and radiotherapy for Hodgkin's disease and the patient had already developed premature ovarian failure before harvesting was performed. Although the presence of a few follicles permitted temporary resumption of ovarian function, it is not surprising that this was not sustained. While the techniques used in these studies provide evidence of the success and safety of the procedures, it is evident that careful selection of patients is necessary. In addition to concerns regarding the potential harbouring of malignant cells in ovarian tissue with the reactivation of disease on reimplanting the tissue, harvesting of cortical strips must be from ovaries where there are likely to be abundant primordial follicles to withstand the procedures and sustain ovarian function for a reasonable period of time following reimplantation. Despite these encouraging results, no pregnancy has occurred to date and the question of whether natural fertility can be restored and healthy offspring produced remains unanswered.

Clinical practice for harvesting gonadal tissue

Harvesting and storage of ovarian cortical tissue from girls and young women before gonadotoxic chemotherapy has been available in a number of centres since the mid 1990s (Brook et al., 2001). The harvesting of ovarian tissue can readily be achieved laparoscopically before potentially sterilizing cytotoxic therapy. The tissue can be safely cryopreserved until required for future use. The Royal College of Obstetricians and Gynaecologists (2000) has provided a report from a working party on the storage of ovarian and prepubertal testicular tissue. This provides standards for best practice in the cryopreservation of gonadal tissue, including the criteria for providing a service, patient identification and selection, standard operating procedures and requirements for safe storage.

Ethical issues

The cryopreservation and subsequent use of prepubertal ovarian tissue presents a number of practical and ethical problems that must be addressed before embarking on any clinical programme (Grundy et al., 2001b; Wallace and Walker, 2001). These include issues of safety relating to the harvesting of the tissue, subsequent use and possible implications for the progeny. Valid consent is necessary for clinical research, rendering potentially harmful interventions both ethical and legal. To be valid, consent must be informed, voluntarily obtained and given by a competent person. In practice, it may be difficult to satisfy these criteria, especially in children with cancer. The information necessary for parents and children to make an informed choice about fertility preservation is inevitably complex and its comprehension cannot be guaranteed. Legal competence to consent requires that the individual giving it is able to understand the information given, believes that it applies to them, retains it and uses it to make an informed choice. Parental anxieties about their child's illness may reduce their competence. It may involve consideration of a future that neither they nor the child can envisage

or have discussed. Therapeutic imperatives may limit the time available for discussion, which in turn imposes constraints on the voluntariness of the consent. The concept of informed consent is also difficult to reconcile when issues of safety are uncertain and the future use of any tissue is entirely experimental. Some of these practical difficulties may be alleviated if obtaining consent is considered as a continuum, which can be divided into two stages. The first stage concerns the harvesting and cryopreservation of the tissue and the second concerns the subsequent use of the tissue. Future use of the tissue also raises a number of issues for both autotransplantation or in vitro maturation of the tissue. Autotransplantation carries a potential risk of reintroducing cancer cells into the patient, while in vitro maturation would involve the development of mature gametes and subsequent use with assisted reproductive techniques. Clearly, subsequent use of the tissue would require separate consent. Issues relating to the use of the tissue in the event of the death of the patient should also be discussed.

The removal of ovarian tissue is an invasive procedure that carries an element of risk, a risk that is augmented in individuals whose health is already compromised by their disease. The subsequent reimplantation of stored tissue may carry as yet unquantified risk, with the potential of reactivating disease in individuals in remission. Given our current lack of knowledge surrounding the issues of safety and future use, it is questionable whether even competent individuals can give fully informed consent. Reiteration of the experimental nature of these procedures is necessary.

As early as 1970, the World Health Organization recognized that it was a fundamental right of every individual to have freedom from organic disorders, disease and deficiencies that interfere with sexual and reproductive function. Therefore, not to offer storage may be an infringement of this right by denying choice at a later stage in life. Success in animals does not guarantee applicability in humans, and optimization of the methodology and refining of storage techniques should be restricted to specialist centres with experience in the cryobiology of reproductive tissue.

Summary

As treatment for childhood cancer has become increasingly successful adverse effects on female reproductive function are assuming greater importance (Box 32.1). It is incumbent upon oncologists that appropriate counselling of patients at risk of impaired ovarian function and infertility forms part of their routine care. Preservation of fertility before treatment must be considered in all young patients at high

---

Box 32.1 Key points

- Successful treatment of childhood cancer may be associated with impaired female reproductive function in adulthood.
- Females are generally less susceptible than males to the deleterious effects of chemotherapy.
- Total body, abdominal or pelvic irradiation may cause ovarian and uterine damage and the degree of impairment is related to the radiation dose, fractionation schedule and age at time of treatment.
- Human primordial follicles survive cryopreservation and return of ovarian hormonal activity has been achieved with reimplantation; however, no pregnancies have yet been reported and this procedure must be considered experimental.
- Best practice in the cryopreservation of ovarian tissue, including the criteria for providing a service, patient identification and selection, standard operating procedures and requirements for safe storage, need to be established.
- Concerns that the offspring of patients successfully treated for cancer might have an increased risk of congenital abnormalities and childhood cancer have not been substantiated.

risk of infertility; however, options for preservation of fertile potential are limited and largely experimental. Limitation of radiation exposure by ovarian transposition should be practised where possible. Harvesting ovarian tissue and cryopreservation of cortical slices are practised in a number of centres, although these procedures remain experimental and future utilization of stored tissue is uncertain. Ultimately, autografting and restoration of natural fertility is the aim of cryopreservation of ovarian tissue, but techniques need to be developed to ensure malignant cells are not transferred in the tissue. Isolation of follicles and in vitro maturation for assisted reproduction is an alternative option that will eliminate any risk of transmission of malignant cells. Even where harvesting of ovarian tissue and subsequent maturation of oocytes, whether in vivo or in vitro, is successful, uterine function will play an important role in determining the success of any pregnancy.

The rapidly advancing experimental techniques of harvesting ovarian tissue must be considered and embarked upon without unrealistic expectations, although future utilization of the tissue is likely to be realized in the next decade and preservation of fertile potential in females treated for childhood cancer will be attainable.

REFERENCES

Abir R, Franks S, Mobberley M A, Moore P A, Margara R A, Winston R M (1997). Mechanical isolation and in vitro growth of preantral and small antral human follicles. *Fertil Steril* 68, 682–688.

Abir R, Fisch B, Raz A, Nitke S, Ben-Rafael Z (1998). Preservation of fertility in women undergoing chemotherapy: current approach and future prospects. *J Assist Reprod Genet* 15, 469–478.

Ahmed Eddiary N A, Lenton E A, Cooke I D (1994). Hypothalamic–pituitary ageing: progressive increase in FSH and LH concentrations throughout the reproductive life in regularly menstruating women. *Clin Endocrinol* 41, 199–206.

Ataya K, Ramahi-Ataya A (1993). Reproductive performance of female rats treated with cyclophosphamide and/or LHRH agonist. *Reprod Toxicol* 7, 229–235.

Ataya K, Rao L V, Lawrence E, Kimmel R (1995a). Luteinizing hormone-releasing hormone agonist inhibits cyclophosphamide-induced ovarian follicle depletion in rhesus monkeys. *Biol Reprod* 52, 365–372.

Ataya K, Pydyn E, Ramahi-Ataya A, Orton C G (1995b). Is radiation-induced ovarian failure in rhesus monkeys preventable by leuteinizing hormone-releasing hormone agonist? Preliminary observations. *J Clin Oncol Endocrinol Metab* 80, 790–795.

Atkinson H G, Apperley J F, Dawson K, Goldman J M, Winston R M (1994). Successful pregnancy after embryo cryopreservation after BMT for CML. *Lancet* 344, 199.

Baird D T, Webb R, Campbell B K, Harkness L M, Gosden R G (1999). Long-term ovarian function in sheep after ovariectomy and transplantation of autografts stored at –196°C. *Endocrinology* 140, 462–471.

Balow J E (1993). Risk for sustained amenorrhoea in patients with systemic lupus erythematosus receiving intermittent pulse cyclophosphamide therapy. *Ann Intern Med* 1, 366–369.

Bath L E, Critchley H O, Chambers S E, Anderson R A, Kelnar C J, Wallace W H (1999). Ovarian and uterine characteristics after total body irradiation in childhood and adolescence: response to sex steroid replacement. *Br J Obstet Gynaecol* 106, 1265–1272.

Bath L E, Anderson R A, Critchley H O D, Kelnar C J H, Wallace W H B (2001). Hypothalamic–pituitary–ovarian dysfunction after prepubertal chemotherapy and cranial irradiation for acute leukaemia. *Hum Reprod* 16, 1838–1844.

Bines J, Oleske D M, Cobleigh M A (1996). Ovarian function in premenopausal women treated with adjuvant chemotherapy for breast cancer. *J Clin Oncol* 14, 1718–1729.

Birkebaek N H, Fisker S, Clausen N, Tuovinen V, Sindet-Pedersen S, Christiansen J S (1998). Growth and endocrinological disorders up to 21 years after treatment for acute lymphoblastic leukaemia in childhood. *Med Pediatr Oncol* 30, 351–356.

Bleyer W A (1990). The impact of childhood cancer on the United States and the world. *Cancer* 40, 355–367.

Block E (1952). Quantitative morphological investigations of the follicular system in women. Variations at different ages. *Acta Anat* 14, 108–123.

(1953). A quantitative morphological investigation of the follicular system in newborn female infants. *Acta Anat* 17, 201–206.

Blumenfeld Z (2000). Ovarian rescue/protection from chemotherapeutic agents (1). *J Soc Gynecol Invest* 8, S60–S64.

Blumenfeld Z, Avivi I, Linn S, Epelbaum R, Ben-Shahar M, Haim N (1996). Prevention of irreversible chemotherapy-induced ovarian damage in young women with lymphoma by a gonadotrophin-releasing hormone agonist in parallel to chemotherapy. *Hum Reprod* 11, 1620–1626.

Blumenfeld Z, Shapiro D, Shteinberg M, Avivi I, Nahir M (2000). Preservation of fertility and ovarian function and minimizing gonadotoxicity in young women with systemic lupus erythematosus treated by chemotherapy. *Lupus* 9, 401–405.

Bosma G C, Custer R P, Bosma M J (1983). A severe combined deficiency mutation in the mouse. *Nature* 301, 527–530.

Boumpas D T, Austin H A III, Vaughan E M, Yarboro C H, Klippel J H, Balow J E (1993). Risk for sustained amenorrhoea in patients with systemic lupus erythematosus receiving intermittent pulse cyclophosphamide therapy. *Ann Intern Med* 1, 366–369.

Brennan B M, Rahim A, Mackie E M, Eden O B, Shalet S M (1998). Growth hormone status in adults treated for acute lymphoblastic leukaemia in childhood. *Clin Endocrinol* 48, 777–783.

Brook P F, Radford J A, Shalet S M, Joyce A D, Gosden R G (2001). Isolation of germ cells from human testicular tissue for low temperature storage and autotransplantation. *Fertil Steril* 75, 269–274.

Brusamolino E, Lunghi F, Orlandi E et al. (2000). Treatment of early-stage Hodgkin's disease with four cycles of ABVD followed by adjuvant radiotherapy:analysis and efficacy and long-term toxicity. *Haematologica* 85, 103–105.

Byrne J, Fears T R, Gail M H et al. (1992). Early menopause in long-term survivors of cancer during adolescence. *Am J Obstet Gynecol* 166, 788–793.

Cain L, Chatterjee S, Collins T J (1995). In vitro folliculogenesis of rat preantral follicles. *Endocrinology* 136, 3369–3377.

Candy C J, Wood M J, Whittingham D G (1995). Follicular development in cryopreserved marmoset ovarian tissue after transplantation. *Hum Reprod* 10, 2334–2338.

(2000). Restoration of normal reproductive life span after grafting of cryopreserved ovaries. *Hum Reprod* 15, 1300–1304.

Carroll J, Gosden R G (1993). Transplantation of frozen-thawed mouse primordial follicles. *Hum Reprod* 8, 1163–1167.

Chatterjee R, Goldstone A H (1996). Gonadal damage and effects on fertility in adult patients with haematological malignancy undergoing stem cell transplantation. *Bone Marrow Transplant* 17, 159–167.

Chapman A M, Marrett L D, Darlington G (1979). Cytotoxic-induced ovarian failure in Hodgkin's disease. I. Hormone function. *J Am Med Assoc* 242, 1877–1881.

Chapman R M, Sutcliffe S B, Malpas J S (1981). Cytotoxic-induced ovarian failure in women treated with MOPP chemotherapy for Hodgkin's disease. *Am J Med* 71, 552–556.

Chiarelli A M, Marrett L D, Darlington G (1999). Early menopause and infertility in females after treatment for childhood cancer diagnosed in 1964–1988 in Ontario, Canada. *Am J Epidemiol* 150, 245–254.

Clark S T, Radford J A, Crowther D, Swindell R, Shalet S M (1995). Cytotoxic induced ovarian failure in women treated for Hodgkin's disease: a comparative study of MVPP and a seven-drug hybrid regimen. *J Clin Oncol* 13, 134–139.

Cox S L, Shaw J M, Jenkin G (1996). Transplantation of cryopreserved fetal ovarian tissue to adult recipients in mice. *J Reprod Fertil* 107, 315–322.

Critchley H O, Buckley C H, Anderson D C (1990). Experience with a 'physiological' steroid replacement regimen for the establishment of a receptive endometrium in women with premature ovarian failure. *Br J Obstet Gynaecol* 97, 804–810.

Critchley H O, Wallace W H, Shalet S M, Mamtora H, Higginson J, Anderson D C (1992). Abdominal irradiation in childhood; the potential for pregnancy. *Br J Obstet Gynaecol* 99, 392–394.

Critchley H O, Wang H, Kelly R W, Gebbie A E, Glasier A F (1998). Progestin receptor isoforms and prostaglandin dehydrogenase in the endometrium of women using a levonorgestrel-releasing intrauterine system. *Hum Reprod* 13, 1210–1217.

Crowne E C, Moore C, Wallace W H B et al. (1992). A novel variant of growth hormone insufficiency following low dose cranial irradiation. *Clin Endocrinol* 36, 59–68.

Eppig J J, O'Brien M (1996). Development in vitro of mouse oocytes from primordial follicles. *Biol Reprod* 54, 197–207.

Eppig D G, Schroeder A C (1989). Capacity of mouse oocytes from preantral follicles to undergo embryogenesis and development to live young after growth, maturation, and fertilization in vitro. *Biol Reprod* 41, 268–276.

Faddy M J, Gosden R G (1996). A model conforming the decline in follicle numbers to the age of menopause in women. *Hum Reprod* 11, 1484–1486.

Faddy M J, Gosden R G, Edwards R (1983). Ovarian follicle dynamics in mice: a comparative study of three inbred strains and an F1 hybrid. *J Endocrinol* 96, 23–33.

Faddy M J, Gosden R G, Gougeon A, Richardson S J, Nelson J F (1992). Accelerated disappearance of ovarian follicles in mid-life: implications for forecasting menopause. *Hum Reprod* 7, 1342–1346.

Familiari G, Caggiati A, Nottola S A, Ermini M, Di Benedetto M R, Motta P M (1993). Ultrastructure of human ovarian primordial follicles after combination chemotherapy for Hodgkin's disease. *Hum Reprod* 8, 2080–2087.

Fisher B, Cheung A Y (1984). Delayed effect of radiation therapy with or without chemotherapy on ovarian function in women with Hodgkin's disease. *Acta Radiol Oncol* 23, 43–48.

Gosden R G (1990). Restitution of fertility in sterilised mice by transferring primordial ovarian follicles. *Hum Reprod* 5, 117–122.

Gosden R G, Baird D T, Wade J C, Webb R (1994a). Restoration of fertility to oopherectomized sheep by ovarian autografts stored at −196°C. *Hum Reprod* 9, 597–603.

Gosden R G, Boulton M I, Grant K, Webb R (1994b). Follicular development from ovarian xenografts in SCID mice. *J Reprod Fertil* 101, 619–623.

Gosden R G, Wade J C, Fraser H M, Sandow J, Faddy M J (1997a). Impact of congenital and experimental hypogonadism on the radiation sensitivity of the mouse ovary. *Hum Reprod* 12, 2483–2488.

Gosden R G, Rutherford A J, Norfolk D R (1997b). Ovarian banking for cancer patients: transmission of malignant cells in ovarian grafts. *Hum Reprod* 12, 403.

Green D M, Hall B, Zevon A (1989). Pregnancy outcome after treatment for acute lymphoblastic leukaemia during childhood or adolescence. *Cancer* 64, 235–244.

Green S H, Smith A U, Zuckerman S (1956). The number of oocytes in ovarian autografts after freezing and thawing. *J Endocrinol* 13, 333–334.

Greenwald G S, Moor R M (1989). Isolation and preliminary characterization of pig primordial follicles. *J Reprod Fertil* 87, 561–571.

Grundy R, Gosden R G, Hewitt M et al. (2001a). Fertility preservation for children treated for cancer (1): scientific advances and research dilemmas. *Arch Dis Child* 84, 355–359.

Grundy R, Larcher V, Gosden R G et al. (2001b). Personal practice: fertility preservation for children treated for cancer (2); ethics of consent for gamete storage and experimentation. *Arch Dis Child* 84, 360–362.

Guanasena K T, Villines P M, Crister E S, Crister J K (1997). Live births with autologous transplant of cryopreserved mouse ovaries. *Hum Reprod* 12, 101–116.

Hawkins M M (1994). Pregnancy outcome and offspring after childhood cancer. *Br Med J* 309, 1034–1040.

Hawkins M M, Smith R A (1989). Pregnancy outcomes in childhood cancer survivors; probable effect of abdominal irradiation. *Int J Cancer* 43, 399–402.

Hawkins M M, Draper G J, Smith R A (1989). Cancer among 1348 survivors of childhood cancer. *Int J Cancer* 43, 975–978.

Holm K, Laursen E M, Brocks V, Muller J (1995). Pubertal maturation of the internal genitalia: an ultrasound evaluation of 166 healthy girls. *Ultrasound Obstet Gynecol* 6, 155–181.

Hovatta O, Silye R, Kraustz T et al. (1996). Cryopreservation of human ovarian tissue by using dimethylsulphoxide and propandiol-sucrose as cryoprotectants. *Hum Reprod* 11, 1268–1272.

Hudson M M, Greenwald C, Thompson E et al. (1993). Efficacy and toxicity of multi agent chemotherapy and low-dose involved-field radiotherapy in children and adolescents with Hodgkin's disease. *J Clin Oncol* 11, 100–108.

Kim S S, Gosden R G, Radford J A et al. (1999). A model to test the safety of human ovarian tissue transplantation after cryopreservation: xenografts of ovarian tissue from cancer patients into NOD/LtSz-scid mice. [*Annual Meeting of the American Society of Reproductive Medicine*, Toronto, Canada.] *Fertil Steril Suppl* p. 3.

Larsen E C, Loft A, Holm K, Muller J, Brocks V, Anderson A N (2000). Oocyte donation in women cured of cancer with bone marrow transplantation including total body irradiation in adolescence. *Hum Reprod* 15, 1505–1508.

Leporrier M, von Theobald P, Roffe J L, Muller G (1987). A new technique to protect ovarian function in young women undergoing pelvic irradiation. Heterotopic ovarian autotransplantation. *Cancer* 60, 2201–2204.

Li F P, Fine W, Jaffe N, Holmes G E, Holmes F F (1979). Offspring of patients treated for cancer in childhood. *J Natl Cancer Inst* 62, 1193–1197.

Li F P, Gimbrere K, Gelber R D et al. (1987). Outcome of pregnancy in survival of Wilm's tumour. *J Am Med Assoc* 257, 216–219.

Littley M D, Shalet S M, Beardwell C G, Ahmed S R, Applegate G, Sutton M L (1989). Hypopituitarism following external radiotherapy for pituitary tumours in adults. *Q J Med* 70, 145–160.

Livesey E A, Brook C G D (1988). Gonadal dysfunction after treatment of intracranial tumours. *Arch Dis Child* 63, 495–500.

Louis L, Lemaryi L R, Best W R (1956). Treatment of chronic granulocytic leukaemia with myleran. *Arch Int Med* 97, 299–308.

Ludwig M, Al-Hasani S, Felderbaum R, Diedrich K (1999). New aspects of cryopreservation of oocytes and embryos in assisted reproduction and future perspectives. *Hum Reprod* 14, 162–185.

Lushbaugh C C, Casarett G W (1976). The effects of gonadal irradiation in clinical radiation therapy: a review. *Cancer* 37, 1111–1125.

Mackie E J, Radford M, Shalet S M (1996). Gonadal function following chemotherapy for childhood Hodgkin's disease. *Med Pediatr Oncol* 27, 74–78.

Matsumoto M, Shinohara O, Ishiguro H et al. (1999). Ovarian function after bone marrow transplantation performed before menarche. *Arch Dis Child* 80, 452–454.

Marcello M F, Nuciforo G, Romeo R et al. (1990). Structural and ultrastructural study of the ovary in childhood leukaemia after successful treatment. *Cancer* 66, 2099–2104.

Meirow D (1999). Ovarian injury and modern options to preserve fertility in female cancer patients treated with high-dose radio-chemotherapy for haemato-oncological neoplasias and other cancers. *Leuk Lymphoma* 33, 65–76.

(2000). Reproduction post chemotherapy in young cancer patients. *Mol Cell Endocrinol* 169, 123–131.

Meirow D, Nugent D, Epstein M et al. (1998). An in vitro study of the effects of chemotherapy on human primordial follicles. *Hum Reprod* A13.

Mok C C, Lau C S, Wong R W (1998). Risk factors for ovarian failure in patients with systemic lupus erythematosus receiving cyclophosphamide therapy. *Arthritis Rheum* 41, 831–837.

Montz F J, Wolff A J, Gambone J C (1991). Gonadal protection and fecundity rates in cyclophosphamide-treated rats. *Cancer Res* 51, 2124–2126.

Moore H C (2000). Following treatment for breast cancer. The incidence of treatment related amenorrhoea is related to patient age and to the treatment regimen. *Curr Oncol Rep* 2, 587–593.

Morita Y, Perez G I, Paris F et al. (2000). Oocyte apoptosis is suppressed by disruption of the acid sphingomyelinase gene or by sphingosine-1-phosphate therapy. *Nat Med* 6, 1109–1114.

Nicholson H S, Byrne J (1993). Fertility and pregnancy after treatment for cancer during childhood or adolescence. *Cancer* 71, 3392–3399.

Nugent D, Meirow D, Brook P F, Aubard Y, Gosden R G (1997). Transplantation in reproductive medicine: previous experience, present knowledge and future prospects. *Hum Reprod Update* 3, 267–280.

Nygaard R, Clausen N, Simes M A et al. (1991). Reproduction following treatment for childhood leukaemia: a population based prospective cohort study of fertility and offspring. *Med Pediatr Oncol* 19, 459–466.

Oktay K (2001). Ovarian tissue cryopreservation and transplantation: preliminary findings and implications for cancer patients. *Hum Reprod Update* 7, 526–534.

Oktay K, Karlikaya G (2000). Ovarian function after transplantation of frozen, banked, autologous ovarian tissue. *N Engl J Med* 342, 1919.

Oktay K, Nugent D, Newton H, Salha O, Chatterjee P, Gosden R G (1997). Isolation and characterization of primordial follicles from fresh and cryopreserved human ovarian tissue. *Fertil Steril* 67, 481–486.

Oktay K, Newton H, Mullan J, Gosden R G (1998). Development of human primordial follicles to antral stages in SCID/hpg mice stimulated with follicle stimulating hormone. *Hum Reprod* 13, 1133–1138.

Oktay K, Karlikaya G G, Aydin B A (2000a). Ovarian cryopreservation and transplantation: basic aspects. *Mol Cell Endocrinol* 169, 105–108.

Oktay K, Newton H, Gosden R G (2000b). Transplantation of cryopreserved human ovarian tissue results in follicle growth initiation in SCID mice. *Fertil Steril* 73, 599–603.

Oktay K, Economos K, Kan M, Rucinski J, Veeck L, Rosenwaks Z (2001). Endocrine function and oocyte retrieval after autologous transplantation of ovarian cortical strips to the forearm. *J Am Med Assoc* 286, 1490–1493.

Parkes A S, Smith A U (1952). Regeneration of rat ovarian tissue grafted after exposure to low temperatures. *Proc Roy Soc Lond* 140, 455–467.

Parrot D M (1960). The fertility of mice with orthotopic grafts derived from frozen tissue. *J Reprod Fertil* 1, 230–241.

Pasqualini T, Escobar M E, Domene H, Muriel F S, Pavlovsky S, Rivarola M A (1987). Evaluation of gonadal function following long-term treatment for acute lymphoblastic leukaemia in girls. *Am J Pediatr Hematol Oncol* 9, 15–22.

Perez G I, Knudson C M, Leykin L, Korsmeyer S J, Tilly J L (1997). Apoptosis-associated signalling pathways are required for chemotherapy-mediated female germ cell destruction. *Nat Med* 3, 1228–1232.

Perez G I, Maravei D V, Trbovich A M, Cidlowski J A, Tilly J L, Hughes F M Jr (2000). Identification of the potassium-dependent and -independent components of the apoptotic machinery in mouse ovarian germ cells and granulosa cells. *Biol Reprod* 63, 1358–1369.

Porcu E, Fabbri R, Seracchioli R, Ciotti P M, Magrini O, Flamigni C (1997). Birth of a healthy female after intracytoplasmic sperm injection of cryopreserved human oocytes. *Fertil Steril* 68, 724–726.

Radford J A, Leibermann B A, Brison D R et al. (2001). Orthotopic reimplantation of cryopreserved ovarian cortical strips after high-dose chemotherapy for Hodgkin's lymphoma. *Lancet* 357, 1172–1175.

Richardson S J, Senikas V, Nelson J F (1987). Follicular depletion during the menopausal transition: evidence for accelerated loss and ultimate exhaustion. *J Clin Endocrinol Metab* 65, 1231–1237.

Robertson C M, Hawkins M M, Kingston J E (1994). Late deaths and survival after children with cancer: implications for cure. *Br Med J* 309, 162–166.

Roy S K, Greenwald G S (1989). Hormonal requirements for the growth and differentiation of hamster preantral follicles in long-term culture. *J Reprod Fertil* 87, 103–114.

Roy S K, Treacy B J (1993). Isolation and long-term culture of human preantral follicles. *Fertil Steril* 59, 783–790.

Royal College of Obstetricians and Gynaecologists (2000). *Storage of Ovarian and Prepubertal Testicular Tissue: Report of a Working Party*. Royal College of Obstetricians and Gynaecologists, London.

Salooja N, Szydlo R M, Socie G et al. (2001). Pregnancy outcomes after peripheral blood or bone marrow transplantation: a retrospective survey. *Lancet* 358, 271–276.

Sanders J E (1991). The impact of marrow transplant preparation regimens on subsequent growth and development. *Semin Hematol* 28, 244–249.

Sanders J E, Hawley J, Levy W et al. (1996). Pregnancies following high-dose cyclophosphamide with or without high-dose busulfan or total-body irradiation and bone marrow transplantation. *Blood* 87, 3045–3052.

Sanger W G, Olson J H, Sherman J K (1992). Semen cryobanking for men with cancer: criteria change. *Fertil Steril* 58, 1024–1027.

Schimmer A D, Quatermain M, Imrie K et al. (1998). Ovarian function after bone marrow transplantation. *J Clin Oncol* 16, 2359–2363.

Shaw J M, Bowles J, Koopman P, Wood E C, Trounson A O (1996). Fresh and cryopreserved ovarian tissue samples from donors with lymphoma transmit the cancer to graft recipients. *Hum Reprod* 11, 1668–1673.

Shaw J M, Cox S L, Trounson A O, Jenkin G (2000). Evaluation of the long-term function of cryopreserved ovarian grafts in the mouse, implications for human applications. *Mol Cell Endocrinol* 161, 103–110.

Sherman B M, West J H, Korenman S G (1976). The menopausal transition: analysis of LH, FSH, estradiol, and progesterone concentrations during menstrual cycles of older women. *J Clin Endocrinol Metab* 42, 629–636.

Siris E S, Leventhal B G, Vaitukaitis J L (1976). Effects of childhood leukaemia and chemotherapy on puberty and reproductive function in girls. *N Engl J Med* 294, 1143–1146.

Snijders M P, de Goeij A F, Debets-Te Baerts M J, Rousch M J, Koudstaal J, Bosman F T (1992). Immunocytochemical analysis of oestrogen receptors and progesterone receptors in the human uterus throughout the menstrual cycle and after the menopause. *J Reprod Fertil* 94, 363–371.

Spears N, Boland N I, Murray A A, Gosden R G (1994). Mouse oocytes derived from in vitro grown primary ovarian follicles are fertile. *Hum Reprod* 9, 527–532.

Stiller C A (1997). Aetiology and epidemiology. In *Paediatric Oncology: Clinical Practice and Controversies*, 2nd edn, Pinkerton C R, Plowman P N, eds., pp. 3–21. Chapman & Hall, London.

Sy Ortin T T, Shostak C A, Donaldson S S (1990). Gonadal status and reproductive function following treatment for Hodgkin's disease in childhood: the Stanford experience. *Int J Radiat Oncol, Biol, Phys* 304, 1377–1382.

Sztein J M, O'Brie M J, Farley J S, Mobraaten L (1998). Cryopreservation and orthotopic transplantation of mouse ovaries: new approach in gamete banking. *Biol Reprod* 58, 1071–1074.

Teinturier C, Hartmann O, Valteau-Couanet D, Benhamou E, Bougneres P F (1998). Ovarian function after autologous bone marrow transplantation in childhood: high dose busulfan is a major cause of ovarian failure. *Bone Marrow Transplant* 22, 989–994.

Thibaud E, Rodriguez-Macias K, Trivin C, Esperou H, Michon J, Brauner R (1998). Ovarian function after bone marrow transplantation. *Bone Marrow Transplant* 21, 287–290.

Thomas P R, Winstanly D, Peckham M J, Austin D E, Murray M A, Jacobs H S (1976). Reproductive and endocrine function in patients with Hodgkin's disease: effects of oopheropexy and irradiation. *Br J Cancer* 33, 226–231.

Thomson A B, Critchley H O D, Kelnar C J H, Wallace W H B (2002). Late reproductive sequelae following treatment of childhood cancer and options for fertility preservation. Adult sequelae of childhood endocrine disorders. *Baillière's Best Pract Res Clin Endocrinol Metab* 16, 311–334.

Torrance C, Telfer E, Gosden R G (1989). Quantitative study of the development of isolated mouse pre-antral follicles in collagen gel culture. *J Reprod Fertil* 87, 367–374.

Wallace W H B (1997). Growth and endocrine function following the treatment of childhood malignant disease. In *Paediatric Oncology: Clinical Practice and Controversies*, 2nd edn, Pinkerton C R, Plowman P N, eds., pp. 706–731. Chapman & Hall, London.

Wallace W H B, Walker D A (2001). Conference consensus statement: ethical and research dilemmas for fertility preservation in children treated for cancer. *Hum Fertil* 4, 69–76.

Wallace W H, Shalet S M, Crowne E C, Morris-Jones P H, Gattamaneni H R (1989a). Ovarian failure following abdominal irradiation in childhood: natural history and prognosis. *Clin Oncol* 1, 75–79.

Wallace W H, Shalet S M, Hendry J H, Morris-Jones P H, Gattamaneni H R (1989b). Ovarian failure following abdominal irradiation in childhood: The radiosensitivity of the human oocyte. *Br J Radiol* 62, 995–998.

Wallace W H B, Shalet S M, Crowne E C, Morris-Jones P H, Gattamaneni H R, Price D A (1989c). Gonadal dysfunction due to cis-platinum. *Med Pediatr Oncol* 17, 409–413.

Wallace W H, Shalet S M, Tetlow L J, Morris-Jones P H (1993). Ovarian function following the treatment of childhood acute lymphoblastic leukaemia. *Med Pediatr Oncol* 21, 333–339.

Wallace W H B, Blacklay A, Eiser C et al. (2001). Developing strategies for long term follow up of survivors of childhood cancer. *Br Med J* 323, 271–274.

Wallace W H B, Thomson A B, Kelsey T W (2003). The radiosensitivity of the human oocyte. *Hum Reprod* 18, 117–121.

Waxman J H X, Terry Y A, Wrigley P F M et al. (1982). Gonadal function in Hodgkin's disease: long-term follow-up of chemotherapy. *Br Med J* 285, 1612–1613.

Weissman A, Gotlieb L, Colgan T, Jurisicova A, Greenblatt E M, Casper R F (1999). Preliminary experience with subcutaneous human ovarian cortex transplantation in the NOD-SCID mouse. *Biol Reprod* 60, 1462–1467.

Wells S A Jr, Ellis G J, Gunnells J C, Schneider A B, Sherwood L M (1976). Parathyroid autotransplantation in parathyroid hyperplasia. *N Engl J Med* 295, 57–62.

Whitehead E, Shalet S M, Blackledge G, Todd I, Crowther D, Beardwell C G (1983). The effect of combination chemotherapy on ovarian function in women treated for Hodgkin's disease. *Cancer* 52, 988–993.

33

Preservation of fertility before cancer therapy

Helen M. Picton[1] and Anthony J. Rutherford[2]

[1] Academic Unit of Paediatrics, Obstetrics and Gynaecology, University of Leeds, Leeds, UK
[2] Assisted Conception Unit, Leeds General Infirmary, Leeds, UK

Introduction

In recent years, the improvement in the diagnosis, management and treatment of a range of solid and haematological childhood malignancies has led to a marked increase in the chances of long-term survival for a significant number of children and adolescents. However the chemo- and radiotherapies for treating cancers are frequently gonadotoxic and can render patients of either sex and any age temporarily or even permanently infertile. Like the malignant cells that are their intended targets, germ cells are highly susceptible to alkylating agents and platinum compounds used in chemotherapy formulations.

At the present time sperm banking remains the only proven method of fertility preservation for postpubertal boys, although hormonal manipulation and cryopreservation of testicular germ cells are possibilities for the future that could also benefit younger boys. The options for the preservation of female fertility are far more limited.

For girls and young women, mature oocyte freezing has many advantages, but it is unreliable. Most recently, the cryopreservation of immature oocytes in situ in small pieces of ovarian cortex followed by storage at low temperatures has been developed as an option to preserve female fertility before cancer treatment commences. Once the patient is in full remission and wishes to have fertility restored, the gonadal tissue can be thawed and either returned to the body as an autograft or, if there is any risk of reintroducing cancer cells in the graft, it may be possible to grow the gametes contained within the tissue to maturity in vitro. Although gonadal freezing has proved effective experimentally, considerable research effort is required to optimize this new approach for different patient age groups and diagnoses.

Furthermore, the efficiency of transplantation techniques must be improved and the safety of in vitro growth strategies must be fully evaluated before the potential of gonadal cryopreservation can be fully realised.

Clinical application of gonadal cryopreservation

Once an entire population of spermatogonial cells in the testis or primordial follicles in the ovary have been lost they cannot be replaced naturally (Apperley and Reddy, 1995; Brook et al., 2001; Meirow and Schenker, 1995). Furthermore, it appears that the extent of gonadal damage induced by irradiation or chemotherapy depends on the patients' gender, age at the time of treatment, radiation dose and/or fractionation schedule, and the total dose and nature of chemotherapy delivered (Grundy et al., 2001a). In boys, for example, future sperm production is susceptible to damage at very low doses of irradiation (> 1.2 Gy), but as Leydig cell function is usually preserved up to 12 Gy, it is possible for males who have sustained some degree of damage to the germinal epithelium to progress through puberty and remain fertile (Grundy et al., 2001a). In contrast, the human oocyte is sensitive to radiation with the dose of radiation required to destroy 50% of the oocytes (LD_{50}) of less than 4 Gy (Wallace et al., 1989), and uterine irradiation has been shown to reduce the efficacy of assisted reproductive technologies (ART) and increase the incidence of nulliparity, fetal loss and small-for-dates infants (Critchley, 1999; Critchley et al., 1992). In addition to the treatment of cancers, high-dose chemotherapy is also being used to treat an increasing number of nonmalignant conditions such as autoimmune diseases and thalassaemias.

Paediatric and Adolescent Gynaecology, ed. Adam Balen et al. Published by Cambridge University Press.
© Cambridge University Press 2004.

416

As the prospect of surviving into adulthood is increasing for these young patients, so premature gonadal failure or total sterility is becoming increasingly unacceptable. While some clinical and experimental studies have attempted to quantify the likelihood of gonadal failure after cancer treatment (Oktay and Yih, 2002), others have indicated that the gonads can be protected from the late effects of oncology treatments by using oral contraceptives and gonadotrophin-releasing hormone (GnRH) agonists or antagonists before the start of chemo- or radiotherapy (Ataya et al., 1995; Chapman and Sutcliffe, 1981). However, there is conflicting evidence of the benefit of this type of approach (Gosden et al., 1997; Howell and Shalet, 2001) and for the most part the data are unconvincing. The mixed results obtained so far may be explained by study design, and there is evidence that reducing blood flow to the ovaries through GnRH analogue use may be effective for certain chemotherapeutic regimens. In this context, it is of interest that programmed cell death (apoptosis) has now been identified as the mechanism responsible for the loss of oocytes that occurs during the normal process of oogenesis, and the oocyte loss induced by anticancer therapies (Morita et al., 1999, 2000). The capacity to control early events in the apoptosis pathway may be of value in the development of new clinical approaches for protecting the gonads of cancer patients from side-effect damage during treatment. However, it is questionable whether overriding apoptosis in germ cells is sensible, if DNA damage has occurred.

Healthcare professionals are, therefore, faced with the challenge of developing and improving technologies not only to protect the individual's wellbeing but also to conserve the fertility of these young patients. Patients receiving substerilizing doses of chemotherapy or radiotherapy are not normally offered fertility conservation even if they are treated with potentially mutagenic alkylating agents, because there is as yet no evidence of excessive birth defects among children born to former cancer patients (Green et al., 1991). For those individuals at high risk of premature sterility, the development and application of gamete and gonadal tissue cryopreservation in association with ART now provide a means both to preserve their germ cells and to restore natural fertility to young cancer patients as well as to girls who have a familial history of premature ovarian failure.

Currently the treatment options available to preserve the fertility of young patients are limited (Figs. 33.1 and 33.2). The most common approach used to preserve the fertility of pubertal boys and young men is to cryopreserve spermatozoa (Lass et al., 2001). In contrast, for adolescent girls and women, apart from gamete donation and surrogacy, the available options include ovarian transposition (Tulandi and Al-Took, 1998) and the collection of mature oocytes and storage of embryos following in vitro fertilization (IVF; Atkinson et al., 1994; Byrd, 2002). While embryo freezing has been used successfully to treat a limited number of women before cancer treatment, the need for large numbers of mature oocytes for IVF and embryo cryopreservation to be successful necessitates a long protocol of drug stimulation before egg retrieval. This may not be possible, as it could delay the onset of cancer therapy. Additionally, IVF treatment is costly and stressful, requires that the patient have a male partner, carries no guarantee of success, and may create "orphan embryos". What is more, the required ovarian hyperstimulation may be contraindicated in the case of steroid-dependent cancers. Perhaps most importantly, this strategy is only suitable for patients of reproductive age and it is clearly not an option for prepubertal girls. With the recent advances in cryobiology, it is now possible to bank immature germ cells at low temperatures so that they can be potentially reimplanted when it is safe. This strategy could be used to conserve the fertility of young children and young adults of both sexes who are diagnosed with cancer when they are too young to have either started or completed their families. While these new techniques could theoretically provide the complete restoration of natural fertility, more realistically they will provide a fertile window of opportunity that will enable an individual to parent a child genetically related to themselves. Options for preserving the fertility of young oncology patients, therefore, range from no medical intervention at all to the use of invasive procedures to harvest tissues or isolate cells. Each method has its own advantages, disadvantages and risks.

While there remains uncertainty amongst professionals on how optimally to preserve the fertility of young patients, there are also specific psychological concerns about the extent to which adolescents should be involved in the decision-making process, and what treatments are available (Grundy et al., 2001b). For young children, the issue of parental consent made on the child's behalf raises problems in deciding what is likely to be in the child's best interests both in the short and the long term. To enable the best advice and care to be given to children undergoing cancer treatments, parents and clinicians must be supported by a close liaison between paediatric oncologists, reproductive medicine specialists and counsellors. This requires evidence derived from multidisciplinary clinical trials involving the long-term follow-up of patients receiving this type of treatment, combined with regular audit of the procedures involved. Clinical guidelines need to be established for the least toxic but effective treatment regimens, appropriate volume of tissue collected and optimal methods of

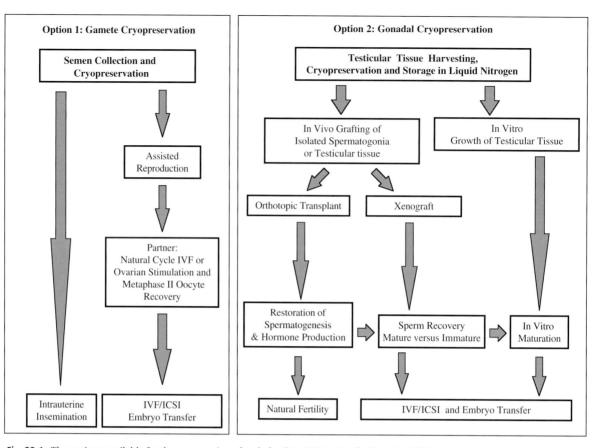

Fig. 33.1. The options available for the preservation of male fertility. IVF, in vitro fertilization; ICSI, intracytoplasmic sperm injection.

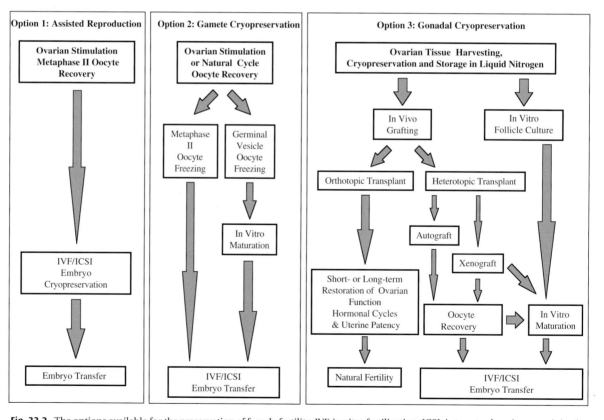

Fig. 33.2. The options available for the preservation of female fertility. IVF, in vitro fertilization; ICSI, intracytoplasmic sperm injection.

Table 33.1. Summary of principles and practices of equilibration and vitrification protocols for cryopreservation of tissues and cells

Equilibration protocols	Vitrification protocols
Slow	Ultrarapid
Extracellular ice formed	Amorphous glass formed
Moderate concentration of cryoprotective agents used	High concentrations of cryoprotective agents used
Expensive apparatus required	No expensive apparatus required
Commonly used for both isolated cells and complex tissues	Used for isolated cells, recently applied to complex tissues
Sealed tubes most commonly used for tissue storage	Both straws and cryoloops used for isolated cells
Protocols require further optimization to improve efficiency for different cell types	Protocols require further optimization to improve efficiency for different cell types
Safety implications for tissue storage in liquid nitrogen apply	Safety implications for tissue storage in liquid nitrogen apply
Storage and handling relatively easy	Freeze fracture of straw/vial contents can occur in storage vessel; storage and handling, therefore, more difficult

storage. Continued research is essential for the development of this new technology.

The principles of cryopreservation

An in depth understanding of the principles and practices of cryopreservation is fundamental to the development of strategies designed to preserve fertility (Pegg, 2002). Cryopreservation protocols for gametes and gonadal tissue can be broadly classified as slow freezing (equilibration protocols) or rapid freezing (vitrification protocols) (Lane et al., 1999; Martino et al., 1996; Rall, 1987; Rall and Fahy, 1985; Vajta et al., 1998) according to the cooling rates and cryoprotective agents (CPAs) used (Table 33.1). While both protocols have been used to freeze mature oocytes, slow freezing protocols are most commonly used to preserve sperm and gonadal tissues. The basic concepts of slow and rapid freezing protocols are the same, as they both aim to protect the cells from the effects of intracellular ice crystal formation, cellular dehydration and drastic changes in solute concentrations at both high and low temperatures (Pegg, 2002). Fundamentally, gamete cryopreservation requires that cells tolerate three nonphysiological conditions: exposure to molar concentrations of CPAs, cooling to subzero temperatures and, finally, removal or conversion of almost all liquid cell water into the solid state. On thawing, most protocols stipulate that gametes and gonadal tissues are thawed rapidly and the CPA is progressively diluted from the tissue by repeated rinses with fresh medium. In general, the cryopreservation procedures used for the slow freezing of oocytes and ovarian cortex are very similar to the procedures designed for storage of cleavage stage embryos.

The freeze storage of spermatozoa, isolated oocytes and ovarian tissue is subject to the usual safety concerns of long-term banking of tissues in liquid nitrogen. Because of the known risks of viral transmission in nitrogen storage tanks (Tedder et al., 1995), it is preferable that patients should be screened for blood-borne viral diseases prior to tissue storage. The possibility of the long-term storage of gonadal tissues from paediatric patients also raises the question of how long banked tissues and gametes should be stored. Little is known about the long-term consequences of cryopreserving ovarian tissue, or oocytes, although semen storage has a proven safety record. In the case of ovarian tissue storage for young cancer patients it is important to ensure that the patient (or guardian) consents to an upper time limit for storage and also to the disposal of tissue in the event of death or mental incapacitation.

Options for fertility preservation in males

The most prevalent malignancies in boys and young men of reproductive age are Hodgkin's disease, testicular cancer and leukaemia. Using modern diagnostic tools and a combination of surgery, chemotherapy and/or radiotherapy, many of these malignancies can be treated successfully. However, these oncological therapies commonly cause testicular dysfunction, as the testis and spermatogenesis are particularly susceptible to cytotoxic damage (Howell and Shalet, 2001). While there is evidence in some cases that the natural fertility of boys and adolescents may not be compromised by cancer treatment (Lass et al., 2001), a majority of these young patients will require fertility preservation in association with ART to enable them to father their own genetic children as spermatogenesis will be compromised. Although DNA damage occurs in spermatozoa immediately following cancer treatments, there is no evidence of an increase in genetic defects or congenital malformations among children conceived naturally to parents who have previously undergone chemotherapy or radiotherapy

(Arnon et al., 2001). However, where the reduction in semen count is such that micromanipulation techniques need to be employed, the risks to the children remains to be quantified. The options available for the conservation of fertility in boys and adolescents have been summarized in Fig. 33.1.

Sperm cryopreservation

Semen banking can be offered to postpubertal boys and young men to preserve their fertile potential prior to cancer treatments. It appears that the procedures routinely used for sperm cryopreservation are not likely to induce structural abnormalities in the frozen gametes or result in altered sex ratios in the offspring produced using frozen–thawed sperm (Leibo et al., 2002). Furthermore, it has been shown that spermatozoa do not deteriorate even when stored for decades in liquid nitrogen (Leibo et al., 1994). Although there is still inherent variability in the level of survival after thawing of spermatozoa from different individuals (Leibo et al., 2002), at the practical level, the advent of intracytoplasmic sperm injection (ICSI) (Palermo et al., 1992) has provided a treatment option even when semen quality is poor after freeze storage. Unfortunately, despite the routine nature of sperm cryopreservation (Agca and Crister, 2002), there may be insufficient time to bank sperm, or even a failure to provide a suitable sample for freezing before the onset of cancer therapy. An alternative for postpubertal boys, which provides acceptable pregnancy rates, is to freeze–thaw testicular spermatozoa obtained after testicular biopsy followed by ICSI (Küpker et al., 2002). Storage of mature spermatozoa is clearly not an option for prepubertal boys, and although testicular biopsy is possible in this younger age group, spermatocytes are only sparsely present in prepubertal testes so relatively large biopsy specimens are required. This option would need careful consideration as there is a significant risk of compromising future testicular endocrine function (Schlegel and Su, 1997).

Cryopreservation of spermatogonia

A more radical approach, which can be applied to both men and young boys, is to preserve spematogonial stem cells rather than mature sperm. Autologous germ cell transplantation of the frozen–thawed spermatogonia could then be used to restore fertility. This means that the patient's own stem cells could be used to repopulate the testis when he has returned to full health and wishes to start a family. The concept of autologous germ cell transplantation is possible in boys and young men because in males the germ cells continue to proliferate and enter into meiosis in the postpubertal adult. This is in marked contrast to the

situation in the ovary, where the full complement of oocytes are established early in fetal life and meiosis is arrested at the diplotene stage of meiosis I in all of the female gametes. In males, the undifferentiated diploid germ cells, the "A" spermatogonia, are located at the basement membrane of the seminiferous tubules in the testis and they develop into differentiating spermatogonia when they undergo several cycles of mitosis. Since the gonadotoxic effects of chemo- or radiotherapies appear to target the spermatogonia, in oncological patients the development of techniques for spermatogonia recovery, cryopreservation and transplantation might be considered a means to preserve testicular function in pre-, peri- and postpubertal patients. However, it is important to consider the optimal timing of testicular biopsy in these cases.

In support of this idea, successful male germ cell transplantation has been reported in laboratory rodents and primates (Schlatt et al., 1999, 2000). In mice, the infusion of either fresh or cryopreserved germ cell preparation into the seminiferous tubules of infertile hosts has led to the repopulation of the testis with donor germ cells and so restored fertility (Schlatt et al., 2000). Results from murine studies show that fertility can be restored to busulphan-sterilized mice after microinjection of suspensions of crude germ cells or spermatogonia, either freshly harvested or frozen–thawed, into the seminiferous tubules at the surface of the testis (Avarbock et al., 1996; Brinster and Avarbock, 1994; Brook et al., 2001). Restoration of donor spermatogenesis was reported in 18% of the genetically germ cell-deficient recipient mice and in 38% of the busulfan-treated mice with the birth of live offspring (Avarbock et al., 1996; Brinster and Avarbock, 1994). Additionally, the xenografic transfer of rat germ cells into mouse testis resulted in the initiation of rat spermatogenesis in mouse testis (Clouthier et al., 1996).

A similar protocol of germ cell transplantation has recently been developed and applied to the restoration of fertility in men (Brook et al., 2001; Hovatta, 2001; Radford et al., 1999; Schlatt et al., 1999). Brook et al. (2001) and Schlatt et al. (1999) have both shown that crude suspensions of spermatogonial stem cells can be extracted from human seminiferous tubules and successfully cryopreserved using protocols that are similar to those used to preserve human ovarian cortex. Following freeze–thaw, these stem cells can be transplanted back into the testis where they migrate to the adluminal compartment of the testis and so restore spermatogenesis. Preliminary results suggest that reimplantation can be achieved by gravity feed into the rete testis, under standard operating room conditions, with the use of ultrasonography to localize the rete testis and the injection needle for guidance in the infusion of germ cells (Brook et al., 2001; Schlatt et al., 1999). The results from all the three species tested so far suggest that successful reimplantation of the testis can only be achieved in either partially involuted or pubertal testes as the back pressure of fluid in fully active testis blocks the deep infusion of the suspension of spermatogonia into the tubules (Brook et al., 2001; Schlatt et al., 1999). This physiological state can be induced in adults by using GnRH agonist or antagonist pretreatment to involute the testes prior to germ cell transplantation. Although it is hoped that this approach will reestablish normal spermatogenesis with the production of mature spermatozoa in vivo, in reality it may still be necessary to use ART to restore fertility.

While germ cell transfer is one way to safeguard the fertility of boys, a simpler alternative to restore spermatogenesis in vivo is to autograft seminiferous tubules from frozen–thawed testicular biopsies. By this approach, it may be possible to obtain sufficient mature spermatozoa for fertilization by ICSI (Gosden and Nagano, 2002).

While germ cell multiplication and differentiation are necessary after cryopreservation and transplantation, they are not sufficient alone to assure restoration of fertility; quality control, protection from environmental damage and elimination of defective cells are also required (Gosden and Nagano, 2002). The successful development of testicular cryopreservation and transplantation as a means to preserve the fertility of young boys, therefore, requires that sophisticated methods are developed that allow in vitro multiplication and manipulation of male germ cell lines. These would support both cryopreservation and in vitro growth of testicular tissue and isolated spermatogonia through the coculture of germ cells and Sertoli cells prior to transplantation. In addition, techniques to assist in the isolation and enrichment of spermatogonia suspensions (Schlatt et al., 2000) prior to either culture or transplantation should be developed. This approach will help to improve the efficiency and hence the success of male germ cell transplantation. Finally, the risk of reimplanting malignant cells in the cryopreserved cell suspension, especially in the case of haematological disease, should not be overlooked. Consequently, techniques should be developed to enable the identification of even small numbers of malignant cells in the suspensions before transplantation.

Options for fertility preservation in females

The unique architecture and the physiology of the ovary make the female gonad particularly susceptible to damage through exposure to contemporary cancer treatments. The documented late effects of pelvic irradiation with or without treatment with alkylating chemotherapy agents for young female patients include reduced pregnancy rates and a high risk of ovarian failure, particularly in women over the age of 30 years (Gosden and Nagano, 2002; Meirow and Nugent, 2001). While cytotoxic-induced damage may be reversible in tissues of rapidly dividing cells such as bone marrow and gastrointestinal tract, it appears to be progressive and irreversible in the ovary, where the number of oocytes is limited, fixed since fetal life, and cannot be regenerated. The fate of follicles in vivo is naturally determined by a balance between survival factors, apoptosis-inducing factors and intracellular mediators of cell survival. When the reserve of follicles, and their contained oocytes, has been exhausted, menopause ensues. On average, this would occur naturally in women around the age of 51 years. This heralds a major life change, with the abrupt losses of ovarian oestrogens, leading to increased risks of a number of debilitating health problems, including cardiovascular disease, osteoporosis and neurological dysfunction. Cancer therapies in young women and girls greatly accelerate oocyte depletion and can result in complete sterilization or premature ovarian failure, with loss of reproductive potential and the onset of these menopause-related health problems (Critchley et al., 1992). Therefore, these young patients may face a future of lifelong hormone replacement therapy as a consequence of their successful cancer treatment.

Oktay and Yih (2002) have reviewed the childhood/youth cancer types where treatment places females at the greatest risk of ovarian failure after chemotherapy, radiotherapy or bone marrow transplantation. These include leukaemia, neuroblastoma, Hodgkin's lymphoma, osteosarcoma, Ewing's sarcoma, Wilms' tumour and nonHodgkin's lymphoma. The authors have also attempted to qualify the relative risks of ovarian metastasis in these childhood/youth diseases. Others have attempted to quantify the relative risk of ovarian failure by different classes of chemotherapy agent and radiation treatment (Table 33.2) (Arnon et al., 2001, Meirow and Nugent, 2001). The risk of premature loss of ovarian function is increased in older patients, who naturally have a reduced ovarian reserve, and is dependent on the type of chemotherapy agent or dose of radiation used to treat the cancer. Where there is a risk of partial or complete ovarian failure following cancer treatment, oocytes and/or ovarian tissue can now be cryopreserved for the patients' later use. The options available for the preservation of female fertility are summarized in Fig. 33.2.

Mature oocyte storage

Mature oocyte freezing has the potential to be an important adjunct to ART in adults and, if successful, has many

Table 33.2. The childhood/youth cancers types where treatment places females at the greatest risk of ovarian failure after chemotherapy, radiotherapy or bone marrow transplantation, but for which patients have a high survival rate

Disease	Relative risk of ovarian failure %	Relative risk of ovarian involvement
Leukaemia	15	High
Neuroblastoma	–	High
Hodgkin's lymphoma	32	Low
NonHodgkin's lymphoma	44	Low
Osteogenic sarcoma	–	Low
Ewing's sarcoma	–	Low
Wilms' tumour	–	Low
Breast cancer	50	Moderate
Adenocarcinoma of uterine cervix	–	Moderate

Source: Data taken from Meirow and Nugent (2001) and Oktay and Yih (2002).

advantages for adolescents and young women at risk of ovarian failure (Paynter, 2000). However, the ease and success of cryopreservation programmes for sperm (Agca and Crister, 2002; Leibo et al., 2002; Trounson and Dawson, 1996) and embryos (Trounson and Dawson, 1996) contrast markedly with the problems associated with freezing human oocytes, as these cells are large and fragile (Shaw et al., 2000). Despite numerous attempts, the results of oocyte freezing are disappointing. The technology has proved unreliable, and few babies have been born worldwide using this method (Picton et al., 2002a). Furthermore, conventional superovulation is required to obtain a large enough cohort of follicles, and oocytes. This process can take precious time to complete as it has to be programmed to the woman's menstrual cycle.

Overall, the results of numerous clinical studies confirm that the survival of human oocytes after cryopreservation can be affected by their stage of maturation, their "quality" and by biophysical factors resulting from the cryopreservation procedures used (Picton et al., 2002; Shaw et al., 2000). Morphological factors such as the presence or absence of the cumulus granulosa cells during the freezing process may also have a direct impact on oocyte survival after thawing. Despite these problems, both denuded and cumulus-enclosed oocytes have been successfully frozen in straws or ampoules after a period of equilibration in an aqueous solution of CPAs and osmolyte(s) (Imoedehme and Sigue, 1992; Ludwig et al., 1999; Picton et al., 2002).

Most of the difficulties encountered in mature oocyte freezing can be attributed to the biological character-

istics of this unique cell. Mature human oocytes show great heterogeneity in the distribution and organization of cytoplasmic organelles as well as their nuclear material. Metaphase II oocytes are particularly vulnerable to cryo-injury because the meiotic spindle, on which the chromosomes align, is acutely temperature sensitive (Al-Hasani and Diedrich, 1995; Gook et al., 1993; Pickering et al., 1990; Vincent and Johnson, 1992; Zenzes et al., 2001). Furthermore, precocious cortical granule release and premature zona hardening can occur in metaphase II oocytes as a direct result of the freeze–thaw process. While this combination of events will undoubtedly compromise normal fertilization, disruption of the cytoskeletal architecture may also lead to abnormal cytokinesis, retention of the second polar body and alterations in the organization and trafficking of molecules and organelles as well as to chromosomal aneuploidies. Alteration in calcium influx and membrane damage can lead to increased incidence of parthenogenetic activation.

The deleterious effects of chilling on the cytoskeleton of metaphase II oocytes can be avoided by cryopreservation of oocytes at the germinal vesicle stage of maturation. These oocytes can be collected using a modification of the conventional oocyte pickup procedure, from small antral stage follicles found in most abundance in the mid-follicular phase of the menstrual cycle. However, at present, the difficulties associated with in vitro maturation of oocytes and their extended culture appear to counteract the potential benefits of oocyte freezing at the germinal vesicle stage. Only a modest number of pregnancies have been achieved after in vitro maturation of human oocytes and even fewer after the initial attempts to cryopreserve full-sized germinal vesicles containing oocytes (Cha et al., 2000). Therefore, for now, cryopreservation of germinal vesicle oocytes offers little or no advantage over that of metaphase II oocytes.

Despite the many potential difficulties associated with mature oocyte banking, recent modifications to both slow freezing (Fabbri et al., 2001) and vitrification protocols (Kuleshova et al., 1999; Yoon et al., 2000) have improved success rates of oocyte cryopreservation and resulted in a resurgence of interest in this technology. However, until these breakthroughs have been fully evaluated and proved to be reliable, metaphase II and germinal vesicle oocyte banking cannot be justified as the sole option for young cancer patients who have only one chance of an oocyte collection before commencing a potentially sterilizing cancer therapy. The development of protocols for this group of patients that optimize the survival, fertilization and developmental rates of fully grown oocytes following exposure to the extreme chemical and physical stresses associated with cryopreservation remains a major challenge.

Immature oocyte storage

An alternative approach to mature oocyte cryopreservation involves the freeze-storage of the outer most layer of the ovary, the ovarian cortex, which contains the earliest staged oocytes within primordial follicles. The primordial follicles and the primordial oocytes they contain represent the reserve from which all preovulatory follicles and mature oocytes will ultimately develop. Ironically, while primordial oocytes are highly susceptible to cytotoxic damage induced by cancer treatments, they also appear to be far less vulnerable to cryo-injury than mature oocytes as they are smaller, lack a zona pellucida and cortical granules, and are relatively metabolically quiescent and undifferentiated. Additionally, primordial follicles are apparently more tolerant to insults such as immersion in CPA solutions and cooling to very low temperatures as their small size makes them less susceptible to damage induced by water movements into and out of the cells during freezing and thawing. Finally, primordial oocytes have more time to repair sublethal damage to organelles and other structures during their prolonged growth phase after thawing. Ovarian cortex contains tens to hundreds of thousands of primordial and primary follicles, depending on the mass of tissue and age of the patient (Faddy et al., 1992) (Fig. 33.3). This tissue can be harvested, either by laparoscopy or laparotomy, in small biopsies or by removal of a whole ovary. The suitability of ovarian tissue for freezing is enhanced by the developmental plasticity of the tissue, as the ovary is capable of functioning even when its complement of follicles has been severely reduced: as naturally occurs during ageing or can occur after partial ablation or injury. The practice of banking primordial follicles in situ, in strips of ovarian cortex, offers the potential to restore natural fertility and conception by autografting the thawed tissue to an orthotopic site, or employing ART after grafting to a heterotopic site (Meirow, 1999; Oktay et al., 2001a). Alternatively, the primordial follicles can be theoretically grown to maturity in vitro (Picton and Gosden, 2000).

Unlike the cryopreservation of isolated cells, freeze-storage of ovarian tissue presents new problems because of the complexity of the tissue architecture. Ovarian freezing protocols must, therefore, strike a balance between the optimal conditions required for each different cell type. Nonetheless, despite the apparent difficulties, the storage of ovarian tissue has proved surprisingly successful, and a number of reports have demonstrated that human primordial follicles can survive cryopreservation after slow cooling to $-196\,^\circ$C in liquid nitrogen (Gosden et al., 1994; Gunasena et al., 1997; Newton et al., 1996, 1998; Oktay and Karlikaya, 2000; Oktay et al., 1998a; Picton et al., 2000; Radford et al.,

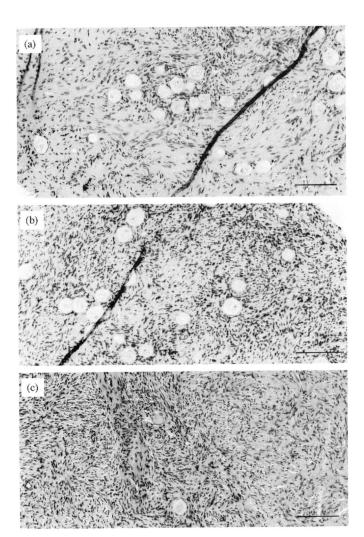

Fig. 33.3. Illustration of the decline in the follicle reserve with advancing ovarian age in human ovarian cortex. Histological preparations of ovarian cortex from a 12-year-old girl (a) and a 17-year-old woman (b), both showing clusters of primordial follicles in the ovarian cortex. (c) A 31-year-old woman where primordial follicles are indicated by the presence of a circular oocyte surrounded by flattened pregranulosa cells. Scale bar represents 100 μm. IVF, in vitro fertilization; ICSI, intracytoplasmic sperm injection.

2001). The current options for the storage of primordial follicles include intact isolated primordial follicles, thin slices of the ovarian cortex (Gosden et al., 1994; Newton et al., 1996; Oktay and Karlikaya, 2000; Radford et al., 2001) and, perhaps more controversially, whole ovary cryopreservation (Revel et al., 2001; Wang et al., 2002). Although yet to be fully optimized, the most commonly used clinical practices involve oophorectomy and removal of the ovarian cortex as thin slices 1–2 mm thick or as multiple ovarian biopsies (Meirow et al., 1999). The tissue is frozen employing a programmed cryostat and a slow-freezing technique, before transfer to nitrogen storage tanks. Like sperm and embryos, it is thought that ovarian tissue can be safely stored in liquid nitrogen for as long as required. Using the slow-freezing approach, it is possible to obtain high acute post-thaw follicle survival rates of 84% and 74% for frozen–thawed human primordial follicles (Newton et al., 1996; Newton et al., 1998) with normal tissue morphology at both light microscopy (Gook et al., 1999) and electron microscopy (Picton et al., 2000) levels. However, it is also clear that the choice of an inappropriate CPA together with poor laboratory practice can lead to extensive cellular damage, which will compromise tissue viability on thawing (Picton et al., 2000). There is a clear need to audit ovarian freezing practices and to develop long term functionality tests such as xenografting (Kim et al., 2001; Oktay et al., 1998b) and/or tissue culture (Picton and Gosden, 2000) to assess the post-thaw survival and developmental potential of cryopreserved ovarian tissue.

While it is relatively easy and cheap to store ovarian tissue, experience suggests that far greater technical problems will be encountered when the stored tissue is thawed and used to restore fertility. On the basis of both animal experiments (Gosden et al., 1994; Kim et al., 2001; Oktay et al., 1998b; Wang et al., 2002) and recent clinical studies (Oktay and Karlikaya, 2000; Oktay et al., 2001b; Radford et al., 2001), it is likely that the first cases of successful fertility restoration using cryopreserved ovarian tissue will be achieved by heterotopic or orthotopic autografting. None of these recent reports was ideal to judge the full potential of ovarian cryopreservation and autografting as a means of restoring fertility, and this whole approach must still be considered experimental until the optimal site for grafting has been identified and a pregnancy achieved. While many questions about the validity of ovarian cryopreservation have yet to be answered, there is little doubt that the lifespan of the grafted tissue will be affected by follicle density, patient age at the time of cryopreservation and prior exposure to chemo- or radiotherapies. Graft longevity will be further reduced by follicle losses associated with freeze–thaw injury and ischaemia following the grafting procedure (Nugent et al., 1997, 1998). Finally, it is important to bear in mind that radiotherapy can also damage the uterus, in a dose-dependent manner, preventing successful implantation.

One significant concern in autografting tissue removed before cancer treatment is the potential for the stored ovarian tissue to contain malignant cells, which may result in reintroduction of the original malignancy (Kim et al., 2001; Shaw and Trounson, 1997). Selectively transplanting tissue where there is a very low risk of ovarian metastasis reduces the possibility of disease transmission (Oktay and Yih, 2002). Safer alternative approaches, such as xenografting the tissue into a secondary host followed by oocyte harvest and ART (Oktay et al., 1998b), or growth of follicles to maturity in vitro (Picton and Gosden, 2000), are also theoretically possible. Following fertilization by IVF or ICSI, embryos, free from contamination, could then be transferred back to the patient. In support of this concept, xenografting has been successfully used as a research tool to investigate the developmental potential of frozen–thawed human ovarian tissues (Oktay et al., 1998b) and may offer some advantages over in vitro follicle culture. However, xenografting may never be an acceptable therapeutic option on ethical grounds; in addition, there is the potential risk of interspecies viral transfer. Much hope, therefore, rests on human follicle culture, particularly as encouraging results suggest that it may soon be possible to grow follicles to antral stages after cryopreservation (Picton and Gosden, 2000). Nevertheless, a considerable amount of research is needed to confirm that gonadal cryopreservation followed by extended follicle culture to maturity is in itself a safe procedure and that it does not induce epigenetic alterations in the oocytes (Duranthon and Renard, 2001; Reik and Walter, 2001; Young and Fairburn, 2000).

Future prospects of fertility conservation

Cryo-storage of gonadal tissue, spermatogonias and mature oocyte has enormous potential as means to treat, restore or prolong fertility of young patients with cancer. However, these technologies are still in their infancy and continued research and ethical scrutiny are required to ensure they do not carry greater risks than freezing spermatozoa and embryos. Improved efficiency of gonadal cryopreservation strategies will only be achieved through intense research effort aimed at increasing the survival rates and development potential of the gametes. While encouraging, the results of gonadal transplantation experiments in animals should not be extrapolated directly to the treatment of humans with cancer. Furthermore, while the viability and functionality of frozen–thawed and transplanted gonadal tissue has been demonstrated in both humans and animal species, the longevity of such transplants in humans is unknown. The timing of gonadal autografting for the restoration of a cancer survivor's fertility is, therefore, critical and should, at the present time, be limited to the acute period of time needed to grow and mature gametes in vivo, to provide the patient with a fertile window. Future research must also focus on testing the safety of these new procedures to ensure that genetically and epigenetically normal embryos and offspring are created from cryopreserved germ cells grown to maturity in vitro or in vivo after grafting (Clyde et al., 2001; Cobo et al., 2001; Márquez et al., 1998). Until such time, the development of techniques to screen the gonadal tissue for the presence of residual disease and so protect the cancer survivor from exposure to occult metastatic cells, if fertility is to be restored through tissue transplantation, remains a priority. Xenotransplantation into secondary hosts, while unacceptable therapeutically, may be a valuable way of screening cryopreserved gonadal tissue for the presence of disease (Kim et al., 2001; Oktay et al., 1998b). If reliable pharmacological alternatives become available, the relative advantages and risks of these treatments versus cryopreservation for preserving genetic parenthood will need to be reassessed.

REFERENCES

Agca Y, Crister J K (2002). Cryopreservation of spermatozoa in assisted reproduction. *Semin Reprod Med* 20, 15–24.

Al-Hasani S, Diedrich K (1995). Oocyte storage. In *Gametes: The Oocyte*, Grudzinskas J G, Yovich J L, eds., Ch. 15. Cambridge, UK: Cambridge University Press.

Apperley J F, Reddy N (1995). Mechanisms and management of treatment related gonadal failure in recipients of high dose chemoradiotherapy. *Blood Rev* 9, 93–116.

Arnon J, Meirow D, Lewis-Roness H, Ornoy A (2001). Genetic and teratogenic effects of cancer treatments on gametes and embryos. *Hum Reprod Update* 7, 36–45.

Ataya K, Rao L V, Lawrence E, Kimmel R (1995). Luteinizing hormone-releasing hormone agonist inhibits cyclophosphamide-induced ovarian follicular depletion in rhesus monkeys. *Biol Reprod* 52, 365–372.

Atkinson H G, Apperley J F, Dawson K, Goldman J M, Winston R M L (1994). Successful pregnancy after embryo cryopreservation after BMT for CML. *Lancet* 344, 199.

Avarbock M R, Brinster C J, Brinster R L (1996). Reconstitution of spermatogenesis from frozen spermatogonial stem cells. *Nat Med* 2, 693–696.

Brinster R L, Avarbock M R (1994). Germline transmission of donor haplotype following spermatogonial transplantation. *Proc Natl Acad Sci USA* 91, 11303–11307.

Brook P F, Radford J A, Shalet S M, Joyce A D, Gosden R G (2001). Isolation of germ cells from human testicular tissue for low temperature storage and autotransplantation. *Fertil Steril* 75, 269–274.

Byrd W (2002). Cryopreservation, thawing, and transfer of human embryos. *Semin Reprod Med* 20, 37–44.

Cha K Y, Chung H M, Lim J M et al. (2000). Freezing immature oocytes. *Mol Cell Endocrinol* 169, 43–47.

Chapman R M, Sutcliffe S B (1981). Protection of ovarian function by oral contraceptives in women receiving chemotherapy for Hodgkin's disease. *Blood* 58, 849–851.

Clouthier D E, Avarbock M R, Maika S D, Hammer R E, Brinster R L (1996). Rat spermatogenesis in mouse testis. *Nature* 381, 418–421.

Clyde J, Gosden R G, Rutherford A J, Picton H M (2001). Demonstration of a mechanism of aneuploidy in human oocytes using Multifluor fluorescence *in situ* hybridisation. *Fertil Steril* 76, 837–840.

Cobo A, Rubio C, Gerli S, Ruiz A, Pellicer A, Remohi J (2001). Use of fluorescent in situ hybridisation to assess the chromosomal status of embryos obtained from cryopreserved oocytes. *Fertil Steril* 75, 354–360.

Critchley H O (1999). Factors of importance for implantation. *Med Pediatr Oncol* 33, 9–14.

Critchley H O, Wallace W H, Shalet S M, Mamtola H, Higginson J, Anderson D C (1992). Abdominal irradiation in childhood; the potential for pregnancy. *Br J Obstet Gynaecol* 99, 392–394.

Duranthon D, Renard J P (2001). The developmental competence of mammalian oocytes: a convenient but biologically fuzzy concept. *Theriogenology* 55, 1277–1289.

Fabbri R, Porcu E, Marsella T, Rocchetta G, Venturoli S, Flamigni C (2001). Human oocyte cryopreservation: new perspectives regarding oocyte survival. *Hum Reprod* 16, 411–416.

Faddy M J, Gosden R G, Gougeon A, Richardson S J, Nelson J F (1992). Accelerated disappearance of ovarian follicles in mid-life: implications for forecasting menopause. *Hum Reprod* 7, 1342–1346.

Gook D A, Osborn S M, Johnston W I (1993). Cryopreservation of mouse and human oocytes using 1,2-propanediol and the configuration of the meiotic spindle. *Hum Reprod* 8, 1101–1109.

Gook D A, Edgar D H, Stern C (1999). Effect of cooling and dehydration on the histological appearance of human ovarian cortex following cryopreservation in 1,2-propanediol. *Hum Reprod* 14, 2061–2068.

Gosden R G, Nagano M (2002). Preservation of fertility in nature and ART. *Reproduction* 123, 3–11.

Gosden R G, Baird D T, Wade J C, Webb R (1994). Restoration of fertility in oophorectomised sheep by ovarian autografts stored at −196°C. *Hum Reprod* 9, 597–603.

Gosden R G, Wade J C, Fraser H M, Sandow J, Faddy M J (1997). Impact of congenital or experimental hypogonadotrophism on the radiation sensitivity of the mouse ovary. *Hum Reprod* 12, 2483–2488.

Green D M, Zevon M A, Lowrie G, Seigelstein N, Hall B (1991). Congenital abnormalities in children of patients who received chemotherapy for cancer treatment in childhood and adolescence. *N Engl J Med* 325, 141–146.

Grundy R, Gosden R G, Hewitt M et al. (2001a). Fertility preservation for children treated for cancer (1): scientific advances and research dilemmas. *Arch Dis Child* 84, 355–359.

Grundy R, Larcher V, Gosden R G et al. (2001b). Fertility preservation for children treated for cancer (2): ethics of consent for gamete storage and experimentation. *Arch Dis Child* 84, 360–362.

Gunasena K T, Villines P M, Critser E S, Critser J K (1997). Live births after autologous transplant of cryopreserved mouse ovaries. *Hum Reprod* 12, 101–106.

Hovatta O (2001). Cryopreservation of testicular tissue in young cancer patients. *Hum Reprod Update* 7, 20–25.

Howell S J, Shalet S M (2001). Testicular function following chemotherapy. *Hum Reprod Update* 7, 5–11.

Imoedehme D G, Sigue A B (1992). Survival of human oocytes cryopreserved with or without the cumulus in 1,2–propanediol. *J Asst Reprod Genet* 9, 323–322.

Kim S S, Radford J, Harris M et al. (2001). Ovarian tissue harvested from lymphoma patients to preserve fertility may be safe for autotransplantation. *Hum Reprod* 16, 2056–2060.

Kuleshova L, Gianaroli L, Magli C, Ferraretti A, Trounson A (1999). Birth following vitrification of a small number of human oocytes: case report. *Hum Reprod* 14, 3077–3079.

Küpker W, Al-Hasani S, Johannisson R et al. (2002). The use of cryopreserved mature and immature testicular spermatozoa for intracytoplasmic sperm injection: risks and limitations. *Semin Reprod Med* 2, 25–36.

Lane M, Bavister B D, Lyons E A, Forest K T (1999). Containerless vitrification of mammalian oocytes and embryos-adapting a proven method for flash-cooling protein crystals to the cryopreservation of live cells. *Nat Biotechnol* 17, 1234–1236.

Lass A, Akagbosu F, Brinsden P (2001). Sperm banking and assisted reproduction treatment for couples following cancer treatment of the male partner. *Hum Reprod* Update 7, 12–19.

Leibo S P, Semple M E, Kroetsch T G (1994). In vitro fertilization of oocytes by 37-year-old bovine spermatozoa. *Theriogenology* 42, 1257–1262.

Leibo S P, Gosden R G, Picton H M (2002). Current status of the cryopreservation of human spermatozoa. In *Medical, Social and Ethical Aspects of Assisted Reproduction*, WHO Technical Bulletin. World Health Organization, Geneva.

Ludwig M, Al-Hasani S, Felberbaum R, Diedrich K (1999). New aspects of cryopreservation of oocytes and embryos in assisted reproduction and future perspectives. *Hum Reprod* 14(Suppl. 1), 162–185.

Márquez C, Cohen J, Munné S (1998). Chromosomal identification in human oocytes and polar bodies by spectral karyotyping. *Cytogenet Cell Genet* 81, 254–258.

Martino A, Songsasen N, Leibo S P (1996). Development into blastocysts of bovine oocytes cryopreserved by ultra-rapid cooling. *Biol Reprod* 54, 1059–1069.

Meirow D (1999). Ovarian injury and modern options to preserve fertility in female cancer patients treated with high dose radio-chemotherapy for haemato-oncological neoplasias and other cancers. *Leuk Lymphoma* 33, 65–76.

Meirow D, Nugent D (2001). The effects of radiotherapy and chemotherapy on female reproduction. *Hum Reprod Update* 7, 59–67.

Meirow D, Schenker J G (1995). Cancer and male infertility. *Hum Reprod* 10, 2017–2022.

Meirow D, Fasouliotis S J, Nugent D, Gosden R G, Rutherford A J (1999). The technique of laparoscopic ovarian cortical biopsies in cancer patients prior to sterilising treatments. *Fertil Steril* 71, 948–951.

Morita Y, Perez G I, Maravei D V, Tilly K I, Tilly J L (1999). Targeted expression of Bcl-2 in mouse oocytes inhibits ovarian follicle atresia and prevents spontaneous and chemotherapy-induced oocyte apoptosis in vitro. *Mol Endocrinol* 13, 841–850.

Morita Y, Perez G I, Paris F et al. (2000). Oocyte apoptosis is suppressed by disruption of the acid sphingomyelinase gene or by sphingosine-1-phosphate therapy. *Nat Med* 6, 1109–1114.

Newton H, Aubard Y, Rutherford A, Sharma V, Gosden R (1996). Low temperature storage and grafting of human ovarian tissue. *Hum Reprod* 11, 1487–1491.

Newton H, Fisher J, Arnold J R, Pegg D E, Faddy M J, Gosden R G (1998). Permeation of human ovarian tissue with cryoprotective agents in preparation for cryopreservation. *Hum Reprod* 13, 376–380.

Nugent D, Meirow D, Brook P F, Aubard Y, Gosden R G (1997). Transplantation in reproductive medicine: previous experience, present knowledge and future prospects. *Hum Reprod Update* 3, 267–280.

Nugent D, Newton H, Gallivan L, Gosden R G (1998). Protective effect of vitamin E on ischaemia-reperfusion injury in ovarian grafts. *J Reprod Fertil* 114, 341–346.

Oktay K, Karlikaya G (2000). Ovarian function after transplantation of frozen, banked autologous tissue. *N Eng J Med* 342, 1919.

Oktay K H, Yih M (2002). Preliminary experience with orthotopic and heterotopic transplantation of ovarian cortical strips. *Semin Reprod Med* 20, 63–74.

Oktay K, Newton H, Aubard Y, Salha O, Gosden R G (1998a). Cryopreservation of immature human oocytes and ovarian tissue: an emerging technology? *Fertil Steril* 69, 1–7.

Oktay K, Newton H, Mullan J, Gosden R G (1998b). Development of human primordial follicles to antral stages in SCID/hpg mice stimulated with follicle stimulating hormone. *Hum Reprod* 13, 1133–1138.

Oktay K, Aydin B A, Karlikaya G (2001a). A technique for laparoscopic transplantation of frozen-banked ovarian tissue. *Fertil Steril* 75, 1212–1216.

Oktay K, Economos K, Kan M, Rucinski J, Veeck L, Rosenwaks Z (2001b). Endocrine function and oocyte retrieval after autologous transplantation of ovarian cortical strips to the forearm. *J Am Med Assoc* 286, 1490–1493.

Palermo G, Joris H, Devroy P, Van Steirtegem A C (1992). Pregnancies after intracytoplasmic injection of single spermatozoon into an oocyte. *Lancet* 340, 17–18.

Paynter S J (2000). Current status of the cryopreservation of human unfertilised oocytes. *Hum Reprod Update* 6, 449–456.

Pegg D E (2002). The history and principles of cryopreservation. *Semin Reprod Med* 20, 5–14.

Pickering S J, Braude P R, Johnson M H, Cant A, Currie J (1990). Transient cooling to room temperature can cause irreversible disruption of the meiotic spindle in the human oocyte. *Fertil Steril* 54, 102–108.

Picton H M, Gosden R G (2000). In vitro growth of human primordial follicles from frozen-banked ovarian tissue. *Mol Cell Endocrinol* 166, 27–35.

Picton H M, Kim S S, Gosden R G (2000). Cryopreservation of gonadal tissue and cells. *Br Med Bull* 56, 603–615.

Picton H M, Gosden R G, Leibo S P (2002). Cryopreservation of oocytes and ovarian tissue. In *Medical, Social and Ethical Aspects of Assisted Reproduction*, WHO Technical Bulletin. World Health Organization, Geneva.

Radford J A, Shalet S M, Lieberman B A (1999). Fertility after treatment for cancer. *Br Med J* 319, 935–936.

Radford J A, Lieberman B A, Brison D R et al. (2001). Orthotopic re-implantation of cryopreserved ovarian cortical strips after high-dose chemotherapy for Hodgkin's lymphoma. *Lancet* 357, 1172–1175.

Rall W F (1987). Factors affecting the survival of mouse embryos cryopreserved by vitrification. *Cryobiology* 24, 387–402.

Rall W F, Fahy G M (1985). Ice-free cryopreservation of mouse embryos at $-196°C$ by vitrification. *Nature* 313, 573–575.

Reik W, Walter J (2001). Genomic imprinting: parental influence on the genome. *Nature Rev Genet* 2, 21–32.

Revel A, Elami A, Bor A, Yavin S, Natan Y, Arav A (2001). Intact sheep ovary cryopreservation and transplantation. *Fertil Steril* 76(Suppl. 1), S42–S43.

Schlatt S, Rosiepen G, Weinbauer G F, Rolf C, Brook P F, Nieschlag E (1999). Germ cell transfer in rat, bovine, monkey and human testes. *Hum Reprod* 14, 144–150.

Schlatt S, von Schönfeldt V, Schepers A G (2000). Male germ cell transplantation: an experimental approach with a clinical perspective. *Br Med Bull* 56, 824–836.

Schlegel P N, Su L-M (1997). Physiological consequences of testicular sperm extraction. *Hum Reprod* 12, 1688–1692.

Shaw J, Trounson A O (1997). Ovarian banking for cancer patients: oncological implications in the replacement of ovarian tissue. *Hum Reprod* 12, 403–405.

Shaw J M, Oranratnachai A, Trounson A O (2000). Fundamental cryobiology of mammalian oocytes and ovarian tissue. *Theriogenology* 53, 59–72.

Tedder R S, Zuckerman M A, Goldstone A H et al. (1995). Hepatitis B transmission from contaminated cryopreservation tank. *Lancet* 346, 137–140.

Trounson A O, Dawson K (1996). Storage and disposal of embryos and gametes. *Br Med J* 313, 1–2.

Tulandi T, Al-Took S (1998). Laparoscopic ovarian suspension before irradiation. *Fertil Steril* 70, 381–383.

Vajta G, Holm P, Kuwayama M (1998). Open pulled straw (OPS) vitrification: a new way to reduce cryoinjuries of bovine ova and embryos. *Mol Reprod Dev* 51, 53–58.

Vincent C, Johnson M H (1992). Cooling, cryoprotectants and the cytoskeleton of the mammalian oocyte. *Oxford Rev Reprod Biol* 14, 72–100.

Wallace W H B, Shalet S M, Hendry J H (1989). Ovarian failure following abdominal irradiation in childhood: the radiosensitivity of the human oocyte. *Br J Radiol* 62, 995–998.

Wang X, Chen H, Yin H, Kim S S, Lin Tan S, Gosden R G (2002). Fertility after intact ovary transplantation. *Nature* 415, 385.

Yoon T K, Chung H M, Lim J M, Han S Y, Ko J J, Cha K Y (2000). Pregnancy and delivery of healthy infants developed from vitrified oocytes in a stimulated in vitro fertilization-embryo transfer program. *Fertil Steril* 74, 180–181.

Young L E, Fairburn H R (2000). Improving the safety of embryo technologies: possible role of genomic imprinting. *Theriogenology* 53, 627–648.

Zenzes M T, Bielecki R, Casper R F, Leibo S P (2001). Effects of chilling to $0°C$ on the morphology of meiotic spindles in human metaphase II oocytes. *Fertil Steril* 75, 769–777.

34

The management of infertility with surrogacy and egg donation

Peter R. Brinsden[1] and Melanie C. Davies[2]

[1]Bourn Hall Clinic, Cambridge, UK
[2]Reproductive Medicine Unit, University College London Hospitals, London, UK

Surrogacy

PETER R. BRINSDEN

Until recently, women born with severe abnormalities of development of the Müllerian duct system have been unable to have their own genetic children. Adoption or childlessness have been their only options. The introduction of gestational or in vitro fertilization (IVF) surrogacy during the 1990s as a treatment option has changed the prognosis for women in this situation. Now, women with congenital absence or severe malformations of the uterus, or hysterectomy and abnormalities of the uterus incurred as a result of trauma or cancer treatment, have a chance of having their own genetic child, albeit gestated by another woman. As IVF surrogacy has become increasingly acceptable as a treatment option, both to the medical profession and to the general public (British Medical Association, 1996; Bromham, 1992, 1995), these young women can now have their own children, provided, as most of them do, they have normally functioning ovaries. However, some who have survived the treatment of a malignancy in childhood may have lost not only their uterine function, but also their ovarian function. This section reviews the indications for IVF surrogacy and the selection and management of women seeking this treatment, particularly relating to those with congenital abnormalities. The following section discusses the use of egg donation.

Indications

The main indications for considering treatment by IVF surrogacy are:

- congenital absence or abnormality of the uterus
- hysterectomy following malignancy or haemorrhage
- recurrent abortion
- severe medical problems precluding pregnancy and childbirth
- repeated IVF failure.

Congenital absence of the uterus and following hysterectomy are the commonest indications for surrogacy. Often forgotten, however, are uterine abnormalities that have arisen following anticancer therapy in childhood, resulting in failure of implantation or recurrent pregnancy loss (Critchley, 1999; Levitt and Jenney, 1998; Waring and Wallace, 2000).

The embryological and genetic developmental abnormalities that may be diagnosed in childhood or early adulthood are described elsewhere in this volume. The large majority of children with Müllerian duct abnormalities will have normal ovarian function in adulthood. Minor abnormalities in uterine development do not normally preclude normal conception, pregnancy and delivery (Rock and Schlaff, 1985; Stein and March, 1990). However, the more severe degrees of uterine, cervical or vaginal dysgenesis or agenesis are likely to be incompatible with conception or gestation, in spite of normal ovulation. If surgical correction of the abnormality is not feasible or not successful, the parents of these teenagers, or the patients themselves if they are young adults, should be fully counselled about the implications of their condition and about the possibility of treatment by IVF surrogacy in the future. Because of the natural desire to have their own genetic children, when this option is put to them and if it is felt to be acceptable and practical to them, they can at least go into their adulthood knowing that it will be possible in

Paediatric and Adolescent Gynaecology, ed. Adam Balen et al. Published by Cambridge University Press.
© Cambridge University Press 2004.

the future. If, ultimately, they decide that IVF surrogacy is not acceptable or a practical option, they will in the future require in-depth counselling about accepting their childlessness or the feasibility of adopting children.

Major improvements in survival rates over recent years following treatment of childhood malignancies have meant that many more children are reaching adulthood and are seeking to have their own families (Nicholson and Byrne, 1993; Waring and Wallace, 2000). It is well recognized that both chemotherapy and radiotherapy in childhood and adulthood may cause sufficient damage as to reduce or destroy ovarian function (Levy and Stillman, 1991), but fewer people realise the harmful effect of radiotherapy during childhood on the future function of the uterus in pregnancy (Critchley, 1999). Failure of implantation and early or mid-trimester pregnancy loss are more frequent after radiotherapy in childhood. Counselling of children or teenagers about the implications of their congenital uterine anomaly or the consequences of their cancer therapy on their long-term prospects of having a child are of course difficult, and having children in 10 or more years time is often the least of their or their parents' concerns. However, appropriate advice and counselling early on can answer many of their concerns. Similarly, good advice to late teenagers or women in their early twenties about the effect of their treatment on their potential for having their own children in the future can be exceptionally beneficial to their morale when undergoing or recovering from treatment or after being told that they have a major uterine abnormality. Informed and supportive counselling is an essential part of the management and treatment of girls and young women with congenital or acquired abnormalities of the genital tract.

Management of the commissioning or "genetic couple"

Most "genetic couples" referred to a tertiary level fertility centre have already been fully assessed by their own gynaecologist. This workup will often have included a laparoscopy and vaginal examination and assessment of the extent of any abnormality in the Müllerian duct system. Pelvic ultrasound scanning will usually indicate the site of the ovaries and whether they are active. This can be confirmed by one or more estimations of serum follicle-stimulating hormone (FSH), luteinizing hormone (LH) and oestradiol. The women themselves will often be aware of cyclical symptoms such as breast tenderness and mood changes, which are helpful in assessing the timing of cycles. Karyotyping is not normally required. The blood groups of both proposed genetic parents are requested and both are

normally tested for hepatitis B (HBV), hepatitis C (HCV) and human immunodeficiency virus (HIV) status. Other investigations may be carried out as necessary on an individual basis.

A semen assessment is carried out for the male partner of the genetic couple and, depending on how soon treatment is likely to be undertaken, one or more samples may be frozen and stored for future use. The Code of Practice of the Human Fertilisation and Embryology Authority (HFEA, 2001a) states that semen used for surrogacy arrangements must be treated as if it is donor semen and a minimum of six months' storage, with reassessment of the HIV status at the end of that time, is required. Alternatively, embryos may be created with fresh semen and the embryos "quarantined" for six months.

Careful counselling and assessment is carried out on all medical and scientific aspects of the treatment, followed by in-depth counselling by an independent counsellor. In our practice, all IVF surrogacy arrangements are referred to the independent Ethics Committee to Bourn Hall Clinic, who have drawn up their own guidelines for the practice of IVF surrogacy (Appendix, p. 438). One of the questions most frequently asked by women with congenital anomalies of the uterus is whether any child that they might have by IVF surrogacy will be normal or whether it will inherit their condition. A recent survey (Petrozza et al., 1997) studied 34 livebirths from 58 women and found no congenital abnormalities of the Müllerian system in 17 female fetuses born to hosts commissioned by women with congenital absence of the uterus. They suggested that congenital absence of the uterus is not inherited as a dominant condition and is probably a rare (estimated 1 in 5000) recessive trait.

In our own practice, treatment of the genetic couple may be started once Ethics Committee approval has been obtained, provided a host has already been identified, counselled and also approved.

The IVF treatment cycle of the female partner of the genetic couple is usually straightforward. A standard ovarian follicular stimulation cycle is begun; monitoring and oocyte recovery techniques are the same as for routine IVF (Macnamee and Brinsden, 1999). Oocyte recovery is occasionally not possible by the vaginal route if there is only a very rudimentary vagina, and transabdominal ultrasound-directed or laparoscopic oocyte recovery may be necessary.

Women with congenital absence or other major anomalies of the uterus tend to respond well to follicular stimulation (Goldfarb et al., 2000) and in our own practice a mean of 10 oocytes are recovered, the same as the overall average for regular IVF. Standard IVF laboratory techniques are used with the oocytes and semen (Elder, 1999).

If semen has not previously been frozen for six months, then any resulting embryos must be frozen for six months, and the negative HIV status of the husband reconfirmed before embryo transfer can be arranged to the host. If sperm has previously been frozen for six months, "fresh" embryo transfer to the host can be arranged. This quarantining of sperm or embryos is mandatory in the UK and should, in our opinion, be considered to be best practice.

Treatment of the host

The law in the UK requires that the commissioning couple must find their own host. Clinics may not act as agencies to put commissioning couples and hosts in contact with each other (Surrogacy Arrangements Act, 1985). Many commissioning couples will have a sister, another relative or a close friend who has volunteered to carry a child for them. Failing this, there are organizations who will put couples who require hosts in contact with women who wish to act as hosts. The best known of these organizations in the UK is COTS (Childlessness Overcome Through Surrogacy) who are a charitable organization founded by Mrs Kim Cotton. They have a great deal of experience in organizing both natural and IVF surrogacy arrangements and they also provide their own counselling services to both parties in surrogacy arrangements.

Surrogate hosts should be normal fit women, generally under the age of 38 years and who have had one or more children. The Independent Ethics Committee to Bourn Hall recommends (Appendix, p. 438) that a host preferably should be married or in a stable heterosexual relationship and that her husband or partner should be made fully aware during the counselling process of the implications of his partner acting as a host.

Minimal investigation of the host is usually necessary, as they are invariably fit, normal healthy fertile young women. Routine testing for HBV, HCV and HIV status is carried out as well as for blood group.

Embryo transfer to the surrogate host may be carried out in a synchronized "fresh" embryo transfer cycle if sperm has previously been frozen, or with frozen/thawed embryos. In our own practice, transfer of a maximum of two embryos is carried out in a natural cycle or, more commonly now, in a hormone-controlled cycle with the use of a gonadotrophin-releasing hormone (GnRH or LHRH) analogue and estradiol valerate in a standard regimen (Marcus and Brinsden, 1999). Luteal phase support with vaginal progesterone is provided in hormone-controlled cycles but not normally in natural cycles. All hosts must be carefully counselled about the need for adequate contraception right up until the start of the treatment cycle, and advice is given about avoiding conception during the treatment cycle.

Complications of treatment

There are relatively few reports of series of women treated by IVF surrogacy. No major clinical complications have been reported. The complications that tend to gain publicity are mainly related to "natural surrogacy" arrangements, when the host, who is the genetic and birth mother of the child, wishes to retain custody of the child. The major court cases involving gestational surrogacy have occurred in the USA. The courts have generally found in favour of the genetic or commissioning couples, who have been granted custody of the babies. Full and in-depth counselling, which is mandatory in most clinics practising IVF surrogacy, has hitherto prevented any major problems arising in our own practice.

Another major concern that is always discussed in the counselling sessions is what would happen in the event of an abnormal child being born to the host, or if an abnormality is found on early pregnancy scanning. Again, in-depth counselling and addressing the issue and agreeing a plan before any treatment is started has prevented any major problems.

Payment of hosts has been another contentious issue. It is perfectly reasonable and right that hosts should have all reasonable expenses covered, including time lost for work, clothing, travel, etc. It has happened in natural surrogacy arrangements that hosts have become pregnant and, part way through that pregnancy, have demanded more money to continue the pregnancy. This, as with the problems mentioned above, has not been a problem with IVF surrogacy arrangements in our own practice.

The long-term effects on both the genetic and the host parents and their respective children has not yet been studied. Early reports (Parkinson et al., 1999; Serafini, 2001) have indicated that there are no major problems, but long-term studies on the children and their parents should be carried out (American Fertility Society Ethics Committee, 1990).

Generally, the ovarian follicular response to stimulation of women with the Rokitansky–Küster–Hauser (RKH) syndrome has been remarkably good. In the series reported by Ben-Raphael et al. (1998) a mean of 14.6 oocytes were collected, with a fertilization rate of 71%. Wood and colleagues (1999) retrieved a mean of 8.7 oocytes, with a 53% fertilization rate. In our own series (Brinsden et al., 2000), women with RKH syndrome have performed better with regard to the number of oocytes recovered than women who have had hysterectomies. Meniru and Craft (1997) reported that 3 of their 11 patients who had hysterectomies failed to respond to ovulation induction and two others produced only very few oocytes, which failed to fertilize.

The British Fertility Society carried out a survey of all licensed clinics in the UK that performed surrogacy (Balen and Hadyn, 1998). They found that 29 of 113 licensed clinics had performed one or more surrogacy treatments and had reported very few problems, the most significant of which were:

- one host initially failed to surrender the baby after the birth but subsequently did so
- one couple separated just before treatment started
- unwelcome newspaper publicity in one case
- a number of couples decided not to pursue treatment having received in-depth counselling (this should still be considered a good outcome, since it is much better to let problems arise before treatment starts rather than after a child is born)
- poor responses to follicular stimulation: noted by several clinics and following Wertheim's hysterectomy was the most common.

Most units responding to this survey felt that, in the UK, there should be much greater control over surrogacy, particularly "natural surrogacy" and that all treatment should be performed in licensed clinics, where suitable counselling, screening and treatment can be provided.

Results of treatment

The largest reported series on IVF surrogacy is by Goldfarb et al. (2000), who looked at 180 treatment cycles in their centre conducted between 1984 and 1999 on 112 couples. The average age of the female partner of the commissioning couple was 34.4 years and the livebirth rate per cycle was 15.8%. They note that in this series the women with RKH syndrome had significantly more oocytes retrieved (15.0 ± 1.2 versus 9.34 ± 1.4 oocytes recovered; $p < 0.006$) and more embryos available for transfer than the other groups, even though the average age was the same. In this series, 11 women had abnormalities arising from DES (diethylstilbestrol) syndrome and 15 had RKH syndrome, which accounted for 23.2% of the total cases. Other less-common abnormalities, some of which could be considered to be congenital include:

autoimmune haemolytic anaemia	2
incompetent cervix	1
antithrombin 3 deficiency	1
progesterone receptor deficiency	1
autoimmunity	3
neurofibromatosis	1
recurrent pregnancy loss of different aetiologies	4
cystic fibrosis	1

These, combined with the patients with DES and RKH syndrome, accounted for more than one-third of the patients in this series.

Utian et al. (1985) were the first group to report a success-

Table 34.1. Summary of results of treatment by in vitro fertilization surrogacy at Bourn Hall Clinic from 1990 to 1998

	Results
Treatment of genetic couples	
No. patients started treatment	49
Mean age at start (years)	32.9 (range 22–40)
Total stimulated cycles	80 (range 1–5)
Mean No. oocytes recovered	10 (range 2–24)
Mean No. embryos frozen	5.4 (range 0–13)
Treatment of host surrogates	
No. hosts started treatment	53
No. cycles to embryo transfer	87
Mean No. embryos transferred	2.1
Mean No. host transfers	1.6
Final outcomes	
Clinical pregnancies/surrogate host	31/53 (58.5%)
Delivered/ongoing pregnancies/host transfer cycle	18/87 (21%)
Delivered/ongoing pregnancies/surrogate host	18/53 (34%)
Clinical pregnancies/genetic couple	31/49 (63%)
Delivered/ongoing pregnancies/genetic couple	18/49 (37%)

Source: From Brinsden et al. (2000). *Br Med J* 320, 924–928; reproduced with permission of the Editor.

ful IVF surrogacy pregnancy and they were the first group to report on the results of a large group of women treated by IVF surrogacy (Utian et al., 1989). Their group achieved a clinical pregnancy rate of 18% in 59 cycles. A more recently reported series from the USA gave an ongoing or delivered pregnancy rate of 36% (172 out of 484 surrogate hosts) (Batzofin et al., 1999) with a mean of 5 ± 1.3 embryos transferred. Corson and colleagues (1998) reported a clinical pregnancy rate of 58% per commissioning couple and 33.2% per embryo transfer in women where the genetic woman was less than 40 years of age.

In our own series of 49 genetic couples treated, we reported livebirth rates of between 37% per commissioning couple and 34% per host surrogate with a mean of two embryos transferred (Brinsden et al., 2000). Table 34.1 gives a more detailed breakdown of the outcome of our own series. Meniru and Craft (1997), also from the UK, reported a series of 22 women, all of whom had had a hysterectomy, and achieved a pregnancy rate of 37.5% per surrogate host and 27.3% per cycle of treatment begun.

Parkinson et al. (1999) reviewed the perinatal outcome of pregnancies from IVF surrogacy and compared them with the outcome of pregnancies resulting from standard IVF. The outcomes of the pregnancies were similar, with similar rates of prematurity owing to multiple gestation as is found in a normal IVF population. Most interestingly, pregnancy-induced hypertension and bleeding in the third trimester of pregnancy was five times as frequent in the surrogate hosts than in the standard IVF patient controls.

Summary

Gestational surrogacy is successful in helping women without a uterus, but with normal functioning ovaries, to have their own genetic children (Batzofin et al., 1999; Brinsden et al., 2000; Utian et al., 1989; Corson et al., 1998). Until the mid 1980s, women with congenital absence or gross abnormalities of the uterus had no option but to adopt a child or to accept their childlessness. Technically, treatment by IVF surrogacy is not complicated and involves no more than standard IVF techniques, but with the transfer of resulting embryos to another woman. The principle difficulties with IVF surrogacy are with setting up the arrangements, which must be done by the commissioning couple themselves, the detailed counselling of all parties, due consideration of all the legal issues and the synchronization of the commissioning and host womans' treatment. At all stages, very careful consideration must be given to the welfare of any child who may be born from a surrogacy arrangement.

Very few ethical or legal problems have arisen out of gestational surrogacy programmes (Batzofin et al., 1999; Corson et al., 1998), including our own (Brinsden et al., 1999, 2000). The majority of problems that have arisen have been in natural surrogacy arrangements, where there is a genetic bond between the child and the host (Annas, 1992; Rothenberg, 1988). Because many, if not most, natural surrogacy arrangements are carried out without professional counselling or medical supervision, it is understandable that more problems might arise from them.

Young girls and women should be counselled at the earliest opportunity after their diagnosis has been made of RKH syndrome or other abnormalities of the uterus likely to preclude conception and gestation of a child in the future. They should be told that it may still be possible for them to have their own genetic children in the future, but through surrogacy. If this "good news" is given to them early, the devastating effects of the "bad news" of their condition is very considerably alleviated.

Egg donation

MELANIE C. DAVIES

Until recently, women with primary ovarian failure had no choice other than to remain childless or consider adoption.

Conventional fertility treatment has nothing to offer if the ovaries do not contain sufficient eggs to respond to gonadotrophin stimulation, either endogenous production from the pituitary gland or exogenous administration. The clinical manifestation of this lack of eggs is amenorrhoea, and elevated gonadotrophins (particularly FSH) in an amenorrhoeic patient are diagnostic of ovarian failure.

The development of IVF in the UK in the 1970s (Steptoe and Edwards, 1976) utilized techniques of oocyte recovery, making it possible to harvest eggs from one woman for implantation in another. The first egg donation treatments were carried out in Australia in the 1980s (Lutjen et al., 1984). Subsequently, egg donation programmes were set up in the late 1980s in the UK, USA and other countries (Abdalla and Leonard, 1988; Asch et al., 1987; Serhal and Craft, 1987; Van Steirteghem et al., 1987), and by the 1990s it was an established technique (Cameron et al., 1989).

There are currently 67 centres in the UK licensed to perform egg donation and approximately 1700 cycles of treatment are undertaken each year (HFEA, 2000). Success rates have risen to yield a livebirth rate nationally above 20% per cycle but surpassing this in specialist centres (HFEA, 2000). An increasing number of these cycles are undertaken for young women with Turner's syndrome or chemotherapy-induced ovarian failure.

Indications for egg donation

Egg donation is appropriate for women with ovarian failure of any cause (Table 34.2). The normal human ovary contains a fixed pool of primordial follicles, maximal at about five months of gestational age (Baker, 1963). This store is depleted by atresia during fetal life, childhood and adulthood, as well as by recruitment of follicles during

Table 34.2. Indications for oocyte donation

Indication	Causes
Ovarian failure	Idiopathic, genetic, autoimmune, infective
Gonadal dysgenesis	Turner's syndrome: 45,X and variants; X chromosome translocation or deletion; Perrault's syndrome; 46,XX gonadal dysgenesis
Iatrogenic ovarian failure	Chemotherapy, radiotherapy, pelvic surgery, gonadectomy
Avoidance of transmissible genetic disease	
Repetitive failure of in vitro fertilization	

menstrual cycles (Faddy and Gosden, 1996). When the store of eggs is exhausted, ovarian failure (menopause) occurs. Early ovarian failure in children and adolescents can occur from congenital or acquired disorders. In Turner's syndrome, the loss of eggs is accelerated and is usually complete before birth. Gonadal dysgenesis may also occur with an XX or XY karyotype. Galactosaemia causes almost universal ovarian failure (Robinson et al., 1984). Cytotoxic damage from chemotherapy and radiotherapy in childhood or adolescence may induce ovarian atrophy. Rarely, childhood surgery may involve bilateral oophorectomy. Autoimmune damage may occur, for example in mumps oophoritis.

In some circumstances there may be absence of the uterus as well as ovarian damage, for example following radical therapy of gynaecological malignancy in childhood. These patients cannot become genetic or biological parents; however with their partner's sperm they could undertake donor surrogacy (Ziegler and Russell, 1995). Uterine damage following pelvic radiotherapy is discussed below.

Egg donation may also be requested by women who are carriers of a serious genetic disease, particularly where prenatal diagnosis is not available, and by women carrying a chromosomal anomaly such as Robertsonian translocation causing recurrent miscarriage (Sauer et al., 1994). Preimplantation genetic diagnosis may be an alternative for these patients (Ogilvie et al., 2001; Snowdon and Green, 1997).

Donors

Selection and recruitment
Donors may be anonymous or known to the recipient. There are several sources of donors.

Known donors. Donation may be from a relative or friend of the recipient, although this may not be recommended for ethical reasons (see below).

Unpaid volunteers. Some women are willing to undergo ovarian stimulation and egg recovery to benefit anonymous recipients for altruistic reasons. In the UK, this has until recently been the main source of donor eggs. Volunteers may be recruited in response to advertisement or through publicity in the media. Donors may also be introduced by recipients attending the clinic, who do not then receive their eggs: a "cross-over" system is instituted whereby the eggs are donated anonymously to a matched recipient on the waiting list.

Paid volunteers. In the USA, this is the main source of donors, who are often college students willing to donate eggs (Lindheim et al., 1998). (Payment for donation is not allowed in the UK.)

IVF donors. IVF patients who are themselves undergoing ovarian stimulation for egg retrieval can donate some of their eggs. This is often termed "egg-sharing" (Ahuja et al., 1996). Although it might disadvantage the donor, who will have fewer eggs available for fertilization for their own use, with careful selection, success rates are unaffected. However, fewer embryos will be available for cryopreservation. The charge made by the clinic to the recipient will support the costs of the donor's cycle and thus both parties benefit (Moomjy et al., 2000). This is an increasingly common source of donation.

Patients undergoing sterilization. This is nowadays rare. Parous women requesting sterilization may be recruited to donate if they are willing to undergo ovarian stimulation and timed admission to hospital for egg harvest and laparoscopy.

Unfortunately, in the UK, the supply of donor eggs is limited and the number of recipients outstrips donors, leading to waiting lists for treatment even in the private sector.

Success rates are correlated with the age of the egg donor (Faber et al., 1997). In addition, the risk of chromosomally abnormal pregnancies and of genetic miscarriage rises with age. Consequently, egg donors should be less than 35 years of age.

Donors should ideally be parous women. Donation from infertile women is less successful than from fertile women (Darder et al., 1996) and so IVF donors need to be carefully selected – for example from couples with male factor infertility – and to undergo testing of ovarian reserve.

Counselling
Every donor should be offered independent counselling before committing herself to donate, and she must be free to withdraw at any time if she changes her mind. The counsellor should be separate from the clinic staff so that the donor does not feel under any pressure to comply. Implications of donation must be explored, including the donor's feelings about being a genetic mother to a child with whom she has no contact, how this might affect her relationship and her own children, and the possibility of her own childlessness.

Counselling is particularly important for known or related donors to consider with regard to future interrelationships and disclosure to the child.

Screening
Donors are medically screened before commencing treatment (American Society for Reproductive Medicine, 1998; Gorrill et al., 2001). A full medical and family history are recorded to exclude any heritable disease. A karyotype is performed. Screening for genetic disease may include

cystic fibrosis screening, sickle cell in Afro-Caribbean donors, haemoglobin electrophoresis in Mediterranean and Afro-Caribbean donors, and Tay–Sachs screening in Jewish donors. Donors are tested for transmissible infections (HIV, HBV, HCV, cytomegalovirus and syphilis serology). Because of the incubation period of HIV infection, some clinics will freeze all embryos resulting from donated eggs and wait for six months before retesting the donor to confirm HIV-negative status. (This quarantine period is universal in donor sperm laboratories.) However, frozen–thawed embryos have roughly half the chance of implanting compared with fresh embryos, and most clinics will undertake serial tests for donors and perform fresh embryo transfer.

For matching donor to recipient, the donor's ethnic background, colour of skin, hair and eyes, height, weight and build are recorded. Blood group is also recorded and matched to the recipient where appropriate (e.g. when the recipient couple are Rhesus negative).

Treatment

The donor must undergo ovarian stimulation and egg harvest. Treatment regimens are standardized and generally use a combination of two drugs. Gonadotrophin administration, either FSH or human menopausal gonadotrophin (hMG, a mixture of FSH and LH) is given by daily injection (subcutaneous or intramuscular) during the "follicular phase" of the cycle to stimulate follicle recruitment and growth. A GnRH analogue – usually in the form of a nasal spray – desensitizes the pituitary gland and prevents premature luteinization or ovulation (Remohi et al., 1995); GnRH antagonists can also be used (Sauer et al., 1997a).

Progress is monitored by transvaginal ultrasound scanning of follicle growth and blood tests for oestrogen measurement. The LH surge that triggers ovulation is mimicked by an injection of human chorionic gonadotrophin (hCG), following which egg harvest is carefully timed (36–38 hours after hCG administration) to collect mature eggs prior to ovulation. This will usually occur on day 14 of the stimulation cycle. Egg pickup is performed as an outpatient or daycase procedure under sedation or anaesthesia. Under ultrasound guidance, a transvaginal needle is passed into each ovarian follicle in turn and the follicular fluid is drained and flushed using a suction pump to extract the oocyte.

The most serious risk to the egg donor is ovarian hyperstimulation. In its severe form, this comprises painful ovarian enlargement, vascular permeability causing ascites, pleural effusions and intravascular volume depletion, leading to a risk of renal failure and thrombosis. This is seen in about 1% of women undergoing IVF cycles but is less

common in donors who do not undergo embryo transfer (Sauer, 2001); it can be minimized by continuation of the GnRH analogue after egg recovery. Other side effects from the drugs are rare; there is controversy over the theoretical effect of ovarian stimulation on subsequent risk of ovarian cancer. The egg collection procedure is rarely complicated by infection or haemorrhage and antibiotic cover is given.

Contraception is essential for non-IVF donors and they must be warned of their increased fertility during the stimulated cycle and either avoid intercourse or use barrier contraception. Donors must avoid smoking, alcohol and recreational drugs.

The risk to the donor of undergoing ovarian stimulation could be avoided if it were possible to collect eggs from unstimulated cycles and mature them in vitro prior to fertilization. This is a relatively new technique (Child et al., 2001) but may hold promise for the future (Hwang et al., 1997).

Recipients

Uterine function

Successful pregnancy depends on the ability of the embryo to implant and the uterus to nurture it. The endometrium must be receptive to the embryo to allow implantation. This occurs around day 7 after ovulation in a natural cycle and depends on endometrial priming with oestrogen and progesterone. Despite years of research, detailed knowledge of the mechanism of implantation is still lacking. In egg donation cycles, physiological or supraphysiological doses of exogenous sex steroids are administered to the recipient and the uterine and endometrial response is assessed by ultrasound and occasionally by endometrial biopsy.

Uterine function may be compromised following radiotherapy that involves the pelvis (for example, total body irradiation, treatment of Wilms' tumour or pelvic sarcoma). Spontaneous pregnancies in irradiated patients have an increased incidence of miscarriage, premature delivery and intrauterine growth retardation. Chemotherapy alone, however, does not carry this risk (Hawkins and Smith, 1989; Li et al., 1987; Nicholson and Byrne, 1993).

Critchley et al. (1992) and Bath et al. (1999) have documented the effect of uterine irradiation and described reduction in uterine volume following prepubertal treatment, presumably reflecting radiation fibrosis and reduced vascularization. They have also studied the effect of physiological hormone replacement therapy (HRT) in young women following total body irradiation for childhood leukaemia, monitoring uterine size and endometrial thickness (Bath et al., 1999, Critchley et al., 1990). The implication for oocyte donation is that patients irradiated in childhood are likely to have a poor outcome from treatment. Few cases have yet been reported, but they include a report of mid-trimester miscarriage in a patient with reduced uterine size (Larsen et al., 2000).

Investigation of uterine function is, therefore, important before treatment commences. Ultrasound scanning is an excellent method of assessing uterine volume, endometrial thickness and endometrial morphology. Blood supply to the uterus is assessed by Doppler scanning of the uterine artery and measurement of resistance to flow. Ultrasound measurement of endometrial thickness correlates with endometrial maturation and in clinical practice a thickness of 7 mm or greater is considered satisfactory for implantation (Hofmann et al., 1996; Noyes et al., 2001).

Endometrial biopsy (usually taken as an outpatient procedure in the "luteal phase" of the HRT cycle) is largely a research tool. Histological dating by light microscopy, ultrastructure on electron scanning microscopy and secretory products identified by immunocytochemistry have all been used to assess endometrial function (Damario et al., 2001; Davies et al., 1990; Navot et al., 1989; Sauer et al., 1997b).

Commonly, a "dummy run" of HRT is given prior to treatment, monitored by ultrasound with or without serum oestradiol levels; results correlate with pregnancy outcome (Remohi et al., 1997). HRT can then be optimized for the treatment cycle (Dmowski et al., 1997).

Fitness for pregnancy

Patients who have undergone chemotherapy and radiotherapy in childhood or adolescence may be at increased risk of cardiac disease, renal impairment, osteopenia and endocrine disturbance. The demands of pregnancy, particularly on cardiac and renal function, must be considered before treatment starts. The help of an obstetric physician may be invaluable both in prepregnancy assessment and in obstetric care. For example, patients who have been exposed to anthracyclines should have echocardiography.

Women with Turner's syndrome may also face medical risks in pregnancy. Cardiac problems of Turner's syndrome include coarctation of the aorta, ventricular and atrial septal defects, and aortic root dilatation. There have been reports of aortic dissection occurring in pregnancy and two maternal deaths have resulted (Nagel and Tesch, 1997). Before fertility treatment, an echocardiogram should be performed and a magnetic resonance image obtained of the aortic arch. Renal anomalies such as horseshoe kidney are also common; if these have not been excluded, a renal ultrasound should be performed. Hypertension is common in Turner's syndrome, as are glucose intolerance and hypothyroidism; consequently, prepregnancy medical screening is important.

The metabolic demands of pregnancy are all increased in multiple gestations, and the number of embryos replaced should be limited for this reason besides others. Fetal reduction may need to be considered in the event of a multiple gestation on the grounds of risk to maternal health.

Pretreatment assessment

Both the egg recipient and her partner need to undergo pretreatment investigation. The male partner's fertility must be assessed with a semen analysis; if this is poor, IVF will involve intracytoplasmic sperm injection of the donated eggs (Borini et al., 1996; Tsirigotis et al., 1995). Both partners should be screened for viral infections (HIV, HBV, HCV) and the egg recipient for cytomegaloviral status and blood group.

Before embryo transfer to the uterus, it is advisable to assess the uterine cavity. Ultrasound scanning is used to measure the length of the cavity and assess its shape. Hysterocontrast sonography, using saline infusion, distends and outlines the cavity and may reveal pathology such as a uterine polyp, fibroid or congenital anomaly. If necessary, hysteroscopy should be performed for confirmation and for treatment of the lesion. If egg transfer to the Fallopian tubes is planned, then tubal patency must be assessed. Hysterocontrast sonography using galactose solution (as an outpatient procedure) can be used as a screening tool but most units perform a hysterosalpingogram (Lindheim and Sauer, 1998).

While waiting for a donor to be recruited for their treatment cycle, egg recipients who are amenorrhoeic must use HRT in a standard cyclical combined preparation to maintain regular menstruation.

Counselling

Before approaching a clinic for egg donation, infertile patients may have undergone numerous investigations and perhaps failure of conventional fertility treatment; they may be helped by supportive counselling. They may need help to come to terms with their inability to be a genetic parent – even though they may have been aware of their medical condition since childhood. Such patients are likely to have positive views of egg donation (Westlander et al., 1998) but they may wish to discuss the ethical or religious aspects of gamete donation. Counselling will also consider the choice of anonymous or known donors (Baetens et al., 2000), and the issue of disclosure.

Treatment cycle

The egg recipient receives HRT to prepare the endometrium as outlined above. The first HRT regimens were designed to give physiological replacement (Lutjen et al., 1984; Navot et al., 1986) but it was soon apparent that a simplified regimen could be used (Serhal and Craft, 1987). Various routes of administration have also been used (Ben-Nun and Shulman, 1997; Toner, 2000; reviewed by Devroey and Pados, 1998). A standard modern regimen used in the UK is to administer oestrogen replacement orally (estradiol valerate 2 mg twice or three times a day) and progesterone by the intramuscular route (progesterone in oil 100 mg daily) or vaginally (800 mg daily). Egg recipients who still have natural menstrual cycles but poor ovarian function need a modified regimen; they receive GnRH analogue to suppress their cycle prior to HRT.

The length of the "follicular phase" of oestrogen can be varied to synchronize with the donor's cycle (Michalas et al., 1996; Yaron et al., 1995). Progesterone is usually added on the morning of the donor's egg collection so that the endometrium is "in phase", and embryo transfer takes place on the third or fourth day of progesterone administration. The "window" of receptivity is short and determined by the duration of progesterone (Prapas et al., 1998) even though pregnancy has been reported with late transfers (Schulte and Serhal, 1996).

On the day of the donor's egg collection, the recipient's partner provides a fresh semen sample, which is used to inseminate the donated eggs. They are kept under standard IVF culture conditions and the resulting embryos are transferred to the recipient. Embryo transfer is usually performed as an outpatient procedure; the cervix is visualized with a speculum and cleansed, the embryos are loaded into a specially designed catheter, which is passed into the uterine cavity under ultrasound guidance, and released. Tubal transfer of eggs and sperm (GIFT) can also be performed by laparoscopy. In the UK, the usual number of embryos transferred now is two (HFEA, 2001b).

Synchronization of the donor and recipient cycle is essential. This can be achieved in several ways: varying the length of the recipient's "follicular phase" of oestrogen replacement, adjusting the recipients cyclical HRT to commence oestrogen three to four days before the donor's period, scheduling the donor's menstrual period with pretreatment (e.g. a combined oral contraceptive pill), or adjusting the duration of downregulation with GnRH analogue. The need to synchronize cycles is avoided if frozen–thawed embryos are used or cryopreserved eggs are donated (Polak de Fried et al., 1998).

Biochemical pregnancy testing is performed 14 days after embryo transfer, and ultrasound scanning is offered at 7 weeks to confirm clinical pregnancy (the presence of a fetal heartbeat) and to identify multiple gestation or ectopic pregnancy. When pregnancy is achieved, the recipient must continue HRT until at least 7 weeks of gestation when the placental output is sufficient to maintain the pregnancy (Schneider et al., 1993). (There are, however, reports of successful pregnancy without support (Lindheim and Sauer, 1999; Stassart et al., 1995).) In practice, HRT is usually continued to 12 weeks. Pregnancy is traditionally dated from the last menstrual period, and in artificial cycles this is calculated as 14 days prior to egg recovery.

Pregnancy outcome

Success rates

The success of egg donation treatment has always outstripped that of "ordinary" IVF. This probably reflects both the appropriate selection of fertile donors and the careful hormonal preparation of the endometrium for implantation. In the UK, all clinics licensed to undertake assisted conception are obliged to report their success rates in a standardized format to the HFEA, which has kept a central database since 1991. Consequently the outcome of egg donation cycles has been reliably documented. The most recently published data from the Authority gives a clinical pregnancy rate of 27.5% per cycle using fresh embryos (HFEA, 2000). "Clinical pregnancy" means that, following a positive pregnancy test, ultrasound scanning has demonstrated an intrauterine pregnancy with a fetal heartbeat. Some pregnancies are subsequently lost in miscarriage or stillbirth, resulting in a livebirth rate of 22.5%. Over 450 babies a year are born in the UK following egg donation (HFEA, 2000).

Success rates may vary between patient groups. It has been suggested that patients with primary ovarian failure do better than others (Abdalla et al., 1990). There are numerous reports of pregnancies in patients with gonadal dysgenesis, both XX and XY (Cornet et al., 1990; Kan et al., 1997; Pados et al., 1992). In Turner's syndrome, there are some conflicting data, with some authors suggesting low pregnancy and implantation rates (Rogers et al., 1992; Yaron et al., 1996) and others reporting a particularly high success rate (e.g. a 46% clinical pregnancy rate being reported by Foudila et al. (1999)) but also a high miscarriage rate of 40–50% (Foudila et al., 1999; Khastgir et al., 1997; Press et al., 1995), which may be related to uterine hypoplasia (Khastgir et al., 1997).

Data on survivors of childhood cancer is still limited (Kavic and Sauer, 2001). Egg donation pregnancies have been reported in survivors of Hodgkin's disease (Anselmo et al., 2001) and bone marrow transplantation with conditioning chemotherapy (Lee et al., 1995). An early report suggested a lower pregnancy rate (Sauer et al., 1994); the effect of uterine irradiation has been discussed above and in Ch. 32. The age of the recipient does not affect the pregnancy rate (Abdalla et al., 1997).

The high success rate of egg donation is reflected in a high proportion of multiple births. Unfortunately, these pregnancies are more likely to miscarry and are highly likely to deliver prematurely. In the UK database, triplets have a risk of stillbirth or neonatal death of 6.0%, compared with 1% of singletons (HFEA, 2000). Higher-order multiple pregnancies from egg donation can be avoided by two-embryo transfer (Licciardi et al., 2001), and single-embryo transfers should be considered in high-risk patients (Foudila et al., 1999).

Pregnancy complications

It is well known that the risks of pregnancy are increased in older mothers and in first pregnancies, and many ovum recipients are in these categories. It has also been suggested that egg donation itself increases the risk of postpartum haemorrhage (Abdalla et al., 1998) and also of hypertension in pregnancy: a rate of 23% was reported by Abdalla and colleagues, and hypertension appears more common than in other IVF pregnancies (Soderstrom-Antilla et al., 1998a) perhaps because of an immunological response (Salha et al., 1999).

Cardiac complications pose the greatest risk for women with Turner's syndrome; two fatal cases of aortic dissection during egg donation pregnancies have been reported (Nagel and Tesch, 1997). There is also a predisposition to hypertension and gestational diabetes in these women.

All pregnant women are now offered antenatal screening for chromosomal anomalies, and egg recipients may wish to consider this; however, the estimates of risk must be based on the age of the donor.

The majority of egg donation pregnancies are delivered by caesarean section. In women with Turner's syndrome this is a consequence of their short stature; in others it may be a response to a "precious pregnancy" or it may reflect a genuine increase in obstetric problems.

Outcome for the child

The majority of children born from donated eggs are entirely healthy (Applegarth et al., 1995). There is increased morbidity among children of multiple pregnancies through prematurity, as discussed above. There may also be an increased incidence of intrauterine growth retardation in egg donation pregnancies (Abdalla et al., 1998).

The psychological outcome for children appears good (reviewed by Soderstrom-Anttila et al., 1998b; Soderstrom-Anttila, 2001) and the relationships and quality of parenting

in assisted conception families is excellent even where there is no genetic link between mother and child (Golombok et al., 1999). The long-term outcome in adulthood is as yet unknown, but parallels may be drawn with the children of sperm donation, where it is recognized that many offspring wish to trace their genetic origin.

Legal aspects

In the UK, assisted conception treatments involving IVF are regulated under the terms of the Human Fertilisation and Embryology Act 1990, and all clinics are inspected and licensed by the HFEA. This is the only country where there is a statutory body. Not all countries have enacted legislation (e.g. USA, Canada, Ireland) (Gunning, 1998). Egg donation is not available in some countries (e.g. Sweden, Germany, Saudi Arabia) (IFFS, 2001).

Under UK law, a woman who gives birth to a child is the mother; therefore, the recipient of donated eggs is legally the child's mother. The donor has no relationship in law with the child nor obligations to or rights over the child. The Act requires that the names and details of all donors are registered with the HFEA; these details, and the names of the couple treated and any children born, are highly confidential – indeed, disclosure of such information is a criminal offence. The HFEA can tell people who enquire (aged 18 or over) whether they were born as a result of egg or sperm donation and whether they could be related to someone they want to marry (aged 16 or over).

There is currently a public consultation in the UK to review the principle of donor anonymity; in some other countries anonymity has been withdrawn (e.g. Austria) or donors may decide whether they wish to disclose their identity (e.g. the Netherlands). However, information that might identify the donor cannot be released under current legislation in the UK.

Ethical issues

Payment to egg donors has raised great debate. Payment for egg or sperm donation is not allowed in the UK; only expenses can be paid. Altruistic donation from volunteers is preferred (Davies, 1996; Johnson, 1997; Shenfield and Steele, 1995). This is the rule in most countries, but in others, notably the USA, payment is given for donation. The number of donors is greatly increased but of course there are concerns that women may donate for the "wrong" reasons or even conceal their medical history in order to donate for money (German et al., 2001). Bringing egg donation into the "marketplace" is also felt to reduce the gift of a child into a commercial transaction.

Recently, it has been possible in the UK for patients undergoing IVF to donate "spare" eggs and to have their treatment cycle funded by the egg recipient. This has raised further debate as the arrangement could be considered a form of payment, but it has the approval of the HFEA (Johnson, 1999).

Anonymous donation from unrelated donors is the norm in the UK. A related donor may be preferred by some couples as the offspring will be genetically closer to the recipient, and in some families and cultures this will be acceptable, but for many it is inadvisable because it will lead to complex family interrelationships. There is also some risk of coercion or family pressure on an unwilling sister to donate.

Disclosure of the identity of unrelated donors is under discussion in the UK, as mentioned above. The right of the child to know his or her genetic identity or origins, which is established already for adopted children, who may trace their biological parents at the age of 18, is denied to the donor child. There is a conflict with the right of the donor to privacy (Pennings, 2001).

Even if identifying information about the donor were available, many donor children might not seek it because they remain unaware of their origins. Many couples seeking treatment do not disclose it to their offspring nor to family or friends. Couples undergoing egg donation are more open than those having donor insemination: 38% of the former intended to tell their offspring (Soderstrom-Anttila et al., 1998b) but only 8.6% of the latter (Golombok et al., 2002). However, secrecy cannot always be maintained, and the implications for the child of later discovery are severe. A more open approach is recommended (McWhinnie, 2001; Shenfield and Steele, 1997).

Finally, the availability of egg donation in most countries is limited to those who can afford the high cost of treatment; inequity of access on financial grounds may be considered an ethical issue.

Summary

In conclusion, egg donation is a highly successful treatment for infertility caused by premature ovarian failure. It allows women without ovarian function to become mothers, although not to their genetic child (Box 34.1). However, it may not be acceptable to all couples for moral or religious reasons. In many countries, the availability of treatment is limited and expensive. Women requiring egg donation for disorders diagnosed in childhood and adolescence need careful medical assessment to reduce risks in pregnancy, and multiple pregnancies should be avoided.

Box 34.1 Key points

- Gestational surrogacy allows a woman to have her own genetic child, although gestated by another woman.
- IVF surrogacy uses standard IVF techniques.
- The principle difficulties with IVF surrogacy lie in the arrangements, counselling and synchronization of treatment.
- Egg donation is a highly successful method of assisted conception and is the only appropriate fertility treatment for premature ovarian failure.
- A uterine response to HRT is essential.
- Egg donation is limited by donor availability and expense.
- Careful medical assessment of recipients reduces the risk in pregnancy; multiple pregnancies should be avoided to reduce risk to mother and offspring.

APPENDIX   **The Bourn Hall Ethics Committee guidelines for surrogacy**

Introduction

Bourn Hall Ethics Committee is prepared to consider IVF surrogacy in cases where an embryo or embryos from the commissioning couple are transferred to the uterus of the host. The use of donor eggs or donor sperm and natural surrogacy may be considered in exceptional circumstances. They consider that surrogacy should only be undertaken as a last resort. The need to safeguard the welfare of any children born as a result of surrogacy arrangement will be a guiding principle.

The Committee considers that every case must be looked at by the Ethics Committee on its own merit, based on information provided by the Clinic.

Procedures

Following examination by a clinician, the prospective genetic parents and host and partner must be counselled by a professional counsellor. If the clinician and counsellor, who are not members of the Ethics Committee, are satisfied they will prepare a report, a copy of which must be submitted to each member of the Ethics Committee. The case will then be considered by the Ethics Committee in consultation with the clinician and counsellor. If they are satisfied that the case falls within the Guidelines and is acceptable, the Ethics Committee will make their recommendations to the Clinic.

The genetic parents and host and her partner will be asked to take independent legal advice and encouraged to take out insurance.

Cases will not be considered if there is any doubt that the genetic couple will comply with the requirements for a parental order under Section 30 of Human Fertilisation and Embryology Act 1990 or subsequent legislation.

Categories acceptable for treatment

1 Total or partial absence of the uterus either of congenital origin or after surgery.
2 Repeated miscarriage.
3 Multiple failure of infertility treatment. The clinicians must be satisfied that there is no reasonable prospect of success in the future.

Motives considered unacceptable

1 Social reasons.
2 Prospective genetic parents with severe health problems. Clinicians and the Committee will need to be satisfied that the strain of bringing up a child might not damage the mother's health so seriously as to jeopardise the welfare of that child and the family.

Considerations which apply to all cases

- The Clinic must not be involved in initiating or making arrangements between genetic and host couples.
- The relationship between genetic couple and host must be carefully considered and avoid creating conflicting family relationships.
- Independent counselling must be available to both genetic and host couples.
- HIV, hepatitis B and hepatitis C antibody tests are required of both genetic and host couples.
- The age of the genetic mother and of the host is important. In view of the HFEA Code of Practice (HFEA, 2001a), the Committee considers that 35 should be the maximum age of the genetic mother unless there are exceptional circumstances; however, the Committee will consider genetic mothers up to and including 38. The host should generally be below 40.
- The principal motive of a prospective host should always be to help an infertile couple.
- A prospective host should have had at least one child before becoming a surrogate.

- The commissioning couple in a surrogacy arrangement should be married. The host should preferably be in a stable relationship. If the host is single then she should be adequately supported.

REFERENCES

Abdalla H, Leonard T (1988). Cryopreserved zygote intra-fallopian transfer for anonymous oocyte donation. *Lancet* i: 835.

Abdalla H I, Baber R, Kirkland A, Leonard T, Power M, Studd J W (1990). A report on 100 cycles of oocyte donation; factors affecting the outcome. *Hum Reprod* 5, 1018–1022.

Abdalla H I, Wren M E, Thomas A, Korea L (1997). Age of the uterus does not affect pregnancy or implantation rates; a study of egg donation in women of different ages sharing oocytes from the same donor. *Hum Reprod* 12, 827–829.

Abdalla H I, Billett A, Kan A K et al. (1998). Obstetric outcome in 232 ovum donation pregnancies. *Br J Obstet Gynaecol* 105, 332–337.

Ahuja K K, Simons E G, Fiamanya W et al. (1996). Egg-sharing in assisted conception: ethical and practical considerations. *Hum Reprod* 11, 1126–1131.

American Fertility Society Ethics Committee (1990). Surrogate gestational mothers: women who gestate a genetically unrelated embryo. *Fertil Steril* 53, 64S-67S.

American Society for Reproductive Medicine (1998). Guidelines for oocyte donation. *Fertil Steril* 70(Suppl. 3), 5S-6S.

Annas G (1992). Using genes to define motherhood: the California solution. *N Engl J Med* 326, 417–420.

Anselmo A P, Cavalieri E, Aragona C, Sbracia M, Funaro D, Maurizi Enrici R (2001). Successful pregnancies following an egg donation program in women with previously treated Hodgkin's disease. *Haematologica* 86, 624–628.

Applegarth L, Goldberg N C, Cholst I (1995). Families created through ovum donation: a preliminary investigation of obstetrical outcome and psychosocial adjustment. *J Assist Reprod Genet* 12, 574–580.

Asch R, Balmaceda J, Ord T et al. (1987). Oocyte donation and gamete intrafallopian transfer as treatment for primary ovarian failure. *Lancet* i: 687.

Baetens P, Devroey P, Camus M, Van Steirteghem A C, Ponjaert-Kristoffersen I (2000). Counselling couples and donors for oocyte donation: the decision to use either known or anonymous oocytes. *Hum Reprod* 15, 476–484.

Baker T G (1963). A quantitative and cytological study of germ cells in the human ovary. *Proc Roy Soc Lond* 158, 417–433.

Balen A H, Hadyn C A (1998). British Fertility Society survey of all licensed clinics that perform surrogacy in the UK. *Hum Fertil* 1, 6–9.

Bath L E, Critchley H O, Chambers S E et al. (1999). Ovarian and uterine characteristics after total body irradiation in childhood and adolescence: response to sex steroid replacement. *Br J Obstet Gynaecol* 106, 1265–1272.

Batzofin J, Nelson J, Wilcox J et al.(1999). Gestational surrogacy: is it time to include it as part of ART? In *Proceedings of the American Society for Reproductive Medicine*, P-017.

Ben-Nun I, Shulman A (1997). Induction of artificial endometrial cycles with s.c. oestrogen implants and injectable progesterone in in-vitro fertilization treatment with donated oocytes: a preliminary report. *Hum Reprod* 12, 2267–2270.

Ben-Raphael Z, Barr-Hava I, Levy T, Orvieto R (1998). Simplifying ovulation induction for surrogacy in women with Mayer–Rokitansky–Kuster–Hauser syndrome. *Hum Reprod* 13, 1470–1471.

Borini A, Bafaro M G, Bianchi L, Violini F, Bonu M A, Flamigni C (1996). Oocyte donation programme: results obtained with intracytoplasmic sperm injection in cases of severe male factor infertility or previous failed fertilization. *Hum Reprod* 11, 548–550.

Brinsden P R (1999). IVF surrogacy. In *A Textbook of in vitro Fertilization and Assisted Reproduction*, Brinsden P R, ed., pp. 361–368. Parthenon, Carnforth, New York.

Brinsden P R, Appleton T C, Murray E, Hussein M, Akagbosu F, Marcus S F (2000). Treatment by in vitro fertilisation with surrogacy – the experience of a single centre in the United Kingdom. *Br Med J* 320, 924–928.

British Medical Association Report (1996). *Changing Conceptions of Motherhood. The Practice of Surrogacy in Britain.* British Medical Association Publications, London.

Bromham D R (1992). Surrogacy: the evolution of opinion. *Br J Hosp Med* 47, 767–772.

(1995). Surrogacy: ethical, legal and social aspects. *J Assist Reprod Genet* 12, 509–516.

Cameron I T, Rogers P A W, Caro C, Harman J, Healy D L, Leeton J (1989). Oocyte donation: a review. *Br J Obstet Gynaecol* 96, 893–899.

Child T J, Abdul-Jalil A K, Gulekli B, Tan S L (2001). In vitro maturation and fertilization of oocytes from unstimulated normal ovaries, polycystic ovaries, and women with polycystic ovary syndrome. *Fertil Steril* 76, 936–942.

Cornet D, Alvarez S, Antoine J M et al. (1990). Pregnancies following ovum donation in gonadal dysgenesis. *Hum Reprod* 5, 291–293.

Corson S L, Kelly M, Braverman A, English M E (1998). Gestational carrier pregnancy. *Fertil Steril* 69, 670–674.

Critchley H O (1999). Factors of importance for implantation and problems after treatment of childhood cancer. *Med Paediatr Oncol* 33, 9–14.

Critchley H O D, Buckley C H, Anderson D C (1990). Experience with a 'physiological' steroid replacement regimen for the establishment of a receptive endometrium in women with premature ovarian failure. *Br J Obstet Gynaecol* 97, 804–810.

Critchley H O D, Wallace W H B, Shalet S M et al. (1992). Abdominal irradiation in childhood; the potential for pregnancy. *Br J Obstet Gynaecol* 99, 392–394.

Damario M A, Lesnick T G, Lessey B A et al. (2001). Endometrial markers of uterine receptivity utilizing the donor oocyte model. *Hum Reprod* 16, 1893–1899.

Darder M C Epstein Y M, Treiser S L, Comito C E, Rosenberg H S, Dzingalla L (1996). The effects of prior gravidity on the outcomes of ovum donor and own oocyte cycles. *Fertil Steril* 65, 578–582.

Davies M C (1996). Oocyte donation. Fools rush in where angels fear to tread. *Hum Reprod* 11, 1154–1156.

Davies M C, Anderson M C, Mason B A, Jacobs H S (1990). Oocyte donation: the role of endometrial receptivity. *Hum Reprod* 5, 862–869.

Devroey P, Pados G (1998). Preparation of endometrium for egg donation. *Hum Reprod Update* 4, 856–861.

Dmowski W P, Michalowska J, Rana N, Friberg J, McGill-Johnson E, DeOrio L (1997). Subcutaneous estradiol pellets for endometrial preparation in donor oocyte recipients with a poor endometrial response. *J Assist Reprod Genet* 14, 139–144.

Elder K T (1999). Laboratory techniques: oocyte collection and embryo culture. In *A Textbook of in vitro Fertilization and Assisted Reproduction*, Brinsden P R, ed., pp. 185–202. Parthenon, Carnforth, New York.

Faber B M, Mercan R, Hamacher P, Muasher S J, Toner J P (1997). The impact of an egg donor's age and her prior fertility on recipient pregnancy outcome. *Fertil Steril* 68, 370–372.

Faddy M J, Gosden R G (1996). A model conforming the decline in follicle numbers to the age of menopause in women. *Hum Reprod* 11, 1484–1486.

Foudila T, Soderstrom-Anttila V, Hovatta O (1999). Turner's syndrome and pregnancies after oocyte donation. *Hum Reprod* 14, 532–535.

German E K, Mukherjee T, Osborne D, Copperman A B (2001). Does increasing ovum donor compensation lead to differences in donor characteristics? *Fertil Steril* 76, 75–79.

Goldfarb J, Austin C, Peskin B, Lisbona H, Desai N, Loret de Mola J R (2000). Fifteen years experience with an in vitro fertilisation surrogate gestational pregnancy programme. *Hum Reprod* 15, 1075–1078.

Golombok S, Murray C, Brinsden P, Abdalla H (1999). Social versus biological parenting: family functioning and the socioemotional development of children conceived by egg or sperm donation. *J Child Psychol Psychiatry* 40, 519–527.

Golombok S, Brewaeys A, Giavazzi M T, Guerra D, MacCallum F, Rust J (2002). The European study of assisted reproduction families: the transition to adolescence. *Hum Reprod* 17, 830–840.

Gorrill M J, Johnson L K, Patton P E, Burry K A (2001). Oocyte donor screening: the selection process and cost analysis. *Fertil Steril* 75, 400–404.

Gunning J (1998). Oocyte donation: the legislative framework in Western Europe. *Hum Reprod* 13(Suppl. 2), 98–104.

Hawkins M M, Smith R A (1989). Pregnancy outcomes in childhood cancer survivors; probable effect of abdominal irradiation. *Int J Cancer* 43, 399–402.

HFEA (Human Fertilisation, Embryology Authority) (2000). *Annual Report*. HFEA, London.

(2001a). *Code of Practice for Clinics Licensed by the Human Fertilisation and Embryology Authority*. HFEA, London.

(2001b). *Embryo Transfer Policy Review*. CH(01)10 HFEA, London.

Hofmann G E, Thie J, Scott R T Jr, Navot D (1996). Endometrial thickness is predictive of histologic endometrial maturation in women undergoing hormone replacement for ovum donation. *Fertil Steril* 66, 380–383.

Hwang J L, Lin Y H, Tsai Y L (1997). Pregnancy after immature oocyte donation and intracytoplasmic sperm injection. *Fertil Steril* 68, 1139–1140.

IFFS (2001). Surveillance 01. *Fertil Steril* 76(Suppl. 2), S16–S18.

Johnson M (1997). Payments to gamete donors: position of the human fertilisation and embryology authority. *Hum Reprod* 12, 1839–1842.

(1999). The medical ethics of paid egg sharing in the UK. *Hum Reprod* 14, 1912–1918.

Kan A K, Abdalla H I, Oskarsson T (1997). Two successful pregnancies in a 46XY patient. *Hum Reprod* 12, 1434–1435.

Kavic S M, Sauer M V (2001). Oocyte donation treats infertility in survivors of malignancies: ten-year experience. *J Assist Reprod Genet* 18, 181–183.

Khastgir G, Abdalla H, Thomas A, Korea L, Latarche L, Studd J (1997). Oocyte donation in Turner's syndrome: an analysis of the factors affecting the outcome. *Hum Reprod* 12, 279–285.

Larsen E C, Loft A, Holm K, Muller J, Brocks V, Anderson A N (2000). Oocyte donation in women cured of cancer with bone marrow transplantation including total body irradiation in adolescence. *Hum Reprod* 15, 1505–1508.

Lee S, Ghalie R, Kaizer H, Sauer M V (1995). Successful pregnancy in a bone marrow transplant recipient following oocyte donation. *J Assist Reprod Genet* 12, 294–296.

Levitt G A, Jenney M E (1998). The reproductive system after childhood cancer. *Br J Obstet Gynaecol* 105, 946–953.

Levy M, Stillman R (1991). Reproductive potential in survivors of childhood malignancy. *Paediatrician* 18, 61–70.

Li F P, Gimbrere K, Gelber R D et al. (1987). Outcome of pregnancy in survival of Wilms' tumour. *J Am Med Assoc* 257, 216–219.

Licciardi F, Berkeley A S, Krey L, Grifo J, Noyes N (2001). A two-versus-three embryo transfer: the oocyte donation model. *Fertil Steril* 75, 510–513.

Lindheim S R, Sauer M V (1998). Upper genital-tract screening with hysterosonography in patients receiving donated oocytes. *Int J Gynaecol Obstet* 60, 47–50.

(1999). Trophoblast persists despite lack of sex-steroid support following ovum donation. *J Assist Reprod Genet* 16, 52–54.

Lindheim S R, Frumovitz M, Sauer M V (1998). Recruitment and screening policies and procedures used to establish a paid donor oocyte registry. *Hum Reprod* 13, 2020–2024.

Lutjen P, Trounson A, Leeton J, Findlay J, Wood C, Renou P (1984). The establishment and maintenance of pregnancy using in vitro fertilisation and embryo donation in a patient with primary ovarian failure. *Nature* 307, 174–175.

Macnamee M C, Brinsden P R (1999). Superovulation strategies in assisted conception. In *A Textbook of in vitro Fertilization and Assisted Reproduction*, Brinsden P R, ed., pp. 91–101. Parthenon, Carnforth, New York.

Marcus S F, Brinsden P R (1999). Oocyte donation. *A Textbook of in vitro Fertilization and Assisted Reproduction*, Brinsden P R, ed., pp. 343–354. Parthenon, Carnforth, New York.

McWhinnie A (2001). Gamete donation and anonymity: should offspring from donated gametes continue to be denied knowledge of their origins and antecedents? *Hum Reprod* 16, 807–817.

Meniru G I, Craft I L (1997). Experience with gestational surrogacy as a treatment for sterility resulting from hysterectomy. *Hum Reprod* 12, 51–54.

Michalas S, Loutradis D, Drakakis P et al. (1996). A flexible protocol for the induction of recipient endometrial cycles in an oocyte donation programme. *Hum Reprod* 11, 1063–1066.

Moomjy M, Mangieri R, Beltramone F, Cholst I, Veeck L, Rosenwaks Z (2000). Shared oocyte donation: society's benefits. *Fertil Steril* 73, 1165–1169.

Nagel T C, Tesch L G (1997). ART and high risk pregnancies. *Fertil Steril* 68, 748–749.

Navot D, Laufer N, Kopolovic J et al. (1986). Artificially induced endometrial cycles and establishment of pregnancies in the absence of ovaries. *N Engl J Med* 314, 806–811.

Navot D, Anderson T L, Droesch K, Scott R T, Kreiner D, Rosenwaks Z (1989). Hormonal manipulation of endometrial maturation. *J Clin Endocrinol Metab* 68, 801–807.

Nicholson H S, Byrne J (1993). Fertility and pregnancy after treatment for cancer during childhood or adolescence. *Cancer* 71, 3392–3399.

Noyes N, Hampton B S, Berkeley A, Licciardi F, Grifo J, Krey L (2001). Factors useful in predicting the success of oocyte donation: a 3-year retrospective analysis. *Fertil Steril* 76, 92–97.

Ogilvie C M, Braude P, Scriven, P N (2001). Successful pregnancy outcomes after pre-implantation genetic diagnosis for carriers of chromosomal translocations. *Hum Fertil* 4, 168–171.

Pados G, Camus M, Van Waesberghe L, Liebers L, Van Steirteghem A, Devroey P (1992). Oocyte and embryo donation: evaluation of 412 consecutive trials. *Hum Reprod* 7, 1111–1117.

Parkinson J, Tran C, Tan T (1999). Perinatal outcome after in-vitro fertilisation: surrogacy (IVF-surrogacy). *Hum Reprod* 14, 671–676.

Pennings G (2001). The right to privacy and access to information about one's genetic origins. *Med Law* 20, 1–15.

Petrozza J C, Gray M R, Davies A J, Reindollar R H (1997). Congenital absence of the uterus and vagina is not commonly transmitted as a dominant genetic trait: outcomes of surrogate pregnancies. *Fertil Steril* 67, 387–389.

Polak de Fried E, Notrica J, Rubinstein M, Marazzi A, Gomez Gonzalez M (1998). Pregnancy after human donor oocyte cryopreservation and thawing in association with intracytoplasmic sperm injection in a patient with ovarian failure. *Fertil Steril* 69, 555–557.

Prapas Y, Prapas N, Jones E E et al. (1998). The window for embryo transfer in oocyte donation cycles depends on the duration of progesterone therapy. *Hum Reprod* 13, 720–723.

Press F, Shapiro H M, Cowell C A, Oliver G D (1995). Outcome of ovum donation in Turner's syndrome patients. *Fertil Steril* 64, 995–998.

Remohi J, Gallardo E, Guanes P P, Simon C, Pellicer A (1995). Donor-recipient synchronization and the use of gonadotrophin-releasing hormone agonists to avoid the premature luteinizing hormone surge in oocyte donation. *Hum Reprod* 10(Suppl. 2), 84–90.

Remohi J, Ardiles G, Garcia-Velasco J A, Gaitan P, Simon C, Pellicer A (1997). Endometrial thickness and serum oestradiol concentrations as predictors of outcome in oocyte donation. *Hum Reprod* 12, 2271–2276.

Robinson A C, Dockeray C J, Cullen M J et al. (1984). Hypergonadotrophic hypogonadism in classical galactosaemia: evidence of defective oogenesis. Case report. *Br J Obstet Gynaecol* 91, 199–200.

Rock A, Schlaff W (1985). The obstetric consequences of uterovaginal anomalies. *Fertil Steril* 43, 681–691.

Rogers P A W, Murphy C B R, Leeton J, Hoise M J, Beaton L (1992). Turner's syndrome patients lack tight junctions between uterine epithelial cells. *Hum Reprod* 7, 883–885.

Rothenberg K H, Baby M (1988). The surrogacy contract, and the healthcare professional: unanswered questions. *Law Med Health Care* 16,113–120.

Salha O, Sharma V, Dada T et al. (1999). The influence of donated gametes on the incidence of hypertensive disorders of pregnancy. *Hum Reprod* 14, 2268–2273.

Sauer M V (2001). Defining the incidence of serious complications experienced by oocyte donors: a review of 1000 cases. *Am J Obstet Gynecol* 184, 277–278.

Sauer M V, Paulson R J, Ary B A, Lobo R A (1994). Three hundred cycles of oocyte donation at the University of Southern California: assessing the effect of age and infertility diagnosis on pregnancy and implantation rates. *J Assist Reprod Genet* 11, 92–96.

Sauer M V, Paulson R J, Lobo R A (1997a). Comparing the clinical utility of GnRH antagonist to GnRH agonist in an oocyte donation program. *Gynecol Obstet Invest* 43, 215–218.

Sauer M V, Paulson R J, Moyer D L (1997b). Assessing the importance of endometrial biopsy prior to oocyte donation. *J Assist Reprod Genet* 14, 125–127.

Schneider M A, Davies M C, Honour J W (1993). The timing of placental competence in pregnancy after oocyte donation. *Fertil Steril* 59, 1059–1064.

Schulte A C, Serhal P (1996). Twin pregnancy following embryo transfer on day 7 of the luteal phase in an oocyte donation programme. *Hum Reprod* 11, 893–894.

Serafini P (2001). Outcome and follow up of children born after IVF-surrogacy. *Hum Reprod* 7, 23–27.

Serhal P F, Craft I L (1987). Ovum donation: a simplified approach. *Fertil Steril* 48, 265–269.

Shenfield F, Steele S J (1995). A gift is a gift is a gift, or why gamete donors should not be paid. *Hum Reprod* 10, 253–255.

(1997). What are the effects of anonymity and secrecy on the welfare of the child in gamete donation? *Hum Reprod* 12, 392–395.

Snowdon C, Green J M (1997). Preimplantation diagnosis and other reproductive options: attitudes of male and female carriers of recessive disorders. *Hum Reprod* 12, 341–350.

Soderstrom-Anttila V (2001). Pregnancy and child outcome after oocyte donation. *Hum Reprod Update* 7, 28–32.

Soderstrom-Anttila V, Tiitinen A, Foudila T, Hovatta O (1998a). Obstetric and perinatal outcome after oocyte donation: comparison with in-vitro fertilization pregnancies. *Hum Reprod* 13, 483–490.

Soderstrom-Anttila V, Sajaniemi N, Tiitinen A, Hovatta O (1998b). Health and development of children born after oocyte donation compared with that of those born after in-vitro fertilization, and parents' attitudes regarding secrecy. *Hum Reprod* 13, 2009–2015.

Stassart J P, Corfman R S, Ball G D (1995). Continuation of a donor oocyte pregnancy in a functionally agonadal patient without early oestrogen support. *Hum Reprod* 10, 3061–3063.

Stein A L, March C M (1990). Pregnancy outcome of women with Müllerian duct anomalies. *J Reprod Med* 35, 411–414.

Steptoe P C, Edwards R G (1976). Reimplantation of a human embryo with subsequent tubal pregnancy. *Lancet* i: 880–882.

Surrogacy Arrangements Act (1985). Her Majesty's Stationery Office, London.

Toner J P (2001). Vaginal delivery of progesterone in donor oocyte therapy. *Hum Reprod* 15(Suppl. 1), 166–171.

Tsirigotis M, Hutchon S, Pelekanos M, Lawrence J, Yazdani N, Craft I L (1995). Experience with oocyte donation and intracytoplasmic sperm injection. *Hum Reprod* 10, 2821–2823.

Utian W H, Sheean L A, Goldfarb J M, Kiwi R (1985). Successful pregnancy after in vitro fertilisation and embryo transfer from an infertile woman to a surrogate. *N Engl J Med* 313, 1351–1352.

Utian W F, Goldfarb J M, Kiwi R et al. (1989). Preliminary experience with in vitro fertilization–surrogate gestational pregnancy. *Fertil Steril* 52, 633–638.

Van Steirteghem A C, Van den Abbeel E, Braeckmans P et al. (1987). Pregnancy with a frozen-thawed embryo in a woman with primary ovarian failure. *N Engl J Med* 317, 113.

Waring A R, Wallace W H (2000). Subfertility following treatment for childhood cancer. *Hosp Med* 61, 550–555.

Westlander G, Janson P O, Tängfors U, Bergh C (1998). Attitudes of different groups of women in Sweden to oocyte donation and oocyte research. *Acta Obstet Gynecol Scand* 77, 317–321.

Wood E, Batzen F, Corson S (1999). Ovarian response to gonadotrophins, optimal method for oocyte retrieval and pregnancy outcome in patients with vaginal agenesis. *Hum Reprod* 14, 1178–1181.

Yaron Y, Amit A, Mani A et al. (1995). Uterine preparation with estrogen for oocyte donation: assessing the effect of treatment duration on pregnancy rates. *Fertil Steril* 63, 1284–1286.

Yaron Y, Ochshorn Y, Amit A, Yovel I, Kogosowki A, Lessing J B (1996). Patients with Turner's syndrome may have an inherent endometrial abnormality affecting receptivity in oocyte donation. *Fertil Steril* 65, 1249–1252.

Ziegler W F, Russell J B (1995). High success with gestational carriers and oocyte donors using synchronized cycles. *J Assist Reprod Genet* 12, 297–300.

35

Dermatological conditions of the female genitalia

Leith A. Banney and Jane C. Sterling

Department of Dermatology, Addenbrooke's Hospital, Cambridge, UK

Introduction

Disorders of the skin in the vulval area can present at any stage of life. A young child may be unable to describe changes in skin sensation and a pubertal child may not be sure what is normal and what is abnormal at a time when so many bodily changes are occurring. Vulval disease in children and adolescents may, therefore, present late and hence be diagnosed slowly. There may be misconceptions that vulval disease is a result of poor hygiene and hence a feeling of shame or embarrassment, which can result in a further delay to presentation. The causes are multiple (Table 35.1).

As in adults, the most common symptoms of vulval disease are itch and pain. In children, these may mainly be noticed by parents as a change in behaviour, for instance a reluctance to go to the toilet, as that produces pain, a wish for certain clothes that do not press on the vulval skin, or rubbing and scratching. Careful examination of the vulval skin, the vagina, where possible, the oral mucosa and the rest of the skin and appendages can give many clues to the possible diagnosis of vulval skin disease. Common and some rare causes of vulval symptoms are listed in Table 35.2 and the signs of vulval disease shown in Table 35.3.

Infections

Streptococcal infection

Definition, epidemiology and aetiology
Streptococcal infection of the vulval area is not uncommon and can present at any age, but most commonly prepuber-

tally (Dhar et al., 1993). In several series of children with vulval symptoms, this infection was present in 10–18% (Dhar et al., 1993; Donald et al., 1991; Fischer and Rogers, 2000; Heller, 1969; Piippo et al. 2000). The responsible organism is usually the beta-haemolytic streptococcus *Streptococcus pyogenes*. A vulvitis with associated abscess formation has been reported with *Streptococcus pneumoniae* (Zeiguer et al., 1992).

Clinical features and prognosis
The predominant symptom is usually pain, variously described as soreness, tenderness or heat in the affected skin. Commonly, when the vulva is affected, the perianal area is also involved and may be the primary site of infection. The skin can be beefy red with skin oedema and sometimes erosions, exudate and crusting. It is usually, but not always, accompanied by a painful vaginitis and a vaginal discharge or anal involvement. Mild and chronic forms also occur and in these, itch may be a more prominent symptom. There may be general malaise, but even in an acute infection, this is frequently absent.

Differential diagnosis
Erythema of the vulva without vaginitis may be caused by seborrhoeic dermatitis and psoriasis. Other infecting organisms causing a vulvovaginitis with similar features to streptococcal infection are *Haemophilus influenzae* in up to 10% of cases (McFarlane and Sharma, 1987; Cox 1997), *Shigella* (Gryngarten et al., 1994), *Gardnerella vaginalis*, *Klebsiella pneumoniae* or *Candida* spp. (Piippo et al., 2000).

Paediatric and Adolescent Gynaecology, ed. Adam Balen et al. Published by Cambridge University Press.
© Cambridge University Press 2004.

Table 35.1. Dermatological conditions of the vulva

Types	Disorders
Infections	
Bacterial	Streptococcal infection
	Staphylococcal infection
	Folliculitis
	Intravaginal foreign body
	Other causes of vulvovaginitis
Viral	Warts
	Vulval intraepithelial neoplasia, grade 3 (Bowenoid papulosis)
	Molluscum contagiosum
	Herpes simplex
	Infectious mononucleosis
Fungal	Candidal infection
	Tinea cruris
Infestations	Scabies
	Pubic lice
	Threadworms
	Schistosomiasis
Inflammation	
Dermatitis	Irritant dermatitis
	Pseudoverrucose papules and nodules
	Allergic contact dermatitis
	Atopic dermatitis
	Seborrhoeic dermatitis
Other inflammatory skin disease	Intertrigo
	Psoriasis
	Lichen sclerosus
	Lichen planus
	Plasma cell vulvitis
	Focal vulvovestibulitis
	Acrodermatitis enteropathica
	Kawasaki disease
	Urticaria
Bullous disease	Epidermolysis bullosa
	Epidermolysis bullosa acquisita
	Chronic bullous disease of childhood
	Dermatitis herpetiformis
	Bullous pemphigoid and cicatricial pemphigoid
	Pemphigus
	Hailey–Hailey disease
	Darier's disease
	Erythema multiforme and Stevens–Johnson syndrome
Ulceration	Aphthous ulcer
	Behçet's disease
	Lipschütz ulcer
Vulval lumps	
	Hidradenitis suppuritiva
	Fox–Fordyce disease
	Crohn's disease
	Histiocytosis
	Lymphangioma
	Haemangioma
	Neurofibromatosis
	Syringomas

Table 35.2. Causes of vulval symptoms

Symptom	Causes
Itch	Lichen sclerosus
	Candidal infection
	Atopic eczema
	Seborrhoeic eczema
	Intertrigo
Pain	Lichen sclerosus
	Intertrigo
	Herpes
	Streptococcal infection
	Focal vulvitis
	Vulval ulceration
	Sexual abuse
Bleeding premenarche	Intravaginal foreign body
	Sexual abuse
	Premature menarche

Investigations

The infecting organism can usually be cultured from the vagina, vulval area or perianal skin. The nose and throat should also be swabbed as these sites may harbour the infection without symptoms (Kokx et al., 1987). After infection, a raised antistreptolysin O titre (ASOT) or anti-DNAse B may help to confirm the diagnosis. A persistent or recurrent infection may be triggered by an intravaginal foreign body.

Treatment

Systemic antibiotics such as penicillin, erythromycin or clarithromycin will be necessary to eradicate the infection. Relapse may occur in up to a third of treated individuals. Topical antibiotics are unlikely to treat vaginal infection adequately.

Staphylococcal infection

Definition, epidemiology and aetiology

Staphylococcal infection can occur alone or in combination with streptococcal infection in the form of impetigo. In the adolescent, superficial infection in the pubic area can cause a deeper folliculitis (see below). Atopy and eczema can predispose to staphylococcal infection.

Clinical features and prognosis

The classical presentation of yellow crusting is frequently not seen in the vulval area; instead, the infection may be seen as patchy erythema with superficial erosions. Occasionally, infection with epidermolytic strains of

Table 35.3. Causes of vulval disease

Disease	Cause
Paediatric vulvovaginitis	Intravaginal foreign body
	Candidal infection
	Haemophilus influenzae infection
	Streptococcal infection
	Staphylococcal infection
	Trichomonal infection
	Gonococcal infection
	Threadworms
Vulval rash	Dermatitis: atopic, seborrhoeic, contact irritant, contact allergic
	Psoriasis
	Candidal infection
	Viral exanthem, especially coxsackie virus
	Impetigo
	Toxic shock
	Tinea cruris
	Syphilis
	Acrodermatitis enteropathica
	Histiocytosis
Vulval ulceration	Herpes simplex infection
	Varicella zoster infection
	Hand, foot and mouth infection
	Infectious mononucleosis
	Lipschütz ulcers
	Behçet's syndrome
	Aphthous ulcer
	Erythema multiforme/ Stevens–Johnson syndrome
	Severe cellulitis
	Drug eruption
	Primary autoimmune blistering disorders: pemphigoid, pemphigus
	Epidermolysis bullosa
Vulval lumps	Molluscum contagiosum
	Warts
	Hidradenitis suppuritiva
	Syringomata
	Bowenoid papulosis
	Schistosomiasis

Staphylococcus aureus can produce transient blistering of the skin, known as bullous impetigo.

Differential diagnosis

Inflammation with erosions may also be caused by infection with *Candida*, *Streptococcus* or *Haemophilus* spp. but the autoimmune blistering disorders of pemphigus and chronic bullous dermatosis of childhood may cause confusion.

Investigations

A surface skin swab should permit culture of the infecting organism. A vaginal swab should also be taken, particularly if there is a discharge. The organism may be harboured in the nose of the child or the parents.

Treatment

The superficial infection of impetigo may respond to topical antibiotics such as mupirocin, polymyxin or short-term gentamicin. If mild, simple measures such as increased ventilation of the vulva and improved hygiene may be adequate to allow clearance. Gentle soaking with warm water will help to remove crusts, and topical antiseptic application will help to prevent reinfection. Flucloxacillin or erythromycin or clarithromycin may be needed in more severe or resistant infection.

Folliculitis

Definition, epidemiology and aetiology

Inflammation of the hair follicles is usually caused by infection with *S. aureus*. It occurs occasionally prepubertally (Fischer and Rogers, 2000), but when hair growth thickens, follicles deepen and skin flora changes, an infection may produce a persistent pustular eruption.

Bacterial folliculitis is more likely to develop if the skin is treated with topical steroid creams or if the area is persistently occluded. Repeated hair removal from the pubic area or in the groins (the "bikini line") either by depilatory methods or shaving can damage the follicles or adjacent skin and provide an easy portal of entry for organisms.

Clinical features and prognosis

The symptoms are of itch or tenderness. Initial signs are of perifollicular erythema and small pustules visible at the openings of the follicles. The hair may be retained, or, if the inflammation is deep and intense, may be lost. Occasional lesions may develop into deeper uncomfortable, hot swellings with abscess formation (Heller et al., 1969).

Differential diagnosis

A pseudofolliculitis following hair removal and subsequent ingrowing hair regrowth can also lead to inflammation centred around follicles.

Investigations

Ideally culture from a pustule should be obtained to establish the infecting organism.

Treatment

Treatment is often slow. Antibiotics may need to be taken for a few weeks to eradicate the infection. Topical agents do not work as effectively as systemic antimicrobial agents. Hair removal methods should be discontinued. Adequate ventilation of the skin by wearing loose clothing will help to prevent high numbers of surface bacteria.

Intravaginal foreign body

Definition, epidemiology and aetiology

A foreign body within the vagina can stimulate a vaginal discharge and act as a focus for infection. Several different items have been reported to be inserted either intentionally or by accident into the vagina by the child. Amongst those retrieved include beads, beans, coins and toilet paper. In a series of 17 children, small wads of toilet paper was the most common foreign body found within the vagina, being the cause in nine children (Pokorny, 1994). In teenagers, a forgotten tampon may be the commonest cause.

Clinical features and prognosis

The first feature is usually a vaginal discharge with an associated irritant vulvitis. The discharge may be purulent and foul-smelling and is occasionally blood stained. Secondary infection in the vagina may occur.

Differential diagnosis

All the causes of vulvovaginitis should be considered.

Investigations

Diagnosis of the presence of such foreign bodies in young children will usually need to be done under a general anaesthetic and with the use of a thin flexible scope, although some objects may be visible during standard examination and able to be retrieved easily.

Treatment

Removal of the foreign body and treatment of any infection should prove sufficient. However, repeated episodes may occur, either because of behavioural difficulties or because of poor use of toilet paper (Pokorny, 1994).

Other causes of vulvovaginitis

Other causes of vulvovaginitis are listed in Table 35.2.

Warts

Definition, epidemiology and aetiology

Warts are thickened and papillomatous benign epidermal tumours caused by infection with human papillomavirus (HPV). In adults and sexually active teenagers, the HPV types responsible for warts in the anogenital area are most commonly HPV types 6 and 11, but common cutaneous

types are also found in prepubertal children. Of these, HPV type 2 is reported most commonly, being present in between 16 and 42% of anogenital warts in children (Cohen et al., 1990; Handley et al., 1997).

Spread of the virus is by direct or indirect contact, so warts in children should always raise the possibility of sexual abuse. Other indicators of abuse should be considered. However, nonsexual acquisition may be the means of transmission (Cohen et al., 1990; Padel et al., 1990) as the virus may be caught by indirect contact or harmless interaction and may be caused by virus types found commonly in common nongenital warts.

Clinical features and prognosis

Warts in the anogenital area of young children often show features similar to warts at other cutaneous sites. They are raised, papillomatous and often hyperkeratotic (Fig. 35.1, colour plate). On mucosal surfaces, they are softer. There may be irritation, signs of scratching and possibly secondary bacterial infection.

Without treatment, anogenital warts will resolve spontaneously in most immunocompetent children. In one study of 41 children, 54% of children had cleared within five years either without treatment or after failed treatment (Allen and Siegfried, 1998). Treatment may help to speed regression.

Differential diagnosis

Vulval papules that may be confused with warts include molluscum contagiosum, epidermal naevi and syringomata. In areas in which schistosomiasis is endemic, vulval granulomatous masses containing schistosomal ova may occur as a response to the pelvic infection.

Investigations

Usually the diagnosis can be made clinically, but confirmation may be necessary by histological examination of a biopsy. Molecular typing of HPV can demonstrate whether the type is that most commonly found in genital lesions or in common skin warts, but this is not a widely used routine investigation.

Treatment

There is no treatment of warts that can guarantee clearance. The virus may be present subclinically in adjacent skin and apparent reinfection may be the result of ongoing infection. A recurrence rate of 27% has been reported in children even after clearance (Armstrong et al., 1998). Destructive or antimitotic approaches are used for cutaneous warts and can be applied to genital warts, although with greater caution especially in the younger child. Virally infected epidermis can be destroyed by cautery, cryotherapy, surgical removal using the scissor-snip technique

(Armstrong et al., 1998) or laser. None of these provides absolute chance of clearance.

Podophyllin has been a useful therapy for adult genital warts for many years. In the younger child, the purified podophyllotoxin would be a better choice as it is less likely to produce severe irritation. However, this product is not licensed for use in children. In adults, it is reported to be effective, resulting in clearance rate of 60% but recurrences are frequent.

Attempts to stimulate the immune response have so far given no conclusive evidence of efficacy. Systemic therapy with immuno modulating effects has been attempted with inosine pranobex and cimetidine. The latter has given some initially promising results (Franco, 2000), but placebo-controlled trials in cutaneous warts have not been supportive (Yilmaz et al., 1995). Stimulation of the immune response locally with the topical agent imiquimod has been reported to induce clearance, but controlled trials are needed.

Bowenoid papulosis (syn. vulval intraepithelial neoplasia grade 3)

Vulval intraepithelial neoplasia grade 3 (VIN 3) is very rare in childhood (Halasz et al., 1986) and only occasionally reported in adolescence. It is often associated with high-risk genital HPV infection (Weitzner et al., 1989). Full-thickness dysplasia of the epidermis may produce papules or plaques on the skin, which can appear erythematous or pigmented and may be velvety or smooth. The risk of progression to squamous cell carcinoma of the vulva should be considered, especially in immunosuppression (Giaquinto et al., 2000).

Molluscum contagiosum

Definition, epidemiology and aetiology
The lesions of molluscum contagiosum are caused by infection with the molluscum contagiosum virus, a member of the poxviruses. It is not an uncommon infection in young children, being most common in nursery and primary school children. Spread is by direct contact. In immunosuppressed individuals, infection may be particularly widespread and prolonged. Molluscum contagiosum may appear in the late stages of infection with the human immunodeficiency virus (HIV).

Clinical features and prognosis
The trunk and limbs are the most common areas of infection, but the anogenital area and upper thighs may be involved. Lesions only in the vulval area should alert the practitioner to the possibility that infection has been acquired by sexual contact (Bargman et al., 1986). In sexually active adolescents, the genital area may be infected primarily, with secondary spread to other sites.

Individual lesions are 1–5 mm in diameter and are domed papules with a characteristic central depression or umbilication (Fig. 35.2, colour plate). The papules are often slightly pale and shiny. In atopic individuals, even if there has been no eczema of infancy, there is often a mild eczema associated with the papules. This causes irritation, with the result that the papules of molluscum may be traumatized. Although in most cases, healing occurs without residual effect, residual scarring may occur on areas of skin above deeper adipose tissue (Fig. 35.3, colour plate). Scarring may also occur in isolated lesions that have had deep inflammation.

The infection will clear spontaneously within 6 to 36 months. Usually, once clearance starts, it proceeds rapidly.

Differential diagnosis
Individual lesions have a classical appearance, but appearances may be masked if the lesions are traumatized or amongst areas of eczema. Other papular lesions that might cause confusion are warts, syringomata or trichoepitheliomata on the face. In immunosuppression, cutaneous cryptococcosis may appear similar to molluscum contagiosum, although vulval lesions would be unusual.

Investigations
Diagnosis can usually be made on the basis of clinical appearance. In uncertain cases, either histological examination of a biopsy sample or microscopical examination of an unstained curetted lesion or expressed central core crushed on a slide will establish the diagnosis. If the infection is unusually widespread or persistent, or with marked involvement of the face, immunosuppression associated with HIV infection should be considered.

Treatment
Many treatments have been tried for molluscum contagiosum, but none is of proven efficacy. Clearance of lesions will probably only occur when an effective immune response against the virus is mounted, but it is possible that this may be stimulated by inflammation around individual lesions. Methods of destruction of the papules have been used for many years and these include curettage, cryotherapy, laser (Amstey and Trombetta, 1985), squeezing or poking a pointed wooden stick into the centre of each lesion. However, many children do not find these methods tolerable, even with the use of a local anaesthetic (Rosdahl et al., 1988) and scarring may occur if the destructive process damages

the dermoepidermal junction (Friedman and Gall, 1987). Causing local inflammation at the site of the mollusca may induce an immune response, and methods to do this include phenol, cantharadin (Epstein, 1989), podophyllin, podophyllotoxin (Syed et al., 1994), tretinoin (Papa and Berger, 1976) and salicylic acid (Ohkuma 1990).

Herpes simplex

Definition, epidemiology and aetiology
Herpes simplex (HSV) infection of the vulval and/or vagina is usually acquired sexually. In a young child, vulval herpes should definitely alert to the possibility of sexual abuse, although it is possible for the infection to have been acquired innocently from transmission via fingers of a parent.

Clinical features and prognosis
Many cases of primary herpetic infection may be subclinical, but when clinical it will usually cause a painful eruption at the site of inoculation. Yellowish blisters develop on an inflammatory base; when they burst, these will discharge serous fluid. There may be general malaise, pyrexia and fatigue. Reactivation episodes occur in up to 95% of individuals (Lafferty et al., 1987). There may be obvious triggers to reactivation such as another viral infection, general debilitation, trauma to the site or inflammation of the site. The clinical features of recurrent episodes are not usually as severe as a primary episode. Recurrences of the infection may occur only rarely or may occur up to monthly. Coincidence with the menstrual cycle is not uncommon.

Differential diagnosis
Small blisters in the vulval area may also be caused by impetigo, in which the infecting organism is an epidermolytic staphylococcal strain. The autoimmune blistering disorders of pemphigus and pemphigoid may occasionally cause confusion and are considered later in this chapter.

Investigations
Accurate diagnosis is important for appropriate treatment and also in cases where abuse is considered a possibility. Blister fluid can be examined rapidly using the electron microscope to detect typical herpetic viral particles. This is only possible in specialist centres. Alternatively, viral culture of the blister fluid will give a result in three to five days. Another rapid method for diagnosis is polymerase chain reaction amplification of DNA extracted from blister fluid or exudate from a blister floor. This permits distinction between HSV-1 and HSV-2. Immunocytochemistry using fluorescent labelled antibodies against HSV-1 or HSV-2 can be performed on cells scraped from the floor of a

deroofed blister. In uncertain cases, a skin biopsy may be taken and should show epidermal cell necrosis, multinucleate giant cell formation within the keratinocytes and an inflammatory cell infiltrate in the upper dermis and epidermis (Fig. 35.4, colour plate).

Treatment
Antiviral agents are of proven effectiveness in shortening the episode. Topical aciclovir cream or ointment may be soothing but does not produce a significant reduction of pain, infection or viral shedding. Oral aciclovir and the more recently developed valaciclovir and penciclovir, if taken early in the course of the disease or reactivation episode, will, in most cases, alleviate the clinical course. Pain relief and local measures may increase comfort. If recurrences are frequent or debilitating, continuous oral antiviral therapy can reduce the frequency of recurrences.

Infectious mononucleosis

Definition, epidemiology and aetiology
Orogenital ulceration can occur during acute infection with Epstein–Barr virus. It may be the major presenting feature of the illness (Hudson and Perlman, 1998). Although infectious mononucleosis is most common in young adults, infection with associated genital ulceration may occur in childhood (Wilson, 1993). The genital ulcers may be part of the spectrum of Lipschütz ulceration (see below).

Clinical features and prognosis
When occurring in the vulval area, an ulcer associated with infectious mononucleosis may occur alone or as part of a group (Sisson and Glick, 1998). The individual lesion may start as a small blister and progress rapidly to a superficial or necrotic ulcer. There is likely to be associated dysuria. Healing is complete within about a week to a month. The other features of infectious mononucleosis such as malaise, tiredness, sore throat and lymphadenopathy are frequently present either before or after the appearance of the ulceration.

Differential diagnosis
Ulceration in the genital area may be caused by aphthous ulceration, HSV infection, chicken pox, staphylococcal infection or autoimmune blistering in pemphigus.

Investigations
Culture of a surface swab will exclude other infective causes of ulceration and indicate whether secondary infection has occurred. If persistent, skin biopsy to exclude autoimmune

blistering is advised. The monospot test and antibody detection should confirm infection with Epstein–Barr virus.

Treatment

No specific treatment is necessary but general measures to reduce pain and the chance of secondary infection may be used.

Candidal infection (syn. moniliasis, thrush, candidiasis)

Definition, epidemiology and aetiology

Candida albicans is a common commensal organism within the vagina in adolescence and adult life but may cause an inflammatory reaction especially during overgrowth of the yeast. Candidal infection is less common before puberty and after the menopause. The organism may be found in vaginal swabs in nearly 10% of prepubertal girls (Cox, 1997) and in 23% of adolescent females with vulvovaginitis (Koumantakis et al., 1997).

Clinical features and prognosis

The main symptom is of irritation, usually both on the vulva and in the vagina. There is frequently a thick white or cream-coloured discharge, and the vulval skin may be erythematous with superficial fissures. Erosions and discomfort may arise after scratching.

In infants, *Candida* within the bowel is not uncommon, and inflammation may start around the anus and spread to affect the nappy area. The affected skin is smoothly erythematous, often with small superficial pustules at the edge of the erythematous area. There may be associated oral thrush. In infants who are inadvertently treated with topical steroids, the candidal infection may develop into a deeper nodular infection, granuloma gluteale infantum (see below).

Investigations

Culture of a swab from the vagina will show the presence of yeasts and culture will give confirmation.

Differential diagnosis

Lichen sclerosus may be misdiagnosed as candidiasis because of the symptom of itch and the whitish appearance of the vulva. Other irritant and eczematous conditions may be initially thought to be caused by *Candida* sp.

Treatment

Imidazoles are the most useful topical agent and should be used to treat both the vulva and the vagina. Vulval treatment alone is likely only to produce temporary relief. In more resistant or recurrent infections, oral fluconazole or itraconazole can be used.

Granuloma gluteale infantum

Definition, epidemiology and aetiology

A deep nodular inflammation in the napkin area may develop when candidal infection in this occluded site is treated inappropriately with topical steroids. The eruption has also been regarded as a variant of irritant napkin dermatitis and has been reported without evidence of candidiasis or steroid use (Konya and Gow, 1996). The condition is rare.

Clinical features and prognosis

The lesions may rarely be seen in infants or older children with incontinence. Dermal nodules within the napkin area are erythematous or purplish, sometimes resembling angiomas (Tappeiner and Pfleger, 1971). They may be slightly tender.

Differential diagnosis

Similar deep nodular area of inflammation or infiltration may be caused by deep fungal infection, panniculitis or a neoplastic infiltrate such as lymphoma.

Investigations

Biopsy may be necessary to exclude other causes of nodules. The changes are of an intense mixed inflammatory cell infiltrate without granulomatous features (Bluestein et al., 1990).

Treatment

Avoidance of possible contributory factors and adequate skin care should lead to a gradual resolution of the localized inflammation.

Tinea cruris (syn. ringworm)

Definition, epidemiology and aetiology

Fungal infection of the skin in temperate climates is usually caused by the dermatophytes *Trichophyton rubrum*, *Trichophyton mentagrophytes* or *Epidermophyton floccosum*.

Clinical features and prognosis

Fungal skin infection may be asymptomatic but is frequently pruritic. In the vulval area, there is a well-defined area of erythema, often spreading from the groin, without symmetry. The edge of the erythema may show flaking. The apex of the flexure is usually involved and may be macerated and sore.

It is very common for the toe-webs to be infected before the groins and so this area should always be examined. Evidence of dermatophyte infection may occasionally be seen elsewhere on the body as ringworm.

Differential diagnosis

Inflammatory rashes in the groin involving the vulva include psoriasis, seborrhoeic dermatitis, intertrigo, atopic eczema and contact eczema.

Investigations

Skin scrapings may show microscopical features of fungal hyphae and can be cultured for fungi.

Treatment

Topical imidazole creams are usually effective for treatment. Occasionally, for resistant or widespread disease or for poor compliance with self-administered cream, systemic therapy with griseofulvin or terbinafine may be needed.

Scabies

Definition, epidemiology and aetiology

Infestation with the *Sarcoptes scabiei* mite causes an intensely itchy response in the skin. The mite is unable to survive for prolonged periods away from the skin and infection between individuals requires skin to skin contact, probably for several minutes. The adult mite is able to burrow into the surface of the epidermis and continues to live within the epidermis throughout life. Eggs laid and faeces deposited within the burrow can elicit an inflammatory response, although it may take up to eight weeks for the allergic response to develop. The allergy is to constituents of mite faeces. In immunosuppressed individuals, the immune response may not elicit itch.

The infestation is spread by contact and in young children this is often a result of sharing a bed with an infected individual. In adolescents, the infestation may be acquired through sexual contact.

Clinical features and prognosis

The first and major symptom is of itch. This is often severe, especially when in bed, and may be of an intensity to wake the patient from sleep. Lesions in the genital area are not uncommon and often develop into firm inflammatory nodules of 0.5–1 cm in diameter.

Extragenital sites such as edges of palms and soles, wrists, elbows and axillary folds are more likely to reveal the characteristic burrows. In these, the female mite may be seen as a tiny dark dot at the deeper end of the skin line. Skin excoriation may lead to secondary bacterial infection. Spontaneous clearance of the infestation is unlikely and it will become chronic if untreated.

Differential diagnosis

Genital nodules may also be caused by candidal infection or staphylococcal folliculitis.

Investigations

Confirmation of the presence of the mite within the skin will facilitate treatment. If a burrow is found, the mite may be carefully extracted with a blunt pin point and viewed under a microscope. Alternatively, a surface skin scraping from an area over possible burrows examined under a microscope may reveal clusters of eggs.

Treatment

The infestation can be treated with topical application of malathion or permethrin. The widely available benzoyl benzoate is effective but application is usually painful. The whole body from neck to toes must be treated and any close contacts treated at the same time. Bedding and clothing should ideally be washed coincidentally. Treatment can be repeated after one week to try to ensure that no mites are missed.

Pubic lice (syn. crab lice, phthiriasis pubis)

Definition, epidemiology and aetiology

The pubic louse, *Pthirus pubis*, is spread from person to person by close contact. It is able to survive in hair of relative sparsity and hence its adaptation to the pubic area. The louse is occasionally found in the eyelashes, eyebrows, margins of scalp hair, body hair or, in men, beard.

Clinical features and prognosis

Adolescents, but not usually prepubertal children, may be at risk of acquiring this infestation and the route of acquisition is usually through sexual contact. Young children may occasionally be infected (Klaus et al., 1994), when close contact through bedsharing may be the route of transmission.

The infected individual will usually complain of irritation in the pubic area and any other infected sites. There may be scratching and skin damage, possibly complicated by secondary bacterial infection. The lice are usually visible on close inspection of the pubic hair. Small bruises, corresponding to the sites of bites, may also be seen in the skin of the affected area. Examination of eyelashes and eyebrows may occasionally reveal lice in these areas too.

Differential diagnosis
Scabies.

Investigations
Diagnosis can be made by close inspection of the pubic hairs. Eggs are laid and cemented onto the hair shafts. Occasionally the louse may be visible, seen as a 1 mm creature with widely splayed legs gripping onto adjacent hairs.

Treatment
Treatment is with the topical application of an aqueous solution of malathion or permethrin cream. These can be very irritant in the eye, so for treatment of eyelash infestation, a thick layer of white soft paraffin will suffocate the lice.

Threadworm infection (syn. Pinworm infection)

Definition, epidemiology and aetiology
Threadworms or pinworms (*Enterobius vermicularis*) are found throughout the world. The infection is more common in areas of overcrowding and poor hygiene. The infection is acquired via orofaecal spread.

Clinical features and prognosis
The most common symptom is of itching around the anus, especially at night. Migration of the worms from the anus to the vulva and vagina may lead to symptoms of itch or pain and soreness in these areas. About 20% of girls with threadworm infection have symptoms of vulval irritation (Altchek, 1981). The features visible on the skin are usually those caused by scratching, with inflammation and excoriation. Secondary bacterial infection may bring signs of impetigo or streptococcal infection.

Differential diagnosis
Bacterial vulvitis and vulvovaginitis can produce a similar picture.

Investigations
Confirmation of infection can be gained by examination of stool for live worms or eggs. The application of clear adhesive tape to the perianal skin after sleep is very likely to trap eggs or live worms, which can be identified microscopically.

Treatment
Eradication of infection, prevention or minimization of reinfection and treatment of local symptoms are all desirable. The infection can only be eradicated by systemic therapy with an antiparasitic such as mebendazole or piperazine, which should ideally also be given to close contacts. Clothing and bedding should be washed after the treatment.

The risk of reinfection can be minimized by attention to hygiene and personal habits. The skin of the vulval and perianal area may be excoriated, sore and secondarily infected. A soothing bland application such as white soft paraffin or zinc and castor oil cream may need to be combined with a topical antibiotic.

Schistosomiasis (syn. bilharzia)

Definition, epidemiology and aetiology
Infection with the parasitic fluke *Schistosoma* spp. causes schistosomiasis. Three species are the common causes of schistosomiasis: *S. haematobium*, *S. mansoni* and *S. japonicum*. The areas of infection are in the tropics and subtropical areas of the world, especially Africa, South America, the Middle East, India and Southeast Asia.

The life cycle of the organism involves the hatching in water of the ovum into a miracidia, which can develop in the aquatic snail into a cercaria. This is able to penetrate the skin of animals, including humans. In the animal host, the cercaria develops in the liver into a fluke, which can spread via the blood throughout the body. In the pelvic veins, the fluke produces eggs, which are shed to the environment. The organism usually spreads from person to person via water, leaving one individual via the faeces or, in the case of *S. haematobium*, via the urine and being acquired via the skin.

Clinical features and prognosis
Skin lesions develop at the site of infection. These are usually areas of itchy eczematous reaction appearing after contact with infected water through swimming or bathing. In areas of high endemicity, especially of *S. haematobium*, perianal and vulval lesions may occur (Adeyemi-Doro et al., 1979; Mawad et al., 1992) most commonly in children. These are a reaction to the spread of ova from the pelvic veins through the tissues to the surface. The early lesions may be small irritating papules or nodules, but these can develop into protuberant masses with sinus formation and ulceration. These may be itchy and sore and associated with a vaginitis. The lesions usually start at the skin/mucosal junction but may gradually spread. Local fibrosis may affect fertility, cause pelvic pain and menstrual irregularity (Leutscher et al., 1998). Other clinical features include dermatitis at the site of skin penetration, urticaria and systemic features. There are potential late complications of liver fibrosis and bladder cancer.

Investigations
The infection is systemic and diagnosis can be made via detection of the ova in faeces or urine. Antischistosoma antibodies are detectable. Skin biopsy of vulval masses will

be helpful to exclude other diagnoses. Schistosomal vulval tumours are granulomatous masses with fissures and sinuses. Ova may be visible within the masses.

Differential diagnosis
The vulval lesion may be confused with anogenital warts (Kingston et al., 2001), lymphogranuloma venereum or malignancy.

Treatment
Eradication of the infection from the body can usually be achieved with antihelminthics such as praziquantel, metrifonate or oxamniquinine. Longer-term clearance of the infecting organism from the environment will be necessary to reduce the risk of reinfection.

Inflammation

Vulval inflammation can be usefully divided broadly into inflammation of the vulva and vagina together (vulvovaginitis) and inflammation of the vulva alone (vulvitis). Although some conditions may never involve the vagina, some are likely to involve both sites. Conditions listed in Table 35.3 are described in greater detail here.

Dermatitis

Definition
Dermatitis or eczema is a pattern of reaction (i.e. inflammation) of the skin and is not, by itself, a diagnosis. There are several forms of dermatitis, varying by their cause, clinical pattern, and, to a lesser extent, treatment.

Irritant dermatitis

Definition, epidemiology and aetiology
Repeated or continuous mechanical or chemical trauma that alters the barrier function of the skin and produces an inflammatory reaction may result in irritant dermatitis. The factors that are likely to produce such a reaction will depend on age (Table 35.4).

Table 35.4. Causes of irritant dermatitis of the vulva

Age	Causative factor
Baby/infant	Urine, faeces, prolonged humidity
Toddler	Sand, bubble baths, prolonged contact with wet clothes
Child	Bubble bath, soap
Adolescent	Hygiene products

Clinical features and prognosis
The skin of the vulva is erythematous and uncomfortable. There may be tenderness to touch and itching. In severe cases, there may be ulceration and occasionally the development of nodular lesions (see pseudoverrucous papules and nodules, below). Prolonged irritation and the development of the habit of scratching can lead to lichen simplex, which is a chronic dermatitis in which the skin appears leathery and thickened.

Investigations
The diagnosis is based mainly on clinical features. A biopsy may help to distinguish the features of dermatitis (lichen simplex) from other causes of itch (Fig. 35.5, colour plate).

Differential diagnosis
Atopic dermatitis, allergic contact dermatitis, seborrhoeic dermatitis, psoriasis and intertrigo may present similarly.

Treatment
Avoidance of the causative agent should eventually lead to clearance. Inflammation can be controlled with a mild or moderate strength topical steroid and the barrier function of the skin is assisted by the use of an ointment emollient. Secondary infection should be considered and treated appropriately.

Pseudoverrucose papules and nodules

Prolonged faecal or urinary incontinence and the associated skin irritation may lead to the development of nodular or warty swellings in the perianal or vulval area (Goldberg et al., 1992; Silverberg and Laude, 1998). The nodular lesions may become ulcerated or friable and there is a risk of secondary infection. Biopsy shows epidermal hyperplasia and hyperkeratosis, with mild to moderate dermal inflammation. The condition may be confused with anogenital warts (raising concerns about abuse (Amiry et al., 2001)), granuloma gluteale infantum, Crohn's disease and other causes of skin papules in the anogenital area.

Allergic contact dermatitis

Definition, epidemiology and aetiology
The development of a contact sensitivity can occur to many agents when applied repeatedly to the skin (Marren et al., 1992). Potential culprits for the vulval skin include perfumes, hygiene products and clothing dyes, which may leach out of new clothes under conditions of occlusion and high humidity. Treatment preparations contain a number of possible allergens, which are the responsible agents in the majority of vulval allergies (Bauer et al., 2000).

Preservatives in creams as well as the active agents such as antibiotics, anaesthetics and steroids can all act as allergens. Latex allergy can develop after contact with condoms.

Clinical features and prognosis

The symptoms are of itch, tenderness or a burning sensation. The skin will be erythematous and possibly flaking. In more severe cases, there may be erosions and weeping of the skin.

Investigations

The most important investigation is thorough and accurate allergy patch testing. The standard battery as well as preservatives in creams and medicaments will cover the most usual allergens.

Differential diagnosis

Atopic and seborrhoeic eczema appear similar and intertrigo and candidal infections may initially give the same picture.

Treatment

Avoidance of the causative allergen will eventually lead to remission. Topical steroids, emollients and treatment of secondary infection may be essential in the acute phase.

Atopic dermatitis (syn. atopic eczema)

Definition, epidemiology and aetiology

Atopic dermatitis forms part of the atopic syndrome of hay fever, asthma and eczema in combination with a raised IgE level and a tendency to form type I hypersensitivity reactions to multiple allergens. Atopic eczema affects up to 15% of infants and young children, but up to 10% of adults (Holden and Parish, 1998). There is a strong genetic tendency to inherit atopy.

Clinical features and prognosis

The main complaints are of itch and possibly soreness. The skin may feel tight and dry. The areas affected are primarily the limb flexures, although in infants and adults, the extensor surfaces of limbs, face and scalp may be involved. Buttock and occasionally groin and vulval skin may show the characteristic signs of dry and flaky skin with erythema and sometimes erosions and secondary infection. The tendency to exhibit one or more of the diseases of atopy will not change with age, although it is not unusual for childhood eczema to fade at puberty.

Investigations

Measurement of serum IgE level will help to establish if the patient is atopic. Skin swabs will frequently show evidence of colonization of the skin with *S. aureus* but in the vulval area other pathogens such as streptococci and yeasts may exacerbate the condition.

Differential diagnosis

Other causes of flexural eczema such as seborrhoeic dermatitis may appear similar.

Treatment

Frequent use of emollients in the affected area will help to maintain barrier function of the skin and reduce dryness. A topical steroid of mild to moderate strength may be indicated for short periods if the skin is inflamed. Secondary bacterial infection should be treated and the possibility of a contributory contact allergy considered. Systemic antihistamine may produce sedation, thus helping to reduce irritation and the tendency to scratch.

Seborrhoeic dermatitis

Definition, epidemiology and aetiology

Seborrhoeic dermatitis is an inflammation of the skin thought to be associated with reaction to surface yeasts and possibly bacteria.

Clinical features and prognosis

It can develop in infancy, frequently in association with the other common manifestation of the condition, cradle cap. In cradle cap, the scalp is covered with rather greasy, adherent scales, affecting the anterior vertex only in mild cases but becoming more extensive in severe cases. The napkin area is often involved, with the skin showing well-demarcated erythema with some flaking.

Seborrhoeic dermatitis is rare in childhood but can appear in adolescence. Once the sebaceous glands are active, it may develop on the face and also flexural sites such as the groins and axillae. In the vulva, the interlabial sulcus is often involved. Seborrhoeic dermatitis in the groin and vulva is not very scaly but is erythematous with a slight yellow-orange shade. It affects the apex of the flexures, where, especially in overweight individuals, the skin may become macerated and eroded, probably as a result of secondary bacterial infection.

Investigations

The diagnosis of seborrhoeic dermatitis is clinical. Surface swabs may be necessary to exclude secondary bacterial or yeast infection.

Differential diagnosis

Candidal infection, psoriasis and intertrigo can produce similar clinical pictures.

Treatment

The best therapeutic response in seborrhoeic dermatitis is usually with a combination of a topical anti-inflammatory steroid plus an agent active against yeasts. A hydrocortisone/imidazole cream is a suitable choice. However, care must be taken in the application of even mild steroids in this occluded flexural site in young children to avoid the side effects of skin thinning and striae formation.

Other inflammatory skin diseases

Intertrigo

Definition, epidemiology and aetiology

Inflammation of the flexures in the presence of some bacterial or yeast growth constitutes the rather ill-defined condition of intertrigo. The condition is more common in overweight and diabetic individuals.

Clinical features and prognosis

Defined areas of flexural skin are erythematous with maceration and some peeling, especially at the apices of the flexures. The groins, natal cleft, axillae, submammary areas and umbilicus may be affected. The skin is frequently sore and uncomfortable, made worse by friction and sweating.

Investigations

Surface skin swab will usually detect bacteria or yeasts. These may be commonly *S. aureus*, group G Streptococci, *Escherichia coli*, *Proteus* spp., *C. albicans* and less commonly beta-haemolytic *Streptococci* or *Pseudomonas aeruginosa*.

Differential diagnosis

There is possibly some overlap with seborrhoeic dermatitis and psoriasis, and eruptions with features of both may be labelled "sebopsoriasis". The soreness of seborrhoeic dermatitis might suggest streptococcal infection.

Treatment

Hygiene with ventilation of the affected area will reduce skin flora. The inflammation will be improved with the use of a mild to moderate topical steroid for a limited period of time. This can be combined with a topical antibiotic or antiseptic to reduce the effect of superficial infection or irritation by surface organisms.

Psoriasis

Definition, epidemiology and aetiology

Psoriasis is a disorder of skin renewal driven by an immunological abnormality. A genetic predisposition plus an environmental trigger is believed to result in the onset of the disease. Psoriasis can become evident at any age, but the onset is rare before two. The disease presents most commonly in the teenage years or early adult life (Farber and Nall, 1974). Both sexes are affected equally, but in childhood, girls are affected more commonly than boys.

Clinical features and prognosis

The onset of psoriasis may be rapid or gradual. When the onset of psoriasis is in infancy, the nappy area is most commonly affected (Farber and Jacobs, 1977) with predominant involvement of the skin in direct contact with the nappy (Warin and Faulkner, 1961). Small pits in the nails may give a clue to the diagnosis as well as the typical scaly lesions of psoriasis elsewhere on the body.

The typical psoriatic lesion is a well-demarcated area of erythematous skin covered with shiny scales. In the flexural areas, including the anogenital region, the scaling is frequently absent and the lesions appear as larger, often confluent areas of erythema with a slightly shiny or glazed surface. If the apex of the flexure is involved, there may be maceration of the skin and some superficial fissuring. The mucous membranes are not involved.

Investigations

Diagnosis is based on clinical signs. A skin biopsy will show epidermal thickening with elongation of the rete ridges, dilated dermal blood vessels and a neutrophilic infiltrate, possibly with microabscesses within the epidermis. When the napkin area is involved in infancy, swabs from this site will frequently show evidence of *Candida* spp. (Rasmussen et al., 1986).

Differential diagnosis

The main possibilities are seborrhoeic dermatitis, intertrigo and candidal infection and indeed, these conditions may overlap with psoriasis. In seborrhoeic dermatitis, other areas commonly affected are the scalp and eyebrows. Atopic eczema and contact allergy may be considered. In infancy, the distinction between napkin psoriasis and a severe irritant napkin dermatitis can be difficult (Neville and Finn, 1975).

Treatment

Treatment of psoriasis of the vulva, as in other flexural sites, is limited by the relatively thin skin and the risk of potential irritation. Bland emollients can help to reduce the frictional irritation, but mild or moderate topical steroids will often be necessary to reduce the ongoing inflammation. Treatments used commonly to treat psoriasis elsewhere on the body, such as tar preparations, dithranol or vitamin D analogues can often be too irritant for use in the occluded skin of a young child. In severe psoriasis, systemic therapy may be required to control the disease.

Lichen sclerosus (syn. lichen sclerosus et atrophicus)

Definition, epidemiology and aetiology

Lichen sclerosus (LS) is an inflammatory, scarring condition with a predilection for the vulva and perianal area. It produces inflammatory hypopigmented plaques that progress to areas of atrophy.

Females are affected with LS ten times more frequently than males, but it is reported at all ages in both sexes. Two age peaks of incidence occur in females. The perimenopausal group is the larger but there is an increasing incidence in premenarchal girls (Powell and Wojnarowska, 2001). Children as young as four weeks have been reported with LS (Lynch and Edwards, 1994). In a study of the Oxford area, UK, an incidence of at least 1 in 900 prepubertal girls was estimated (Powell and Wojnarowska, 2001). In a review of vulval disorders presenting in a paediatric dermatology clinic, LS accounted for 18% of cases (Fischer and Rogers, 2000). Caucasians form the majority of cases. An English study of 350 patients with LS included only three Asian women and no Blacks (Ridley, 1989). In this series, 31 of these 350 had onset in childhood.

LS is most likely multifactorial in origin. Genetic variation may predispose to the disease and local factors such as hormones, infection and trauma may act as precipitants.

Autoimmunity

There is an increased incidence of both autoantibodies and autoimmune disease. In two series of 30 and 70 paediatric cases, 4% and 14%, respectively, had associated autoimmune disease (Fischer and Rogers, 2000; Powell and Wojnarowska, 2001). A family history of autoimmunity was seen in over 50% of affected individuals. Autoimmune diseases reported in association with LS include thyroid disease, pernicious anaemia, diabetes mellitus, alopecia areata and vitiligo, systemic lupus erythematosus, CREST (calcinosis, Raynaud phenomenon, oesophageal involvement, sclerodactyly and telangiectasia syndrome) and primary biliary cirrhosis (Meyrick Thomas et al., 1988; Rowell and Goodfield, 1998). An increased incidence of certain HLA (human leukocyte antigen) loci are seen. In particular, the association with HLA DQ7 is higher in paediatric compared with adult-onset LS, although there is a significant association in all age groups. DQ7 occurred in 66% of

30 children with LS, in 51% of affected adult female and 31% of controls. The presence of HLA DQ7 is seen as associated with early age of onset of LS. Other HLA associations have been reported but not always confirmed with subsequent studies. These include HLA A2, A29, B40, B44, as well as DQ8 and DQ9 (Rowell and Goodfield, 1998).

Hormones

Onset in prepubertal and perimenopausal females leads to the concept of LS susceptibility in persons without adult female oestrogen levels. The resolution of some cases at puberty adds further credence to this. However, it is increasingly recognized that resolution at puberty is uncommon. In a series of 37 patients, 36 still had signs of LS after puberty although many had no remaining symptoms.

Infection

Vaginitis has preceeded LS in some women. The significance of this is unclear, however, as an inflammatory and sometimes erosive condition may itself provide a fertile ground for secondary infection. *Borrelia burgdorferi* DNA has been reported in tissue from areas of LS, but no definite association has been made (Fujiwara et al., 1997).

Trauma

The "Koebner" phenomenon, in which new lesions evolve at a site of trauma, is well described in LS. LS has been reported to develop in vaccinations, radiotherapy and burn scars. It has even occurred in grafts of normal skin used in the vulval area. However, vulval skin grafted to the thigh has been reported to return to normal (Ridley, 1988).

Clinical features and prognosis

The presentation of LS in children varies. Symptoms vary from distressing pruritus and pain through to completely asymptomatic disease. When present, the commonest symptom is pruritus, but soreness, dysuria and surface bleeding also occur. Perianal symptoms such as painful bowel movements and constipation owing to fissures may also occur.

Clinically, LS has a "figure of eight" distribution around the vulva and the perianal areas. LS does not extend to involve the vagina. Ivory-coloured atrophic plaques and papules, often with superimposed telangiectasia and purpura, are seen (Fig. 35.6, colour plate). Classically, the white plaques show a fine surface wrinkling and shiny hue. Follicular plugging may be present in hair-bearing areas. With progressive atrophy of the skin, fragility, fissures and erosions, even frank ulceration, can develop. Secondary bacterial infection may develop affecting both the skin and the genitourinary tract. In very inflammatory cases, complete separation can occur between the epidermis and dermis, leading to blister formation (Fig. 35.7, colour plate). Bullae may contain serosanguinous fluid. With progressive disease, there may be distortion of the normal vulval architecture. In severe disease, this can even lead to resorption of structures such as the labia, with narrowing of the introitus and adhesion formation. Urinary obstruction and loss of sexual function can occur as late sequelae.

Up to 10% of children have extragenital lesions of lichen sclerosus. These tend to be ivory plaques and papules, usually between 0.5 and 5 cm in diameter. They are at first thickened and then become atrophic, sometimes leading to areas of hyper- as well as hypopigmentation. The same spectrum of changes is seen in extragenital and genital lesions (i.e. purpura, telangiectasia, erosions, bullae, fissures, follicular plugging and secondary infection). The extragenital lesions are commonest on the upper trunk, breasts, neck, volar wrists and face.

In addition to infection, several other secondary changes are known to occur. Lichen simplex chronicus (i.e. thickening of skin owing to rubbing and scratching) is seen in many cases, but if typical changes of LS are seen, the diagnosis should not be difficult. Dysplasia and squamous cell carcinoma are well known to occur in areas of chronic inflammation.

Investigations

Usually clinical examination is the only necessary diagnostic procedure. If secondary infection is suspected, swabs should be taken, and biopsy will be needed if the presentation is unusual or any areas suggestive of malignancy are seen.

Histological examination shows a progression of changes. In early disease, a layer of oedema develops in the upper dermis with an associated infiltrate of lymphocytes along the dermoepidermal junction. Later, the lymphocytic infiltrate is displaced below the band of altered collagen and in advanced disease, the lymphocytes dissipate and no longer feature (Fig. 35.8, colour plate). Dilatation of small blood vessels in the upper dermis occurs and these are poorly supported owing to the surrounding damaged collagen. The blood vessels often rupture, leading to purpura and ecchymoses. When severe inflammation occurs, there may even be separation and bulla formation between the dermis and the epidermis. The epidermis (skin surface) is at first thickened and follicular plugging may be seen in hair-bearing areas. Later the epidermis thins and is prone to splits, erosions and infection.

The autoimmune associations with LS mean that screening for diabetes, pernicious anaemia, thyroid and connective tissue disease is a sensible approach. In children who are completely well and have no signs or symptoms of these conditions, it is reasonable for the caring doctor to investigate on an as needed basis. Once old enough to

tolerate blood testing without distress, autoantibody screening may be helpful to indicate those at risk of subsequent disease.

Differential diagnosis

The main differential diagnoses of LS in paediatric patients are

- eczematous conditions: atopic eczema, seborrheic eczema or dermatitis, contact dermatitis (irritant and allergic)
- psoriasis
- vulvovaginitis
- lichen simplex chronicus
- sexual abuse/trauma
- morphoea
- lichen planus
- vitiligo
- histiocytosis X (Langerhans' cell histiocytosis).

Most important in children is the misdiagnosis of LS as sexual abuse. Because of symptoms of soreness, itch and bleeding, as well as the clinical appearance of purpura, this is a common mistake. Recently, three cases of LS wrongly managed as cases of abuse were reported (Wood and Bevan, 1999). Also in a series of 72 girls with LS, it was found that the possibility of sexual abuse had been raised by either the GP or a family member in 77% of these (Powell and Wojnarowska, 2001). LS and sexual abuse could of course coexist, and LS will koebnerize into areas of trauma. If real signs of sexual abuse are seen, full investigation is necessary.

As well as systemic autoimmune disease, several cutaneous disorders are associated with LS and may cause diagnostic problems. Morphoea (localized scleroderma) has often been described as overlapping LS, and many believe they form a spectrum of the same disease. Morphoea results in hypopigmented inflammatory plaques, often with a violaceous border. These classically affect the trunk, and there is no involvement of the perineum in most cases. Extragenital lesions of LS are often indistinguishable from morphoea. The histology findings differ in these diseases and Ackerman believes that, despite clinical similarity, the diseases are entirely different (Patterson and Ackerman, 1984).

Lichen planus is also reported in association with LS (Connelly and Winkelman, 1985) and, again, many would consider these disorders a spectrum. Extragenital LS lesions often mimic lichen planus. Pathology may distinguish these diseases.

Treatment

There are three important issues in management of LS: (i) symptom and disease control, (ii) awareness of the association with disorders of autoimmunity, and (iii) the potential for the rare development of squamous cell carcinoma (SCC) in affected areas of chronic inflammation. Symptomatic control is usually easily achieved with the use of topical corticosteroids. It has recently been shown that not only do topical corticosteroids resolve symptoms but they can also resolve disease clinically (Fivozinsky and Laufer, 1998). In a series of 11 girls aged 3–11 with LS, response to potent topical corticosteroids included complete clinical resolution in nine cases over four months. The other two patients were asymptomatic but still had some clinical disease. Only three girls required maintenance with a lower strength topical corticosteroid (Fischer and Rogers, 1997). Various studies concur, with an approximately 90% complete resolution of symptoms with the use of potent topical corticosteroids (Chari et al., 1994; Fischer et al., 1995; Sinha et al., 1999). Unfortunately, symptoms respond better than does clinical and histological evidence of disease. In a retrospective study of 81 cases, 22% were clinically unchanged yet only 5% had unchanged symptoms with potent topical corticosteroids. At the other end of the spectrum, 31.5% had clinical remission, versus a total of 77% with a symptomatic remission (Bracco et al., 1993).

Initially, the steroid strength should be adequate to control symptoms and halt ongoing inflammation. Use of topical corticosteroids of inadequate strength is a common mistake in treatment and leads to an overall longer treatment period, necessitating larger amounts of total steroid used. In adults and all but the mildest cases in children, potent topical steroids will be needed initially, for example clobetasone propionate 0.05%. A soap substitute such as aqueous cream is a good idea to avoid drying and irritation of an already sensitive area.

Tapering the strength of steroid should be done once symptoms have abated and gross signs of inflammation are settling. Hopefully, the disease will enter a remission, but more often than not it will wax and wane, requiring intermittent or graduated use of topical steroids over many months. Side effects from the use of topical corticosteroids in LS are extremely rare. Prolonged continuous use of potent topical corticosteroids will result in atrophy and should be avoided. However, LS is a potentially scarring condition with a small but definite risk of SCC in chronic disease, and this means that treatment should be tailored to the individual. Other side effects are contact irritant (or far less commonly allergic) dermatitis, telangiectasia and rarely acneiform skin eruptions.

In particularly troublesome areas of LS, injected corticosteroids have a role. In particular, areas of intense pruritus and painful cracks and erosions may respond well. There is no role for oral corticosteroids in LS as this would mean the develop of often significant systemic side effects. Absorption of topical treatments in the perineum is excellent.

Apart from topical corticosteroids, multiple other treatments have been used. There is now believed to be little benefit from topical testosterone, progesterone and oestrogen preparations. Trials have not proven the value of these treatments, although topical testosterone is still used widely in adults (Pincus and McKay, 1993). One controlled trial has clearly shown superiority of clobetasol 0.05% topically compared with 2% testosterone in petrolatum, 2% progesterone in petrolatum and placebo (Bracco et al., 1993). Systemic androgenization has been reported with topical testosterone, including hirsutism, voice deepening, acne and increased libido. Some of these have been permanent and, consequently, its use in children cannot be considered safe (Lynch and Edwards, 1994). Other management strategies have included retinoids in the form of oral etretinate, cryotherapy, oral potassium *para*-aminobenzoate and the use of the flashlamp-pulsed dye and carbon dioxide (resurfacing) lasers. None of these can be considered reliable or desirable treatments.

With respect to the complication of SCC in adults with chronic LS, retrospective studies suggest an incidence of 4–5% (Hart et al., 1975; MacLean, 1993; Meyrick Thomas et al., 1988). No prospective studies have been done and this is possibly an overestimate of positive findings. Certainly, there have not been cases of SCC in affected children with LS. However, an advanced vulval SCC has been reported in a woman aged 32 with a childhood history of LS (Powell et al., 2001). This patient had improvement of symptoms at puberty and was lost to follow-up. Awareness of the risks of SCC is necessary, for both the clinician and patient, and cessation of symptoms should not necessarily mean the end of follow-up.

Owing to its link with SCC, LS has been treated in the past as a premalignant condition and vulvectomies performed. Commonly, recurrence of disease occurs in scars of surgery (Koebner phenomenon), and with other locally destructive treatments. Surgery should be avoided unless frank malignancy develops. Occasionally, labial adhesions or other local complications may need to be dealt with surgically.

Lichen planus

Definition, epidemiology and aetiology

Lichen planus is an inflammatory condition of unknown aetiology that can affect individuals of any age. The disease occurs worldwide.

Clinical features and prognosis

Lichen planus is most common in adult life. Onset in childhood or adolescence accounts for 1–2% of cases (Samman, 1961). The characteristic lesion of lichen planus is a skin papule or plaque with a purplish hue. The surface may show whitish streaks, known as Wickham's striae. The buccal mucosa is frequently affected coincidentally with skin lesions or alone; at this site, the whitish streaks often produce an interlacing pattern that may be more obvious than any signs of inflammation. The vulval area can be affected and also the vaginal mucosa.

Lichen planus affecting the labia is usually very itchy and produces some thickening of the skin with a purplish colour. If the vagina is involved, the predominant complaint is of soreness and pain. The vagina is very inflamed and the surface friable. The prolonged intense inflammation may result in scarring and narrowing of the vagina (Edwards, 1989). Erosive lichen planus of the vagina and vulva can coexist with oral lesions and has been described as the vulvovaginal–gingival syndrome (Pelisse, 1989). The course of the disease is frequently chronic, especially if mainly mucosal. Skin lichen planus often resolves spontaneously after many months.

Differential diagnosis
The mucosal lesions may appear similar to pemphigus or mucosal erythema multiforme. On external genital skin, other diagnoses to consider are LS, psoriasis, intertrigo and seborrhoeic dermatitis.

Investigations
Biopsy of affected skin or mucosa will show features of a band-like chronic inflammatory cell infiltrate in the dermis and changes at the basal epidermis with necrotic cells or colloid bodies (Fig. 35.9, colour plate). In the mucosa, there is frequently erosion of the epidermal surface.

Treatment
Anti-inflammatory agents are the most useful approach to lichen planus. Topical steroids of potent strength may be required for skin disease as a means of subduing the sensation of itch. Intravaginal erosive lichen planus is more difficult to treat. Prednisolone suppositories or liquid or foam steroid preparations used to treat rectal inflammation can be used in the vagina. Systemic immunosuppression with prednisolone or ciclosporin may be considered if local measures are unsuccessful.

Plasma cell vulvitis (syn. vulvitis circumscripta plasmacellularis)

Definition, epidemiology and aetiology
Plasma cell vulvitis is mainly a disease of adults, but it can rarely present in the teenage years.

Clinical features and prognosis
Discomfort of a tender or burning sensation may be well localized to the involved skin. The vaginal introitus is a common site, especially anteriorly. The appearances may be of a rather nonspecific erythema, but there is usually a moderately well-defined area of yellow–orange discolouration, sometimes with purpura or some friable surface blood vessels.

Differential diagnosis
Other causes of vulval erythema and soreness should be considered. The erythema, purpura and soreness may suggest child abuse (Albers et al., 2000).

Investigations
Plasma cell vulvitis is essentially a histological diagnosis. The appearances are of a dense upper dermal infiltrate of mixed inflammatory cells including many plasma cells. There is frequently dermal oedema and telangiecteses. Red cell extravasation and haemosiderin deposition in the dermis are frequently also apparent.

Treatment
Treatment is first with a moderate or potent topical steroid (Scurry et al., 1993). Intralesional steroid injection may also reverse signs and symptoms (Yoganathan et al., 1994). Topical oestrogen cream may help, although this has only been reported after the menopause (Scurry et al., 1993) and there may be improvement with a systemic retinoid (Robinson et al., 1998).

Vulvovestibulitis (syn. focal vulvitis, vestibular adenitis)

Definition, epidemiology and aetiology
Patchy inflammation at the vaginal introitus associated with discomfort or pain on light to moderate touch are the main features of this syndrome of unknown cause. An increased baseline of electromyographic activity has been reported in individuals with vulvovestibulitis although it is not certain if this is prior or secondary to the pain (White et al., 1997). Vulvovestibulitis is most common in young adults, sometimes starting as early as puberty.

Clinical features and prognosis
The most common symptom is of variable pain at the introitus. This may be limited to dyspareunia or may be associated with tampon use, physical activities such as riding or cycling, or may be experienced as constant burning or tenderness. The most common site for tenderness and erythema is at each side of the posterior introitus at the openings of the Bartholin's glands, although the whole introitus

may be affected. The mucosa may appear erythematous and sometimes has easy bleeding on touch. Areas of affected mucosa may occur at other areas of the introitus and occasionally in the lower half of the vagina.

The onset of the disorder may be sudden and may seem to be linked to an inflammatory event affecting the vulva or vagina, such as a vaginal infection, a urinary tract infection, a contact dermatitis or local surgery. It is usually a chronic disorder lasting months to years, but in most cases will eventually fade.

Differential diagnosis

The erythema and friable inflammation of the lower vagina may suggest erosive lichen planus. If accompanied by a discharge, a vaginal infection may be a possible cause of these symptoms.

Investigations

Vaginal swabs will be necessary to search for a vaginal infection. A mucosal biopsy will show nonspecific inflammation of lymphocytes and plasma cells, but will be helpful in excluding lichen planus.

Treatment

No treatment has yet been reported as uniformly effective. Many therapies have been tried and there are useful benefits reported with topical steroids, intralesional steroid injection, topical clindamycin cream, surgery and laser ablation (Reid et al., 1995). In addition, dietary oxalate reduction is felt by some to be beneficial (Baggish et al., 1997). As dyspareunia can be severe, the occasional prior application of a local anaesthetic cream may permit intercourse. The use of low-dose tricyclic or selective serotonin reuptake inhibitor antidepressant can help as a "pain modifier", permitting adaptation to chronic pain and augmentation of effect of standard analgesics (McKay, 1993). Psychosexual support may be needed.

Acrodermatitis enteropathica

Definition, epidemiology and aetiology

Inflammation and superficial erosions, predominantly in the perioral and anogenital skin, associated with systemic zinc deficiency constitute acrodermatitis enteropathica. It may occur in malabsorption or during a diet with prolonged insufficient zinc, such as parenteral nutrition.

Clinical features and prognosis

The perimucosal skin is the major site affected, with variable involvement of flexural areas. The skin is erythematous, peeling and frequently raw and eroded.

Investigations

The serum zinc can be measured, although this does not always accurately reflect tissue levels.

Differential diagnosis

Flexural inflammation caused by intertrigo or seborrhoeic dermatitis may produce a similar appearance. Cutaneous histiocytosis also causes an inflamed and sometimes eroded eruption.

Treatment

Oral or parenteral zinc replacement should lead to improvement within days and clearance within weeks. Local measures such as emollients and mild topical steroids will keep the skin more comfortable until clearance occurs.

Kawasaki disease (syn. mucocutaneous lymph node syndrome)

Definition, epidemiology and aetiology

The cause of this rare acute febrile illness with vascular inflammation is unknown although viral and bacterial agents have been proposed as triggers. Kawasaki disease occurs mainly in young children, but rarely in older children, adolescents and adults. There is geographical variation, with the majority of cases occurring in East Asia.

Clinical features and prognosis

The disorder is characterized by fever for at least 5 days plus other features, which include perineal and palmoplantar erythema that evolves over a few days to peeling. Other clinical signs of conjunctival inflammation, oropharyngeal inflammation, a polymorphic eruption, cervical lymphadenopathy as well as coronary artery involvement may be present to complete the diagnosis (Nasr et al., 2000).

Differential diagnosis

Many disorders can be indistinguishable from Kawasaki disease initially. These include infectious and connective tissue diseases.

Investigations

The diagnosis of Kawasaki disease is mainly clinical with nonspecific markers of inflammation. Investigation of the coronary arteries and cardiac function is important in order to identify these complications.

Treatment

Successful treatment has been reported with aspirin (Kawasaki, 1995) and intravenous immunoglobulin (Neuberger et al., 1986)

Urticaria and angio-oedema

Definition, epidemiology and aetiology
Itchy weals with flare may occur together with or independently from deeper subcutaneous swelling of angio-oedema. The junctions between mucous membrane and skin, such as the lips and external genitalia, are common sites for angio-oedema. Although in many cases there is no obvious precipitating factor, the attacks can be linked in some to ingestion of specific foods or salicylic acid, or to physical trauma such as pressure or cold or heat. Congenital or acquired abnormality of C1 esterase enzyme of the complement pathway may be the cause in a small minority of affected individuals. Other possible causes of urticaria and angio-oedema include thyroid disease, myeloma and connective tissue disease.

Clinical features and prognosis
Vulval angio-oedematous swelling may be asymptomatic but there is usually variable irritation, tingling or discomfort (Lambiris and Greaves, 1997). The swelling of angio-oedema can take several hours to clear. Recurrent attacks can occur every day or less frequently. The disorder is frequently chronic.

Investigations
Exclusion of possible underlying disease as a cause for urticaria is necessary.

Differential diagnosis
Acute vulval swelling may be caused by infection, especially streptococcal, or inflammation in hidradenitis suppuritiva; more chronic swelling may be caused by lymphangioma.

Treatment
Oral antihistamine will improve the irritation but is less effective against oedematous swelling. In severe cases, systemic immunosuppression with prednisolone or ciclosporin may reduce severity of attacks.

Bullous (blistering) disorders

The spectrum of bullous disorders affecting children and adults differ. Inherited disorders will be diagnosed in childhood, and acquired (usually immune mediated) bullous disorders are less common than in adults. Bullous disorders usually require biopsy as clinical signs overlap greatly between diseases and the correct treatment of each condition can be quite different.

Those bullous diseases with a predilection for the genital region include chronic bullous dermatosis of childhood, dermatitis herpetiformis (buttock area) and a rare presentation of pemphigoid, which has been described as childhood vulval pemphigoid (De Castro et al., 1985; Farrell et al., 1999; Guenther and Shum, 1990; Haustein, 1988).

Flexural distribution of blistering is seen in pemphigus, and the rare Fox–Fordyce disease. Flexural erosions occur in Darier's disease and Hailey–Hailey disease.

Bullous disorders of the genital region in paediatric patients include
- infections: candida, HSV, staphylococci (including bullous impetigo, staphylococcal scalded skin), scabetic pustular lesions, hand foot and mouth disease, varicella and cytomegalovirus (see above sections)
- mechanobullous disease: epidermolysis bullosa
- autoimmune bullous disease: including chronic bullous dermatosis of childhood, dermatitis herpetiformis, pemphigoid, pemphigus
- trauma: chemical or thermal injury.

Epidermolysis bullosa

Definition, epidemiology and aetiology
Epidermolysis bullosa is the name given to a group of inherited defects of the basement membrane zone of skin.

Clinical features and prognosis
Epidermolysis bullosa usually presents with widespread blistering in the neonate, not localized to perineal structures. The exception to this would be a breech delivery or infant with trauma to the perineum. The severity of the disease depends upon which element of the basement membrane is abnormal. Generally speaking, the more superficial the defect, the less severe the condition. Blisters are mechanobullous, that is occur at sites of trauma and friction. Epidermolysis bullosa ranges from localized nonscarring forms through to generalized scarring of skin and mucous membranes, including oesophagus and gut (Petersen et al., 1996). The most severe forms are usually lethal in infancy and result in blindness; loss of hair, teeth and nails; and strictures of mucosal surfaces. Scarring in the vulva can lead to difficulty with menstruation (Steinkampf et al., 1987). Small cell carcinoma occurs in areas of chronic ulceration.

Differential diagnosis
The differential diagnosis includes HSV, staphylococcal scalded skin syndrome and other bullous conditions (discussed below).

Investigations

Biopsies are necessary to diagnose the level of split (or blistering) and immunofluorescence and electron microscopy studies on skin can assist in clarifying the defect and aid in providing prognostic information.

Treatment

Of utmost importance in the management of patients with epidermolysis bullosa is the avoidance of skin friction and trauma. No adhesive dressing should be used, handling needs to be minimized and sheets and bedding should be soft and seamless. When the patient is in hospital, appropriate signage of the hospital bed prevents staff from unsafe handling of the child. For a more detailed discussion, the reader is referred to dermatology texts (Atherton, 2000; Eady, 1998).

Epidermolysis bullosa acquisita

Epidermolysis bullosa acquisita (EBA) mimics inherited epidermolysis bullosa or bullous pemphigoid but is an acquired blistering disorder with autoantibodies to collagen VII: part of the dermoepidermal junction (basement membrane of skin). Although rare, around 16 cases are so far described in children (Henk Sillevis Smitt, 2000). Involvement of the perineum would be limited. Biopsy and specific immunofluorescence studies would be needed for diagnosis.

Chronic bullous dermatosis of childhood

Definition, epidemiology and aetiology

Chronic bullous dermatosis of childhood is the usual name given to the childhood form of linear IgA disease. There is much overlap in these diseases but the childhood form tends to resolve by puberty whereas linear IgA disease persists. Chronic bullous dermatosis of childhood is occasionally known as linear IgA disease of childhood.

Clinical features and prognosis

Characteristically, the blister pattern known as the "string of pearls" or "crown of jewels" occurs. This is an arrangement of small (approximately 5 mm) blisters at the periphery of a polycyclic or annular inflammatory plaque. Itchy urticated papules and plaques also occur. Mucous membrane involvement is common, with oral blistering, conjunctivitis and nasal and pharyngeal symptoms. Mucosal lesions can rarely result in scarring. Bullae may contain serous or haemoserous fluid and may leave milia as they heal. Blistering has a predilection for the genitals and face.

Onset is in the preschool group and the disease is most severe initially, waxing and waning with resolution over several years. A minority have disease persisting into adult life. Two studies have found a mean disease duration of approximately 3.5–4 years (Collier and Wojnarowska, 2000). The authors estimate 65% of cases remit. There are reports of HLA associations but no significant risk of autoimmune disease (Collier and Wojnarowska, 1992).

Drug-induced disease is reported in the adult form, most notably with vancomycin, diclofenac and penicillin. Preceeding infections (and vaccinations) may possibly trigger the disease, and history prior illness was found in 38% of patients in one series (Leigh et al., 1988; Wojnarowska et al., 1988). An unusual association with building work carried out in the home has been described, with nearly three-quarters of cases having exposure to this within 3 months before disease onset (Collier and Wojnarowska, 1993).

Investigations

A skin biopsy is necessary to distinguish chronic bullous dermatosis of childhood from dermatitis herpetiformis, pemphigoid, pemphigus and epidermolysis bullosa. The linear deposition of IgA is seen at the basement membrane on direct skin immunofluorescence, confirming the diagnosis. Biopsy should be of a fresh lesion and preferably from a covered site, as forearm biopsies have been reported to show false-negative immunofluorescence. Indirect immunofluorescence (i.e. detection of circulating IgA antibodies to basement membrane), is usually positive.

Treatment

Response to dapsone or sulfamethoxypyridazine is generally good but the expected spontaneous remission over several years means that treatment should not be overly aggressive. Mild cases may respond to topical corticosteroids. Oral corticosteroids are effective, but their side-effect profile cannot be justified and the treatment of choice is either dapsone or sulfamethoxypyridazine.

Dermatitis herpetiformis

Definition, epidemiology and aetiology

Dermatitis herpetiformis is a vesiculobullous disorder affecting predominantly extensor surfaces of the body, associated in all cases with a gluten-sensitive enteropathy. Most commonly this is asymptomatic and, therefore, although a gluten-free diet is helpful in disease control, compliance is poor. Slow disease response and the restrictive nature of the gluten-free diet means that most patients will require medical treatment, at least initially. (Gluten or gliadin is a protein found in wheat, barley, rye and oats. It should be noted that only a small minority of gluten-sensitive individuals (i.e. coeliac disease sufferers) will manifest dermatitis herpetiformis) (Hervonen et al., 2000). HLA associations and increased risk of autoimmune disease are known to occur with dermatitis herpetiformis (Leonard, 2000).

Clinical features and prognosis

Lesions are seen on the buttocks and sacrum as well as other extensor surfaces including elbows, knees, posterior neck and scalp. Intense pruritus is common and often no intact blisters remain as excoriations leave only patchy erosions in a characteristic distribution. Urticated papules and plaques are common; these are also seen in chronic bullous dermatosis of childhood and in bullous pemphigoid. Mucous membrane lesions and the formation of milia are rare, which can be clinical clues to diagnosis.

Onset is after weaning and requires exposure to gluten. Of 57 affected children in one series, females were more commonly affected and the average age of onset was seven years (Reunala et al., 1984). Diagnosis is greatly facilitated by serology, although a skin biopsy is still desirable. Both antigliadin and antiendomysial antibodies are found but the latter is far more sensitive and specific (Peters and McEvoy, 1989). The titre of these will fall with a gluten-free diet.

Investigations

The skin biopsy in dermatitis herpetiformis will show granular deposits of IgA in the papillary dermis as well as splitting at the dermoepidermal junction and filling of the dermal papillae with neutrophils (so-called papillary microabscesses). Only the direct immunofluorescence findings are unique to dermatitis herpetiformis and the immunoglobulin type and granularity of deposits help to separate this disease from chronic bullous dermatosis of childhood and bullous pemphigoid.

Before skin biopsy and serology were available, several challenge tests were known to be helpful in diagnosis. Gluten loading will cause a flare of disease in many patients, as will exposure to iodine (either in seafood or when used as a medicament). Even topical iodine can provoke skin lesions. Lastly, dermatitis herpetiformis is exquisitely responsive to treatment with dapsone or sulfapyridine, and this has been used as a diagnostic test.

Treatment

Management is of the skin disease as well as any gastrointestinal problems. The majority of affected patients have no bowel symptoms and do not have malabsorption. Reunala et al. (1984) found that, unlike coeliac disease, dermatitis herpetiformis is not associated with short stature. A gluten-free diet does slowly reduce disease activity and in some cases is eventually curative. The time course for this improvement is slow, but 8 of 12 paediatric cases on a strict diet were able to stop dapsone after a time course ranging from 5 to 24 months (Reunala et al., 1984). Those unable to stop dapsone can usually reduce their required dose. Apart from disease control, another important reason to remain gluten free is the probable increased risk of bowel lymphoma with continued exposure (Lewis et al., 1996). Medical treatment involves the use of either dapsone or sulfapyridine. Doses needed for control are often very small, in particular in conjunction with gluten avoidance. Even dosage every second or third day may be effective. Reductions in dosage should be attempted at least several times yearly, to minimize the amount of drug needed. Screening for associated autoimmune disease should be undertaken on an individual basis.

Bullous pemphigoid and cicatricial pemphigoid

Definition, epidemiology and aetiology

Although classically affecting elderly persons, around 40 cases of pemphigoid and 15 of cicatricial pemphigoid (mostly female) have now been reported in children (Henk Sillevis Smitt, 2000). Rare in absolute numbers, these cases are important to separate from other bullous diseases as treatment and prognosis will be different.

As mentioned above, *localized vulvar pemphigoid* is a recognized condition with approximately 12 cases to date (Farrell et al., 1999; Henk Sillevis Smitt, 2000). Clinically, it presents identically to classic bullous pemphigoid but is localized to the vulva only. Its prognosis and the reason for involvement of this particular area is unclear. It does seem to be controllable with topical corticosteroids.

Clinical features and prognosis

Classic bullous pemphigoid presents with tense blisters and erythematous plaques, which may appear urticarial. Bullous pemphigoid antibodies are directed against components of the hemidesmosome in the dermoepidermal junction. Waves of blisters form and affected areas are pruritic. Milia may form as blisters resolve and erosion of oral mucosa is common. Fortunately the prognosis is relatively good and blistering will cease in most of those affected within two years.

Cicatricial pemphigoid may involve the same antibodies as seen in bullous pemphigoid as well as antibodies to laminin 5. Blistering and subsequent scarring is directed at mucous membrane sites. Consequently, the vulval, perianal, conjunctival and oropharyngeal mucosae are progressively damaged. Prognostically, this form of pemphigoid has a bleaker outlook. The disease in children seems to continue into adult life and the scarring can be devastating. Vision can be damaged and painful erosions occur in the mouth and perineum. Strictures can form, with dysphagia and involvement of the respiratory tract.

Investigations

In bullous pemphigoid, eosinophilia and circulating antibodies to the basement membrane are seen. Diagnosis is confirmed with the demonstration of a subepidermal blister and the presence of IgG and less often C3 found along the dermoepidermal junction.

The histological and immunofluorescence findings in cicatricial pemphigoid mimic bullous pemphigoid except for the presence of scarring and the presence of IgA in some cases as well as IgG.

Treatment

Treatment of bullous pemphigoid is with corticosteroids either as a potent topical application or given orally in more resistant disease. Dapsone or sulfapyridine are effective in some but not all. They are worth trying as steroid-sparing agents. Also reported is the combination of erythromycin and niacinamide. Adult treatments such as tetracyclines, azathioprine, ciclosporin and cyclophosphamide are best avoided in children.

Treatment of cicatricial pemphigoid is difficult and must be multidisciplinary. Topical corticosteroids should be trialled but may be ineffective and oral treatment will be required. Dapsone and sulfapyridine may help.

Pemphigus

Definition, epidemiology and aetiology

Pemphigus is a rare autoimmune blistering disorder that occurs uncommonly in childhood. It differs from other bullous diseases clinically, producing more superficial, flaccid blisters and erosions. Its course is also more aggressive. Antibodies are to either desmoglein 1 or 3 and less consistently to other antigens. These are components of intercellular desmosomes of the epidermis.

Clinical features and prognosis

Four main forms of pemphigus occur. *Pemphigus vulgaris* (the commonest form) and *pemphigus vegetans* form a suprabasal split: just above the basal cells of the epidermis. *Pemphigus foliaceous* and *pemphigus erythematosus* form higher splits, at the level of the stratum granulosum, and intact blistering is rarely seen.

Pemphigus vularis forms the largest group and usually presents with painful oral erosions. The skin then becomes involved with blisters and erosions. The course is variable, but most will be reliant on oral immunosuppressives

for many years. The minority will respond to topical corticosteroids alone. Resistant disease may require pulsed intravenous methylprednisolone or the addition of other immunosuppressives. The use of gold, dapsone, plasmapheresis and intravenous gammaglobulin may be preferable in childhood disease rather than the conventional adult treatments such as azathioprine, ciclosporin and cyclophosphamide.

Pemphigus vegetans is specific for its clinical picture of "vegetating" (i.e. thickened and eroded) inflammatory plaques. These occur in flexural sites. The prognosis, histology and treatment is the same as pemphigus vulgaris.

Pemphigus foliaceous is more superficial than the above forms and spares the mucous membranes. It is more often induced by drugs and is particularly reported with amoxicillin in children (Escallier et al., 1991). In adults, pemphigus foliaceous is more responsive to topical corticosteroids than is pemphigus vulgaris. Certainly this should be the first line of treatment, although oral immunosuppressives as described above may be needed. An endemic form of pemphigus foliaceous is seen in Latin America: known as fogo selvagem or Brazilian wildfire. In absolute numbers, this is commoner than all other forms of pemphigus, although its mechanism of spread is unclear. Children are often affected, in particular those living near rivers and those whose family members already have the disease. If untreated with immunosuppressives, chronic skin lesions and growth retardation supervene. The minority undergo spontaneous remission.

As an autoimmune disease, transplacental spread of antibodies in pemphigus can occur and the neonate may be affected. This is known as *pemphigus neonatorum*. Stillbirth has been reported (Terpstra et al., 1979), but in livebirths, the condition is self limited and resolves within weeks. There is not always active disease in the mother at the time of presentation (Storer et al., 1982). *Paraneoplastic pemphigus* has been reported twice in children with lymphoproliferative disease (Rybojad et al., 1993; Lemon et al., 1997). Treatment is that of the underlying malignancy.

Investigations

Antibodies can be demonstrated indirectly on serum and directly on skin biopsy. Skin biopsy is the usual method of diagnosis.

Treatment

Prior to effective treatment being available, pemphigus was considered relentlessly progressive and fatal. Currently morbidity and mortality is related to treatment side effects, rather than pemphigus per se. Significant levels of immunosuppression are required for control and so side effects are almost inevitable. If the disease is allowed to recur by cessation of, or reduction in, immunosuppression, "rebound" may occur with marked deterioration.

Hailey–Hailey disease

Hailey–Hailey disease is an autosomal dominant skin disorder with variable penetrance. This results in the development of eroded plaques of skin affecting the groin and axillae. Other flexural sites may also be involved. Onset is often in adolescence but may occur later. Diagnosis combines the clinical picture, family history and biopsy findings. Treatment is difficult but topical antibiotics and anti-inflammatories (i.e. topical corticosteroids) can help. Recently, carbon dioxide laser resurfacing has shown promise (Christian and Moy, 1999).

Darier's disease (syn. keratosis follicularis)

Darier's disease is an uncommon autosomal dominant disorder with variable penetrance producing keratotic papules that become eroded and often secondarily infected. The first signs of the disease usually appear around puberty and are initially mild (Burge, 1992). Although often worst on the upper body, some patients have a flexural distribution with significant perineal involvement. Rarely, the disease may be limited to the vulval area (Salopek et al., 1993). Clinical findings and skin biopsy confirm the diagnosis. Nail changes or red and white longitudinal bands plus V-shaped nicks at the free nail edge are seen. Palmar pitting may occur. Keratotic papules over the dorsa of the hands and involving the oral mucosa ("oral cobblestoning") are characteristic. Mild disease requires only avoidance of trigger factors (i.e. sunlight and infection), plus topical emollients and antiseptics. More stubborn cases respond well to retinoids.

Erythema multiforme and Stevens–Johnson syndrome

Definition, epidemiology and aetiology
Erythema multiforme is a pattern of reaction in the skin in which intense inflammation and necrosis of the epidermis presents as a florid erythematous and purpuric eruption. The characteristic lesion of the eruption is a target-shaped area of zoned degrees of inflammation. Involvement of the mucous membranes by the process, quite often without much skin eruption, is Stevens–Johnson syndrome. Many precipitating causes have been described for this spectrum of reaction and the commonest are HSV infection (recurrent), connective tissue disease, therapies such as sulphonamides, and internal malignancy.

Clinical features and prognosis
The eruption of erythema multiforme is most common on extensor surfaces of the limbs, but it can affect the trunk and head. Mucous membrane involvement produces painful erosions that weep and crust. Difficulties with eating, drinking and passing urine are common.

Differential diagnosis
Blistering or ulceration of the vulva or vagina may be caused by autoimmune blistering disorders, HSV infection, aphthous ulceration or erosive lichen planus (see Table 35.3). Vulval erythema as in the early stages of erythema multiforme may cause confusion with Kawasaki disease or streptococcal cellulitis.

Investigations
A biopsy of affected skin is important to establish the histological features of erythema multiforme or exclude other causes of similar erosions.

Treatment
Removal of any precipitating cause is essential, plus local measures to decrease pain and encourage healing. Topical steroid application can help. In some cases, systemic steroids or other immunosuppressive agents may be used, but in severe disease with widespread skin or mucosal erosion, such agents may increase the risks of complications.

Vulval ulceration

Aphthous ulceration

Definition, epidemiology and aetiology
Small oral ulcers occur occasionally in most people. The cause is unknown, but more persistent or recurrent lesions have been associated with streptococcal infection, vitamin deficiency and malabsorption. Major aphthae, in which larger, deeper ulcers occur, are uncommon. There may be a family history with major ulceration.

Clinical features and prognosis
Both minor and major ulceration may occur on the vulva. The ulcer develops over the course of approximately a day, from an area of tenderness to an ulcer of 2–20 mm edged with a ring of erythema. Initially, the floor of the ulcer may be lined with a greyish membrane. The degree of pain will depend on the size of the ulcer and, to a lesser extent, the exact site affected. Each lesion is self-healing within a few days.

Investigations

Usually the diagnosis is clear, but other diagnoses may need to be excluded by skin biopsy, surface swabs and blood tests.

Differential diagnosis

Diseases with a similar presentation include Behçet's disease, pemphigus, and Crohn's disease. Oral HSV infection should be excluded.

Treatment

Treatment may not be necessary as healing can be rapid. Pain control with analgesics or nonsteroidal anti-inflammatory agents can relieve discomfort. Topical steroid applications may speed time to healing. Frequency of recurrence of episodes may be reduced by several months of treatment with penicillin or tetracycline. Other agents that have been used to treat major aphthae include thalidomide and systemic immunosuppression.

Behçet's disease (syn. Behçet's syndrome)

Definition, epidemiology and aetiology

Behçet's syndrome is an inflammatory disease of unknown cause that can affect many organs. It was originally defined by a triad of oral and genital ulceration with iridocyclitis, but frequently it involves many body systems. It is a rare disease affecting approximately 1 in 500 000 in Europe with highest numbers in the Middle East.

Clinical features and prognosis

The first signs of Behçet's syndrome may begin in adolescence or adult life, but it may rarely start in childhood. The cutaneous features of ulceration and pustule formation often occur at sites of skin trauma. A pustule developing at the site of venepuncture is a classical sign, known as pathergy. Mucous membrane involvement is common, affecting the eyes, nose, mouth and anogenital areas. Involvement of the skin or anogenital mucosa occurs in about one-third of patients with the disease (Uziel et al., 1998). Ulceration may rarely be limited to the vulva.

Other organs are frequently involved and the patient may have general malaise, fever and arthralgia. The course of the disease is prolonged but remission may occur after several years (Rakover et al., 1987).

Investigations

Histology of affected skin is often nonspecific, but neutrophil infiltrate and necrosis are usual.

Differential diagnosis

Aphthous ulceration, Lipschütz ulcers and autoimmune blistering disorders may present similarly.

Treatment

Topical corticosteroids are of limited benefit in treatment of vulval ulceration. Systemic therapies that have been tried include glucocorticoids, colchicine and chlorambucil.

Lipschütz ulcer (syn. ulcus vulvae acuta)

Definition, epidemiology and aetiology

Acute vulval ulceration in adolescence was first described in 1903 and again over the following decades (reviewed by Berlin, 1965). Subsequent recognition of Behçet's syndrome and infectious mononucleosis as causes for some of these cases has still left a proportion without identifiable cause. It is rare.

Clinical features and prognosis

The first symptom may be of vulval irritation, followed rapidly by pain and intense discomfort on micturition. After a short phase of vulval swelling and erythema, ulceration, usually of the labia minora, occurs within a day or two (Fig. 35.10, colour plate). The ulcers are initially covered with a greyish membrane and the edge is ragged and slightly undermined. The ulcers heal over about two weeks.

Differential diagnosis

Possible causes of ulceration include major aphthous ulceration, Behçet's syndrome, mononucleosis, HSV infection, streptococcal infection and pyoderma gangrenosum.

Investigations

Vulval biopsy will help to distinguish other causes of ulceration. Swabs should be taken to check for infectious causes.

Treatment

Symptomatic care will include pain control and local measures such as gentle bathing, topical soothing antiseptic or antibiotic ointment or cream. Catheterization may be necessary to allow urine passage.

Vulval lumps

Hidradenitis suppuritiva

Definition, epidemiology and aetiology

Inflammation, frequently purulent, of the apocrine glands can occur in the groins, buttocks, axilliary, and submammary areas. One or more of these areas may be affected in each individual. There may be a familial tendency for the disease (Von der Werth et al., 2000), but it is also associated with obesity and is more common in females than males. Contributory factors to the pathogenesis are follicular occlusion (Yu and Cook, 1990) and end-organ response to androgens (Boer and Weltevredem, 1996; Lewis et al., 1993).

Clinical features and prognosis

The inflammatory lesions may first present in adolescence or later and may run a variable but often persistent course (Palmer and Keefe, 2001). It is rare before puberty but can occur (Mengesha et al., 1999). Initially, relatively superficial pustules and boils may develop into chronic discharging sinuses, with fibrosis and scarring. Features of comedones and bridged scarring are more common as the disease becomes chronic.

Investigations

Surface swabs as well as culture of pus from discharging lesions should be performed. Diabetes should be excluded.

Differential diagnosis

Staphylococcal boils can appear very similar to early hidradenitis suppuritiva.

Treatment

In adolescents, the disease is not usually severe as it often tends to become more chronic and severe with age. Treatment should include good local hygiene and topical antiseptic use. Persistence of painful inflamed lesions may require long courses of oral antibiotics, but response is often suboptimal. Acutely inflamed lesions may benefit from local immunosuppression such as injected triamcinolone and occasionally systemic immunosuppression with oral glucocorticoids. Oral retinoids or cyproterone acetate can be of benefit (Brown et al., 1988; Mortimer et al., 1986). Excision of affected skin may remain an option if the disease is localized, but when the groins, vulva and natal cleft are involved, surgery would be mutilating.

Fox–Fordyce disease

Definition, epidemiology and aetiology

Fox–Fordyce disease is a condition of unknown cause in which there is dysfunction of the apocrine sweat glands. Its onset only after the glands become active and its usual abatement after the menopause suggest hormonal control.

Clinical features and prognosis

The condition is first apparent at or soon after the onset of puberty. All areas of apocrine gland distribution can be affected, namely the axillae, the groins and vulva, and around the areolae of breasts. Itch is the main symptom, coming on when the glands are active. As the disease progresses, inflammation may bring discomfort and visible papules, giving the skin a rough, cobblestone surface.

Investigations

The diagnosis is usually made on clinical grounds. A biopsy of affected skin will show inflammation, rupture and ultimately plugging of the apocrine duct.

Differential diagnosis

Other conditions producing thickened or roughened skin in the apocrine areas may be considered, such as hidradenitis suppuritiva and acanthosis nigricans.

Treatment

No easy treatment options are available and in some patients relief can only be obtained from surgical removal of the affected areas. However, there are reports of symptom relief from treatments that encourage exfoliation, such as ultraviolet light (Pinkus, 1973) and retinoids (Giacobetti et al., 1979; Tkach, 1979), from topical antibiotics (Feldman et al., 1992) and from hormonal manipulation (Kronthal et al., 1965).

Crohn's disease

Definition, epidemiology and aetiology

Crohn's disease is a chronic inflammatory disease of the gastrointestinal tract. Onset is usually in adult life but can occur in childhood.

Clinical features and prognosis

Anogenital Crohn's disease may occur in the absence of intestinal symptoms or in combination with more usual manifestations such as diarrhoea, abdominal pain and malabsorption. Perianal involvement is the most common area of anogenital Crohn's, occuring in over half of children affected with Crohn's disease (Tuffnell and Buchan, 1991), but the vulva alone may be affected (Werlin et al., 1992). The involved skin may show swelling, induration, papules and tags, plus fissuring and erosions and sometimes sinus formation. Large ulcers may occasionally develop. Oral ulceration is a possible associated finding.

Investigations

Biopsy of vulval or perianal Crohn's disease should reveal noncaseating granulomatous inflammation. Erosion and secondary infection may lead to a prominent neutrophilic infiltrate. Blood investigations may show evidence of malabsorption and raised markers of inflammation. Radiological examination of the bowel is important to establish the extent of the disease.

Differential diagnosis

Swelling and fissures of the vulval or perianal skin may suggest sexual abuse (Sellman et al., 1996; Stratakis et al., 1994).

Treatment

Therapy will depend on the extent and severity of the disease. Systemic immunosuppression and dietary measures may be used for bowel disease and will also affect extra-intestinal disease of the vulva and perianal areas.

Langerhans' cell histiocytosis (syn. histiocytosis X, Hand–Schuller–Christian disease, Letterer–Siwe disease)

Definition, epidemiology and aetiology

Langerhans' cell histiocytosis is a spectrum of reactive disorders in which the skin or other organs are infiltrated with Langerhans' cells, with resultant tissue damage. The onset is usually in infancy or early childhood, but it can occur later. The aetiology is unknown.

Clinical features and prognosis

The disease is usually multisystem and most commonly affects bone, skin and lymph nodes. In the skin, the scalp and flexures are usually involved with rough and thickened erythematous patches, frequently covered with crusts and scales. Indurated areas and ulceration may occur.

Differential diagnosis

The major differential diagnosis is seborrhoeic dermatitis, but infected atopic eczema or psoriasis may present similarly.

Investigations

A skin biopsy is essential to make a diagnosis by identification of the infiltrating cells within the skin.

Treatment

Treatment is dependent upon the severity of the disease and the degree of organ involvement; in mild disease, no specific treatment may be necessary. In severe disease, topical or systemic chemotherapy may produce improvement and sometimes clearance.

Benign tumours

A variety of benign tumours not already described may present as vulval swellings or lumps. These include haemangiomas, lymphangiomas, epidermal naevi, neurofibromas (Nogita et al., 1990), lipomas, mucous cysts (Lorrmann et al., 1985), syringomas (Scherbenske et al., 1988) and sebaceous glands as Fordyce spots.

Summary

Vulval skin disorders in children and adolescents can have many causes (Table 35.1) and produce overlapping, and embarrassing, symptoms. Consequently, investigation can be difficult (Box 35.1) and requires awareness of the incidence of various disorders and their differential diagnosis (Box 35.2).

Box 35.1 Recommendations for practice

- Infection with *Streptococcus*, *Staphylococcus* or *Haemophilus* spp. should be sought in all children with inflammation of the vulva.
- Infection with herpes, warts or molluscum contagiosum localized to the anogenital area in children should prompt consideration of sexual acquisition.
- Lichen sclerosus treatment with potent topical steroids produces good symptomatic relief and may also reduce the risks of vaginal introital stenosis and adult squamous cell carcinoma.
- Blistering or ulceration in the vulval area requires histological diagnosis.

Box 35.2 Key points

- Bacterial infection is a common cause of vulvovaginal inflammation in prepubertal children and may be related to an intravaginal foreign body.
- Anogenital warts in children may be an indicator of abuse but may also be acquired innocently.
- Irritant dermatitis most commonly arises from prolonged contact with urine or faeces but may also be related to excessive detergent use.
- Lichen sclerosus is rising in incidence and may present with many different features.
- Acute vulval ulceration may be associated with Epstein–Barr virus infection.

REFERENCES

*Indicates key references.

Adeyemi-Doro F A B, Osoba A O, Junaid T A (1979). Perigenital cutaneous schistosomiasis. *Br J Vener Dis* 55, 446–449.

Albers S E, Taylor G, Huyer D, Oliver G, Krafchik B R (2000). Vulvitis circumscripta plasmacellularis mimicking child abuse. *J Am Acad Dermatol* 42, 1078–1080.

Allen A L, Siegfried E C (1998). The natural history of condylomata in children. *J Am Acad Dermatol* 39, 951–955.

Altchek A (1981). Vulvovaginitis, vulval skin disease, and pelvic inflammatory disease. *Pediatr Clin North Am* 28, 397–431.

Amiry S A, Pride H B, Tyler W B (2001). Perianal pseudoverrucose papules and nodules mimicking condylomata acuminata and child sexual abuse. *Cutis* 67, 335–338.

Amstey M S, Trombetta G C (1985). Laser therapy for vulvar molluscum contagiosum infection. *Am J Obstet Gynecol* 153, 800–801.

Armstrong D K B, Bingham E A, Dinsmore W W, Swann A, Handley J M (1998). Anogenital warts in prepubertal children: a follow-up study. *Br J Dermatol* 138, 544–564.

Atherton D J (2000). Epidermolysis Bullosa. In *Textbook of Pediatric Dermatology*, Harper J, Oranje A, Prose N, eds., pp 1075–1100. Blackwell Science, Oxford.

Baggish M S, Sze E H, Johnson R (1997). Urinary oxalate excretion and its role in vulvar pain syndrome. *Am J Obstet Gynecol* 177, 507–511.

Bargman H (letter); Schachner L, Hankin D (reply) (1986). Is genital molluscum contagiosum a cutaneous manifestation of sexual abuse in children? *J Am Acad Dermatol* 14, 847–849.

Bauer A, Geier J, Elsner P (2000). Allergic contact dermatitis in patients with anogenital complaints. *J Reprod Med* 45, 649–654.

Berlin C (1965). The pathogenesis of the so-called ulcus vulvae acutum. *Acta Dermatol Venereol* 45, 221–222.

Bluestein J, Furner B B, Phillips D (1990). Granuloma gluteale infantum: case report and review of the literature. *Pediatr Dermatol* 7, 196–198.

Boer J, Weltevreden E F (1996). Hidradenitis suppuritiva or acne inversa. A clinicopathological study of early lesions. *Br J Dermatol* 135, 721–725.

Bracco G L, Carli P, Sonni L, Maestrini G, De Marco A, Taddei G L, Cattaneo A (1993). Clinical and histological effects of topical treatments of vulvar lichen sclerosus. *J Reprod Med* 38, 37–40.

Brown C F, Gallup D G, Brown V M (1988). Hidradenitis suppuritiva of the anogenital region: response to isotretinoin. *Am J Obstet Gynecol* 158, 12–15.

Burge S M (1992). Darier's disease: the clinical features and pathogenesis. *Clin Exp Dermatol* 19, 193–205.

Chari S P, Connolly P, Shafi M I, Luesley D M (1994). The treatment of lichen sclerosus et atrophicus and squamous cell hyperplasia with graduated topical steroids. *J Obstet Gynecol* 14, 172–174.

Christian M M, Moy R L (1999). Treatment of Hailey–Hailey disease using short pulsed and short dwell time carbon dioxide lasers. *Dermatol Surg* 25, 661–663.

Cohen B A, Honog P, Androphy E (1990). Anogenital warts in children. Clinical and virological evaluation for sexual abuse. *Acta Dermatol* 126, 1575–1580.

Collier P M, Wojnarowska F (1992). MHC class I and II antigens in linear IgA dermatosis. *J Invest Dermatol* 98, 526.

*(1993). Linear IgA disease and chronic bullous disease of childhood. *Eur J Dermatol* 3, 623–634.

(2000). Chronic bullous disease of childhood. In *Textbook of Pediatric Dermatology*, Harper J, Oranje A, Prose N, eds., pp. 711–723. Blackwell Science, Oxford.

Connelly M G, Winkleman R K (1985). Coexistence of lichen sclerosus, morphoea and lichen planus. Report of 4 cases and review of the literature. *J Am Acad Dermatol* 12, 844–851.

*Cox R A (1997). Haemophilus influenzae: an underrated cause of vulvovaginitis in young girls. *J Clin Pathol* 50, 765–768.

DeCastro P, Jorizzo J, Rajaraman S, Solomon A R Jr, Briggaman R A, Raimer S S (1985). Localized vulvar pemphigoid in a child. *Paediatr Dermatol* 2, 302–307.

Dhar V, Roker K, Adhmi Z, McKenzie S (1993). Streptococcal vulvovaginitis in girls. *Pediatr Dermatol* 10, 366–367.

Donald F E, Slack R C B, Colman G (1991). Streptococcus pyogenes vulvovaginitis in children in Nottingham. *Epidemiol Infect* 106, 459–465.

Eady R A J (1998). Epidermolysis Bullosa. In *Textbook of Dermatology*, 6th edn, Champion R H, Burton J L, Burns D A, Breathnach S M, eds., pp. 1817–1844. Blackwell Science, Oxford.

Edwards L (1989). Vulval lichen planus. *Arch Dermatol* 125, 1677–1680.

Epstein E (1989). Cantharidin treatment of molluscum contagiosum. *Acta Derm Venereol* 69, 91–92.

Escallier F, Gaudard S, Boulitrop-Morvan C et al. (1991). Pemphigus superficiel de l'enfant. *Ann Dermatol Venereol* 118, 381–384.

Farber E M, Jacobs A H (1997). Infantile psoriasis. *Am J Dis Child* 131, 1266–1269.

Farber E M, Nall M L (1974). The natural history of psoriasis in 5600 patients. *Dermatologica* 148, 1–18.

Farrell A M, Kirtschig G, Dalziel K L et al. (1999). Childhood vulval pemphigoid: a clinical and immunopathological study of five patients. *Br J Dermatol* 140, 308–312.

Feldman R, Misouyé I, Chavaz R, Saurat J H (1992). Fox–Fordyce disease: successful treatment with topical clindamycin in alcoholic propylene glycol solution. *Dermatology*, 184, 310–313.

*Fischer G, Rogers M (1997). Treatment of childhood vulvar lichen sclerosus with potent topical corticosteroids. *Pediatr Dermatol* 14, 235–238.

*(2000). Vulvar disease in children: a clinical audit of 130 cases. *Pediatric Dermatol* 17, 1–6.

Fischer G, Spurrett B, Fischer A (1995). The chronically symptomatic vulva. Aetiology and management. *Br J Obstet Gynaecol* 102, 773–779.

Fivozinsky K B, Laufer M R (1998). Vulvar disorders in prepubertal girls. A literature review. *J Reprod Med* 43, 763–773.

Franco I (2000). Oral cimetidine for the management of genital and perigenital warts in children. *J Urol* 164, 1074–1075.

Friedman M, Gal D (1987). Keloid scars as a result of CO_2 laser for molluscum contagiosum. *Obstet Gynecol* 70, 394–396.

Fujiwara H, Fujiwara K, Hashimoto K et al. (1997). Detection of *Borrelia burgdorferi* (*B. garnii* or *B. afzelii*) DNA in morphoea and lichen sclerosus et atrophicus tissues of German and Japanese but not of US patients. *Arch Dermatol* 133, 41–44.

Giacobetti R, Caro W A, Roenigk H H (1979). Fox–Fordyce disease: control with tretinoin cream. *Arch Dermatol* 115, 1365–1366.

Giaquinto C, Del Mistro A, De Rossi A et al. (2000). Vulval carcinoma in a 12-year-old girl with vertically acquired human immunodeficiency virus infection. *Pediatrics* 106, e57.

Goldberg N S, Esterly N B, Rothman K F (1992). Perianal pseudoverrucous papules and nodules in children. *Arch Dermatol* 128, 240–242.

Gryngarten M G, Turco M D, Escobar M E, Woloj M G, Bergada C (1994). Shigella vulvovaginitis in prepubertal girls. *Pediatr Gynecol* 7, 86–89.

Guenther L, Shum D (1990). Localized childhood vulvar pemphigoid. *J Am Acad Dermatol* 22, 762–764.

Halasz C, Silvers D, Crum C P (1986). Bowenoid papulosis in a three year old girl. *J Am Acad Dermatol* 14, 326–330.

Handley J, Hanks E, Armstrong K et al. (1997). Common association of HPV 2 with anogenital warts in prepubertal children. *Pediatric Dermatol* 14, 339–343.

Hart W R, Norris H J, Helwig E B (1975). Relation of lichen sclerosus et atrophicus of the vulva to the development of carcinoma. *Obstet Gynecol* 45, 369–377.

Haustein U F (1988). Localized nonscarring bullous pemphigoid of the vagina. *Dermatologica* 176, 200–201.

Heller R H, Joseph J M, Davis H J (1969). Vulvovaginitis in the premenarcheal child. *J Pediatr* 74, 370–377.

Henk Sillevis Smitt J (2000). Pemphigus, pemphigoid and epidermolysis bullosa acquisita. In *Textbook of Pediatric Dermatology*, Harper J, Oranje A, Prose N, eds., pp 731–753. Blackwell Science, Oxford.

Hervonen K, Karell K, Holopainen P, Collin P, Partanen J, Reunala T (2000). Concordance of dermatitis herpetiformis and celiac disease in monozygous twins. *J Invest Dermatol* 115, 990–993.

Holden C A, Parish W E (1998). Atopic dermatitis. In *Textbook of Dermatology*, 6th edn, Champion R H, Burton J L, Burns D A, Breathnach S M, eds., pp. 681–708. Blackwell Science, Oxford.

Hudson L B, Perlman S E (1998). Necrotising genital ulcerations in a pre-menarcheal female with mononucleosis. *Obstet Gynecol* 92, 642–644.

Kawasaki T (1995). Kawasaki disease. *Acta Pediatr* 84, 713–715.

Kingston M, Warren C, Carlin E (2001). Tropical warts. *Lancet* 358, 808.

Klaus S, Shvil Y, Mumcuoglu K Y (1994). Generalised infection of a 3 1/2 year old girl with the pubic louse. *Pediatr Dermatol* 11, 26–28.

Kokx N P, Comstock J A, Facklam R R (1987). Streptococcal perianal disease in children. *Pediatrics* 80, 659–663.

Konya J, Gow E (1996). Granuloma gluteale infantum. *Aust J Dermatol* 37, 57–58.

Koumantakis E E, Hassan E A, Deligeoroglou E K, Creatsas G K (1997). Vulvovaginitis during childhood and adolescence. *J Pediatr Adolesc Gynecol* 10, 39–43.

Kronthal H L, Pomeranz J R, Sitomer G (1965). Fox–Fordyce disease. *Arch Dermatol* 91, 243–245.

Lambiris A, Greaves M W (1997). Dyspareunia and vulvodynia: unrecognised manifestations of symptomatic dermographism. *Lancet* 349, 28.

Lafferty W E, Coombs R W, Benedetti J, Critchlow C, Corey L (1987). Recurrences after oral and genital herpes simplex virus infection. *N Engl J Med* 316, 1444–1449.

Leigh G, Marsden R, Wojnarowska F (1988). Linear IgA dermatosis with severe arthralgia. *Br J Dermatol* 119, 789–792.

Lemon M A, Weston W L, Huff J C (1997). Childhood paraneoplastic pemphigus associated with Castleman's tumour. *Br J Dermatol* 136, 115–117.

Leonard J N (2000). Dermatitis herpetiformis. In *Textbook of Pediatric Dermatology*, Harper J, Oranje A, Prose N, eds., pp. 724–730. Blackwell Science, Oxford.

Leutscher P, Ravaoalimalala V E, Raharisolo C et al. (1998). Clinical findings in female genital schistosomiasis in Madagascar. *Trop Med Int Health* 3, 327–332.

Lewis F, Messenger A G, Wales J K (1993). Hidradenitis suppuritiva as a presenting feature of premature adrenarche. *Br J Dermatol* 129, 447–448.

Lewis H M, Renaula T L, Garioch J J et al. (1996). Protective effect of a gluten free diet against development of lymphoma in dermatitis herpetiformis. *Br J Dermatol* 135, 363–367.

Lorrmann H, Cendron J, Bavieral E (1985). Kystes vulvaires à révélation néonatale. A propos de 6 cas. *Ann Urol* 19, 259–262.

Lynch P J, Edwards L (1994). White patches and plaques. In *Genital Dermatology*, Lynch P J, Edwards L, eds., pp. 149–162. Churchill-Livingstone, New York.

MacFarlane D E, Sharma D P (1987). *Haemophilus influenzae* and genital tract infections in children. *Acta Paediatr Scand* 76, 363–364.

MacLean A B (1993). Precursors of vulva cancers. *Curr Obstet Gynecol* 3, 149–156.

Marren P, Wojnarowska F, Powell S (1992). Allergic contact dermatitis and vulvar dermatoses. *Br J Dermatol* 126, 52–56.

Mawad N M, Hassanein O M, Mahmoud O M, Taylor M G (1992). Schistosomal vulval granuloma in a 12 year old Sudanese girl. *Trans Roy Soc Trop Med Hyg* 86, 644.

McKay M (1993). Dysesthetic ('essential') vulvodynia. Treatment with amitriptyline. *J Reprod Med* 38, 9–13.

Mengesha Y M, Holcombe T C, Hansen R C (1999). Prepubertal hidradenitis suppuritiva: Two case reports and review of the literature. *Pediatr Dermatol* 16, 292–296.

Meyrick Thomas R H, Ridley C M, McGibbon D H, Black M M (1998). Lichen sclerosus et atrophicus and autoimmunity: a study of 350 women. *Br J Dermatol* 118, 41–46.

Mortimer P S, Dawber R P R, Gales M A, Moore R A (1986). A double-blind controlled cross-over trial of cyproterone acetate in females with hidradenitis suppuritiva. *Br J Dermatol* 115, 263–268.

Nasr I, Tometzki A J P, Schofield O M V (2000). Kawasaki disease: an update. *Clin Exp Dermatol* 26, 6–12.

Neuberger J W, Takahashi M, Burns J C et al. (1986). The treatment of Kawasaki's disease with intravenous gamma globulin. *N Engl J Med* 315, 341–347.

Nevill E A, Finn O A (1975). Psoriasiform napkin dermatitis: a follow-up study. *Br J Dermatol* 92, 279–285.

Nogita T, Kawabata Y, Tsuchida T et al. (1990). Clitoral and labial involvement of neurofibromatosis. *J Am Acad Dermatol* 5, 937–938.

Ohkuma M (1990). Molluscum contagiosum treated with iodine solution and salicylic acid plaster. *Int J Dermatol* 29, 443–445.

Padel A F, Venning V A, Evans M F, Quantrill H M, Fleming K A (1990). Human papillomavirus in anogenital warts in children. *Br Med J* 300, 1491–1494.

Paek S C, Merritt D F, Mallory S B (2001). Pruritus vulvae in prepubertal children. *J Am Acad Dermatol* 44, 795–802.

Palmer R A, Keefe M (2001). Early-onset hidradenitis suppuritiva. *Clin Exp Dermatol* 26, 501–503.

Papa C M, Berger R S (1976). Venereal herpes-like molluscum contagiosum: treatment with tretinoin. *Cutis* 18, 537–540.

Patterson J A K, Ackerman A B (1984). Lichen sclerosus et atrophicus is not related to morphoea. *Am J Dermatopathol* 6, 323–335.

Pelisse M (1989). The vulvo-vaginal–gingival syndrome: a new form of erosive lichen planus. *Int J Dermatol* 28, 381–384.

Peters M S, McEvoy M T (1989). IgA antiendomysial antibodies in dermatitis herpetiformis. *J Am Acad Dermatol* 21, 1225–1231.

Petersen C S, Brocks K, Weisman K, Kobayasi T, Thompsen H K (1996). Pretibial epidermolysis bullosa with vulvar involvement. *Acta Dermatovenereol* 76, 80–81.

*Piippo S, Lenko H, Vuento R (2000). Vulval symptoms in paediatric and adolescent patients. *Acta Paediatr* 89, 431–435.

Pinkus H (1973). Treatment of Fox–Fordyce disease. *J Am Med Assoc* 223, 924.

Pincus S H, McKay M (1993). Lichen sclerosus et atrophicus. In *Dermatology in General Medicine*, 4th edn, Fitzpatrick T B, Eisen A Z, Wolff K, Freedberg I M, Austen, K F, eds., pp. 1469–1470. McGraw-Hill, New York.

Pokorny F (1994). Long-term intravaginal presence of foreign bodies in children. A preliminary study. *J Reprod Med* 39, 931–935.

Powell J, Wojnarowska F (2001). Childhood vulval lichen sclerosus: an increasingly common problem. *J Am Acad Dermatol* 44, 803–806.

Powell J, Wojnarowska F, Winsey S, Marren P, Welsh K (2000). Lichen sclerosus premenarche: autoimmunity and immunogenetics. *Br J Dermatol* 142, 481–484.

Powell J, Wojnarowska F, Shafi M, Laird E (2001). Childhood-onset lichen sclerosus and vulval squamous cell carcinoma. *Br J Dermatol* 145(Suppl. 59), 124–125.

Rakover Y, Adar H, Tal I, Lang Y, Kedar A (1987). Behçet disease: long term follow-up of three children and review of literature. *Pediatrics* 83, 986–992.

Rasmussen H B, Hagdrup H, Schmidt H (1986). Psoriasiform napkin dermatitis. *Acta Derm Venereol* 66, 534–536.

Reid R, Omoto K H, Precop S L et al. (1995). Flashlamp-excited dye laser therapy of idiopathic vulvodynia is safe and efficaceous. *Am J Obstet Gynecol* 172, 1684–1701.

Reunala T, Kosnai L, Karpati S, Kuitunen P, Torok E, Savilahti E (1984). Dermatitis herpetiformis: jejunal findings and skin response to gluten free diet. *Arch Dis Child* 59, 517–522.

Ridley C M (1988). General dermatological conditions and dermatoses of the vulva. In *The Vulva*, Ridley C M, ed., p. 138. Churchill Livingstone, Edinburgh.

(1989). Lichen sclerosus et atrophicus. *Semin Dermatol* 8, 54–63.

Robinson J B, Im D D, Simmons-O'Brian E, Rosenshein N B (1998). Etretinate: therapy for plasma cell vulvitis. *Obstet Gynecol* 92, 706.

Rosdahl I, Edmar B, Gisslen H, Nordin P, Lillieborg S (1988). Curettage of molluscum contagiosum in children: analgesia by topical application of a lidocaine/prilocaine cream (EMLA®). *Acta Derm Venereol* 68, 149–153.

Rowell N R, Goodfield M J D (1998). Lichen sclerosus. In *Textbook of Dermatology*, 6th edn, Champion R H, Burton J L, Burns D A, Breathnach S M, eds., pp. 2547–2553. Blackwell Science, Oxford.

Rybojad M, Leblanc T, Flageul B et al. (1993). Paraneoplastic pemphigus in a child with a T-cell lymphoblastic lymphoma. *Br J Dermatol* 128, 418–422.

Salopek T G, Krol A, Jimbow K (1993). Case report of Darier's disease localised to the vulva in a 5 year old girl. *Pediatr Dermatol* 10, 146–148.

Samman P D (1961). Lichen planus: an analysis of 200 cases. *Trans Rep St John's Hosp Dermatol Soc*, 46, 36–38.

Scherbenske J M, Lupton G P, James W D, Kirkle D B (1988). Vulval syringomas occurring in a 9 year old child. *J Am Acad Dermatol* 19, 575–577.

Scurry J, Dennerstein G, Brenan J, Ostor A, Mason G, Dorevitch A (1993). Vulvitis circumscripta plasmacellularis. A clinicopathological entity? *J Reprod Med* 38, 14–18.

Sellman S P, Hupertz V F, Reece R M (1996). Crohn's disease presenting as suspected abuse. *Pediatrics* 97, 272–274.

Silverberg N B, Laude T A (1998). Jacquet diaper dermatitis: a diagnosis of etiology. *Pediatr Dermatol* 15, 489.

Sinha P, Sorinola O, Luesley D M (1999). Lichen sclerosus of the vulva. Long term steroid maintenance therapy. *J Reprod Med* 44, 621–624.

Sisson B A, Glick L (1998). Genital ulceration as a presenting manifestation of infectious mononucleosis. *J Pediatr Adolesc Gynecol* 11, 185–187.

Steinkampf M P, Reilly S D, Ackerman A B (1987). Vaginal agglutination and hematometra associated with epidermolysis bullosa. *Obstet Gynecol* 69, 519–521.

Storer J, Galen W K, Nesbitt L T, DeLeo V A (1982). Neonatal pemphigus vulgaris. *J Am Acad Dermatol* 6, 929–932.

Stratakis C A, Graham W, DiPalma J, Leiowitz I (1994). Misdiagnosis of perianal manifestations of Crohn's disease. Two cases and a review of the literature. *Clin Pediatr* 33, 631–633.

Syed T A, Lundin S, Ahmad M (1994). Topical 0.3% and 0.5% podophyllotoxin cream for self-treatment of molluscum contagiosum in males. *Dermatology* 189, 65–68.

Tappeiner S, Pfleger L (1971). Granuloma gluteale infantum. *Hautartz* 22, 383–388.

Terpstra H, de Jong M C J M, Klokke A H (1979). In vivo bound pemphigus antibodies in a still born infant. *Arch Dermatol* 115, 316–319.

Tkach J R (1979). Tretinoin treatment of Fox–Fordyce disease. *Arch Dermatol* 15, 1285.

Tuffnell D, Buchan P C (1991). Crohn's disease of the vulva in childhood. *Br J Clin Pract* 45, 159–160.

Uziel Y, Brik R, Padeh S et al. (1998). Juvenile Behçet's disease in Israel. The Pediatric Rheumatology Study Group of Israel. *Clin Exp Rheumatol* 16, 502–505.

Von der Werth J M, Williams H C, Raeburn J A (2000). The clinical genetics of hidradenitis suppuritiva revisited. *Br J Dermatol* 142, 947–953.

Warin R P, Faulkner K E (1961). Napkin psoriasis. *Br J Dermatol* 73, 445–450.

Weitzner J M, Fields K W, Robinson M J (1989). Pediatric Bowenoid papulosis: risks and management. *Pediatr Dermatol* 6, 303–305.

Werlin S L, Esterly N B, Oechler H (1992). Crohn's disease presenting as unilateral labial hypertrophy. *J Am Acad Dermatol* 27, 893–895.

White G, Jantos M, Glazer H (1997). Establishing the diagnosis of vulvar vestibulitis. *J Reprod Med* 42, 157–160.

Wilson R W (1993). Genital ulcers and mononucleosis. *Pediatr Infect Dis J* 12, 418.

Wojnarowska F, Marsden R, Bhogal B, Black M (1988). Chronic bullous disease of childhood, childhood cicatricial pemphigoid and linear IgA disease of adults, a comparative study demonstrating clinical and immunopathological overlap. *J Am Acad Dermatol* 19, 792–805.

Wood P L, Bevan T (1999). Child sexual abuse enquiries and unrecognised vulval lichen sclerosus et atrophicus. *Br Med J* 319, 899–900.

Yilmaz E, Alpsoy E, Basaran E (1995). Cimetidine therapy for warts: a placebo-controlled, double-blind study. *J Am Acad Dermatol* 34, 1005–1007.

Yoganathan S, Bohl T G, Mason G (1994). Plasma cell balanitis and vulvitis (of Zoon). *J Reprod Med* 39, 939–944.

Yu C C, Cook M G (1990). Hidradenitis suppuritiva: a disease of follicular epithelium rather than apocrine glands. *Br J Dermatol* 122, 763–769.

Zeiguer N J, Galvano A, Comparato M R, Guelfand L, Benitez M (1992). Vulvar abscesses caused by streptococcus pneumonia. *Pediatr Infect Dis J* 11, 335–336.

36

Vaginal discharge

Rosamund Cox and Paul Wood

Kettering General Hospital, Kettering, UK

Vaginal discharge in childhood

Vaginal discharge is the most common gynaecological complaint in young girls. The majority are managed by general practitioners (primary care physicians) and referral to a gynaecologist tends to occur only if the patient fails to respond to treatment. It is, therefore, important that all those involved in the management of vaginal discharge in children understand the causes, so that the condition can be adequately investigated and treated.

History

The history is usually provided by the child's mother whose anxiety may be fuelled by concerns over the implications of abnormal vaginal discharge and the association with pelvic inflammatory disease (PID) recognized in older subjects. Such fears need to be allayed since there is no such proven association in prepubertal girls with vaginal discharge. Alternatively, family members may be concerned about a potential sexual abuse situation, although they perhaps will volunteer these fears less frequently. The child should be engaged in general conversation and asked questions about her complaints. In this way she can be involved in the consultation, can acknowledge that she is an important part of the process and can appreciate the need for an examination.

The duration, frequency and quantity of the discharge, its colour and associated odour need to be established along with details of previous treatments received. An offensive odour indicates anaerobic bacterial involvement. The presence of a blood-stained or offensive discharge is significant and warrants examination of the upper vagina and cervix

to exclude a foreign body or tumour, either through direct visualization in the outpatient setting or vaginoscopy using a hysteroscope with carbon dioxide insufflation under light general anaesthesia.

A resume of hygiene habits can prove helpful, with enquiry about frequency of bathing, continence, wiping technique after defaecation, and correct positioning during urination (avoiding close apposition of the child's knees). A history of frequent handling of the genitalia, scratching and complaints of soreness should be elicited. A general medical and family history should be taken along with details of any current medication. Enquiries should be made of the exposure to any potential irritants to the vulva such as perfumed soaps or deodorants.

Examination of the prepubertal girl

Examination must be carried out with the greatest care because the unoestrogenized prepubertal female genitalia does not readily tolerate instrumentation, and even the normal cotton-tipped swabs, used for collecting samples for culture, may be abrasive and painful.

For a child who has a benign history of vulvitis and minimal vaginal discharge (Fig. 36.1, colour plate), a brief external genital examination in the frog-leg (supine) position (Fig. 36.2) may be sufficient. Any child who experiences persistent, purulent, recurrent or bloodstained vaginal discharge, or about whom there are concerns about sexual abuse, requires a complete gynaecological assessment.

Following a general examination, the perineum and vaginal introitus are inspected with the child in the frog-leg position (Fig. 36.2). The labia can be separated and retracted gently to allow visualization of the hymen and

Paediatric and Adolescent Gynaecology, ed. Adam Balen et al. Published by Cambridge University Press.
© Cambridge University Press 2004.

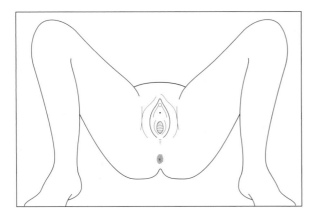

Fig. 36.2. The "frog-leg" (supine) position.

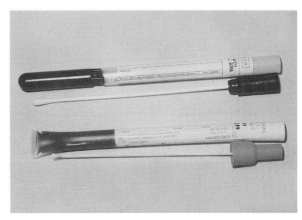

Fig. 36.5. Small wire cotton-tipped swab (lower swab) shown with normal-sized swab (upper swab) for comparison.

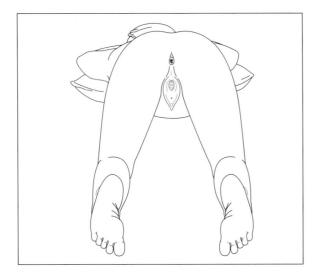

Fig. 36.4. The knee–chest position for examination.

lower vagina (Fig. 36.3, colour plate). The child is then asked to assume the knee-chest position. The buttocks are held apart laterally and slightly upwards (Fig. 36.4). As the child takes several deep breaths, the vaginal orifice falls open and by using an ordinary otoscope head (without a speculum) the vagina and cervix can be visualized in most prepubertal girls. Examination under anaesthesia may be necessary if the hymen is microperforate or the child is uncooperative (Vandeven and Emans, 1993).

Specimens of vaginal secretions are best obtained with the child in the frog-leg position. The catheter-in-a-catheter technique (Pokorny, 1992) allows samples to be obtained using a soft bladder catheter. Alternatively, a small wire cotton-tipped swab should be used (Fig. 36.5).

Physiological vaginal discharge before puberty

Most female babies have a physiological vaginal discharge during the neonatal period. The neonatal vagina is hy-

pertrophied and the stratified squamous epithelial cells contain glycogen as a result of placental and maternal hormonal stimulation. The relatively glycogen-rich environment encourages colonization with lactobacilli. The shedding of these epithelial cells plus the mucus production of a stimulated cervix results in a neonatal vaginal discharge (Wald, 1984). The discharge may occasionally be bloodstained owing to withdrawal bleeding secondary to in utero endometrial stimulation by oestrogen. This physiological leukorrhoea of the newborn tends to disappear within seven to ten days, and after two to three weeks the vaginal mucosa becomes anoestrogenic.

Rare, noninfective causes of vaginal discharge

Before considering the well-recognized infective causes of vaginal discharge, there are a number of less-common, noninfective conditions, which need to be excluded.

If the discharge is bloodstained, causes such as trauma (including sexual abuse), vaginal foreign bodies, urethral prolapse and single organ prolapse need to be considered. Congenital malformations, such as retroperitoneal cavernous lymphangioma, may present with a vaginal discharge (Allen-Davis et al., 1996), as can congenital abnormalities of the Müllerian system such as hemivagina with a double uterus (Perone, 1997). Congenital abnormalities of the urinary system can also result in a presenting complaint of vaginal discharge. Urological abnormalities such as duplicated collecting systems with ectopic upper-pole ureters opening into the introitus are a rare cause of discharge but should be included in the differential diagnosis (See and Mayo, 1991).

Rare tumours such as sarcoma botryoides (embryonal rhabdomyosarcoma), endodermal carcinoma and mesonephric carcinoma may produce vaginal bleeding in young girls (see also Ch. 31). Clear cell adenocarcinoma of the vagina or cervix is another neoplasm that may present as a bloodstained discharge. This tumour was associated with intrauterine exposure of the mother to diethylstilbestrol, which was first available commercially in 1938. The drug has been banned in the USA since 1971. There have been over 5000 reported cases in the literature associated with exposure in utero to synthetic oestrogens. The median age at presentation was 19 years and 60% of the vaginal lesions were accompanied by lesions on the ectocervix. The passage of time means that cases associated with diethylstilbestrol are no longer being seen de novo.

Chylous reflux is a manifestation of primary or secondary lymphatic obstruction. Leakage of chyle into the vagina can occasionally occur with either form of obstruction and the symptom of a chylous vaginal discharge may be the presenting complaint (Shahlaee et al., 1997). Chylous discharge should be considered in a child with chronic vaginal discharge and swelling of her lower extremities. Treatment can be effected by the division and ligation of the retroperitoneal lymphatics (Zelikovski et al., 1989).

Endocrine changes caused by premature or precocious puberty, oestrogen ingestion and oestrogen-producing cysts or tumours may cause unexpected bleeding and an increase in vaginal discharge (Cowan and Morrison, 1991; Pokorny, 1992).

Predisposing factors for vulvovaginitis

The commonest cause of vaginal discharge in young girls is vulvovaginitis. It order to interpret the results of swabs taken from prepubertal girls with vulvovaginitis, it is necessary to understand the factors that predispose the juvenile vagina to infection: the anatomy of the young female genitalia, the histology of the vagina, the influence of hormones and the normal microbial flora.

The genitalia of prepubertal girls are relatively unprotected because of a lack of labial fat pads and pubic hair. The labia minora are small and tend to open when the child squats, uncovering the more sensitive tissues within the hymenal ring. The proximity of the anus risks faecal bacterial contamination, which may be promoted by wiping from "back to front" (Arsenault and Gerbie, 1986).

The squamous epithelium of the prepubertal vagina is undifferentiated (is thin and atrophic), leaving it more susceptible to invasion by bacterial pathogens. The pH is in the neutral range of 6.5–7.5. Oestrogen promotes the differentiation of squamous epithelium into the basal, intermediate and superficial cell layers characteristic of the vaginal mucosa present during reproductive years.

Normal vaginal flora in the prepubertal child

The largest study to be published on the normal vaginal flora was that of Hammerschlag et al. in Boston (1978). One hundred healthy girls, aged two months to 15 years of age, were routinely examined for normal and potentially pathogenic organisms. Only 59 girls had cultures examined for aerobic and facultatively anaerobic bacteria. Diphtheroids and *Staphylococcus epidermidis* were the most frequently isolated organisms, followed by streptococci (alpha-haemolytic and nonhaemolytic), lactobacilli and coliforms. Lactobacilli were isolated most frequently from older girls, whereas enteric organisms were isolated from the younger girls. *Gardnerella vaginalis*, yeast species and genital mycoplasmas were isolated from 13.5%, 28%, and 28% of the girls, respectively, none of whom had symptoms. This study did, however, suffer from three major limitations. First, eight of the children in the study were postmenarche, which means that although this was a study of vaginal flora in children, they were not exclusively premenarche. Second, the culture methods used did not include atmospheric conditions suitable for the isolation of fastidious anaerobes. Finally, the paediatric walk-in clinic served a disadvantaged inner city population, so the findings may not be transferable to other paediatric populations.

Paradise et al. (1982) studied children attending outpatient clinics at Philadelphia's Children's Hospital. Like Hammerschlag's group, these were predominantly of low socioeconomic status. However, this group included anaerobic culture of vaginal secretions and identified various species of *Bacteriodes* in 11 of their 40 asymptomatic control children.

A more recent study, from the Royal Children's Hospital, Melbourne (Jaquiery et al., 1999) sampled vaginal flora in children over two years of age undergoing surgery. Children who were previously known to have a history of sexual abuse, current antibiotic treatment or vulvovaginitis were excluded. Mixed anaerobes, diphtheroids and coagulase-negative staphylococci (*S. epidermidis*) were the commonest organisms detected (Table 36.1).

Abnormal vaginal discharge in prepubertal girls

A number of studies have been published either comparing symptomatic subjects with age-matched controls, (Jaquiery et al., 1999; Paradise et al., 1982), or attempting to identify putative pathogens in symptomatic children (Cox, 1997; Donald et al., 1991; Jones, 1996; Pierce and Hart, 1992). No specific infective cause was identified in the majority of children studied. This has given rise to the concept of "nonspecific" vaginitis associated with mixed bacterial flora (usually commensal flora derived from the bowel), which, it is suggested, gives rise to inflammation of the

Table 36.1. Microbiology of the genital tract in girls over two years of age who were asymptomatic ($n = 50$)

Organism	Number	Percentage
Anaerobes	46	92
Diphtheroids	31	62
Coagulase-negative staphylococci	28	56
Escherichia coli	17	34
Streptococcus viridans	14	28
Enterococcus sp.	5	10
Haemophilus influenzae	2	4
Streptococcus pneumoniae	1	2
Group G streptococcus	1	2
Group B streptococcus	1	2
Lactobacilli	2	4
Proteus sp.	1	2
Staphylococcus aureus	1	2
Enterobius sp.	1	2

Source: From Jaquiery et al. (1999).

vulva and lower vagina. This is said to be attributable to poor hygiene, (Jones, 1996; Pierce and Hart, 1992). However, the theory that poor hygiene practices are a contributory factor has recently been challenged (Jaquiery et al., 1999). This group also made the important observation that vulvovaginitis associated with specific pathogens tends to cause moderate or severe inflammation as well as vaginal discharge.

Vaginitis associated with specific bacterial pathogens

Group A beta-haemolytic streptococci

The commonest infective cause of vulvovaginitis in prepubertal girls is the group A beta-haemolytic streptococci (Fig. 36.6, colour plate). This organism has constituted 11–18% of isolates in various studies (Cox, 1997; Dhar et al., 1993; Donald et al., 1991; Pierce and Hart, 1992). The epidemiology of this vulvovaginitis is unclear and merits further study. Dhar et al. (1993) speculated that the streptococci are transmitted from throat to vulva on the child's fingers. Straumanis and Bocchini (1990), in a 20 year review of the literature, found that 9 out of 12 identified cases also had throat cultures positive for group A beta-haemolytic streptococci, although only a quarter of children reported symptoms of upper respiratory tract infection. Sixty five per cent vulvovaginitis associated with group A streptococci occurred between September and January, in contrast to the peak incidence of associated pharyngitis, which occurs in late winter and spring in temperate climates. The mean (SD) (± 2.2) age was 5.0 years (range, 2.5–12 years).

The onset of symptoms is abrupt, with a seropurulent vaginal discharge (Fig. 36.7a, colour plate). The child often complains of dysuria as a result of urine passing over the inflamed vulva. Perineal inflammation has also been described, both with and without accompanying vulvovaginitis (Mogielnicki et al., 2000). In this series of 23 children observed over a year, the average age was again five years but the peak incidence was in late winter and early spring. Proctitis has also been described in two five-year-old children (Figueroa-Colón et al., 1984; Guss and Larsen, 1984).

Group A streptococci are always sensitive to penicillin, so a well-absorbed oral beta-lactam antibiotic, such as amoxicillin, is the treatment of choice. Erythromycin is a suitable alternative if the patient is hypersensitive to penicillin. The optimal duration of treatment is unknown, but traditionally penicillin is given for 10 days for streptococcal pharyngitis (Bisno, 2001).

Haemophilus influenzae

Non-capsulate strains of *Haemophilus influenzae* have been identified as the second most common cause of juvenile vulvovaginitis, after group A streptococci (Cox, 1997; Donald et al., 1991; Jones; 1996). In one study, this species even outnumbered group A streptococci (Pierce and Hart, 1992). In the UK, there seems to be little appreciation of the important role of this organism amongst doctors treating these patients (Cox, 1997). This may be because *H. influenzae* is fastidious in its growth requirements and requires the inclusion of selective/enrichment media to isolate it from specimens that contain large numbers of less nutritionally demanding bowel flora. The noncapsulate strains should not be confused with *H. influenzae* type b, the cause of paediatric meningitis and epiglottitis, against which the Hib vaccine has proved so effective.

Although most strains of *H. influenzae* remain sensitive to amoxicillin, resistance is increasing, so treatment should be guided by the results of sensitivity tests.

Candida *spp.*

Although candidal infection is the commonest cause of vulvovaginitis in women of childbearing age, it is uncommon in prepubertal girls (Cox, 1997; Jaquiery et al., 1999; Pierce and Hart, 1992). In one study (Paradise et al., 1982), candidiasis occurred exclusively in girls who were pubertal. In another study (Pierce and Hart, 1992), all but one of the girls with candidiasis were less than two years old or were pubertal. Predisposing factors include a recent course of antibiotics, diabetes mellitus or the wearing of nappies (diapers). Two studies (de Jong, 1985; Steele and de San Lazaro, 1994) have suggested that candidal vaginitis is associated with sexual abuse.

The clinical diagnosis is suggested by the symptoms of pruritus and a curd-like discharge, which does not smell offensive. Inflammation of the vulva and perianal region is common; satellite lesions may be present, and white plaques adherent to the vagina are often present.

Treatment with a topical antifungal agent such as clotrimazole or miconazole is usually effective.

Enterobius vermicularis
Threadworms or pinworms are a well-recognized cause of vaginal itching and discharge in school-age girls. Pierce and Hart (1992) in Liverpool identified threadworms in 43/200 (21%) of the children in their study, whereas Jaquiery et al. (1999) studying patients in Melbourne, Australia, identified only one symptomatic child (2%). Diagnosis is relatively straightforward. Eggs can be collected by pressing a piece of sticky tape (Sellotape; Scotch tape) onto the perianal area in the early morning. This must then be applied to a glass slide and examined by microscopy.

The treatment of choice for children over two years of age is mebendazole, 100 mg given as a single dose. The entire family should be treated and all bedclothes washed in hot water. As reinfection is common, a second dose may be given after two to three weeks. Children under two may be given piperazine, but this has a number of uncommon, unpleasant side effects, and children dislike the taste.

Other streptococci
The beta-haemolytic streptococci groups C and G have a similar pathogenic potential to group A streptococci but are less-common causes of vulvovaginitis. Group G is more common than group C, causing 4–8% of cases in various studies, compared with 1–6% for group C streptococci (Cox 1997; Donald et al., 1991; Jaquiery et al., 1999).

Similarly, *Streptococcus pneumoniae* is an uncommon but well-recognised cause of juvenile vulvovaginitis, causing 1–10% of infections in the studies quoted above.

The role of *group B beta-haemolytic streptococci* is harder to define. Although identified in symptomatic patients in a number of studies (Jaquiery et al., 1999; Pierce and Hart, 1992) their role as a primary pathogen is yet to be established. Vaginal carriage in pregnant women is extremely important in the aetiology of neonatal disease, but the organisms are not a recognized cause of vaginal discharge in either adult women or prepubertal girls. As bowel carriage of group B streptococci is common, it may be part of the mixed bowel flora associated with nonspecific vaginitis.

Staphylococcus aureus
Staphylococcus aureus has been identified in both symptomatic and asymptomatic children (Hammerschlag et al., 1978; Jaquiery et al., 1999; Jones, 1996; Pierce and Hart, 1992). As the perineum is the second most common site of staphylococcal carriage after the nose, it is difficult to distinguish incidental carriage from true pathogenic potential.

Shigella sonnei
Shigella sonnei is an uncommon cause of vulvovaginitis in Western countries but is more common in the tropics. The vaginal discharge is usually chronic (sometimes persisting for months), purulent, blood-streaked and foul smelling (Sanders and Wasilauskas, 1973). Most patients have not had acute diarrhoea or dysentery immediately before or at the time of presentation (Murphy and Nelson, 1979).

Yersinia enterocolitica
Another enteric pathogen, *Yersinia enterocolitica*, has been reported as the cause of vulvovaginitis in a four-year-old girl. This was part of a large community outbreak of gastroenteritis associated with the consumption of contaminated tofu (Watkins and Quan, 1984).

Virus infections in prepubertal girls
Human papillomavirus and genital warts
Genital warts (condylomata acuminata) are caused by the human papillomavirus (HPV). There are over 40 types of HPV, which have been characterized by DNA hybridization techniques. In adults and children, anogenital warts are most commonly caused by HPV types 6 or 11, but occasionally other types are found, including type 16, the type associated with cervical carcinoma in adult women.

Children may acquire genital warts in a number of ways. HPV can be transmitted perinatally, leading to laryngeal papillomatosis as well as genital warts. As many cases of juvenile-onset laryngeal papillomatosis do not become clinically obvious until the child is several years old, the same may well apply to genital warts in children.

Sensitive HPV detection techniques, such as DNA detection by Southern blot, have shown that asymptomatic and transient carriage of HPV is relatively common at birth (Hammerschlag, 1998). HPV DNA has been found in oral mucosal scrapings of healthy girls, so the possibility of genital warts resulting from autoinoculation also exists. Transmission from an adult to child during bathing has been recorded (Oriel, 1988). Sexual abuse is also an established mode of transmission. Condylomata have been reported in 1–2% of abused children; 50–70% of cases of genital warts in children reported in the literature appear to be the result of abuse (Hammerschlag, 1998).

In children, condylomata acuminata do not have the typical cauliflower, hyperkeratotic appearance seen in physiologically mature individuals. They may form flesh-coloured lesions, which are difficult to see on the unoestrogenized mucosa of the prepubertal child. Small red punctations (the tips of the capillaries that extend through each papule) may cause the lesions to bleed. Sometimes, however, the papilloma may present as large, exophytic lesions (Pokorny, 1992).

If a child has clinically evident condylomata acuminata before the age of two, the condylomata should be symptomatically managed because they often resolve spontaneously. In the older child, large condylomata can become inflamed, producing an irritative discharge. In these circumstances, treatment is indicated. This usually involves examination under anaesthesia, excisional biopsy (with optional determination of the DNA type) and ablation of the lesion.

Herpes simplex

Herpes simplex virus can cause infection at the cervix, vagina or vulva, or simultaneously at multiple sites. The lesions, notable for their discomfort, present as 2–3 mm vesicles on an erythematous base, which go on to ulcerate. The diagnosis is made by virus culture or by antigen detection using immunofluorescence or enzyme-linked immunoassay.

Common noninfective causes of vulvovaginitis in prepubertal girls

Foreign bodies

Probably the most common noninfective cause of vulvovaginitis in young girls is a retained foreign body. It is particularly important to exclude this in girls who have a bloodstained or chronic discharge. Small pieces of tissue paper seem to be a common finding in this situation (Farrington, 1997; Pierce and Hart, 1992; Pokorny, 1992). These may become embedded into the atrophic mucosa of the vaginal walls and it may be necessary to remove them under a general anaesthetic. Other objects, including a lead pencil, have been described (Dahiya et al., 1999).

Allergy and contact dermatitis

Allergic reactions to bath additives, clothing materials and washing powder are often quoted as causes of vaginal discharge in children, but case reports are hard to find. It has been suggested that the common practice of shampooing children's hair while bathing can contribute to the problem (Brown, 1989). In the study of Jaquiery et al. (1999), children with vaginal discharge were *more* likely to wear cotton underwear and were *less* likely to have used bubble bath than asymptomatic controls. There are single case reports of vulvovaginitis induced by house dust mite allergy (Moraes, 1998) and vaginal pruritus resulting from allergy to ragweed (Dhaliwal and Fink, 1995).

Skin diseases

Local skin diseases such as eczema and psoriasis have been described in children who presented with vulvovaginitis (Jaquiery et al., 1999; Pierce and Hart, 1992). The most important skin condition is lichen sclerosus et atrophicus (see

Ch. 35), which, if unrecognized, may lead to misdiagnosis of child sexual abuse (Wood and Bevan, 1999). It causes itching and soreness, rather than vaginal discharge. Treatment with potent topical steroids leads to rapid resolution of symptoms (Powell and Wojnarowska, 2000).

Idiopathic vulvovaginitis

If examination and cultures are negative, the most likely cause of the child's symptoms is "nonspecific" vaginitis. Reassurance and advice on simple hygiene measures are all that are required. A written advice sheet may be helpful (Box 36.1).

Box 36.1 Patient information sheet for vulvovaginitis in children

Vulvovaginitis is a term for a fairly common condition which affects little girls. The usual presentation is that of redness and soreness between the legs with possible itching and there is often a yellow or green vaginal discharge which may stain the pants.

The condition is commonest between the ages of three and ten years when children have more control over their own personal hygiene. For this reason, it is important to teach and practise good personal hygiene at home, playgroup, nursery or school.

In order to prevent the worsening or recurrence of this condition the following measures are advised:

1 Good toilet hygiene. Always wipe from front to back after using the toilet and ensure that the toilet paper is clean before completing the exercise.
2 Ensure urination takes place with the child's legs spread apart.
3 A daily warm bath is advised. Unscented bubble baths and plain unperfumed soaps may be used. The area should be dried carefully by patting with a soft towel.
4 It is advisable to wear cotton pants and to avoid tight clothes such as leggings or jeans.
5 Avoid wearing pants in bed.
6 Do not apply creams or lotions unless prescribed by your doctor.

If the condition worsens, or should there be blood in the discharge, please inform your doctor as further investigations are indicated. An appointment can then be made at the Paediatric and Adolescent Gynaecology clinic.

If the swabs taken today reveal the presence of an infection, we shall inform you and your own doctor so that a course of antibiotics may be prescribed.

Reproduced with permission of the authors: T. Bevan and P. Wood.

Vaginal discharge and child sexual abuse

The possibility of childhood sexual abuse should be considered when evaluating a child with vulvovaginitis.

Sexual abuse may be difficult to diagnose because the majority of children who are abused have no physical complaints related to either trauma or infection. A study from Boston (Emans et al., 1987) reported on the appearance of the external genitalia inspected using magnification with either a colposcope or a paediatric otoscope in a large group of girls aged 1–14 years who had a history of sexual abuse. Sexually molested girls were more likely than asymptomatic control girls to have increased friability of the posterior fourchette, attenuation of the hymen, scars and synechiae from the hymen to the vagina. However, the majority of sexually abused girls under 10 years had normal findings on genital examination. A history of vulvovaginitis or urinary symptoms was also uncommon, occurring in only 13% of subjects.

The prevalence of sexual abuse in children is difficult to estimate and transmission of sexually transmitted disease (STD) in this situation is generally low, with reported prevalence rates ranging from 0 to 13% (Hammerschlag et al., 1978, 1985; Paradise et al., 1982; Robinson et al., 1998; Steele and de San Lazaro, 1994). Transmission varies according to the type of assault, the site, the prevalence of STD in the abusing population and whether single or multiple episodes have occurred (Hammerschlag, 1998; Robinson et al., 1998).

Robinson and coworkers in London (1998) found a low prevalence (3.7%) of sexually transmitted organisms (*Neisseria gonorrhoeae*, *Chlamydia trachomatis* and *Trichomonas vaginalis*) in a group of 159 girls who were suspected to be the victims of sexual abuse. The authors concluded that screening for infection should be mandatory for presumed sexually abused girls with vaginal discharge and ideally should be undertaken in all children attending for evaluation of sexual abuse.

This leads to the difficult question as to which microorganisms should be regarded as sexually transmitted and, therefore, markers of sexual abuse when isolated from the vaginal secretions of young girls. Unfortunately, no single microorganism can be regarded as an absolute marker of sexual abuse. Children who have not been abused can acquire STDs by vertical transmission or, more rarely (and more questionably), by nonsexual contact such as fomites or nonsexual acts.

An appreciation of the likelihood of various microorganisms being sexually transmitted is extremely important because the question may be raised by the unexpected isolation of such an organism in a child with a vaginal discharge in whom sexual abuse has not been suspected until that moment. When *N. gonorrhoeae* or *C. trachomatis* are isolated in these circumstances, there is a strong likelihood that they are sexually transmitted. Similarly, *T. vaginalis* is very rare in prepubertal girls in the absence of sexual activity. The situation regarding *G. vaginalis*, the genital mycoplasmas and the other anaerobes, which contribute to the abnormal flora of bacterial vaginosis, is much less clear. Different studies have produced conflicting results, but there is some evidence that they are not part of the normal flora of the prepubertal vagina and that the change in the vaginal flora occurs predominantly in those who are sexually active. The evidence for this is examined in more detail below.

Sexually transmitted infections in prepubertal girls

Neisseria gonorrhoeae in prepubertal girls

Studies of gonorrhoea in children demonstrate that there is a history of sexual abuse in the majority of children who have this infection (Folland et al., 1977; Ingram et al., 1982). Mother-to-infant transmission of *N. gonorrhoeae* can occur during childbirth and may result in a purulent ophthalmitis (ophthalmia neonatorum), which responds well to appropriate antibiotic treatment. Nonvenereal transmission has been described (Altchek, 1972; Shore and Winkelstein, 1971), but there is some doubt whether the authors of these earlier reports were sufficiently rigorous in excluding the possibility of child sexual abuse. Ris (1978) pointed out that *N. gonorrhoeae* is a fragile, fastidious organism that is extremely sensitive to drying and is, therefore, unlikely to survive on bedclothing. He quoted two studies of young girls with gonococcal vaginitis in which nearly all the children disclosed a history of sexual abuse.

The reported prevalence of gonorrhoea in studies of prepubertal girls with vulvovaginitis varies from 0 to 11% (Hammerschlag et al., 1978; Jaquiery et al., 1999; Paradise et al., 1982; Pierce and Hart, 1992). All the studies emphasized the higher prevalence in girls who have a discharge compared with those who do not, and in those who have a history of sexual abuse compared with those who do not.

Shapiro et al. (1999) noted the high prevalence of unsuspected gonorrhoea in its area and the importance of culturing for *N. gonorrhoeae* when investigating young girls with vaginal discharge. In their group of 43 girls, four (9%) had gonorrhoea, even though they excluded children who gave a history of sexual abuse. Siegel et al. (1995) studied the prevalence of STD in children who had been sexually abused. They found that 11% of prepubertal girls with vaginal discharge, and none of those without discharge, had a positive culture for *N. gonorrhoeae*. Again, this underlines the importance of investigating sexually abused children with symptoms for possible STDs.

Diagnosis and treatment is extremely important because of the risk of later development of PID. In sexually active young women, PID is more common in teenagers that in older women (Bell and Holmes, 1984). First coitus before the menarche is also a risk factor for PID (Duncan et al., 1990).

As many strains of gonococcus are resistant to penicillin, cephalosporins such as ceftriaxone or cefuroxime are the agents of choice for treatment. Single-dose intramuscular spectinomycin therapy (40 mg/kg) has also been shown to be effective in this age group (Rettig et al., 1980).

Chlamydia trachomatis in prepubertal girls

The isolation of *C. trachomatis* from genital swabs from a child suspected to be the victim of sexual abuse has important medicolegal implications. While sexual transmission is the most likely route of acquisition, *C. trachomatis*, like *N. gonorrhoeae*, can be transmitted perinatally from mother to child. Perinatal transmission most commonly presents as ophthalmia neonatorum. Symptoms occur a little later than those caused by *N. gonorrhoeae*: at 3–13 days of age. A later clinical manifestation, interstitial pneumonia, may occur at 4–12 weeks (Oriel and Ridgway, 1982). Unlike *N. gonorrhoeae*, carriage of *C. trachomatis* can persist for as long as six years (Stenberg and Mårdh, 1986; Thompson et al., 2001). Consequently, the finding of *C. trachomatis* in a child suspected of being sexually abused will always be accompanied by the doubt that the organism may have been acquired perinatally, even if the child is no longer an infant.

A second problem associated with the detection of *C. trachomatis* in cases of sexual abuse is the method used for diagnosis. Most laboratories now employ automated antigen detection methods such as enzyme immunoassay or the newer molecular methods. Many practitioners in this field had hoped that the recently developed molecular amplification methods, with their increased sensitivity, would play a role here. The fact that urine samples, rather than swabs, can be tested makes them an even more attractive option. However, the difficulties associated with validating these techniques in a population where the prevalence is low has delayed their introduction. A recent study (Embree et al., 1996) has indicated that the polymerase chain reaction (PCR) may well increase the sensitivity of *Chlamydia* detection in young girls. Using a vaginal wash technique combined with PCR, and comparing this with culture of swabs, they found that PCR detected both children whose swabs were culture positive for *Chlamydia* and identified two further girls whose swabs were culture negative.

Studies of children with prepubertal vaginal discharge have shown that *C. trachomatis* is only occasionally encountered in children who do not have a history of known sexual abuse (Hammerschlag et al., 1978; Pierce and Hart, 1992).

A higher prevalence has been found in children who are either sexually active or who are suspected to be subjects of sexual abuse. Siegel et al. (1995) identified 11 children with *C. trachomatis* in their study group of 14 sexually abused children. Nearly all were pubertal, not prepubertal. Rettig and Nelson (1981) examined 23 prepubertal children with nongonococcal urethritis and vaginitis and 31 with gonococcal anogenital infection. *C. trachomatis* was not found in the 12 males and 11 females with nongonococcal urethritis and vaginitis but 9 of the 33 episodes of gonorrhoea (27%) were complicated by concurrent or subsequent chlamydial infection.

Diagnosis and treatment is extremely important because asymptomatic carriage may result in the later development of PID.

Trichomonas vaginalis in prepubertal girls

Although *T. vaginalis* is a common cause of vaginal discharge in adult women, it is an extremely uncommon cause of vaginal discharge in prepubertal girls. In the studies that sought this organism in children with vaginal discharge, (Hammerschlag et al., 1978; Steele and de San Lazaro, 1994) the only children in whom it was found were those over 10 who were sexually active or who had been sexually abused. The subject is well reviewed by Ross et al. (1993), who described the dilemma that confronts clinicians when this organism is isolated from girls at risk of sexual abuse.

T. vaginalis can be acquired during the passage through the birth canal, but this is uncommon (Al-Salihi et al., 1974). Infection acquired in this way may persist in the infant's vagina, while under the influence of maternal oestrogen, but it does not persist beyond the first year of life. Routes other than sexual contact are possible as the organism can remain viable on toilet seats for up to 45 minutes and on wet clothes for up to 23 hours (Burch et al., 1959; Whittington, 1957).

Bacterial vaginosis in prepubertal girls

Bacterial vaginosis is the most frequent cause of vaginal discharge in adult women, but its existence in children is the subject of conflicting reports. It is characterized by a malodorous, frothy, off-white discharge, which produces a fishy odour when potassium hydroxide is added to vaginal fluid. The presence of "clue cells" on microscopy (squamous epithelial cells covered with Gram-variable coccobacilli), may be used for diagnosis. Bacterial vaginosis occurs when lactobacilli (which are the predominant flora in the adult vagina) are replaced by anaerobes such as *Mobiluncus* sp., *Mycoplasma* sp. and *G. vaginalis*.

De Jong (1985) seems to have been the first to draw attention to the association of *G. vaginalis* with vaginitis in children who had been sexually abused. This was supported by the results of a large study in Newcastle (Steele and de San Lazaro, 1994). *G. vaginalis* was the commonest organism recovered from transhymenal cultures in young girls who were known to have been sexually abused (19%) compared with those where there was only the suspicion of sexual abuse (3%) or those who had vulvovaginitis but no suspicion of sexual abuse (2%). In this study, 32 of the 34 girls were over nine years of age. These findings were confirmed in a similar study by Bartley et al. (1987), who found a prevalence of 14.6% in the abuse group of girls compared with 4.2% in the control group. However, a large study from North Carolina, USA, did not confirm the higher prevalence of *G. vaginalis* in children evaluated for sexual abuse (Ingram et al., 1992). Three groups of children were studied: girls who gave a history of sexual contact and/or had proven infection with *N. gonorrhoeae* or *C. trachomatis* (group 1), a group evaluated for possible sexual abuse who proved not to have such a history or infection with *N. gonorrhoeae* or *C. trachomatis* (group 2), and a control group consisting of healthy girls (children of the authors' friends; Group 3). *G. vaginalis* was found in 5.3% of group 1, 4.9% of group 2 and 6.4% of group 3.

As bacterial vaginosis is caused by the overgrowth of a number of different species, it may be misleading to rely on *G. vaginalis* as the sole indicator of this condition. *G. vaginalis* is part of the normal adult vaginal flora and there is some evidence that it is part of the vaginal flora of young girls (Hammerschlag et al., 1978) although not all studies have confirmed this (Jaquiery et al., 1999).

Hammerschlag and colleagues (1985) modified the criteria used for the diagnosis of adult bacterial vaginosis when comparing vaginal wash specimens from abused with those from non-abused children. They scored children as having "definite" bacterial vaginosis if vaginal secretions contained clue cells and gave off a fishy odour after the addition of 10% potassium hydroxide and "possible" if they had odour only. They found a low prevalence in both non-abused children and abused children examined within 48 hours of the abuse episode. However, the prevalence of both "definite" and "possible" bacterial vaginosis rose to 13% in girls examined more than seven days after the episode of abuse or rape. This is quite persuasive evidence that this condition can develop as the result of sexual activity.

There are also individual case reports and clinical studies that report the association of other anaerobic bacteria such as *Mycoplasma hominis* with vaginitis in young patients who have been evaluated for possible sexual abuse (Robinson et al., 1998; Waites et al., 1983).

The microbiological investigation of child sexual abuse

The detection of a sexually transmitted pathogen in a child raises the possibility of child sexual abuse. As this diagnosis has far-reaching medical, psychosocial and legal implications, it is essential that all microbiological techniques are performed to the highest standard and that every procedure is meticulously documented (Dyson and Hosein, 1996.) A recent report (Royal College of Physicians' Working Party, 1997) has recommended investigation for *N. gonorrhoeae*, *C. trachomatis*, *T. vaginalis* and *Treponema pallidum* in all cases. Vaginal, rectal and pharyngeal swabs are recommended for *N. gonorrhoeae*, vaginal and rectal specimens for *C. trachomatis* and a vaginal specimen only for *T. vaginalis*. *T. pallidum* is investigated by serology.

It is essential that a "chain of evidence" supports all specimens. This is a record of the transfer of specimens from the time of collection to receipt by the laboratory. This is most easily achieved by attaching a preprinted label to the laboratory request card, which can be signed by each person in the "chain". A copy of the record used in the authors' microbiology department is shown in Box 36.2. Only qualified staff working to written protocols should undertake examination of the specimens and all test results must be carefully documented.

Box 36.2 Laboratory record for "chain of evidence"

PG SCREEN CHLAMYDIA

Delivered:	Date:	Time:
Received:	Date:	Time:
Labelled:		
Stained:	Date:	
Micro by:	Date:	
Checked:	Date:	
Reported:	Date:	Time:

PG SCREEN, paediatric–gynaecology screen.

Culture remains the gold standard for the detection of *N. gonorrhoeae* and *T. vaginalis* as well as *C. trachomatis*. This achieves maximum test specificity and also offers high sensitivity. The antigen detection tests for *N. gonorrhoeae* and *C. trachomatis*, which are widely used for adults, have not been licensed for use in children.

These arrangements for transport and laboratory examination of specimens in cases of possible child sexual abuse require close liaison between paediatrician, gynaecologist and microbiologist. All staff should be made aware of the need for a very high standard of documentation and the importance of adhering to written protocols.

Vaginal discharge in adolescence

History and examination

An adolescent presenting with a history of vaginal discharge may require not only an explanation and treatment for her presenting symptom but also help and advice on additional issues such as contraception and sexual health. A description of the discharge can be helpful along with the menstrual history and accompanying hygiene issues. The extent of sexual activity should be explored frankly and the adolescent should see this as being nonjudgemental and nondirectional. The adolescent is best given an opportunity to talk about such matters in private, whether or not a parent or guardian has accompanied them to the consultation. Under these circumstances, the clinician can ask to speak to the adolescent alone for at least a brief period in the course of the overall consultation.

An explanation of the examination procedure is important since for most this will be their first clinical gynaecological examination. A general examination to include secondary sexual characteristics and an abdominal examination is recommended, prior to inspection of the vulva for signs of inflammation or any lesions. A Cusco's speculum examination, using a suitably sized instrument, will allow for the taking of vaginal and cervical swabs and inspection of the upper vagina and cervix in appropriate cases, depending on the clinical history, patient compliance, previous tampon usage and previous sexual history.

Vaginal discharge in adolescents who have passed puberty may be physiological (leukorrhoea) or may be caused by the same infectious agents that cause this symptom in adult women. As with prepubertal girls, an understanding of vaginal physiology, histology and microbial flora is important when investigating a complaint of vaginal discharge.

Changes in the vaginal flora at menarche

At the onset of the cyclic ovarian activity that precedes menarche, the vagina once again develops a glycogen-filled epithelium and cervical secretions increase. The desquamated vaginal cells and cervical secretions are the cause of the so-called physiological leukorrhoea seen at puberty.

The pH of the vagina becomes substantially more acidic, accounting for some of the differences in manifestations of infection.

The epithelial cell changes are particularly important at the cervix, since persistence of columnar epithelium in young women appears to significantly increase their vulnerability to STDs. Although cervical columnar epithelium eventually recedes completely, to be replaced with squamous epithelium, this is a gradual process continuing well into adulthood. Typically, the cervix in the adolescent still displays areas of exposed columnar epithelium (ectopy). This is significant because *C. trachomatis* infects columnar not squamous epithelium. The presence of ectopy also seems to predispose to infections with *N. gonorrhoeae* and is associated with the adverse outcomes of both infections (Berman and Hein, 1991).

Normal vaginal flora after the menarche

Following puberty, major changes take place in the microbial flora that makes up the ecosystem of the vagina. Oestrogen increases glycogen in the vaginal epithelium, which in turn is metabolized to glucose and then to lactic acid by the microbial flora, which by then consists mainly of lactobacilli. This results in a low pH, which selectively favours colonization by acid-tolerant species such as lactobacilli (Hill et al., 1984).

Although anaerobes such as *Bifidobacterium*, *Peptostreptococcus*, *Porphyromonas* and *Prevotella* spp. are readily detected when appropriate anaerobic culture techniques are used (Murray, 1999), the normal vaginal flora is predominantly aerobic. As well as large numbers of lactobacilli (with counts up to 10^8 colony-forming units (cfu)/g), coryneforms and coagulase-negative staphylococci are present, with counts of 10^5–10^6 cfu/g (Masfari et al., 1986).

The vagina is not a single environment. The flora of the lower vagina consists of a mixture of organisms from the vagina, perineum and introitus, whereas the flora of the cervix and fornices more closely resembles true vaginal flora.

The vaginal ecosystem is subject to many changes. The state of the mucosa and secretions change with age, within each menstrual cycle and with pregnancy.

Causes of vaginal discharge in adolescents

Vaginal discharge is a common complaint in adolescent girls. In a primary care setting, 60% of teenagers between 15 and 19 years of age presenting with a spontaneous complaint of vaginal discharge had experienced earlier episodes (Bro, 1989).

Noninfective conditions

Noninfective conditions may cause vaginal discharge. Foreign bodies, particularly forgotten tampons, may result in a foul-smelling and sometimes blood-streaked vaginal discharge. Removal of the tampon followed by bathing is all that is usually required.

Specific infective causes of vulvovaginitis in adolescents

Candidal infection

Candidal vulvovaginitis becomes more common in girls as puberty approaches (Paradise et al., 1982; Pierce and Hart, 1992) and is a common cause of vaginal infection in postpubertal girls and adult women. Predisposing factors include diabetes, antibiotic use, oral contraceptives, steroids, obesity and tight-fitting garments (Wald, 1984).

The most prominent symptom is pruritus, with a white, curdy discharge. The patient often complains of dysuria. On examination, the vulva is erythematous and may be fissured. Not all women with candidiasis have pruritus and confirmation of the diagnosis by culture is recommended (Oriel et al., 1972). A preliminary diagnosis can be obtained by swabbing the vaginal secretions with a cotton-tipped swab, which is then rolled on a glass slide. A drop of 10% potassium hydroxide and saline are added and the preparation is covered with a coverslip. On microscopy, the characteristic budding yeasts and hyphae are seen. Laboratory techniques for the isolation of yeast species include culture on Sabouraud's agar (Fig. 36.8a). After 48 hours of incubation, large creamy colonies characteristic of *Candida* spp. can be seen. *Candida albicans* is by far the commonest yeast to cause vulvovaginitis (over 80% in one series), followed by *Candida* (*Torulopsis*) *glabrata* (16%) (Oriel et al., 1972). Traditionally *C. albicans* was identified by its ability to produce "germ tubes" when incubated with horse serum at 37°C for 1 hour (Fig. 36.8b). It is not necessary routinely to identify *Candida* to the species level. In cases when it is necessary, for example following treatment failure with fluconazole, the newer carbohydrate utilization tests (e.g. Candida API) are more suitable for this purpose.

Most young women with vaginal candidiasis respond to topical treatment with imidazole agents such as clotrimazole or miconazole, which are available as creams and pessaries. The triazoles fluconazole and itraconazole are effective as short-term oral treatments for vaginal candidiasis. Fluconazole is given as a single dose of 150 mg and itraconazole as two 200 mg doses 8 hours apart. They are more expensive than topical treatments, but compliance is improved and oral treatment is less painful to administer if the vulva is very inflamed (Working Group of the British Society for Medical Mycology, 1995).

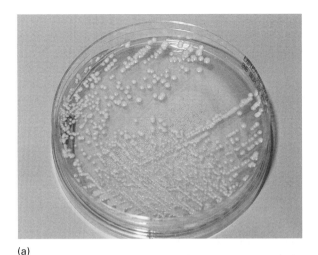

(a)

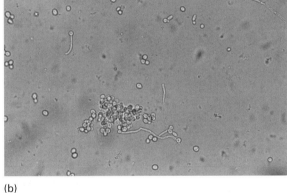

(b)

Fig. 36.8. Candidal infection. (a) Creamy colonies on Sabouraud's agar after 48 hours of incubation at 37°C. (b) Microscopy of a wet preparation showing germ tube.

Trichomonas vaginalis

T. vaginalis, a flagellate protozoon (Fig. 36.9), is the cause of one of the commonest STDs worldwide (Anon., 2000). The only prevalence study undertaken in the UK in the past 10 years detected a prevalence of 0.1% among women requesting cervical smears (Waghorn et al., 1998). In other countries, studies undertaken in settings such as clinics for STDs have detected prevalence of 6–8% (Bowden and Garnett, 2000).

Clinically, *T. vaginalis* infection is characterized by a frothy, yellowish-green discharge with an unpleasant odour. On speculum examination, the cervix typically displays "strawberry" spots. The diagnosis is most readily undertaken by examining vaginal fluid in a drop of saline on a slide (the wet mount technique). *T. vaginalis* is easily recognized by an experienced observer, and the use of phase-contrast microscopy may enhance the sensitivity of

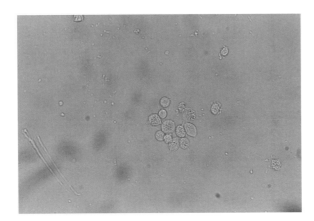

Fig. 36.9. Trophozoites of *Trichomonas vaginalis* in a wet preparation.

this method. Other nonculture techniques such as acridine orange and fluorescent antibody staining have sensitivities that are higher than the wet mount but lower than culture (Bickley et al., 1989.) The use of various culture media may improve the sensitivity of detection (Poch et al., 1996). There is one report of microscopy of spun urine for detection of *T. vaginalis* in adolescent women (Blake et al., 1999). Although microscopy of urine alone (64%) was less sensitive than microscopy of vaginal fluid (75%), microscopy on both specimens improved diagnosis by 12%. *T. vaginalis* is often diagnosed incidentally in asymptomatic women whose cervical smears are examined by Papanicolaou's method as part of a cervical screening programme. This is superior in sensitivity to wet film microscopy and to many culture methods (Clay et al., 1988).

Infection usually responds to oral metronidazole. Rarely, strains are encountered that have increased resistance to metronidazole. These may respond to higher doses of metronidazole given topically and orally. Persistent infection with metronidazole-resistant *T. vaginalis* has been successfully treated with paromomycin (Nyijesy et al., 1995).

Bacterial vaginosis

Bacterial vaginosis is a polymicrobial syndrome associated with a change in the vaginal flora from the dominant hydrogen peroxide-producing lactobacilli to a mixed flora, which includes strict and facultative anaerobes such as *Mobiluncus* sp., *G. vaginalis*, *Bacteroides* sp. and *Mycoplasma hominis*. Although bacterial vaginosis is often associated with STDs, it can occur in monogamous and sexually abstinent women. It is now the commonest cause of vaginal discharge in women in their reproductive years. In the UK, a prevalence of 12% and 28% has been reported from stud-

ies of antenatal and termination of pregnancy clinics, respectively (Blackwell et al., 1993; Hay et al., 1994). A recent study in primary care in the UK reported a prevalence of 9% (Lamont et al., 2000).

The condition was originally called nonspecific vaginitis. This was superseded by the term anaerobic vaginosis (Blackwell et al., 1983), but this was later replaced by the name bacterial vaginosis.

The principal symptom is an offensive, fishy smell, which is usually accompanied by an off-white vaginal discharge. Sometimes the odour is more offensive after sexual intercourse and during menstruation. The smell is caused by volatile amines such as cadaverine and putrescine (Chen et al., 1979).

Most clinical studies of bacterial vaginosis have used Amsel's criteria for diagnosis (Amsel et al., 1983). This requires the presence of three out of the following four features: (i) vaginal pH greater than 4.5, (ii) characteristic homogeneous discharge, (iii) a strong fishy odour on adding 10% potassium hydroxide to vaginal fluid (positive amine or "whiff" test), (iv) presence of "clue cells" (vaginal epithelial cells heavily coated with bacilli) on wet microscopy. These criteria are subject to considerable variation between centres and attempts have been made to replace Amsel's criteria with a standardized method of Gram film interpretation (Nugent et al., 1991). A simplified scoring system, ranging from grade 1 (normal), showing predominantly lactobacilli (Fig. 36.10a, colour plate) to grade 3 as the most abnormal, with few or no lactobacilli, the presence of many other bacteria and clue cells (Fig. 36.10b, colour plate), has been suggested (Hay et al., 1994).

It is important to recognize and treat bacterial vaginosis because it may cause a number of complications. It has been associated with first-trimester miscarriage, preterm birth, low birth weight, postabortal endometritis, intraamniotic infection and postpartum endometritis (Eschenbach et al., 1988; Hay et al., 1994). Trials of antimicrobial treatment in pregnancy to reduce preterm birth have shown conflicting results (Carey et al., 2000; Hauth et al., 1995).

Bacterial vaginosis usually responds readily to oral metronidazole (400 mg twice daily for seven days.) A single 2 g dose has also been shown to be effective and free of major side effects in adolescent girls (Minkowski et al., 1983). Topical metronidazole (0.75%) is available as a gel in packs with five applicators for once nightly intravaginal dosing. An alternative is the more expensive clindamycin cream, which is supplied as a pack with seven applicators for nightly intravaginal dosing (Hay, 1998). Relapse is common after all treatments. There does not seem to be any benefit of treating male partners of women with bacterial vaginosis.

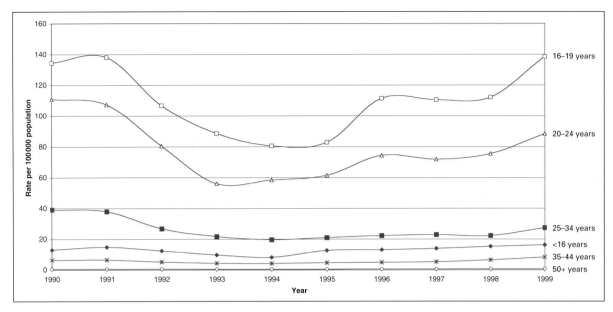

Fig. 36.11. Rates of uncomplicated gonorrhoea seen in genitourinary medicine clinics by age group for women in the UK, 1990–1999.

It has been suggested that women undergoing termination of pregnancy should be screened for bacterial vaginosis as well as for *C. trachomatis* and treated if either is found (Blackwell et al., 1993.)

Sexually transmitted diseases in adolescents

Both *N. gonorrhoeae* and *C. trachomatis* are important causes of STDs in adolescents and both may lead to PID and its sequelae of ectopic pregnancy and infertility. *C. trachomatis* tends to be the major cause of PID in the developed world and *N. gonorrhoeae* in the underdeveloped world.

For rates of STD to reflect risk among those who are sexually experienced, appropriate denominators should include only the number of individuals in the demographic group who have had sexual intercourse. Most population-based rates of STDs underestimate the risk of STDs for sexually active adolescents, because the rate is inappropriately expressed as cases of disease divided by the number of individuals in that age group. Whereas nearly all 20- to 24-year-olds have had sexual intercourse, this is true only of 50% of women in the 15–19 year age group (Berman and Hein, 1999).

Weström et al. (1982) defined age-specific attack rates of PID in Lund, Sweden, in this way during the early 1970s. They found that the risk of PID declined with age and that the risk of PID in sexually active 15-year-old adolescents was ten times that in sexually active 25-year-old women. An analysis of data from the USA between 1971 and 1976 showed similar trends for syphilis, gonorrhoea and PID. Rates of all three diseases were highest for adolescents and declined exponentially with increasing age (Bell and Holmes, 1984). In the UK, rates of gonorrhoea fell in the decade between 1985 and 1995, but increased in the five years between 1995 and 1999 (Fig. 36.11). The proportion of cases in young women under the age of 20 increased from 37 to 43% of the total, and the highest rate in 1999 was in women aged 16 to 19 years (www.phls.co.uk/facts/STI).

Neisseria gonorrhoeae

Gonorrhoea is a serious and increasingly frequent infection in sexually active adolescents. It may present as cervicitis, with a purulent vaginal discharge, or as PID, characterized by lower abdominal pain, adnexal tenderness, dyspareunia and sometimes fever, in addition to a purulent discharge.

Diagnosis of gonococcal infection in adolescents is the same as for adult women. Endocervical (not high vaginal) swabs are essential to maximize the likelihood of detecting *N. gonorrhoeae*. Swabs should also be taken from the rectum and pharynx if the clinical history suggests infection at these sites. An initial indication of infection may be obtained from the Gram stain of the endocervical smear, which typically shows Gram-negative diplococci within pus cells (Fig. 36.12, colour plate). As commensal species of *Neisseria* also produce this appearance, it is essential that the diagnosis is confirmed by culture. This is achieved either by inoculating agar plates immediately in the clinic or by sending swabs in Amies' or charcoal transport medium to the laboratory without delay. The use of a selective/enrichment process is essential for cervical specimens to prevent overgrowth with normal flora. The most commonly used media are Thayer–Martin or New York City agar with antibiotic supplements such as VCNT (vancomycin–colistin–nystatin–trimethoprim) or LCAT (lincomycin–colistin–amphotericin B–trimethoprim). After 48 hours incubation in 5–10% carbon dioxide, *N. gonorrhoeae* produces small, shiny, grey colonies. Suspect colonies that are Gram negative and oxidase positive should be confirmed as gonococci by sugar utilization tests or a coagglutination test such as Phadebact (MacSween and Ridgway, 1998).

As many strains of *N. gonorrhoeae* are resistant to penicillin, this is no longer the treatment of choice. In adult women, several cephalosporins and quinolones, such as ciprofloxacin, are widely used and are very effective (Moran and Levine, 1995). However, there is still some concern about the possible development of ciprofloxacin-induced arthropathy in children and adolescents, although ciprofloxacin has been used safely in some children long term (Black et al., 1990). The current consensus is that ciprofloxacin should be used in selected situations where efficacy outweighs the risk (Redmond, 1997). As cephalosporins offer a readily available and safe alternative, these are the drugs of choice. The Centers for Disease Control and Prevention (CDC) recommend a number of treatment options (CDC, 1998a), including intramuscular ceftriaxone and the oral drugs cefixime and cefpodoxime.

The diagnosis of gonorrhoea in an adolescent girl should always prompt a referral to a genitourinary medicine spe-

cialist. Investigation for other STDs such as *C. trachomatis* is mandatory as the two often occur together. Contact tracing is also essential, partly as a public health disease prevention exercise but partly to prevent reinfection of the index case. Follow-up of the individual to ensure that treatment has been successful is also important. In some areas, referral to a specialist has been improved by instituting a system where the microbiology laboratory automatically informs the genitourinary medicine clinic of all new cases of gonorrhoea and chlamydial infection identified by local departments of obstetrics and gynaecology (Haddon et al., 1998).

Chlamydia trachomatis

Genital infection caused by *C. trachomatis* is similar to that caused by *N. gonorrhoeae* in a number of respects: both infections may occur together (Osser and Persson, 1982); both infections may result in infertility as a consequence of PID; both occur predominantly in young, sexually active women; both are increasing in frequency (particularly in the developed world); and both may cause asymptomatic infection.

C. trachomatis is the most commonly diagnosed bacterial STD in the developed world. In 1999, over 32 000 cases of uncomplicated genital chlamydial infection were diagnosed in women attending genitourinary medicine clinics in the UK. This represents an increase of 80% over the number diagnosed five years earlier. The number of cases in the 16–19 year age group has been increasing sharply since 1993, reaching 11 000 in 1999 (Fig. 36.13). The rate per

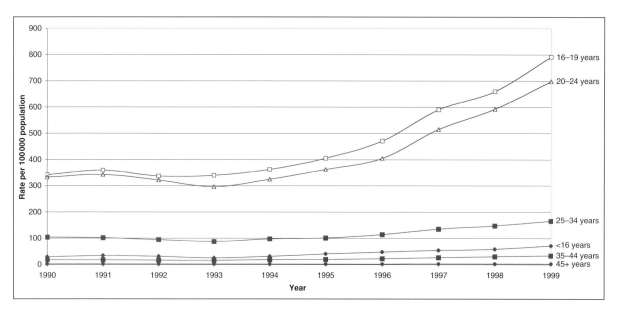

Fig. 36.13. Rates of uncomplicated genital chlamydial infection seen in genitourinary medicine clinics by age group for women in the UK, 1990–1999.

100 000 population in females more than doubled between 1993 and 1999, from 340 to 791 (www.phls.co.uk/facts/STI). It is estimated that cases diagnosed in genitourinary medicine clinics only represent 10% of all cases. These data indicate that there is a huge potential epidemic of chronic chlamydial infection, with its associated sequelae of PID, ectopic pregnancy and infertility.

As most infections are asymptomatic (70%), there is a great deal of debate over screening for this condition and the results of two pilots recently undertaken in the UK are awaited (Catchpole, 2001). In the USA, there has been a call for screening adolescent girls at six monthly intervals (Burstein et al., 1998).

The prevalence of chlamydial infection depends upon the population studied. Rates vary from 3–4% in women screened in primary care (Stokes, 1997) to 8–12% in those attending termination of pregnancy clinics (Webb and Chandioc, 1989; Southgate et al., 1989) to 10% in those attending genitourinary medicine clinics (Webb and Chandioc, 1989).

Even when symptoms are present, they are often mild and nonspecific (Ridgway, 1986). As with gonococcal infection, patients may complain of a vaginal discharge. They may present with established PID, which is characterized by less-severe symptoms than gonococcal disease but has a more protracted course (Kristensen et al., 1985). *C. trachomatis* may present with symptoms outside the genital tract. Manifestations of chlamydial infection include conjunctivitis, reactive arthritis, perihepatitis (Fitz–Hugh–Curtis syndrome) and peritonitis.

The most serious complication of *C. trachomatis* infection is PID. This results from ascending infection (Osser and Persson, 1982) by *C. trachomatis*, which is rapidly followed by secondary infection by the mixed anaerobic flora associated with bacterial vaginosis, which inflicts further damage (McCormack, 1994).

Diagnosis of *C. trachomatis* was originally based on culture of endocervical secretions in cycloheximide-treated McCoy cells. Infected cells were identified by the presence of intracytoplasmic inclusion bodies (Fig. 36.14, colour plate). Cell culture remains the "gold standard", particularly for medicolegal cases, but it is labour intensive, time consuming and technically demanding. In the early 1980s, direct immunofluorescence kits were introduced. These use a monoclonal antibody that detects either a major outer membrane protein (MOMP) epitope or genus-specific antigen present on elementary bodies. This technique meant that detection of *Chlamydia* sp. was possible in routine microbiology laboratories that did not have cell culture facilities. However, it was still labour intensive and subject to problems with specificity. In the mid-1980s, enzyme immunoassay tests were introduced and this made it practicable to screen large numbers of samples. There were problems with both the sensitivity and specificity of these tests, but the major problem of specificity was overcome when confirmatory tests were adopted for positive results.

Since the early 1990s, nucleic acid amplification tests (NAAs), such as the ligase chain reaction (LCR), PCR, transcription-mediated amplification (TMA) and strand displacement modification (SDA) have been introduced. Studies comparing NAAs with the earlier diagnostic tests indicate that the molecular tests have greater sensitivity and specificity (Davies and Ridgway, 1997; de Barbeyrac et al., 1998). This means that they can detect the low organism load in female urine, although a combination of urine and vaginal flush samples gives maximum sensitivity (Östergaard et al., 1996). However, endocervical swabs are still required to detect concurrent *N. gonorrhoeae* infection. False-positive results from sample contamination and false-negative results from the presence of inhibitors (Jensen et al., 1997) are problems that are yet to be completely resolved. Urinary inhibitors of LCR may increase during the latter part of the menstrual cycle (Horner et al., 1998), a time when other diagnostic tests indicate that the chlamydial load usually increases (Crowley et al., 1997).

Once the diagnosis of chlamydial infection is confirmed, it is essential that the patient be referred to a genitourinary medicine clinic for treatment, contact tracing and post-treatment test of cure. It has been claimed that effective antibiotic treatment can halve the rate of PID (Scholes et al., 1996).

Tetracyclines such as doxycycline, have been the mainstay of treatment for chlamydial infection for over 20 years (Ridgway, 1997). If coinfection with *N. gonorrhoeae* is detected, tetracycline cannot be relied upon to eradicate both organisms as the prevalence of tetracycline-resistant *N. gonorrhoeae* has increased dramatically in recent years (www.phls.co.uk).

The usual dose of doxycycline is 100 mg twice daily for 7 days. Erythromycin is an alternative to doxycycline and is given in a dose of 500 mg 6 hourly for seven days. However, gastrointestinal side effects are common and patients may prefer 500 mg twice daily for 10 days. The newer macrolide azithromycin shows promise as a single-dose treatment and has been advocated as empirical treatment to eradicate chlamydial infection prior to termination of pregnancy.

Amoxicillin is recommended by the CDC (500 mg orally three times a day for 7–10 days) for pregnant women who are unable to tolerate erythromycin.

Ofloxacin, which has the additional benefit of activity against *N gonorrhoeae*, is highly effective in eradicating *C. trachomatis*. The optimal dosage and length of course is still to be determined (Walker et al., 1993).

Treatment of pelvic inflammatory disease

Treatment regimens must provide empiric, broad-spectrum coverage of likely pathogens including *N. gonorrhoeae*, *C. trachomatis*, anaerobes, Gram-negative facultative bacteria (such as *E. coli*) and streptococci. There are no efficacy data comparing parenteral and oral regimens, although there are a number of randomized trials demonstrating the efficacy of different regimens in terms of clinical and microbiological cure (Walker et al., 1993). Information on intermediate and long-term outcomes is less readily available.

A number of parenteral and oral regimens are recommended (CDC, 1998b). Most employ metronidazole or a cephalosporin to cover anaerobes, together with doxycycline or ofloxacin. A total of 14 days of treatment is recommended. An adolescent who seeks medical advice for a complaint of vaginal discharge provides an excellent opportunity for the clinician to offer guidance on the risks and consequences of STDs.

Summary

Until recently, the causes of vaginal discharge in both children and adolescents have been a source of confusion for many clinicians (Box 36.3). The possibility that this may have resulted from sexual abuse has sometimes impeded thorough investigation and delayed appropriate treatment (Box 36.4). With improved understanding of this condition, the patient's anxieties and physical symptoms can be managed with reassurance and sensitivity.

Box 36.3 Key points

Childhood
- Vaginal discharge is the most common gynaecological complaint in young girls.
- The commonest cause of prepubertal vaginal discharge is vulvovaginitis; rarer conditions are congenital malformations, tumours, trauma, skin diseases and hormonal influences.
- Often a specific infective cause cannot be identified for vulvovaginitis; the commonest organism identified is group A beta-haemolytic streptococcus, followed by noncapsulate *H. influenzae*.
- Sexually transmitted organisms in young girls usually indicate sexual abuse but are not absolute markers.

Adolescence
- In the UK, rates of *N. gonorrhoeae* and *C. trachomatis* infection have increased rapidly in teenagers (data available up to 1999).
- Two-thirds of *C. trachomatis* infections are asymptomatic.
- Adolescents are at greatest risk for STDs because they frequently have unprotected intercourse, are biologically susceptible to infection and may face obstacles to accessing healthcare.
- The risk of PID in sexually active 15 year olds is 10 times that of sexually active 25 year olds.

Box 36.4 Recommendations for practice

- Any child who experiences persistent, purulent, recurrent or bloodstained vaginal discharge requires a complete gynaecological assessment. This also applies to children where there are concerns about sexual abuse.
- Laboratories should include culture media appropriate for *H. influenzae* when examining vaginal swabs from young girls as this is a common cause of juvenile vulvovaginitis.
- Screening for STDs is mandatory for presumed sexually abused girls and should ideally be undertaken in all children attending for evaluation of sexual abuse.
- For medico-legal purposes, culture for *N. gonorrhoeae* and *C. trachomatis* is the diagnostic method of choice. The examination of all specimens must be supported by a "chain of evidence" recording the transfer and handling of specimens.
- An adolescent who presents with a history of vaginal discharge should be given the opportunity to see the clinician without a parent or guardian present to enable discussion of sexual activity, contraception and sexual health.
- The diagnosis of gonorrhoea or chlamydial infection in an adolescent girl should prompt referral to a genitourinary medicine specialist for investigation of other STDs, contact tracing and follow-up of the index case.

REFERENCES

*Indicates key references.

Allen-Davis J T, Russ P, Karrer F M, Shroyer K, Ruyle S, Odom L F (1996). Cavernous lymphangioma presenting as a vaginal discharge in a six-year-old female: a case report. *J Pediatr Adolesc Gynecol* 9, 31–34.

Al-Salihi F L, Curran J P, Wang J-S (1974). Neonatal *Trichomonas vaginalis*: report of three cases and review of the literature. *Paediatrics* 53, 196–200.

Altchek A (1972). Pediatric vulvovaginitis. *Pediatr Clin North Am* 19, 559–580.

Amsel R, Totten P A, Spiegel C A, Chen K C, Eschenbach D, Holmes K K (1983). Non-specific vaginitis. Diagnostic criteria and microbial and epidemiologic associations. *Am J Med* 74, 14–22.

Anon. (2000). Sexually transmitted infections quarterly report: bacterial vaginosis. *Trichomonas vaginalis* and candidiasis in England and Wales. *CDR Wkly (Online)* 10, 350–352.

Arsenault P S, Gerbie A B (1986). Vulvovaginitis in the preadolescent girl. *Pediatr Ann* 15, 577–585.

Bartley D L, Morgan L, Rimsza M E (1987). *Gardnerella vaginalis* in prepubertal girls. *Am J Dis Child* 141, 1014–1017.

Bell T A, Holmes K K (1984). Age-specific risks of syphilis, gonorrhea, and hospitalized pelvic inflammatory disease in sexually experienced US women. *Sex Transm Dis* 11, 291–295.

*Berman S M, Hein K (1999). Adolescents and STDs. In *Sexually Transmitted Diseases*, 3rd edn, Holmes K K, Mårdh P- A, Sparling P F et al., eds., pp. 129–142. McGraw Hill, New York.

Bickley L S, Krisher K K, Punsalang A, Trupei M A, Reichman R C, Menegus M A (1989). Comparison of direct fluorescent antibody, acridine orange, wet mount and culture for detection of *Trichomonas vaginalis* in women attending a public sexually transmitted diseases clinic. *Sex Transm Dis* 16, 127–131.

Bisno A L (2001). Acute pharyngitis. *N Engl J Med* 344, 205–211.

Black A, Redmond A O B, Steen H J, Oborska I T (1990). Tolerance and safety of ciprofloxacin in paediatric patients. *J Antimicrob Chemother* 26(Suppl. F), 25–29.

Blackwell A L, Fox A R, Phillips I, Barlow D (1983). Anaerobic vaginosis (non-specific vaginitis): clinical, microbiological and theraputic findings. *Lancet* ii, 1379–382.

Blackwell A L, Thomas P D, Wareham K, Emery S J (1993). Health gains from screening for infection of the lower genital tract in women attending for termination of pregnancy. *Lancet* 342, 206–210.

Blake D R, Duggan A, Joffe A (1999). Use of spun urine to enhance detection of *Trichomonas vaginalis* in adolescent women. *Arch Pediatr Adolesc Med* 153, 1222–1225.

Bowden F J, Garnett G P (2000). *Trichomonas vaginalis* epidemiology: parameterising and analysing a model of treatment interventions. *Sex Transm Infect* 76, 248–256.

Bro F (1989). Patients with vaginal discharge in general practice. *Acta Obstet Gynecol Scand* 68, 41–43.

Brown J L (1989). Hair shampooing technique and pediatric vulvovaginitis. *Pediatrics* 83, 146.

Burch T A, Rees C W, Reardon L V (1959). Epidemiological studies on human trichomoniasis. *Am J Trop Med Hyg* 8, 312–318.

Burstein G R, Gaydos C A, Diener-West M, Howell M R, Zenilman J M, Quinn T C (1998). Incident *Chlamydia trachomatis* infections among inner-city adolescent females. *J Am Med Assoc* 280, 521–526.

Carey J C, Klebanoff M A, Hauth *et al.* (2000). Metronidazole to prevent preterm delivery in pregnant women with asymptomatic bacterial vaginosis. *N Engl J Med* 342, 534–540.

Catchpole M (2001). Sexually transmitted infections: control strategies. *Br Med J*, 322, 1135–136.

*CDC (Centers for Disease Control and Prevention) (1998a). Guidelines for treatment of sexually transmitted diseases. *MMWR* 47, 61–62.

(1998b). Guidelines for treatment of sexually transmitted diseases. *MMWR* 47, 79–84.

Chen K C, Forsyth P S, Buchanan T M, Holmes K K (1979). Amine content of vaginal fluid from untreated and treated patients with nonspecific vaginitis. *J Clin Invest* 63, 828–835.

Clay J C, Veeravahu M, Smythe R W (1988). Practical problems of diagnosing trichomoniasis in women. *Genitourin Med* 64, 115–117.

Cowan B D, Morrison J C (1991). Management of abnormal genital bleeding in girls and women. *N Engl J Med* 324, 1710–1715.

Cox R A (1997). *Haemophilus influenzae*: an underrated cause of vulvovaginitis in young girls. *J Clin Pathol* 50, 765–768.

Dahiya P, Sangwan K, Khosla A, Seth N (1999). Foreign body in vagina: an uncommon cause of vaginitis in children. *Indian J Pediatr* 66, 466–467.

Davies P O, Ridgway G L (1997). The role of polymerase chain reaction and ligase chain reaction for the detection of *Chlamydia trachomatis*. *Int J STD AIDS* 81, 731–738.

de Barbeyrac B, Rodriguez P, Dutilh B, Le Roux P, Bébéar C (1995). Detection of *Chlamydia trachomatis* by ligase chain reaction compared with polymerase chain reaction and cell culture in urogenital specimens. *Genitourin Med* 71, 382–386.

de Jong A R (1985). Vaginitis due to *Gardnerella vaginalis* and to *Candida albicans* in sexual abuse. *Child Abuse Negl* 9, 27–29.

Dhaliwal A K, Fink J N (1995). Vaginal itching as a manifestation of seasonal allergic disease. *J Allergy Clin Immunol* 95, 780–782.

Dhar V, Roker K, Adhami Z, McKenzie S (1993). Streptococcal vulvovaginitis in girls. *Pediatr Dermatol* 10, 366–367.

Donald F E, Slack R C B, Colman G (1991). *Streptococcus pyogenes* vulvovaginitis in children in Nottingham. *Epidemiol Infect* 106, 459–465.

Duncan M E, Tibaux G, Pelzer A *et al.* (1990). First coitus before menarche and risk of sexually transmitted disease. *Lancet* 335, 338–340.

*Dyson C, Hosein I K (1996). The role of the microbiology laboratory in the investigation of child sexual abuse. *J Med Microbiol* 45, 313–318.

Emans S J, Woods E R, Flagg N T, Freeman A (1987). Genital findings in sexually abused, symptomatic and asymptomatic, girls. *Pediatrics* 79, 778–785.

Embree J E, Lindsay D, Williams T, Peeling R W, Wood S, Morris M (1996). Acceptability and usefulness of vaginal washes in premenarcheal girls as a diagnostic procedure for sexually transmitted diseases. *Pediatr Infect Dis J* 15, 662–667.

Eschenbach D A, Hillier S, Critchlow C, Stevens C, DeRouen T, Holmes K K (1988). Diagnosis and clinical manifestations of bacterial vaginosis. *Am J Obstet Gynecol* 158, 819–828.

Farrington P F (1997). Pediatric vulvovaginitis. *Clin Obstet Gynecol* 40, 135–140.

Figueroa-Colón R, Grunow J E, Torres-Pinedo R, Rettig P J (1984). Group A streptococcal proctitis and vulvovaginitis in a prepubertal girl. *Pediatr Infect Dis* 3, 439–442.

Folland D S, Burke R E, Hinman A R, Schaffner W (1977). Gonorrhoea in preadolescent children: an enquiry into source of infection and mode of transmission. *Pediatrics* 60, 153–156.

Guss C, Larsen J G (1984). Group A beta-haemolytic streptococcal proctocolitis. *Pediatr Infect Dis* 3, 442–443.

Haddon L, Heason J, Fay T, McPherson M, Carlin E M, Jushuf I H A (1998). Managing STIs identified after testing outside genitourinary medicine departments: one model of case. *Sex Transm Infect* 74, 256–257.

*Hammerschlag M R (1998). Sexually transmitted diseases in sexually abused children: medical and legal implications. *Sex Transm Infect* 74, 167–174.

Hammerschlag M R, Alpert S, Rosner I *et al.* (1978). Microbiology of the vagina in children: normal and potentially pathogenic organisms. *Pediatrics* 62, 57–62.

Hammerschlag M R, Cummings M, Doraiswamy B, Cox P, McCormack W M (1985). Nonspecific vaginitis following sexual abuse in children. *Pediatrics* 75, 1028–1031.

Hauth J C, Goldenberg R L, Andrews W W, DuBard M B, Copper R L (1995). Reduced incidence of preterm delivery with metronidazole and erythromycin in women with bacterial vaginosis. *N Engl J Med* 333, 1732–1736.

Hay P E (1998). Therapy of bacterial vaginosis. *J Antimicrob Chemother* 41, 6–9.

Hay P E, Lamont R F, Taylor-Robinson D, Morgan D J, Ison C, Pearson J (1994). Abnormal bacterial colonisation of the genital tract and subsequent preterm delivery and late miscarriage. *Br Med J* 308, 295–298.

Hill G B, Eschenbach D A, Holmes K K (1984). Bacteriology of the vagina. In *Bacterial Vaginosis*. Mårdh, P-A, Taylor-Robinson D, eds., pp. 23–39. Almqvist & Wiksell, Stockholm, Sweden.

Ingram D L, White S T, Durfee M F, Pearson A W (1982). Sexual contact in children with gonorrhoea. *Am J Dis Child* 136, 994–996.

Ingram D L, White S T, Lyna P R *et al.* (1992). *Gardnerella vaginalis* infection and sexual contact in female children. *Child Abuse Negl* 16, 847–853.

*Jaquiery A, Stylianopoulos A, Hogg G, Grover S (1999). Vulvovaginitis: clinical features, aetiology and microbiology of the genital tract. *Arch Dis Child* 81, 64–67.

Jensen I P, Thorson P, Müller B R (1997). Sensitivity of ligase chain reaction assay of urine from pregnant women for *Chlamydia trachomatis*. *Lancet* 349, 329–330.

Jones R (1996). Childhood vulvovaginitis and vaginal discharge in general practice. *Fam Pract* 13, 369–372.

Kristensen G B, Bollerup A C, Lind K *et al.* (1985). Infections with *Neisseria gonorrhoea* and *Chlamydia trachomatis* in women with acute salpingitis. *Genitourin Med* 61, 179–184.

Lamont R F, Morgan D J, Wilden S D, Taylor-Robinson D (2000). Prevalence of bacterial vaginosis in women attending one of three general practices for routine cervical cytology. *Int J STD AIDS*, 11, 495–498.

MacSween K F, Ridgway G L (1998). The laboratory investigation of vaginal discharge. *J Clin Path* 51, 564–567.

Masfari A N, Duerden B I, Kinghorn G R (1986). Quantitative studies of vaginal bacteria. *Genitourin Med* 62, 256–263.

McCormack W M (1994). Pelvic inflammatory disease. *N Engl J Med* 330, 115–119.

Minkowski W L, Baker C J, Alleyne D, Baghai M, Friedlander L, Schultz B (1983). Single oral dose metronidazole therapy for *Gardnerella vaginalis* vaginitis in adolescent females. *J Adolesc Health Care* 4, 113–116.

Mogielnicki N P, Schwartzman J D, Elliott J A (2000). Perineal group A streptococcal disease in a pediatric practice. *Pediatrics* 106, 276–281.

Moraes P S A (1998). Allergic vulvovaginitis induced by house dust mites: a case report. *J Allergy Clin Immunol* 101, 557–558.

Moran J S, Levine W C (1995). Drugs of choice for the treatment of uncomplicated gonococcal infections. *Clin Infect Dis* 20(Suppl. 1), S47–S65.

Murphy T V, Nelson J D (1979). Shigella vaginitis: report of 38 patients and review of the literature. *Pediatrics* 63, 511–516.

Murray P R (1999). Human Microbiota. In. *Topley and Wilson's Microbiology and Microbial Infections*, 9th edn, Collier L., Balows A, Sussman M, eds., Vol. 2: *Systematic Bacteriology*, Balow A, Duerden B I eds., pp. 295–306. Arnold, London.

Nugent R P, Krohn M A, Hillier S L (1991). Reliability of diagnosing bacterial vaginosis is improved by a standardized method of gram stain interpretation. *J Clin Microbiol* 29, 297–301.

Nyirjesy P, Weitz M V, Gelone S P, Fekete T (1995). Paromomycin for nitromidazole-resistant trichomoniasis. *Lancet* 346, 1110.

Oriel D, Partridge B M, Denny M J, Coleman J C (1972). Genital yeast infections. *Br Med J* 4, 761–764.

Oriel J D (1988). Anogenital papillomavirus infection in children. *Br Med J* 296, 1484–1485.

Oriel J D, Ridgway G L (1982). Neonatal infection. In *Genital Infection by* Chlamydia trachomatis, pp. 68–73. Arnold, London.

Osser S, Persson K (1982). Epidemiologic and serodiagnostic aspects of Chlamydial salpingitis. *Obstet Gynecol* 59, 206–209.

Östergaard L, Müller J K, Andersen B, Olesen F (1996). Diagnosis of urogenital *Chlamydia trachomatis* infection in women based on mailed samples obtained at home: multipractice comparative study. *Br Med J* 313, 1186–1189.

Paradise J E, Campos J M, Friedman H M, Frishmuth G (1982). Vulvovaginitis in premenarcheal girls: clinical features and diagnostic evaluation. *Pediatrics* 70, 193–198.

Perone N (1997). Rare urogenital anomaly causing discharge and pain. A case report. *J Reprod Med* 42, 593–596.

Pierce A M, Hart C A (1992). Vulvovaginitis: causes and management. *Arch Dis Child* 67, 509–512.

Poch F, Levin D, Levin S, Dan M (1996). Modified thioglycolate medium: a simple and reliable means for detecting *Trichomonas vaginalis*. *J Clin Microbiol* 34, 2630–2631.

Pokorny S F (1992). Prepubertal vulvovaginopathies. *Obstet Gynecol Clin North Am* 19, 39–58.

Powell J, Wojnarowska F (2000). Childhood vulval lichen sclerosis and sexual abuse are not mutually exclusive diagnoses. *Br Med J* 320, 311.

Redmond A O (1997). Risk–benefit experience of ciprofloxacin use in pediatric patients in the United Kingdom. *Pediatr Infect Dis J* 16, 147–149.

Rettig P J, Nelson J D (1981). Genital tract infection with *Chlamydia trachomatis* in prepubertal children. *J Pediatr* 99, 206–210.

Rettig P J, Nelson J D, Kusmiesz H (1980). Spectinomycin therapy for gonorrhoea in prepubertal children. *Am J Dis Child* 134, 359–363.

Ridgway G L (1986). Chlamydial infections in man. *Postgrad Med J* 62, 249–253.

(1997). Treatment of chlamydial genital infection. *J Antimicrob Chemother* 40, 311–314.

Ris H W (1978). Nonvenereal transmission of gonococcal vaginitis. *Pediatrics* 61, 144–145.

Robinson A J, Watkeys J E M, Ridgway G L (1998). Sexually transmitted organisms in sexually abused children. *Arch Dis Child* 79, 356–358.

Ross J D C (2001). Outpatient antibiotics for pelvic inflammatory disease. *Br Med J* 322, 251–252.

Royal College of Physicians' Working Party (1997). *Physical Signs of Sexual Abuse in Children*, 2nd edn. RCP, London.

Sanders D Y, Wasilauskas B L (1973). Shigella vaginitis. clinical notes on two childhood cases. *Clin Pediatr* 12, 54–55.

Scholes D, Stergachis A, Heidrich F E, Andrilla H, Holmes K K, Stamm W E (1996). Prevention of pelvic inflammatory disease by screening for cervical chlamydial infection. *N Engl J Med* 334, 1362–1366.

See W A, Mayo M (1991). Ectopic ureter: a rare cause of purulent vaginal discharge. *Obstet Gynecol* 78, 552–555.

Shahlaee A H, Burton E M, Sabio H, Plouffe L, Teeslink R (1997). Primary chylous vaginal discharge in a 9-year-old girl: CT-lymphangiogram and MR appearance. *Pediatr Radiol* 27, 755–757.

Shapiro R A, Schubert C J, Siegel R M (1999). *Neisseria gonorrheae* infections in girls younger than 12 years of age evaluated for vaginitis. *Pediatrics* 104, e72, 1378.

Shore W B, Winkelstein J A (1971). Nonvenereal transmission of gonococcal infections to children. *J Pediatr* 79, 661–663.

Siegel R M, Schubert C J, Myers P A, Shapiro R A (1995). The prevalence of sexually transmitted diseases in children and adolescents evaluated for sexual abuse in Cincinnati: rationale for limited STD testing in prepubertal girls. *Pediatrics* 96, 1090–1094.

Southgate L, Treharne J, Williams R (1989). Detection, treatment and follow up of women with *Chlamydia trachomatis* infection seeking abortion in inner city general practices. *Br Med J* 299, 1136–1137.

Steele A M, de San Lazaro C (1994). Transhymenal cultures for sexually transmissible organisms. *Arch Dis Child* 71, 423–427.

Stenberg K, Mårdh P-A (1986). Persistent neonatal chlamydial infection in a 6-year-old girl. *Lancet* ii, 1278–1279.

Stokes T (1997). Screening for *Chlamydia* in general practice: a literature review and summary of the evidence. *J Public Health Med* 19, 222–232.

Straumanis J P, Bocchini J A (1990). Group A beta-haemolytic streptococcal vulvovaginitis in prepubertal girls: a case report and review of the past twenty years. *Pediatr Infect Dis J* 9, 845–848.

Thompson C, Macdonald M, Sutherland S (2001). A family cluster of *Chlamydia trachomatis* infection. *Br Med J* 322, 1473–1474.

Vandeven A M, Emans S J (1993). Vulvovaginitis in the child and adolescent. *Pediatr Rev* 14, 141–147.

Waghorn D J, Tucker P K, Chia Y, Spencer S, Luzzi G A (1998). Collaborative approach to improve the detection and management of trichomoniasis in a low prevalence district. *Int J STD AIDS* 9, 164–167.

Waites K B, Brown M B, Stagno S et al. (1983). Association of genital mycoplasmas with exudative vaginitis in a 10 year old: a case of misdiagnosis. *Pediatrics* 71, 250–252.

Wald E R (1984). Gynecologic infections in the pediatric age group. *Pediatr Infect Dis* 3(Suppl. 3), S10–S13.

Walker C K, Kahn J G, Washington A E, Peterson H B, Sweet R L (1993). Pelvic inflammatory disease: metaanalysis of antimicrobial regimen efficacy. *J Infect Dis* 168, 969–978.

Watkins S, Quan L (1984). Vulvovaginitis caused by *Yersinia enterocolitica*. *Pediatr Infect Dis* 3, 444–445.

Webb A M C, Chandioc S (1989). *Chlamydia trachomatis* infection. *Br Med J* 299, 1527.

Weström L, Svensson L, Wølner-Hansen P, Mårdh P-A (1982). Chlamydial and gonococcal infections in a defined population of women. *Scand J Infect Dis Suppl* 32, 157–162.

Whittington M J (1957). Epidemiology of infections with *Trichomonas vaginalis* in the light of improved diagnostic methods. *Br J Vener Dis* 33, 80–88.

Wood P L, Bevan T (1999). Child sexual abuse enquiries and unrecognised vulval sclerosus et atrophicus. *Br Med J* 319, 899–900.

Working Group of the British Society for Medical Mycology (1995). Management of genital candidiasis. *Br Med J* 310, 1241–1244.

Zelikovski A, Mimouni M, Shuper A, Haddad M, Zer M (1989). Primary chylocolporrhea successfully managed by division and ligation of retroperitoneal lymphatics. *Lymphology* 22, 132–134.

37

Psychological gender development in individuals born with ambiguous genitalia

Melissa Hines

Department of Psychology, City University, London, UK

Introduction

Gonadal hormones play an important role in sexual differentiation of the external genitalia. In addition, in nonhuman mammals, gonadal hormones have profound influences on brain development; consequently, alterations in levels of these hormones during critical periods of prenatal or neonatal development exert permanent influences on behaviour. This suggests that children born with ambiguous genitalia might also experience hormone-induced changes in behaviour, particularly in regard to behaviours related to sex. This chapter reviews what is known about psychosexual development in individuals born with intersex conditions or otherwise exposed during early development to unusual hormone environments.

Causes of genital ambiguity

The most common cause of genital ambiguity is the genetic disorder congenital adrenal hyperplasia (CAH) in XX individuals. Females with CAH are born with partially to completely virilized genitalia, caused by prenatal exposure to excess androgen from the adrenal glands. Other causes of genital ambiguity include:

- androgen insensitivity syndrome (AIS) in XY infants (in the complete form of AIS (CAIS) the genitalia appear to be essentially female at birth because of complete inability of cells to respond to androgen; in partial AIS (PAIS) the genitalia are typically ambiguous, because the cells show some ability to respond to androgen)
- disorders in XY individuals involving enzymes needed to produce hormones in the androgen pathway (e.g. defi-

ciency of 5α-reductase or of 17β-hydroxysteroid dehydrogenase); both deficiencies result in genitalia that look more like those of females than males at birth but which virilize at puberty.

- maternal ingestion, during pregnancy, of hormones that stimulate or block receptors for gonadal steroids (the genitalia of exposed females are often virilized to some degree, although this is not always the case, depending on the hormone prescribed and the time period during which it was taken).

Situations producing genital ambiguity typically involve an abnormality in the level or activity of gonadal hormones beginning prenatally, and it is this prenatal hormonal aberration that causes the genital ambiguity. In addition, there are situations where XY individuals are exposed to normal levels of testicular hormones prenatally but are reassigned as girls because their external genitalia are improperly formed. These conditions include aphallia (or absence of the penis) and cloacal exstrophy (a defect of midline development in which the penis is typically absent or bifid and small). Sex reassignment has also occurred in some instances following severe genital damage in male infants (e.g. during circumcision). In these cases, the testes have been removed, and the formerly male infant has been reared subsequently as a girl.

To understand the role of hormones in the development of genital ambiguity, it is useful to consider the processes involved in sexual differentiation. During normal development, genetic information on the Y chromosome instructs the primordial gonads, initially identical in XX and XY individuals, to become testes. This occurs at about week 6 of gestation in humans; soon thereafter the testes begin to secrete testosterone and other hormones. These testicular

Paediatric and Adolescent Gynaecology, ed. Adam Balen et al. Published by Cambridge University Press.
© Cambridge University Press 2004.

hormones then cause the external genitalia to develop as penis and scrotum, and the internal genitalia to develop from the Wolffian ducts into vas deferens, seminal vesicles and prostate. Without instruction from the Y chromosome (e.g. when there are two X chromosomes), the same primordial gonads differentiate as ovaries. In addition, in the absence of testicular hormones, the external genitalia differentiate into clitoris, labia and lower vagina, while, internally, the Müllerian ducts develop into the Fallopian tubes, uterus and upper vagina.

The same hormones that accomplish sexual differentiation of the external genitalia also influence sexual differentiation of certain brain regions, at least in nonhuman mammals. There are androgen and other steroid receptors in circumscribed regions of the brain during prenatal development, notably in the hypothalamus, amygdala and cerebral cortex. In addition, manipulating testosterone prenatally or neonatally alters the structure and function of these neural regions, and, as a consequence, permanently alters behaviour (De Vries and Simerly, 2002). The behaviours that are influenced by the early hormone environment are those that show sex differences, meaning that they differ on the average for males and females of the species (Collaer and Hines, 1995). In rodents, the affected behaviours include sexual initiation and sexual responses, as well as some nonsexual behaviours, such as rough-and-tumble play, maze learning, aggression and activity levels. Similar effects of hormones have been seen in Rhesus monkeys, at least for sexual behaviours and rough-and-tumble play. These permanent behavioural influences of the early hormone environment are thought to occur because gonadal hormones influence development in neural regions containing the appropriate steroid receptors. Hormonal manipulations influence the number of neurons that live or die in these brain regions, their patterns of anatomical connectivity with other neural regions and their neurochemical characterization (e.g. Arnold and Gorski, 1984; De Vries and Simerly, 2002).

Thus, humans with ambiguous genitalia have been exposed to unusual levels of gonadal hormones prenatally. As similar hormonal alterations in other mammals cause permanent changes in brain regions and behaviours that show sex differences, it is possible that syndromes involving genital ambiguity (and early hormonal abnormalities) in humans also cause behavioural changes. This possibility is relevant to basic theoretical questions regarding sexual differentiation (e.g. do hormones influence development of the human brain and behaviour in a manner similar to that documented in other mammals?). These theoretical implications are discussed fully in Hines (2002). Of more relevance to the current chapter is information on hormones and human development that can contribute to an understanding of psychological gender development in individuals with ambiguous genitalia, and, perhaps, aid in decisions related to genital surgery and gender assignment. The current chapter draws to some degree on information in the theoretically oriented chapter (Hines, 2002) and interested readers are referred there for additional information. In addition, both theoretical and clinical implications of hormonal influences on human neural and behavioural sexual differentiation are discussed in detail in Hines (2004), and readers interested in additional information in these areas are referred to that volume as well.

Gender and human behaviour

Gender-related behaviours in humans are typically conceptualized in three domains: core gender identity (the sense of self as male or female), sexual orientation (the direction of erotic interest, in same sex individuals, opposite sex individuals or both) and gender role behaviours (characteristics that are culturally assigned to males and females or that show sex differences in a given culture). Each of these three areas will be discussed in turn.

Core gender identity

Most people born with ambiguous genitalia appear to develop a sense of self that accords with their gender assignment and sex of rearing, regardless of the cause of their genital ambiguity and regardless of whether they are assigned as males or females.

For instance, XX individuals with CAH are usually assigned and reared as females, even if their genitalia are so virilized at birth as to be essentially indistinguishable from those of a male infant. In addition, in almost all cases where gender assignment is female, gender identity in adulthood is female. There are exceptions, however. One study (Meyer-Bahlberg et al., 1996) reported that four XX individuals with CAH in the New York area who had been assigned and reared as females were living as men. The probability that this occurred by chance was estimated as 1 in 420 million. A second study (Zucker et al., 1996) found that 1 of 53 XX patients with CAH who had been seen at one clinic was now living as a man, despite assignment and rearing as a female. The authors calculated the odds that this coincidence of gender dysphoria and CAH had occurred by chance as 1 in 608. So, although the vast majority of XX individuals with CAH who are assigned as females develop a female core gender identity, some do not. As a consequence, the incidence of gender dysphoria, although extremely low, appears to be higher than in the general population.

There is relatively little information on sexual identity in XX individuals who were raised as males following genital virilization caused by CAH. Reports on small numbers of cases suggest successful male identity with male assignment and rearing (Money and Dalery, 1976; Zucker, 1999). The degree of ambiguity in XX individuals with CAH varies from an essentially female appearance through every degree of combined female and male appearance to an essentially male appearance. Individuals assigned as male are probably those with the most masculinized genitalia at birth. It is not known what the outcome would be if females with less-severe virilization were assigned as males. Also, assignment of an XX female with CAH as male has generally been avoided, in part, because XX individuals with CAH have female internal genitalia and the potential for successful pregnancy.

Ambiguity of the external genitalia owing to enzymatic deficiencies (e.g. 5α-reductase deficiency and 17β-hydroxysteroid dehydrogenase deficiency) also appears to be associated with flexibility in the development of gender identity. In some cultures, individuals with these deficiencies are assigned as girls in infancy but virilize physically at puberty under the influence of the high levels of androgen produced at that time. In these cases, a change in gender identity from female to male has been reported to accompany the physical virilization (Imperato-McGinley et al., 1979a,b; Rosler and Kohn, 1983). In contrast, in other settings, where gender assignment is female and the gonads are removed prior to puberty, physical virilization does not occur. In these cases, gender identity reportedly remains female (see Wilson et al., 1993; Zucker 1999). Consequently, gender identity in these disorders appears to correspond most closely to the appearance of the external genitalia from puberty on. Cultural factors may also be important. In the settings where virilization occurs at puberty, and the individuals adopt a male role beginning at this time, infertile females have low status. It is not known how successful similar individuals would be in cultures where infertile females are less stigmatized. Also, information on psychological satisfaction in those who choose to live as males following physical virilization at puberty is limited.

Individuals with PAIS are sometimes assigned and reared as females and sometimes as males. The direction of assignment probably corresponds to some extent with the degree of physical virilization, with those who are most virilized being assigned as males and those who are least virilized as females. However, there is no formal documentation of this presumed association between degree of virilization and direction of gender assignment. Also, factors other than the degree of physical virilization can influence the direction of gender assignment. Cultural factors are again important. Parents in some cultures value male infants more than female infants and may request this direction of assignment for XY babies with PAIS, regardless of the appearance of the external genitalia. As in the case of XX individuals with CAH, XY individuals with PAIS, or other causes of a severely underdeveloped penis at birth, are generally content with their sex of assignment, whether that assignment was as female or as male (Wisniewski et al., 2001; Migeon et al., 2002). However, this is not always the case, although, again, neither female assignment nor male assignment appears to be more likely to be associated with a satisfactory outcome overall (Migeon et al., 2002).

Some reports on XY individuals who have been surgically feminized and reared as girls because of cloacal exstrophy, penile agenesis or aphallia suggest a high incidence of gender identity problems (e.g. Reiner, 1999; Reiner et al., 1999). However, others do not (e.g. Schober et al., 2002). As yet, published reports on these situations are limited, making it impossible to determine which perspective (dramatically increased gender dysphoria in XY individuals reared as females, versus generally good gender identity and psychological development) will prove more accurate.

Evidence regarding the role of androgen in the development of core gender identity has also come from cases where gender reassignment has occurred in early life, without the presence of an underlying disorder, following penile ablation. One widely publicized case involved identical XY twins, one of whom was sex reassigned because of a surgical accident during a phimosis repair at the age of 8 months. Reassignment as female occurred sometime before the age of 17 months. Although the reassignment was reportedly successful during early childhood (Money and Ehrhardt, 1972), by adulthood this individual was living as a man and was said to have been unhappy as a female for many years (Diamond, 1982; Diamond and Sigmundson, 1997). Although this might be interpreted to suggest that early exposure to testicular hormones determines male gender identity, this individual was reared as a male for at least the first 8 months of life. We also have few data on the rearing environment after the child was reassigned to the female sex and do not know how well the parents (or others) adapted to treating a child, who had previously been a boy, as a girl. A second, similar case produced a different outcome. This time the penis was damaged during electrocautery circumcision at the age of 2 months and the child was reassigned as female sometime before the age of 7 months. She was evaluated at the age of 16 years and 26 years and found to have a female core gender identity with no evidence of gender dysphoria (Bradley et al., 1998). The different outcomes in the two cases could have resulted from differences in the age at sex reassignment or from other factors, such as the social or cultural environment.

Therefore, data from clinical syndromes and from individuals who experienced sex reassignment following surgical accidents suggest that the gonadal hormone environment influences the development of gender identity but does not completely determine it. The risk of gender dysphoria in individuals reared as females is increased following early androgen exposure, but it is still relatively rare. Most individuals assigned and reared as females are content with that identity, even if they were exposed to higher than normal levels of androgens prenatally. Males with enzymatic disorders that impair androgen production sometimes choose to live as men after virilizing puberty, despite having been reared as females, whereas others with the same diagnoses remain living as females, particularly if virilizing puberty has not occurred. This argues that factors other than the prenatal hormone environment influence the formation of gender identity. There are two well-documented cases where the complete male hormonal cascade has been present prenatally and neonatally. In both cases, sex reassignment as female occurred after a period of postnatal socialization as a male. In one case, female reassignment was successful, but in the other it was not. Obviously, more information is needed before strong conclusions can be made about the likelihood of successful sex change in these difficult cases where severe penile damage occurs, or where the external genitalia are severely undervirilized at birth. However, the ability of an XY infant, exposed to normal levels of testicular hormones prenatally and in early infancy and reared as a boy for at least the first two months of life, to be reared subsequently as a girl and maintain a female gender identity into adulthood is noteworthy. It suggests that human gender identity is not determined completely by the early hormone environment but also can be dramatically influenced by socialization. In fact, the most obvious conclusion based on data from these two sex-reassigned infants, as well as on individuals born with ambiguous genitalia, is that, given the right social environment, it is possible for an XY individual to develop a female gender identity, despite exposure to high levels of androgenic hormones during early development.

Sexual orientation

As is the case for gender identity, sexual orientation in XX individuals with CAH usually accords with expectations based on the sex of rearing. Most such individuals are assigned and reared as girls, and most have a heterosexual orientation as adults (i.e. their primary erotic interest is in males). However, as for gender identity, there are exceptions, and sexual orientation in females with CAH is more likely to be bisexual or homosexual than would be expected in the general population.

In one study (Money et al., 1984), 7 of 30 women with CAH were noncommittal about their sexual orientation; 12 said they were heterosexual and 11 said they were bisexual or homosexual. This differed from 27 controls who had either CAIS or Rokitansky syndrome (a syndrome involving abnormalities of the external genitalia, but no hormonal disorder). All 27 controls were willing to reveal their sexual orientation, and 25 said they were exclusively heterosexual. A second study (Dittman et al., 1992) compared 34 females with CAH with 14 of their unaffected sisters. Among those old enough to have had sexual experiences, none of the controls and 44% of the females with CAH desired or had experienced sexual relations with other women. Also, on inventories of sexual orientation, the women with CAH scored higher on homosexual interest, and lower on heterosexual interest and general sexual interest, than did their sisters. A third study (Zucker et al., 1996) found reduced heterosexual activity and reduced general sexual activity in 30 women with CAH compared with unaffected female relatives. A fourth (Kuhnle and Bullinger, 1997) again found reduced sexual activity in women with CAH compared with matched controls, as well as reduced experience in relationships. However, self-report of homosexuality appeared similar in the two groups. The lack of a relationship between CAH and sexual orientation in this last study could reflect methodological differences. Unlike the other studies, it included women with late-onset CAH, whose hormonal disorder was likely to have begun after the presumed prenatal or neonatal critical period for hormonal influences on sexual differentiation. In addition, it assessed whether the women with CAH called themselves homosexual and lived with a female partner, whereas the other studies included information on desires and fantasies, as well as actual behaviour, to assess sexual orientation.

As noted earlier, girls with CAH are born with ambiguous genitalia, and this, as well as possible hormonal influences on the developing brain, could influence their sexual behaviour. Following surgical feminization early in life, the genitalia of women with CAH often are not identical to those of other women, and the surgeries can have consequences that make intercourse difficult or painful (Schober, 1999). In addition, the knowledge of virilization at birth and experience with genital surgery could themselves influence sexual behaviour.

Data on women exposed to diethylstilbestrol (DES), because their mothers were prescribed this hormone during pregnancy, could help to determine whether alterations in sexual orientation in women with CAH reflect a hormonal influence on the developing brain. DES is a synthetic oestrogen that promotes masculine-typical brain development and behaviour in female rodents (Hines et al., 1987), without virilizing the external genitalia. This occurs because testosterone in the normal male animal is converted to oestrogen before interacting with neural oestrogen receptors to produce male-typical brain development; DES and other oestrogens do not virilize the external genitalia because this is accomplished by testosterone itself or by its product dihydrotestosterone, both of which act through androgen receptors.

DES-exposed women, like women with CAH, show elevated bisexuality or homosexuality. This has been reported in three samples studied by one group of researchers (Ehrhardt et al., 1985; Meyer-Bahlburg et al., 1995). The first included 30 DES-exposed women, 12 unexposed sisters and 30 unexposed controls recruited from the same source as the DES-exposed group (a doctor treating women with abnormal smears in Papanicolaou (PAP) tests). (This control group was used because prenatal DES exposure often causes abnormal smears.) The DES-exposed women were more likely than the controls to indicate a homosexual or bisexual orientation (24% versus 0%). Among the 12 sister pairs, 42% of the DES-exposed group versus 8% of the unexposed sisters indicated a homosexual or bisexual orientation. The second sample included a new group of 30 DES-exposed women, eight of their unexposed sisters and 30 controls matched for demographic background. The DES-exposed women again were more likely than the matched controls to indicate a lifelong homosexual or bisexual orientation (35% versus 13%). Among the eight sister pairs, the DES-exposed women also were more likely to report a lifelong homosexual or bisexual orientation (36% versus 0%). The final sample included 37 women identified from medical records of their mothers' pregnancies indicating treatment with at least 1000 mg DES. They were matched to women of similar age who were identified from the same medical practice but whose records indicated no DES treatment. In this study, 16% of DES-exposed women and 5% of controls indicated a lifelong homosexual or bisexual orientation.

Therefore, sexual orientation in women appears to be influenced by the prenatal hormone environment, with exposure to high levels of androgen or oestrogen increasing the likelihood of bisexuality or homosexuality. As was the case for core gender identity, however, the relationship is not one-to-one. Although an increased percentage of hormone-exposed women are bisexual or homosexual, compared with women not exposed to hormones, most are primarily or exclusively heterosexual. This suggests that the prenatal hormone environment is only one of the factors influencing variability in sexual orientation among women.

Do hormones also influence sexual orientation in men? Reports on sexual orientation in XY individuals with enzymatic deficiencies producing reduced androgen exposure are somewhat sketchy, but those who change to live as men after puberty also appear to adopt a sexual orientation toward women (Wilson et al., 1993; Zucker, 1999). This suggests that reduced androgen during early development does not prevent erotic interest in females in adulthood. In cases where the testes have been removed before puberty in individuals with the same enzymatic deficiencies, sexual orientation, like core gender identity, usually resembles that of women in general (Wilson et al., 1993; Zucker, 1999). Again, the conflicting outcomes in different settings suggest that sexual orientation, although perhaps influenced by the early hormonal environment, is not determined by it and can be influenced by other factors as well.

The influence of prenatal exposure to DES (or other oestrogens and progestins taken by pregnant women) on sexual orientation in males has also been examined. These studies have been based in part on the assumption that oestrogen, and other so-called "female" hormones, would feminize developing males. We now know that oestrogen has little, if any, feminizing influences on XY individuals during development. On the contrary, as mentioned above, it seems to play a role in masculine-typical development. However, oestrogen can sometimes interfere with the action of androgen, and oestrogen was sometimes prescribed in combination with progestins, some of which act as antiandrogens, providing a basis for predicting a demasculinizing or feminizing influence on sexual differentiation in males. (Some progestins also have androgenic effects, however, complicating the interpretation of studies involving varied progestins.)

Men exposed to DES or to progestins prenatally do not appear to differ in sexual orientation from other men. One study (Kester et al., 1980) compared four groups of hormone-exposed men with matched controls. One group was exposed to DES alone ($n = 17$), one to DES plus progesterone (a hormone that can act as an antiandrogen $n = 21$), one to progesterone alone ($n = 10$) and one to progestins alone ($n = 13$). None of the hormone-exposed groups differed in sexual orientation in fantasy or behaviour from male controls matched for demographic background. A second study, comparing two groups of DES-exposed men with matched controls, produced similar findings (Meyer-Bahlburg et al., 1987). Sexual orientation in fantasy or behaviour was similar in 31 men identified from maternal records indicating DES treatment during pregnancy and in 29 men whose records did not indicate DES treatment.

Similarly, 34 DES-exposed men and 15 controls recruited from a urological practice did not differ on the same assessments of sexual fantasy and behaviour.

The two cases where boys were reassigned as girls following damage to the penis differed in outcomes for sexual orientation, as well as outcomes for gender identity. The child for whom the damage occurred at 8 months of age was erotically interested exclusively in women as an adult (Diamond and Sigmundson, 1997), whereas the child for whom the damage occurred at 2 months of age was bisexual (Bradley et al., 1998). Despite this difference in specific outcomes, both cases suggest that early exposure to masculine-typical levels of testicular hormones influences sexual orientation away from a primary, or exclusive, erotic interest in men.

Consequently, the early hormone environment appears to influence sexual orientation. Exposure of XX individuals to high levels of androgens, because of CAH, or to high levels of oestrogen, because DES was prescribed to their mothers during pregnancy, results in less-exclusive interest in males. Genetic males exposed to the complete male hormonal cascade, but sex reassigned and reared as females because of penile damage early in life, appear to develop either bisexual interest or erotic interest in women. In men, prenatal exposure to oestrogens, such as DES, or to progestins does not appear to relate to sexual orientation. Individuals with enzymatic deficiencies that impair production of certain androgens appear capable of developing erotic interest in women when spontaneous virilization occurs at puberty. However, when the testes are removed prior to puberty, and virilization does not occur, erotic interest appears to be in men. Whether this difference in outcome relates to cultural differences, the influence of hormones at puberty or other factors is not known. Regardless, it appears that although the early hormone environment contributes to sexual orientation, it is not the only factor determining it.

Gender role behaviour

The term gender role behaviour is sometimes used to refer to traits that are thought to be culturally associated with being male or female. However, the term also can be used to refer to behaviours that show sex differences, meaning that they differ on the average for males and females. This latter definition will be used here.

There has been some debate as to exactly which human behaviours show sex differences, and it is not as easy to reach conclusions in this area as might be thought. A major difficulty is the tendency to analyse for male/female differences routinely but to publish findings only when a significant difference is found (Maccoby and Jacklin, 1974). This leads to an overreporting of sex differences, and renders single reports of sex differences potentially unreliable. Therefore, I will focus on behaviours for which numerous studies suggest a sex difference. In addition, where possible, I will use meta-analytic data (which allows information from a number of studies to be combined) to estimate the size of sex differences. Size estimates will be provided in standard deviation units (SD). To provide a familiar characteristic for comparison, the size of the sex difference in height is 2.0 SD (Tanner et al., 1966).

Behaviours that show reliable sex differences include childhood play (toy, activity and playmate preferences), certain cognitive abilities (e.g. mental rotations ability, some aspects of mathematical ability, verbal fluency, perceptual speed and accuracy) and some personality characteristics (e.g. aggression, nurturance).

Childhood play

Boys and girls tend to prefer different toys. If observed in a playroom, boys spend more time on average with vehicles, weapons and building toys, whereas girls spend more time with dolls, cosmetics and kitchen paraphernalia. Similar differences are found on questionnaires measuring toy preferences (e.g. Berenbaum and Hines, 1992; Sutton-Smith et al., 1963). Boys and girls also prefer different playmates. The vast majority of girls' playmates (80–90%) are other girls and a similar percentage of boys' playmates are other boys (Hines and Kaufman, 1994; Maccoby, 1988). Finally, play-styles of boys and girls tend to differ, with boys preferring rough, active play involving body contact and girls preferring calmer play-styles (DiPietro, 1981; Hines and Kaufman, 1994; Maccoby, 1988). Meta-analyses of the size of the sex differences in play behaviour are not available. However, individual studies suggest that sex differences in toy preferences are large for behavioural sex differences ($d > 0.8$), whereas those in play-styles are small to moderate ($d = 0.3$–0.5) (e.g. Hines, 2002, 2004). (Behavioural differences of 0.8 SD or larger are generally considered large, those of about 0.5 moderate, those of 0.3 small, and those smaller than 0.2 negligible (Cohen, 1988).)

Personality (aggression and nurturance)

Sex differences in aggression have been noted across cultures and in children as well as adults. Studies have assessed aggression in fantasy, in imitation of aggressive models, in the frequency of verbal insults and in interviews or on questionnaires. Males are more aggressive than females (Maccoby and Jacklin, 1974), and meta-analytic results suggest that the sex difference is moderate in size ($d = 0.50$). It also may be larger in children than in adults ($d = 0.58$ versus 0.27), although the apparent age difference could reflect the use of different measures in different age groups (Hyde, 1984). Regarding nurturance, questionnaire measures generally show a sex difference favouring females (Feingold, 1994). Interest in infants also shows a sex difference (Berman, 1980), again measurable using questionnaires. Questionnaires suggest bigger sex differences than behavioural observation (Berman, 1980), and part of the sex difference on this and other self-report personality measures may be artifactual (e.g. Feingold, 1994). That is, females and males know that certain characteristics, such as interest in infants, are more valued in one sex than the other and may, therefore, respond to questionnaires in a way that is more sex typed than their actual behaviour. In addition, the sex difference in interest in infants changes over the lifespan (Berman, 1980). It is largest in young adults, perhaps because issues related to parenting are most salient at that age.

Cognition

General intelligence does not differ in males and females (e.g. Collaer and Hines, 1995). However, some measures of specific cognitive abilities show sex differences. These include subtypes of visuospatial, mathematical and verbal abilities, and perceptual speed and accuracy.

Visuospatial abilities

Mental rotations (the ability to rotate two- or three-dimensional stimuli in the mind) shows a sex difference favouring males. The difference is present in children (Linn and Petersen, 1985) and adults (Voyer et al., 1995) and may increase with age, although it is hard to be certain because different tasks are used with different age groups. The sex difference on three-dimensional tasks ($d = 0.92$) appears to be larger than that on two-dimensional tasks ($d = 0.26$) (Linn and Petersen, 1985; Voyer et al., 1995). Tests of spatial perception also show sex differences favouring males. These tasks require accurate positioning of a stimulus (e.g. a line) within a distracting array (e.g. a tilted frame). As for mental rotations, the sex difference in spatial perception appears to be larger in adults than children ($d = 0.56$ versus 0.38), but the tests may be too difficult for children, resulting in uniformly low scores that reduce the apparent sex difference (Voyer et al., 1995). In contrast to mental rotations and spatial perception tasks, measures of a third aspect of visuospatial ability, spatial visualization, do not show appreciable sex differences (Linn and Petersen, 1985; Voyer et al., 1995). These tasks require complex, sequential manipulation of spatial information and typically have more than one solution strategy. Measures include tests requiring identification of simple figures within complex

designs and imagining what unfolded shapes would look like when folded to form three-dimensional objects. Sex differences on these types of task are negligible ($d = 0.16$).

Mathematical abilities

The overall sex difference in mathematical abilities is negligible and favours females ($d = -0.05$) (Hyde et al., 1990). However, measures of problem solving show small sex differences favouring males, particularly among older, highly selected samples, such as college students ($d = 0.32$). In childhood, tests of computational skills show small sex differences favouring females ($d = -0.21$). There are no sex differences in computational skills in adults ($d = 0.00$) or in understanding of mathematical concepts at any age ($d = -0.06$).

Verbal abilities

Girls and women show a negligible advantage for general verbal ability ($d = -0.11$; Hyde and Linn, 1988). However, males show a negligible advantage on analogies ($d = 0.16$; Hyde and Linn, 1988), and females show a small advantage on speech production ($d = -0.33$; Hyde and Linn, 1988) and a moderate advantage on verbal fluency (e.g. the ability to generate words that meet certain constraints, such as beginning with specified letters: $d = -0.53$; Kolb and Wishaw, 1985; Spreen and Strauss, 1991). There are essentially no sex differences for vocabulary ($d = -0.02$) or reading comprehension ($d = -0.03$).

Perceptual speed and accuracy

Among high-school students, there is a sex difference favouring females in perceptual speed and accuracy. Estimates of its size range from $d = 0.29$ to $d = 0.66$ (mean $= 0.48$), at least as assessed using the clerical speed and accuracy subtest of the Differential Aptitudes Test (DAT) (Feingold, 1988). Sex differences of similar size have been observed on other measures of perceptual speed and accuracy ($d = 0.49$; Ekstrom et al., 1976). The magnitude of the sex difference on the DAT appears to have declined over time, from a mean of 0.62 in 1947 to 0.34 in 1980 (Feingold, 1988).

Change in sex differences with time

Sex differences in some other cognitive abilities also may be declining. Feingold (1988) presented data on various measures of specific cognitive abilities from the 1940s to the 1980s, showing that sex differences declined linearly over the decades. One exception is algebraic problem solving, on which males consistently outperformed females. Another exception was three-dimensional mental rotations, on which the sex difference favouring males was stable from the 1970s to the 1990s (Sanders et al., 1982; Voyer et al., 1995). The reduction in sex differences on some tests does not seem to be caused by test revision aimed at removing sex differences, since the decline is linear, not stepwise (Feingold, 1988). However, despite the declines, which could have resulted from social and educational changes, sex differences in performance have not disappeared, and the portion that remains could be related, at least in part, to other factors, including hormones.

Hormones and gender role behaviour

Childhood play

The early hormone environment appears to influence childhood play behaviours. Girls with CAH, although surgically feminized in infancy, treated to normalize hormones postnatally and raised unambiguously as girls, show increased interest in masculine-typical toys, activities and playmates and reduced interest in feminine-typical toys, activities and playmates. These findings come from studies in which these girls and their mothers have been interviewed or have completed questionnaires about their behaviour, as well as from studies where their behaviour has been observed directly. For instance, when videotaped in a playroom with a variety of toys, girls with CAH spend more time with boy-preferred toys and less time with girl-preferred toys compared with their unaffected sisters and female cousins (Berenbaum and Hines, 1992). Similar results (of more masculine-typical play behaviour in girls with CAH) have been obtained using questionnaire and interview measures in a number of different cultural settings including the USA (Ehrhardt and Baker, 1974; Ehrhardt et al., 1968; Hines and Kaufman, 1994; Money and Ehrhardt, 1972), Canada (Zucker et al., 1996), Germany (Dittman et al., 1990a,b), Sweden (Nordenstrom et al., 2002) and the UK (Hines et al., 2003a). The behaviours that are influenced include playmate preferences (increased preferences for boys), rough, active play and toy preferences.

Convergent evidence suggesting that the enhanced male-typical play behaviour in girls with CAH is caused by androgen exposure, rather than other aspects of the disorder, comes from studies of girls whose mothers were prescribed androgenic progestins during pregnancy for medical reasons. These girls show masculinized play behaviour similar to that seen in girls with CAH (Ehrhardt and Money, 1967). Also, girls whose mothers were prescribed the antiandrogen, medroxyprogesterone acetate show less masculine-typical and more feminine-typical play (Ehrhardt et al., 1977). The effects of medroxyprogesterone appear to be smaller than those seen following

androgen exposure, perhaps because there is limited scope for further feminization or demasculinization in genetic females. Finally, normal variability in testosterone levels during pregnancy has been found to relate to sex-typed play behaviour in female offspring (Hines et al., 2002), suggesting that androgen exposure may contribute to individual differences in sex-typical behaviour among healthy girls.

There is less information regarding hormonal influences on play in boys than in girls. In addition, the information that does exist as boys is equivocal. Boys with CAH do not generally show alterations in play behaviour, although one study found them to show reduced rough-and-tumble play (Hines and Kaufman 1994), but no alterations in playmate preferences or toy choices (Berenbaum and Hines, 1992; Hines and Kaufman, 1994). In contrast, another report found them to show an increased intensity of energy expenditure in outdoor play and sports (Ehrhardt and Baker, 1974). In regard to progestins, there is some evidence that exposure to the anti-androgen medroxyprogesterone acetate is associated with minor reductions in some aspects of male-typical play (Meyer-Bahlburg et al., 1977, 1988). However, a study of boys exposed to 17-α-hydroxyprogesterone caproate, a different antiandrogenic progestin, found no evidence of reduced male-typical play (Kester, 1984). A third study of boys exposed to oestrogen and progestins reported reduced athleticism at six years of age but no changes in other aspects of sex-typical play and no reduction in athleticism at age 16 (Yalom et al., 1973). There is little information on childhood play behaviour in individuals with CAIS or in individuals with enzymatic deficiencies resulting in reduced androgen exposure. Summary comments and retrospective assessments suggest that both groups show normal female gender role behaviour as children (Imperato-McGinley et al., 1979a,b; Hines et al., 2003b; Wisniewski et al., 2000), but no detailed prospective data have been published.

Therefore, individuals reared as girls following exposure to higher than normal levels of androgen prenatally show increased male-typical, and reduced female-typical play behaviour. This has been reported for XX individuals with CAH and in girls exposed prenatally to androgenic progestins. Also, girls exposed to antiandrogenic progestins prenatally show behavioural changes in the opposite direction, and maternal testosterone during pregnancy has been found to predict sex-typed play behaviour in female offspring. All of this evidence suggests that hormones, particularly androgens, present during prenatal development contribute to sex-typed childhood behaviour. There are fewer data on boys than on girls exposed prenatally to unusual hormone environments, and the few studies that do exist have produced inconsistent results.

Personality

Aggression

Several studies have used questionnaires to assess aggressive response tendencies or other aspects of aggression in children and adults exposed prenatally to unusual hormone environments. One reported increased aggressive response tendencies in children exposed prenatally to androgenic progestins (Reinisch, 1981). Seventeen girls and eight boys (ages 6 to 18 years) whose mothers had been prescribed hormones during pregnancy were compared with their 17 sisters and eight brothers born from pregnancies where hormones were not prescribed. When aggression-promoting situations were described (e.g. someone pushes in front of you in a line), both hormone-exposed boys and girls indicated that they would be more likely to react with physical aggression. Possible confounding influences of genital virilization were not a problem, because the hormone-exposed children were born with normal-appearing genitalia. In a second study, females with CAH (aged 17–34 years) gave more masculine-typical responses than matched controls on measures of Indirect Aggression and Detachment, two of eight personality measures that showed sex differences in controls in the same study (Helleday et al., 1993). Similar differences were not seen in CAH males compared with controls. A third report presented data for three samples of CAH patients and three samples of relative controls (Berenbaum and Resnick, 1997). One group of 18 female adolescents and adults with CAH showed enhanced aggressive response tendencies compared with 13 female controls in the same age range, but no such difference was observed in a second group of 11 females with CAH of similar age compared with five control females. The first sample also showed the expected sex differences in 13 female versus 11 male controls, whereas sex differences in the second sample of 5 female and 10 male controls were not significant. For children, ages almost 3 to almost 13 years, the expected sex difference was seen in 10 female versus 20 male controls, but not between 20 girls with CAH and the 10 female controls. Males with and without CAH did not differ in any of the three samples.

Fighting in girls with CAH has been assessed in two studies using interviews. Neither study found differences. One compared 15 girls with CAH, aged 5 to 16 years, and 15 matched controls (Ehrhardt et al., 1968). The second compared 17 females with CAH (aged 4–20 years) with 11 sisters of CAH individuals (aged 6–25 years) (Ehrhardt and Baker, 1974).

Therefore, studies of aggression following prenatal exposure to atypical hormone environments, particularly those involving androgen exposure, provide some evidence of increased tendencies to aggressive responses on personality inventories, although this has not always been found. In addition, it is not clear that these response tendencies translate into increased aggressive behaviour. Firm conclusions await research using larger samples and more sensitive measures.

Nurturance

As noted above, girls with CAH show reduced interest in toys typically preferred by girls, including dolls (Berenbaum and Hines, 1992; Ehrhardt and Baker, 1974; Ehrhardt et al., 1968). In addition, three studies suggest that girls with CAH show reduced interest in babysitting and other aspects of childcare, including plans to have children (Dittman et al., 1990a,b; Ehrhardt and Baker, 1974; Ehrhardt et al., 1968). The reduced interest in childcare may be more apparent in CAH girls older than 16 (Dittman et al., 1990a). These studies relied on a few questions, sometimes even a single question, from an interview. A more extensive questionnaire assessment of 23 girls and 16 boys with CAH compared with 12 female and 22 male relatives (all aged 3 to 12 years) produced equivocal results (Leveroni and Berenbaum, 1998). The questionnaire was completed by parents of the children and showed the expected sex difference among controls; girls showed more interest in infants than boys. The CAH girls also received lower scores than control girls on the questionnaire, but when items related to doll play were removed, the difference was no longer significant ($p > 0.05$, one-tailed). Also, the girls with CAH scored lower on interest in pets, although control girls and boys did not differ on this measure. Boys with CAH did not differ from male relatives in regard to interest in either infants or pets.

As with other sex-typed behaviours, CAH girls' and their parents' knowledge of their condition and their intersex genitalia could contribute to apparent psychological differences. Because of this, researchers have also investigated interests related to parenting and nurturance in women exposed prenatally to the synthetic oestrogen DES, since DES does not masculinize the external genitalia. As noted above, DES-exposed women have been reported to be more likely to be bisexual or homosexual than other women. However, their interest in parenting appears unaltered. The same researchers who studied sexual orientation also administered questionnaires (completed by the women as well as their mothers) that provided retrospective assessments of childhood behaviour, including interest in parenting. An initial study suggested reduced interest in parenting in DES-exposed women (Ehrhardt et al., 1989), but the study had included a large number of dependent variables making it likely that the finding was a chance result. This was confirmed when two subsequent studies found no association between prenatal DES exposure and interest in parenting (Lish et al., 1991, 1992).

Therefore, some data suggest that early exposure to higher than normal levels of androgen prenatally decreases interest in parenting in females, but findings are not consistent. Findings from oestrogen-exposed women suggest that, if androgen influences the development of interest in parenting, it does not do so after conversion to oestrogen. As with other sex-typed behaviours, methodological issues, such as small samples, prevent definitive conclusions.

Cognition

General intelligence

Early reports concluded that individuals exposed to androgen prenatally had elevated intelligence compared with the population norm (Ehrhardt and Money, 1967; Money and Lewis, 1966). Prenatal exposure to natural progesterone was also claimed to enhance intelligence, based on reports of increased academic achievement in the offspring of mothers given progesterone for pregnancy difficulties (Dalton, 1968, 1976). Because natural progesterone acts as an antiandrogen, these latter results contradict those reported following prenatal androgen exposure. Subsequently, it was concluded that high intelligence in the androgen-exposed individuals and academic excellence in those exposed to progesterone related to factors other than hormones. When patients with CAH were compared with their relatives or with controls matched for demographic background, there were no differences in intelligence (Baker and Ehrhardt, 1974; McGuire and Omenn, 1975; Perlman, 1973; Wenzel et al., 1978). The elevation compared with the population norm probably resulted from selection biases; individuals with high intelligence were more likely to enrol in the research project. In regard to prenatal progesterone exposure, inappropriate statistical analyses contributed to the apparent academic enhancement; re-analyses of the original data (and subsequent research) found no evidence of academic enhancement (Lynch and Mychalkiw, 1978; Lynch et al., 1978; see Collaer and Hines (1995) for further discussion). Other studies of individuals exposed to a variety of progestins, to oestrogen and progestin or to DES also have found no differences on measures of general intelligence (Hines and Sandberg, 1996; Hines and Shipley, 1984; Reinisch and Karow, 1977). In retrospect, the lack of an influence of gonadal steroids on general intelligence is not surprising, since general intelligence does not show a sex difference, and research in other species suggests that only characteristics that show sex differences are likely to be influenced by gonadal hormones (Collaer and Hines, 1995).

Visuospatial abilities

Certain visuospatial abilities show sex differences and so would be more likely candidates than general intelligence for hormonal influences. However, prenatal exposure to high levels of androgen, because of CAH, appears to have little, or no, influence on most visuospatial abilities, including mental rotations, spatial visualization and spatial perception, in females (Baker and Ehrhardt, 1974; Hampson et al., 1998; Helleday et al., 1994; Hines et al., 2003a; McGuire et al., 1975; Resnick et al., 1986). Although two of these studies have reported that females with CAH show enhanced visuospatial abilities (Hampson et al., 1998; Resnick et al., 1986), the others have not found this, and one study found that women with CAH performed worse on a visuospatial task (Helleday et al., 1994). The two studies that reported increased visuospatial abilities did not use particularly large samples. One included 17 girls with CAH and 13 unaffected female relatives and the second included seven girls with CAH and six unaffected sisters. In fact, the sample size in these studies tended to be smaller than those in the studies finding no effect or impaired spatial ability in CAH females. In those studies, sample sizes ranged from 17 to 40 females with CAH compared with 11 to 29 unaffected female relatives. Similarly, the tasks found to differ in the two positive studies were not necessarily those that show the largest sex differences. Consequently, increased experimental power does not seem a likely explanation for the findings. More likely, these were spurious effects, deemed publishable, despite the small samples, because the results appeared to fit an expectation. In general, research on relatively rare endocrine disorders, such as CAH, may be particularly susceptible to the "file drawer problem" (e.g. Maccoby and Jacklin, 1974), wherein results that are significant are published, even if they are based on a small sample, while those that are not are left unpublished (in the file drawer).

Another difficulty in evaluating hormonal influences on human cognition is that sex differences on these tasks are not as large as those in core gender identity, sexual orientation or even childhood play behaviour. Although meta-analytic data are not available, sex differences in core gender identity, sexual orientation and childhood play behaviours appear to be at least three times as large as the sex difference on three-dimensional mental rotations ability, the cognitive task that shows the largest difference between males and females (Hines, 2004). Perhaps consistent with this explanation of the largely negative results, targeting, a task that includes a motor component as well as a spatial component and shows a sex difference almost as large as the sex difference in height, does appear to relate to the prenatal androgen exposure. A sample of 40 adolescent and adult females with CAH have been found to be more accurate at throwing both balls and darts at a target than a group of 29 unaffected female relatives (Hines et al., 2003a).

There are fewer data on cognitive performance in males with CAH than females with CAH, and the data that are available are based on even smaller samples. However, two studies have observed impaired visuospatial performance in males with CAH (Hampson et al., 1998; Hines et al., 2003a). Although other studies have not reported similar outcomes (Baker and Ehrhardt, 1974; McGuire et al., 1975; Resnick et al., 1986), one of the studies that found impairment was particularly strong methodologically. It had the largest sample of all the studies and used measures of mental rotations that show particularly large sex differences (Hines et al., 2003a). Cognitive and other behavioural outcomes in males with CAH have not been studied extensively and merit additional investigation.

Tasks at which females excel, such as verbal fluency and perceptual speed and accuracy, have generally not been found to be altered in either males or females with CAH (Baker and Ehrhardt, 1974; McGuire et al., 1975; Resnick et al., 1986; Sinforiani et al., 1994). Most of the studies of visuospatial abilities also measured verbal fluency, or perceptual speed and accuracy, or both. A single study reported impaired performance on a measure of perceptual speed and accuracy in girls with CAH (Hampson et al., 1998). Given the small sample (seven girls with CAH and six female controls), and the lack of similar findings in other studies, this could be a spurious finding. Alternatively, because the sex difference in perceptual speed and accuracy is relatively small, larger samples than those used in virtually all studies to date might be needed to detect it consistently.

Some studies have reported impaired computational ability in CAH children. One found impairment in girls with CAH but not boys (Perlman, 1973), one in both girls and boys (Baker and Ehrhardt, 1974) and one in a combined group of boys and girls with CAH (Sinforiani et al., 1994). These findings are surprising. Although females are better at computational ability, the sex difference is small and seen only in young children (Hyde et al., 1990). No studies have reported enhanced mathematical performance in girls or boys exposed to androgen prenatally, despite speculations that males outperform females on standardized tests of mathematical ability because of their higher prenatal androgen exposure (Benbow, 1988; Benbow and Stanley, 1983). However, tests of mathematical abilities that show large sex differences have not been studied in hormone-exposed individuals.

Studies of women exposed to DES prenatally have found no alterations in cognitive performance. Two studies from one research group compared the performance of

DES-exposed women and their unexposed sisters on tasks that show sex differences. The first found no differences between 25 sister pairs (where one in each pair had been exposed to DES for at least 20 weeks prenatally and one had not been exposed at all) on a two-dimensional mental rotations task or on a measure of verbal fluency (Hines and Shipley, 1984). The second found no differences between a second sample of 42 DES-exposed women and their 26 unexposed sisters on three-dimensional mental rotations, spatial perception, perceptual speed and accuracy or verbal fluency (Hines and Sandberg, 1996). Both of these studies also found no differences between DES-exposed and unexposed women on measures of vocabulary or general intelligence. A third study, from a different research group, investigated cognitive abilities in DES-exposed men and women who had participated in a true experiment (i.e. pregnant women were assigned at random to treatment with DES or placebo. The study was designed to evaluate the usefulness of DES in preventing miscarriage). American College Testing subtest scores were compared in 325 female offspring (175 DES-treated and 150 placebo-treated) and 347 male offspring (172 DES-treated and 175 placebo-treated). Four subtests showed sex differences, but none differed in DES-exposed versus placebo-exposed females (Wilcox et al., 1992). Males exposed to DES scored higher than males exposed to placebo on the social sciences subtest, a test at which males typically outperform females, but not on other subtests, and the authors attributed this single unpredicted finding to chance. Another study found that 10 boys exposed prenatally to DES showed impaired performance compared with 10 unexposed brothers on a composite of three spatial subtests from the Wechsler scales (Picture Completion, Object Assembly and Block Design), tests that show small-to-negligible sex differences. The 10 pairs of brothers did not differ on composites of verbal or sequencing tasks (Reinisch and Sanders, 1992). Similarly, a study of 20 16-year old boys exposed to oestrogen and progesterone prenatally also reported that they scored worse than matched controls on the Embedded Figures Test, a result that approached statistical significance ($p < 0.10$, one-tailed). This test, however, is also one that does not show a substantial sex difference. In addition, over 100 statistical comparisons were conducted in the study, and this was one of only a handful reported to approach significance. Consequently, it could have been a chance finding. Consistent with this, a third study of 22 men exposed prenatally to DES and natural progesterone and 17 men exposed prenatally to DES alone did not find any differences from matched controls in performance on the Embedded Figures Test.

Therefore, reports that prenatal exposure to testosterone enhanced intelligence have proved erroneous, as have reports linking prenatal progesterone exposure to academic performance. Hormonal influences on specific cognitive abilities that show sex differences are theoretically more likely. However, research to date has produced inconsistent, and largely negative, findings. Most studies have used small samples, causing two problems. First, the likelihood of negative findings is increased, even if a hormone–behaviour relationship exists. Second, significant results that occur by chance are likely to be overreported, since nonsignificant findings could be attributed to the small sample. A second problem has been the use of measures that do not show appreciable sex differences and so would be unlikely to relate to hormones.

To date, the clearest data on hormones and human cognition have come from studies of DES-exposed women, which have had a combination of relatively large samples, measures that show reliable sex differences and, in one study, placebo-treated controls. These studies suggest that prenatal exposure to DES does not influence the development of either general intelligence or specific abilities that show sex differences. These negative findings include the cognitive ability that shows the largest sex difference: three-dimensional mental rotations ability. Therefore, it appears that prenatal exposure to higher than normal levels of oestrogen does not influence human cognitive development. However, definitive conclusions as to whether hormones make any contribution to sex differences in human cognition await studies of larger samples using measures that show substantial sex differences.

It is also possible that hormonal influences on at least some aspects of human cognition could occur neonatally rather than prenatally. Because DES was prescribed for pregnancy maintenance, exposure in humans was limited to the prenatal period. Similarly, most girls with CAH are diagnosed soon after birth and treated with corticosteroids to normalize hormones postnatally. It is possible that hormonal influences on cognitive abilities occur during infancy. The cortical systems on which these abilities depend are still developing during the first year of postnatal life, and males have high levels of androgen during the first six months of postnatal life (Smail et al., 1981). Oestrogen levels are also high in females shortly after birth (Bidlingmaier et al., 1974, 1987). Therefore, the neonatal period, rather than (or in addition to) the prenatal period, could be important for hormonal influences on human cognition. Reports of impaired visuospatial ability in men with idiopathic hypogonadotropic hypogonadism (IHH) (Buchsbaum and Henkin, 1980; Cappa et al., 1988; Hier and Crowley, 1982) are consistent with this speculation. Males with IHH do not have genital ambiguity at birth but are thought to have lower than normal levels of testicular

hormones neonatally. However, additional evidence on IHH and other syndromes that involve neonatal hormone alterations are needed to evaluate fully any possible influences of the neonatal hormone environment on human cognition.

Neural mechanisms underlying hormonal influences on behaviour and neural correlates of gender identity

Influences of the early hormone environment on human behaviour are assumed to involve hormone-induced changes in brain structure, similar to those seen in other mammals following prenatal or neonatal hormone manipulations. In addition, several regions of the human brain have been reported to show sex differences. They include subregions of the corpus callosum, the medial amygdala, bed nucleus of the stria terminalis (BNST) and anterior hypothalamic/preoptic area (see Hines (2002, 2004) for additional discussion). The most consistently replicated of these sex differences is located in the anterior hypothalamic preoptic area. A sex difference in a nucleus within this area, called the third interstitial nucleus of the anterior hypothalamus (INAH-3), has been reported by three independent groups of researchers (Allen et al., 1989; Byne et al., 2000; LeVay, 1991). Hormone-related changes in behaviour could occur because hormones alter development of this, or other, neural regions that vary in males and females. In addition, such neural sex differences could relate to sex-related psychological characteristics.

In addition to being larger in men than in women, the volume of INAH-3 is greater in heterosexual men than in homosexual men (Byne et al., 2000; LeVay, 1991). However, the second of these studies found that, although INAH-3 was smaller in homosexual men than in heterosexual men, there was no difference between the groups in the number of cells in the nucleus (Byne et al., 2000), raising questions about the functional significance of the volumetric difference. A separate study reported that the central subregion of the BNST (BNSTc) shows a sex difference and that the volume of this region relates to core gender identity, but not sexual orientation (Zhou et al., 1995). The volume of BNSTc was larger in 15 men with typical gender identity than in 12 women or in 6 men with strong, long-standing feelings of being psychologically female (i.e. male to female transsexuals). In contrast, the volume of BNSTc was similar in the 15 nontranssexual (and presumed heterosexual) men compared with nine homosexual men, suggesting that the BNSTc relates to core gender identity (i.e. transsexualism), but not sexual orientation (i.e. heterosexuality versus homosexuality). Because male to female transsexuals can be either heterosexual (preferring women as sexual partners), or homosexual (preferring men as sexual partners), it was also possible to relate sexual orientation to BNSTc volume within the transsexual group. No relationship was seen, providing further support for a relationship only to core gender identity.

To date, no studies have examined either INAH-3 or BNSTc in the brains of individuals who developed in atypical hormone environments. This is probably because these neural sex differences can be seen only in brain tissue itself (e.g. obtained at autopsy) and not by using imaging technologies, such as magnetic resonance or positron emission tomography that allow visualization of the living brain. Several sex differences have been reported in human brain structure or function using these imaging techniques, but findings are inconsistent, and a clear picture of exactly where and under what conditions these sex differences can be seen has yet to emerge (see Hines (2004) for additional discussion). Nevertheless, the identification of replicable neural sex differences, and information on similar patterns of neural structure and function following atypical hormone exposure, is an area of active research interest and is likely to provide new information on the neural mechanisms involved in psychosexual development, both in those with and in those without intersex conditions.

Summary

There is substantial evidence that childhood play behaviours are altered in girls born with ambiguous genitalia, following prenatal androgen exposure. For instance, numerous studies, using a variety of methodologies and conducted in several different countries, have found that XX individuals with CAH show more masculine-typical toy, activity and playmate preferences than do matched controls or unaffected relatives of the same sex. Similar findings have been reported for girls exposed to androgenic progestins prenatally, as well as in a study relating prenatal variability in hormones to postnatal behaviour in healthy girls. In all cases, masculine-typical play behaviours are elevated in girls with higher androgen exposure prenatally. There is less evidence of alterations in other aspects of gender role behaviour, such as personality characteristics and cognitive abilities, following prenatal androgen exposure. However, the possibility that other behaviours are influenced cannot be excluded because studies using sufficiently large samples and the most sensitive measures generally have not been conducted.

Alterations in the early hormone environment, including some that cause ambiguous genitalia, have also been found to relate to sexual orientation. High levels of androgen (or oestrogen) in XX individuals promote interest in female sexual partners. However, the influence of hormones is not uniform, and, although females exposed to high levels of androgen or oestrogen are more likely than other women to show interest in same-sexed erotic partners, most hormone-exposed women are heterosexual.

Of the three categories of gender-related behaviour considered in this chapter (core gender identity, sexual orientation and gender role behaviour), core gender identity appears to be the least vulnerable to hormonal influence, despite showing the largest sex difference. In the great majority of cases, XX individuals with CAH develop a female core gender identity, even though their childhood behaviour, and to some extent their sexual orientation, is more masculine-typical than would otherwise be the case. Similar results have generally been reported for individuals with other syndromes who have been assigned and reared as females, even if they have an XY chromosomal make-up and have been exposed to high levels of male-typical hormones prenatally (e.g. individuals with cloacal exstrophy, PAIS, aphallia or sex reassignment owing to penile damage). In other cases, where the sex of assignment and rearing is male, individuals with the same disorders and similar genital ambiguity at birth have developed a male gender identity. Also, XY individuals who have enzyme deficiencies that cause severely undervirilized genitalia at birth appear to be able to change to the male gender role and gender identity at puberty, despite having been reared as girls, if their external genitalia virilize at puberty and if they are in an appropriate cultural setting. In other cases, where physical virilization at puberty is prevented by removal of the testes, individuals with the same diagnosis appear content with the female identity and role, again particularly when the social and cultural environment encourages this.

Consequently, human beings appear to be remarkably flexible in terms of gender identity development. Nevertheless, despite overall success, there are some individuals for whom the sex of assignment appears to be unsatisfactory. This has been noted in some XX individuals with CAH who were assigned to the female sex, and in a small, but significant, minority of XY males assigned to the female sex because of penile problems such as those related to surgical accidents, PAIS, micropenis or cloacal exstrophy. Further research is needed to determine if there are more undetected cases where gender assignment has been unsuccessful. In addition, an important question for the future is why gender assignment in a particular direction leads to a satisfactory outcome for some individuals but not for others with the same diagnosis. Research to date suggests that genital appearance at birth is not a strong predictor of outcome in terms of gender role behaviour or sexual orientation. For instance, for girls with CAH, the degree of genital virilization at birth does not predict the degree of behavioural masculinization, at least for childhood play behaviours or sexual orientation (e.g. Berenbaum and Hines, 1992; Dittman et al., 1990a,b). However, further examination of the relationship between virilization at birth and core gender identity (as opposed to sexual orientation or gender role behaviour) would be useful. Other factors that merit additional investigation in relationship to gender assignment and psychosexual development include the family environment, communication between medical personnel and patients/families, and the degree and nature of involvement by psychologists or other mental health professionals with patients and their families to facilitate psychosexual development. Finally, future research developments are likely to include more detailed information on structural and functional sex differences in the human brain and their relationship to psychological development, particularly in the area of core gender identity. It is conceivable that neonatal neural assessments might someday augment genetic, hormonal, psychological and other information to inform considerations related to gender assignment in individuals born with ambiguous genitalia.

REFERENCES

Allen L S, Hines M, Shryne J E, Gorski R A (1989). Two sexually dimorphic cell groups in the human brain. *J Neurosci* 9, 497–506.

Arnold A P, Gorski R A (1984). Gonadal steroid induction of structural sex differences in the central nervous system. *Annu Rev Neurosci* 7, 4113–4424.

Baker S W, Ehrhardt A A (1974). Prenatal androgen, intelligence and cognitive sex differences. In *Sex Differences in Behavior*, Friedman R C, Richart R N, van de Wiele R L, eds., pp. 53–76. Wiley, New York.

Benbow C P (1988). Sex differences in mathematical reasoning ability in intellectually talented preadolescents: their nature, effects and possible causes. *Behav Brain Sci* 11, 169–232.

Benbow C P, Stanley J C (1983). Sex differences in mathematical reasoning ability: more facts. *Science* 222, 1029–1031.

Berenbaum S A, Hines M (1992). Early androgens are related to childhood sex-typed toy preferences. *Psychol Sci* 3, 203–206.

Berenbaum S A, Resnick S M (1997). Early androgen effects on aggression in children and adults with congenital adrenal hyperplasia. *Psychoneuroendocrinology* 22, 505–515.

Berman P W (1980). Are women more responsive than men to the young? A review of developmental and situational variables. *Psychol Bull* 88, 668–695.

Bidlingmaier F, Versmold H, Knorr D (1974). Plasma estrogens in newborns and infants. In *Sexual Endocrinology of the Perinatal Period*, Forest M and Bertrand J, eds., pp. 299–314. Institut National de la Sante et de la Recherche Medicale, Paris.

Bidlingmaier F, Strom T M, Dorr G, Eisenmenger W, Knorr D (1987). Estrone and estradiol concentrations in human ovaries, testes and adrenals during the first two years of life. *J Clin Endocrinol Metab* 65, 862–867.

Bradley S J, Oliver G D, Chernick A B, Zucker K J (1998). Experiment of nurture: ablatio penis at 2 months, sex reassignment at 7 months, and a psychosexual follow-up in young adulthood. *Pediatrics* 102, E91–E95.

Buchsbaum M S, Henkin R I (1980). Perceptual abnormalities in patients with chromatin negative gonadal dysgenesis and hypogonadotropic hypogonadism. *Int J Neurosci* 11, 201–209.

Byne W, Lasco M S, Kemether E et al. (2000). The interstitial nuclei of the human anterior hypothalamus: an investigation of sexual variation in volume and cell size number and density. *Brain Res* 856, 254–258.

Cappa S F, Guariglia C, Papagno C et al. (1988). Patterns of lateralization and performance levels for verbal and spatial tasks in congenital androgen deficiency. *Behav Brain Res* 31, 177–183.

Cohen J (1988). *Statistical Power Analysis for the Behavioral Sciences*, 2nd edn. Lawrence Erlbaum, Hillsdale, NJ.

Collaer M L, Hines M (1995). Human behavioral sex differences: a role for gonadal hormones during early development? *Psychol Bull* 118, 55–107.

Dalton K (1968). Ante-natal progesterone and intelligence. *Br J Psychiatry* 114, 1377–1382.

  (1976). Prenatal progesterone and educational attainments. *Br J Psychiatry* 129, 438–442.

De Vries G J, Simerly R B (2002). Anatomy, development, and function of sexually dimorphic neural circuits in the mammalian brain. In *Hormones, Brain and Behavior*, Vol. 4, Pfaff D W, Arnold A P, Etgen A M, Fahrbach S E, Rubin R T, eds., pp. 137–191. Academic Press, San Diego, CA.

Diamond M (1982). Sexual identity, monozygotic twins reared in discordant sex roles and a BBC follow-up. *Arch Sex Behav* 11, 181–185.

Diamond M, Sigmundson K (1997). Sex reassignment at birth: long-term review and clinical implications. *Arch Pediatr Adolesc Med* 151, 290–304.

Diamond M C, Dowling G A, Johnson R E (1981). Morphologic cerebral cortical asymmetry in male and female rats. *Exp Neurol* 71, 261–268.

DiPietro J A (1981). Rough and tumble play: a function of gender. *Dev Psychol* 17, 50–58.

Dittman R W, Kappes M H, Kappes M E et al. (1990a). Congenital adrenal hyperplasia II: gender-related behavior and attitudes in female salt-wasting and simple virilizing patients. *Psychoneuroendocrinology* 15, 421–434.

  (1990b). Congenital adrenal hyperplasia I: gender-related behavior and attitudes in female patients and sisters. *Psychoneuroendocrinology* 15, 401–420.

Dittman R W, Kappes M E, Kappes M H (1992). Sexual behavior in adolescent and adult females with congenital adrenal hyperplasia. *Psychoneuroendocrinology* 17, 153–170.

Ehrhardt A A, Baker S W (1974). Fetal androgens, human central nervous system differentiation, and behavior sex differences. In *Sex Differences in Behavior*, Friedman R C, Richart R N, van de Wiele R L, eds., pp. 33–52. Wiley, New York.

Ehrhardt A A, Money J (1967). Progestin-induced hermaphroditism: IQ and psychosexual identity in a study of ten girls. *J Sex Res* 3, 83–100.

Ehrhardt A A, Epstein R, Money J (1968). Fetal androgens and female gender identity in the early-treated adrenogenital syndrome. *Johns Hopkins Med J* 122, 165–167.

Ehrhardt A A, Grisanti G C, Meyer-Bahlburg H F L (1977). Prenatal exposure to medroxyprogesterone acetate (MPA) in girls. *Psychoneuroendocrinology* 2, 391–398.

Ehrhardt A A, Meyer-Bahlburg H F L, Rosen L R et al. (1985). Sexual orientation after prenatal exposure to exogenous estrogen. *Arch Sex Behav* 14, 57–77.

Ehrhardt A A, Meyer-Bahlburg H F L, Rosen L R et al. (1989). The development of gender-related behavior in females following prenatal exposure to diethylstilbestrol (DES). *Horm Behav* 23, 526–541.

Ekstrom R B, French J W, Harmon H H (1976). *Manual for Kit of Factor-Referenced Cognitive Tests*. Educational Testing Service, Princeton, NJ.

Feingold A (1988). Cognitive gender differences are disappearing. *Am Psychol* 43, 95–103.

(1994). Gender differences in personality: a meta-analysis. *Psychol Bull* 116, 429–456.

Hampson E, Rovet J F, Altmann D (1998). Spatial reasoning in children with congenital adrenal hyperplasia due to 21-hydroxylase deficiency. *Dev Neuropsychol* 14, 299–320.

Helleday J, Edman G, Ritzen E M, Siwers B (1993). Personality characteristics and platelet MAO activity in women with congenital adrenal hyperplasia (CAH). *Psychoneuroendocrinology* 18, 343–354.

Helleday J, Bartfai A, Ritzen E M, Forsman M (1994). General intelligence and cognitive profile in women with congenital adrenal hyperplasia (CAH). *Psychoneuroendocrinology* 19, 343–356.

Hier D B, Crowley W F (1982). Spatial ability in androgen-deficient men. *N Engl J Med* 306, 1202–1205.

Hines M (2002). Sexual differentiation of human brain and behavior. In *Hormones, Brain and Behavior*, Vol. 4, Pfaff D W, Arnold A P, Etgen A M, Fahrbach S E, Rubin R T, eds., pp. 425–462. Academic Press, San Diego.

Hines M (2004). *Brain Gender*. Oxford University Press, New York.

Hines M, Collaer M L (1993). Gonadal hormones and sexual differentiation of human behavior: developments from research on endocrine syndromes and studies of brain structure. *Annu Rev Sex Res* 4, 1–48.

Hines M, Kaufman F R (1994). Androgen and the development of human sex-typical behavior: rough-and-tumble play and sex of preferred playmates in children with congenital adrenal hyperplasia (CAH). *Child Dev* 65, 1042–1053.

Hines M, Sandberg E C (1996). Sexual differentiation of cognitive abilities in women exposed to diethylstilbestrol (DES) prenatally. *Horm Behav* 30, 354–363.

Hines M, Shipley C (1984). Prenatal exposure to diethylstilbestrol (DES) and the development of sexually dimorphic cognitive abilities and cerebral lateralization. *Dev Psychol* 20, 81–94.

Hines M, Alsum P, Roy M, Gorski R A, Goy R W (1987). Estrogenic contributions to sexual differentiation in the female guinea pig: influences of diethylstilbestrol and tamoxifen on neural, behavioral and ovarian development. *Horm Behav* 21, 402–417.

Hines M, Chiu L, McAdams L A, Bentler P M, Lipcamon J (1992). Cognition and the corpus callosum: verbal fluency, visuospatial ability and language lateralization related to midsagittal surface areas of callosal subregions. *Behav Neurosci* 106, 3–14.

Hines M, Johnston K, Golombok S and the ALSPAC Study Team (2002). Prenatal stress and gender role behavior in girls and boys: a longitudinal study. *Horm Behav* 42, 126–134.

Hines M, Fane B A, Pasterski V L, Mathews G A, Conway G S, Brook C (2003a). Spatial abilities following prenatal androgen abnormality: targeting and mental rotations performance in individuals with congenital adrenal hyperplasia. *Psychoneuroendocrinology* 28, 1010–1026.

Hines M, Ahmed S F, Hughes I A (2003b). Psychological outcomes and gender-related development in complete androgen insensitivity syndrome. *Arch Sex Behav* 32, 93–101.

Hyde J S (1984). How large are gender differences in aggression? A developmental meta-analysis. *Dev Psychol* 20, 722–736.

(1990). *Understanding Human Sexuality*. McGraw Hill, New York.

Hyde J S, Linn M C (1988). Gender differences in verbal ability: a meta-analysis. *Psychol Bull* 104, 53–69.

Hyde J S, Fennema E, Lamon S J (1990). Gender differences in mathematics performance: a meta-analysis. *Psychol Bull* 107, 139–155.

Imperato-McGinley J, Peterson R E, Gautier T, Sturla E (1979a). Androgens and the evolution of male-gender identity among male pseudohermaphrodites with 5 alpha reductase deficiency. *N Engl J Med* 300, 1233–1237.

Imperato-McGinley J, Peterson R E, Stoller R, Goodwin W E (1979b). Male pseudohermaphroditism secondary to 17-beta-hydroxysteroid dehydrogenase deficiency: gender role change with puberty. *J Clin Endocrinol Metab* 49, 391–395.

Kester P A (1984). Effects of prenatally administered 17 alpha hydroxyprogesterone caproate on adolescent males. *Arch Sex Behav* 13, 441–455.

Kester P, Green R, Finch S J, Williams K (1980). Prenatal 'female hormone' administration and psychosexual development in human males. *Psychoneuroendocrinology* 5, 269–285.

Kolb B, Whishaw I Q (1985). *Fundamentals of Human Neuropsychology*, 2nd edn. Freeman, New York.

Kuhnle U, Bullinger M (1997). Outcome of congenital adrenal hyperplasia. *Pediatr Surg Int* 12, 511–515.

LeVay S (1991). A difference in hypothalamic structure between heterosexual and homosexual men. *Science* 253, 1034–1037.

Leveroni C L, Berenbaum S A (1998). Early androgen effects on interest in infants: evidence from children with congenital adrenal hyperplasia. *Dev Neuropsychol* 14, 321–340.

Linn M C, Petersen A C (1985). Emergence and characterization of sex differences in spatial ability: a meta-analysis. *Child Dev* 56, 1479–1498.

Lish J D, Ehrhardt A A, Meyer-Bahlburg H F L et al. (1991). Gender-related behavior development in females exposed to diethylstilbestrol (DES) in utero: an attempted replication. *J Am Acad Child Adolesc Psychiatry* 30, 29–37.

Lish J D, Meyer-Bahlburg H F L, Ehrhardt A A, Travis B G, Veridiano N P (1992). Prenatal exposure to diethylstilbestrol (DES): childhood play behavior and adult gender-role behavior in women. *Arch Sex Behav* 21, 423–441.

Lynch A, Mychalkiw W (1978). Prenatal progesterone II. Its role in the treatment of pre-eclamptic toxaemia and its effect on the offspring's intelligence: a reappraisal. *Early Hum Dev* 2, 323–339.

Lynch A, Mychalkiw W, Hutt S J (1978). Prenatal progesterone I. Its effect on development and on intellectual and academic achievement. *Early Hum Dev* 2, 305–322.

Maccoby E E (1988). Gender as a social category. *Dev Psychol* 24, 755–765.

Maccoby E E, Jacklin C N (1974). *The Psychology of Sex Differences*. Stanford University Press, Stanford, CA.

McGuire L S, Omenn G S (1975). Congenital adrenal hyperplasia I: family studies of IQ. *Behav Genet* 5, 165–173.

McGuire L S, Ryan K O, Omenn G S (1975). Congenital adrenal hyperplasia II: cognitive and behavioral studies. *Behav Genet* 5, 175–188.

Meyer-Bahlburg H F L, Grisanti G C, Ehrhardt A A (1977). Prenatal effects of sex hormones on human male behavior: medroxyprogesterone acetate (MPA). *Psychoneuroendocrinology* 2, 383–390.

Meyer-Bahlburg H F L, Ehrhardt A A, Whitehead E D, Vann F H (1987). Sexuality in males with a history of prenatal exposure to diethylstilbestrol (DES). In *Workshop on Psychosexual and Reproductive Issues Affecting Patients with Cancer*. American Cancer Society, New York.

Meyer-Bahlburg H F L, Feldman J F, Cohen P, Ehrhardt A A (1988). Perinatal factors in the development of gender-related play behavior: sex hormones versus pregnancy complications. *Psychiatry* 51, 260–271.

Meyer-Bahlburg H F L, Ehrhardt A A, Rosen L R et al. (1995). Prenatal estrogens and the development of homosexual orientation. *Dev Psychol* 31, 12–21.

Meyer-Bahlburg H F L, Gruen R S, New M I et al. (1996). Gender change from female to male in classical congenital adrenal hyperplasia. *Horm Behav* 30, 319–332.

Migeon C J, Wisniewski A B, Gearhart J P et al. (2002). Ambiguous genitalia with perineoscrotal hypospadias in 46,XY individuals: long-term medical, surgical, and psychosexual outcome. *Pediatrics* 110, e31.

Money J, Dalery J (1976). Iatrogenic homosexuality: gender identity in seven 46,XX chromosomal females with hyperadrenocorti-

cal hermaphroditism born with a penis, three reared as boys, four reared as girls. *J Homosex* 1, 357–371.

Money J, Ehrhardt A (1972). *Man and Woman: Boy and Girl*. Johns Hopkins University Press, Baltimore, MD.

Money J, Lewis V (1966). IQ, genetics and accelerated growth: adrenogenital syndrome. *Johns Hopkins Hosp Bull* 118, 365–373.

Money J, Schwartz M, Lewis V (1984). Adult erotosexual status and fetal hormonal masculinization and demasculinization: 46 XX congenital virilizing adrenal hyperplasia and 46 XY androgen-insensitivity syndrome compared. *Psychoneuroendocrinology* 9, 405–414.

Nordenstrom A, Servin A, Bohlin G, Larsson A, Wedell A (2002). Sex-typed play behavior correlates with the degree of prenatal androgen exposure as assessed by CYP21 genotypes in girls with congenital adrenal hyperplasia. *J Clin Endocrinol Metab* 87, 5119–5124.

Perlman S M (1973). Cognitive abilities of children with hormone abnormalities: screening by psychoeducational tests. *J Learn Disabil* 6, 21–29.

Reiner W G (1999). Psychosocial concerns in classical and cloacal exstrophy patients. *Dialog Pediatr Urol* 22, 3.

Reiner W G, Gearhart J P, Jeffs R (1999). Psychosexual dysfunction in males with genital anomalies: late adolescence, Tanner stages VI to VI. *J Am Acad Child Adolesc Psychiatry* 38, 865–872.

Reinisch J M (1981). Prenatal exposure to synthetic progestins increases potential for aggression in humans. *Science* 211, 1171–1173.

Reinisch J M, Karow W G (1977). Prenatal exposure to synthetic progestins and estrogens: effects on human development. *Arch Sex Behav* 6, 257–288.

Reinisch J M, Sanders S A (1992). Effects of prenatal exposure to diethylstilbestrol (DES) on hemispheric laterality and spatial ability in human males. *Horm Behav* 26, 62–75.

Resnick S M, Berenbaum S A, Gottesman I I, Bouchard T (1986). Early hormonal influences on cognitive functioning in congenital adrenal hyperplasia. *Dev Psychol* 22, 191–198.

Rosler A, Kohn G (1983). Male pseudohermaphroditism due to 17 beta-hydroxysteroid dehydrogenase deficiency: studies on the natural history of the defect and effect of androgens on gender role. *J Steroid Biochem* 19, 663–674.

Sanders B, Soares M P, D'Aquila J M (1982). The sex difference on one test of spatial visualization: a nontrivial difference. *Child Dev* 53, 1106–1110.

Schober J (1999). Feminizing genitoplasty for intersex. In *Pediatric Surgery and Urology: Long Term Outcomes*, Stringer M D, ed., pp. 549–558. Saunders, London.

Schober J M, Carmichael P A, Hines M, Ransley P G (2002). The ultimate challenge of cloacal exstrophy. *J Urol* 167, 300–304.

Sinforiani W, Livieri C, Mauri M et al. (1994). Cognitive and neuroradiological findings in congenital adrenal hyperplasia. *Psychoneuroendocrinology* 19, 55–64.

Smail P J, Reyes F I, Winter F S D, Faiman C (1981). The fetal hormonal environment and its effect on the morphogenesis of the genital system. In *Pediatric Andrology*, Kogan S J, Hafez E S E, eds., pp. 9–19. Martinus Nijhoff, The Hague.

Spreen O, Strauss E (1991). *A Compendium of Neuropsychological Tests*. Oxford University Press, New York.

Sutton-Smith B, Rosenberg B G, Morgan E F, Jr (1963). Development of sex differences in play choices during preadolescence. *Child Dev* 34, 119–126.

Tanner J M, Whitehouse R H, Takaishi M (1966). Standards from birth to maturity for height, weight, height velocity and weight velocity: British children, 1965. *Arch Dis Child* 41, 454–471.

Voyer D, Voyer S, Bryden M P (1995). Magnitude of sex differences in spatial abilities: a meta-analysis and consideration of critical variables. *Psychol Bull* 117, 250–270.

Wenzel U, Schneider M, Zachmann M et al. (1978). Intelligence of patients with congenital adrenal hyperplasia due to 21-hydroxylase deficiency, their parents and unaffected siblings. *Helv Paediatr Acta* 33, 11–16.

Wilcox A J, Maxey J, Herbst A L (1992). Prenatal hormone exposure and performance on college entrance examinations. *Horm Behav* 24, 433–439.

Wilson J D, Griffin J E, Russell D W (1993). Steroid 5 alpha reductase 2 deficiency. *Endocr Rev* 14, 577–593.

Wisniewski A B, Migeon C J, Meyer-Bahlburg H F L et al. (2000). Complete androgen insensitivity syndrome. Long-term medical, surgical, and psychosexual outcome. *J Clin Endocrinol Metab* 85, 2664–2669.

Wisniewski A B, Migeon C J, Gearhart J P et al. (2001). Congenital micropenis: long-term medical, surgical and psychosexual follow-up of individuals raised male or female. *Horm Res* 56, 3–11.

Yalom I D, Green R, Fisk N (1973). Prenatal exposure to female hormones: effect on psychosexual development in boys. *Arch Gen Psychiatry* 28, 554–561.

Zhou J, Hofman M, Gooren L, Swaab D (1995). A sex difference in the human brain and its relation to transsexuality. *Nature* 378, 68–70.

Zucker K J (1999). Intersexuality and gender identity differentiation. *Annu Rev Sex Res* 10, 11–69.

Zucker K J, Bradley S J, Oliver G, Blake J, Fleming S, Hood J (1996). Psychosexual development of women with congenital adrenal hyperplasia. *Horm Behav* 30, 300–318.

38

Eating disorders in adolescence

Nadia Micali[1], Peter Webster[1] and Janet Treasure[2]

[1]Maudsley Hospital, London, UK
[2]Guys Campus, London, UK

Introduction

The main eating disorders so far described are anorexia nervosa, bulimia nervosa and binge-eating disorder. This chapter will concentrate, for reasons of space, on the first two.

Historically, the eating disorders have all suffered from being seen as a "backwater" of psychiatry and medicine, as seen by the late acceptance of all of them as illnesses, the still prevalent view of anorexia and bulimia nervosa as "slimmers' diseases" and the fact that binge-eating disorder has only established itself as a diagnosable disorder in the fourth edition of *The Diagnostic Standard Manual* (DSM-IV; American Psychiatric Association, 1994). This has occurred despite the description of anorexia nervosa as an illness since the 1860s (Gull, 1874; Lasegue, 1873) and bulimia nervosa since 1979 (Russell, 1979).

Two other profound discrepancies exist between the emphasis that these illnesses have been afforded and the reality regarding them. Anorexia has the highest morbidity and mortality of any psychiatric illness (Nielsen et al., 1998) and presents a similar burden of care to that of severe psychoses (Treasure and Serpell, 2001).

Both anorexia and bulimia present primarily, but not exclusively, as disorders of adolescence for a number of postulated reasons (see below); however, as the illnesses often run a chronic course, professionals in all disciplines, beyond childhood, will see "graduate" cases as well as those of primary onset. Consequently, paediatricians and psychiatrists managing adolescents (traditionally puberty–adult; usually considered as 14–18 years) will see prepubertal-onset child "graduates" and pre- and postpubertal adolescent-onset patients.

As shall be seen, paediatricians play a key role in the identification, management and reduction in delay in diagnoses of both disorders as sufferers, particularly of anorexia nervosa, often present initially because of medical complications; in addition, many aspects of management, such as refeeding and acute rehydration, involve medical care. Gynaecological aspects are particularly relevant as both anorexia and bulimia nervosa commonly present with menstrual or endocrine abnormalities. In fact, in one study, 52% of children presenting with determined food avoidance spent some time on a paediatric ward (Fosson et al., 1987).

Definitions

The defining criteria for eating disorders are provided by both main classificatory systems, ICD-10 (World Health Organization, 1992) and DSM-IV (American Psychiatric Association, 1994).

Anorexia nervosa is defined as follows.

1. Weight loss, leading to a body weight at least 15% below the expected for age and height. The weight (kg): height^2 (m) ratio (body mass index (BMI)) is also used; the normal range being 20–25 kg/m^2. Anorexia is defined by this ratio being less than 17.5 kg/m^2 and severe anorexia by less than 13.5 kg/m^2. In children and adolescents, this is most evident by failure to grow at a normal rate.
2. The weight loss is self-induced by avoidance of "fatty foods".
3. An intrusive dread of fatness, leading to a self-imposed weight threshold.
4. A widespread endocrine disorder involving the hypothalamic–pituitary–gonadal axis is manifest in

Paediatric and Adolescent Gynaecology, ed. Adam Balen et al. Published by Cambridge University Press.
© Cambridge University Press 2004.

women as amenorrhoea and in men as a loss of sexual interest and potency. In prepuberty this is seen as its delayed onset.

DSM-IV subtypes the illness into restricting and binge-ing/purging.

Bulimia nervosa is defined as follows.

1 Recurrent episodes of overeating (at least twice a week over three months) where large amounts of food are consumed in short periods of time.

2 Persistent preoccupation with eating and a strong craving to eat.

3 Partial attempts to counteract the "fattening" effects of food by at least one of the following: self-induced vomiting, self-induced purging, alternating periods of starvation, use of drugs (e.g. appetite suppressants, thyroid preparations, diuretics, insulin therapy neglect in diabetics).

4 Self-perception of being too fat, with an intrusive dread of fatness (usually leading to underweight).

Bulimia nervosa is divided by DSM-IV into the subtypes *purging* and *non-purging*.

Although these conditions are regarded as distinct disorders, the possibility exists of an overlap; however, if both occur, then anorexia nervosa is considered the primary diagnosis. If not all of these criteria are met, the particular illness is defined as atypical or as "eating disorder not otherwise specified".

DSM-IV also includes a definition of "binge eating disorder", which is similar to bulimia nervosa without compensatory strategies.

Recently, some concerns have been raised regarding the inclusion in the diagnosis of anorexia the criteria of fat phobia or elements of body image disorder. Some authors have suggested that this is a perspective restricted to a Western culture (Katzmann and Lee, 1997). This may be supported by the fact that patients' attributions for not eating are diverse across cultures and can include abdominal bloating, loss of appetite, no hunger, fear of food, distaste for food or "don't know" (Lee et al., 2001).

Epidemiology

The incidence of anorexia nervosa is approximately 7/100 000, with a prevalence in women of 0.1–1%. Bulimia nervosa has approximately twice these rates, and both illnesses are ten times more common in women at present. Both present mostly in late adolescence, with a median onset of 17–18 years, but early- and late- onset cases certainly do occur, in childhood and in later life, although both

disorders are very rare below the age of eight years. A number of demographic misunderstandings about eating disorders exist, mostly a consequence of theorizing by the media. First, there is no clear evidence of increasing rates in anorexia nervosa, but there has certainly been striking rise in bulimia nervosa since its description in 1979, although equally in men and women. A striking fact is how universal anorexia nervosa is across the globe, with equal prevalence in non-Western countries; bulimia in contrast does seem restricted to western cultures. Contrary to popular belief, there is only a slightly overrepresentation in upper and middle social classes, but certain occupational groups, combining an emphasis on perfection, competition and looks, such as modelling and dancing, certainly do have higher rates (Hoek, 1991).

Aetiology

Throughout the years, much effort has been put into trying to understand the causality of eating disorders. Psychological, biological and social theories have been postulated. It would appear that one causal factor is not sufficient. Eating disorders are multidetermined and the result of a vast range of interacting factors. Biological, psychological, familial, sociocultural and personality factors are all relevant contributing elements. These factors also emerge at different times in life. Consequently it is important to distinguish between:

- predisposing factors, which are necessary for the disorder to occur
- precipitating factors, which act as triggers
- maintaining factors, which perpetuate the disorder once developed.

Biologically, genetic risk factors are definitely significant in developing an eating disorder. Family aggregation studies show a fourfold risk of anorexia in the daughter of an affected parent (Treasure & Holland, 1995) and a significantly higher risk of developing an eating disorder in female first-degree relatives compared with control subjects (Strober et al., 1990). Twin and adoption studies have shown a concordance for anorexia nervosa in monozygotic twins to be around ten times greater than for dizygotic twins (Holland et al., 1998; Treasure & Holland, 1990).

In bulimia nervosa, concordance seems also to be significantly higher for monozygotic than dizygotic twins (Kendler et al., 1991).

Some other biological factors have been thought to be relevant in the causation of eating disorders, although it is difficult to demonstrate if they play a role in the aetiology or are only secondary to the physiological and metabolic alterations that characterize these conditions.

Some authors have suggested that neuroendocrine dysfunctions in the hypothalamus might be relevant, particularly in the realm of cortisol function and regulation (Weiner, 1985). Some older studies indicated that abnormalities in the serotonergic system and its functioning might contribute to the pathogenesis of both disorders (Treasure et al., 1997), whereas more recent interest has focused on other neurotransmitters possibly involved in the regulation of appetite, such as vasoactive peptide, somatostatin, neurotensin and cholecystokinin (Wakeling, 1985). The most recent interest has focused on leptin, a hormone secreted by adipose tissue that causes inhibitory effects on appetite and increased activity (see Ch. 6).

Psychologically, several explanations have been sought for the development of an eating disorder. Early experiences and mother–child interactions have been closely analysed in anorexia nervosa (Bruch, 1973). Research has recently shown that individuals with eating disorders have high rates of insecure attachment, mainly of the dismissive type (Ward et al., 2000). The incidence of obstetric complications in the child, features of overconcerned mothering and maternal grief is higher in individuals with anorexia nervosa compared with controls (Shoebridge and Gowers, 2000). In both illnesses, higher levels of developmental stress have been evidenced, but more so in bulimia, mainly in the form of child neglect, abuse and sexual trauma.

Familial dysfunction in interaction and communication has been postulated as having an important role in the pathogenesis of eating disorders but controversy has existed whether abnormal family dynamics are causal or subsequent to the disorders (Selvini Palazzoli, 1974; Kog and Vandereycken, 1998). There is, however, empirical evidence of predisposing features in maternal parenting style and perinatal experience (Shoebridge and Gowers, 2000).

Some personality traits are believed to increase the vulnerabilities, namely rigidity, perfectionism and obsessionality in anorexia nervosa and impulsivity and risk-taking in bulimia nervosa.

The role of specific life events as triggers should not be dismissed, especially interpersonal ones. Bereavements, family changes, episodes of illness or other adverse events are often found to be associated with the onset in 70% of those affected in both illnesses (King, 1990).

Puberty is often regarded as a time when eating disorders are very likely to surface. Hormonal changes with subsequent pubertal development and rapid growth all contribute as important precipitating factors. There is also a requirement for the adolescent girl to adapt to a new psychosocial role, which can be a significant factor.

Presentation

Eating disorders often present late because of their covertness, insidiousness and, in anorexia, the regular presence of insightlessness. However, in adolescence, it is usually via their concerned family, school or peer group. As eating disorders, more than any other illnesses, form such a unique kaleidoscope of concurrent psychiatric and physical symptoms, presentation can be in the form of the primary illness or any of the psychiatric or physical complications. Because of this wide spectrum, initial presentation can occur in primary care and in almost all medical and psychiatric specialities, most notably endocrinology, gastoenterology, renal medicine, rheumatology, orthopaedics and child and adolescent or general psychiatry. In adolescence, these generally condense to paediatricians and paediatric endocrinology. Although some features are clear, the more discriminatory features can often be subtle.

Medical presentation

Anorexia nervosa will present with the primary effects of malnutrition and any subsequent medical complication (Fig. 38.1 and Table 38.1) (Hall and Beresford, 1989). The most obvious primary features are weight loss, or delayed/arrested growth, and primary or secondary amenorrhoea or delayed puberty. Other features are dry hair and skin, fine body hair, heightened cold sensitivity and teeth loss caused by gum shrinkage. Any secondary medical complication, however, may precipitate presentation (e.g. bone fracture secondary to osteoporosis).

Bulimia nervosa is physically much better disguised, but third parties may express concern over hearing vomiting, the patient spending too long in the bathroom or going there after every meal. There may also be some suspicion of compensatory behaviours such as purging with laxatives or diuretics, or behaviours such as overexercising. Physical signs are the smell of vomitus, swollen parotid glands (Fig. 38.5, colour plate), rotting teeth and callused knuckles from self-induced vomiting (Russell's sign; Fig. 38.6, colour plate). The medical consequences, however, can at times be serious and can occasionally present as a medical crisis. The most concerning of these is low potassium secondary to vomiting, which can cause potentially fatal cardiac arrhythmias. Patients can, however, have chronically profoundly low potassium levels and, therefore, care must be taken to rectify levels slowly.

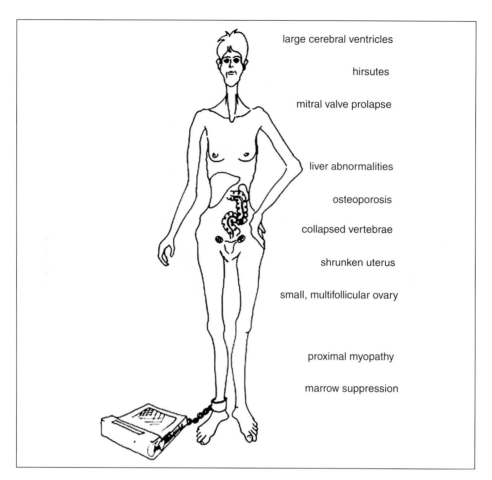

large cerebral ventricles

hirsutes

mitral valve prolapse

liver abnormalities

osteoporosis

collapsed vertebrae

shrunken uterus

small, multifollicular ovary

proximal myopathy

marrow suppression

Fig. 38.1. The physical side effects of anorexia nervosa. (Courtesy of Professor J. Treasure.)

Psychological presentation

In anorexia nervosa, the patient will be typically female and will usually present with the primary psychological symptoms, such as overconcern with weight-gain avoidance and with varying levels of insight as to whether her behaviour and beliefs are abnormal. She will typically be emaciated, covered in layers of baggy clothes (for warmth and to cover her perceived fat) and there will often be reduced eye contact and a poor rapport. Most will be withdrawn and depressed, with the biological symptoms of depression such as disturbed sleep, low energy and motivation and loss of pleasure in life. On fuller assessment they may have associated syndromes such as obsessive compulsive disorder or social phobia and may show evidence of personality disorder. Suicidality is a concern and needs a full assessment as it is a major cause of death in these patients.

Bulimia nervosa is more subtle, but suspicion is usually aroused as the compensatory strategies are frequent and less disguisable. The patients will, as for anorexia, present with psychological features characteristic of bulimia nervosa. Usually a girl, she will not look emaciated but her parotid glands are often visibly enlarged. She will also seem more insightful and less withdrawn. Depression often presents associated with bulimia nervosa, as well as substance and alcohol abuse, risk-taking behaviours and impulsivity disorders. Often associated are a history of self-harm and suicide attempts. There is also a higher rate of emotionally unstable personalities amongst patients with bulimia.

Medical complications of anorexia nervosa

The malnutrition, weight loss and associated behaviours in adolescent anorexia nervosa affect every organ system and aspect of normal development. Furthermore, as fat supplies are lower in younger patients and they dehydrate more rapidly, the effects can be more concerning. Important effects are summarized in Table 38.1.

Table 38.1. Medical complications of anorexia nervosa and bulimia nervosa

System	Complications (anorexia nervosa, unless stated)
Dental	Gum erosion
	Loosened teeth
	Osteoporosis of the jaw
	Tooth erosion (bulimia)
	(Fig. 38.2, colour plate)
Musculoskeletal	Osteoporosis
	Pathological fractures
	Proximal myopathy
	Reduced respiratory function
Central nervous system	Decreased pituitary size and function
	Decreased total brain substance
	Cerebral oedema (in extreme malnutrition)
Cardiovascular	Decreased cardiac size and function
	Peripheral oedema and cyanosis (Figs. 38.3 and 38.4, colour plates)
	Valvular impairment
	Arrhythmias
	QT elongation on electrocardiograph
Reproductive	Decreased fertility,
	Decreased plasma oestrogen, progesterone, follicle-stimulating hormone, luteinizing hormone
	Decreased birth weight
	Increased perinatal mortality
Gastrointestinal	Salivary gland hypertrophy (bulimia) (Fig. 38.5, colour plate)
	Peptic ulceration
	Pancreatitis (bulimia: rare)
	Impaired liver function: severe malnutrition
	Hypoglobulinaemia
Haematological	Bone marrow dysfunction: pancytopenia
	Macrocytosis of red cells: vitamin B_{12} deficiency
	Petechial rash (severe end-stage malnutrition)
	Reduced immune function
Metabolic	Decreased potassium (vomiting), glucose
	Abnormal sodium, urea
	Increased cholesterol
	Metabolic alkalosis if purging
Endocrine	Increased cortisol
	Decreased triiodothyronine

Endocrine abnormalities

Abnormalities are seen across the endocrine spectrum, as the primary dysfunction is in the hypothalamic–pituitary axis, which shows a pan-dysfunction. This used to be thought of as aetiological, but it is now seen as more secondary to weight loss. It is significant, however, that some effects, such as amenorrhoea, show some independence of weight levels; a third of patients present with amenorrhoea before weight loss (Theander, 1970) and an association has been shown between return of menstruation and psychological improvement (Van Binsbergen et al., 1990). Further, more ovarian maturation on recovery is not fully correlated with weight gain.

As in other starvation states, plasma cortisol is raised and the diurnal variation is lost. There is a reduction in cortisol metabolism and impairment in the dexamethasone suppression test (Newman and Halmi, 1988). Growth hormone (GH) is similarly raised in approximately half of patients with an associated reduction in somatomedin C (Argente et al., 1997). Consequently, the feedback control of GH is impaired, an effect that seems to be mediated by the hypothalamus as there seems to be no dysfunction in GH stimulation tests (Muller et al., 1987).

Thyroid function varies in anorexia nervosa. Whereas thyroxine levels are consistently normal, triiodothyronine levels are related to weight and are low (low triiodothyronine syndrome). Normalization of this only occurs after considerable weight gain has occurred. Interestingly, the levels of thyroid-stimulating hormone are not secondarily raised.

Sexual development

The gonadotrophins follicle-stimulating hormone and luteinizing hormone universally show attenuation in their levels. Their pattern of secretion becomes similar to a prepubertal one, even after stimulation with exogenous gonadotrophic-releasing hormone (Sherman et al., 1975). In low-weight children this will go unnoticed; however, as there is inhibition of the commencement of nocturnal gonadotrophin pulsatile secretion – the primary event of puberty – patients will present with delayed onset of puberty.

More common, particularly in adolescence, is postpubertal onset, in which case these hormone changes present as primary or secondary amenorrhoea, depending on the time of onset.

The ovaries and uterus show a marked reduction in size in girls with secondary amenorrhoea, and the ovaries characteristically become quiescent with no follicular activity.

Weight gain leads to normalization of many physical characteristics of anorexia nervosa; however it has been reported that some deficits might persist, for example decreased bone density (Ward et al., 1997). Low levels of sex steroids during a time of development probably impacts not only on bone formation but also on growth and healthy development of secondary sexual characteristics.

Growth

There is still some debate on the consequences of anorexia nervosa on growth. Danziger et al. (1994), in a study on early-onset anorexia, suggested that the occurrence of anorexia nervosa in the pubertal and peripubertal period commonly resulted in growth arrest. Onset earlier in puberty has probably the most relevant consequences on growth, given that the pubertal growth spurt occurs at the earlier stages in puberty.

There are few studies on bone age in early-onset anorexia nervosa, although it has been shown that chronic malnutrition leads to a delay in bone age (Dreizen et al., 1967).

Bone density

Osteoporosis was described as a complication of anorexia nervosa in 1984 (Rigotti et al., 1984) and is now one of the major concerns regarding the long-term outcome of patients with eating disorders. In children, this is an important issue, given that bone mass is developing. Oestrogens play a fundamental role in bone formation and this is the reason why restoration of the menstrual cycle is one of the first goals in the treatment of anorexia nervosa. Moreover, maximal bone accretion and formation happens during puberty. It seems also that an adequate peak bone mass might not be reached if the amounts of sex steroids are reduced during puberty.

Other organs

The effects of prolonged starvation on the heart can lead to a decrease in cardiac muscle mass, which can result in peripheral oedema and hypotension. Patients often present with bradycardia, which is compensatory; arrhythmias can also occur, commonly when hypokalaemia is present.

The gastrointestinal tract often shows no significant abnormalities on examination. Patients often have a slower gastric emptying rate for solids and liquids (McCallum et al., 1985).

Increases in serum creatinine levels and low creatinine clearance may result from microvascular changes in the kidneys and muscle mass reduction.

Dehydration and renal stones occur as a consequence of low fluid intake, vomiting and laxative or diuretic abuse.

The liver has been shown to develop fatty changes in severe malnutrition, and this has been confirmed in anorexia nervosa.

Assessment

Assessment of eating disorders usually is performed first by GPs or primary carers (King, 1990). The parents usually have an important role in helping the clinician to understand how the problem developed. Assessment of both anorexia and bulimia nervosa relies on many common aspects. A full psychological and physical assessment is often not necessary in a medical setting, there are though some key features that are essential, mainly in regard to important physical complications. This is essential, given that the physical conditions of an adolescent with an eating disorder can range from life threatening to normal. The following is an outline of essential information needed in assessing a patient with an eating disorder.

History of the eating disorder

The following factors are important:
- age
- height (m) and weight (kg): BMI
- onset, course and symptomatology
- current eating pattern and caloric intake
- techniques used to reduce and avoid gaining weight (see above): include precipitants, frequency and severity
- lowest, highest and ideal weights.

Illness dimensions

The dimensions of the illness can be considered in four groups:
- physical/medical (as outlined above): mainly amenorrhoea, fractures
- psychological: in particular taking into consideration features characteristic of the disorders (described above) plus associated features (i.e. depression and associated suicidal risk, obsessional compulsive disorder (OCD) symptoms, low self-esteem)
- family: this is crucial, especially looking at reactions to illness and concerns about this, but also involvement in management and support for the adolescent
- insight/capacity: the ability to recognize the illness and accept help for it.

Physical examination

The following areas are assessed:
- height, weight and BMI (kg/m^2)
- blood pressure and pulse rate (sitting and standing)
- proximal myopathy (e.g. standing unassisted from a squatting position)
- neurological complications: peripheral myopathy from thiamine deficiency
- skin: purpura, Raynaud's syndrome, lesions from compulsive hand-washing.

Laboratory findings

The following tests should be carried out on serum:
- electrolytes: sodium increased in dehydration; potassium decreased if there is vomiting, laxative and diuretic misuse
- urea: increased if there is dehydration
- creatinine: increased if dehydration is extreme
- amylase: raised serum amylase is a sign of "refeeding pancreatitis"; raised salivary amylase is associated with vomiting
- glucose: levels are low in patients with anorexia nervosa, fluctuating in patients with bulimia
- protein: usually normal unless very chronic malnutrition
- phosphate: low.

The following blood analyses are useful:
- red blood cell count: anaemia is usually mild, associated with iron deficiency
- white blood cell count: leukopenia is possible
- eosinophil sedimentation rate: can be raised in bulimia nervosa if associated with oesophageal inflammation.

Liver function tests include:
- alanine and aspartate amino transferases and alkaline phosphatase: usually raised
- gamma-glutamyl transferase: raised less frequently
- total bilirubin: usually normal
- albumin levels: low or normal.

Assessment of sexual development

The assessment of pubertal status is very important in adolescents with eating disorders in order to evaluate the presence of developmental and growth delay caused by the illness. Pubertal delay is usually determined by assessing the Tanner stage and comparing this with data for normal ranges, pelvic ultrasound, discrepancy between bone age and chronological age and suppression of gonadotrophins.

Pelvic ultrasound is a very useful means to evaluate disorders of sexual development in girls. It is based on an accurate knowledge and assessment of both ovarian and uterine size and development during childhood and adolescence. In patients with primary amenorrhoea, ultrasound will show prepubertal ovaries and uterus; in secondary amenorrhoea there is a regression of the uterus and ovaries.

Pelvic ultrasound has become a very useful clinical tool also in determining when a "target weight" has been reached (Lai et al., 1994).

Bone density

Bone mineral density is used as a measure of the degree of osteoporosis. This is characterized by a decrease in bone mass and an increased bone fragility, resulting in an augmented risk of fractures.

Bone mineral density is measured with a dual energy X-ray absorptiometry (DEXA), which measures both bone and soft tissue composition. Normal values for bone mineral content and bone mineral density for children and adolescents are available; the assessment has to take into account growth.

Investigations

The following investigations are essential:
- full blood cell count
- urea and electrolytes (sodium, potassium, calcium, magnesium, phosphate)
- serum proteins
- liver function tests
- electrocardiography.

The following investigations are additional to be used where required:
- vitamin B_{12}, folate
- DEXA scan
- thiamin
- bone markers
- thyroid function tests
- eosinophil sedimentation rate.

Management

Eating disorders are very common disorders in adolescence. They are protean in presentation, have a multifaceted pathogenesis and are potentially life threatening.

Management, therefore, needs to be comprehensive, integrated and to take into account a biopsychosocial perspective.

Management usually involves three different levels of care: primary (GP and psychiatric community team), secondary (psychiatric, medical and surgical) and tertiary (specialist eating disorders services). A comprehensive approach requires:

1 the appropriate diagnostic measures (including medical investigations)
2 treatment of the disorder, in the form of adequate nutrition (i.e. refeeding) and psychological therapies; the co-existing medical complications; and the comorbid psychiatric conditions
3 decision-making regarding the appropriate location of treatment.

All of this requires the integration of several disciplines and a multidisciplinary approach: assessment and treatment should be provided by nurses, psychologists, social workers, dieticians, physiotherapists and occupational therapists.

An essential component during the first stages is giving clear information and education to the adolescent about the illness and its complications without a judgemental but with an empathic approach. Parents need to be involved in the management from an early stage, and the understanding of their child's condition, including its implications, has to be shared with them (Bryant-Waugh and Lask, 1999).

In adolescent anorexics, in fact, three aspects are very relevant: the lack of insight, the potentially severe physical risk, and the battle for control. The teenager does not usually recognize the extent of the illness and has little insight into it; she may be at risk of severe damage to her health and still fiercely fighting for control over her eating. It is, therefore, of primary importance to support the parents in taking responsibility for their child and in taking decisions regarding the child's health and in joining in management decisions (Treasure, 1997).

Location of treatment for patients with eating disorders varies. Some are best treated as outpatients; others require inpatient treatment. Usually inpatient treatment becomes necessary in those with severe malnutrition (i.e. BMI below the 3rd centile); serious medical complications such as dehydration, electrolyte imbalance, circulatory failure, arrythmias, haematemesis; deliberate-self-harm, suicidal risk or severe comorbid depression; or failure to gain weight during outpatient treatment. It is clear that this applies mainly to anorexia nervosa (Honig and Sharman, 2000).

Outpatient treatment

Outpatient treatment can be provided in different settings and at different levels.

Primary care

Eating disorders in adolescents present very often in a primary care setting; recognition, consequently, is a necessary early step to improve access to appropriate treatment. Many authors believe that the sooner the treatment, the better.

Physical assessment is crucial to stimulate suspicion of an eating disorder. Weight loss or failure to reach expected weight for age and height, amenorrhoea and dehydration should help the clinician to consider the possibility of anorexia nervosa. By comparison, bulimia is often more covert; smell of vomit or swollen parotid glands might be indicative. Appropriate clinical investigations and gathering of information from the patient become key elements.

Further steps should then be taken to ensure parental involvement, the motivation and insight of the adolescent and to evaluate the risk or severity of physical complications, before referral to specialist service is made. The clinician involved in primary care takes on the significant role of ensuring regular monitoring of weight, blood tests and blood pressure. Practice nurses and community dieticians are often involved in the management of patients in this setting.

Secondary care

Milder eating disorders can be managed in standard psychiatric care by general adolescent teams. Usually this requires the involvement of a CPN (Community Psychiatric Nurse) or a psychologist attached to the team. Usually, weight and medical monitoring are done in this setting.

Tertiary care

Specialist services usually offer outpatient treatment as well as day-hospital facilities. Patients with low-risk eating disorders are often treated as outpatients. This involves a careful integration of different aspects of management: psychological and educational, and requires liaising with primary and secondary care teams to provide an adequate consistent care.

Bulimia nervosa and mild anorexia are usually managed as outpatients.

Inpatient treatment

Inpatient treatment can be offered in general paediatric wards, adolescent psychiatric units taking different patients or in specialized eating disorder units. It is generally considered that admission should be restricted to life-threatening situations, when there is severe medical or psychiatric risk. These are outlined in Table 38.2. However, because of the centrality of the family in the overall

Table 38.2. Indications for inpatient admission

Risk	Indications
Life-threatening conditions	
Medical	Body mass index $< 13.5\,\text{kg}/\text{m}^2$ or rapid fall $> 20\%$ in 6 months
	Proximal myopathy
	Syncope
	Hypoglycaemia
	Severe electrolyte disturbance (e.g. $K^+ < 2.5$; $Na^+ < 130$)
	Poor diabetic control
	Petechial rash and significant platelet suppression
Psychiatric	High risk of suicide
	Severe psychiatric comorbidity (e.g. severe depression or obsessive compulsive disorder)
Compromised community treatment	
Weight gain	Failure to gain weight as out-patient
Social situation	Extreme isolation, lack of support
	Intolerable family situation (e.g. high expressed emotion, abuse, collusion)

management of these problems, the length of admission should be minimized.

Paediatric wards have the advantage of offering medical care. Young people with eating disorders who have severe or life-threatening medical complications or require artificial feeding are best treated in this setting.

Psychiatric adolescent units are in almost all areas the only specialist inpatient care that can be offered; although they have the advantage of providing a peer group who are much less concerned with eating, they can lack the specific skills to ensure adequate refeeding. The usual other option of an adult eating disorder unit is the reverse of this situation. This makes a strong case for units that specialize for children and adolescents with eating disorders but these are very rare. Ideally, they should offer staff who have the skills and experience to manage both physical and psychological aspects. The other benefit is peer support, which is often beneficial, although this environment has the potential to create feelings of competition amongst patients (Garfinkel et al., 1985).

The primary focus of inpatient treatment is to facilitate weight gain as well as to provide adequate support and psychological help to the patient. This usually involves collaborating with families and offering them support and therapeutic work. During inpatient management of adolescents with eating disorders, parents need to be consulted, involved in the decision-making process and encouraged in actively participating with the treatment. They also need

to be helped to enhance their problem-solving skills and to become empowered as parents (Le Grange et al., 1992).

Refeeding

The refeeding process is clearly a crucial part of treatment, given that weight gain has an important bearing on the medical and psychiatric well-being of this group of patients. Depending on the severity of the patient's medical condition, it will occur on a medical or psychiatric unit and, therefore, the paediatrician should be aware of the medical issues in refeeding and liaise closely with dieticians and mental health staff. This is accomplished in different ways in different units. Usually behavioural methods are used, such as rewards, group eating with fixed eating times and boundaries. Refeeding is systematic and should be monitored by a dietician. The initial aim for weight gain is 1 kg/week, which requires a caloric intake of around 3000 kcal/day. This is generally divided into moderate size meals and snacks.

When the refeeding needs to be immediate because of the adolescent's physical condition and this cannot be achieved orally, nasogastric feeding should be considered. This is accomplished liaising with a medical team and a dietician. The adolescent and the family should be included in planning for this. Sometimes this procedure gives rise to concerns regarding the rights of the individual who is being fed; however, given the nature of the illness, the Mental Health Act has to be used at times (see below).

Another important aspect of the refeeding programme is establishing a target weight range. This triggers different reactions depending on the type of eating disorder, but, given that weight gain is the main preoccupation both in bulimia and anorexia nervosa, reaching a normal BMI is accompanied by several negotiations. Compromise BMIs are reached considering several metabolic and endocrine elements. Pelvic ultrasound scanning is often used to determine whether the appropriate size of pelvic organs has been reached for a certain age and whether they are mature, and thus whether the weight reached is appropriate for age (Adams, 1993).

Specific medical treatments

The basis of almost all medical treatments is refeeding, and this is also true of all gynaecological symptoms.

Osteoporosis

As described above, the issue of osteoporosis in eating disorders is complex but a very relevant area of concern for long-term complications.

Several treatments have been advocated, including oestrogens, calcium, bisphosphonates, and insulin-growth factors (IGF) (Grinspoon et al., 1997).

The use of oestrogen replacement is still controversial, mainly in young people, given that the goal of treatment is currently to reach a maximum peak bone mass through weight restoration and appropriate nutrition (Nicholls et al., 2000). In young people, oestrogen prevents further growth by fusing the epiphyses. One randomized controlled trial of osteoporosis treatment in women with anorexia nervosa has been published (Klibanski et al., 1995). This studied a population of adult women and the effect of the contraceptive pill or other oestrogen supplementation. Only partial or no protection was provided by either of these.

Recently a prospective study on calcium supplementation in women with a history of anorexia nervosa failed to find an effect of supplementation on bone mineral density (Serpell et al., unpublished data). A randomized control trial is currently in progress to study the efficacy of calcium supplementation in children and adolescents with anorexia nervosa (Treasure and Serpell, 2001).

Bisphosphonates and IGF are unlikely to be useful in treatment given that the former are not recommended in pregnancy (because of possible teratogenic effects), and the latter requires constant glucose monitoring to prevent hypoglycaemia.

Psychological treatments

Psychological treatments are used both in inpatient and outpatient settings and include self-help books, individual, group and family therapy.

Self-help manuals aim to give nutritional information, help refeeding and provide information on the nature and the course of the disorders.

Individual therapies include:
- cognitive-behavioural therapy
- psychodynamic psychotherapy
- other therapies (e.g. cognitive analytic therapy).

Cognitive-behavioural therapy

Usually, cognitive-behavioural techniques are very useful for patients with bulimia nervosa, even though research on outcome has mainly been done with adults (Fairburn, 1997). The aim of this therapy is to achieve changes in behaviour accompanied by changes in the way the adolescent thinks; this is done in a collaborative and empowering way.

Psychodynamic psychotherapies

Psychodynamic psychotherapy is sometimes useful for individuals who have found it difficult to develop their abilities to own and contain their emotions through family therapy (Magagna, 2000). However, these therapies are costly and difficult to complete in the short term.

Group therapy

Group work is useful in helping young people with eating disorders to share concerns and have mutual support.

Family work

Working with the family of an individual who has an eating disorder has a fundamental role in the management of this age group. Children and adolescents do better in treatment with their family compared with individual therapy; in adults it is the reverse (Russell et al., 1987).

However to have family therapy might mean for some parents that their family is dysfunctional and that they might have caused their child's illness. It is for this reason important to move away from the idea of blame, and to aid families in recognizing their way of functioning. Different kinds of intervention can be used to involve families in treatment, from simple counselling to family therapy.

The basis of family work is the idea that it is useful in these disorders to focus not only on the teenager intrapsychic processes but also on the family context and how this reinforces and maintains the illness in the child. Empowering parents and actively involving them in their child's illness helps parents to offer their children adequate support and to be able to manage difficult situations at home.

Medication

The use of psychotropic drugs in eating disorders is fairly limited. Fluoxetine has been shown to be useful in reducing bulimic behaviours (Goldstein et al., 1999). Recently, there have been reports of olanzapine, an atypical antipsychotic, causing resolution of anorexic cognitions (Hansen, 1999; Jensen and Mejhede, 2000).

Medication, mainly tranquillizers and antidepressants, can help in the reduction of agitation and levels of arousal.

Legal and ethical aspects

Anorexia nervosa sometimes presents the clinician with a patient who, to varying levels of understanding of the medical implications, argues the case that they have the right to refuse to eat. This can occasionally be further complicated by parental collusion. In the past, clinicians have allowed such patients to die owing to a misunderstanding of the nature of the illness.

As our understanding of eating disorders has grown, its psychopathology has been deeper understood and increasingly it has been appropriately seen as a mental illness. Consequently, the above arguments are seen as occurring in a state of impaired capacity and the management has been changed accordingly. Therefore, feeding the anorexic patient is considered primary psychiatric treatment for the condition. In practical terms, this means that patients who put their lives in danger by refusing to eat enough can be fed against their will (Audit Commission, 1997). This moves management into the realm of treatment under parental consent in the case of minors and use of the Mental Health Act, usually in those over 16 years. Occasionally, parents refuse treatment, in which case the social worker will need to approach the courts. Needless to say, all these situations need to be handled with extreme sensitivity and only used when absolutely necessary.

Feeding a patient orally against their will using behavioural methods should always be distinguished from feeding with a nasogastric tube against their will. Although the same legal procedures apply in both cases, the latter is much rarer and should only be used in extreme circumstances as it can be countertherapeutic. However, it is necessary at times and should not be baulked from when necessary, despite its unpleasantness. It is these patients that often involve the skills of the paediatrician and their specialist dieticians; nasogastric feeding, whether voluntary or involuntary, often occurs on paediatric wards because of the medical status of the patient. Close liaison with psychiatrists and if necessary legal advisors is essential.

Summary

The eating disorders in adolescence are severe and complex disorders that have a high rate of physical morbidity and mortality. They, therefore, represent a challenge for clinicians. The impact of an eating disorder on many different aspects and systems of healthy body functioning contributes to the crucial importance of contributions from clinicians in different specialties (Box 38.1). For many years, the eating disorders have been neglected and considered disorders of "spoiled young girls", and this has contributed to poor understanding and knowledge of these illnesses.

Many advances are being made in disentangling the different aetiological factors and in the development of effective treatments (Box 38.2). There is, however, a continuous need to implement new therapeutic strategies and to evaluate the effectiveness of particular treatments.

Box 38.1 Recommendations for practice

- Adolescents with eating disorders often deny problems and are notoriously ambivalent about treatment; the clinician needs to address this and attempt to build a therapeutic alliance, rather than just respond to a medical urgency.
- Initial management always needs investigations for and treatment of any medical complications.
- The family needs to be involved at every stage of management including assessment and needs to play an important role in care provision.
- Eating disorders cause high rates of physical morbidity and mortality; they, therefore, need a careful and comprehensive approach.

Box 38.2 Key points

- Prevalence of anorexia nervosa in adolescence is 0.5–1% and for bulimia nervosa it is 1–3%.
- Both anorexia and bulimia often present in adolescence with endocrine and/or menstrual abnormalities.
- Medical complications are very common in both disorders, but can be life-threatening in anorexia nervosa.
- Eating disorders can be managed at different levels; however a multidisciplinary approach is essential.

REFERENCES

*Indicates key references.

Adams J (1993). The role of pelvic ultrasound in the management of paediatric endocrine disorders. In *Clinical Paediatric Endocrinology*, Brook C G D, eds., pp. 675–691. Blackwell Science, Oxford.

American Psychiatric Association (1994). *Diagnostic and Statistical Manual of Mental Disorders* 4th edn. American Psychiatric Association, Washington DC.

Argente J, Caballo N, Barrios V et al. (1997). Multiple endocrine abnormalities of the growth hormone and insulin-like growth factor axis in patients with anorexia nervosa: effects of short and long term weight recuperation. *J Clin Endocrinol Metab* 82, 2084–2092.

Audit Commission (1997). Department of Health, London.

Bruch H (1973). *The Golden Cage: The Enigma of Anorexia Nervosa.* Open Books, London.

Bryant-Waugh R, Lask B (1999). *Eating Disorders in Childhood and Adolescence: A Parent's Guide.* Penguin, London.

*Danziger Y, Mukamel M, Zeharia A, Dinari G, Mimouni M (1994). Stunting of growth in anorexia nervosa during the prepubertal and pubertal period. *Israeli J Med Sci* 30, 581–584.

Dreizen S, Spirakis C, Stone R (1967). A comparison of skeletal growth and maturation in undernourished and well nourished girls before and after menarche. *J Paediatr* 70, 256–263.

Fairburn C G (1997). Eating disorders. In *Science and Practice of Cognitive Behaviour Therapy*, Clark D M, Fairburn C G, eds., pp. 209–241. Oxford University Press, Oxford.

Fosson A, Knibbs J, Bryant-Waugh R, Lask B (1987). Early onset anorexia nervosa. *Arch Dis Child* 62, 114–118.

Garfinkel P E et al. (1985). Special problems of inpatient management. In *Handbook of Psychotherapy for Anorexia Nervosa and Bulimia*, Garner D M, Garfinkel P E, eds., pp. 344–359. Guilford Press, New York.

Goldstein D J, Wilson M C, Ascroft R C, Al-Banna M (1999). Effectiveness of fluoxetine therapy in bulimia nervosa regardless of co-morbid depression. *Int J Eating Disord* 25, 19–27.

Grinspoon S, Herzog D, Klibanski A (1997). Mechanisms and treatment options for bone loss in anorexia nervosa. *Psychopharmacol Bull* 33, 399–404.

Gull W W (1874). Anorexia nervosa (apepsia hysterica, anorexia hysterica). *Trans Clin Soc Lond* 7, 22.

Hall R C W, Beresford T P (1989). Medical complications of anorexia and bulimia. *Psychiatr Med* 7, 165–192.

Hansen L (1999). Olanzapine in the treatment of anorexia nervosa. *Br J Psychol* 175, 592.

Hoek H W (1991). The incidence and prevalence of anorexia nervosa and bulimia nervosa in primary care. *Psychol Med* 21, 455–460.

Holland A, Sicotte N, Treasure J (1998). Anorexia nervosa: evidence for a genetic basis. *J Psychosom Res* 32, 549–554.

Honig P, Sharman W (2000). Inpatient treatment. In *Anorexia Nervosa and Related Eating Disorders in Childhood and Adolescence*, Lask B, Bryant-Waugh R, eds., pp. 265–288. Psychology Press, Hove, UK.

Jensen V S, Mejlhede A (2000). Anorexia nervosa: treatment with olanzapine. *Br J Psychol* 177, 87.

Katzmann M, Lee S (1997). Beyond body image: the integration of feminist and transcultural theories in the understanding of self starvation. *Int J Eating Disord* 22, 385–394.

Kendler K S, MacLean C, Neale M, Kessler R, Heath A, Eaves L (1991). The genetic epidemiology of bulimia nervosa. *Am J Psychiatry* 148, 1627–1637.

*King M B (1990). Eating disorders in general practice. *J Roy Soc Med* 83, 229–232.

Klibanski A, Biller B, Shoenfeld D et al. (1995). The effects of oestrogen administration on trabecular bone loss in young women with anorexia nervosa. *J Clin Endocrinol Metab* 80, 898–904.

Kog E, Vandereycken W (1998). The facts: a review of research data on eating disorder families. In *The Family Approach to Eating Disorders: Assessment and Treatment of Anorexia Nervosa and Bulimia*, van der Eycken W, Kog E, Vanderlinden J, eds., pp. 25–26. PMA, New-York.

Lai K Y, de Bruin R, Lask B, Bryant-Waugh R, Hankins M (1994). Use of pelvic ultrasound to monitor ovarian and uterine maturity in childhood onset anorexia nervosa. *Arch Dis Child* 71, 228–231.

Lasegue C (1873). De l'anorexie hysterique. *Arch Gen Med* 21, 385–403.

Le Grange D, Eisler I, Dare C, Hodes M (1992). Family criticism and self starvation: a study of expressed emotion. *J Fam Ther* 14, 190.

Lee S, Lee A, Ngai E, Dominic T S, Wing Y K (2001). Rationales for food refusal in Chinese patients with anorexia nervosa. *Int J Eating Dis* 29, 224–229.

Magagna J (2000). Individual psychotherapy. In *Anorexia Nervosa and Related Eating Disorders in Childhood and Adolescence*, Lask B, Bryant-Waugh R, eds. Psychology Press, Hove, UK.

McCallum R W, Grill B B, Lange R, Planky M, Glass E E, Greenfeld D G (1985). Definition of a gastric emptying abnormality in patients with anorexia nervosa. *Acta Paedopsychiatr* 52, 1–11.

Muller E E, Cavagnini F, Panerai A E, Massironi R, Ferrari E, Brambilla F (1987). Neuroendocrine measures in anorexia nervosa: comparisons with primary affective disorders. *Adv Biochem Psychopharmacol* 43, 261–271.

Newman M M, Halmi K A (1988). The endocrinology of anorexia nervosa and bulimia nervosa. *Neurol Clin* 6, 195–212.

*Nicholls D, deBruyn R, Gordon I (2000). Physical assessment and complications. In *Anorexia Nervosa and Related Eating Disorders in Childhood and Adolescence*, Lask B, Bryant-Waugh R, eds. Psychology Press, Hove, UK.

Nielsen S, Moller-Madsen S, Isager T, Jorgensen J, Pagsberg K, Theander S (1998). Standardized mortality in eating disorders: a quantitative summary of previously published and new evidence. *J Psychosom Res* 44, 413–434.

Rigotti N A, Nussbaum S R, Herzog D B, Neer R M (1984). Osteoporosis in women with anorexia nervosa. *N Engl J Med* 311, 1601–1606.

Russell G (1979). Bulimia nervosa: an ominous variant of anorexia nervosa. *Psychol Med* 9, 429–448.

Russell G, Szmukler G, Dare C, Eisler I (1987). An evaluation of family therapy in anorexia nervosa and bulimia nervosa. *Arch Gen Psychiatry* 44, 1047–1056.

Selvini Palazzoli M (1974). *Self-starvation.* Chancer, London.

Sherman B M, Halmi K A, Zamudio R (1975). LH and FSH response to gonadotropin-releasing hormone in anorexia nervosa: effect of nutritional rehabilitation. *J Clin Endocrinol Metab* 41, 135–142.

Shoebridge P, Gowers S G (2000). Parental high concern and adolescent-onset anorexia nervosa. A case control study to investigate direction of causality. *Br J Psychol* 176, 132–137.

Strober M et al. (1990). A controlled family study of anorexia nervosa: evidence of familial aggregation and lack of shared transmission with affective disorders. *Int J Eating Disord* 1, 28–43.

Theander S (1970). Anorexia nervosa: a psychiatric investigation of 94 female patients. *Acta Psychiatr Scand Suppl* 214, 1–194.

Treasure J, Holland A J (1995). Genetic factors in eating disorders. *The Eating Disorders: Handbook of Theory Treatment and Research*, Szmukler G, Dare C, Treasure J, eds., pp. 65–82. Wiley, Chichester, UK.

Treasure J, Serpell L (2001). Osteoporosis in young people: research and treatment in eating disorders. *Psychiatr Clin North Am* 24, 359–370.

Treasure J, Holland A (1990). Genetic vulnerability to eating disorders: evidence in twin and family studies. In *Anorexia Nervosa*, Remschmidt H, Schmidt M, eds., pp. 59–69. Hargrefe & Huber, Toronto, Canada.

Treasure J, Collier D, Campbell I (1997). Ill fitting genes: the biology of weight and appetite control. *Psychol Med* 27, 505–508.

Treasure J (1997). *Anorexia Nervosa. A Survival Guide for Sufferers and Those Caring for Someone with an Eating Disorder*. Psychology Press, Hove, UK.

*Van Bisbergen C J M, Bennink H J T C, Odink J, Haspels A A, Koppeschaar H P F (1990). A comparative and longitudinal study on endocrine changes related to ovarian function in patients with anorexia nervosa. *J Clin Endocrinol Metab* 71, 705–711.

Ward A, Brown N, Treasure J (1997). Persistent osteopenia after recovery from anorexia nervosa. *Int J Eating Dis* 22, 71–75.

Ward A, Ramsay R, Treasure J (2000). Attachment research in eating disorders. *Br J Med Psychol* 73, 35–51.

*Weiner H (1985). The physiology of eating disorders. *Int J Eating Disord* 4, 347–388.

World Health Organization (1992). *International Classification of Diseases*, 10th edn. World Health Organization, Geneva.

39

Nutritional amenorrhoea: long-term sequelae

Joanna L. Fried, Russalind Ramos and Michelle P. Warren

Columbia Presbyterian Medical Center, New York, USA

Introduction

The amenorrhoea associated with energy deficit or nutritional imbalance has far-reaching long-term effects, including reduced bone density, stress fractures, osteopenia, osteoporosis, and infertility. This can be illustrated by referring to EG, a 54-year-old woman. She is a former professional ballet dancer who has performed on stages all over the world. Today, she relies on a walker in order to get from place to place. After a lifelong struggle with anorexia nervosa, she suffers from severe osteoporosis. She has suffered numerous fractures in the last 20 years and today her bone mineral density (BMD) is comparable to that of an 80-year-old woman. This is an extreme, though not uncommon, result of long-term nutritionally induced amenorrhoea.

Figure 39.1 shows the BMD scans for three women: a normal 25-year-old woman with regular periods; a 25-year-old woman who has had amenorrhoea for 5 years and has 30% lower total bone mass than most women her age; and a woman in her thirties with a 15 year history of amenorrhoea and osteoporotic bones.

There are a number of different environmental stressors thought to be associated with hypothalamic amenorrhoea (HA). Reproductive function may be affected by weight loss, exercise, nutritional deprivation or emotional stress. Recent research suggests that it may be an adaptive response to chronic low energy intake, and that metabolic factors may mediate reproductive adaptations in response to nutritional insults. It is more and more widely accepted that poor nutrition or an energy deficit with an adaptation to large caloric needs is fundamentally linked with a prolonged amenorrhoeic state (Couzinet et al., 1999; Warren et al., 1999; Zanker, 1999).

Hypothalamic amenorrhoea

Amenorrhoea is defined as the lack of regular menstrual periods. It may be classified as primary or secondary. Primary amenorrhoea is a delay in menarche beyond the age of 16 years. Secondary amenorrhoea is the absence of menstruation for more than six months in women who were previously cyclical (Constantini and Warren, 1994; see also Ch. 26). Premenopausal women may develop amenorrhoea for a number of reasons, among them premature ovarian failure, androgen excess, intensive physical training, nutritional restriction and stress. We will focus here on HA, which is most often associated with undernutrition and energy imbalance. HA is manifested clinically as primary amenorrhoea, secondary amenorrhoea and ovulatory dysfunction characterized by prolonged follicular or shortened luteal phases (Al-Othman and Warren, 1998).

Women with low body weight and low body fat as a result of excessive exercise or disordered eating frequently develop HA (Locke and Warren, 2000), and body composition has been hypothesized to be predictive of amenorrhoea (Warren and Shangold, 1997). Menstrual irregularity is more common in female athletes than in nonathletic women (Constantini and Warren, 1994): in the general adult population, menstrual irregularities have an estimated prevalence of 1.8–5% (Pettersson et al., 1973; Singh, 1981) while studies of adult athletes report a prevalence as high as 79% (Abraham et al., 1982). Long-distance runners, gymnasts, dancers and other athletes are often pressured to keep their body fat below 10% of their total body weight. This amenorrhoea is similar to that seen in women with eating disorders, particularly anorexia nervosa. Anorexia nervosa in young women is associated with

Paediatric and Adolescent Gynaecology, ed. Adam Balen et al. Published by Cambridge University Press.
© Cambridge University Press 2004.

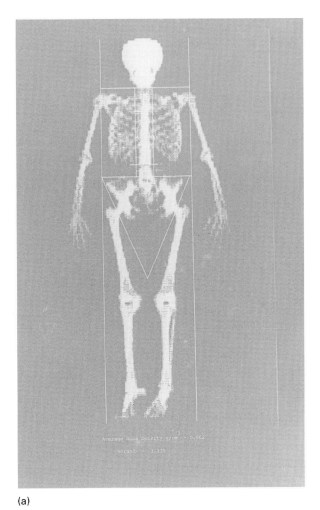

(a)

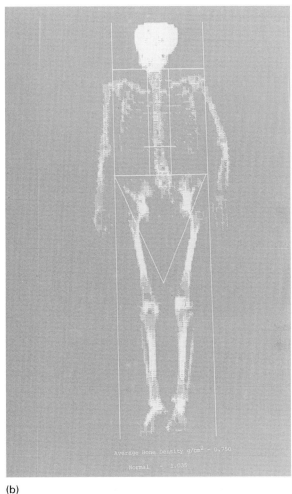

(b)

Fig. 39.1. Bone density scans. (a) A normal 25-year-old woman with regular periods. (b) A 25-year-old woman who has had amenorrhoea for 5 years and has 30% lower bone mass than most women her age. (c) The osteoporotic bones of a woman in her thirties who has a 15 year history of amenorrhoea.

severe weight loss and amenorrhoea, which often reverses with weight gain (see Ch. 38). Amenorrhoea also occurs in at least 50% women with bulimia nervosa without any loss of body mass (Pirke et al., 1987).

Functional HA is HA of unknown aetiology in normal-weight, nonathletic women and is often thought to be psychogenic, caused by stress. However, mounting evidence suggests the possibility that this so-called idiopathic amenorrhoea is actually a response to nutritional restriction and the resulting endocrine and metabolic response (Laughlin, 1999; Schweiger, 1991; Warren et al., 1994, 1999; Zucker and Zucker, 1961). There is evidence of subclinical eating disorders in weight-stable, nonathletic women with functional HA, and unbalanced nutrient intake in psychogenic functional HA has been associated with multiple endocrine–metabolic alterations (Laughlin et al., 1998). While stress

may contribute to the disordered eating, which, in turn, may cause amenorrhoea, it is unlikely that the stress itself is directly responsible for menstrual dysfunction in women with functional HA.

Even in women without clinically defined eating disorders, excessive dieting or nutritional imbalances often cause hormonal abnormalities similar to those seen in anorexics or athletes. Reduced ovarian function is one of the first adaptations associated with caloric reduction (Schweiger et al., 1987). One 1992 study (Schweiger et al., 1992) compared a group of restrained eaters with a group of controls matched for age, age of menarche, absolute height and weight, and body mass index (BMI) and found significant differences in menstrual cyclicity. Restrained eaters demonstrated reduced caloric intake, avoidance of fat, increased intake of artificial sweeteners and diet

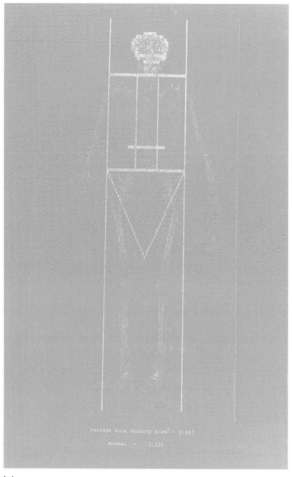

(c)

Fig. 39.1. (*Cont.*)

Table 39.1. Nutritional patterns of amenorrhoeic and normally cycling women

	Amenorrheics	Controls	p-value
Number	18	34	
Weight (lb)	110.30 ± 13.00	125.00 ± 11.10	< 0.001
Percentage of ideal weight	89.77 ± 10.11	97.20 ± 13.61	< 0.05
Percentage body fat	20.79 ± 4.48	27.06 ± 3.96	< 0.001
Anorexia	8	1	< 0.001
Bulimia	4	2	NS
Energy expended (Kcal/day)	2303.73 ± 438.50	2576.72 ± 370.21	< 0.05
Energy intake (Kcal/day)	1936.61 ± 675.07	1712.67 ± 500.57	NS
Fibre intake (g/day)	26.14 ± 13.25	14.69 ± 9.36	< 0.001
Fat intake (g/day)	20.70 ± 4.48	27.10 ± 3.96	< 0.001
Percentage engaging in intense physical activity	85	58	< 0.05

Source: Data are presented as mean $\pm$ SD; NS, not significant. Adapted from Warren et al., 1994.

1996). Table 39.1 illustrates the results of a study of amenorrhoeic and normal women, matched for age and height. The amenorrheics engaged in more aerobic activity despite expending fewer calories per day, ate twice as much fibre and less fat, and, although they denied them, had a higher incidence of eating disorders (Warren et al., 1994).

Consequently, while amenorrhoeic women have varied backgrounds, psychiatric profiles and professions, it is increasingly agreed that nutritional restriction and disordered eating play a central role in the development of all causes of HA.

Aetiology

Normal menstrual cyclicity is the result of a number of different endocrine systems working together. Puberty is initiated when the hypothalamus at the base of the brain is activated to secrete gonadotrophin-releasing hormone (GnRH) (see also Chs. 4 and 5). Released in pulses occurring every 60 to 90 minutes, GnRH signals the anterior pituitary to release bursts of gonadotrophins (luteinizing hormone (LH) and follicle-stimulating hormone (FSH)), which in turn stimulate the ovary to release the mature follicle. The rhythm of the GnRH pulse is controlled by a pulse generator located in the arcuate nucleus in the medial central area of the hypothalamus. The pulses of

products and increased variability of food intake. The restrained eaters also demonstrated a higher rate of irregular menstrual cycles, with reduced or shortened progesterone production during the luteal phase (Schweiger et al., 1992).

Evidence of subclinical eating disorders has been found in weight-stable, nonathletic women with functional HA as well as a significant restriction of dietary fat intake (Laughlin and Yen, 1996). While women with functional HA have been found to have caloric intakes comparable to normally cycling women, they consume 50% less fat and significantly more carbohydrates and fibre: an unbalanced nutrient intake that is associated with multiple endocrine–metabolic alterations (Laughlin et al., 1998). The same imbalance in dietary intake has been observed in women with exercise-associated amenorrhoea (Laughlin and Yen,

GnRH activate a sequence of events in the reproductive tract via the hypothalamic–pituitary–ovarian (HPO) axis. In turn, the ovaries secrete oestrogens (mostly oestradiol), progestins (mostly progesterone) and androgens. These steroids regulate the HPO axis through a feedback mechanism by acting directly on the pituitary or indirectly on the hypothalamic GnRH pulses (Ferin et al., 1993).

The physiological basis for HA is the disruption of the hypothalamus' pulsatile secretion of GnRH. The pulse generator appears to be very sensitive to stress and metabolic factors and is highly sensitive to environmental insults, particularly weight loss. GnRH secretion also appears to be sensitive to decreased energy intake, particularly when expenditure of exercise exceeds the dietary intake (Warren and Shangold, 1997). GnRH inhibition then lowers the anterior pituitary's secretion of LH and FSH, which shuts down or limits ovarian stimulation and oestradiol production. A prolonged follicular phase, or the absence of a critical LH or oestradiol surge mid-cycle, results in the mild or intermittent suppression of menstrual cycles frequently observed in athletes. Lack of pituitary stimulation results in delayed menarche, or primary or secondary amenorrhoea (Loucks et al., 1989; Warren, 1980).

Early research focused on body composition and the stress of exercise as possible causes of amenorrhoea in athletes. However, more recent evidence suggests that the primary factor in reproductive dysfunction is the energy deficit women incur when their daily caloric intake is insufficient for the level of their activity (Loucks and Heath, 1994; Loucks et al., 1995; Myerson et al., 1991; Warren et al., 1999). Moreover, a significant amount of recent research suggests that a decrease in resting metabolic rate is associated with a negative energy balance and with menstrual dysfunction (Kaufman et al., 2002; Salisbury et al., 1995; Tuschl et al., 1990). Metabolic rate may remain depressed in individuals who maintain a body weight lower than their normal or genetically predetermined weight (Leibel et al., 1995), as observed in recovered anorectics (Brooks-Gunn et al., 1987) and amenorrhoeic runners (Myerson et al., 1987). Even women who maintain a normal weight may suffer an energy deficit; their normal weight is likely maintained by a decrease in metabolic rate (Myerson et al., 1991).

The metabolic adaptation to energy deficit or starvation is evident in a number of factors including lowered tri-iodothyronine (and occasionally thyroxine) levels and clinical signs of hypothyroidism (Fowler et al., 1972; Kiyohara et al., 1989; Moshang and Utiger, 1977; Warren and van de Wiele, 1973). Metabolism of certain steroids like testosterone is similar to that seen in hypothyroidism (Boyar and Bradlow, 1977). Maximal aerobic power (volume of oxygen utilized) and heart rates are reduced, indicating an adaptation to low caloric intake (Fohlin, 1975). Basal growth hormone levels are elevated above normal levels, and insulin-like growth factor-1 (IGF-1) is suppressed; both of these abnormalities resolve with nutritional therapy (Newman and Halmi, 1988). Mean levels of cortisol are elevated, and 24-hour studies of women with HA have found that episodic and circadian rhythms are normal but levels are elevated (Boyar et al., 1977), suggesting that a new set-point has been determined by the hypothalamic–pituitary–adrenal (HPA) axis.

In addition to metabolic alterations, HA is associated with a constellation of neuroendocrine secretory disturbances. Low body fat or body weight appears to be associated with the neuroendocrine controls concerned with the maintenance of normal menstrual cycles in exercising women (Warren, 1983; Vigersky et al., 1977). Some of the neuropeptides involved in the control of GnRH release are opioids, neuropeptide Y and corticotrophin-releasing factor; neurotransmitters that may play a role include noradrenaline, dopamine, serotonin (5-hydroxytryptamine), melatonin and gamma-aminobutyric acid (Genazzani et al., 1998). However, because neurohormones cannot be accurately measured in the peripheral circulation, their roles in the aetiology of HA are not yet well defined (Ferin et al., 1993).

New research on amenorrhoea and body composition was prompted after the 1994 discovery of leptin, a polypeptide of 167 amino acid residues secreted primarily by the adipocyte (Ducy et al., 2000; Zhang et al., 1994; see also Ch. 6). Leptin levels appear to be regulated by total energy intake and fat stores and correlate significantly with BMI in humans (Macut et al., 1998). Studies have shown that leptin-deficient rodents tend to be amenorrhoeic and infertile (Legradi et al., 1997, 1998). Low leptin levels have been associated with amenorrhoea (Miller et al., 1998; Warren et al., 1999) and with disordered eating (Warren et al., 1999); it appears that if leptin falls below a critical level, menstruation will not occur (Kopp et al., 1997). Because leptin is a hormone regulator of the basal metabolic rate, it is thought to be a particularly important indicator of nutritional status (Maffei et al., 1995); consequently, leptin may be a significant mediator of reproductive function in that it responds to a negative energy balance found in women with exercise-induced HA (Laughlin and Yen, 1997). Leptin receptors are found on hypothalamic neurons thought to be involved in control of the GnRH pulse generator, suggesting that it may trigger changes in GnRH pulsatility (Cheung et al., 1997).

Leptin also plays a role in thyroid function and the initiation of puberty; in the presence of nutritional deficiencies, alterations in leptin levels are directly associated with thyroid hormone changes (Warren et al., 1999). Thus, leptin may act not only as a regulator of metabolic rates but also as a mediator of menstrual status, responding to starvation by slowing metabolism and possibly returning a woman to a prepubertal-like state.

Bone

HA during adolescence in young women is associated with reduced bone accretion or premature bone loss (Biller et al., 1989; Dhuper et al., 1990; Drinkwater et al., 1984; Jonnavithula et al., 1993; Lindberg et al., 1984; Marcus et al., 1985; Rigotti et al., 1984, 1991; Warren et al., 1991, 1986), placing them at high risk for fractures, significant osteopenia and severe osteoporosis at menopause. Recent research suggests that poor nutrition or an energy deficit with an adaptation to large caloric needs is fundamentally linked not only with a prolonged amenorrhoeic state but also with osteopenia (Tsafriri et al., 1982; Zanker, 1999; Zanker and Swaine, 1998a,b).

Bone density is responsive to mechanical loading, and exercise is beneficial in preserving and increasing bone mass; in postmenopausal women, exercise will offset the loss of bone mass associated with hypooestrogenism and may even increase BMD above baseline. However, studies of hypooestrogenic ballet dancers suggest that they may not accumulate bone in response to mechanical stress (Warren et al., 1991) and amenorrhoeic athletes consistently exhibit spinal BMD 10–20% lower than their eumenorrhoeic counterparts (Bennell et al., 1997; Fisher et al., 1986; Lindberg et al., 1984; Lloyd et al., 1986; Wolman et al., 1990). When peak bone mass is not attained, the relative osteopenia in weight-bearing bones results in a higher risk for injury. A high incidence of stress fractures (61%), directly related to delayed menarche, has been reported in young ballet dancers (Warren et al., 1986); one study of ballet dancers found that the incidence of both scoliosis and stress fractures rose with each year of delayed menarche (Khan et al., 1999). High-impact activity appears to have a beneficial effect on BMD primarily at the hip (Khan et al., 1999). Amenorrhoea in athletic women affects trabecular and cortical bone, and studies have shown that spinal BMD is particularly affected in amenorrhoeic athletes (Rutherford, 1993): amenorrhoeic athletes' vertebral BMD has been found to be up to 25% lower than athletes with normal menstrual cycles (Gibson et al., 1999). Weight-

bearing physical activity does not completely compensate for the side effects of reduced oestrogen levels even in weight-bearing bones in the lower extremities and the spine (Pettersson et al., 1999).

Two homeostatic mechanisms act on bone simultaneously: hormones and mechanical stress. In normal circumstances, these homeostatic mechanisms maintain both skeletal integrity and serum calcium levels. However, with ageing or menstrual disturbance, factors such as diet, hormonal levels and mechanical strain cause bones to become more vulnerable to fracture and osteoporosis (Smith and Gilligan, 1994).

At least 40% of bone mass is formed during adolescence and young adulthood, making this period critical to women's health (Kreipe, 1992; Kreipe and Forbes, 1990; Ott, 1990; Riggs and Eastell, 1986; Warren and Shangold, 1997). The amount of bone attained during adolescence is a major determinant for fractures and osteoporosis later in life. As the skeleton enlarges in children and adolescents, bones are constantly growing; bones model as bone mass is added to areas of high loading or stress, and remodel as fatigue-damaged bone is resorbed and replaced by new bone (Barr and McKay, 1998). Women who fail to reach peak bone mass (the maximal amount of bone tissue accrued in individual bones and the whole skeleton) are at an increased risk for osteoporosis later in life, and the reduction of bone mass accretion during adolescence may be a major cause of low BMD and fracture in old age (Bass and Myburgh, 2000). This is a significant problem for women with HA. After the age of 40, bone mass begins to decline (Arnaud, 1996).

It is unclear what changes in bone metabolism cause osteoporosis in women with HA. One 1999 study of women with anorexia nervosa suggested that bone formation is reduced while bone resorption remains normal (Soyka et al., 1999), while another suggested that bone formation is decreased and bone resorption increased (Bruni et al., 2000). Further analyses of bone turnover indices in women with HA and anorexia nervosa have also produced inconsistent results, with some data suggesting normal bone turnover, while others suggest low bone formation that is uncoupled from bone resorption (Grinspoon et al., 1999; Kreipe et al., 1993). Results of a 1998 study of amenorrhoeic long-distance runners demonstrated reductions in bone turnover and, in particular, bone formation (Zanker and Swaine, 1998a). The reduced bone formation was linked to a low BMI and oestrogen deficiency (Zanker and Swaine, 1998b). While the effects of prolonged oestrogen deficiency on adolescents are not fully understood, recent research suggests that hypooestrogenism in young

Table 39.2. Bone density in amenorrhoea in a 2-year longitudinal study

Bone density	Amenorrhoeic ($n = 44$)	Resumption of menses ($n = 7$)	Normal ($n = 67$)
Spine			
Baseline (g/cm^2 ± SE)	1.16 ± 0.04	0.99 ± 0.05	1.27 ± 0.03
24 months (g/cm^2 ± SE)	1.20 ± 0.04	1.16 ± 0.06	1.31 ± 0.02
Change (%)	4.05 ± 1.95	$17.47 \pm 4.93^*$	4.08 ± 1.14
Wrist			
Baseline (g/cm^2 ± SE)	0.61 ± 0.02	0.59 ± 0.05	0.66 ± 0.01
24 months (g/cm^2 ± SE)	0.62 ± 0.03	0.67 ± 0.03	0.67 ± 0.01
Change (%)	3.40 ± 2.20	$17.54 \pm 8.75^*$	2.89 ± 1.39
Foot			
Baseline (g/cm^2 ± SE)	0.84 ± 0.03	0.76 ± 0.03	0.87 ± 0.02
24 months (g/cm^2 ± SE)	0.83 ± 0.02	0.81 ± 0.03	0.86 ± 0.01
Change (%)	-0.83 ± 2.84	7.05 ± 4.79	-0.70 ± 1.60

$^*p < 0.001$.
Source: From Warren et al. (2002).

women decreases bone density and increases the risk of stress fractures and osteoporosis (Warren and Shangold, 1997), causing serious bone loss similar to that which occurs after artificial or spontaneous menopause (Cann et al., 1984; Rigotti et al., 1984).

A recent study (Warren et al., 2002) followed 111 subjects, 44 of whom had HA and 54 of whom were dancers. Both exercising and nonexercising amenorrhoeics showed reduced BMD in the spine, wrist and foot (Table 39.2). During the course of the study, seven of the amenorrhoeic women resumed menses, and while these seven showed an increase in spine and wrist BMD of 17%, they did not achieve normalization of BMD, suggesting that reduced bone accretion may result in a permanent failure to achieve peak bone mass. This underscores the importance of intervention in HA, either preventative or therapeutic (Warren et al., 2002).

Early bone loss and osteoporosis are well-documented and common complications of anorexia nervosa (Biller et al., 1989; Brotman and Stern, 1985; Hay et al., 1992; Rigotti et al., 1984; Salisbury and Mitchell, 1991). Up to one-third of females who recovered from anorexia nervosa during adolescence were found to have persistent osteopenia (Bachrach et al., 1991). Young women with anorexia nervosa may suffer irreversible developmental and growth retardation; older chronic anorectics are at a higher risk for pathological fractures (Hartman et al., 1999).

Other nutritionally regulated processes may underlie the osteopenia. Hypercortisolaemia (Ding et al., 1988; Loucks et al., 1989; Prior et al., 1990), hypoprogestinaemia (Prior et al., 1990), IGF-1 deficiency (Zanker, 1999) or other metabolic adaptations seen in amenorrhoeic women may contribute to osteopenia. Undernutrition lowers bone formation markers (triiodothyronine and IGF-1) in amenorrhoeic runners but not in controls (Zanker, 1999). A study of ballet dancers showed normal vitamin D and parathyroid levels, suggesting that these may not be the causal factors in the bone loss (Warren et al., 1986). In past studies of women with anorexia nervosa, levels of IGF-1 and triiodothyronine, two nutritionally dependent hormones, predicted the change in trabecular bone mass with oestrogen–progestin therapy (Klibanski et al., 1995).

New research has suggested that amenorrhoeic women with anorexia nervosa have significantly lower serum testosterone levels compared with normal controls, and that this androgen deficiency is a determinant of bone density BMD (Miller et al., 2001). The pathophysiology of testosterone deficiency and the possible effects of androgen replacement have yet to be explored, but these findings raise new questions about testosterone's role in reduced BMD.

Reproduction

Patients who are partially recovered from anorexia nervosa tend to have exaggerated responses to GnRH (Beaumont et al., 1976; Mecklenburg et al., 1974; Warren et al., 1975). This hyperreactive phase is characterized by a greatly increased LH response. As weight is gained, the normal response ratios return: the LH response is much greater than that of FSH (Fritz and Speroff, 1983). When an anorectic patient attains normal weight, GnRH secretion is released from inhibition and reproductive hormones and ovarian morphology retrace their way through pubertal development (Kanders et al., 1988; van Binsbergen et al., 1990; Warren et al., 1975). However, HA and reproductive dysfunction may persist if disordered eating is present, suggesting the persistence of metabolic factors inhibiting reproduction that may be independent of weight.

One of the intriguing occurrences in anorexia nervosa is the persistence of the amenorrhoea despite a return to normal weight, which may occur in up to 10–30% of recovered anorectics (Falk and Halmi, 1982; Kohmura et al., 1986; Kreipe et al., 1989a). This persistence has been tied to disordered eating (Kreipe et al., 1989b) and suggests that metabolic abnormalities may persist despite a return to normal weight. In fact, an immature pattern of LH secretion may occur in this group despite a normal weight (Katz et al., 1978), suggesting that a factor other than weight is responsible for the hypothalamic dysfunction.

It has been suggested that women with nutritionally induced HA may have a higher incidence of psychosexual dysfunction than normal controls (Hamann and Matthaei, 1996), but a more thorough investigation into this aspect of amenorrhoea is needed before conclusions can be drawn.

While patients with anorexia nervosa can become pregnant despite amenorrhoea by induction of ovulation, it is negligent to provide such therapy. For although ovulation may be easily induced there is a high rate of miscarriage, intrauterine growth retardation and stillbirth in women who are undernourished: as after all this is "nature's way" of preventing pregnancy (Nagatani et al., 1998). Women who have recovered weight after anorexia may have an increased incidence of infertility if they still have an active eating disorder (Bulik et al., 1999; Conti et al., 1998; Franko and Walton, 1993). Some may still have menstrual disturbance and anovulation despite a gain in weight as a consequence of underlying polycystic ovary syndrome (see also Chs. 6 and 27).

Treatment recommendations

Ideally, women should not develop long-term amenorrhoea. In women with amenorrhoea, a physical and pelvic examination is indicated to exclude androgenization, galactorrhoea and hyperprolactinaemia, as well as pregnancy. A careful history of weight loss and eating disorders should also be taken; eating disorders can often be missed, and often a standardized scale or diagnostic interview will be helpful in making the diagnosis (Warren and Shangold, 1997). In women with nutritional imbalances or disordered eating, one of the most important aspects of treatment is addressing and reversing unhealthy eating behaviours. A history of amenorrhoea as an adolescent or young adult may be the only causal event in women presenting with osteoporosis or osteopenia later in life.

The current mode of treatment for patients suffering from nutritional amenorrhoea should aim at improving diet, maintaining a positive energy balance and achieving weight gain (although this is admittedly difficult, especially among patients whose lifestyles demand low weight). Assessment of nutritional intake, including calcium and vitamin D, should be part of the management of the patient, and calcium supplements at 1500 mg daily and vitamin D supplements at 400 mg daily may be given. Often, patients with nutritional amenorrhoea are resistant to changing restrictive eating patterns, and nutritional and/or psychiatric counselling may be necessary. Weight gain is particularly important in the management of these patients, and a 1–2 kg increase in body weight is recommended. If weight gain is not observed within three months, a progesterone challenge may be performed. The patient will not experience a withdrawal bleed after progesterone if she is hypooestrogenic, although some patients, particularly as they near recovery, will experiences menses with this challenge. An ultrasound scan of endometrial thickness will also help with the assessment of oestrogenization. If the progesterone challenge does not result in resumption of menstruation, oral contraceptives are then used to restore menses and possibly prevent bone loss, but their use is controversial. In our experience, oral contraceptives have not been convincing useful therapy, but one randomized trial did show benefit on BMD among women with HA (Hergenroeder et al., 1997).

Because adolescent patients with anorexia nervosa are at high risk of reduced BMD, densitometry is often recommended to determine the degree of osteopenia (Barash et al., 1996). It is important to note that bone age should be measured in younger patients with a radiograph of the wrist, and that oral contraceptives or hormone replacement therapy should only be prescribed when bone growth is completed or adequate. Although oestrogen therapy and weight gain may not fully restore BMD in patients recovering from HA, upon restoration of menses, bone mass can probably be preserved.

Administration of short-term recombinant IGF-1, a bone trophic hormone, has been found to increase markers of bone turnover in patients with anorexia nervosa (Gordon et al., 1999; Grinspoon et al., 1996). Given that undernutrition appears to be directly linked to subnormal IGF-1 levels, it is speculated to be a major contributor to the pathogenesis of osteopenia in anorexia nervosa and potentially in all forms of HA. Short-term supplementation of the adrenal steroid dehydroepiandrosterone, speculated to be linked to low BMD among patients with anorexia nervosa, has been shown to significantly decrease levels of bone resorption and increase markers of bone formation (Gordon et al., 1999). These recent developments are important in that they could redirect the focus of treatment towards correcting the metabolic abnormalities and androgen deficiencies that impact bone formation and thereby decrease the risk for osteopenia and osteoporosis. Both IGF-1 and dehydroepiandrosterone have therapeutic potential; however, further investigation is warranted before specific recommendations can be made.

Summary

A complete understanding of the causes and mechanisms of HA remain unknown, and continuing research on metabolic rate, leptin and other factors will ultimately answer many of the outstanding questions and will help to create even better tools for treating this disorder. In the meantime, when treating patients for nutritionally induced amenorrhoea, it is important to identify contributing factors such as metabolic insufficiency, disordered eating and nutritional restriction and to treat these factors in order to prevent such long-term effects as osteopenia, osteoporosis, stress fractures and reproductive problems.

REFERENCES

Abraham S F, Beumont P J V, Fraser I S, Llewellyn-Jones D (1982). Body weight, exercise and menstrual status among ballet dancers in training. *Br J Obstet Gynaecol* 89, 507–510.

Al-Othman F N, Warren M P (1998). Exercise, the menstrual cycle, and reproduction. *Infertil Reprod Med Clin North Am* 9, 667–687.

Arnaud C D (1996). Osteoporosis: Using 'bone markers' for diagnosis and monitoring. *Geriatrics* 51, 24–30.

Bachrach L K, Katzman D K, Litt I F, Guido D, Marcus R (1991). Recovery from osteopenia in adolescent girls with anorexia nervosa. *J Clin Endocrinol Metab* 72, 602–606.

Barash I A, Cheung C, Weigle D S et al. (1996). Leptin is a metabolic signal to the reproductive system. *Endocrinology* 137, 3144–3147.

Barr S I, McKay H A (1998). Nutrition, exercise, and bone status in youth. *Int J Sports Med* 8, 124–142.

Bass S L, Myburgh K H (2000). The role of exercise in the attainment of peak bone mass and bone strength. In *Contemporary Endocrinology: Sports Endocrinology*, Warren M P, Constantini N W, eds., pp. 253–280. Humana Press, Totowa, NJ.

Beaumont P J V, George G C W, Pimstone B L, Vinik A L (1976). Body weight and pituitary response to hypothalamic releasing hormone in patients with anorexia nervosa. *J Clin Endocrinol Metab* 43, 487.

Bennell K L, Malcolm S A, Wark J D et al. (1997). Skeletal effects of menstrual disturbances in athletes. *Scand J Med Sci Sports* 7, 261–273.

Biller B M K, Saxe V, Herzog D B, Rosenthal D I, Holzman S, Klibanski A (1989). Mechanisms of osteoporosis in adult and adolescent women with anorexia nervosa. *J Clin Endocrinol Metab* 68, 548–554.

Boyar R M, Bradlow H L (1977). Studies of testosterone metabolism in anorexia nervosa. In *Anorexia Nervosa*, Vigersky R, ed., p. 271. Raven Press, New York.

Boyar R M, Hellman L D, Roffwarg H et al. (1977). Cortisol secretion and metabolism in anorexia nervosa. *N Engl J Med* 296, 190–193.

Brooks-Gunn J, Warren M P, Hamilton L H (1987). The relation of eating problems and amenorrhea in ballet dancers. *Med Sci Sports Exerc* 19, 41–44.

Brotman A W, Stern T A (1985). Osteoporosis and pathological fractures in anorexia nervosa. *Am J Psychiatry* 142, 495–496.

Bruni V, Dei M, Vicini I, Beninato L, Magnani L (2000). Estrogen replacement therapy in the management of osteopenia related to eating disorders. *Ann N Y Acad Sci* 900, 416–421.

Bulik C M, Sullivan P F, Fear J L, Pickering A, Dawn A, McCullin M (1999). Fertility and reproduction in women with anorexia nervosa: a controlled study. *J Clin Psychiatry* 60, 130–135.

Cann C E, Martin M C, Genant H K, Jaffe R B (1984). Decreased spinal mineral content in amenorrheic women. *J Am Med Assoc* 251, 626–629.

Cheung C C, Clifton D K, Steiner R A (1997). Proopiomelanocortin neurons are direct targets for leptin in the hypothalamus. *Endocrinology* 138, 4489–4492.

Constantini N W, Warren M P (1994). Physical activity, fitness, and reproductive health in women: clinical observations. In *Physical Activity, Fitness, and Health: International Proceedings and Consensus Statement* Bouchard C, Shephard R J, Stephens T, eds., pp. 955–966. Human Kinetics, Champaign.

Conti J, Abraham S, Taylor A (1998). Eating behavior and pregnancy outcome. *J Psychosom Res* 44, 465–477.

Couzinet B, Young J, Brailly S, Le Bouc Y, Chanson P, Schaison G (1999). Functional hypothalamic amenorrhoea: a partial and reversible gonadotrophin deficiency of nutritional origin. *Clin Endocrinol* 50, 229–235.

Dhuper S, Warren M P, Brooks-Gunn J, Fox R P (1990). Effects of hormonal status on bone density in adolescent girls. *J Clin Endocrinol Metab* 71, 1083–1088.

Ding J H, Sheckter C B, Drinkwater B L, Soules M R, Bremner W J (1988). High serum cortisol levels in exercise-associated amenorrhea. *Ann Intern Med* 108, 530–534.

Drinkwater B L, Nilson K, Chesnut C H, III, Bremner W J, Shainholtz S, Southworth M B (1984). Bone mineral content of amenorrheic and eumenorrheic athletes. *N Eng J Med* 311, 277–281.

Ducy P, Amling M, Takeda S et al. (2000). Leptin inhibits bone formation through a hypothalamic relay: a central control of bone mass. *Cell* 100, 197–207.

Falk J R, Halmi K A (1982). Amenorrhea in anorexia nervosa: examination of the critical body weight hypothesis. *Biol Psychiatry* 17, 799–806.

Ferin M, Jewelewicz R, Warren M P (1993). *The Menstrual Cycle*, Oxford University Press, New York.

Fisher E C, Nelson M E, Frontera W R et al. (1986). Bone mineral content and levels of gonadotropins and estrogen in amenorrheic running women. *J Clin Endocrinol Metab* 62, 1232–1236.

Fohlin L (1975). Exercise, performance, and body dimensions in anorexia nervosa before and after rehabilitation. *Acta Med Scand* 204, 61.

Fowler P B S, Banim S O, Ikram H (1972). Prolonged ankle reflex in anorexia nervosa. *Lancet* ii, 307.

Franko D L, Walton B E (1993). Pregnancy and eating disorders: a review and clinical implications. *Int J Eat Disord* 13, 41–47.

Fritz M A, Speroff L (1983). Current concepts of the endocrine characteristics of normal menstrual function: the key to diagnosis and management of menstrual disorders. *Clin Obstet Gynecol* 26, 647–689.

Genazzani A R, Petraglia F, Bernardi F et al. (1998). Circulating levels of allopregnanolone in humans: gender, age, and endocrine influences. *J Clin Endocrinol Metab* 83, 2099–2103.

Gibson J H, Mitchell A, Reeve J, Harries M G (1999). Treatment of reduced bone mineral density in athletic amenorrhea: a pilot study. *Osteoporos Int* 10, 284–289.

Gordon C M, Grace E, Emans S J, Goodman E, Crawford M H, Leboff M S (1999). Changes in bone turnover markers and menstrual function after short-term oral DHEA in young women with anorexia nervosa. *J Bone Min Res* 14, 136–145.

Grinspoon S, Baum H, Lee K, Anderson E, Herzog D, Klibanski A (1996). Effects of short-term recombinant human insulin-like growth factor I administration on bone turnover in osteopenic women with anorexia nervosa. *J Clin Endocrinol Metab* 81, 3864–3870.

Grinspoon S, Miller K K, Coyle C (1999). Severity of osteopenia in estrogen-deficient women with anorexia nervosa and hypothalamic amenorrhea. *J Clin Endcrinol Metab* 68, 402–411.

Hamann A, Matthaei S (1996). Regulation of energy balance by leptin. *Exp Clin Endocrinol Diabetes* 104, 293–300.

Hartman D, Crisp A, Rooney B, Rackow C, Atkinson R, Patel S (1999). Bone density of women who have recovered from anorexia nervosa. *Int J Eat Disord* 28, 107–112.

Hay P, Delahunt J W, Hall A, Mitchell A W, Harper G, Salmond C (1992). Predictors of osteopenia in premenopausal women with anorexia nervosa. *Calcif Tissue Int* 50, 498–501.

Hergenroeder A C, O'Brian Smith E, Shypailo R et al. (1997). Bone mineral changes in young women with hypothalamic amenorrhea treated with oral contraceptives, medroxyprogesterone, or placebo over 12 months. *Am J Obstet Gynecol* 176, 1017–1025.

Jonnavithula S, Warren M P, Fox R P, Lazaro M I (1993). Bone density is compromised in amenorrheic women despite return of menses: A 2-year study. *Obstet Gynecol* 81, 669–674.

Kanders B, Dempster D W, Lindsay R (1988). Interaction of calcium nutrition and physical activity on bone mass in young women. *J Bone Miner Res* 3, 145–149.

Katz J L, Boyar R M, Roffwarg H, Hellman L, Weiner H (1978). Weight and circadian luteinizing hormone secretory pattern in anorexia nervosa. *Psychosom Med* 40, 549–567.

Kaufman B A, Warren M P, Dominguez J L, Wang J, Heymsfield S B, Pierson R N (2002). Bone density and amenorrhea in ballet dancers is related to a decreased resting metabolic rate. *J Clin Endocrinol Metab* 87, 2777–2783.

Khan K M, Warren M P, Stiehl A, McKay H A, Wark J D (1999). Bone mineral density in active and retired ballet dancers. *J Dance Med Science* 3, 15–23.

Kiyohara K, Tamai H, Takaichi Y, Nakagawa T, Kumagai L F (1989). Decreased thyroidal triiodothyronine secretion in patients with anorexia nervosa: influence of weight recovery. *Am J Clin Nutrit* 50, 767–772.

Klibanski A, Biller B M K, Schoenfeld D A, Herzog D B, Saxe V C (1995). The effects of estrogen administration on trabecular bone loss in young women with anorexia nervosa. *J Clin Endocrinol Metab* 80, 898–904.

Kohmura H, Miyake A, Aono T, Tanizawa O (1986). Recovery of reproductive function in patients with anorexia nervosa: A 10-year follow up study. *Eur J Obstet Gynaecol Reprod Biol* 22, 293–296.

Kopp W, Blum W F, von Prittwitz S et al. (1997). Low leptin levels predict amenorrhea in underweight and eating disordered females. *Mol Psychiatry* 2, 335–340.

Kreipe R E (1992). Bones of today, bones of tomorrow. [Editorial]. *Am J Dis Child* 146, 22–25.

Kreipe R E, Forbes G B (1990). Osteoporosis: a 'new morbidity' for dieting female adolescents? *Pediatrics* 86, 478–480.

Kreipe R E, Churchill B H, Strauss J (1989a). Long-term outcome of adolescents with anorexia nervosa. *Am J Dis Child* 143, 1322–1327.

Kreipe R E, Strauss J, Hodgeman C H, Ryan R M (1989b). Menstrual cycle abnormalities and subclinical eating disorders: a preliminary report. *Psychosom Med* 51, 81–86.

Kreipe R E, Hicks D G, Rosier R N, Puzas J E (1993). Preliminary findings on the effects of sex hormones on bone metabolism in anorexia nervosa. *J Adolesc Health* 14, 319–324.

Laughlin G A (1999). The role of nutrition in the etiology of functional hypothalamic amenorrhea. *Curr Opin Endocr Diabetes* 6, 38–43.

Laughlin G A, Yen S S C (1996). Nutritional and endocrine: metabolic aberrations in amenorrheic athletes. *J Clin Endocrinol Metab* 81, 4301–4309.

(1997). Hypoleptinemia in women athletes: absence of a diurnal rhythm with amenorrhea. *J Clin Endocrinol Metab* 82, 318–321.

Laughlin G A, Dominguez C E, Yen S S C (1998). Nutritional and endocrine-metabolic aberrations in women with functional hypothalamic amenorrhea. *J Clin Endcrinol Metab* 83, 25–32.

Legradi G, Emerson C H, Ahima R S, Flier J S, Lechan R M (1997). Leptin prevents fasting-induced suppression of prothyrotropin-releasing hormone messenger ribonucleic acid in neurons of the hypothalamic paraventricular nucleus. *Endocrinology* 138, 2569–2576.

Legradi G, Emerson C H, Ahima R S, Rand W M, Flier J S, Lechan R M (1998). Arcuate nucleus ablation prevents fasting-induced suppression of proTRH mRNA in the hypothalamic paraventricular nucleus. *Neuroendocrinology* 68, 89–97.

Leibel R L, Rosenbaum M, Hirsch J (1995). Changes in energy expenditure resulting from altered body weight. *N Engl J Med* 333, 343–347.

Lindberg J S, Fears W B, Hunt M M, Powell M R, Boll D, Wade C E (1984). Exercise-induced amenorrhea and bone density. *Ann Intern Med* 101, 647–648.

Lloyd S J, Triantafyllou S J, Baker E R et al. (1986). Women athletes with menstrual irregularity have increased musculoskeletal injuries. *Med Sci Sports Exerc* 18, 374–379.

Locke R J, Warren M P (2000). How to prevent bone loss in women with hypothalamic amenorrhea. *Womens Health Primary Care* 3, 270–278.

Loucks A B, Heath E M (1994). Induction of low-T_3 syndrome in exercising women occurs at a threshold of energy availability. *Am J Physiol* 266, R817–R823.

Loucks A B, Mortola J F, Girton L, Yen S S C (1989). Alterations in the hypothalamic–pituitary–ovarian and the hypothalamic–pituitary–adrenal axes in athletic women. *J Clin Endocrinol Metab* 68, 402–411.

Loucks A B, Brown R, King K, Thuma J R, Verdun M (1995). A combined regimen of moderate dietary restriction and exercise training alters luteinizing hormone pulsatility in regularly menstruating young women. In *Proceedings of the 77th Endocrine Society Annual Meeting* Washington DC, pp. 558–558.

Macut D, Micic D, Pralong F P, Bischof P, Campana A (1998). Is there a role for leptin in human reproduction? *Gynecol Endocrinol* 12, 321–326.

Maffei M, Halaas J, Ravussin E et al. (1995). Leptin levels in human and rodent: measurement of plasma leptin and ob RNA in obese and weight-reduced subjects. *Nat Med* 1, 1155–1161.

Marcus R, Cann C E, Madvig P et al. (1985). Menstrual function and bone mass in elite women distance runners. *Ann Intern Med* 102, 158–163.

Mecklenburg R S, Loriaux D L, Thompson R H (1974). Hypothalamic dysfunction in patients with anorexia nervosa. *Medicine* 53, 147.

Miller K K, Parulekar M S, Schoenfeld E et al. (1998). Decreased leptin levels in normal weight women with hypothalamic amenorrhea: the effects of body composition and nutritional insults. *J Clin Endocrinol Metab* 83, 2309–2312.

Miller K K, Klibanski A, Grinspoon S K (2001). Androgen deficiency in women with anorexia nervosa. In *Proceedings of the 83rd Endocrine Society Annual Meeting*, pp. 394–394.

Moshang T Jr, Utiger R D (1977). Low triiodothyronine euthyroidism in anorexia nervosa. In *Anorexia Nervosa* Vigersky R, ed., p. 263. Raven Press, New York.

Myerson M, Gutin B, Warren M P et al. (1987). Energy balance of amenorrhea and eumenorrheic runners. *Med Sci Sports Exer* 19(Suppl.), S37.

Myerson M, Gutin B, Warren M P et al. (1991). Resting metabolic rate and energy balance in amenorrheic and eumenorrheic runners. *Med Sci Sports Exer* 23, 15–22.

Nagatani S, Guthikonda P, Thompson R C, Tsukamura H, Maeda K I, Foster D L (1998). Evidence for GnRH regulation by leptin: leptin administration prevents reduced pulsatile LH secretion during fasting. *Neuroendocrinology* 67, 370–376.

Newman M M, Halmi K A (1988). The endocrinology of anorexia nervosa and bulimia nervosa. *Neurol Clin* 6, 195–212.

Ott S M (1990). Editorial: Attainment of peak bone mass. *J Clin Endocrinol Metab*, 71, 1082A–1082C.

Pettersson F, Fries H, Nillius S J (1973). Epidemiology of secondary amenorrhea: Incidence and prevalence rates. *Am J Obstet Gynecol* 7, 80–86.

Pettersson U, Stalnacke B, Ahlenius G, Henriksson-Larsen K, Lorentzon R (1999). Low bone mass density at multiple skeletal sites, including the appendicular skeleton in amenorrheic runners. *Calcif Tissue Int* 64, 117–125.

Pirke K M, Fichter M M, Chlond C et al. (1987). Disturbances of the menstrual cycle in bulimia nervosa. *Clin Endocrinol* 27, 245–251.

Prior J C, Vigna Y M, Schechter M T, Burgess A E (1990). Spinal bone loss and ovulatory disturbances. *N Engl J Med* 323, 1221–1227.

Riggs B L, Eastell R (1986). Exercise, hypogonadism and osteopenia. *J Am Med Assoc* 256, 392–393.

Rigotti N A, Nussbaum S R, Herzog D B, Neer R M (1984). Osteoporosis in women with anorexia nervosa. *N Engl J Med* 311, 1601–1606.

Rigotti N A, Neer R M, Skates S J, Herzog D B, Nussbaum S R (1991). The clinical course of osteoporosis in anorexia nervosa: A longitudinal study of cortical bone mass. *J Am Med Assoc* 265, 1133–1138.

Rutherford O M (1993). Spine and total body bone mineral density in amenorrheic endurance athletes. *J Applied Physiol* 74, 2904–2908.

Salisbury J J, Mitchell J E (1991). Bone mineral density and anorexia nervosa in women. *Am J Psychiatry* 148, 768–774.

Salisbury J J, Levine A S, Crow S J, Mitchell J E (1995). Refeeding, metabolic rate, and weight gain in anorexia nervosa: a review. *Int J Eat Disord* 17, 337–345.

Schweiger U (1991). Menstrual function and luteal-phase deficiency in relation to weight changes and dieting. *Clin Obstet Gynecol* 34, 191–197.

Schweiger U, Laessle R, Pfister H et al. (1987). Diet-induced menstrual irregularities: effects of age and weight loss. *Fertil Steril* 48, 746–751.

Schweiger U, Tuschl R J, Platte P, Broocks A, Laessle R G, Pirke K M (1992). Everyday eating behavior and menstrual function in young women. *Fertil Steril* 57, 771–775.

Singh K B (1981). Menstrual disorders in college students. *Am J Obstet Gynecol* 1210, 299–302.

Smith E L, Gilligan C (1994). Bone Concerns. In *Women and Exercise: Physiology and Sports Medicine*, Shangold M M, Mirkin G, eds., pp. 89–101. F.A. Davis, Philadelphia, PA.

Soyka L A, Grinspoon S, Levitsky L L, Herzog D B, Klibanski A (1999). The effects of anorexia nervosa on bone metabolism in female adolescents. *J Clin Endcrinol Metab* 84, 4489–4496.

Tsafriri A, Dekel N, Bar-Ami S (1982). The role of oocyte maturation inhibitor in follicular regulation of oocyte maturation. *J Reprod Fertil* 64, 541–551.

Tuschl R J, Platte P, Laessle R G, Stichler W, Pirke K M (1990). Energy expenditure and every day eating behavior in healthy young women. *Am J Clin Nutrit* 52, 81–86.

van Binsbergen C J M, Coelingh Bennink H J T, Odink J, Haspels A A, Koppeschaar H P F (1990). A comparative and longitudinal study on endocrine changes related to ovarian function in patients with anorexia nervosa. *J Clin Endocrinol Metab* 71, 705–711.

Vigersky R A, Andersen A E, Thompson R H, Loriaux D L (1977). Hypothalamic dysfunction in secondary amenorrhea associated with simple weight loss. *N Engl J Med* 297, 1141–1145.

Warren M P (1980). The effects of exercise on pubertal progression and reproductive function in girls. *J Clin Endocrinol Metab* 51, 1150–1157.

    (1983). The effects of undernutrition on reproductive function in the human. *Endocr Rev* 4, 363–377.

Warren M P, Shangold M M (1997). *Sports gynecology: Problems and Care of the Athletic Female*, Blackwell Science, Cambridge, MA.

Warren M P, van de Wiele R L (1973). Clinical and metabolic features of anorexia nervosa. *Am J Obstet Gynecol* 117, 435–449.

Warren M P, Jewelewicz R, Dyrenfurth I, Ans R, Khalaf S, van de Wiele R L (1975). The significance of weight loss in the evaluation of pituitary response to LH-RH in women with secondary amenorrhea. *J Clin Endocrinol Metab* 40, 601–611.

Warren M P, Brooks-Gunn J, Hamilton L H, Warren L F, Hamilton W G (1986). Scoliosis and fractures in young ballet dancers: Relation to delayed menarche and secondary amenorrhea. *N Engl J Med* 314, 1348–1353.

Warren M P, Brooks-Gunn J, Fox R P et al. (1991). Lack of bone accretion and amenorrhea: Evidence for a relative osteopenia in weight bearing bones. *J Clin Endocrinol Metab* 72, 847–853.

Warren M P, Holderness C C, Lesobre V, Tzen R, Vossoughian F, Brooks-Gunn J (1994). Hypothalamic amenorrhea and hidden nutritional insults. *J Soc Gynecol Invest* 1, 84–88.

Warren M P, Voussoughian F, Geer E B, Hyle E P, Adberg C L, Ramos R H (1999). Functional hypothalamic amenorrhea: hypoleptinemia and disordered eating. *J Clin Endocrinol Metab* 84, 873–877.

Warren M P, Brooks-Gunn J, Fox R P et al. (2002). Osteopenia in exercise-induced amenorrhea using ballet dancers as a model: a longitudinal study. *J Clin Endocrinol Metab* 87, 3162–3168.

Wolman R L, Clark P, McNally E, Harries M, Reeve J (1990). Menstrual state and exercise as determinants of spinal trabecular bone density in female athletes. *Br Med J* 301, 516–518.

Zanker C L (1999). Bone metabolism in exercise associated amenorrhoea: the importance of nutrition. *Br J Sports Med* 33, 228–229.

Zanker C L, Swaine I L (1998a). Bone turnover in amenorrhoeic and eumenorrhoeic distance runners. *Scand J Med Sci Sports* 8, 20–26.

    (1998b). The relationship between bone turnover, oestradiol, and energy balance in women distance runners. *Br J Sports Med* 32, 167–171.

Zhang Y, Proenca R, Maffei M, Barone M, Leopold L, Friedman J M (1994). Positional cloning of the mouse *obese* gene and its human homologue. *Nature* 372, 425–432.

Zucker L M, Zucker T F (1961). Fatty, a new mutation in the rat. *J Hered* 52, 275–278.

40

How to set up a service: how to teach and train

Jane MacDougall

Current Chair of the British Society for Paediatric and Adolescent Gynaecology and
Addenbrooke's Hospital, Cambridge, UK

Introduction

Preceding chapters have discussed the specialist management of paediatric and adolescent patients with gynaecological problems. They have also addressed some of the generic issues associated with their care. When many of us began to be interested in this area of gynaecological care, we did not fully appreciate its breadth. Adolescent and paediatric gynaecology covers any gynaecological condition presenting in a girl less than 19 years of age and includes intersex, developmental and endocrine disorders as well as menstrual dysfunction, infection, vulval disorders and the sequelae of oncological treatment of childhood tumours.

In the past, children with complex problems who outgrew the paediatric clinic were either discharged to their general practitioners (GPs) or care was transferred to a variety of adult clinics. Many of these adolescents have gynaecological problems. These require a specific approach, both in consultation and subsequent management, that involves an understanding of both gynaecology and the specific needs of adolescents. The adolescent gynaecologist acts as a transitional carer between the paediatricians and the adult physician and needs to act in liaison with both. Some adolescents with gynaecological problems, and in particular those with genetic problems, also need to see a variety of other specialists. A lack of coordinated care and multiple visits has negative implications both socially and emotionally. Throughout this book we have, therefore, advocated a multidisciplinary approach to our patients.

Setting up a service

Setting up a paediatric and adolescent gynaecological service requires a clear vision of what you are aiming for, and then a marshalling of people and facilities to make it happen. You may be starting from scratch or building on preexisting services. The first step is to identify a local or regional need for such a service. As we have discussed in this book, paediatric and adolescent gynaecology does benefit from a multidisciplinary approach and above all you need to know the expertise available locally and obtain the support of key individuals. National and regional guidelines can be used as a driver for setting up a service. It is important to look at other units to see how they organize themselves. There needs to be a discussion with managers at a senior level; there may well be cross-speciality support for such an initiative. Once the clinic is open it is important to put together a database and audit outcomes.

Adolescent clinics provide a transition from paediatric to adult care and are a relatively new concept, at least in the UK. There are barriers to their development, but their importance is being increasingly recognized (Viner, 2001a). The House of Commons Select Committee on Health (1997) concluded: "services for adolescents should be given greater focus and priority. The transfer of young people, particularly those with special health needs, from child to adult services requires specific attention."

The needs of patients and parents were discussed in Ch. 15. Adolescent medical needs include learning to take responsibility for their own health as well as managing their current illness. This may be an individual's first

Paediatric and Adolescent Gynaecology, ed. Adam Balen et al. Published by Cambridge University Press.
© Cambridge University Press 2004.

contact with the health service. It is also an opportunity for health education. The adolescent has other, more general, needs as well; these include educational, recreational and social needs and a right to privacy. An individual's medical needs should determine the service provided, be it in primary care, secondary care or tertiary care in a teaching hospital setting. In the UK, the first will be focused around general practitioner (GP) surgeries and involve advice on family planning, contraception and menstrual dysfunction. At secondary level, more complex cases can be managed by one gynaecologist in the hospital who has a particular interest in this age group. At tertiary level, additional areas may include intersex services, the management of complex endocrine problems and the sequelae of paediatric malignancies. Specific multidisciplinary clinics, aimed at particular conditions (for example Turner's syndrome or congenital adrenal hyperplasia) and a specialist adolescent unit or adolescent inpatient facility may also be included. It is important to develop a service in liaison with surrounding hospitals to avoid duplication.

Once a decision has been made on the form of service to offer, how is it organized? It is often easier to start a service, in the absence of clear additional funding, by reorganizing previous arrangements. All adolescents with gynaecological problems can be seen by a consultant with training and expertise in this area. This obviously requires cooperation from other gynaecological colleagues and local GPs. At the same time, links should be made with consultants in other specialities, for example paediatrics, surgery, genetics and plastics.

The advantages and disadvantages of multidisciplinary clinics have already been discussed at several points in this book; they do provide a forum for developing guidelines for the management of teenagers in hospital, but attention must be paid to management and administrative issues. Advantages for patients include a reduced number of visits, consultant-based care, the opportunity to see experts in each area who understand adolescent needs and better standards of care. Patients also have an opportunity to see nonclinical experts in their particular area, for example psychologists. The disadvantages for patients include reduced flexibility for appointments and often longer waiting times for clinic appointments, as less patients can be seen per clinic and clinics are infrequent. A group of doctors can be intimidating to an individual patient and care must be taken to avoid this in the way clinics are organized. This type of clinic is often only viable in tertiary care and this may involve long journeys for patients.

As far as clinicians are concerned, multidisciplinary clinics can be enormously educational, both for the experts and

attendant trainees, and this will be discussed in more detail below. They do provide an opportunity for discussion of general patient management issues in addition to the discussion of often difficult and complex cases. They also provide the opportunity for coordinated research on rare conditions so that an evidence base can be generated and act as a driver for the development of guidelines. Funding can be problematic, as this is often across directorate boundaries. However, the authors have not found this a major problem provided colleagues from other specialities are committed and interested.

Organisation of clinics abroad and in UK

It can be helpful to look at other units in this country and abroad to see what they do and how they organize services.

In the USA, adolescent units were established in the 1970s and 1980s. By the mid 1990s, there were 40–60 units (MacFarlane & Blum, 2001). As in the UK, these may just be sections within other wards. The Society of Adolescent Medicine in the USA advocates "the continuation and establishment of adolescent inpatient units in both paediatric and general hospitals as an optimal approach to the delivery of developmentally appropriate health care to hospitalized adolescents" (Watson, 1998).

In the UK, in contrast to North America and Australia, the use of health services by adolescents has been largely ignored until recently (Byron & Madge, 2001; House of Commons Select Committee on Health, 1997; Viner, 1999, 2001a) despite the Platt report in 1959, which acknowledged that the "requirements of adolescents differed from those of adults and children and ideally adolescents need their own accommodation" (Watson, 1998). Viner argues that the care of adolescents is becoming a quality issue for the National Health Service in the UK (NHS). In a subsequent paper (Viner, 2001b), he calculated that adolescents aged 12–19 years occupied an average of 18 inpatient beds and 2.2 day-case beds in a district general hospital that served 250 000 people (this excluded obstetric, mental health and learning disabilities). The use of hospital beds increases during adolescence and he calculated that 12.8 inpatient beds are needed for each 10 000 adolescents (Viner, 2001b).

The accompanying editorial in the same issue of the *British Medical Journal* (MacFarlane & Blum, 2001) concluded that, even if it is not possible to establish an inpatient unit, "a multidisciplinary approach for health professionals with interest and expertise in adolescent health is still feasible in every hospital". The best way of achieving this may be via the establishment of guidelines for managing teenagers in hospital. Additionally, they stressed the importance of providing training for all health professionals.

There is at present no coherent policy in the UK for adolescents (Aynsley-Green et al., 2000). It is difficult to know who, if anyone, is speaking for children and adolescents and their health at policy level. Demographics suggest that increasing numbers of the ageing population will in future drain resources from children's services even further (Hall, 1999). Children and young people are a nation's most precious resource; their health is vital for the future success of our society. Despite this, improving the health of children in the UK is not a key government target; only 1 in 10 Health Authorities have any policies on adolescent physical health. The government supports the UN's Convention on the Rights of the Child, yet there is no specific national or government body or individual specifically charged with protecting the rights of children or assessing the impact of policies formulated by different ministeries on children or young people (Aynsley-Green et al., 2000). In general, improving child health is not seen as a high priority for local service delivery. In Scotland the situation is a little different from England, with a minister for children. The health of children has been one of four key UK health priorities for 2000–3.

Training

Why should we bother to train postgraduates in adolescent and paediatric gynaecology? It can be argued that one way to deliver comprehensive services to adolescents is to provide appropriate training to health professionals in both primary and secondary care so that optimal care is given (McFarlane & Blum, 2001). In the field of paediatric and adolescent gynaecology, provision for such training is somewhat limited, at least in the UK. Gynaecologists have been largely trained as adult physicians and surgeons; some may have spent an elective training period in neonatology but this hardly equips them for consultations with children, adolescents and their parents. Although all will have come in contact with the management of menstrual problems, this will usually be in an older age group where the management emphasis may be rather different. Few will have seen patients with intersex disorders or with endocrine problems such as ovarian failure following treatment for childhood cancer. As has been demonstrated in this book, management of such cases is often not surgical but medical and requires expertise outwith the experience of the average gynaecologist.

So what should we be aiming for? This section will discuss, briefly, some principles of adult learning and then apply this knowledge to teaching within the clinic at both undergraduate and postgraduate level (the process). A discussion of what needs to be taught at each level (the content) will be included.

Principles of adult learning

Sir Walter Scott, writing to J.G. Lockhart in 1830, said: *"All men who have turned out worth anything have had the chief hand in their own education".*

Adult educational theory suggests that teaching should be learner centred and should encourage self-motivation. This is based on an understanding of how adults learn and yet there continues to be considerable debate in educational circles about how adults actually do learn and whether this is different from children (Hanson, 1996; Knowles, 1996). Nowadays, medical practice is continually changing as a result of technological advances and this, together with a move over recent years to evidence-based practice, means that education for doctors must be lifelong and in the main self-directed. This fits well with learner centred and self-motivated adult educational theory.

Knowles (1996) argued that adults differ from children: they are usually voluntary learners, they have a greater reservoir of experience, they are self-directing rather than dependent, their readiness to learn is related to their role in society and they are more interested in problem solving than in subject matter per se. This theory of adult learning is generating new ways of educating adults, which has been described as "andragogy" (the art and science of helping adults to learn, in contrast to "pedagogy", the art and science of teaching children). Proponents of this approach argue that these differences in how adults learn have major implications for how their education should be organized. They need to be treated with respect and encouraged to take responsibility for their own learning. Adults will be better motivated if they set their own agenda; this requires them to identify their learning needs. The teacher's role is to facilitate this process. Knowles described the teacher as a catalyst and a guide. He argued that because the adult learner brings experience to the teaching situation greater emphasis can be placed on small group work, role play, skill practice exercises and problem solving, and considerably less on "transmission" techniques such as lectures.

There are those who disagree with this approach. Hanson (1996) argued that this view is too simplistic and utopian. The imposition of curriculum detracts from the concept of self-directed learning; the adult learner can no longer set the agenda, there are targets to be achieved, examinations to pass. This is, of course, particularly true of medical education where the acquisition of a specific body of knowledge is considered important by students, medical teachers and the general public. Hanson argued that the experience of adult learners may, in fact, be a hindrance rather than a help in their learning as they become set in their ways.

The assumption by Knowles (1996) that adults are different from children has also been challenged; surely it is more of a continuum? Perhaps the practical approach lies somewhere between the two viewpoints. Further examination of how adults learn has led to the gradual replacement of the familiar, traditional transmission model of teaching, in which learners play passive roles, in favour of the so-called constructivist model. In this model, learners assume a more active and interactive role (Dart, 1997). One of the early proponents of this type of approach was Abercrombie, who described a project that involved medical students and looked at how they made judgements (Abercrombie, 1969). This was and still is a highly influential study that aimed to increase the autonomy and responsibility of learners by making them question their basic assumptions. Students were encouraged to participate actively in their own learning and that of others via discussion groups and to improve practice by integrating this with theory (Nias, 1987). It is undoubtedly important, particularly in medicine, to encourage students to think for themselves. Abercrombie's study demonstrated that medical students were more than capable of doing this and were able to challenge their own and others' perceptions.

There are two main strands of "modern" medical teaching, sometimes referred to as the "New Path"; problem-based learning and small group teaching. Learning may be an individual process, but in reality teaching often takes place in small groups; on the job training in medicine can of course be one to one (Hargreaves, 1997). Smaller groups allow interaction between members while the group can provide a supportive environment for learning, a challenge to the learner (no dozing in the back row of the lecture theatre) and the opportunity to use more complex structures for learning.

Adults will tend only to engage in learning if they can see that what they are learning is useful to them. The medical teacher's role, therefore, is to encourage self-directed learning while checking that the curriculum is covered.

In the model proposed by educationalists specializing in adult teaching, the effectiveness of teaching depends on the learner. The focus has, therefore, moved from the teacher to the learner and learning drives the teaching. The teacher has become the facilitator of learning rather than the giver of information. An old proverb says, "Tell me and I will forget, show me and I may not remember, involve me and I will understand".

In medicine, clinical students and young doctors do learn by (supervised) doing and apprenticeship still plays an important part in medical training (Ashley, 2000). As Grant (1998) wrote, medical education "is about learning to be a doctor by being a doctor, caring for patients under controlled conditions of safety and care".

Learning needs in paediatric and adolescent gynaecology: what to teach (the content)

There are three areas of learning needs (the so-called "domains" of learning); trainees need to acquire the appropriate knowledge, skills and attitude. A hierarchy of learning needs can be developed dependent on the role of an individual. For example, the learning needs of medical students will be different from those of GPs and general gynaecologists, whilst those gynaecologists planning to practise paediatric and adolescent gynaecology as a special interest (either as part of subspeciality training in reproductive medicine or independent of this) will require more detailed knowledge. Then there is nurse training and counselling, which has been dealt with elsewhere in this book.

It could be argued that all medical students should be aware that children and adolescents can present with gynaecological problems; the emphasis at this level should be on family planning, obstetric care and menstrual dysfunction.

Similarly, potential GPs should have further training in these areas. They should, in addition, be aware of endocrine problems and be clear about management of amenorrhoea and oligomenorrhoea and when to refer patients on.

All gynaecologists should have the above understanding and be able to recognize the more complex problems that need onward referral. Those planning to practise paediatric and adolescent gynaecology at subspeciality or special interest level require an in-depth knowledge of management of simple as well as more complex patients. Only a few gynaecologists in selected teaching centres need the surgical expertise necessary for management of complex intersex cases. Such cases are not appropriately managed by the occasional operation by the average gynaecologist.

All of these groups should have some knowledge and experience of generic issues such as consultation skills in this age group.

Different methods of teaching: how to teach (the process)

Acquiring the necessary knowledge, skills and attitude should primarily take place "on the job" in the presence of patients. All three areas of learning can be enhanced by additional work away from patients. The optimal place to learn about paediatric and adolescent gynaecology is in the clinic, sitting in with a gynaecologist who is an expert in this area. With the reduction in the length of training (Calmanization) in the UK and reduction in working hours (New Deal) there are increasing demands to improve the quality of training by making it as focused and relevant as possible. Hargreaves et al. (1997) discussed ways in which clinics can be structured in order to facilitate training. They quote S. K. Calman, Chief Medical Officer, who said in 1993: "We need to look again at how doctors learn and how teaching methods can be improved in order that time spent in education can be used efficiently. Supervision and feedback are crucial . . . the integration of theoretical teaching with practical work, progressive assessment and feedback to teachers and trainees is essential." They also quoted the medical educators D. A. West and A. Kaufman, who said in 1981: "The guiding principle of education in the clinic must be that of flexibility".

Hargreaves et al. (1997) described four models of training in the clinic: (i) sitting in, (ii) service-led training, (iii) service delivery with follow-up training, and (iv) planned training within service delivery. The first model is typically used for medical students and junior trainees; when the consultant gets on with the service work and the trainee sits in and listens. Its advantages include a large amount of teaching and the opportunity to see a full range of cases. However, there are disadvantages; trainees get bored by just watching and there is limited hands on experience. Training can often deteriorate into that obtained by osmosis only.

Service-led training occurs when trainees sit in a separate consulting room and see their own patients. This is a commonly used model for registrars and senior house officers and certainly increases the numbers of patients seen, but not necessarily the quality of clinical management. There are several disadvantages; trainees may only see simple cases and be reluctant to seek advice and, therefore, patients get a suboptimal service with little training taking place.

The third model involves service delivery by the trainee with an opportunity to discuss all or some cases at the end of the clinic; this has some advantages: it tends to be efficient and teaching at the end is often very valuable. However, training tends to lack structure and does not necessarily address trainees' learning needs. There is also a tendency to forgo the postclinic discussion if the clinic is busy.

In the final model (considered ideal, but probably not very practical, by Hargreaves et al., 1997) the trainee sees cases within his/her competence as "service" and is given training on other subjects when competence or experience is lacking. This involves the trainee in selecting a training menu for a particular clinic (for example a trainee attending a paediatric and adolescent gynaecology clinic might have on his/her training menu the management of intersex). If a patient presents who is on the "training menu", then trainer and trainee meet to discuss the case. This model supports trainee progression and is more focused. It also gives the trainee an opportunity to read up beforehand and be more prepared. This obviously requires some forethought and a certain amount of organization.

A further model has been described by a local consultant and in certain circumstances may work well, particularly in larger clinics attended by a number of trainees. The consultant has no patient list of his own and acts as a "true" consultant. He/she moves from trainee to trainee discussing cases and advising on management. There are ample opportunities for training en route. The consultant can also observe history taking and examination technique.

Whichever model is used, guiding principles should include the application of an appropriate clinic model to match the trainees' learning needs and the use of training menus. It is important to ensure that nursing and managerial staff are aware of why and which model is being used and that in the long term this does speed up service.

There are particular difficulties associated with teaching adolescent and paediatric gynaecology in the clinic; one is of male students and doctors. Young adolescent girls in particular are often embarrassed enough: the presence of a youngish male only adds to this. It is important always to introduce everyone who is sitting in the room and to ask both patients and parents if they mind having them there. If information has been sent out prior to the clinic visit, most will be prepared. It is important to be as positive as possible and explain the importance of teaching. A compromise may involve the observers being present for the history, but not for the examination.

However, although the clinic is probably the best place to learn, training opportunities in dedicated adolescent gynaecology clinics tend to be limited in the UK at present. Family planning clinics and adolescent obstetric clinics, where they exist, may be useful. Some alternative strategies have been proposed.

One suggestion is the use of simulated patients (Blake & Greaven, 1999), particularly for teaching generic skills such as consultation. The use of adult simulators has become common practice, particularly for the teaching of communication skills (Kurtz et al., 1998) but few medical schools have tried to use adolescent simulators. One argument against has been that asking adolescents to simulate illness may adversely affect their psychosocial development or interfere with schoolwork or extracurricular activities. These fears may be unfounded.

Blake & Greaven (1999) describe the use of adolescent girls as simulators of medical illness; they were paired with simulated mothers and provided with training for their roles. A matched control group was also recruited. They found no evidence of adverse effects from role playing reported by schools, parents or by the girls themselves, and in fact the role-playing experience was viewed positively by the adolescent participants. Benefits may include learning about medical illnesses, adolescent issues and use of the health service, as well as an increase in confidence levels. Although small and preliminary, this study does suggest that this may prove a useful way of teaching consultation skills in adolescent gynaecology.

Specialist knowledge and skills can be augmented by training days and seminars, away from patients. The newly formed British Society of Paediatric and Adolescent Gynaecology (BritSPAG; www.britspag.org.uk) includes as one of its aims "to provide a network of appropriate education and training for clinicians, nurses, counselors, psychologists and other health professionals working in this clinical area". Training days such as those being planned by this society may be helpful. In addition the Royal College of Obstetricians and Gynaecologists (RCOG) organizes occasional meetings on the subject. Conferences organized by groups such as BSPAG, the North American Society of Pediatric and Adolescent Gynecology (NASPAG), the British Fertility Society (BFS), the American Fertility Society (AFS) and the European Society for Human Reproduction and Embryology (ESHRE) are also valuable sources of education.

On the job training in theatre

Surgical teaching in paediatric and adolescent gynaecology will tend to be limited as it is only relevant to those aiming to practise this specialist interest at subspeciality level. General principles of teaching in theatre apply (Hargreaves et al., 1997). These should include preplanning, the use of training menus, encouraging trainees to ask questions and the provision of specific feedback after each case (often usefully done over coffee between cases).

General training issues

Training in general can be enhanced by teachers using techniques such as questioning and feedback. Trainees should be encouraged to take responsibility for their own learning; there is a useful booklet entitled *Getting the Most out of Your Training* (Hargreaves et al., 1998) that describes the use of training menus, asking for feedback and the use of critical self-reflection. The aim is to move away from training "as osmosis" towards training "as partnership".

Summary

The approach to health care is changing rapidly; we need to encourage young doctors to be self-directed learners who work well in multidisciplinary teams. This is not easily achieved by using traditional didactic teaching to separate professional groups. We need to consider altering the ways in which we deliver their education. Postgraduate medical education is becoming increasingly multidisciplinary in its approach and this approach can be extended to teaching paediatric and adolescent gynaecology, a subject that, as the preceding chapters show, lends itself to a multidisciplinary approach (Box 40.1).

Box 40.1 Teaching

- Providing health professionals with appropriate training will improve the quality of adolescent clinical services.
- Paediatric and adolescent gynaecology can and should be taught using a multidisciplinary approach.
- Training should be learner centred.
- Teachers should act as facilitators of learning rather than givers of information. They do need to check that the curriculum is covered.
- Teachers should encourage trainees to become self-directed learners who work well in multidisciplinary teams.
- Learning should primarily take place "on the job" and particularly in clinics.

This is reflected in how clinics are organized. There are four different areas that need to be covered under the umbrella of paediatric and adolescent gynaecology, whether this is at primary, secondary or tertiary level. Balen et al. (2002) identified these as sexual health (contraception, family planning, sexually transmitted disease), pregnancy (wanted and unwanted), gynaecological complaints (menstrual cycle dysfunction, pelvic pain and ovarian cysts) and disorders of sexual differentiation (complex or rare endocrine and developmental disorders of sexual differentiation and puberty including intersex). It has been suggested that specialist units should provide contact with gynaecologists with a special interest in reproductive endocrinology, ovarian function, paediatric and adolescent gynaecological development, reconstructive and endoscopic surgery and infertility (Balen et al., 2002). In addition, there should be access to a clinical psychologist trained in adolescent psychology, nurse specialists with training to supervise the use of vaginal dilators, consultant plastic surgeons with experience in reconstructive surgery, consultant adult and paediatric urologists with experience in surgery for developmental anomalies of the renal tract, bladder and urethra, and consultant paediatric surgeons with an interest in the management of complex intersex and reproductive endocrine conditions. Access to a consultant psychiatrist with a special interest in adolescence and psychosexual medicine and disorders of sexuality is helpful as is a consultant geneticist for genetic advice and counselling. Additional useful links include a consultant radiologist and chemical pathologist.

In the UK now, a national network is beginning to emerge that should provide a framework for the appropriate care of complex patients and also appropriate training and education of professionals involved in these and more straightforward problems (Balen et al., 2000). These are two of the aims of BritSPAG. There is also a clear need for better data collection and designated facilities for adolescent and gynaecological problems.

Children are vital for the future strength and success of our society, yet one in three lives in poverty, which has major deleterious effects on health. Much adult disease has its origins in early life, and events in adolescence have long-term sequelae that determine adult well-being. Many key indicators for youth health are going in the wrong direction: obesity, smoking, suicide, reduction in exercise. Adolescents should be on the health agenda (Box 40.2). Care needs to be given by appropriately trained staff at every level in order to improve the quality of care. We need to aim to provide a high-quality service that addresses adolescent needs both related to their health and to their use of healthcare systems. We should acknowledge that their needs are different from those of adults.

Being an adolescent is never easy, and health problems only compound this. Our challenge is to address the health needs of young people in a sensitive and comprehensive manner.

Box 40.2 Key points

- Adolescents have different needs to adults and children. The needs of adolescent patients should determine the services provided.
- Clinicians working in this field need an understanding of gynaecology and of the generic needs of adolescents.
- Adolescents with gynaecological problems benefit from a multidisciplinary approach.
- Adolescent clinics provide a transition from paediatric to adult care; there is a need for designated facilities for adolescents with gynaecological problems.

REFERENCES

Abercrombie M L J (1969). *The Anatomy of Judgement.* Free Association, London.

Ashley E A (2000). Medical education-beyond tomorrow? The new doctor – Asclepiad or Logiatros? *Med Educ* 34, 455–459.

Aynsley-Green A, Barker M, Burr S et al. (2000). Who is speaking for children and adolescents and for their health at the policy level? *Br Med J* 321, 229–232.

Balen A H, Fleming C, Robinson A (2000). Health needs of adolescents in secondary gynaecological care: results of a questionnaire survey and a review of current issues. *Human Fertil* 5, 127–132.

Blake K, Greaven S (1999). Adolescent girls as simulators of medical illness. *Med Educ* 33, 702–703.

Byron M, Madge S (2001). Transition from paediatric to adult care: psychological principles. *J Roy Soc Med* 94(Suppl. 40), 5–7.

Dart B (1997). Learners' metacognitive behaviour in higher education. In *Adult Learning: A Reader*, Sutherland P, ed., pp. 30–57. Kogan Page, London.

Grant J (1998). Training the Trainers. *Lancet* 352(Suppl IV), 19.

Hall D M B (1999). Children in an ageing society. *Br Med J* 319, 1356–1358.

Hanson A (1996). The search for a separate theory of adult learning. Does anyone really need andragogy? In *Boundaries of Adult Learning*, Edwards R, Hansom A, Raggatt P, pp. 99–108. Routledge, London.

Hargreaves D H, Bowditch M G, Griffin D G (1997). *On the Job Training for Surgeons.* Royal Society of Medicine Press, London.

Hargreaves D H, Stanley P, Ward S (1998). *Getting the Best out of your Training. A Practical Guide for Trainees.* Association for the Study of Medical Education, Edinburgh.

House of Commons Select Committee on Health (1997). *Fifth Report: Hospital Services for Children and Young People.* HMSO, London.

Knowles M (1996). Andragogy. An emerging technology for adult learning. In *Boundaries of adult learning*, Edwards R, Hansom A, Raggatt P, pp. 82–98. Routledge, London.

Kurtz S, Silverman J, Draper J (1998). *Teaching and Learning Communication Skills in Medicine*, pp. 186–91. Ratcliffe Medical Press, Abingdon, UK.

MacFarlane A, Blum R W (2001). Do we need specialist adolescent units in hospitals? [Editorial] *Br Med J* 322, 941–942.

Nias J (1987). *Seeing Anew: Teachers' Theories of Action*. Deakin University Press, Victoria.

Viner R (1999). Transition from paediatric to adult care. Bridging the gaps or passing the buck? *Arch Dis Child* 81, 271–275.

(2001a). National survey of use of hospital beds by adolescents aged 12–19 in the United Kingdom. *Br Med J* 322, 957–958.

(2001b). Barriers and good practice in transition from paediatric to adult care. *J Roy Soc Med* 94(Suppl. 40), 2–4.

Watson S (1998). A ward of their own. *Nurs Stand* 12, 12.

Index